Therapy

Editors

Rosemary M. Scully, Ed.D., P.T.
Associate Professor and Chair
Department of Physical Therapy
University of Pittsburgh
School of Health-Related Professions
Pittsburgh, Pennsylvania

Marylou R. Barnes, Ed.D., P.T.
Professor of Physical Therapy
Georgia State University
School of Allied Health Sciences
Atlanta, Georgia

With 76 contributors

Associate Editors

Judith S. Canfield, Ed.D., P.T.
Associate Professor and Director
School of Physical Therapy
Children's Hospital of Los Angeles/Chapman College
Los Angeles, California

Marilyn Moffat, Ph.D., P.T.
Professor of Physical Therapy
New York University
New York, New York

Katherine F. Shepard, Ph.D., P.T.
Associate Professor
Director of Graduate Physical Therapy
Temple University
Philadelphia, Pennsylvania

Sponsoring Editor: Richard Winters
Manuscript Editor: Virginia Barishek
Indexer: Barbara Littlewood
Design Coordinator: Ellen C. Dawson

Cover Designer: Joe Netherwood
Production Manager: Carol A. Florence
Production Supervisor: Charlene Squibb
Compositor: TSI, Inc.
Printer/Binder: R.R. Donnelley & Sons
Company

1   3   5   6   4   2

Library of Congress Cataloging-in-Publication Data

Physical therapy.

   Includes bibliographies and index.
   1. Physical therapy. I. Scully, Rosemary M.
II. Barnes, Marylou R. [DNLM: 1. Physical Therapy.
WB 460 P5777]
RM700.P473 1989   615.8'2   88-32607
ISBN 0-397-50798-4

The authors and publisher have exerted every effort to ensure that drug selection and dosage set forth in this text are in accord with current recommendations and practice at the time of publication. However, in view of ongoing research, changes in government regulations, and the constant flow of information relating to drug therapy and drug reactions, the reader is urged to check the package insert for each drug for any change in indications and dosage and for added warnings and precautions. This is particularly important when the recommended agent is a new or infrequently employed drug.

Physical Therapy

Physical

J.B. LIPPINCOTT COMPANY   Philadelphia

Cambridge   New York   St. Louis   San Francisco
London   Singapore   Sydney   Tokyo

Contributors

Joyce L. Adcock, M.A., P.T.
Director of Physical Therapy
Jenkintown Rehabilitation Services
Jenkintown, Pennsylvania

Susan A. Bemis, Ed.D., P.T.
Associate Professor
University of New England
Biddeford, Maine

Marlene L. Bonham, P.T.
Formerly, Education Coordinator
Department of Physical Therapy
Pacific Presbyterian Medical Center
San Francisco, California

Barbara Bourbon, Ph.D., P.T.
Adjunct Assistant Professor
Department of Physical Therapy
Philadelphia College of Pharmacy and
    Science;
Co-Director
The Philadelphia Institute for Physical
    Therapy
Philadelphia, Pennsylvania;
Adjunct Assistant Professor
Graduate Program in Physical Therapy
Beaver College
Glenside, Pennsylvania

Marybeth Brown, Ph.D., P.T.
Assistant Professor of Physical Therapy
Washington University
St. Louis, Missouri

Judith S. Canfield, Ed.D., P.T.
Associate Professor and Director
School of Physical Therapy
Children's Hospital of Los
    Angeles/Chapman College
Los Angeles, California

George E. Carvell, Ph.D., P.T.
Associate Professor
Department of Physical Therapy
School of Health-Related Professions
University of Pittsburgh
Pittsburgh, Pennsylvania

Catherine M. E. Certo, Sc.D., P.T.
Associate Professor and Chairman
Department of Physical Therapy
Sargent College of Allied Health
    Professions
Boston University
Boston, Massachusetts

Emily L. Christian, Ph.D., P.T.
Associate Professor
Department of Physical Therapy
College of Allied Health Professions
Temple University
Philadelphia, Pennsylvania

Richard A. Clendaniel, M.S., P.T.
Instructor
Division of Physical Therapy
School of Health-Related Professions
University of Alabama at Birmingham;
Senior Physical Therapist
Department of Physical Therapy
University of Alabama Hospital
Birmingham, Alabama

Jack D. Close, M.A., P.T.
Director
Las Vegas Institute of Physical Therapy
  and Sports Medicine
Las Vegas, Nevada

Peggy Clough, M.S., P.T.
Supervisor
Physical Therapy Division
University of Michigan Hospitals
Ann Arbor, Michigan

Janet C. Cookson, M.A., P.T.
Guest Lecturer
Kaiser Orthopedic Physical Therapy
  Curriculum
Hayward, California

Linda Crane, M.M.Sc., P.T.
Instructor
Division of Physical Therapy
School of Medicine
University of Miami
Miami, Florida

Carolyn A. Crutchfield, Ed.D., P.T.
Professor
Department of Physical Therapy
Georgia State University
Atlanta, Georgia

Vincent L. Eldridge, P.T.
Director of Rehabilitation
Cincinnati Sports Medicine and
  Orthopaedic Center
Cincinnati, Ohio

Corinne Ellingham, M.S., P.T.
Assistant Professor
Program in Physical Therapy
University of Minnesota
Minneapolis, Minnesota

M. Katie Gillis, M.S., P.T.
Clinical Specialist
UCLA Outpatient Physical and
  Occupational Therapy Department
University of California, Los Angeles
Los Angeles, California

Carol A. Giuliani, Ph.D., P.T.
Assistant Professor
Division of Physical Therapy
University of North Carolina at Chapel Hill
Chapel Hill, North Carolina

Jay M. Goodfarb, P.T.
Private Practice
Phoenix, Arizona

Ann Hallum, M.S., P.T.
Ph. D. Candidate (A.B.D.), Counseling and
  Health Psychology
Stanford University;
Formerly, Senior Lecturer
Stanford University School of Medicine
Stanford, California

Timothy P. Heckmann, A.T.C., P.T.
Clinical Instructor
Department of Physical Therapy
Virginia Commonwealth University
  Medical College of Virginia
School of Medicine
Richmond, Virginia;
Clinical Instructor
Department of Physical Therapy
College of Applied Health Professions
University of Kentucky
Lexington, Kentucky;
Director of Rehabilitation
Cincinnati Sports Medicine and
  Orthopaedic Center
Cincinnati, Ohio

Carolyn B. Heriza, Ed.D., P.T.
Associate Professor
Department of Physical Therapy
School of Allied Health Professions
St. Louis University
St. Louis, Missouri

Ellen Hillegass, M.M.S., P.T., C.C.S.
Fitness and Wellness Cardiac Rehabilitation
Atlanta, Georgia

Fay B. Horak, Ph.D., P.T.
Assistant Scientist
Department of Neuro-otology
Good Samaritan Hospital and Medical
   Center
Portland, Oregon

Janet Bower Hulme, M.A., P.T.
Associate Professor
University of Montana
Missoula, Montana

Susan J. Isernhagen, P.T.
President
Isernhagen & Associates Consultation and
   Education
Duluth, Minnesota

Gail M. Jensen, Ph.D., P.T.
Assistant Professor
Division of Physical Therapy
School of Health-Related Professions
University of Alabama
Birmingham, Alabama

Diane U. Jette, M.S., P.T.
Associate Professor of Physical Therapy
Simmons College
Boston, Massachusetts

Joseph Kahn, Ph.D., P.T.
Clinical Assistant Professor
State University of New York
Stony Brook, New York;
Adjunct Associate Professor
Touro College
Huntington, New York;
Clinical Associate
New York University
New York, New York;
Adjunct Clinical Professor
Daemen College
Amherst, New York

Timothy L. Kauffman, M.S., P.T.
Clinical Assistant Professor
Hahnemann University
Philadelphia, Pennsylvania;
Private Practice
Lancaster, Pennsylvania

Glenda L. Key, P.T.
Founder and President
Key Functional Assessments, Inc.
Minneapolis, Minnesota

Claire P. Kispert, Ph.D., P.T.
Assistant Professor of Physical Therapy
The University of Texas
Southwestern Medical Center
Dallas, Texas

David E. Krebs, Ph.D., P.T.
Associate Professor
MGH Institute of Health Professions
Massachusetts General Hospital
Boston, Massachusetts

Susan Paulsen Layfield, P.T.
Private Practice
Encino, California

Susan A. Liska, P.T.
Cardiopulmonary Physical Therapist
Massachusetts General Hospital
Boston, Massachusetts

Elizabeth H. Littell, Ph.D., P.T.
Associate Professor and Director
Program in Physical Therapy
Idaho State University
Pocatello, Idaho

Robert Mangine, M.Ed., P.T., A.T.C.
Clinical Instructor
Virginia Commonwealth University
   Medical College of Virginia
School of Medicine;
Clinical Coordinator
Deaconess Hospital Center for Sports
   Medicine and Cardiovascular
   Rehabilitation
Cincinnati, Ohio

Tink Martin, M.A.Ct., P.T.
Associate Professor
Department of Physical Therapy
University of Evansville
Evansville, Indiana

Susan J. Middaugh, Ph.D., P.T.
Associate Professor of Physical Medicine
and Rehabilitation
College of Medicine
Medical University of South Carolina
Charleston, South Carolina

Mary Moffroid, Ph.D., P.T.
Associate Professor
Department of Physical Therapy
University of Vermont
Burlington, Vermont

Thomas Mohr, Ph.D., P.T.
Associate Professor
Department of Physical Therapy
University of North Dakota
Grand Forks, North Dakota

Carolee Moncur, Ph.D., P.T.
Associate Professor
Division of Physical Therapy
Adjunct Associate Professor
Division of Rheumatology
University of Utah
Salt Lake City, Utah

Matthew C. Morrissey, M.A., P.T.
Clinical Assistant Professor
Department of Physical Therapy
Sargent College of Allied Health
Professions
Boston University
Boston, Massachusetts

James R. Morrow, Ph.D., P.T.
Professor
Physical Therapy Educational Department
Medical University of South Carolina
Charleston, South Carolina

Garvice G. Nicholson, M.S., P.T.
Assistant Professor
Division of Physical Therapy
School of Health-Related Professions
University of Alabama;
Supervisor
Orthopaedic Physical Therapy
Department of Physical Therapy
University of Alabama Hospital
Birmingham, Alabama

Vickie Nixon, P.T.
Private Practice
San Diego, California

Linda O'Connor, P.T., A.C.C.E.
Physical Therapist and Patient Instructor
Fem-Health Inc.
Fremont, California

Leonard Paré, M.S., R.P.T.
Clinical Education
Physical Therapy and Sport Medicine
Associates of Central Connecticut
New Britain, Connecticut

Dorothy Pinkston, Ph.D., P.T.
Professor
Division of Physical Therapy
School of Health-Related Professions
University of Alabama
Birmingham, Alabama

Linda M. Pipp, P.T.
Clinical Instructor in Obstetrics and
Gynecology
Physical Therapy Program
Oakland University
Rochester, Michigan;
Guest Lecturer in Obstetrics and
Gynecology
Physical Therapy Program
Wayne State University
Detroit, Michigan;
Physical Therapist
Providence Hospital
Southfield, Michigan

Rebecca E. Porter, M.S., P.T.
Associate Professor
Director of Physical Therapy
Division of Allied Health Sciences
Indiana University School of Medicine
Indianapolis, Indiana

Helen Price, M.S., P.T.
Associate Professor and Program Director
Department of Physical Therapy
School of Allied Health Professions
Louisiana State University Medical School
Shreveport, Louisiana

Ruth B. Purtilo, Ph.D., P.T.
Henry Knox Sherrill Professor of Medical
Ethics
MGH Institute of Health Professions
Massachusetts General Hospital
Boston, Massachusetts

Martha L. Rammel, M.H.Ed., P.T.
Associate Professor
University of New England
Biddeford, Maine

Kathryn E. Roach, M.H.S., P.T.
Instructor
Program in Physical Therapy
Washington University;
Supervisor, Home Health Physical Therapy
Service
Barnes/IWS Home Health Agency
St. Louis, Missouri

H. Steven Sadowsky, M.S., P.T.-C.C.S., R.R.T.
Assistant Clinical Professor
University of California;
Clinical Coordinator
Physical Therapy
Rehabilitation Services Department
Washington Hospital
San Francisco, California

H. Duane Saunders, M.S., P.T.
Private Practice
Minneapolis, Minnesota

Beverly J. Schmoll, Ph.D., P.T.
Associate Professor
University of Michigan
Flint, Michigan

Marion B. Schoneberger, M.S., P.T.
Supervisor II
Rancho Los Amigos Medical Center
Downey, California

Carol Schunk, Psy.D., P.T.
Administrator
Associated Health Focus
Oregon/Washington
Portland, Oregon

Katherine F. Shepard, Ph.D., P.T.
Associate Professor
Director of Graduate Physical Therapy
Temple University
Philadelphia, Pennsylvania

Anne Shumway-Cook, Ph.D., P.T.
Director
Balance Disorders Program
Emanuel Rehabilitation Center
Portland, Oregon

Susan S. Smith, M.S., P.T.
Assistant Professor
Department of Physical Therapy
The University of Texas
Southwestern Medical Center
Dallas, Texas

Steven R. Tippett, P.T., A.T.C.
Director of Sports Medicine
Saint Francis Medical Center
Peoria, Illinois

Janice Toms, M.Ed., P.T.
Professor and Chairman
Department of Physical Therapy
Simmons College
Wyland, Massachusetts

Philip Paul Tygiel, P.T.
Director
Tygiel Physical Therapy
Tucson, Arizona

Linda Van Dillen, M.H.O., P.T.
Instructor
Program in Physical Therapy
Consultant to Irene W. Johnson Institute of
Rehabilitation
Washington University
St. Louis, Missouri

Candice Van Iderstine, P.T.
President
Community Therapy Service, Inc.
Davidsonville, Maryland

Jessie M. Van Swearingen, M.S., P.T.
Assistant Professor
Department of Physical Therapy
School of Health-Related Professions
University of Pittsburgh
Pittsburgh, Pennsylvania

Cheryl Wardlaw, P.T.
Supervisor of Physical Therapy
Emory University Hospital
Stone Mountain, Georgia

Susan L. Whitney, M.S., P.T., A.T.C.
Assistant Professor and Assistant
Chairman
Department of Physical Therapy
School of Health-Related Professions
University of Pittsburgh
Pittsburgh, Pennsylvania

George A. Wolfe, Ph.D., P.T.
Associate Professor
School of Physical Therapy
Children's Hospital of Los
Angeles/Chapman College
Los Angeles, California

Russell M. Woodman, M.S., P.T., F.S.O.M.
Associate Professor
Quinnipiac College
Hamden, Connecticut;
Staff Physical Therapist
Yale-New Haven Hospital
New Haven, Connecticut

James E. Zachazewski, M.S., P.T., A.T.C.
Director of Athletic Training and
Rehabilitation
Department of Intercollegiate Athletics
University of California at Los Angeles
Los Angeles, California

Nancy Zimny, M.S., P.T.
Assistant Professor
University of Vermont
Burlington, Vermont

Preface

We undertook the writing of *Physical Therapy* with the hope of providing a conceptual framework for articulating the knowledge and skills for the general practice of physical therapy, as well as providing a foundation for the development of specific areas of clinical expertise. The book was intended primarily for the entry-level student in the latter part of the professional education program, the therapist just beginning practice, the therapist studying for reentry, the "generalist" who wishes to update and expand knowledge and skills, and the "clinical specialist" who wishes to maintain general knowledge and skills.

As we developed the objectives for and the structure of this book, we realized that we had to try to describe the knowledge and skills common to all physical therapists regardless of practice setting, geographical area of practice, and individuals to whom care is rendered. Thus five premises emerged to guide the development of *Physical Therapy*.

The first premise was that the goal of the physical therapist is the enhancement of human movement and function, which is accomplished by the assessment, prevention, and treatment of movement dysfunction and physical disability.

The second premise was that the physical therapist uses a clinical reasoning process that uniquely blends the biologic, kinesiologic, pathologic, psychologic, social, and clinical sciences.

Third, the physical therapist is guided in this clinical reasoning process by an understanding of these disciplines and their relationship to movement, function, movement dysfunction, and physical disability. When the theoretical framework for assessment or intervention has not been articulated or verified, experiences may dictate clinical practice. Thus, the theoretical bases of practice are being developed continually.

Fourth, in the delivery of physical therapy, the therapist uses both science and art to select, combine, and apply various theories, facts, perceptions, judgments, and skills that are appropriate to each consumer.

The fifth premise was that professional activities also may include consultation, education, research, management, and referral.

The authors were asked to incorporate relevant information showing the relationship of these premises to clinical practice within their chapters.

Physical Therapy is divided into six parts. The contributors to Part I wrote of our profession from an historical vantage, described what the future may bring, dealt with ethical considerations confronting each therapist, and defined the process of clinical reasoning.

The authors of Part II, representing many disciplines and content areas, present the theoretical foundations of human movement and function over the life cycle, whereas in Part III, physiologic changes and pathologic conditions affecting bodily functions and the resulting movement dysfunctions and disabilities are described.

Detailed in Part IV are the tests and measurements used by the physical therapist to analyze movement dysfunction and disability from a body systems' point of view and in the context of everyday functioning. The writers in Part V follow with intervention strategies that may be used to prevent, diminish, or correct the problems found through analysis.

For the final section of the book, we asked ten "master clinicians" each to select a patient for evaluation and treatment and then to record for us, as nearly as possible, what went through their minds and what they said and did to the patient, the patient's response, and the ultimate result of the patient–therapist relationship. The resulting nine clinical management studies furnish the reader with an insightful glimpse into the minds of experts as they act to meet the goals for various patients.

The reader who is interested in a specific movement dysfunction or disability problem involving a body system should read the appropriate chapters on that system in Parts III through VI of the book. For example, a cardiopulmonary problem may be studied by reviewing the causes of the problem in Chapters 12 and 13, an analysis of the problem in Chapters 29 and 30, possible interventions in Chapters 42 and 49, and some strategies for dealing with the problem in Chapters 64 and 65.

In our attempt to provide comprehensive coverage of the profession, three prominent physical therapists, Judith Canfield, Marilyn Moffat, and Katherine Shepard, agreed to serve as associate editors. They helped to develop the conceptual framework and the premises for the book, and each took editorial responsibility for a section of the book. Seventy-six authors, each a physical therapist with recognized expertise in a particular area of practice, agreed to be contributors. We would like to thank the associate editors and the contributors for sharing their talents and making their expertise available to all physical therapists.

We would like to dedicate this book to physical therapists past and present for their devotion to patient care and for their continuing search for knowledge and skills with which we all may improve and enhance human movement and function. The editors would especially like to remember Barbara A. Cossoy, who, at the time of her death, was an associate editor of *Physical Therapy* and an enthusiastic advocate of this project.

Rosemary M. Scully, Ed.D., P.T.
Marylou R. Barnes, Ed.D., P.T.

Contents

Part IV   **Analysis of Movement Dysfunction and Physical Disability**
▬▬▬   *Katherine F. Shepard, Editor*

Part V   Physical Therapy Intervention
Marilyn Moffat, Editor

Part VI   **Clinical Managment Studies**
           Judith S. Canfield, Editor

Physical Therapy

PART I

The Practice of Physical Therapy

Evolution of the Practice of Physical Therapy in the United States

1

DOROTHY PINKSTON

I want to take you back with me to England. Here it was I received my education and my background in physical therapy. After two years in college where I was working toward a B.A. degree I decided to [enter]. . . . a two-year course in physical education, or "physical culture and corrective exercise" as it was called. . . . At the completion of the course I felt the need of a better understanding of pathological conditions. I went to London and took some special courses in neuroanatomy, neurology, and psychology. . . . My first job was in Children's Hospital [Liverpool], where the usual polio and spastic conditions and scoliosis were present.

(MARY McMILLAN, 1946)

There is no better way to begin thinking about the evolution of the practice of physical therapy in the United States than with the words of Mary McMillan, who has been identified throughout the twentieth century as the first physical therapist in this country (Fig. 1-1). Her description of background events includes critical elements in the practice of physical therapy that have remained, with varying degrees of focus, throughout its evolution: human movement and biological, clinical, and social sciences. The words of Mary McMillan remind us of our reason for being: to assess, prevent, and treat movement dysfunction and physical disability, with the overall goal of enhancing human movement and function.

The evolution of physical therapy encompasses events that span the twentieth century. The magnitude of these events can be grasped by comparing definitions from the past and the present. Definitions from the 1920s refer to physical therapists as "educated trained assistants to the members of the established medical profession in the following agencies: (a) muscle training, (b) therapeutic massage, (c) electrotherapy, (d) light therapy, (e) mechanotherapy, (f) hydrotherapy" guided by policy to "practice only under the prescription of a licensed physician." Today the physical therapist is described as a practitioner who "may where permitted by law be the entry point into the health care system for evaluation, treatment, preventive programs, and consultation within the scope of his or her knowledge, experience, and expertise." Both definitions are from documents of the American Physical Therapy Association, the body that is viewed as "organized physical therapy" in today's society.

Contrast and similarities between the earliest years of the practice of physical therapy in the United States and the contemporary years could be seen vividly if each student of physical therapy could study McMillan's *Massage and Therapeutic Exercise* along with this textbook, *Physical Therapy*. Few will have such an opportunity, but perhaps you will find in this chapter the stimulus to search for other sources of information that can strengthen your understanding of the forces that have been at play during the evolution of the practice of physical therapy in the United States.

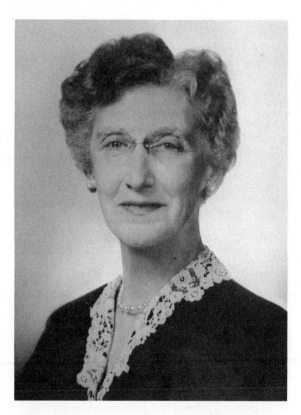

Figure 1-1. Mary McMillan (1880–1959). *(Courtesy of American Physical Therapy Association)*

A NEW OCCUPATION IN EARLY TWENTIETH-CENTURY AMERICA (1900–1930)

SOCIETAL INFLUENCES

Epidemics of Infantile Paralysis

In the United States, the use of physical therapy as a specialty area of therapeutic intervention dates back to the late years of the nineteenth century with an increase in application occurring in the early 1900s. Physical modalities and procedures applied for therapeutic purposes were first used systematically in this country in the treatment programs for infantile paralysis. These early efforts were centered in the New England states, where the incidence of acute anterior poliomyelitis, referred to then as infantile paralysis, reached epidemic proportions during the 1890s and the first two decades of the twentieth century.

The numbers of persons who were stricken during the epidemics of the summers of 1914 and 1916 were particularly high in Vermont. In an attempt to provide treatment and follow-up care to patients throughout the state, teams of workers were organized under the direction of Robert W. Lovett, M.D. The teams included physicians, nurses, and other nonphysician personnel (Fig. 1-2). The physicians who participated in this organized effort were local general practitioners as well as others in the same medical specialty as Dr. Lovett, orthopedic surgery. Among the nonphysician personnel on these teams were those who came to be known as physical therapists.

These individuals—Wilhelmine Wright, Janet Merrill, and Alice Lou Plastridge—had similar educational and experiential backgrounds prior to receiving special training in massage, muscle training, and corrective exercise from Dr. Lovett. Wright's earliest education and training were completed in Germany and included study of massage and exercise. Merrill was a graduate of Sargent College of Physical Education in Boston, Massachusetts. Plastridge was a junior gymnasium assistant in the Boston office of Dr. Lovett and some previous study in exercise or gymnastics must be assumed for one who occupied such a position. These three women figured prominently in the treatment programs for infantile paralysis, and shortly thereafter each became a leader in establishing the occupation of physical therapy in the United States.

Even though the occupation of physical therapy was not at that time a distinct entity, the foundations were being laid. The place of muscle training as a therapeutic procedure and the contributions of one of those earliest physical therapists is acknowledged by Lovett in the preface of the first edition of the classic textbook, *Treatment of Infantile Paralysis.*

> It has seemed desirable also to dwell at some length on the subject of muscle training because all experienced surgeons are today agreed that the operative treatment of infantile paralysis should not be undertaken

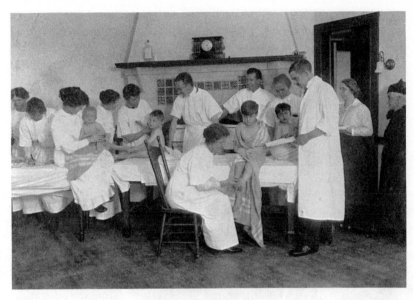

Figure 1-2. Physician and nonphysician personnel with children at a poliomyelitis clinic in New England, 1916. Some of the nonphysician personnel came to be known as physical therapists. *(Courtesy of American Physical Therapy Association)*

until at least two years after the onset and during these two years, when the most rapid progress is to be made, the treatment must needs be a non-operative one. As muscle training in my opinion constitutes the most important of the early therapeutic measures it has been somewhat emphasized. The material for the chapter on this subject has been furnished by my senior assistant in private practice, Miss Wilhelmine G. Wright, who has for some years devoted practically her whole time to this department of physical therapeutics and who has already published an article on the subject. I am greatly indebted to her for formulating for me the exercises and tests.

World War I

Systematization of methods in physical therapeutics was impelled by forces inherent in the needs of a nation at war; manpower needs during World War I forced attention on the use of multiple and combined methods of restoring physical function in members of both the military forces and the civilian work force. Formalized activities in clinical care and in training practitioners of physical therapy in the United States are related specifically to the establishment of the Division of Special Hospitals and Physical Reconstruction in the Office of The Surgeon General, U.S. Army, in 1917. Vogel (1968) reports use of the following definition and description for certain components of the Division:

> Physical reconstruction was defined as maximum mental and physical restoration of the individuals achieved by the use of medicine and surgery, supplemented by physical therapy, occupational therapy or curative workshop activities, education, recreation, and vocational training. Physical therapy was described as consisting of hydrotherapy, electrotherapy, and mechanotherapy, active exercise, indoor and outdoor games, and massage.

Through recognition of the applicability of physical therapeutics to the needs of another patient population—military personnel—the occupation known today as physical therapy received a major impetus for becoming a clearly identifiable occupation (Fig. 1-3).

An Industrial Society After World War I

During the earliest years in the evolution of physical therapy, preservation of human resources was of utmost importance. Attention that had been directed toward preserving, restoring, and maintaining a fighting force was

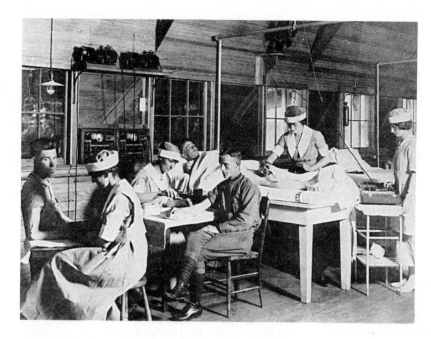

Figure 1-3. Reconstruction Aides treating soldiers at Fort Sam Houston, Texas, 1919. *(Courtesy of American Physical Therapy Association)*

directed toward preserving and maintaining a working force. The early issues of the journal now titled *Physical Therapy* repeatedly refer to the industrial problems of civil life and to the use of physical therapeutics to solve some of these problems. The extent to which the purpose of care for persons with injuries focused on the role of an individual in an industrial society is elaborated in a paper by Ruth E. Winch presented at the Convention of the International Society for Crippled Children in 1931.

> We realize that the crippled individual must adapt himself to an industrial world in which he bears a heavier burden than his fellows. He can scarcely evade this burden for the modern world accepts almost as axiomatic the theory that through work alone can self-expression and enduring satisfaction be found. Idleness is corrosive, work is needed for restorative as well as economic reasons.

Even though the importance of "self-expression" and "enduring satisfaction" for the individual is entertained by Winch, the expressions are used in the context of the work ethic and the economic needs of society.

Intermingled with the complexities of civil life in the early years of an industrial society were interests in the welfare of crippled children. As early as the 1880s, organizations focused on the interests of crippled children were becoming prominent, and state legislation had been enacted prior to 1900 to provide for education and treatment of crippled children. Whether those and similar efforts were motivated out of interest for the children or for the economic welfare of society is debatable. Speaking in 1930 about the Association for the Crippled and Disabled, Rachel Farnsworth made this observation:

> Human nature is much the same whether it be wrapped in a splendid physique or in a broken body. Back of the handicapped is the man, possessing the same instincts as his able-bodied neighbor, and seeking the same legitimate means of self-expression. Our ideal is to enable him to do his share and thus conferring a benefit upon the whole of citizenry.

Humanitarian purposes can be assumed for a portion of the interest expressed in crippled children, but purposes of the industrial society clearly were evident.

FORMALIZED TRAINING FOR EARLY PRACTITIONERS

Mary McMillan, recognized as the first physical therapist in this country, received her training in England and worked there for a number of years before returning to the United States in 1915 (Fig. 1-4). Other early practitioners in the United States provided the needed services without formal education and training specific to physical therapy.

The high number of personnel needed to

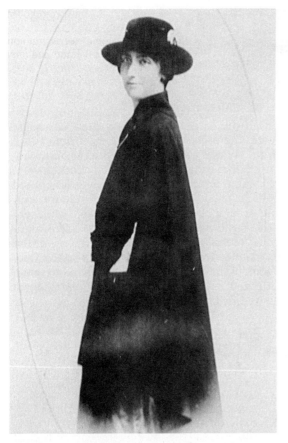

Figure 1-4. Mary McMillan wearing her Reconstruction Aide uniform. *(Courtesy of American Physical Therapy Association)*

provide care to members of the military forces focused attention on formalizing the preparation of those who would render services in physical therapeutics. Preparation for this expanded use of physical therapy fell under the guidance of individuals whose backgrounds were similar to those of practitioners who played a significant role in the early treatment efforts for polio victims. Marguerite Sanderson, a graduate of Wellesley College and the Boston Normal School of Gymnastics, assisted in the planning and organization activities that would make physical therapeutics a part of the care provided for Army personnel. She did so through an assignment to the Office of The Surgeon General of the Army in a position that carried no military status. By April 1918, outlines for a course to be used in training programs had been developed and cooperative efforts between personnel in the Office of The Surgeon General and personnel in civilian institutions were underway to prepare practitioners who would serve, in civilian capacity, as Reconstruction Aides in the recently established Division of Special Hospitals and Physical Reconstruction (Fig. 1-5). Even in the brief three-month program, content that would serve as the foundation for the practice of physical therapy was obvious: human anatomy and exercise (Table 1-1 and Fig. 1-6). Preference for applicants with high scholastic standing in the fundamentals of physical education demonstrated the importance that was placed on knowledge of human movement.

Earlier practitioners had rendered valuable services to the victims of infantile paralysis and many of these practitioners joined the ranks of the Reconstruction Aides. By name and number, the Reconstruction Aides hold the spotlight in the early history of physical therapy in the United States (Fig. 1-7).

A TITLE FOR THE PRACTITIONERS

The establishment in 1917 of the Division of Special Hospitals and Physical Reconstruction in the Office of The Surgeon General, U.S. Army was the initial force for a title and formal preparation for the practitioners. Personnel

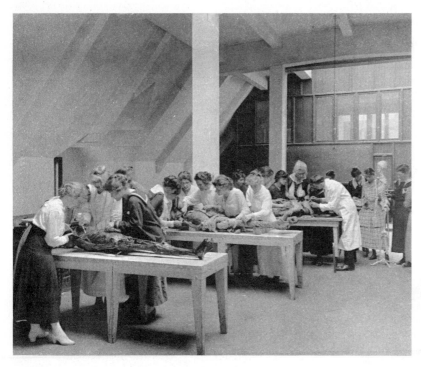

Figure 1-5. Students in training to become Reconstruction Aides studying in the anatomy dissection laboratory at Reed College, Portland, Oregon, 1918. *(Courtesy of American Physical Therapy Association)*

who completed the emergency courses were given the title Reconstruction Aide. Those who had experience in using physical therapeutics in civilian life also were recruited for service with the military as Reconstruction Aides. Practitioners rendering similar service in civilian facilities were referred to as physiotherapy aides, physiotherapy technicians, physical therapy technicians, and, in some instances, physician's assistant. Designation as assistant was used particularly by those physicians who personally trained individuals to work in their private offices.

The precedent was set for the occupational role by the earliest formal title, Reconstruction Aide. The role of aide or assistant was perpetuated by the view held by many who were instrumental in the initial organizational efforts for this occupational group. The original Objects of the American Women's Physical Therapeutic Association expressed the view thusly: "to make available efficiently trained women to the medical profession." Even though the role of practitioners in this new occupation had not

been clarified, the more definitive statements were slanted strongly toward a role that was supportive to the physician, truly that of an assistant. To overlook these realities in our history would not serve us well in trying to understand the evolution of physical therapy.

NATIONWIDE ORGANIZATION BY THE PRACTITIONERS

Organizational efforts, founding, and early development of the national organization that we know as the American Physical Therapy Association (APTA) are described in several publications. Elson addresses the early history in "The Legacy of Mary McMillan," and development throughout the first 25 years is described by Hazenhyer in "A History of the American Physiotherapy Association," published in 1946, the 25th anniversary year of the founding of the organization. Many elements of the history of the Association have been eloquently summarized and beautifully depicted in the January 1976 issue of *Physical Therapy*.

Table 1-1. Required Subjects, Clock Hours, and Percentages* of Total Clock Hours Designated in Emergency Course (1918), Minimum Curriculum Adopted by American Physiotherapy Association (1928), and Minimum Curricula Adopted by American Medical Association (1936, 1955)

REQUIRED SUBJECTS	EMERGENCY COURSE, 1918		APA, 1928		AMA, 1936		AMA, 1955	
	hr	%	hr	%	hr	%	hr	%
Biological and Physical Sciences								
Anatomy	99	16	300	25	210	18	210	13
Physiology	32	5	72	6	75	6	150	9
Chemistry			81	7				
Physics			81	7				
Kinesiology	6	1	36	3				
Social Science								
Psychology	10	2	18	2	15	1	15	1
Ethics†	2	§	6	1	5	§	30	2
Clinical Science (Physical Therapy)								
Electrotherapy	6	1	72	6	75	6		
Exercise‡	117	19	228	19	105	9	210	13
Hydrotherapy	4	1	24	2	20	2		
Light Therapy			45	4				
Massage	112	18	90	8	60	5		
Thermotherapy			3	§				
Physical Agents							165	10
Tests and Measurements							105	7
Clinical Science (Medical)							90	6
Medicine					45	4		
Neurology					25	2		
Orthopedics			72	6	45	4		
Surgery	15	2	36	3	45	4		
Pathology	26	4	36	3	30	3	30	2
Clinical Experience	163	26			400	33	600	37
Other	28	5						
Electives					45	4		
Total	620		1200		1200		1605	

*Not all percent columns equal 100% because numbers were rounded off.
†History, Administration, and Professional Relationships (1955).
‡Assistive Devices included 1955.
§Less than 1%.

The American Women's Physical Therapeutic Association, founded in 1921, was a direct outgrowth of relationships and mutual understanding that had developed among those who served with the U.S. Army as Reconstruction Aides. The earliest practitioners of physical therapy who were instrumental in founding this organization, and who volunteered untold hours toward its ultimate success, repeatedly expressed their beliefs about the need for a foundation in understanding human movement. Reconstruction Aides were the charter members, and a focus on a background in physical education along with training and experience in massage and therapeutic exercise was expressed in the qualifications for "active" membership. During the early years of the Association, membership was opened to nurses who had additional training and specific types of clinical experiences, but the change in requirements for membership was not accomplished without heated debate. Portions of Hazenhyer's series, editorials in the official journal of the Association, and verbatim

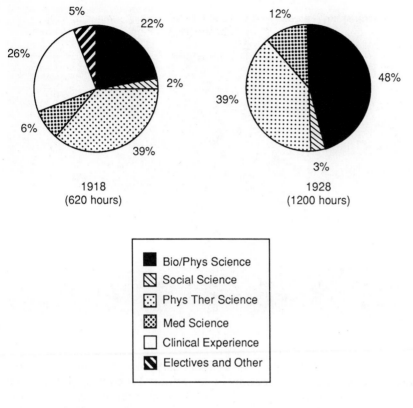

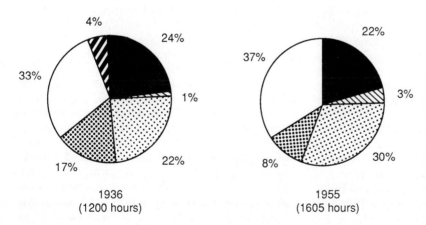

Figure 1-6. Percentage of time devoted to major content areas in the minimum curriculum for physical therapy at key points in the history of physical therapy education: emergency course for training of Reconstruction Aides, 1918; Minimum Standards for Schools of Physical Therapy, APA, 1928; Essentials of an Acceptable School for Physical Therapy Technicians, AMA, 1936; and Essentials of an Acceptable School of Physical Therapy, AMA, 1955. Not all percentages equal 100% because percentages were rounded off.

minutes in files of the Archives Collection (APTA) provide a sense of the intensity of feelings that were expressed in those debates.

The name of the organization was the subject of much debate during the early years, debates that were fueled by the fact that physi-

cians were using the title "physical therapist" in their practice of physical therapy. The terms *physiotherapy, physical therapy, physiotherapist,* and *physical therapist* were used in the United States until the fifth decade of this century to refer to a medical specialty and to the physi-

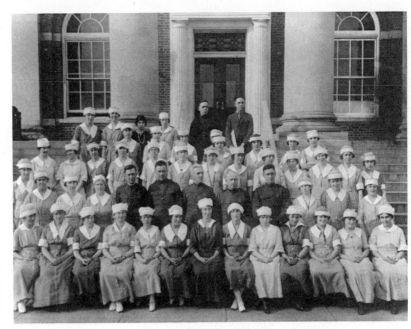

Figure 1-7. Mary McMillan, other Reconstruction Aides, and physicians on steps of Walter Reed General Hospital, Washington, D.C., circa 1919. *(Courtesy of American Physical Therapy Association)*

cians who practiced that specialty. From 1929 until 1933, an American Physical Therapy Association existed as an organization that was formed through merger of two organizations of physicians, the Western Association of Physical Therapy and the American Electrotherapeutic Association. In 1922, the name of the American Women's Physical Therapeutic Association was changed to American Physiotherapy Association (APA) and subsequently, in 1947, to American Physical Therapy Association (APTA).

The history of the APTA and the evolution of physical therapy in the United States are interwoven. Certain intricacies in the relationship of historic events in the development of the APTA and the evolution of physical therapy are included with discussion of subsequent topics.

BORN OF THE TIMES

Physical therapy as an occupation in the United States is clearly an occupation of the twentieth century. It emerged from a need for a specific kind of health service related to the restoration of locomotor function of the human body. At a point now slightly more than one decade from the close of the twentieth century, physical therapy is listed routinely among the occupations related to health care and often is referred to as an emerging profession. The evolution of physical therapy reflects the society in which the occupation evolved and includes five key features: (1) establishment of standards for education and practice; (2) reactions to and involvement in national and international events; (3) response to philanthropic activities; (4) efforts toward clarifying the scope of practice; and (5) endeavors toward professionalization of the occupation. At times progress has been slow, but it has never halted; at times the focus has been dimmed, but it has never been obscured. With each renewal of focus on understanding human movement as a basis for alleviating or correcting movement dysfunction, the services of the physical therapist have been enhanced and the contributions that physical therapists can make to human well-being have been magnified.

PHYSICAL THERAPY IN AMERICAN SOCIETY (1920–1986)

National crises and societal pressures spawned and supported the development of this new occupation in early twentieth-century America. The early practitioners demonstrated quite clearly that an understanding of normal locomotor functions of the human body could play a part in modifying the outcomes of disease and injury. The need for such services was not unique to either the segments of society ravaged by polio or the members of the fighting forces who had sustained injuries.

SCOPE AND SUBSTANCE OF PRACTICE AND PRACTICE SETTINGS

The efforts that were concentrated on training personnel during World War I provided a greater number of physicians and nonphysicians who were knowledgeable about the potential benefits of physical therapeutics. The use of physical modalities in therapeutic intervention spread to a variety of settings throughout the country. Practitioners who would come to be known as physical therapists were employed in special schools and hospitals for crippled children, industrial settings and the related curative workshops and vocational rehabilitation centers, special diagnostic clinics and outpatient treatment centers for crippled children, as well as in private offices of physicians and in general hospitals. The expertise of the physical therapy technician became known in many segments of the American society, particularly those segments touched by such organizations and agencies as the Crippled Children's Division of the Children's Bureau, U.S. Department of Labor; state and federal vocational rehabilitation programs; Visiting Nurses Associations in cities throughout the country; the National Society for Crippled Children and Adults; and the National Foundation for Infantile Paralysis.

In 1921, Mary McMillan referred to four distinct branches in physical therapeutics: massage, therapeutic exercise, electrotherapy, and hydrotherapy. Other authors use more elaborate categories to describe the methods of physical therapy, and often these classify procedures under the following headings: thermotherapy, light therapy, electrotherapy, hydrotherapy, and mechanotherapy. Textbooks from early years of the twentieth century document the application of physical therapy for problems related to the entire scope of systems addressed in this book: musculoskeletal, neuromuscular, cardiovascular, pulmonary, integumentary, reproductive, renal, and psychogenic. The therapeutic procedures used by physical therapy technicians during the post-World War I years usually were chosen by physicians according to the needs of their patient population and the characteristics of individual practice settings. At times the focus was on electrotherapy, and at times on therapeutic exercises. Often a set of procedures became customary treatment in the clinical practice of physical therapy. Specific regimens in physical therapeutics were developed, and often carried the name of the founder or the institution where developed. The regimens in some cases combined heat and exercise, and in other cases were a specific set of exercises to be used for problems related to a given disease or injury. Those who have entered the practice of physical therapy during the past 15 or so years might be hard pressed to describe, much less use, regimens requested by the following names: Klapp's creeping exercises; Kenny's definitive muscle re-education; or Buerger's exercises for the lower extremity. Some of the early eponyms linger in use, such as Frenkel's coordination exercises and Codman's shoulder routine, but rarely are these regimens used today in the original form.

In the 1940s, the value of physical therapy was tested through circumstances reminiscent of those that had stimulated the initial recognition: epidemics of polio and a world at war. Continued epidemics of polio and the outbreak of World War II placed serious demands on the limited number of qualified physical therapy technicians. The challenges were met by combining forces from the civilian and military sectors, and the practice of physical therapy was propelled through a major growth period.

Major concepts related to approaches for rehabilitation—physical, psychological, vocational, and emotional—were introduced in treating the survivors of World War II. The principles of muscle training applied in treating polio were found to be ineffective for treating many of the problems associated with war-related injuries. New frontiers in the neurosciences were being investigated by scientists of many fields and in many countries throughout the world. Physicians and physical therapists turned their attention toward a more extensive application of neurophysiologic principles in rehabilitation efforts. Once again regimens were developed for specific types of problems, and once again the regimens were known by the names of the founders. Along with the new set of eponyms, abbreviations and other shortcuts to labeling the techniques became a part of our vocabulary: DeLorme's routine, PRE, and PNF. Some treatment approaches proposed during the 1940s and 1950s were based soundly in neurophysiology and in principles of neuromuscular physiology. These have been further developed during the intervening years and are in use still. Other approaches were discarded when shown to be more fanciful than factual.

Another area of practice that began a major growth period during the years of World War II was the medical specialty focusing on the use of physical therapeutics: physical medicine. In 1944, the name of the medical specialty officially became *physical medicine;* in 1945, the physicians in the specialty formally adopted the title *physiatrist.* As physicians dropped the title physical therapist, the practitioner title of physical therapy *technician* could be discarded by members of our occupation and the title of *physical therapist* used without hesitation. Even so, the identity of the occupation was far from clear. Physical medicine had been defined as a specialty that includes the employment of the physical and other effective properties of light, heat, cold, water, electricity, massage, manipulation, exercise, and mechanical devices for physical and occupational therapy in the diagnosis and treatment of disease. Two distinct occupations were subsumed in the definition of

physical medicine, one being physical therapy. Elements in the potential confusion about roles and titles can be illustrated rather vividly with a review of changes made in the names of two organizations: American Congress of Rehabilitation Medicine, formerly American Congress of Physical Medicine and Rehabilitation (1953–1966), formerly American Congress of Physical Medicine (1945–1952), formerly American Congress of Physical Therapy (1930–1944), formerly American College of Physical Therapy (1926–1929), originally American College of Radiology and Physiotherapy (1923–1925); and American Academy of Physical Medicine and Rehabilitation, formerly American Society of Physical Medicine and Rehabilitation (1952–1955), formerly American Society of Physical Medicine (1946–1951), originally Society of Physical Therapy Physicians (1939–1945).

The rehabilitation concepts introduced in treating those wounded in World War II fostered the growth of the new specialty of physical medicine. The title became interchangeable with rehabilitation and rehabilitation medicine, and departments under one of the three titles—physical medicine, rehabilitation, or rehabilitation medicine—were established in medical centers throughout the country. The embryonic practice of physical therapy had been nurtured through a close working relationship between the practitioners and physicians, physicians who were specializing in orthopedics as well as physicians in other specialty areas of medical practice, including the general practice of medicine. With the continued development of the specialty of physical medicine came a different combination of personnel in the area of physical therapeutics. In institutions where a department of physical medicine was included among the medical departments, services of the physical therapist were available only through referral to the physiatrist by the attending physician. This arrangement was not accepted readily by physicians who at one time were those closest to the physical therapist and the services that the physical therapist could render for the benefit of their patients. The problem of having a single physician specialty placed between all other referring physicians and the physical therapist was approached in a variety of ways. One approach was to include physical therapists on the staff of other departments in the institution, particularly orthopedics. Another approach was to include one or more physical therapists in the private office staff. Regardless of the approach taken by individual physicians, physical therapists were placed in a position quite different from that of earlier practitioners. All too often, the services that could be provided by the physical therapist as therapeutic intervention for a wide variety of problems were simply ignored.

The scope of practice for the physical therapist was sorely challenged in the environment of departmental organizations for physical medicine, rehabilitation, and rehabilitation medicine. Facing the challenge meant answering key questions about the future of the occupation. Were physical therapy services to be available to all medical specialists who wished to use physical therapy in the overall care of their patients? Were future practitioners to be prepared to work under the direction and supervision of members of one medical specialty? The answers have been formulated slowly during the last 25 years for the occupation; for some individual practitioners, the answers are yet to come. The scope of practice for the physical therapist who serves as an entry point into the health care system—for evaluation, treatment, preventive programs, and consultation within the scope of the practitioner's knowledge, experience, and expertise—includes treatment of patients being cared for by any medical specialist and makes the services available to all segments of society.

The procedures used by physical therapists today still are within those four distinct branches that were identified earlier in the century: massage, therapeutic exercise, electrotherapy, and hydrotherapy. Where each of those branches fits in the practice of physical therapy today is the substance of this book and best left to the chapters that follow. The evolution of physical therapy has come to the point that the House of Delegates of the American

Physical Therapy Association adopted, in 1986, the following definition as one that is appropriate for inclusion in dictionaries, medical and otherwise:

> Physical therapy: (a) treatment by physical means; (b) the profession which is concerned with health promotion, with prevention of physical disabilities, and with rehabilitation of persons disabled by pain, disease, or injury; and which is involved with evaluating patients, and with treating through the use of physical therapeutic measures as opposed to medicines, surgery, or radiation.

The definition reminds us that the principles that undergird our occupation can serve in promotion of health and in prevention of disabilities as well as in therapeutic intervention. And the definition includes a component of our practice that heretofore was seldom included in widespread publications of the public domain: the evaluative, or analytical, skills that serve as a foundation for other components of the practice. Although advances in science and technology have made available to us the means for greater understanding of human movement and function and more refined methods for assessment, the matters that receive our attention today are those that have received the attention of physical therapists for over 65 years. Titles of lead papers presented by invited speakers at annual conferences of the APTA over the years illustrate the point quite well (Fig. 1-8).

The hospital has continued to be the primary setting for the services of therapeutic intervention provided by a physical therapist. Today, however, approximately 50% of the active physical therapists practice in settings other than the hospital. Special schools and hospitals for crippled children, rehabilitation centers, private offices of physicians, and special diagnostic clinics and outpatient treatment centers remain among the settings where physical therapy is practiced. Private offices of physical therapists, extended-care facilities and nursing homes, home health agencies, residential care facilities, academic institutions, fitness and wellness centers, research centers, and prepaid health care organizations as well as governmental and voluntary health agencies also are among the settings where physical therapists work today. Changes in the list of settings reflect expansion that has occurred in the role of the physical therapist and changes in types of health care facilities found in our society.

As the practice of physical therapy has evolved, so have elements in the practice that are distinct from that of the physical therapist as clinician. Rudiments in the role of physical therapist as educator, as consultant, as administrator, and as researcher have been in evidence since the earliest days of the recognizable occupation.

For the most part, the earliest practitioners were first teachers—of physical education or physical culture, gymnastics, and corrective exercises. Teaching was at the very heart of the services rendered for those who had been striken by infantile paralysis. Practitioners taught members of the family and other members of the community how to care for the victims. Some of these early practitioners were called on for classroom and laboratory teaching once formal programs were available to train future practitioners. The physical therapist as consultant was basic to the relationship between many early practitioners and the physicians with whom they worked. This element is demonstrated in the earlier quotation from Lovett's textbook, *Treatment of Infantile Paralysis,* and the physical therapist as consultant has developed in concert with the overall development of the occupation. The understanding of human motion that served as a resource for the contributions that were made in treating victims of polio served similarly in posture clinics and in preventive care in industrial settings. In a consultative role during polio epidemics, physical therapists worked toward the solutions of multiple problems that faced communities throughout this nation and in other countries. With such titles as Supervisor of Reconstruction Aides, Chief Head Aide, and Senior Physiotherapy Technician, supervision and management came into the role of early practitioners. The keen observations of muscle function and of the effects of muscle weakness on human movement made by those who provided care for the victims of infantile paralysis

---

First Annual Convention, 13–16 September 1922, Boston, Massachusetts

Treatment Used for Patients with Infantile Paralysis
Posture Training
Physiotherapy and Its Relation to Industrial Accident Cases
(One morning devoted to inspecting electrotherapy work at Boston City Hospital)

Twenty-first Annual Conference, 28 June–3 July 1942, Lake Geneva, Wisconsin

Infantile Paralysis: Discussion Groups

Acute and Subacute Stages
  Clinical Symptoms and Pathology; Aims of Physical Treatment; Types of Physical Treatment (measures for controlling body alignment, heat, exercise, proprioceptive training, passive and active movement); Records
Convalescent Stage
  Clinical Symptoms and Pathology; Modalities for Stimulation of Circulation and Their Effect upon Normal and Affected Muscles; Therapeutic Exercises: Objectives, techniques
Chronic Stage
  Teaching Functional Activities: Institution or outpatient clinic; In curative workshop; In home
General Session: Treatment of Infantile Paralysis in the Acute Stage—Sister Elizabeth Kenny

War Injuries: Discussion Groups

Peripheral Nerve Injuries; Peripheral Nerve Injuries of the Upper Extremity; Electrical Muscle Stimulation
Surgical Aspects of Amputations; Physical Therapy Treatment in Amputations
Therapy of Burns in Wartime
The After Treatment of War Injuries by Physical Therapy
Fractures of the Calcaneous; The Use of Short Wave in Healing Fractures
Occupational Therapy
Applied Anatomy: Discussion Group

(continued)

might be viewed as the earliest research activities of physical therapists. These observations were recorded and subsequently provided a foundation for the occupation. From those less formal research activities, physical therapists have proceeded to more formal endeavors that can enhance the scientific basis of practice. In addition to providing an obvious option for practice today, each of these elements can enhance the services of the clinician and thus the occupation.

Clinical Specialties

Specialization in clinical practice has been inherent in the evolution of the occupation. In 1978, the House of Delegates of the APTA took action to facilitate the identification and development of clinical specialties and the certification and recertification of physical therapy specialists. A document titled "Essentials for Certification of Physical Therapy Specialists" was adopted by the House of Delegates and mechanisms were put into place to advance this aspect of practice further. Six specialty areas in physical therapy are recognized currently by the American Board of Physical Therapy Specialties (ABPTS): cardiopulmonary, clinical electrophysiology, neurology, pediatrics, orthopaedics, and sports. The first clinical specialists were certified in 1985 in the area of Cardiopulmonary Physical Therapy and the number of physical therapists certified as clinical specialists reached 42 in April 1987.

Supportive Personnel

As the practice of physical therapy and the role of the physical therapist have evolved, so have the roles of supportive personnel in providing physical therapy services. The supply of qualified physical therapists, or physical therapy

---

Thirty-ninth Annual Conference, 17–22 June 1962, San Francisco, California

Legislation and Medical Responsibility
Development of Motor Behavior
Use of Sequential Motor Development
Elements of Motor Learning
Implication of Research in Motor Learning
Muscles and How They Are Used in Human
   Locomotion

Assessment of Motor Abilities
   Testing Methods and Instrumentation
   Recording and Interpretation of Test Data
   Use of Information
   A Basis for Planning
Demonstrations of Developmental Activities
   Cerebral Palsy; Above-Knee Amputee;
   Hemiplegia; Arthritis; Paraplegia

Fifty-ninth Annual Conference, 19–23 June 1982, Anaheim, California

Instructional Courses
   Cost Analysis for Physical Therapists
   Sensory Integration in Physical Therapy
   Rehabilitation of the Surgical Knee
   Basic Life Support: CPR Course
Is Your Body Machinery Tuned Properly?
Journey from Darkness: An Enlightening Review of
   Neuroscience
Role of Diaphragmatic Fatigue in Respiratory Failure:
   Is There a "Digitalis" for the Diaphragm?
Functional Electrical Stimulation
Possible Determinants of Attrition from the Profession
   of Physical Therapy
Art of "Laying-on-of-Hands" Healing: Scientific
   Interdisciplinary Evidence and Implications

Clinical Applications of Motion Analysis
Health and Well-Being of the Young Athlete
Evaluation of Physical Work Capacity in Multiple
   Disabilities
Clinical Neurophysiology
Anatomy of Exercise
Practical Aspects of Clinical Research
Controversies in Cardiac Rehabilitation
Scoliosis
Influence of Kinesiological Principles of Therapeutic
   Exercise
Clinical Education Module for Advanced Training in
   Orthopedic Manual Therapy
Why and How of Trigger Points Demonstrated
Lumbar Spine: Mechanical Diagnosis and Treatment

Figure 1-8. Major topics from programs at four annual conferences held by the organization now known as the American Physical Therapy Association. *(Courtesy of American Physical Therapy Association)*

technicians, has seldom if ever been equal to the demand for services. Aides, attendants, and volunteers provided valuable assistance in direct care for the large numbers of persons who had polio during the epidemics, particularly in the acute care settings. The duties of these supportive, or nonprofessional, personnel in physical therapy were specific to the employment setting, but often there were common elements from setting to setting. Among the common elements in job responsibilities were assisting patients before and after treat-employment setting, but often there were common elements from setting to setting. Among the common elements in job responsibilities were assisting patients before and after treatment, general housekeeping involved with preparing treatment areas and equipment prior to and following a treatment session, and routine maintenance of equipment and supplies. In addition, supportive personnel assisted with routine aspects of treatment. The training for aides, attendants, and volunteers was a responsibility of the facility staff and concentrated on the tasks to be done at the individual facility. Similar patterns continue today in the training and use of aides and attendants, and often volunteers, in the practice of physical therapy.

The 1960s brought profound changes for health care in the United States, and the practice of physical therapy was no exception. Public expectations for health services had been heightened and attention from many sectors was focused on finding ways to meet the expectations. The projected needs in numbers of health care personnel far exceeded the capacity of the educational system; attention was turned to new types of personnel and new approaches to training. These are the forces that stimulated planning for an additional category of personnel in the practice of physical therapy, the physical therapist assistant.

In a span of approximately 20 years, the physical therapist assistant has become a part of the staffing pattern for physical therapy in most areas of the United States. Preparation of the physical therapist assistant includes a minimum of two years of college work, usually in a community college or affiliated institution, and leads to an associate degree. Programs for the

assistant are offered in 28 states and in Puerto Rico and the total number of programs now exceeds 70. Of some interest is the fact that the rate of growth for assistant programs has far exceeded that of the programs for initial preparation of the physical therapists. Over 50 years had passed before the programs for the physical therapist reached similar numbers in the mid-1970s.

The physical therapist assistant, as a technical health care worker, is prepared to function in the application of specific physical therapy procedures to patients and in performing routine administrative procedures. Both areas of function are under the direction and supervision of a physical therapist. Staffing patterns that appropriately incorporate the physical therapist assistant offer the potential for extending the capabilities of the physical therapist severalfold. With the potential for extending capabilities come demands for additional skills in delegating and supervising on the part of the physical therapist. Regardless of the practice setting, the responsibility for the quality of physical therapy services rests ultimately with the physical therapist.

STANDARDS FOR PRACTICE AND PRACTITIONER CREDENTIALS

Founders of the American Women's Physical Therapeutic Association expressed clear intent related to standards for practice in the new occupation: "The purpose of this Association shall be to establish and maintain a professional and scientific standard for those engaged in the profession of physical therapeutics." Modalities that were used in physical therapeutics also were used by members of cults, and in the hands of charlatans were among the fads of early twentieth-century American society. If the new occupation was to be recognized as a respectable type of work, one of the early basic tenets—prescription and direction of a licensed physician—was of particular importance in establishing standards for both practice and education. Standards for practice and practitioner credentials have taken several forms during the evolution of physical therapy in the United States.

AMERICAN PHYSIOTHERAPY ASSOCIATION

Code of Ethics and Discipline
Adopted June 1935

I. Professional Practice

  A. Diagnosing, stating the prognosis of a case, and prescribing treatment shall be entirely the responsibility of the physician. Any assumption of this responsibility by one of our members shall be considered unethical.

  B. The patient shall be referred back to the physician for periodical examinations.

  C. A member shall not attempt to criticize the physician or dictate technique or procedure.

II. Advertising

  A. Members shall not procure patients by means of solicitors, agents, circulars, displays, or advertisements inserted in commercial products.

  B. Announcements in medical journals or business cards, not stating fees, are permissible. A statement that the work is medically supervised should appear on the announcement.

  C. A member may use the term "Physiotherapist" or "Physical Therapist" on an office door.

III. Behavior

  A. Members shall not indulge, before patients, in criticism of doctors, co-workers, or predecessors who have handled the case.

  B. It is well to bear in mind that our reputation as individuals and a group depends upon professional accomplishments and upon adherence to the standards of our organization.

IV. Discipline

  A. Charges and evidence against offenders will be weighed and acted upon by the Executive Committee.

Figure 1-9. First set of ethical principles of the American Physiotherapy Association as adopted in 1935 by the members of the Association. *(Courtesy of American Physical Therapy Association)*

Ethical Principles

A formal set of ethical principles was first adopted by members of the Association over 50 years ago (Fig. 1-9). Even though binding only on members of the Association, ethical principles adopted by the APA and then the APTA have had significant influence on the evolution of physical therapy. The influence has been manifest directly through the behavior of the members and indirectly through standards of practice included in the legal regulations for practice.

The initial Code of Ethics and Discipline, adopted in 1935, addressed the expected behavior in therapeutic intervention and the exclusive responsibilities of the physician for diagnosis, prognosis, and prescription. For the early practitioners to focus on the therapeutic values of physical modalities and the relationship to the physician was critical in establishing the legitimacy of the work. To use their skills with corrective exercises apart from the practice of medicine was tantamount to working as a "drugless healer", a name to be avoided if the occupation was to flourish. Similar statements about the responsibilities of the physician for diagnosis, prescription, and prognosis were included in the Code of Ethics adopted in 1948 and amended in 1952 and 1957 (Fig. 1-10). The document sets forth the ethical principles related to the functions of a technician in carrying out prescribed procedures. Evidence that the practice of physical therapy was evolving beyond a technical level is found in the Code of Ethics adopted in 1968 and amended in 1969 (Fig. 1-11): "2. The physical therapist should accept and seek full responsibility for the exercise of judgment within the area of his compe-

AMERICAN PHYSICAL THERAPY ASSOCIATION
CODE OF ETHICS
Adopted May 1948
Amended June 1952, June 1957

Ethics for the Physical Therapist of the American Physical Therapy Association

Article I. General Principles

Section 1. Physical therapy is a medical service and therefore is regarded as an integral part of this field. The physical therapist shall carry on the techniques of the profession only with adequate and specific medical direction.

Section 2. The profession of physical therapy is devoted to the best welfare of the patient. The physical therapist shall keep this basic principle in view and be guided by it at all times.

Section 3. In entering the profession of physical therapy, an individual assumes definite responsibilities toward his associates and commits himself to the upholding of professional ideals. It shall be well understood by each physical therapist that he acts as a representative of the whole profession and as such shall conduct himself with honor and integrity.

Article II. Responsibility of the Physical Therapist to the Physician

Section 1. Diagnosis of the patient's disability and the prescription of physical therapy are the responsibility of the physician. In no instance shall the physical therapist assume this responsibility.

Section 2. Before treating a patient the physical therapist shall obtain from the physician clear and adequate information regarding diagnosis, instructions for treatment, and, if possible, re-examination date.

Section 3. The physical therapist shall not continue treatment beyond a stated re-examination date without further orders from the physician. Changes of any consequence in the patient's condition occurring between interim visits shall be reported to the physician in charge without delay.

Section 4. The physical therapist shall have a definite statement from the physician regarding termination of treatment and shall comply with this direction.

Article III. Responsibility of the Physical Therapist to the Patient

Section 1. Information of a confidential nature regarding patients gained from any source whatsoever shall be considered a serious trust by the physical therapist. Such confidences shall be well guarded at all times.

Section 2. The physical therapist shall be discreet and tactful in all dealings with the patient and he shall avoid all actions or statements which in any way might be construed by the patient as criticism of the physician in charge or his handling of the case. Likewise, disparaging remarks or implications concerning professional co-workers, particularly those who previously have dealt with the patient, shall be studiously avoided.

Section 3. Specific statements concerning the patient's prognosis shall be made only by the physician in charge. Such statements from the physical therapist may prove detrimental to the welfare of the patient.

Section 4. All suggestions regarding medical referral are the responsibility of the physician and shall not be made by the physical therapist.

Section 5. The physical therapist should not accept gratuities.

Section 6. The direct sale or rental of equipment, supplies, or publications as a part of physical therapy service is unethical except in those instances where the patient cannot readily procure these items; any such sale or rental must be without exploitation of the patient, or net profit to the physical therapist.

(continued)

Article IV. Responsibility of the Physical Therapist to Co-workers, Employers, the Profession, and the Professional Organization

Section 1. The physical therapist shall give his full loyalty and support to the organization and individuals with whom he is professionally associated.

Section 2. A physical therapist shall not solicit patients either through his own efforts, through an agent, or by circulating printed matter in any form other than announcements to the medical profession.

Section 3. In addition to applying techniques of the profession to the best of his ability, the physical therapist should constantly strive to improve his knowledge and proficiency.

Section 4. The physical therapist may patent appliance and equipment or copyright publications, methods, or procedures. However, retarding or inhibiting research or restricting the benefits which may be derived from such patents or copyrights is unethical.

Section 5. The physical therapist should willingly participate in educational programs which promote the welfare of the profession but shall in no wise associate himself with any program which misrepresents to its students the rights and privileges which shall be accorded to them upon completion of their training or which permits utilization of his skills and knowledge to the detriment of the profession.

Section 6. The physical therapist should give his full loyalty and support to the professional organization in its effort to attain its objective.

Section 7. It is the duty of the physical therapist to disclose to the proper authorities any knowledge he may have concerning unethical practice being carried on by any member of this profession and to testify in an investigation of such charges upon request. Only through the integrity of each individual member can the highest purpose of the profession be served.

Figure 1-10. Code of Ethics of the American Physical Therapy Association as adopted by the House of Delegates in 1948 and amended by the House of Delegates in 1952 and in 1957. *(Courtesy of American Physical Therapy Association)*

tence and should require referral by a physician or dentist in providing direct patient services." The continuing evolution of practice is reflected clearly in both the 1977 revision (Fig. 1-12) and the ethical principles set forth in the current Code of Ethics (Fig. 1-13), adopted in 1981. Neither Code mentions the referral relationship with physicians or other practitioners. Each of the most recent revisions does address compliance with the law and Association policies governing the practice of physical therapy, accepting responsibility for the exercise of professional judgment, and maintaining standards of professional practice.

Additional evidence of the evolution of practice related to ethical principles can be found in the companion document to the Code, the Guide for Professional Conduct. The Guide, developed and issued by the Judicial Committee of the APTA, accompanies the Code of Ethics and assists in interpreting the Code for application to specific situations in practice.

Adherence to ethical principles also is expected of the physical therapist assistants who are members of the Association. These principles are included in Standards of Ethical Conduct for the Physical Therapist Assistant (Fig. 1-14), adopted by the House of Delegates of the APTA in 1982. Interpretations in terms of contemporary practice are found in the companion document, Guide for Conduct of the Affiliate Member, also the responsibility of the Judicial Committee.

Registration

For a number of years, membership in the American Physiotherapy Association was viewed by members of the American Medical Association as sufficient credential for identifying qualified physical therapy technicians. In 1934, the American Registry of Physical Thera-

---

AMERICAN PHYSICAL THERAPY ASSOCIATION
CODE OF ETHICS
Adopted July 1968, Amended July 1969

The physical therapist as a member of the American Physical Therapy Association accepts this Code of Ethics as the basis for the practice of his profession. Individually and collectively, the members of this Association are responsible for promoting and maintaining the highest ethical standards of practice.

This Code of Ethics shall be binding on the membership. There shall always be a Guide for Professional Conduct to assist in the interpretation of the Code of Ethics. This Guide, taking reference from the Code of Ethics, shall be subject to monitoring, interpretation, and timely revision by the Association's Judicial Committee.

1. The physical therapist should respect the human dignity of each individual with whom he is associated in his profession, being guided at all times by his concern for the welfare of the patient and by his responsibilities to his associates and colleagues.

2. The physical therapist should accept and seek full responsibility for the exercise of judgment within the area of his competence and should require referral by a physician or dentist in providing direct patient services.

3. The physical therapist should comply with existing laws governing the practice of physical therapy and should maintain acceptable standards of professional practice.

4. The physical therapist should respect the confidentiality of all privileged information and should voluntarily share such information only as it serves the welfare of the patient.

5. The physical therapist should accept responsibility for services to patients referred to him and is obligated to provide continuing supervision when any portion of the service is delegated to supportive personnel. He should not delegate to a less qualified person any service which requires the skill and judgment of the physical therapist.

6. The physical therapist should not solicit patients, should avoid the use of advertisement or any form of self-aggrandizement, and should not seek to obtain more than just and professionally appropriate remuneration for his service.

7. The physical therapist should not permit his name to be used in connection with advertisement of products, and should not dispense or supply physical therapy equipment unless it is in the best interest of the patient.

8. The physical therapist should assume responsibility for the interpretation of his profession to all segments of society so that his services may be appropriately and effectively employed in meeting current health needs and to assure the future growth of the profession.

9. The physical therapist should accept responsibility for exposing incompetence and illegal or unethical conduct to the appropriate authority.

10. The physical therapist should give his loyalty and support to the American Physical Therapy Association in its efforts to attain its objectives.

Figure 1-11. Code of Ethics of the American Physical Therapy Association as adopted by the House of Delegates in 1968 and amended by the House of Delegates in 1969. *(Courtesy of American Physical Therapy Association)*

py Technicians (ARPTT) was established by the American Congress of Physical Therapy, the organization of physicians specializing in the use of physical therapy. The practice of using membership in the Registry as a qualification for employment followed; no longer was membership in the APA a sufficient credential for qualified practitioners.

For a limited period of time, members of the APA were permitted registration with the ARPTT without examination. Once the period for waiver of written examination had ended, taking the written examination for membership in the ARPTT became the final step in the educational process for physical therapy technicians. With satisfactory performance on the

AMERICAN PHYSICAL THERAPY ASSOCIATION
CODE OF ETHICS
PRINCIPLES
Adopted June 1977

Preamble

The physical therapist member of the American Physical Therapy Association accepts this Code of Ethics as the basis for the practice of his profession. Individually and collectively, these members of the Association are responsible for promoting and maintaining the highest ethical standards.

There shall always be a Guide for Professional Conduct to assist in the interpretation of the Code of Ethics. This guide, taking reference from the code, shall be subject to monitoring and timely revision by the Association's Judicial Committee.

This Code of Ethics and the Guide for Professional Conduct shall be binding on the physical therapist members.

Principle 1. The physical therapist should respect the dignity of each individual with whom he is associated in the practice of his profession.

Principle 2. The physical therapist should comply with the law and Association policies governing the practice of physical therapy.

Principle 3. The physical therapist should accept responsibility for the exercise of professional judgment.

Principle 4. The physical therapist should maintain optimal standards of professional practice.

Principle 5. The physical therapist should respect the confidences imparted to him in the course of his professional activities.

Principle 6. The physical therapist should seek reasonable, deserved, and fiscally sound remuneration for his services.

Principle 7. The physical therapist should provide accurate information to the consumer about the profession and services provided.

Principle 8. The physical therapist should not engage in any form of self-aggrandizement.

Principle 9. The physical therapist should accept responsibility for reporting alleged incompetence, illegal activities, and/or unethical conduct to the appropriate authority.

Principle 10. The physical therapist should so conduct himself in all of his affairs as to avoid discredit to the Association and to the profession.

Principle 11. The physical therapist should give his loyalty and support to the American Physical Therapy Association in its efforts to attain its objectives.

Figure 1-12. Code of Ethics of the American Physical Therapy Association as adopted by the House of Delegates in 1977. *(Courtesy of American Physical Therapy Association)*

AMERICAN PHYSICAL THERAPY ASSOCIATION
CODE OF ETHICS
Adopted June 1981

Preamble

This Code of Ethics sets forth ethical principles for the physical therapy profession. Members of this profession are responsible for maintaining and promoting ethical practice. This Code of Ethics, adopted by the American Physical Therapy Association, shall be binding on physical therapists who are members of the Association.

Principle 1. Physical therapists respect the rights and dignity of all individuals.

Principle 2. Physical therapists comply with the laws and regulations governing the practice of physical therapy.

Principle 3. Physical therapists accept responsibility for the exercise of sound judgment.

Principle 4. Physical therapists maintain and promote high standards in the provision of physical therapy services.

Principle 5. Physical therapists seek remuneration for their services that is deserved and responsible.

Principle 6. Physical therapists provide accurate information to the consumer about the profession and about those services they provide.

Principle 7. Physical therapists accept the responsibility to protect the public and the profession from unethical, incompetent, or illegal acts.

Figure 1-13. Code of Ethics of the American Physical Therapy Association as adopted by the House of Delegates in 1981. *(Courtesy of American Physical Therapy Association)*

written examination came membership in the American Registry of Physical Therapy Technicians (later the American Registry of Physical Therapists) and the right of a physical therapy technician to identify herself as *registered.* Examination and certification of qualified practitioners through this national registry continued for over 30 years. Even today use of the designation Registered Physical Therapist (RPT) for registrants with the American Registry of Physical Therapists can be confused with similar legal terminology, ie, RPT as permitted by law for those who have met the statutory requirements for the practice of physical therapy.

Licensure

During the earliest years of the occupation in the United States, concerns related to state legislation were focused most often on protecting the practitioners from being included in undesirable licensure or registration acts. State legislation that required licensure or registration for persons engaged in healing fads and cults was common during that period, and there seemed to be an ever-present danger of physical therapy being included in legislation for drugless healers.

Licensing of practitioners in any field of work is considered to have two protective purposes: (1) to protect the public from the un-

AMERICAN PHYSICAL THERAPY ASSOCIATION
STANDARDS OF ETHICAL CONDUCT FOR THE PHYSICAL THERAPIST ASSISTANT
Adopted June 1982

Preamble

Physical therapist assistants are responsible for maintaining and promoting high standards of conduct. These Standards of Ethical Conduct for the Physical Therapist Assistant shall be binding on physical therapist assistants who are affiliate members of the Association.

Standard 1. Physical therapist assistants provide services under the supervision of a physical therapist.

Standard 2. Physical therapist assistants respect the rights and dignity of all individuals.

Standard 3. Physical therapist assistants maintain and promote high standards in the provision of services.

Standard 4. Physical therapist assistants provide services within the limit of the law.

Standard 5. Physical therapist assistants make those judgments that are commensurate with their qualifications as physical therapist assistants.

Standard 6. Physical therapist assistants give welfare of patients their highest regard.

Figure 1-14. Standards of Ethical Conduct for the Physical Therapist Assistant as adopted by the House of Delegates of the American Physical Therapy Association in 1982. *(Courtesy of American Physical Therapy Association)*

qualified practitioners by identifying through licensure those persons who are qualified to perform the designated tasks of an occupation; and (2) to protect the individuals who have gained the necessary knowledge and skills by not permitting the unqualified to present themselves as qualified. By the 1950s, efforts toward having state legislation enacted were widespread, but the stringency of legislation related to the practice of physical therapy in individual states was quite varied. In some states, all persons who wished to engage in the practice of physical therapy were required by law to obtain a license to practice (mandatory practice acts). The qualifications of practitioners were established in the legislative practice acts, and practice without meeting the qualifications and obtaining a license was prohibited. In other states, legislation was enacted that permitted the use of the title of registered physical therapist (RPT) by practitioners who had applied for and been granted registration (permissive practice acts). These practice acts set forth qualifications that had to be met in order to present oneself as "registered", but the practice of physical therapy was not restricted to persons who had applied for and met the qualifications for registration.

Mandatory acts have replaced permissive legislation through the years. Ultimately, legislation that set forth the legal standards for the practice of physical therapy was enacted in every state, first with a prescriptive relationship required between physical therapist and physician, and later a referral relationship. By mid-1988, practice without referral was legal in

20 states, permitting direct access to physical therapy services. In addition to the legislative regulation of the practice of the physical therapist throughout the United States, practice of the physical therapist assistant is now regulated in 33 states through legislation that requires licensure, registration, certification, or a combination of these.

Efforts toward enactment of legislation and toward continued development of the occupation at times have been rendered counterproductive by the focus and scope of the legal definitions of physical therapy. Ethical principles stated in the Code of Ethics of the APTA have been used in drafting proposed legislation, and the prescriptive or referral relationship with other practitioners became a part of legislative acts. Until recently, definitions of the practice of physical therapy included in the practice acts tended to be focused on the therapeutic elements in the occupation. Routinely, definitions such as the following were incorporated in legislation that regulated the practice of physical therapy.

> Physical Therapy means the treatment of a human being by the use of exercise, massage, heat or cold, air, light, water, electricity or sound, for the purpose of correcting or alleviating any physical or mental condition or preventing the development of any physical or mental disability, or the performance of tests as an aid to the diagnosis or treatment of any human condition, provided, however, that physical therapy shall be practiced only under the prescription of a physician licensed to practice medicine and surgery and shall not include radiology or electro-surgery.

Boundaries established by law have limited the continued development of the preventive aspects of our work. Too often in our history, scenarios have developed where participation by a physical therapist in programs for assessment and prevention of movement dysfunction would be considered illegal and unethical in the absence of physician involvement, and the program would then be left in the hands of someone less qualified than the physical therapist.

Additional Sources of Standards

The commitment to high standards that was expressed by early practitioners has been reiterated in many ways throughout the years of evolution of physical therapy. Apart from standards related to ethical principles and those established by law, physical therapists who are members of the APTA are expected to meet the standards adopted by the Association. "Standards of Practice for Physical Therapy," revised as recently as 1985, describes the conditions and performance that are considered by members of the Association essential for quality physical therapy services. In most health care institutions today, the physical therapy unit is distinct from other units in the institution and, as such, is judged on standards appropriate to the types of services. Physical therapists practicing in institutional settings are expected to meet standards for services established by accrediting agencies.

Persons who are preparing to enter the practice will do well to avail themselves of the guidance that is available for establishing and maintaining a practice of high quality.

EDUCATION AND TRAINING OF THE PHYSICAL THERAPIST

The emergency courses for training of Reconstruction Aides were phased out following the end of World War I in 1918, but ground had been broken and seeds planted. By the close of the following decade, approved programs were offered by 12 institutions, a number that increased steadily during the next 50 years and has now reached well over 100.

Training and education of the physical therapist is another topic in which the history of the development of the APTA and the evolution of the practice of physical therapy in the United States are interwoven. The founding members and others in leadership roles during the early years of the APTA were diligent in their pursuit of establishing, and maintaining, high standards for education in physical therapy as well as high standards for practice. In 1927, the constitution of the Association was revised and with the revision came the clearly stated intent to work toward standardization of the "schools". By 1928 a minimum course of study was agreed upon by the executive committee. The "Minimum Standards for Schools of Physical Therapy", published in 1928, identified the subjects to be studied and the minimum number of clock hours to be devoted to study of theory and to laboratory practice for each subject where applicable. A comparison can be made between the minimum course of study adopted in 1928 and the curriculum used in the emergency courses of 1918 using Table 1-1 and Figure 1-6.

Standards and Standardization

By the time the first minimum course of study was published in 1928, eight institutions were known to be offering programs and others were well along in planning for such a program. A report submitted by the Special Committee on School Investigation (APA) in 1930 includes curricular details for nine programs surveyed following adoption of the minimum course of study. The early programs had several characteristic features. Among the significant features that I identified when studying the development of physical therapy education were the variety of subjects included and the variation in the number of hours devoted to subjects. In most instances, the variation can be related to one or more of the following: special competencies and interests of physicians and physical therapy technicians associated with the program, views of the occupational role, and needs of society or of a segment of society. Where physicians were investigating the therapeutic use of electricity, an emphasis in electrotherapy was seen in the curriculum. One program reported 26 lecture hours and 200 laboratory hours in electrotherapy; another program reported 180 laboratory hours. Similar emphasis on hydrotherapy was seen in those curricula associated with institutions where therapeutic use of water was emphasized, and a program located in a children's hospital showed an emphasis in behaviorism, or psychology. With standards for education and the

efforts toward enforcing those standards came standardization in the curricula and a trend toward uniformity. The variety that was typical of the earliest curricula gave way to a uniform set of course titles and clock hours devoted to the subjects. Standardization of the curricula would play a larger part in the evolution of practice during the 40 years that followed.

The American Physiotherapy Association held sole responsibility for enforcing standards in education until 1936. In 1934 the members of the APA requested that the responsibilities of establishing minimum standards and inspecting schools be assumed by the American Medical Association (AMA). Leadership of the APA had experienced support of physicians for the development of the occupation and saw in the AMA both the authority and financial resources for enforcing educational standards. There appears to be little doubt that the request was made in what seemed to be the best interest of future physical therapists and services to be rendered to society, but the years that followed yielded evidence to the contrary. Once the AMA took action in 1936 to assume the responsibility, curricular changes that might be reflected nationwide were no longer under the control of members of the occupation. Decision making for curriculum development was subjected to bureaucratic deterrence or left entirely in the hands of individuals who were involved in the educational programs. The documents that served to set the standards for training and education of physical therapists remained under the purview of the AMA and the House of Delegates of the AMA from 1936 until 1977.

The first set of standards adopted by the AMA was published in 1936 as "Essentials of an Acceptable School for Physical Therapy Technicians." The minimum curriculum that was included had been developed in cooperation with members of the APA. The importance of biological and physical sciences was reflected even though not to the extent envisioned by those members of the APA who planned the minimum curriculum that was published in 1928 (see Table 1-1 and Fig 1-6). The minimum curriculum of 1936 remained virtually unchanged for almost 20 years until a major revision was accomplished in 1955. Revisions in other sections of the "Essentials" (eg, Preamble, Organization, Faculty, Facilities, Administration) during that period are obscure without close reading. However, these revisions were significant in the continuing development of education and training for the practitioners and in the evolution of the practice of physical therapy. An underlying purpose of using educational standards to control the practice of physical therapy and the role of the practitioners was expressed in two ways in the AMA "Essentials" that were published in 1949: "Therapists are being trained in these schools to work under the direction of qualified physicians and not as independent practitioners of physical therapy;" and "Students shall not be sent to private offices of physicians for clinical practice." Neither the "Essentials" nor the mechanism for putting them into practice were designed to encourage growth and advancement for the occupation. The criteria set forth established minimum standards, and the minimum standards became the end point for curriculum development.

Effecting Change

During the 1940s, the APTA assumed a more active role in effecting change in physical therapy education. The increased activity was related directly to events similar to ones that figured prominently in the earliest years of development of the occupation: epidemics of infantile paralysis and the need for practitioners. Through funds granted to the Association by the National Foundation for Infantile Paralysis (NFIP) a central office was established for the organization, an executive secretary employed, a Department of Educational Services was established, and an educational secretary was employed. The Association was no longer in a position of relying primarily on volunteer services of the members. The School Section, now known as the Section for Education, was becoming an organized special interest group within the Association and, again through funds granted by the NFIP, those who were

serving as program directors were establishing the Council of Physical Therapy School Directors. These are but highlights of organizational changes that occurred during the 1940s; the importance of these highlights lies in the fact that additional means were available to create influences on the educational programs and thus on the evolution of physical therapy.

A chief concern later in the 1940s was the minimum curriculum that had remained in the "Essentials" unchanged since 1936. Newly initiated programs were being approved yearly and the primary source of guidance was the 1936 minimum curriculum. Planning for revision of the "Essentials" was initiated by the APTA and, following an abundance of correspondence and numerous meetings attended by appointed representatives of the AMA and APTA, revised "Essentials" were adopted by the AMA in 1955. Notable in the revision are the increase in hours and percentage of time for physiology, exercise, and clinical practice and a clearly identifiable requirement in tests and measurements (see Table 1-1). Apart from the changes in hours and percentages of time were changes in the titles used for content areas.

The curricula of the 1960s took on features that were characteristic of the revisions in titles for content areas. The course title of Clinical Medicine replaced the previously used Physical Therapy as Applied to Orthopedics, Medicine, Surgery, and Neurology and the broad title of Physical Agents replaced individually identified Electrotherapy, Hydrotherapy, and Massage. In addition to course titles reflecting changes in the "Essentials," content areas not included there appeared with increasing frequency: neuroanatomy, neurophysiology, scientific inquiry and research, public health and community health, education principles, psychosocial aspects of patient care, and management or administration. The "Essentials" that were adopted in 1955 also included for the first time the following statement: "When preparatory training is properly integrated with professional training in a collegiate school of physical therapy, such training will lead to a baccalaureate degree in physical therapy." Semester credits were indicated along with minimum clock hours for each of the content areas. In 1960, the House of Delegates of the APTA adopted the following resolution: "that the American Physical Therapy Association consider attainment of a baccalaureate degree the minimum education qualification of a physical therapist."

Changes that were taking place as a part of the evolution of the practice of physical therapy were reflected in the content additions to the minimum curriculum. The role of the physical therapist had developed beyond that of a skilled technician and was expanding into domains other than that of direct patient services. Expectations in performance demanded that the practitioner not only be skilled in use of the basic procedures of physical therapy but also understand the rationale for application. Therapeutic intervention that had been based in physics of motion and, in some instances, physics of electricity now included neuroanatomic and neurophysiologic foundations. The traditional foundation in gross anatomy and kinesiology was no longer sufficient as a basis for understanding the methods of therapeutic intervention. An increase in the breadth and depth of the foundations of the occupation was being realized.

The 1950s and 1960s were years of major transition for the administrative and academic structure of physical therapy education as well as the physical setting. Programs initially approved, or accredited, during those years were located predominantly in colleges and universities rather than in hospitals or other health care institutions, and physical therapists held the primary administrative positions. Satisfactory completion of the programs led primarily to baccalaureate degrees rather than certificates. By the early 1970s satisfactory completion led to a master's degree at six institutions.

The move away from health care institutions removed long-standing resources for instructing and socializing students into the role of service providers and lead players in a helping relationship. Patient-centered demonstrations for dramatic illustration of therapeutic techniques now required specific and time-consuming planning and coodination with a health care facility. Patients, physicians, nurses, and other personnel related to the therapeutic environment were no longer a routine part of the surroundings for the students. Behaviors that at one time could be taught by example and learned by frequent use as a part of everyday activities became themes for course content and for scheduled events in clinical activities. The transition to an academic setting was achieved for physical therapy education but, in the process, new and different challenges arose that were related to curricular content and administrative structure.

Funding by the federal government and organizational expediency in institutions of higher education fueled the rapid expansion of administrative structures that were given a title such as School of Allied Health Professions, College of Allied Health Professions, School of Allied Health Sciences, or some variation of those titles. A cursory review of a list of physical therapy programs in the latter 1980s will confirm the predominance of such administrative structures as the parent administrative unit for our educational efforts today. The Allied Health Personnel Training Act of 1966 and subsequent amendments to that federal legislation have had profound influences on the evolution of physical therapy in the United States. For the most part, the influences have not yet been analyzed.

In June 1974, the House of Delegates of the APTA adopted "Essentials of an Accredited Educational Program for the Physical Therapist," a document that represented a dramatic departure from course titles, clock hours, and semester hours as included in the 1955 "Essentials". Attention had been turned to the purpose of the educational process and the intended product. Guidance for curriculum planning was stated as the competencies expected of the students upon completion of the program: competencies in individual patient services, communication, administration, and professional growth. A similar approach is found in the "Standards for Accreditation of Physical Therapy Educational Programs," adopted in June 1978 and currently under review for revisions: "As a professional health care provider the physical therapist will be able to: . . . (a) determine the physical therapy needs of any patient referred for treatment; . . . (b) design a physical therapy plan of care; . . . (e) modify physical therapy goals or plan; . . . (o) assume responsibility for personal professional growth and development."

Signal Events

Even if all significant actions and events related to the changes in physical therapy education could be identified, space would not permit even summary attention. However, hallmarks must be included quite briefly and directly. The APTA was recognized as an independent accrediting agency in 1977, by both the U.S. Commissioner on Accreditation, U.S. Office of Education and the Council on Postsecondary Accreditation. Six years later, in 1983, the APTA became the only accrediting agency for physical therapist and physical therapist assistant education. Resolutions were adopted by the House of Delegates of the APTA in 1979 and revised in 1980 that read as follows: "that the American Physical Therapy Association adopt the policy that entry-level education for the physical therapist be that which results in the award of a postbaccalaureate degree"; and "that all educational programs for the physical therapist and all developing educational programs for the physical therapist shall comply with the policy on entry-level education in this resolution by December 31, 1990." These events, or actions, are contemporary and serve quite appropriately to close this portion of the considerations of the evolution of physical therapy in the United States.

CONCLUSION

Sociologic studies of the evolution of the practice of physical therapy are rare, but in-depth study is not required to see a relationship between this evolution and specific factors. The outstanding historical and sociologic events in the evolution of physical therapy include the following:

- Military conflicts: World Wars I and II, the Korean War, and the military action in Vietnam.

- Health and provision of health care: polio epidemics and continuing outbreaks of the 1950s and 1960s, and postpolio syndrome noted in the 1980s; concerns about birth defects, particularly those related to thalidomide; efforts to make comprehensive health care available to all segments of society; programs directed toward the general welfare of the elderly; and changing concepts of health and wellness.
- Legislation: the 1965 amendments to the Social Security Act that initiated the Federal Health Insurance Program for the Aged; federal legislation intended to increase health care manpower (including physical therapists and related supportive personnel); and federal programs focused on combating heart disease, cancer, and stroke.
- Education and recreation: popularity of community colleges and their role in preparing health care manpower; institutional and specialized accreditation in education; and the rise of organized amateur and professional sports.

Perhaps one of the readers using this book will accept the challenge to study the evolution of physical therapy in relation to one or more of these topics.

PHYSICAL THERAPY ON THE CONTINUUM OF PROFESSIONALIZATION

Our occupation—physical therapy—is our profession. The earliest practitioners viewed their work similarly and repeatedly affirmed such views. The continued professionalization of the occupation is in our hands. Certain characteristics of physical therapy are clearly among the characteristics usually considered to be attributes of a profession, whereas others are equivocal.

The *Code of Ethics* that is subscribed to by members of the American Physical Therapy Association, a *national organization* that represents the majority of practitioners in this country, publicly affirms the ethical position supported by a large segment of the occupation. The genesis of the occupation lies in the *service orientation* of a few individuals who found that their understanding of human movement could make a difference in the quality of life experienced by others, and that orientation has been sustained. If these were the only characteristics to be considered, we could speak of the profession of physical therapy unequivocally. But there are others that must be considered.

What can we say about the *body of theoretical knowledge* unique to the occupation of physical therapy? Is extensive *specialized education and training* required to prepare practitioners of the future? And what is the level of *autonomy* exercised by the practitioners in making judgments about those matters that pertain to the practice of physical therapy? We can pose these questions somewhat differently. Do we have a service to offer that is not only beneficial but also available uniquely from physical therapists, based on the special nature of the preparation that is required to enter the practice of physical therapy? Do we make the decisions about the preparation of practitioners and about the substance and scope of our practice? Do we hold the responsibility for making judgments within our scope of practice about patient care?

Answers to these questions have placed physical therapy in the category of a moderately professionalized occupation, or an emerging profession. There are events throughout the evolutional years that pointed to the current status of the occupation. The closing decade of the twentieth century promises to hold key determinants for the place that physical therapy will hold on the occupations-professions continuum for the twenty-first century.

ANNOTATED BIBLIOGRAPHY

Ad Hoc Committee to Study the Utilization and Training of Nonprofessional Assistants: Report to 1967 House of Delegates. Phys Ther 47 (11, Part 2): 31, 1967 (Summary of APTA and Ad Hoc Committee activities related to supportive personnel in physical therapy and proposed policy statement on physical therapy assistant.)

Bouman HD (ed): Proceedings: An exploratory and analytical survey of therapeutic exercise, Northwestern University. Am J Phys Med 46:3, 1967 (Papers from Northwestern University-Special Therapeutic Exercise Project. [NU-STEP].)

Elson MO: The legacy of Mary McMillan. Phys Ther 44:1067, 1964 (Mary McMillan's role in establishing the occupation of physical therapy in the United States and in founding the organization known today as the American Physical Therapy Association.)

Farnsworth R: The Association for the Crippled and Disabled. Physiother Rev 10:287, 1930 (Summary of activities of organization.)

Grunewald LR: A study of physiotherapy as a vocation. Physiother Rev 8(4):37; 8(5):33; 9:60; 104; 139, 1928 and 1929 (Introduced as the first thesis on physiotherapy; includes results of a questionnaire study and conclusions about standardizing educational requirements.)

Hazenhyer IM: A history of the American Physiotherapy Association. Physiother Rev 26:3; 66; 122; 174, 1946 (A series of four articles that describes events that preceded the founding of the Association in 1921 and development of the organization, 1921–1946.)

Lovett RL: The Treatment of Infantile Paralysis 2nd ed. p ix. Philadelphia, P Blakiston & Son Co, 1917 (Description of therapeutic measures used in United States, particularly in New England states, during polio epidemics of 1900–1920.)

Kovacs R: A Manual of Physical Therapy, 4th ed. Philadelphia, Lea & Febiger, 1949 (Typical of textbooks of that period intended for use in training physicians and technicians.)

McMillan M: Massage and Therapeutic Exercise, 2nd ed. Philadelphia, WB Saunders, 1925 (First edition published in 1921; first book written by a physical therapist to be published in this country.)

McMillan M: Physical therapy on three continents. Physiother Rev 26:254, 1946 (Mary McMillan shares events from her work as a physical therapist in Europe, America, and Asia.)

Mock HE, Pemberton R, Coulter JS (eds): Principles and Practice of Physical Therapy. Hagerstown, MD, WF Prior, 1938 (Published in three looseleaf volumes: I, Applications in Medicine; II, Applications in Surgery; III,

Technics of Physical Therapy.)

Nelson PA (ed): Archives of Physical Medicine and Rehabilitation Cumulative Index: 1920–1969 Including 50-Year History. Chicago, Westlake Press, 1970 (Includes early history of organizations of physicians who specialized in practice of physical therapy.)

Pinkston D: A History of Physical Therapy Education in the United States: An Analysis of Development of the Curricula. Doctoral Dissertation. Cleveland, OH, Case Western Reserve University, 1978 (Includes profile of programs 1920s–1972, salient features of change, and documents related to standards in physical therapy education 1928–1971. Provided a basis for portions of this chapter.)

The Archives Collection of the American Physical Therapy Association, Alexandria, VA (Directory for materials contained in the Archives of the APTA. The Archives, open to APTA members and the general public by appointment, houses the official records of the Association and other historical materials.)

Vogel EE: Physical Therapists Before World War II (1917–40). In Lee HS, McDaniel ML (eds): Army Medical Specialist Corps, p 41. Washington DC, Office of the Surgeon General, Department of the Army, 1968 (Chapter details early history; book includes history of physical therapists in the Army 1917–1960.)

Winch RE: Correcting. Physiother Rev 11:159, 1931 (Provides a sense of the place of the disabled in society during that period.)

2 Physical Therapy Today and in the Twenty-first Century

BEVERLY J. SCHMOLL

The environment in which physical therapists practice is subjected to the push and pull of multiple forces. Our effectiveness in the context of today's world rests in large measure with our recognition of the forces that have influenced our profession in the past, forces that influence our profession today, and forces that can be anticipated to influence our profession in the future. We must recognize these forces and identify their potential impact on physical therapy practice. Without an awareness of the dynamic forces acting upon today's environment, we may fail to make foresighted decisions and thus become powerless to influence the environment in which we desire to practice tomorrow.

FORCES AFFECTING PHYSICAL THERAPY PRACTICE

Two broad categories of forces (societal and technological) act upon our environment, singly and collectively. The prevalent forces are societal beliefs and values; population demographics; economic conditions; governmental legislation, rules, and regulations; actions of public and private organizations and agencies; scientific advances; technological advances; and actions of health care disciplines. The nature of these forces and potential impact of each will be described briefly as a background for reviewing the premises of physical therapy practice and the significance of today's environment for physical therapists.

SOCIETAL BELIEFS AND VALUES

For our purposes, the expectations of health care consumers provide a barometric reading of prevalent societal beliefs and values. Consumers generally are disenchanted with "all-knowing" and "trust-me" attitudes of health care practitioners (Ferguson). Increasingly, consumers are knowledgeable about factors influencing their health (Ferguson; Naisbitt).

Consumers seek information and programs to prevent illness and disability. When confronted with illness or disability, they desire a partnership with health care practitioners (Ferguson). Personalized, quality health care that withstands the rigors of accountability, cost-effectiveness, and consumer satisfaction can be expected to remain as the standard for determining the acceptability of health care services (Naisbitt).

Involvement of our clients in all aspects of the therapeutic process is essential for assuring attainment of realistic therapeutic outcomes. The efficacy of physical therapy intervention rests in large measure with the nature of interactions between therapists and clients.

POPULATION DEMOGRAPHICS

According to Hodgkinson, in 1983, persons over the age of 65 years outnumbered teenagers, a condition that is expected to continue well into the next century. Moreover, by the year 2000, one third of the American population will be black, Hispanic, or Asian. According to the same source, increasing numbers of children will be born to teenage mothers; many of these babies will be premature, with a greater likelihood of being at risk developmentally.

The demand for physical therapists to work with geriatric and pediatric populations can be expected to grow. If we practice in the south, fluency in Spanish will be necessary (Naisbitt). Regardless of where we practice, we must be attuned to cultural differences and recognize the potential impact of these differences on the therapeutic relationship.

THE ECONOMY

The cost of health care in relation to the perceived benefits of health care has been and continues to be a strong force influencing the practice of physical therapy. The advent of Medicare and Medicaid increased the availability of physical therapy services. Prospective payment for health care services (DRGs) has modified the settings in which physical therapy services are rendered.

In attempts to remain economically competitive, national and multinational corporations have evolved that embrace smaller, decentralized, regional organizations for delivering a variety of health care services in multiple settings at costs acceptable to fiscal intermediaries and consumers (Toffler, 1983). We can expect the structures in which physical therapy services are delivered to be modified as societal and technological forces emerge and shift. Our relationships with employers, fiscal intermediaries, other health care practitioners, and clients can be expected to change.

We will continue to find ourselves balancing competing forces. Our desire to provide quality care will be countered by demands for high productivity and efficiency. In our attempts to manage and promote scientific and technological advances, we will increase specialization. Economy-minded health care organizations, however, will seek practitioners who have multiple areas of expertise and who can overlap functions effectively to minimize health care costs.

GOVERNMENTAL LEGISLATION, RULES, AND REGULATIONS

State legislation dictates in large measure the levels of responsibility we are sanctioned to assume. State legislation and accompanying rules and regulations influence our roles as entry points into health care and the nature of our relationships with clients and other health care practitioners. Ultimately, reimbursement for our services hinges on governmental actions.

It is imperative that we become knowledgeable and involved in legislative activity that influences the practice of physical therapy. In addition, we can expect to be called upon more frequently to serve as advocates for legislation affecting client populations we serve.

The halls of government may seem remote and governmental lobbying may appear to be beyond our scope of practice. However, it behooves us to be cognizant of the array of legislative activity that influences our practice.

PUBLIC AND PRIVATE ORGANIZATIONS AND AGENCIES

Fiscal intermediaries (private and public), self-help groups, special interest groups, and federal funding agencies constitute a category of forces influencing physical therapy practice. Fiscal intermediaries will continue to focus on cost-benefit as a basis for establishing policy for reimbursement of health care services. Self-help groups will continue to flourish and advocate ready access to services, accountability, and involvement in health care decision making.

Special interest groups (eg, Easter Seal Society, March of Dimes) will influence physical therapy by raising the consciousness of consumers about health, disease, and intervention. They will select and promote areas of needed research, which they will fund. Similarly, federal funding agencies can be expected to continue to influence advances in all segments of health care by establishing priorities for education, training, and research. These organizations and agencies influence our accessibility to clients and the provision of quality care by competent practitioners. In addition, they serve as resources for enabling us to expand our body of knowledge through research.

SCIENTIFIC ADVANCES

Naisbitt states, "Biology is replacing physics as the dominant metaphor of the society." Many of the scientific advances in biology undoubtedly will have tremendous impact on physical therapy practice.

Cetron and O'Toole have forecasted a number of scientific advances. The human life span may be 150 to 200 years in the twenty-first century. Central nervous system regeneration, structurally and functionally, is anticipated for persons with single penetrating injuries. The removal of abnormal genes and splicing of healthy genes in their place will become routine in managing an array of genetic diseases and disorders. A nonaddictive opiate will be developed to control chronic pain. Brain research will result in a clearer understanding of the processes associated with perception, learning, and regeneration (Ferguson; Cetron and O'Toole).

The possible implications of these advancements immediately become evident. Our clients will live longer with fewer of the ailments that are now common to the elderly. We will be challenged to develop new approaches for facilitating the regeneration of neural pathways in the central nervous system. Both the identified and unknown futures of scientific advancements promise great challenges and opportunities for advancements in physical therapy.

TECHNOLOGICAL ADVANCES

Technological advances in telecommunications will continue to influence physical therapy practice. Cetron and O'Toole forecast the routine use of computers in combination with two-way cable television in the delivery of health care services. We can expect most therapeutic equipment to be computerized and mobile,

and pocket telephones to become devices we use in our daily practice.

The advances in telecommunications will increase our capacity to access and disseminate information. Our accessibility by patients and others also will be increased. Our ability to collect objective data and analyze the data as it is being collected will become routine. Collaborative studies and consultation will be expanded and enhanced without regard for barriers of distance or time.

HEALTH CARE DISCIPLINES

Specialization will increase within our profession and within other health care disciplines in reaction to mounting knowledge and as a means of expanding knowledge. New health care disciplines can be expected to emerge as knowledge and specialization grow.

We can expect existing health care disciplines to resist changes that will diminish their societal value or status. Practitioners within health care disciplines will continue to seek an exclusive niche to perpetuate the discipline and protect its future. The degree to which each discipline will be successful will depend upon its ability to demonstrate a need for continuation and evidence the need is worth the cost to society. The disciplines that vigorously pursue research to demonstrate efficacy in the therapeutic milieu and those willing to accept opportunities to demonstrate accountability are most likely to grow and flourish.

The aims, ethics, and standards of practice of physical therapy represent our desire and willingness to demonstrate our value in health care. The challenge remains for each of us to be willing to invest in ourselves and our profession through research, quality assurance, and accountability measures to ensure a tomorrow of our choosing.

IMPLICATIONS FOR PHYSICAL THERAPY

As we examine the practice of physical therapy in relation to the forces described in the previous section, we find that physical therapy appears to be well grounded in the realities of today's world.

The goal of the physical therapist is to enhance human movement and function and to assess, prevent, and treat movement dysfunction and physical disability. This goal is clearly compatible with present and anticipated forces. Our roles may change in terms of the nature of our interventions, but the need for physical therapy remains viable.

The bodies of knowledge that we will draw upon in practice to engage in clinical decision making will continue to expand. Technology will enable us to access information and to manage and use information better. We will accept increased specialization within our profession and greater numbers of emerging health professions, or adapt to alternative models for health care professionals working together.

Our ability to engage in clinical research will continue to expand. Eventually, all physical therapists will actively pursue clinical research. Technological advances will ease the collection and analysis of data and allow ready access and dissemination of information. We will have the capacity to collect data on multiple populations in multiple settings and subject the data to comparative analyses. The findings will result in the development of theory that will be regarded as highly relevant because of its genesis in the practice setting.

The delicate balance between the use of technology and one-on-one interactions will be heightened. The close personal contact between patient and physical therapist represents a unique aspect of physical therapy practice. Societal values suggest this relationship will continue to be sought and valued and, in fact, will help to ensure the continued demand for our services. We will use science to support our art.

Our role as physical therapists will change in regard to consumer populations, practice settings, and interactions with other health care disciplines, agencies, and organizations. We will become stronger advocates for consumers. Increasingly, our professional role will encompass that of an educator: "If I treat you, it's for today. If I teach you, it's for a lifetime."

IMPACT ON PHYSICAL THERAPISTS

"Minds are like parachutes. They only work when they are open" (Cetron and O'Toole).

The dynamic forces that have an impact on the environment of physical therapy require us to be open minded, flexible, and receptive to the host of possibilities that may become realities. If the premises and goals of physical therapy (as sketched under Implications) are to remain valid, we do not have the choice of ignoring the forces that influence our practice. We can choose to anticipate the future and exercise our adaptability. Alternatively, we can choose to engineer our future and exercise our creativity and innovativeness. In either case, we can plan and make foresighted decisions. Our actions today will influence physical therapy tomorrow.

ANNOTATED BIBLIOGRAPHY

Cetron M, O'Toole T: Encounters with the Future: A Forecast of Life into the 21st Century. New York, McGraw-Hill, 1983 (Comprehensive account of forecasts and trends related to the economy, politics, social and cultural affairs, health and medicine, and science and technology.)

Ferguson M: The Aquarian Conspiracy: Personal and Social Transformation in the 1980s. Los Angeles, JP Tarcher, 1980 (Provocative description of transformations occurring within our society. Includes discussion of the emerging health paradigm and brain research.)

Hodgkinson HL: All One System: Demographics of Education—Kindergarten Through Graduate School. Washington, DC, Institute for Educational Leadership, 1985 (Comprehensive account of major demographic trends and factors influencing high school and college completion. Provides a model for viewing education from a holistic perspective.)

Naisbitt J: Megatrends: Ten New Directions Transforming Our Lives. New York, Warner Books, 1982 (Highly readable description of forces and trends that have been transforming our society and shaping the future.)

Toffler A: The Third Wave. New York, William Morrow & Co, 1980 (Comprehensive description of the processes of change that are responsible for transitions in society.)

Toffler A: Previews and Premises. New York, William Morrow & Co, 1983 (Toffler shares his most recent views about society and technology.)

3 Ethical Considerations in Physical Therapy

RUTH B. PURTILO

Physical therapists have always been concerned about the ethics of their profession. The first code of ethics in physical therapy appeared in 1935. It focused almost solely on the physical therapist's duty to show respect and deference to the physician. Although everyone can applaud the desirability of showing respect to one's professional colleagues, such suggestions as promising never to question a physician's judgment sound oddly foreign within today's health care context. The sophistication and timeliness of the current American Physical Therapy Association Code of Ethics stands in stark contrast to these earlier guidelines.

A code is important as a set of broad moral guidelines and as a public document "professing" a group's moral commitments at a period in time. But a profession's ethical code is by no means the only—or best—indicator of a profession's awareness of its moral obligations. Much more telling are a profession's policies and practices, and the behavior and attitudes of its members. In other words, the individual physical therapist's commitment to upholding high standards are the best indicators of how a profession itself will be judged by society.

MORALS AND ETHICS

In commenting on another's attitudes and behaviors, sometimes one hears such statements as, "That's the *moral* and *ethical* thing for the physical therapist to do." Although this phrase is not necessarily incorrect, often people are using the terms "moral" and "ethical" interchangeably, which is incorrect. What is the distinction between the two?

Morals or "moral norms" are the attitudes and behaviors that a society agrees upon as desirable and necessary for maximizing the realization of things cherished most in that society. At one end of this spectrum are minimal rules, designed to keep the society from self-destructing; at the other end are ideals toward which members can strive in trying to create a perfect society. Adhering to the rules and ideals helps to preserve and foster the conditions for living together peacefully and harmoniously. While some rules and ideals have changed, others have had exceptional staying power.

Philosophers, political scientists, theologians, and others have long been interested in understanding and studying these morals. Morals can be grouped into several categories such as duties, rights, responsibilities, character traits, and conditions of justice.

Within health care, some of the basic moral norms are especially important because of the nature of the health professional and patient relationship. Among them are *duties* to do no harm, keep one's promises to patients, and tell the truth; *rights* include the right of patients to their life and autonomy, and the right of health professionals to be free to make the best judgments possible. Additionally, there are *responsibilities* of health professionals, patients, and society that ought to be taken into account, and *character traits* such as compassion, honesty, and conscientiousness that are valued. Of course, many of these moral norms are directly or indirectly referred to in professional codes, but no code embraces all of them.

How, then, are morals and ethics related? Ethics is the study of morals and moral judgments. Philosophers have developed numerous theories about how morals should be interpreted and weighed. Ethical theories function to enable an individual to reflect on and find resolution to conflicts of duties, rights, or responsibilities. In some important regards, ethics resembles a science: There are theories, concepts, and methodologies that one can follow. Often I think of the moral norms (such as duties or rights) as "elements" of ethical analysis, each with its own unique qualities and weight. These elements can be observed, weighed, and compared.

Ethical dilemmas are one of the most perplexing forms of ethical problems. In a dilemma the situation is similar to a classic Greek tragedy in which one cherished norm will have to be compromised whatever one does: One is situated between the proverbial "devil and the deep blue sea" so that to act in accord with one moral norm means that another will necessarily be forfeited. As physical therapists know, there are many of these "no win" situations in health care decision making. For instance, the decision to honor a patient's wishes to have information about his or her condition may be in direct conflict with the physician's expressed wish that the patient not be told. Or a decision to spend an extra 20 minutes with a patient who really needs attention may mean cutting corners with the next one. This description of morals and ethics should help the physical therapist better understand why it is possible to act *morally* in most situations, but still occasionally be confronted with *ethical* dilemmas that demand ethical reflection and analysis.

Ethical Analysis of Moral Problems

Sometimes health professionals say to me, "In an ethical dilemma, there is no right answer. It's all a matter of opinion, and yours is as valid as mine." This is not completely accurate. While no one answer may allow for all cherished values to be honored equally, careful analysis can help to sort out the least harmful or most beneficial course of action from among the various alternatives. The allegation that no agreement exists fails to give credit to the many areas of consensus about the moral life that have been made evident through our laws, policies, professional standards statements, and common practices. Therefore, ethical reflection on moral problems should include the search for existing guidelines. For example, institutional informed consent policies may be very useful to the physical therapist at times, even though there is no departmental requirement that a formal consent be gained. One can find rich discussion about such issues in health care literature, and glean a summary of the recent thinking on a subject in the *Encyclopedia of Bioethics*. Although departure from broad norms and guidelines may be feasible and justifiable in rare cases, the burden of proof of why broadly accepted policies or other guidelines are rejected falls on the shoulders of the person rejecting them.

Whenever a physical therapist is faced with a moral problem that does not lend itself to resolution by reference to existing guidelines, at least four areas of consideration should be taken into account in trying to decide what to do: (1) What are the relevant *facts* of the case? Does the physical therapist know exactly what happened? What is the source of the information? Is the information reliable? Is it complete? (2) Given the facts, what makes this a moral problem? That is, what duties, rights, character traits, and responsibilities are in conflict? (3) Once the nature of the conflict is identified, one can begin to set priorities among the moral norms. (4) Finally, one settles on a course of action.

To identify the type of conflict and set priorities among the moral norms, one must engage in ethical analysis of the problem. Identifying the type of conflict requires knowledge of the range of duties, rights, character traits, and responsibilities present in the situation. Then one can go about assigning weight to the various norms in the task of resolving the conflict. There are two major approaches to the weighing process. A brief case example helps to illustrate the two approaches.

> Mr. C.L. suffered a severe stroke six weeks ago. The physical therapist, M.K., judges that continued intensive rehabilitation is fully indicated for Mr. C.L. at this time. However, Mr. C.L.'s insurance coverage has run out and he is due to be discharged from the unit. M.K. is faced with a moral problem: His duty to try to do what is best for his patient (ie, continue treatment) is in conflict with his duty to act in accordance with equitable policies, that is, assuming M.K. believes that the hospital's policy to discharge such patients when reimbursement is exhausted is, overall, an equitable approach.

The *utilitarian* approach to M.K.'s problem is to give top priority to whatever norms will help to bring about the best consequences for all involved. Taking this approach, M.K. well may decide that the best course of action in this tragic situation is to comply with the policies designed to be equitable for all future stroke patients as well as for Mr. C.L. In other words, in the utilitarian approach the most defensible course of action is that which brings about the most good for the most people. A second approach is the *formalist* or *deontologist* approach. Here the therapist's task is to identify certain moral norms that will always hold more weight, and to be governed by them in deciding a course of action. The formalist approach deeply pervades the ethos of health care. It can be seen in the most ancient oaths and codes, beginning with the Hippocratic Oath, and continues to be expressed in many ways today. Specifically, in this approach M.K.'s duty is to the patient above all else. Morally speaking, almost all health professionals would feel more compelled to try to act in the best interests of Mr. C.L., and especially to avoid harm to him, rather than to discontinue therapy at this critical juncture on the basis of future patients who may need the resources. Of course, even though the more morally justifiable course of action may be clear, M.K. is faced with the practical problem of whether to try to "buck the system" by keeping Mr. C.L. for further treatment.

In actual practice many of us think both about the individual patient's predicament and the consequences that will be brought about by our decisions. Recent innovations in health care, emphasizing cost constraints, have forced health professionals to be more cognizant than ever before of the broader environmental considerations. However, as I have illustrated in the above story, usually the therapist cannot have it both ways in the end. Therefore, it is imperative that M.K. be mindful of which moral norms are *governing* his thinking because the course of action he chooses will reflect those norms.

In addition to considerations about how to decide what to do, ethics also addresses questions related to what kind of persons we ought to strive to be. Aristotle was an early proponent of the idea that if a person cultivates good character, he necessarily will act in ways that will foster a good society. The role in health care of "virtues," or desirable character traits, long has been discussed. Many writings throughout history have supported the idea that health professionals should exhibit such traits as compassion, devotion to the patient, wisdom, and justice. At the same time, the trait of honesty or forthrightness long has been disputed on the basis that telling the patient the truth may dispel the patient's hope. Only in recent years in the United States have the ideas that the patient has a right to know, and that the "truth sets free" led to a departure from this cloak of secrecy surrounding the patient's diagnosis or prognosis. Underlying such discussions is the idea that the health professional should exhibit certain traits of character, as well as do her duty.

ETHICAL ISSUES IN PHYSICAL THERAPY

Physical therapists face a wide range of moral problems confronting the health professions today. In their professional role, they may not be directly involved in some morally complex situations, such as abortion or discontinuing life supports; however, the therapist is by no means exempt from many others. I will list a few, and you can elaborate on them and add others.

1. *Confidentiality.* The age-old idea that the health professional has a duty to keep secret the harmful, shameful, or embarrassing information revealed by a patient continues to be cherished by patients. Some writers have suggested that confidentiality is an outdated or even, as Siegler puts it, a "decrepit" concept. They cite such factors as computerized data systems and the fragmentation of health care delivery approaches as dealing a crushing blow to this ideal. Surely their worries are not without substance. In the health care context, the commitment to honoring confidences can be a momentous challenge, especially when a patient is being seen over a long period of time and by a multitude of professionals.

2. *Informed Consent.* Mechanisms for securing informed consent are many, but they, too, are challenged by long term and the often complex nature of some health care programs. Seldom does a patient consent initially to become a part of a particular program. For example, seldom does the candidate for rehabilitation give consent for the many different kinds of interventions that are tried in the overall goal of "rehabilitating" him. I suggest that today more than ever before, physical therapy treatment and evaluation procedures should be guided by the moral principles and legal constraints that have led to implementation of the mechanism of informed consent (1984).

3. *Interprofessional Issues.* These issues give rise to other types of moral dilemmas for the therapist. For instance, many physical therapists justifiably are worried that the practice of working in a physician-managed or other privately owned physical therapy clinic entails built-in conflicts of interest. The move toward practice independent of physician referral, too, has raised voices of concern regarding the effect such an arrangement may have on the physician-therapist relationship (a relationship believed by some to be designed to best uphold patients' interests). At the same time, therapists are examining ways in which each of these arrangements can be designed to preserve interprofessional integrity while better meeting the needs of patients.

4. *Justice Issues.* The therapist is not exempt from being involved in agonizing decisions about how to distribute scarce resources according to some acceptable standard of fairness and equity. Increasingly, physical therapists are being forced to become more involved in policy and government to help assure that just policies and practices are supported.

Therapists are equipping themselves better than ever before to deal with difficult ethical problems. Most physical therapy teaching programs now include a course or unit in ethics. Some physical therapists attend continuing education sessions or are participants in the summer institutes sponsored by the National Endowment for the Humanities or other groups. Ever-increasing numbers of therapists are making a formal study of ethics in higher education programs or writing ethics articles in journals. With a growing literature in ethics and other educational opportunities geared directly to rehabilitation and therapy, all physical therapists can gain a basic understanding of ethics and how to respond well to complex and difficult issues.

Therapists also are contributing to the understanding of ethical problems in health care through membership on committees designed to create or review ethics policies. Some sit on local hospital ethics committees where difficult cases are reviewed and policies are promulgated. Research regarding the perception of ethical problems by physical therapists is among the types of inquiry being carried out. While physical therapists will not have to become ethicists in the strict sense anymore than they will have to become lawyers, they do have to continue to take seriously the ethical dimensions of their practice. Fortunately there is every reason to believe that recent trends towards more cognizance of the issues, more sensitivity about how to respond to the issues, and more experience in actual decision making about the issues will continue.

ANNOTATED BIBLIOGRAPHY

Guccione A: Ethical issues in physical therapy practice: A survey of physical therapists in New England. Phys Ther 60(11):1264, 1980 (A 1980 survey of the ethical issues that New England physical therapists judged to be the most important in their day-to-day practice. A helpful discussion is presented for consideration by the reader.)

Purtilo RB, Cassel CC: Ethical Dimensions in the Health Professions, 220 pp. Philadelphia, WB Saunders 1981 (A textbook containing the fundamental concepts and theories of ethics as they apply to decision making in the health professions. Major topics include truth telling, confidentiality, care of incurably ill persons, physician-allied health professional relationships, whistle blowing, and allocation of scarce resources.)

Purtilo RB: Ethics in allied health education. J Allied Health 12(3):210, 1983 (Reviews the "state of the art" of instructional offerings in ethics in allied health curricula. The author addresses reasons why ethics is important as a curriculum issue and speculates regarding the relevance of such courses for allied health professionals.)

Purtilo RB: Informed consent: Ethical and legal issues for physical therapists. Phys Ther 64(6):934, 1984 (Specifies treatment and evaluation situations in which physical therapists may be required, ethically or legally, to gain informed consent for procedures. Includes underlying moral and legal principles as well as practical guidelines.)

Purtilo RB: Professional responsibility in physiotherapy. Physiotherapy 72(12):579, 1986 (The keynote address for the 1986 annual meeting of the British Chartered Society of Physiotherapy. The author details the progress of physical therapy in the United States and Britain, showing how it has become a profession in the full ethical sense of the term. Primarily the move has been realized through the profession's acceptance of responsibility for its own excellence in patient care and research.)

Reich W: Encyclopedia of Bioethics, Vol I–IV. New York, MacMillan and Free Press, 1978 (A major reference resource by leaders in the field of bioethics. Still the most complete and useful source for basic history and contemporary thinking regarding bioethics issues. 1933 pages, including appendices of major ethical codes.)

Siegler M: Confidentiality: A decrepit concept? N Engl J Med 307(24):1510, 1982 (Concise but provocative article by a physician delineates the range of problems confronting health professionals who wish to honor the age-old ethical guideline of confidentiality. The author provides rationale for why confidentiality is still important, and suggests mechanisms for protecting it in today's information-rich health care environment.)

Sim J: Ethical considerations in physiotherapy. Physiotherapy 69(4):119, 1983 (A British physiotherapist's view of the status of physiotherapy ethics. A good companion piece to Guccione's or Purtilo's [1983] article, for gaining insight into United States-British similarities and differences.)

Sim J: Truthfulness in the therapeutic relationship. Physiotherapy Pract 2:121, 1986 (A thorough analysis of the concept of truthfulness in the health care context with an emphasis on how problems arise in the physician-physiotherapist relationship. The author is a British physiotherapist whose insights are useful for health professionals anywhere.)

4 Clinical Reasoning in Physical Therapy

JUDITH S. CANFIELD

As you pause outside your new patient's hospital room door, you hear a moan from within. Or, you notice a person sitting in the reception area of your private practice who is wearing a Lennox Hill brace on his right knee. Or, before you leave the base office to make your home visits, you read the referral on your new patient. With the perception of one or more pieces of patient data, the physical therapist begins a process by which information is selected, sorted, grouped, retrieved, combined, and confirmed. It is through such mental activities that the therapist arrives at a diagnosis, determines the treatment goals, selects therapeutic interventions, and modifies a treatment plan. These mental activities are examples of rational thought and are frequently referred to as *reasoning*.

DISCIPLINES EXPLORING RATIONAL THOUGHT

In an attempt to explain why and how various physical phenomena occurred, primitive peoples developed myths. With the passage of time, the need for more accurate methods of observing and describing these occurrences was recognized. Methods by which phenomena could be studied and understood evolved. One of the oldest models of such rational thought is the scientific method. This logical step-by-step process provides a valid and reliable method by which to test theories and principles in the basic sciences and to describe research methodology and findings in professional literature.

As people came to understand and interact with their world, they began to harness and use its resources. With time, however, they recognized that resources such as time, materials, and people must be utilized efficiently. To do so meant that the results of actions had to be considered before the actions were taken. This gave rise to a second model of rational thought called decision analysis, which emerged from the field of management. Decision analysis was developed in an attempt to improve the validity and reliability of decision making by identifying the up side and down side of potential decisions. The process allows for the examination of the relationship between alternative decisions and subsequent events that they could produce over time. Through this process costly, unwanted, ineffective events and the decisions that produce them may be avoided. The worst case can occur and be analyzed on paper, not in reality.

A third field, artificial intelligence, has provided another model of rational thought. As society moved into the information age, more efficient and effective mechanisms were needed to accommodate the processing of increasing amounts of information. The field of artificial intelligence began in 1958 for the purpose of developing machines that could mimic the human mind. In order to mimic the human mind, researchers first had to identify the processes of thought. Processes of pattern recognition, list processing, and recursive problem

41

solving were identified and have been successfully applied in computer use. Pattern recognition has led to the development of "expert systems," some of which even assist the physician with diagnosis.

The use of computers and other forms of artificial intelligence allow humans to process some types of information more accurately and in far less time. However, people continue to be responsible for processing vast quantities of data. In many professions, especially in human services, one person may be responsible for processing the data from initial client contact through delivery of service. Students entering such professions must learn how to proceed rapidly from intake of data to provision of care. In order to acquire this skill, students initially need a guide or scheme to follow. Although this was not the main thrust of researchers in the field of cognitive psychology, they have identified and described methods of human thought that can serve as guides, such as the rational-logical model, the hypothetico-deductive model, and the problem typology. All of these will be discussed later.

MODELS OF MENTAL DATA PROCESSING

To begin to provide service to a client, the physical therapist must arrive at a diagnosis through selective, accurate, and timely data acquisition and analysis. The activities and processes through which the therapist arrives at the diagnosis are similar to those described in the medical literature dealing with clinical medicine and clinical problem solving. The most widespread form of problem solving, and the one that is generally taught to students, is the traditional rational-logical approach. This approach includes the recognition of a problem, the compilation of an extensive data base, the selection and grouping of clues from the data base, and finally the determination of a solution or diagnosis based on the previous three steps. Although tedious and time consuming, it may be the approach of choice when confronted with an ambiguous situation.

Unlike the scientific method and the traditional rational-logical approach, the hypothetico-deductive model was developed following observations of how "expert" and less skilled physicians actually made clinical decisions. The results were published in 1978 by Elstein, Shulman, and Sprafka in the seminal work entitled *Medical Problem Solving: An Analysis of Clinical Reasoning*. The resulting four-step model included the discovery that solutions were not developed after careful data collection, but that hypotheses were generated early in the problem-solving process and subsequent data were gathered to evaluate each hypothesis. The four steps included cue acquisition, early hypothesis generation, cue interpretation to confirm or disconfirm each hypothesis, and hypothesis evaluation through which the choice is made from the alternatives.

Elstein and his colleagues felt that the difference between expert and less skilled problem solvers was not in the process used but in the repertoire of experiences available in the long-term memory. This finding seems to correspond with the distinction between analytical and intuitive thought put forth by Bruner in his 1960 book entitled *The Process of Education*. Bruner describes analytical thought as the traditional approach that proceeds through explicit steps one at a time. Intuitive thought does not proceed through a series of careful, well-defined steps. Bruner felt that through the intuitive thought process, the thinker arrived at an answer without really being aware of the process by which he got there. The thinker is unaware of the cues to which he is specifically responding, or why he touches on only a few aspects in his knowledge base before reaching a solution. To use intuitive thinking, a person must have a solid grasp of the knowledge base involved in the problem.

Barrows and Tamblyn, in their 1980 publication entitled *Problem Based Learning: An Approach to Medical Education*, elaborated on the Elstein work by describing a five-step process that they term "clinical reasoning." They note that most health care problems cannot be solved, and that the more usual pattern of care is to analyze and manage the problem. The first step is the formulation of an initial concept of the patient's problem. Then there occurs a rapid generation of from two to five hypotheses, which guide the interview and examination of the patient. Multiple hypotheses are subsequently processed in a parallel form, not sequentially. This parallel processing is efficient and prevents premature conclusions that might occur if hypotheses were analyzed one at a time. A search and scan approach rather than comprehensive data gathering is used to verify each hypothesis. As data are added, problem formulation occurs through which a clearer, more concise picture of the problem evolves. The final step is the "therapeutic decision" whereby the evaluation is finished and the next action decided.

Both the Elstein and Barrows models, like the majority of models discussed in the medical literature, pertain to the formulation of diagnosis. Once the physical therapist has established a diagnosis, she proceeds to manage the case by setting goals, deciding which therapeutic interventions to implement, and adjusting the program as needed based on the reactions of the patient. Some diagnoses or health care problems can be "solved." For example, the epicondylitis resulting from the annual tennis match can be "cured" by the physical therapist through therapeutic intervention and patient education. However, for most health care problems with which physical therapists deal, there are no solutions. Problems that cannot be solved must be managed. For example, there currently is no solution for the problem of asensitive areas of the body following complete transection of the spinal cord. Even though mechanisms exist by which the patient may be taught to compensate for this sensory loss, the problem still exists and must be managed. On the opposite end of the treatment spectrum are the clients for whom problems do not yet exist. Physical therapists continue to be more involved in health promotion and preventive care. With this, they encounter clients such as the healthy pregnant woman, the middle-aged man whose job predisposes him to back injury, or the premenopausal woman who wishes to begin regular exercises to retard osteoporosis,

all of whom need some type of direction in their activities so that problems do not arise. This ongoing attention to a patient's chronic or permanent problems and to the prevention of problems is clinical management.

One of the most important clinical management activities is decision making. This activity should involve the patient, and frequently involves practitioners in other disciplines. Decision making has evolved through various methods. One of the oldest group decision making processes is the advocacy approach, in which "who said" is more important than "what is said." The caveman with the biggest club, or the chief surgeon, usually got his way. Many excellent and creative decisions went ignored and were not implemented when this model was used. As decision makers became more sophisticated, they resorted to the decide-and-justify model. With this approach, decisions were made and the rationales for the decisions were developed later, on the basis of the results of the actions taken. The danger here is that through hindsight, even poor decisions can be justified in such a way that they are continued while good decisions, which produced less than good results because of external factors, are discarded.

With an increasing emphasis on accountability and efficient use of resources, decision makers needed more systematic and reliable methods of analyzing decisions before implementing them. Algorithms, dendrograms, and decision trees were developed as modes of decision making. Each of these is a variation of decision analysis that uses a branching approach to decision making. The first step in each approach is to narrow the focus and delineate the elements of the problem. The second step is to diagram the various alternative decisions and the events resulting from each decision. Each approach begins with the known facts and proceeds to the selection of the "best" decision. These models frequently serve as guides for the practitioner, as teaching strategies for use with students in the professions, and as methods to decrease health care costs by allowing for accurate and timely case management decisions.

It has long been recognized in patient management that events occurring in one system of an organism, such as diabetes, can have devastating effects on other systems within the same organism, such as a neuropathy or retinopathy. Similarly, the decisions made about and implemented in one system of the body can produce significant alterations in the functioning of other systems: For example, increased work load placed on the musculoskeletal system through exercise will increase the demand on the cardiovascular and pulmonary systems. When the physical therapist evaluates and treats, this relationship of all the parts of the whole (all of the systems to the entire body) must be kept in mind. However, we must not focus only on these internal systems or microsystems. Consideration must also be given to the macrosystems or containing systems external to the organism. Such external systems as the environment, cultural values, and economics have far-reaching effects on the organism or client.

The systems analysis approach to management was developed as a means for simultaneously considering the internal and external influences that could affect the results of a decision. A systems analysis approach is being applied to health care management when the physical therapist considers not only the bodily systems of the patient when deciding on a treatment program, but also takes into account the patient's daily routine, psychological support mechanisms, and ethnic background.

DEALING WITH THE MAZE OF MODELS

In recent years some of the models of mental processing have come under attack. Some are believed to serve well as teaching mechanisms and aids for practitioners, but are not seen as being representative of the scientific method. Other models are thought to be incomplete because they deal only with one type of problem. Some are believed to be too general, resulting in incorrect conclusions because the process does not allow for adequate interaction with a knowledge base. One begins to wonder why so many models of information processing have emerged over the years and from so many different disciplines. Perhaps it is because there are many different kinds of problems.

This is the concept that Getzels puts forth. He suggests a problem typology that consists of four categories of problems. The first type is the situation where both the problem and solution are known by the problem solver. This type of problem may require only simple pattern recognition for the solution to be identified and implemented. In the second classification, the problem is unknown but, once identified, the solution is clear. This type of problem may require hypothesis testing or the hypothetico-deductive method to identify the problem, at which point the solution is obvious. In the third type, identification of problems, management of solutions, or both are not standard or known to the solver. One or more problems may simultaneously exist, of which one cannot be identified or for which the solutions are mutually exclusive. Such a complex situation may require the use of decision analysis techniques so that the most effective solution may be reached. The fourth category consists of problems, such as a new disease entity or syndrome, for which a solution may or may not be currently available.

To clarify this problem typology further, the following will exemplify how the typology could be seen in clinical practice:

1. The patient exhibits pain, swelling, and tenderness in the lateral aspect of the ankle secondary to a sudden athletic injury with the foot in plantar-flexion and inversion.
   - Process: pattern recognition
   - Known problem: anterior talofibular ligament sprain
   - Known solution: ice, compression, and elevation
2. The patient has symptoms as above, but in addition, exhibits pain and swelling on the medial malleolus.
   - Process: hypothetico-deductive
   - Possible problems: fracture or avulsion of the malleolus

- Known solutions: same as above, plus immobilization
3. The patient has symptoms as above, but in addition, exhibits muscle weakness, hypermobility of the ankle joint, and recurrent sprain.
   - Process: decision analysis
   - Multiple problems: as above
   - Multiple solutions: as above, plus strengthening of muscles, re-education proprioceptively, evaluate and advise on footwear
4. The patient complains of knee and hip problems secondary to running in a new shoe. Acute-care hospitals are now seeing this new patient problem.
   - Process: systems analysis
   - New problem: the new running shoe with a medial wedge prevents calcaneus from pronating. However, this also locks the foot so it does not accommodate to the ground.
   - New solutions need to be created.

(The above example was contributed by Debbie Nawoczenski, MED, PT, Temple University.)

The search for the definitive model of problem solving has led to the description of not one but many methods for and approaches to processing data and information. Each model seems appropriate for application with only a few of the different classifications of problems. As the physical therapist proceeds from data acquisition to the management of a patient care program, various problems and situations emerge. These various activities do not require the use of all of these mental processes. Establishment of a diagnosis may pose a different type of problem than deciding on treatment goals or determining when treatment should be terminated. Therefore, the therapist must be able to utilize a variety of data processing techniques. The new graduate will be competent in the use of some of these techniques, but will require experience to gain skill in those and competence in others.

Within the world of music there exist virtuosos, and within the field of physical therapy there exist master clinicians. These are the individuals who have the ability to retain and to retrieve data easily. They not only exhibit high levels of skill in processing information but also demonstrate the ability to combine information creatively to develop the most effective outcome. Few of us will achieve this expert mastery level of clinical performance, but we all can develop the ability to assess our patients safely and effectively, and manage their care efficiently through the use of the processes of clinical reasoning.

Neither students nor clinicians in physical therapy should be seduced into using a single model for processing the thousands of knowledge bits they encounter daily. Each of us is a unique human being. We bring to physical therapy our knowledge, compassion, and technical skills as well as our resourcefulness in coping with all the unknowns inherent in patient care. And our patients and their families are equally unique. To treat each patient effectively we must use both intuitive and analytical thought. Sometimes we solve their problems; more often, we manage problems through a process of clinical reasoning. To do this, we must thoroughly understand the structure and function of the human body as well as the psychological, social, and spiritual needs that all people have. We must recognize the limits of our practice, as well as the rapidly changing social and environmental milieu in which we practice.

ANNOTATED BIBLIOGRAPHY

Barrows H, Tamblyn R: Problem-Based Learning: An Approach to Medical Education. New York, Springer-Verlag, 1980 (Thorough discussion of a five-step clinical reasoning process and its application in education).

Bruner J: The Process of Education. Cambridge, MA, Harvard University Press, 1960 (Classic text on philosophy of education and the nature of learning.)

Culter P: Problem Solving in Clinical Medicine: From Data to Diagnosis, 2nd ed. Baltimore, Williams & Wilkins, 1985 (Excellent, easily read discussion of problem solving as used to reach a medical diagnosis. Written as a text, with two thirds of the text devoted to examples.)

Elstein A, Shulman L, Sprafka S: Medical Problem Solving: An Analysis of Clinical Reasoning. Cambridge, MA, Harvard University Press, 1978 (Seminal work describing the four-step hypothetico-deductive process resulting from observations of physician problem solvers. Focus is on diagnostic reasoning although questions of treatment and clinical management are addressed.)

Getzels J: The problem of the problem. In Hogarth R (ed): New Directions for Methodology of Social and Behavioral Science: Question Framing and Response Consistency (No. 1), pp 37–49. San Francisco, Jossey-Bass, 1983 (Thorough discussion of the problem typology.)

Payton O: Clinical reasoning process in physical therapy. Phys Ther 65:924, 1985 (Comparison of clinical reasoning process used by physical therapists to that used by physicians.)

Roth W. Problem Solving for Managers. New York, Praeger, 1985 (Thorough discussion of social, technical, and socio-technical systems and the systems approach to achievement of goals and objectives. Examines difference between synthesis and analysis.)

Rothstein J, Echternach J: Hypothesis-oriented algorithm for clinicians: A method for evaluation and treatment planning. Phys Ther 66:1388, 1986 (Presents a two-part process to aid in clinical decision making and patient management.)

Weinstein M, Fineberg H: Clinical Decision Analysis. Philadelphia, WB Saunders, 1980 (Thorough discussion of the application of the process of decision analysis to health care.)

Wolf S: Clinical Decision Making in Physical Therapy. Philadelphia, FA Davis, 1985 (Discussion of general considerations of decision making and applications to clinical subspecialties within physical therapy.)

PART II

Biological, Kinesiological, and Social Foundations of Human Movement and Function

5 Embryology and Evolution of Movement and Function

EMILY L. CHRISTIAN

EMBRYONIC DEVELOPMENT

FERTILIZATION AND CLEAVAGE

Development of the human form is nothing short of miraculous. It begins with fertilization, which is defined as the union of an ovum and spermatozoon. In addition to initiating cleavage, fertilization restores the diploid number of chromosomes, determines the sex of the developing organism, and contributes to species variation. The cleavage stage of development terminates with formation of the *blastocyst* (Figs. 5-1, 5-2*A*). Fertilization and initial cleavage normally occur within the fallopian tube, after which the blastocyst becomes implanted within the uterus, with its inner cell mass oriented towards the endometrium (see Fig. 5-1).

FORMATION OF GERM LAYERS

Further differentiation of the blastocystic inner cell mass results in formation of a *bilaminar embryonic disk,* consisting of the epiblast oriented towards the amniotic cavity and the hypoblast on the side of the yolk sac (see Figs. 5-1, 5-2*B*). At approximately day 10, the embryo becomes completely embedded beneath the endometrial surface, and by day 15 gastrulation commences. Gastrulation is the process by which the *trilaminar embryonic disk* is formed, composed of the three germ layers from which all tissues are derived, the ectoderm, mesoderm, and endoderm. Formation of the *noto-*chord from mesoderm during gastrulation results in delineation of the primitive axis of the embryo (see Figs. 5-2*C*, 5-2*D*). Furthermore, the notochord is the central structure around which the vertebrae form and the inducer for formation of the central nervous system from surface ectoderm. Mesoderm on either side of the notochord subdivides into paraxial, intermediate, and lateral columns (Fig. 5-3*A*). Further transverse subdivision of the paraxial mesoderm gives rise to the somites, from which are formed the bones of the appendicular skeleton as well as the muscles, bones, and connective tissue of the axial skeleton (excluding the skull) (see Figs. 5-3*B*, 5-8*A*; and Table 5-1). Cavitation of the lateral column of the mesoderm separates it into dorsal (somatic) and ventral (visceral) layers (see Fig. 5-3*C*).

EMBRYONIC PERIOD

During the embryonic period, from four to eight weeks, all of the organ systems begin to develop from the three germ layers. (Refer to Table 5-1 for germ layer derivatives.) Initially, the embryo is straight, with visible dorsal, cuboidal swellings marking the positions of the somites. The embryo then begins to fold on itself in both the sagittal and transverse planes, producing a dorsal convexity and ventral concavity. Growth and development of the cranial end of the embryo exceeds that of the caudal end, primarily because of rapid growth of the brain. The limb buds appear during this stage, the upper limb bud prior to the lower limb bud,

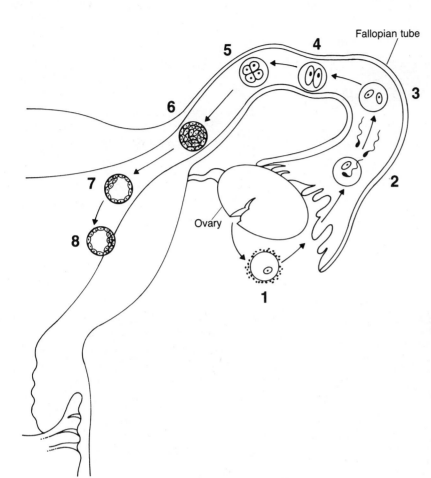

Figure 5-1. Rupture of the ovarian follicle is followed by passage of the ovum into the fallopian tube, fertilization, development, and implantation: *(1)* oocyte after ovulation; *(2)* fertilization; *(3)* male and female pronuclei just prior to DNA replication; *(4)* two-cell stage; *(5)* four-cell stage; *(6)* morula stage; *(7)* blastocyst stage; *(8)* early stage of implantation, with inner cell mass directed towards the endometrium.

and undergo considerable regional differentiation. At the end of the embryonic period, each part of the limbs is identifiable, including digits of the hands and feet. Primordia for the eye and ear (ie, the earliest discernible accumulation of cells for these organs) also become apparent during this period, and the embryo takes on human characteristics.

FETAL PERIOD

Growth and differentiation of embryonic tissues and organs highlight the fetal period, from nine weeks to birth. The rate of growth is greatest from the 9th to the 20th week, and weight gain is greatest in the final weeks before birth. By the end of the 12th week the sex of the fetus is distinguishable and the limbs have grown almost to their relative lengths, although growth of the lower limbs is slightly behind that of the upper limbs. Reflex motor activity in response to external stimuli occurs at this time, but is not usually felt by the mother until a few weeks later. By the end of the 16th week, skeletal ossification can be demonstrated on x-ray film. Surfactant production by the lungs begins at 24 weeks, and the lungs are capable of gaseous exchange as early as 26 weeks. In addition, the central nervous system is sufficiently developed so as to control breathing and maintain body temperature. The 30-week-old fetus exhibits a pupillary light reflex; at 35 weeks, the fetus grasps firmly and spontaneously orients to light. Birth is ex-

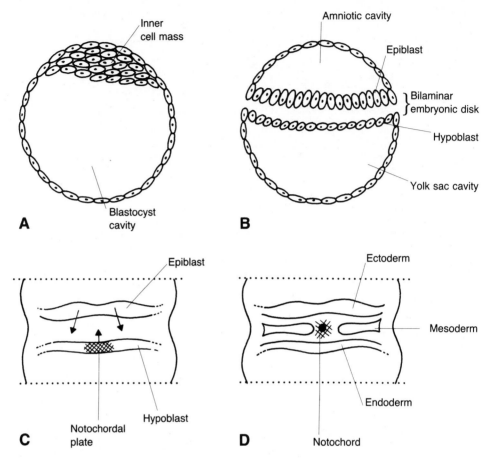

Figure 5-2. Formation of the bilaminar and trilaminar embryonic disks. *(A)* Blastocyst stage. *(B)* Formation of the bilaminar embryonic disk from the blastocyst. *(C, D)* Formation of the trilaminar embryonic disk from the bilaminar disk. Cells from the epiblast migrate deep to give rise to the mesoderm and endoderm. The notochord becomes centrally positioned along the long axis of the embryo.

Table 5-1. Derivatives of the Three Primary Germ Layers of the Trilaminar Embryo

GERM LAYER	SUBDIVISIONS	ADULT DERIVATIVES
Ectoderm	Surface ectoderm	Epidermis, skin appendages, adenohypophysis, inner ear, lens of the eye
	Neuroectoderm	
	Neural tube	Brain, spinal cord, neurohypophysis, retina of the eye
	Neural crest	Sensory and autonomic ganglia of spinal and cranial nerves
Mesoderm	Paraxial mesoderm	Muscles, bones, and connective tissue of the axial skeleton (excluding skull); bones of the appendicular skeleton
	Intermediate mesoderm	Urogenital system
	Lateral mesoderm	Muscles and connective tissue of the limbs and viscera; blood and lymphatic cells
	Head mesoderm	Muscles, bones, and connective tissue of the skull
Endoderm		Visceral epithelium; most visceral organs

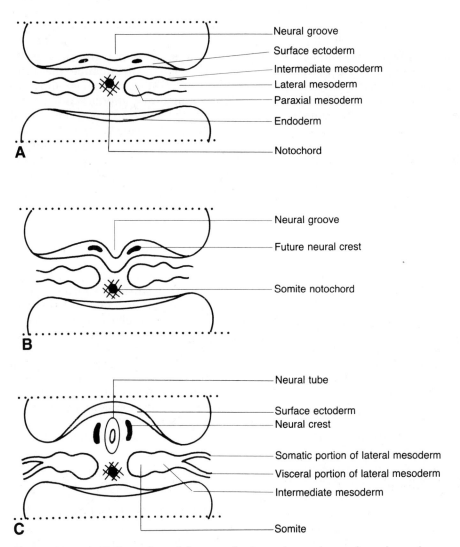

Neural groove
Surface ectoderm
Intermediate mesoderm
Lateral mesoderm
Paraxial mesoderm
Endoderm
Notochord

A

Neural groove
Future neural crest
Somite notochord

B

Neural tube
Surface ectoderm
Neural crest
Somatic portion of lateral mesoderm
Visceral portion of lateral mesoderm
Intermediate mesoderm
Somite

C

Figure 5-3. *(A–C)* Formation of the neural tube and neural crest from the surface ectoderm and subdivision of the mesoderm to form paraxial (somites), intermediate, and lateral columns.

pected to occur at 38 weeks after fertilization or 40 weeks after the last menstrual period.

DEVELOPMENT OF THE NERVOUS SYSTEM

The overlying ectodermal layer of the trilaminar embryo is induced to form the *neural plate* (neuroectoderm) by the notochord and paraxial mesoderm beginning at approximately 18 days

of development. Midline invagination of the neural plate produces a longitudinal *neural groove,* and closure of this groove results in the formation of a *neural tube* and *neural crest* (neurulation) (see Figs. 5-3*A* to *C*). The neural tube gives rise to the central nervous system (brain and spinal cord), while the neural crest cells differentiate into the major components of the peripheral nervous system. Openings at either end of the neural tube, the *rostral* and *caudal neuropores,* temporarily communicate with the amniotic cavity. As dictated by cephalocaudal development, the cranial neuropore closes at approximately day 25 and the caudal neuropore remains open an additional two days. Furthermore, the cranial two thirds of the neural tube, as far caudal as the fourth somite, becomes the brain, while the caudal one third differentiates into the spinal cord. The lumen of the cranial portion of the neural tube represents the future ventricular system, whereas that within the caudal portion becomes the central canal of the spinal cord.

In the fourth week, following closure of the rostral neuropore, the cranial end of the neural tube expands into three *primary brain vesicles:* the prosencephalon, mesencephalon, and rhombencephalon (Fig. 5-4A). Subsequent subdivision of the primary brain vesicles in the fifth week of development results in formation of five *secondary brain vesicles:* the telencephalon, diencephalon, mesencephalon, metencephalon, and myelencephalon (see Fig. 5-4B). (Refer to Table 5-2 for derivatives of the primary and secondary brain vesicles.)

Spinal Cord

The walls of the neural tube caudal to the fourth pair of somites thicken to form the spinal cord. Neuroepithelial cells in this region proliferate and differentiate into all the neurons and macroglial cells of the spinal cord. During this process, the lumen of the neural

tube is reduced to a narrow *central canal* (Fig. 5-5A to C). At approximately six weeks in development, a longitudinal groove appears on the medial wall of the neural tube (the *sulcus limitans*), thus delineating dorsal *alar* and ventral *basal plates,* the future afferent and efferent regions of the spinal cord. (see Fig. 5-5B) Hence, cells of the alar plate become the future *dorsal horn* and those of the basal plate represent the *ventral* and *lateral horns.* As growth continues, central processes of unipolar cells of the dorsolaterally positioned neural crest (the future *dorsal root ganglion*) enter the spinal cord to end in the dorsal horn or ascend the spinal cord to the brain; peripheral processes of neural crest cells are destined to establish functional contact with somatic or visceral receptors. Axons of cells of the basal plate exit the spinal cord and are destined to contact somatic muscle or other peripheral neurons (in ganglia), which will eventually end on visceral motor structures (smooth muscle, cardiac muscle, or glands). Union of fibers entering and leaving the neural tube forms the mixed spinal (segmental) nerves of the spinal cord. (see Fig. 5-5C) Myelination of fibers in the spinal cord begins during fetal development and is completed at approximately one year after birth, generally considered to be coincident with ambulation in the infant.

Brain

The rapidly developing cranial two thirds of the neural tube expands into primary, then sec-

Table 5-2. Adult Derivatives of the Walls and Cavities of the Embryonic Brain Vesicles

PRIMARY BRAIN VESICLES	SECONDARY BRAIN VESICLES	ADULT DERIVATIVES OF VESICLE WALLS	ADULT DERIVATIVES OF VESICLE CAVITIES
Prosencephalon	Telencephalon	Cerebral hemispheres, including cortex, corpus striatum, and medullary center	Lateral ventricles
	Diencephalon	Thalamus, epithalamus, subthalamus, and hypothalamus	Third ventricle
Mesencephalon	Mesencephalon	Midbrain	Cerebral aqueduct of Sylvius
Rhombencephalon	Metencephalon	Pons and cerebellum	Rostral portion of fourth ventricle
	Myelencephalon	Medulla oblongata	Caudal portion of fourth ventricle

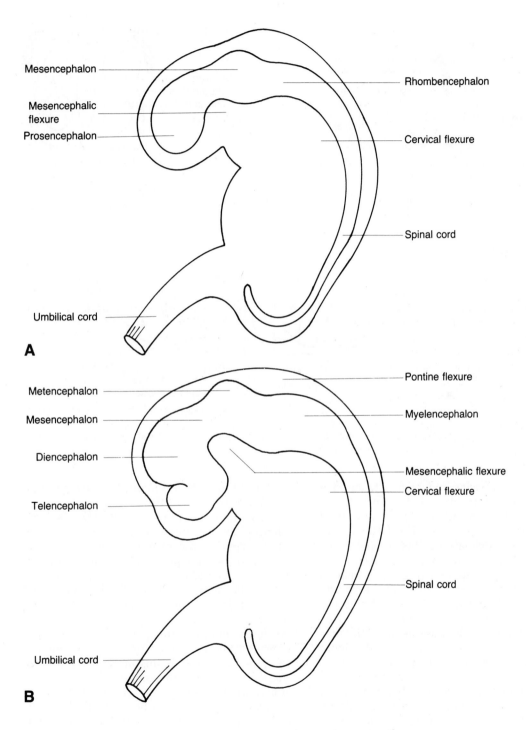

Figure 5-4. Formation of the primary *(A)* and secondary *(B)* brain vesicles.

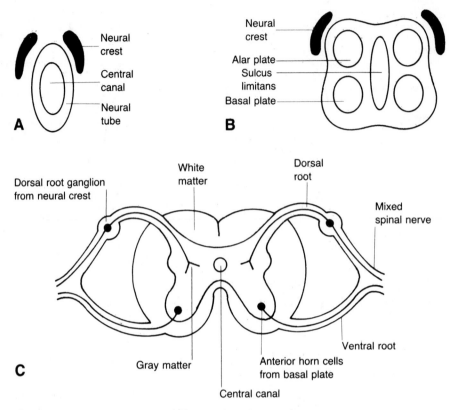

Figure 5-5. *(A–C)* Formation of the spinal cord and peripheral components from the neural tube and neural crest.

ondary, brain vesicles and begins to bend in the sagittal plane, resulting in the formation of pronounced ventral mesencephalic and cervical flexures (see Fig. 5-4A). The latter flexure marks the approximate position of the spinal cord-medulla oblongata junction. Later, a dorsal pontine flexure appears (Fig. 5-6A; also see Fig. 5-4B), resulting in thinning of the rhombencephalic roof and formation of a bulge that represents the future cerebellum. Rostral extension of the sulcus limitans as far as the mesencephalon preserves the spinal cord orientation of dorsal afferent structures and ventral efferent structures in all portions of the brain stem except that of the pons and open medulla. In the latter, thinning of the roof of the rhombencephalon pushes afferent nuclei lateral to efferent nuclei (see Fig. 5-6B). Hence, the spinal

cord and brain stem remain the least differentiated components of the neuraxis.

Evagination of the anterolateral ends of the telencephalon results in formation of the *telencephalic vesicles*, the primordia of the cerebral hemispheres, whose walls expand rapidly in all directions and cover the diencephalon (Fig. 5-7A). The floors of the cerebral hemispheres are essentially tethered, and do not expand with the walls, due to the presence of bulges in the floors marking the position of the *corpus striatum* (see Fig. 5-7B) Consequently, the developing cerebral hemispheres become C-shaped and impart this same shape to the lateral ventricles developing within.

Differentiation of cortical cells leads to formation of numerous axons leaving and entering the cortex with subsequent separation of

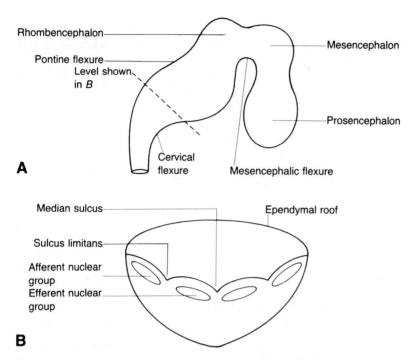

Figure 5-6. (A) The three primary brain vesicles of the developing brain. (B) Cross section at the level indicated by broken line in A. The sulcus limitans of the brain stem delimits afferent and efferent nuclear groups.

the caudate and lenticular nuclei by aggregation of these fibers in the internal capsule. Other cortical fibers accumulate in large bundles that interconnect similar cortical regions, thus forming the *commissures* of the brain, of which the *corpus callosum* is the largest. Initially, the surface of the cerebral hemispheres is smooth (lissencephalic), but rapid growth and differentiation results in the formation of numerous gyri and sulci (gyrencephalic). This process of growth by convolution makes possible a tremendous increase in the surface area of the cerebral cortex without a significant increase in the size of the cranial cavity.

DEVELOPMENT OF THE SKELETAL AND ARTICULAR SYSTEMS

By day 20 of development, the paraxial mesoderm begins to segment into blocks of cells on either side of the midline to form the *somites* (Fig. 5-8A). Typical somites further differentiate into three parts: a superficial dorsolateral mass, the *dermatome*; a deeper dorsolateral mass, the *myotome*; and a ventromedial mass, the *sclerotome* (see Figs. 5-8B and C). The sclerotome consists of loosely packed mesenchymal cells that give rise to the bone, cartilage, and connective tissue of most of the skeletal elements. Mesenchymal cells are said to be pluripotential; that is, they are capable of differentiating into fibroblasts, chondroblasts, osteoblasts, or myoblasts.

Bone formation occurs by two different methods: *intramembranous* or *endochondral ossification*. Bones that form by intramembranous ossification develop directly from mesenchymal cells. However, the majority of the bones of the body form by endochondral ossification, which involves replacement of a preexisting cartilaginous model by bone.

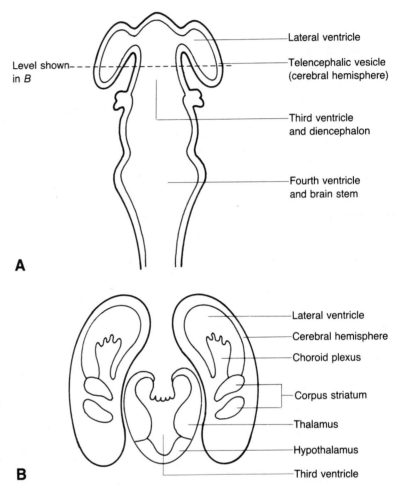

Figure 5-7. *(A)* Development of derivatives of the prosencephalon, the cerebral hemispheres, corpus striatum, and diencephalon. *(B)* Cross section at the level indicated by broken line in *A*.

Axial Skeleton

During the fourth week of development, the paired sclerotomes move medially and appear as condensations of mesenchyme around the notochord and developing spinal cord. During this migration, the sclerotomes retain traces of their metameric or segmental origin. Cranial portions of each sclerotomic segment remain loosely arranged and form the intervertebral disks. Ventral portions of the remaining blocks of sclerotome cells condense to form the cartilaginous models for the vertebral bodies, while those cells surrounding the spinal cord form the vertebral arches (see Fig. 5-8C). Mesenchymal costal processes on either side of thoracic

vertebrae develop into the ribs. Cartilaginous sternal plates develop on the ventral, growing ends of the ribs; fusion of the two plates in the midline results in formation of the sternum.

The skull develops in a complicated fashion from mesenchyme surrounding the brain and will not be described in detail here. It should be sufficient to state that the bones of the cranial vault, the *neurocranium*, develop in a manner different from those of the face, the *viscerocranium*.

Appendicular Skeleton

The upper and lower limb buds, appearing on days 26 and 28 of development, initially consist

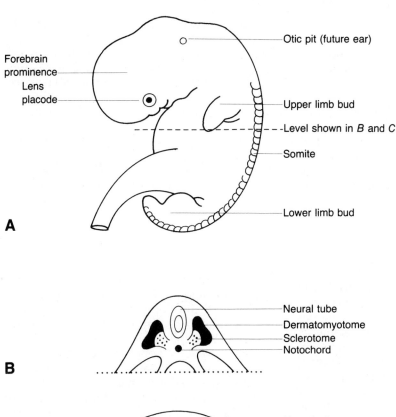

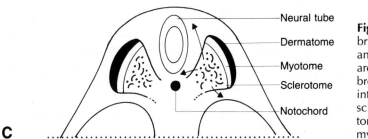

Figure 5-8. *(A)* Lateral view of the embryo indicating the position of the somites and upper and lower limb buds; *B* and *C* are cross sections at the level indicated by broken line in *A*. *(B)* The somites divide into dorsal dermatomyotomes and ventral sclerotomes. *(C)* Later, the dermatomyotomes subdivide into dermatomes and myotomes.

of a mesenchymal core covered with ectoderm. An *apical ectodermal ridge* functions as an inducer of mesenchymal growth and differentiation, in a proximal-to-distal direction (see Fig. 5-8A). Mesenchymal condensations of the limb buds undergo chondrification beginning in the sixth week, and ossification begins as early as the eighth week. As a general rule, bones of the limb girdles form by endochondral ossification, and the largest bones are the first to chondrify

and the first to ossify. The clavicle of the upper limb girdle is apparently an exception; it forms by intramembranous ossification, and it is the first bone to ossify in the body. Prior to birth, primary centers of ossification have appeared in all of the bones of the limbs, with the exceptions of the patellae, carpals, naviculars, and cuboids. Furthermore, the only secondary centers of ossification present at birth are in the distal femoral and proximal tibial epiphyses.

Joints

Skeletal elements develop from condensations of mesenchyme; fibrous connective tissue, cartilaginous connective tissue, or synovial membranes develop between bones at points of articulation.

Amphiarthrodial and *synarthrodial* joints (connected by ligaments or cartilage) are those which allow little or no movement, and will only be mentioned here. Undifferentiated mesenchymal cells interposed between the ends of developing bones later develop into ligaments or cartilage.

Freely movable *diarthrodial* (synovial) joints are characterized by joint cavities lined with synovial membranes and filled with synovial fluid. Furthermore, most diarthrodial joints derive from articulations between endochondral bones. Primordia of the future synovial joints do not appear until after the cartilaginous models differentiate. Soon after, mesenchyme between the ends of the cartilaginous elements forms an *interzone,* which is continuous on either end with the perichondrium of the cartilage model. Cartilaginous growth compresses the interzone while its circumference cavitates. A distinct joint cavity appears as cells in the center of the interzone disappear. Mesenchyme continuous with the perichondrium and surrounding the developing joint differentiates into the joint capsule, while ligaments develop from local thickenings of the capsule. Mesenchymal cells covering the ends of the cartilage models and lining the capsule differentiate into mesothelial cells to form the synovial membrane. Once joint movement occurs, mesothelial cells covering the articular surfaces disappear.

DEVELOPMENT OF THE MUSCULAR SYSTEM

Striated, voluntary, skeletal muscle originates from several sources. Axial musculature develops from *myotomal mesoderm* of the somites, whereas appendicular musculature derives from *mesenchyme* of the limb buds (see Figs. 5-8A to C). In addition, many of the muscles of the head and neck develop from the *branchiomeric arches.* Only the former will be considered here.

Differentiation of mesenchymal cells into *myoblasts* (precursors of muscle cells) is followed by fusion of myoblasts to form the elongated, cylindrical, multinucleated structural element of skeletal muscle, the *muscle fiber.* Later, the specialized organelles of striated muscle appear, the *myofilaments* (actin and myosin).

At birth, most skeletal muscle fibers have already developed; the remainder appear by the end of the first year of life. Subsequent increase in muscle fiber size results from an increase in the number of myofilaments; by this mechanism, muscle fibers increase in diameter.

Axial Muscles

Metamerism of the paraxial mesoderm is established early and is a fundamental characteristic of chordate development. This mesodermal segmentation is also apparent in the brain and spinal cord. In the developing human embryo, there are usually 4 occipital, 8 cervical, 12 thoracic, 5 lumbar, 5 sacral, and 10 coccygeal somites. The first cervical and the last seven or eight coccygeal somites undergo early retrogression. As already indicated, the paraxial somite subdivides into a sclerotome, a dermatome, and a myotome (see Figs. 5-8A to C). The dermatomes extend beneath the overlying ectoderm and are destined to become the *dermis* and *hypodermis.* The myotomes, consisting of embryonic muscle cells, or myoblasts, subsequently give origin to the striated musculature of the trunk.

The myotomes enlarge rapidly both dorsally and ventrally and make contact with the appropriate spinal nerve; once established, this connection is permanent. Between the fifth and sixth weeks, the myotome subdivides along the long axis of the embryo to form a dorsal *epaxial division* and a much larger ventral *hypaxial division* (Fig. 5-9). The spinal nerve also divides, sending a dorsal *primary ramus* to the epaxial portion of the myotome, and a larger *ventral primary ramus* to the hypaxial portion. Most of the developing trunk muscles are nonsegmental, reflecting a migration of the myoblasts away from the midline myotomes; a few,

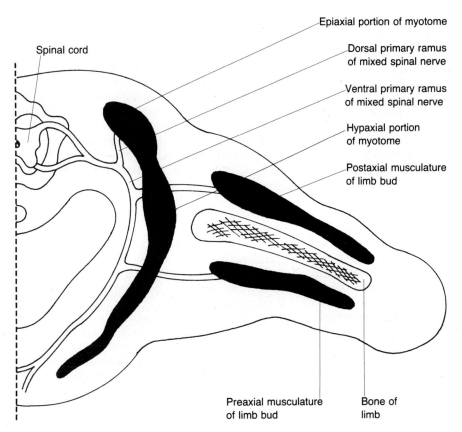

Figure 5-9. Migration of portions of the segmental myotome to form dorsal and ventral trunk musculature. Muscles of the limbs develop from mesoderm of the limb buds. As the mesodermal cells migrate to the appropriate positions, they carry with them branches of the segmental nerves, as indicated.

such as the intercostals, remain segmented.

Muscles derived from the epaxial division of the myotome include the long and short extensors of the vertebral column. Prevertebral, scaleni, geniohyoideus, infrahyoidei, anterolateral trunk, and quadratus lumborum musculature originate from the hypaxial portion of the myotome.

Appendicular Muscles

The limb buds appear early in development, at the end of the fourth week, with the upper limb bud preceding that of the lower limb by a few days. Growth and differentiation of the limbs is under the inductive influence of an *api-cal ectodermal ridge* on the tip of each limb bud (see Fig. 5-8*A*). Striated musculature of the limbs derives in situ from the somatic portion of the lateral mesoderm as condensations of mesenchyme around the developing bones; the myotomes do not contribute to formation of the appendicular musculature.

The limb buds elongate laterally from the long axis of the embryo; the upper limb buds are positioned opposite the lower cervical and upper thoracic somites and the lower limb buds lie opposite the lumbar and upper sacral segments. As the future limbs elongate, extensor musculature is oriented dorsally and flexor muscles are positioned ventrally. Furthermore, the developing dorsal muscles carry with them *postaxial fibers* of the ventral primary rami, whereas ventral muscles are innervated by *preaxial fibers* (see Fig. 5-9). Formation of complicated plexuses of nerve fibers innervating the limbs results in mixing of the preaxial and postaxial fibers; however, these fibers are later sorted and terminate on the respective original ventral (flexor) or dorsal (extensor) muscles. Beginning in the seventh week, the limb buds begin to direct themselves ventrally; in addition, the upper limbs rotate laterally 90 degrees and the lower limbs undergo a medial rotation of 90 degrees. Hence, the elbows are directed posteriorly and further medial rotation, adduction, and extension of the lower limb postnatally result in anterior projection of the knee. These directional changes of the limbs both prenatally as well as postnatally have a significant impact on function later, especially with respect to assumption of the upright posture.

EVOLUTION

The remarkable dominance of human beings in biological and cultural evolution can be traced to a finite number of interrelated developments: an increase in the size and weight of the vertebrate brain from fewer than 100 mg to approximately 1350 g in humans; development of a truly opposable thumb, reflected in greater use of the hand; and assumption of the upright posture with subsequent development of bipedal gait.

UPRIGHT POSTURE

Anatomical changes in the human form that made possible assumption of the upright posture include those related to the vertebral column, pelvis, and lower limb. Initially, the vertebral column develops with a dorsal convexity and a ventral concavity. When the infant raises its head and stands erect, the spine reverses its curve in the cervical and lumbar segments; hence, dorsal concavities appear in the cervical and lumbar regions, with preservation of the dorsally convex thoracic and sacrococcygeal

segments. Concomitant prenatal lower limb medial rotation amounting to approximately 90 degrees, and additional postnatal medial rotation, adduction, and extension bring the lower limb into a weight-bearing position. Several anatomical changes in pelvic morphology then had to occur in order to support the weight of the entire trunk in bipedal stance as compared to only the weight of the hindquarters as exemplified by quadripeds. Paramount among such changes include increasing the stability of the direct union between the pelvic girdle and sacrum, as well as the articulation between the femur and acetabulum of the pelvis. To accomplish increased sacroiliac stability, heavy sacroiliac and sacroischiac ligaments developed. In addition, the three bones of the pelvis fused and formed a direct ventral articulation at the symphysis pubis; articulation with the axial skeleton moved dorsally, reflecting the need for stability instead of mobility. The structure of the hip joint is also indicative of the function of the lower limb; both the depth and diameter of the acetabulum are increased, resulting in enclosure of more than a hemisphere of the femoral head.

UPPER LIMB

Once humans assumed the upright posture, the upper limbs were emancipated from functioning as supporters of weight in stance and locomotion. Indeed, increasing complexity of the hand is believed to be a contributor to human bipedal stance. Hence, the upper limbs became sensory organs, informing the individual regarding the environment, as well as organs useful in manipulating and grasping. Anatomical changes necessary to accomplish these aims included (1) development of an upper limb with increased mobility; (2) an increase in the number of afferent endings and a decrease in the size of the motor unit in the upper limbs, especially the hands; and (3) development of a truly opposable thumb. Whether these changes resulted in an increase in the size of the brain, or the brain dictated these changes in the upper limb, remains a point of disagreement.

BRAIN

Evolutionary changes in the brain offer more information to explain the dominance of humans than any other organ of the body. Humans have developed no new neural structures per se; the brain, however, has grown to an exceptionally large size. This is primarily the result of *telencephalization,* the process whereby higher centers of the central nervous system develop and assume control over the lower centers in the brain stem and spinal cord, and *corticalization,* represented by an increase in the cortical mass.

Central nervous system structures especially large and well developed in humans include the cerebellum with its afferent pathways, thalamus, corpus striatum, red nucleus, and cerebral cortex. Especially noteworthy is the *neopallium,* the portion of the cerebral cortex that is most highly evolved based on organization and stratification. Hence, not only is the volume of the cerebral cortex increased secondary to convolution, but the absolute numbers of cortical neurons are increased and there is increased arborization of pyramidal neurons. In addition, the primary motor and sensory cortical areas are significantly enlarged in humans, and the highly specific lemniscal pathway and direct pyramidal tract are found exclusively in mammals and primates, respectively. Finally, association of cortical areas reach peak development in humans.

Regarding the motor structures in particular, the corpus striatum is an older telencephalic structure phylogenetically and is found in all vertebrates. On the other hand, the neopallium is rudimentary in lower vertebrates, and the direct corticospinal pathway is present only in mammals. Hence, in submammalian forms stereotyped, instinctive activities such as locomotion, defense, feeding, and mating are largely dependent upon the corpus striatum. Evolution of the neopallium in humans resulted in subordination of the functions of the corpus striatum to those of the cerebral cortex. Subsequently, the newer motor system functions in performance of nonstereotyped activities, while the older system is maintained for the well-patterned movements concerned with posture, defense, and feeding.

In closing, it is appropriate to include a discussion of the mechanisms for increasing the size of the brain in response to sensory stimuli, especially those parts of the brain related to the development of motor function. As already indicated, it is not known whether the brain increased in size as a result of functional use of the hand, or if a highly developed hand influenced brain enlargement. A good case can be made for the latter. Vertebrates probably developed, in this order, tactile sensations, followed by senses of smell, vision, taste, and balance, with audition being a more recent acquisition. With increasing complexity, organisms were required to centrally integrate the newly acquired sensation with other sensations. Hence, the need for relative and absolute increases in brain size. However, progressive evolution did not proceed upwards at all points. For instance, the need for a keen sense of olfaction decreased when humans stood upright and began to depend more on vision and the upper limbs for information regarding the environment.

Once again, the biological and cultural success of humans is largely dependent upon an increase in brain size, resulting in (or from) improved hand function and bipedal gait. In addition, the dominance of humans can be related to intelligence, acquisition of new sensory and motor capabilities, and increasingly novel and useful products of cerebral activity.

ANNOTATED BIBLIOGRAPHY

Beuttner-Janusch J (ed): Evolutionary and Genetic Biology of Primates, Vol 1. New York, Academic Press, 1963 (Basic primate evolution, including the peripheral and central nervous systems.)

Beuttner-Janusch J (ed): Evolutionary and Genetic Biology of Primates, Vol 2. New York, Academic Press, 1964 (Basic primate evolution, including comparative anatomy of the hand.)

Crosby EC, Schnitzlein HN (eds): Comparative Correlative Neuroanatomy of the Vertebrate Telencephalon, New York, McMillan, 1982 (A detailed discourse on the comparative neuroanatomy of vertebrates, including the motor systems.)

Hamilton WJ, Mossman HW: Human Embryology: Prenatal Development of Form and Function, 4th ed. Baltimore, Williams & Wilkins, 1972 (Considered to be the finest human embryology text ever written; advanced.)

Moore KL: The Developing Human: Clinically Oriented Embryology, 4th ed. Philadelphia, WB Saunders, 1988 (An excellent embryology text for the beginning student with abundant clinical application.)

Reynolds E: The evolution of the human pelvis in relation to the mechanics of the erect posture. Papers of the Peabody Museum of American Archaeology and Ethnology, Harvard University XI(5):249, 1931 (An in-depth look at anatomical changes in the pelvis as related to assumption of the upright posture.)

Sarnat HB, Netsky MG: Evolution of the Nervous System, 2nd ed. New York, Oxford University Press, 1981 (One of the best texts available on comparative neuroanatomy and evolution of the nervous system; includes a final chapter relating evolutionary changes to motor function and behavior.)

Wake MH (ed): Hyman's Comparative Vertebrate Anatomy, 3rd ed. Chicago, University of Chicago Press, 1979 (A general textbook of comparative vertebrate anatomy for the beginning student.)

Williams PL, Warwick R (eds): Gray's Anatomy, 36th British Edition. Philadelphia, WB Saunders, 1980 (The finest anatomy text available today, including gross anatomy, neuroanatomy, histology, and embryology, with consideration of evolutionary aspects of development.)

Normal Development of Movement and Function:
6 Neonate, Infant, and Toddler

TINK MARTIN

He who sees things grow from the beginning will have the finest view of them.

(ARISTOTLE)

The development of movement is one of the most fascinating scenarios in biological science. The process of regulated growth and differentiation of the structures of the body involves physical changes in size and shape. Internal physiological changes occur in all body systems in order to provide a substrate for movement. Nervous system maturation occurs in the presence of a continually changing musculoskeletal system. Conversely, movement shapes the body's joints, influences the quality of muscle contractions, and readies body parts for stabilizing or mobilizing functions. Movement is the first form of communication with the environment.

Development of movement requires that growth, maturation, and adaptation occur in all systems of the body. Because these changes happen within the environment, they involve learning as well as maturation. The process of development is interactive and dynamic, but is not totally understood. Knowledge of normal movement development is the basis for movement analysis. Analysis of movement is an integral part of the physical therapist's evaluation and treatment of movement dysfunction.

In assessing patients with disorders of posture and movement, the physical therapist's findings are interpreted in view of certain assumptions about the development of normal posture and movement. These assumptions are predicated on developmental theories, concepts, and models of motor control.

THEORIES OF DEVELOPMENT

Theories that are important for an understanding of movement development include the continuity and discontinuity theories, principles of similitude and complementarity, and the law of anticipatory function. These were chosen for review because they provide a foundation for our current understanding of motor development.

The continuity theory states that development occurs along a continuum from infancy to adulthood. Motor patterns change from one to another, prenatally to postnatally, with each change dependent on what came before. These changes are quantitative in nature. You could think of it as a tower of blocks.

Given the appropriate experiences, motor development will proceed along a predictable course. The sequence is universal in the first two years of life, with some individual differences in rate and quality. At this time we do not know if one part of the sequence must be present for the next one to occur. The developmental sequence has provided the most consis-

63

tent base for almost all treatment approaches used by physical therapists.

The discontinuity theory states that at each higher level of motor development, a new characteristic appears that was not previously present. Development would then be viewed as a series of qualitative changes that are discontinuous, or in "stages." This theory does not exclude building on what came before. You could think of it as a pyramid of blocks.

Fishkind and Haley (1986) concluded that achieving independent sitting is a continuous developmental process rather than a stage. Development of independent sitting was more consistent with the pattern of motor development described by Gilfoyle (1982). This three-step process involves a primitive phase, a transition phase, and a mature phase of motor skill acquisition.

The principle of similitude refers to form changing proportionately with size. As bones and muscles increase in length and mass, there must be proportional changes in the muscular force needed to start or stop motion. Changes must also occur in the reactive forces generated. Developmental changes previously explained by neurological maturation may be more simply explained in terms of weight changes of a limb or limbs.

Bohr's principle of complementarity postulates that reflexes alone cannot account for the complexity of infant motor behavior. The infant's brain must have the capacity to generate rhythmical and phasic motor patterns, and must have the capacity for adaptive behavior. Identification of stereotypic infant movement patterns, as well as the increasingly strong connection between social interactive behavior and the acquisition of postural control, support the principal of complementarity.

Carmichael's law of anticipatory function states that systems mature before they are needed. For example, the movement patterns required in kicking are present long before walking is possible. The motor patterns in kicking are thought to be generated by a specific group of cells in the spinal cord (Thelen, 1981). Posture is present before movement control (Haley, 1986).

CONCEPTS OF DEVELOPMENT

All of the following concepts of motor development have formed the basis for treatment strategies. Posture and movement develop in certain anatomical directions (cephalocaudal, proximal-distal, and gross-fine) in the maturing organism. However, one must not assume that the only way to treat abnormal development or motor dysfunction is in the same directional manner.

One long-held assumption about motor development is that it proceeds in a specific direction, cephal to caudal. Actually, it begins in the cervical region and goes both cephally and caudally in ever-widening circles (Fig. 6-1). This parallels the prenatal closure of the neural tube, which begins at C4 and goes both cephally and caudally. Sensory development in utero proceeds cephalocaudally. However, the maturation of the nervous system prenatally is caudal-cephalic, as seen in the pattern of tone development.

Development may still be characterized as cervicocephalocaudal because the postnatal development of motor milestones mirrors the rippling effect seen in Figure 6-1. Head control develops before sitting; sitting develops before standing. Although head control normally begins with head lifting in prone, postural control of the head can be assisted more easily in the sitting position during treatment. The latter is less difficult because of the relationship of the head to the pull of gravity.

Proximal to distal development is another directional concept that states that the areas of the body closer to the midline are controlled before the periphery. Midline control of the axial skeleton occurs before control of either the shoulder or pelvic girdles. The neck and mouth develop first to provide head and oral control, respectively. Proximal shoulder stability necessary to support upper extremity function is achieved by the age of 9 months. Pelvic stability occurs several months later in preparation for independent ambulation. Development of the shoulder and pelvic girdles occurs prior to mature muscular control of distal parts of extremities (*eg*, hands and feet).

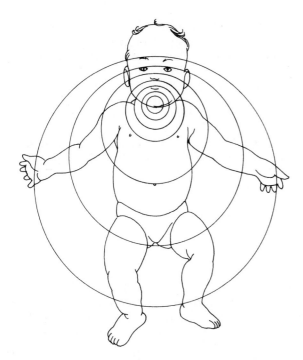

Figure 6-1. Cervicocephalocaudal development.

With increasing maturity gross movement patterns break up into finer, more selective patterns that allow parts of the body to move independently of each other. This process is called dissociation. Whole body responses are noted early in the infant's repertoire, then single limb movements, and finally very specific isolated movements such as a neat pincer grasp. In general, large muscle movements precede fine or small muscle movements. In gross motor development, for example, the milestones of head control, rolling, and sitting occur before the development of a neat pincer grasp. Whole limb movements precede single joint movements. In dissociation of the head from the shoulders, the infant learns to turn his head in all directions without affecting the body as a whole.

The last two concepts deal with kinesiological aspects of movement development: extension-flexion and mobility-stability.

In utero, development of the fetus goes from relative extension to more and more flexion at term. The ability to move against gravity is inherent in the acquisition of upright posture and locomotion. The development of extension against gravity precedes the development of antigravity flexion. Development of lateral neck and trunk flexion is dependent on a balance of neck and trunk flexor and extensor strength. This lateral flexion precedes the development of rotation.

Mobility and movement initiation generally occur before holding movements. Stability, or holding, is seen first at the end of range, then in the midline, and finally anywhere in the available range of motion. Once the separate mobility-stability functions of the neuromusculoskeletal system are initiated, they begin to be combined in various weight-bearing and non-weight-bearing situations. Depending on the posture that is being developed, the distal part of an extremity may be fixed while the proximal part moves, which produces mobility superimposed on stability in weight bearing. This is seen developmentally as weight shifting within postures, and begins in prone. Control in weight bearing is followed by control in space. When the extremity or trunk is no longer supported, it is free to move with the proximal parts, providing stability.

MOTOR CONTROL AND LEARNING

Motor control is the term used to describe the functions that govern posture and movement. The development of movement control begins with control of self movements, and proceeds to the control of movements in relationship to changing conditions. Control of self movements is largely due to the development of the neuromotor system, whereas the latter is due to perceptual-cognitive abilities.

Motor learning occurs concurrently with the acquisition of motor control. The infant learns to move, recognizes appropriate movement, and learns to control movement. Motor development is the end product of the growth, maturation, and learning of the human organism. The acquisition of motor abilities and the learning of new motor skills occur throughout the life span.

TRADITIONAL MODELS OF MOTOR CONTROL

The classical model of motor control is the reflex-hierarchical model. It is a top-to-bottom model predicated on increasing corticalization and inhibition of lower-level reflexes. It is seen in the concept of righting reactions integrating tonic reflexes. Tonic reflexes, such as the asymmetrical tonic neck reflex, are suppressed by the maturation of the neck righting reactions. In the classical model, the reflex is considered as the basic unit of movement.

Another model of motor control is the information processing model, with open- and closed-loop systems. The closed-loop system uses sensory information as feedback to improve the efficiency and accuracy of the movement produced. Movement control is seen first in closed situations, such as in visually directed reaching. This concept operates in early motor learning. An open-loop system uses no sensory guidance, and relies on already programmed patterns of movement. One advantage of this system is speed, as seen in the infant who has mastered creeping and can get across the room faster than the adult who is walking. The infant may be so intent on her destination that she moves over objects in her path rather than going around them.

The processing model partially explains some facets of motor control, but does not reflect the complex interplay of the myriad of sensory and motor subsystems. The human body is not merely a computer that processes incoming stimuli from external and internal sources. Neither the processing nor the classical model totally accounts for the variability of normal movement. Therapists have always considered variability to be the hallmark of normal movement. Even within a well-defined sequence, there are variations on the basic theme.

SYSTEMS MODEL OF MOTOR CONTROL

One recent theory of motor control is a dynamic systems perspective on motor behavior. It incorporates the concept of muscle synergies and the biomechanics of moving segments with the lack of a one-to-one correspondence between neuron firings and motor outcome. Motor outcome is determined by a complex interplay of active and passive forces. Function, not instructions, determines movement (Thelen, 1986).

In the systems model, circular interactions between systems are possible. Stability and mobility are programmed as one system using a feedforward mode. Every movement has a point of stability and a point of mobility. In this way, voluntary movement and posture are integrated. Synergies package the timing, amplitude, and force relationships of muscle groups needed for a certain movement. The choice of synergies makes the motor behavior adaptable to different sensory environments (surrounds). Several different sensory stimuli can produce the same motor response, or one sensory stimulus can produce three different motor responses.

The postural system is cued before the movement begins, in the same way we might think of having a positive mind-set before a test. Next, the movement pattern is chosen and executed with feedback for accuracy. In cases where there is no time for feedback and speed is of the essence, the body can go on automatic pilot. One initiates the movement and the synergy takes over. After years of never having played, your fingers can pick out that long-forgotten piano piece, or the baseball pitcher can fire his favorite pitch.

Motor learning is context dependent. A child does not learn to walk in a sitting position. He must be upright, bearing weight on his lower extremities. Similarly, one learns a skill within the surround, or the context of the situation, and then generalizes it to other situations. A child may learn to tandem walk a line but may not be able to tandem walk on a balance beam without practice. Movement is learned in a postural set or sensory surround. Then it may be generalized or applied to a new situation.

The 6-month-old infant can roll segmentally, but cannot get herself into a sitting position using trunk rotation, or demonstrate trunk rotation when sitting. The trunk rotation must be relearned in the new posture. The child who has learned to go up and down steps with alternating feet on a closed staircase may revert to going one tread at a time on an open staircase because the conditions are changed.

Physical activity is necessary for motor development. An infant must actively move to acquire the basic motor skills of rolling, coming to sit, creeping, and walking. Training is different from physical activity. Training of motor skills such as running or jumping is task specific. Early motor development is a combination of maturation and learning.

Development of postural control in children occurs in stages corresponding with their ability to integrate sensory information. Vision dominates from 1 to 3 years of age. Vision is a strong force in establishing and preserving upright orientation. During this time the proprioceptive system provides only simple and imprecise information. Practice is necessary to fine-tune the somatosensory system so that it uses proprioceptive input effectively.

There is an increased use of somatosensory and vestibular input in children 4 to 6 years of age. This is the onset of adaptational abilities. Adult-like responses are seen in the 7- to 10-year-old child. In response to movement of the base of support in standing, there is a set pattern of muscle activation. This is called an *ankle strategy*. The body is then balanced like an inverted pendulum by a series of muscular interactions. If this strategy is not sufficient to maintain balance, a hip strategy is initiated. The primary source of postural stability in adults and children is somatosensory (Forssberg and Nashner, 1982).

Reflexes

Movement patterns at birth are continuous with fetal movement patterns. These spontaneously generated movement patterns become linked with sensory stimuli on exposure to the environment. Some authorities believe that the most significant role of reflexes may be in the learning of movement. The pairing of sensory and motor components establishes feedback.

Antigravity postures are not observed until 8 to 10 weeks of age. Until this time, the newborn exhibits primitive reflexes. The reflex responses depend on the infant's physiological state, have variable expression, and will habituate with repeated stimulation.

Parmelee and Sigman concluded from their studies of infants that after the first few months of life, it is very difficult to relate neurologic changes directly to the development of movement and behavior (Keogh and Sugden, 1985). General movements and reflexes give way to voluntary and adaptive motor control. Postural control is established first and forms the basis for movement within the physical environment. Movement coordination comes about with the sequencing of movement components.

Sensation

Sensation was once thought to be necessary for movement. We now know that it is possible for movement to occur without sensory input; even in utero, the motor part of the reflex arc functions first. Sensory input is important in learning to move. We learn how it feels to move, and the nervous system recognizes appropriate ways of moving. Sensory input is a part of that learning process. Sensory stimuli are first associated with movement in a stimulus-response mode, as in a reflex. Then the sensory input provides feedback for movement accuracy, as in hand placement during creeping. Finally, sensory input is used as feedforward as an anticipatory cue prior to movement, such as in lifting a heavy weight.

Experience

Experience is vital in the development of the special senses. Specific critical periods for development have been identified in the visual and auditory systems. The visual and auditory cortex respond to stimulation with increased tissue differentiation. Infant kittens deprived of light become blind. Infants and children with chronic serous otitis media can develop functional hearing losses and subsequent language processing problems.

Experience is also vital in the development of the neuromuscular system. The contractile properties of skeletal muscle are influenced by the way they are used. Infants are born with equal amounts of slow- and fast-twitch muscle fibers. Table 6-1 lists physiologic characteristics of muscle fibers. The development of the "slow" fiber characteristics appears to be dependent on their use in tonic or holding movements. If the appropriate movement experiences do not occur postnatally, the infant's slow-twitch fibers do not acquire the adult slow contractile properties. Maturation of skeletal muscle depends on its use and innervation.

Newborns are limited by the amount of movement information, both internal and external, that they can process. At an early age, the child is concerned with the movement. Later, he is concerned with using the movement to explore the environment. Development of movement takes place within the context of the infant's own biological and psychological environment. Development, as a process of change, reflects the transactional nature of the infant's interaction with the environment. Learning occurs as a function of the developmental state.

Wolff (1982) states that "controlled movements are our only means for maintaining posture against gravity, moving in space, changing the environment, and communicating by speech and gesture." Certain parallels can be drawn between movement and language. In the same way that letters combine to make words, muscle strength, range of motion, speed, and endurance combine to form synergies or motor programs.

FACTORS AFFECTING DEVELOPMENT OF MOVEMENT

Biological changes that influence movement development occur structurally in bones, muscle, and fatty tissue. Biological changes also occur functionally in the musculoskeletal, cardiopulmonary, and neuromuscular systems. The mechanical laws of physics that deal with motion and the effect of forces on bodies must be included as factors influencing movement development. Efficiency in movement (force production) is measured by strength, endurance, speed, and accuracy. The neuromotor

Table 6-1. Physiologic Characteristics of Muscle Fibers

CHARACTERISTICS	SLOW	FAST
Contraction velocity	Slow	Fast
Rate of relaxation	Slow	Fast
Time to peak	Long	Short
Time to half decay	Long	Short
Maximum tension	Low	High
Resistance to fatigue	High	Low
Sag	No	Yes

(Slaton D: Muscle fiber types and their development in the human fetus. Phys Occup Ther Pediatr 1(3):51, 1981)

system has been called the basic resource for movement, with other biological and processing systems exerting an influence on movement.

MUSCULOSKELETAL FACTORS

Structural Changes

The musculoskeletal system can only produce movement within its structural constraints. Most bones, with the exception of the skull, are formed in cartilage first. Cartilage is then replaced with bone. The appearance of ossification centers follows a timetable that can be used to establish skeletal maturity prenatally and postnatally. Girls are skeletally more mature in utero and during infancy.

Changes in height and weight are examples of continuous developmental functions. Height can be used as a measure of biological maturity because each child has a consistent pattern. Rate of height change declines from birth to 3 years of age. The height of a 2-year-old child is half her adult height.

Different parts of the body grow at different rates, and proportions change over time. The neonate's head is 70% of its adult size at birth, and will double in size from birth to maturity. The trunk grows the fastest during the first year of life, contributing about 60% of the increase in body length. No wonder head and trunk control are so critical to development of upright posture and locomotion. After the first year, the legs are the fastest growing part of the body.

Functional Significance

Developmental biomechanics is the study of the effects of forces on the musculoskeletal system. The mechanical factors that affect movement abilities are divided into two categories (Keogh and Sugden, 1985). Internal forces include the center of gravity, base of support, and line of gravity. These change relative to the mass of the body parts and body position. The center of gravity is above the umbilicus in the young child and gradually ascends to its adult placement. The base of support defines the limit of stability. External forces include gravity, inertia of the body segment, and ground reaction.

The development of the spinal curves is well documented. The cervical curve increases as the prone infant lifts his head with the erector spinae muscles. As sitting and crawling are attempted, the lumbar lordosis develops. The lordosis is the result of incomplete elongation of the hip flexors as the hips extend to assume an erect posture, as in high kneeling.

The inherent properties of the structures involved in musculoskeletal articulations such as joint play, joint range, ligamentous range, and muscle tension contribute to the acquisition of the physical properties of movement and development of maximal performance. Newborns have hip extension limitation of up to 46 degrees and show limitation in range until 2 years of age (Walker, 1984). Movement and the development of hip extension is limited to the available range.

The skeletal and limb articulations make possible kinematic chains. Open chains such as the free arm produce mobility. Closed chains such as a supporting arm produce stability. Each joint has at least one degree of freedom. The additive effect of the combinations of movement possible in any joint or grouping of joints is called *degrees of freedom.*

Movement can be thought of as a diagram of muscular and nonmuscular forces drawn on many degrees of freedom, such as in gait. The stance leg has fewer degrees of freedom than the swing leg. The gait characteristics depend on force generated, available range, and environmental conditions. Walking to get a lollipop may produce a different gait pattern than walking into the physical therapy department.

Muscle tissue is elastic and springs back if stretched. In kicking, extension of the leg is like stretching a spring: the leg recoils in flexion. As the leg gets bigger, there is less recoil, so more force is needed to move. An infant stops kicking not because of maturation, but because the leg is too heavy (Thelen, 1986).

Strength and endurance follow the development of movement. Postural control requires appropriate development of muscular strength and endurance against gravity. Gravity is the first resistance the newborn experiences. Studies of strength have been limited by quantifiable means of measurement. However, a correlation has been found between height and strength in school-age children. Height and weight also correlate with strength in certain body types, mesomorphs being stronger than ectomorphs. Earlier maturing boys and girls show an earlier increase in strength development. Toddlers in the 95th percentile for height and weight often perform better on tests of gross motor development.

CARDIOPULMONARY FACTORS

The basic purpose of the cardiovascular and pulmonary systems is to provide the fuel for movement. But, the pulmonary system also includes important postural muscles and the breath control for behavioral expression through sound production. The first major adaptation to extrauterine life is made by the pulmonary system. With the application of large force, the lungs open for the first breath. It takes about 40 minutes after birth for the lungs to reach near normal compliance. Pulmonary function tests of healthy infants showed that newborns have proportionately larger airways relative to lung volumes, with female infants demonstrating a greater relative difference. However, when infants' air flow rates are corrected for size, they are similar to rates in children and adults.

Respiratory rates change with age. The average respiratory rate for an awake infant is 30 to 40 breaths per minute. The rate declines rapidly to 25 to 30 breaths per minute during the second year of life. The functional residual capacity of the infant is only half that of the adult. Vital capacity increases steadily with body size, with no gender differences until adolescence. New alveoli are added until 8 years of age. As the surface area increases, so does the diffusion capacity of the lungs.

The ribs of a neonate at birth are essentially horizontal in relationship to the trunk. Only after the infant is exposed to gravity in a sitting position do the ribs take on their adult orientation, rotating downward and slightly outward, thus increasing the size of the thoracic cavity. This increased space coupled with an increasing vital capacity allows for longer phonation. By 13 to 15 months of age, the toddler has developed most of the respiratory control necessary for mature speech production. These structural changes of the chest also allow for a functional change in the more efficient use of the abdominal muscles and development of the oblique muscles. If this change in chest configuration does not occur, the abdominals cannot work effectively.

Circulatory adjustments that occur at birth or shortly thereafter include closure of the foramen ovale, ductus arteriosus, and ductus venosus. All are necessary to switch from fetal circulation to circulation through the lungs. Pressure gradient changes and constriction of muscular walls of the ducts provide the mechanisms for closure. Systemic vascular resistance doubles at birth, with blood no longer going through the placenta. Also, the pulmonary vascular resistance increases tremendously because of the expansion of the lungs.

The newborn has a cardiac output and metabolic rate twice that of an adult. The mean resting heart rate decreases 15 to 20 beats from 2 to 10 years of age. Pulse pressures increase with age, as does blood volume. The basal metabolic rate declines continuously from birth.

Literature dealing with cardiovascular endurance of children under 3 years of age is extremely limited. The few sources report a range of maximum heart rates for children from 180 to 234 bpm. Children's capacity for aerobic work develops early, and their abilities are similar to those of adults when corrected for body size. Problems in research design have been cited in separating physical activity from physical training and accounting for the continually changing variables of body size and functional capacity.

NEUROMOTOR FACTORS

The development and maturation of the nervous system has the most significant impact on the development of movement and function. Structurally, there are changes in the size of the brain, with the rate of growth being greatest at birth. Rapid growth occurs during the first 6 months of life. During this period the brain reaches 50% of its adult weight. The rate then slows so that the brain's maximum weight is achieved by 6 years of age. Different parts of the brain grow at different rates related to their functioning. The vestibular system is functional at birth, whereas the visual system undergoes rapid growth and differentiation as it is exposed to light.

The process of myelination is very important for the nervous system because it results in an increased speed of conduction of nerve impulses. Myelination of nerve fibers begins at the end of the third month of fetal development. Motor fibers are myelinated before sensory fibers. Therefore, the motor part of the reflex arc can function prior to sensory input. Arm withdrawal occurs before leg withdrawal; therefore, reflex connections develop cephalocaudal. All the peripheral nerves are myelinated at birth, whereas the rest of the nervous system continues to myelinate on its own orderly timetable until 7 years of age. Some association fibers and cerebellar tracts continue to myelinate into adulthood.

Fetal movement patterns have been studied with ultrasound. These patterns of movement, which are called primary movement patterns (PMP), begin at 10 weeks' gestation. They increase in number and variety and are described as means of fetal locomotion and propulsion. The propulsion patterns are postulated as triggering or assisting delivery. All movement patterns are developed in utero by

20 weeks. Lack of these movements would indicate nervous system damage. The presence of such movement patterns in utero lends strong support to the concept of the preprogrammed nature of movement. This concept holds that control comes only after the effect of the external environment has been experienced and mastered.

During a study of spontaneous infant behavior, 47 rhythmical stereotypies were identified (Thelen, 1979). These simple rhythmical behaviors generated by the nervous system precede more complex activities or appear just as the infant is gaining postural control over a new position. Most of the stereotypies of the limbs are simple flexion-extension movements. Others involve repetitive weight shift in a position. The most familiar one is rocking on hands and knees. Stereotypic behavior is replaced by goal-directed movement. These stereotypies manifest a significant developmental trend in the first year of life, with peak performance at 24 to 42 weeks (6 to 10 months). This corresponds with the belief that all components of movement are established by 6 months.

Kicking in 1-month-old infants was studied (Thelen and co-workers, 1981). The morphological and temporal structure of the activity was found to be similar to single-limb movement in locomotion. This supports the probability that human locomotion is controlled by a central program, or pattern generator.

Well-coordinated kicking is seen as early as 1 month, with a peak of activity at 5 to 7 months. Kicking declines as crawling and walking begin. These highly organized nonreflexive motor patterns occur before voluntary control has matured. The pattern generators, one for each leg, are functional before the behavior appears, in keeping with Carmichael's law of anticipatory function. Spontaneous kicking and early reflexive stepping may be forerunners of mature locomotion. Other pattern generators have been identified for respiration, heart rate, sucking, swallowing, and mastication.

Early sensorimotor experience is crucial in developing a feedback system for the refinement of movement. The motor system allows exploration of sensory and perceptual information. Movement verifies perceptions. Through movement, the infant develops a sense of the who, what, when, where, and how of her own movements. Kinesthesia allows the baby to differentiate herself from the environment, recognize her body parts, and know her movements. Visual development gives the child the spatial coordinates of the environment. According to Folio and Fewell (1983), "As a child matures, perception becomes a more dominant system than motor behavior for operating on and interacting with the environment."

PSYCHOSOCIAL FACTORS

Personal-social behavior affects participation in movement experiences, and can therefore increase or limit motor development. Between 2 and 4 months of age, the infant undergoes reorganization in many systems and the transition is made from neonatal behavior to "mature" infant behavior.

From birth to 4 months, changes occur physiologically that reflect a rapid organization of inhibition and controlling mechanisms. According to Keogh and Sugden (1985), these changes are manifest in (1) sustained sleep greater than four hours; (2) more organization of sleep states with a doubling of quiet sleep; (3) a closer association of electroencephalogram patterns and sleep states; (4) a sharp decrease in crying during waking hours; (5) a suppression of primitive reflexes; (6) an increase in alertness; and (7) the rapid development of a social smile. The most dramatic changes occur between 4 and 8 weeks after birth.

The concept of state has been described as a means of categorizing the level of alertness in the newborn period. Behavioral state must be taken into account when testing the newborn because his state will affect the quality of his response. Sleep state has a profound organizing effect on respiratory control. The newborn spends half of the time he is asleep in rapid eye movement (REM) sleep. Cerebral blood flow and protein synthesis are increased in REM sleep. By 6 months of age, the infant has the adult pattern of 80% quiet sleep, 20% REM (Bryan and Bryan, 1979).

Wakefulness has been viewed as a self-organizing condition in the infant. The establishment of a 24-hour circadian rhythm occurs around 2 to 4 months of age. Other physiological systems that show circadian rhythms are temperature, pulse rate, and sodium and potassium excretion. It is not clear if these rhythms are initiated by environmental influences and then come under internal control, or if they are internally triggered.

The infant becomes more responsive at 2 months. With the improvement of postural control of the head, the eyes are allowed to change the direction of gaze. This permits the infant to manipulate social interaction. At the same time, major changes are seen in visual functioning in the areas of acuity, accommodation, and contrast sensitivity.

Cognitive processes in infancy involve information processing and organization of adaptive responses. These have been measured by visual attention to novelty. Habituation of attention, recognition memory, and temperament show evidence of stability of individual differences between infancy and childhood (Berg and Sternberg, 1985).

MOTOR DEVELOPMENT

Development has been viewed as a spiraling continuum of spatiotemporal adaptation. Primitive patterns of posture and movement are modified and integrated into more complex movement strategies. Movement for movement's sake, and primitive postures and movement strategies are adapted to purposeful behavior such as rolling, sitting, and creeping. Once the behavior is learned the movement becomes automatic, allowing adaptation to the environment and further learning. This sequential development of motoric behavior has been described as "postural strategies controlling movement and movement strategies giving rise to purposeful action" (Holt, 1975).

Milestones

The developmental sequence consists of certain motor milestones for both gross and fine motor development. The milestones of gross motor development are head control, rolling, sitting, creeping, standing, and walking. Ages for acquiring them are head control, 4 months; rolling segmentally, 6 to 8 months; sitting alone, 8 months; crawling, 8 to 9 months; pulling to stand, 9 months; creeping, 9 to 10 months; and walking alone, 12 to 18 months. Fine motor development is characterized by the following milestones: raking, 5 months; palmar grasp, 6 months; radial digital prehension, 9 months; inferior pincer prehension, 11 months; and neat pincer prehension, 12 months.

Although the sequence of milestones appears to be universal, the age at which a given child may attain the milestones is influenced by child-rearing practices and cultural differences. As with other individual differences, the rate of acquisition may vary.

COMPONENTS OF MOVEMENT

The biomechanical, kinesiological, and sensory variables that combine to produce head control, trunk control, and trunk rotation are the components of movement. These basic components are present in a normal infant by 6 months of age (Bly, 1983).

Normal movement of the head and trunk requires the ability to produce the following movements in the stated positions:

1. Prone—bilateral symmetrical extension against gravity with concurrent elongation of the antagonist flexors.
2. Supine—bilateral symmetrical flexion against gravity with concurrent elongation of the antagonist extensors.
3. Sidelying—unilateral symmetrical contraction of trunk flexors and extensors on one side with the concurrent elongation of the antagonist trunk flexors and extensors.

Stated simply, the infant must learn to extend against gravity in prone, flex against gravity in supine, and laterally flex against gravity in sidelying (Bly, 1983).

Additionally, the range of motion, appropriate arthrokinematics, and vestibular, tactile, and visual inputs and connections are needed to produce normal head and trunk movements. Visually impaired infants can achieve head and trunk control, but do so at later ages.

RIGHTING, PROTECTIVE, AND EQUILIBRIUM REACTIONS

As the infant learns to move against gravity, postural reactions develop. Righting reactions occur in response to several sensory inputs. Gravity and change of head or body position elicit the most frequently used righting reactions. The purpose of righting reactions is to keep the correct orientation of the head and the body in relation to the ground. Protective reactions show a sequence of appearance: (1) downward lower extremity (LE), 4 months; (2) forward upper extremity (UE), 6 to 7 months; (3) sideways UE, 7 to 8 months; (4) backwards UE, 9 months; and (5) protective staggering LE, 15 to 17 months. These should not be confused with propping on extended arms, in which the infant either pushes herself into the position or is placed there by someone else.

Protective reactions are extremity responses to rapid displacements of the body by horizontal or diagonal forces. By extending one or both extremities, the infant attempts to stop the movement.

Equilibrium reactions permit the whole body to adapt when the center of gravity is changed either by movement of the supporting surface or of the body. There are three expected responses: (1) lateral head and trunk righting away from the weight shift; (2) abduction of the arm and leg away from the weight shift; and (3) trunk rotation away from the weight shift (Bly, 1983). Equilibrium reactions allow the infant to regain the position. The other possibilities are protecting or falling.

Equilibrium reactions appear in an orderly sequence beginning in (1) prone at 6 months, (2) supine at 7 to 8 months, (3) sitting at 7 to 8 months, (4) four point at 9 to 12 months, and (5) standing at 12 to 21 months. These reactions mature when the child has moved on to work at a higher postural level. For example, sitting equilibrium reactions mature when the child is creeping; four-point reactions mature when the child is standing.

Some righting reactions may begin at birth, but most are seen between 4 and 6 months of age. Their maximum influence occurs around 10 to 12 months of age. Technically they persist until 5 years of age, when a child can come to stand from supine without trunk rotation.

The role of righting, support, and protective reactions has been described as providing differentiated strategies for "moving or not moving." Additionally they allow "weight shift sets" to emerge and free the extremities to move in space.

Keogh and Sugden (1985) reinforce the concept that head and upper trunk control is a necessary but not a sufficient condition for changing position: "Postural control requires more than righting reflexes to maintain equilibrium and changing a position requires postural control as well as movement skill." Righting reactions establish static equilibrium. Continuous movement of the body requires motion stability as opposed to positional stability. The latter is acquired from postural alignment of the skeleton along the line of gravity.

A posture must be controlled before other body movement can be controlled. Postural stability may come from the relationship of body parts to one another, such as in ring sitting. The infant has positional stability and maintains an upright trunk because of the wide base of support from the position of the legs. If the legs are brought together in a long sitting position, the infant may require the use of one or both hands for balance and the trunk may or may not remain upright. The ability to maintain a posture, such as sitting, may not mean the infant can get into or out of the position with control.

Dynamic stability is required during continuous movement as in a sequence of moving from prone to sitting. According to Keogh and Sugden (1985), "Motion stability means that the body's movement can have either stable or unstable qualities, and it can exist even when the body positions at many points in the motion would not be stable if there was not motion."

Speed is necessary to establish motion stability. Initially, the infant cannot use speed to control his posture. Early movement development is concerned with sequencing the movement of specific body parts with the appropriate amount of force to form a whole movement. Once there is internal movement consistency and better spatio-temporal accuracy, the infant can manipulate the environment. By the age of 2 years, the infant has mastered the basics of posture, locomotion, and manipulation.

The relationship between the sequence of weight shifting and the type of rotation may indicate the infant's ability to control rotation with flexion before rotation with extension. According to Bly's (1983) descriptive analysis of protective extension sideways, the infant rotates to one side, then shifts weight, resulting in rotation with flexion. In a sitting equilibrium reaction, the weight shift occurs before the rotation, resulting in rotation with extension. This has not been supported by any research to date.

The components of the infant's automatic postural adjustment system are acquired in the following order: (1) righting, (2) protective, and (3) equilibrium. Head and trunk control in its mature form is followed by extremity control, and finally total body control. That is, the toddler will first compensate for a weight shift by righting, then abducting extremities, then will either rotate the trunk to regain balance, or protect, or fall.

DEVELOPMENT OF MOVEMENT

Neonate (0 to 10 Days)

The newborn has routinely been characterized as having "physiological" flexor tone. However, no difference has been identified in resistance to passive movement between flexors and extensors. It is surmised that the preferred flexed posture of newborns might be of muscular origin.

The newborn is able to use capital and neck extensors in prone to lift and rotate the head to the opposite side. Head lifting is the first step in the development of antigravity extension and weight shifting. While the newborn is supine, the head is turned to the side because there is not enough muscular control to maintain it in the midline. Touwen (1976) discovered that the newborns in his study were all able to balance their heads for more than three seconds when tested in sitting. In standing, the newborn demonstrates primary standing and automatic walking.

Infant

1 to 3 Months

The infant gradually begins to extend against gravity over the next few months. Internal physiologic processes are stabilizing. Periods of sleep and wake become more established.

The infant's posture in prone becomes more symmetrical as the head is able to be lifted higher and weight is borne on the forearms. By 3 months of age, the head can be lifted to 90 degrees. The puppy position of forearm weight bearing requires the functioning of both the extensors and flexors of the trunk, with the latter acting on the humeri. The relative position of the upper extremities, specifically the amount of abduction, will affect the amount of upper trunk elevation. When the head and trunk are extended, the pelvis stays flat with the legs abducted and externally rotated. As Bly (1983) notes, "The marked hip external rotation during spinal extension in prone is initiating the background mobility for lumbar spine hyperextension and anterior pelvic tilting." These will be important for development of the normal lumbar curve and erect sitting.

In supine, the head is turned to one side and the presence of an asymmetrical tonic neck reflex may be evident. Lateral vision and eye-hand regard is observed in the 2-month-old infant. The 3-month-old infant holds her head more often in midline in preparation for true midline play, which is seen in the 4-month-old infant.

When pulled to sitting from supine, the head lags behind the body. Antigravity flexor neck control is not yet present. In sitting, the 2-month-old infant shows head bobbing with no trunk control. At 3 months of age, the head can be maintained in upright but this will be accompanied by shoulder elevation and a forward head posture. The back continues to be rounded.

4 Months

The 4-month-old infant is characterized by symmetry in all postures. Midline orientation is established. When the hands come together in the midline for the first time an "aha" phenomenon may be observed. Bilateral forward reaching begins. The head is kept in line with the body during a pull-to-sit maneuver.

In prone, the arms assume the pivot prone position of head, neck, and trunk extension accompanied by scapular adduction. Scapular adduction reinforces spinal extension. This pattern of movement reoccurs in the development of sitting, standing, and walking. Spinal extension is balanced by flexor activity during forearm weight bearing. The infant plays between pivot prone and forearm weight bearing. With any asymmetrical weight shift, the infant may roll to the side. If the lower extremities are too widely abducted, or "frogged," the weight shift is prevented biomechanically, and rolling cannot occur.

The supine infant "gathers self together" by getting hands, eyes, and knees together in midline. In the lower extremities, increased hip extension increases anterior pelvic tilting. Conversely, active hip and knee flexion decreases the anterior pelvic tilt, and this interplay initiates anteroposterior pelvic mobility. Random

pushing with the legs also provides pelvic rotation and leads to lateral weight shifts.

Sidelying provides asymmetrical proprioceptive and tactile input. It also stimulates lateral head righting. Lateral head movements are only possible when there is a balance of neck flexor and extensor muscles.

5 Months

The 5-month-old infant practices frequent weight shifting and lateral head and trunk righting. Equilibrium reactions begin in prone. The infant is able to push up on extended arms. From forearm weight bearing, the infant can now weight shift laterally and reach forward with one arm. Again, with too much weight shift, the infant will roll over.

Abdominal and hip flexor control allows the supine infant to lift his legs and bring his feet to his mouth and hands (Fig. 6-2). Elongation of the hamstrings prepares for long sitting. Use of the lower abdominals in bottom lifting prepares for the pelvic control needed for sitting. The infant shows antigravity flexor control by lifting his head off the supporting surface (Fig. 6-3), which allows the head to lead the movement during pull to sit.

In sitting, the 5-month-old infant continues to lean forward from the hips. The abducted position of the lower extremities provides positional stability. During a pull to sit, the infant may pull all the way to stand, using strong knee extension and ankle plantarflexion.

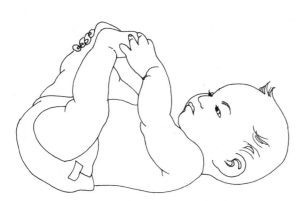

Figure 6-2. Bottom lifting and exploration of feet.

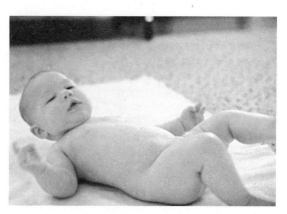

Figure 6-3. Head lifting in supine position.

6 Months

Although the milestone of head control is achieved by 4 months, it is not until 6 months of age that the infant has the ability truly to extend, flex, and laterally flex the head against gravity. The extension that began with the head and neck has progressed down the back to the point where it can be said to go over the hips. When the Landau reflex is tested, the infant's legs extend against gravity. This final stage in the development of extension can only occur if the legs are relatively adducted. Biomechanically, it is very difficult to extend at the hip if the legs are widely abducted and externally rotated.

In prone, the infant now has enough shoulder girdle control to weight shift on extended arms and reach forward. Lateral head and trunk righting are present in response to the weight shift. If weight is shifted too far, an equilibrium reaction may occur, which will bring the infant back to prone and prevent him from falling over. Dissociation of upper and lower extremities is apparent, and the infant can pivot while prone (Fig. 6-4).

Antigravity flexion control continues to get stronger in supine as evidenced by chin tucking and posterior neck elongation with independent forward head lifting. The infant can lift extended legs above the trunk while in supine by contracting the abdominals and hip flexors. She then can reach out to play with her feet in a lower-upper extremity mid-range holding pattern.

Segmental rolling occurs first from prone to supine and later from the more challenging supine to prone. In rolling supine to prone, the movement usually begins with flexion of a body part. Flexion dominates until the infant reaches sidelying, when extension takes over. The infant reaches prone with his head oriented in space. Trunk rotation is essential for development of transitional control. This enables the infant to make the transitions between developmental postures (ie, sitting, four point, standing) with control.

When pulled to sit, the child initiates this action with the arms while tucking the head and flexing the legs. Halfway up, the knees extend while the hips stay flexed, in preparation for sitting. The head and trunk are erect while sitting. Scapular adduction is no longer needed to reinforce spinal extension, freeing the arms for play or protective reactions. Initially, the infant will need to use the arms extended out in front for support.

The 6-month-old infant bears weight on both legs in standing and will bounce. This is one of the rhythmical stereotypies mentioned earlier. Bouncing and rocking in a position appears to occur when a new posture is attained. Reinforcement of the new posture occurs by

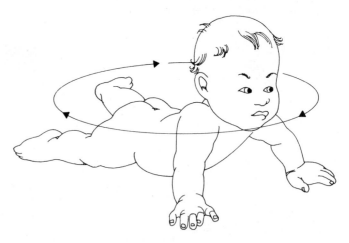

Figure 6-4. Pivoting in a circle while prone.

means of proprioceptive and vestibular input.

By the end of the sixth month, the sequences of movement available to the infant are varied: prone to sitting; prone to four point; prone to runner's position; prone to plantigrade or bear position; and prone to four point to sitting. Figures 6-5 through 6-7 illustrate an actual movement sequence in a 5-month-old infant who was demonstrating movement patterns typical of a 6-month-old infant. She was also in the 95th percentile for height and weight.

7 to 8 Months

The preferred position for the 6-month-old infant is prone, but the 7-month-old infant enjoys sitting for longer periods of time. Equilibrium reactions are seen in supine and are beginning in sitting. The 7-month-old infant demonstrates trunk rotation in sitting, with one or both arms free to play. The legs are still somewhat abducted and extended for positional stability, although trunk control is sufficient to handle small lateral weight shifts. Protective extension sideways is evident (Fig. 6-8).

Some form of pre-walking progression emerges during the seventh month. It may be belly crawling, which has the same components of movement as creeping on hands and knees. These components are upper trunk weight shifting with one arm reaching, combined with lower trunk weight shifting with the opposite leg flexing.

Pushing back in prone, the infant can move into a four-point or a bear position. The abdominal muscles work in the four-point position, with the hip and thigh muscles working in the bear position. As abdominal control gets better, the hip extensors get stronger. The abdominal muscles must develop to produce a stable

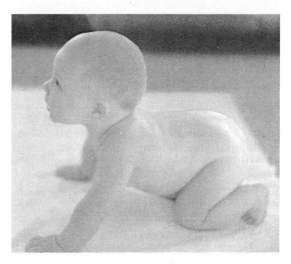

Figure 6-6. Pushing up to four-point position.

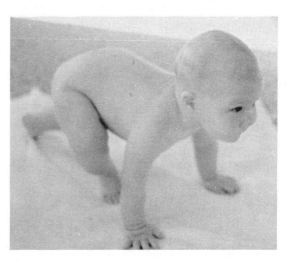

Figure 6-7. Runner's position.

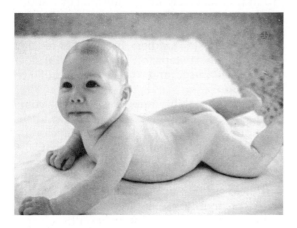

Figure 6-5. Prone on elbows.

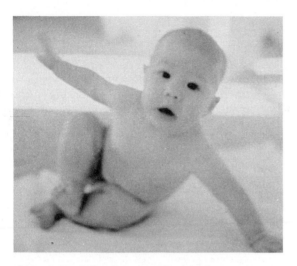

Figure 6-8. Sideways protective reaction.

pelvis from which the gluteal muscles can produce hip extension. Once the four-point position can be maintained, rocking occurs in four point in all directions: forward, backward, and diagonally. This rhythmical stereotypy might be interpreted as heralding the development of postural control in the four-point position.

At 8 months of age, the infant has full equilibrium reactions in sitting. From sitting the infant can now use trunk rotation to make the transition to four-point position by moving over a flexed, abducted, externally rotated leg. The weight-bearing hip is used as the axis of the movement.

9 to 11 Months
The movement components acquired in the first six months of life continue to be refined from 9 to 11 months of age. The transition from independent sitting to being independent in upright begins in earnest. The 9-month-old infant is functional in sitting and plays with various leg positions such as long, tailor, and half-tailor sitting. Because lower extremity external rotation is no longer needed to maintain pelvic stability, the infant can side sit.

Purposeful straight-line movement requires reciprocal movements of the shoulder and pelvis. Bly (1983) states that creeping occurs when the trunk has sufficient control to allow counterrotation of the shoulder girdle and the opposite pelvis. If trunk control is not sufficient, homolateral creeping is observed. The 9- to 10-month-old infant uses creeping as a primary means of locomotion.

Independent mobility by creeping is followed by coming to kneeling. The infant also pulls to stand through the half-kneeling position. When cruising, the trunk is turned partially in the direction of the movement and he practices certain maneuvers (Fig. 6-9). By 11 months, the infant can rise to standing without pulling with his arms. He may stoop to recover a fallen object and stand back up. The 12-month-old infant comes to stand using the following movement sequence: kneeling, half kneeling, weight shift forward, squat, then upright.

Toddler

12 to 18 Months
Initially, independent walking in the toddler is evidenced by a wide base of support. The widely abducted legs help to keep the center of gravity low. The arms are in "high" guard (Fig. 6-10). Weight shift is more side to side, with the toddler moving forward by total lower extremity flexion. The hip joint remains externally rotated throughout the gait cycle. Ankle movements are minimal, with the whole foot on the ground. Limb instability is indicated by a shortened duration of single-limb stance. The following gait characteristics have been described for a 1-year-old toddler: high cadence, 180 steps/min; short steps, on average 20 cm; slow velocity, 60 cm/sec; and a cycle duration of 0.68 seconds.

As trunk stability improves, the legs come farther under the pelvis. The hips and knees are more extended, and the feet are developing plantarflexion. Some authorities state that 50% of all children will walk backwards and sideways by 15 months, and go up and down stairs with help by 16 months of age.

Most toddlers exhibit a reciprocal arm swing and heel strike by 18 months of age. They walk well and will demonstrate a "run-

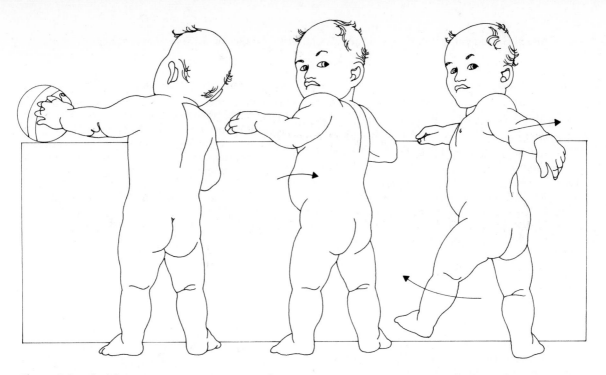

Figure 6-9. Cruising maneuvers.

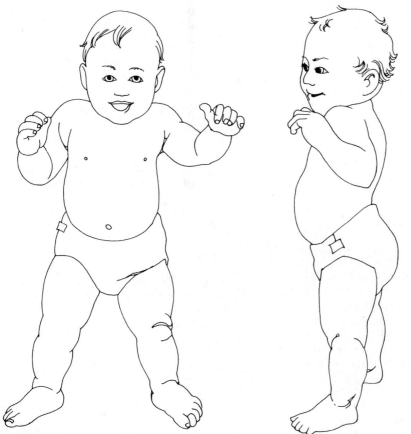

Figure 6-10. Initial independent standing.

ning like'' walk. They jump off low objects by stepping down with one foot, and can momentarily stand on either foot.

24 to 36 Months

The gait of a 2-year-old child is marked by decreased pelvic tilt, hip abduction, and external rotation. Walking velocity increases steadily with age, as does step length, while cadence decreases. The percentage of the gait cycle spent in a single-limb stance increases quickly until 2.5 years of age. Other motor skills of a 2-year-old child include jumping off a step with a two-foot take off; true running with difficulty starting and stopping quickly; kicking a ball; 1- to 3-second single-foot standing balance; and going up and down stairs one tread at a time.

Slaton (1985) measured the gait cycle duration of 3-year-old children to be 0.74 seconds. This compares to findings in 1- and 5-year-old children of 0.68 second and 0.96 second, respectively, which supports the idea that duration increases with age. The most rapid changes occur between 1 and 3 years of age. The cycle duration continues to increase after the age of 3 years, but at a slower rate. Because a mature gait pattern is well established by 3 years of age, the gait cycle duration may be used as a gauge for the acquisition and refinement of mature gait characteristics.

ANNOTATED BIBLIOGRAPHY

Attermeier S: Normal and abnormal development. Presented at CATCH 86, Milwaukee, WI, July 1986

Berg CA, Sternberg RJ: Response to novelty: Continuity versus discontinuity in the developmental course of intelligence. In Reese HW (ed): Advances in Child Development and Behavior, Vol 19. New York, Academic Press, 1985

Bernstein N: Co-ordination and Regulation of Movements. New York, Pergamon Press, 1967

Bishop B, Craik RL: Neural Plasticity pp 1–23. Washington, DC, American Physical Therapy Association, 1982 (Discusses the concept of neural plasticity, critical periods, maturational phenomenon, and the effects of experience on the development of function.)

Bly L: Components of Normal Movement During the First Year of Life and Abnormal Development, pp 1–40. Chicago, Neurodevelopmental Treatment Association, 1983 (The many factors affecting the development of movement have been summarized in this chapter. The continued interaction of these factors supports the further development of movement skills throughout the life span.)

Brooks V: Motor control: How posture and movements are governed. Phys Ther 63:664, 1983

Bryan AC, Bryan MH: Control of respiration in the newborn. In Thibeault DW, Gregory GA: Neonatal Pulmonary Care, pp 2–12. Menlo Park, CA, Addison-Wesley, 1979

Cailliet R: Low Back Pain Syndrome. Philadelphia, FA Davis, 1976

Carmichael L: Onset and early development of behavior. In Mussen PH (ed): Carmichael's Manual of Child Psychology, pp 447–564. New York, John Wiley & Sons, 1970

Connolly KJ, Prechtl HFR: Maturation and Development: Biological and Psychological Perspectives. Clinics in Developmental Medicine 77/78. Philadelphia, JB Lippincott, 1981

Cunningham DA et al: The development of the cardiorespiratory system with growth and physical activity. In Boileau RA (ed): Advances in Pediatric Sport Sciences, Vol 1, Biological Issues, pp 85–116. Champaign, IL, Human Kinetics Publishers, 1984

DeCesare J: Physical therapy for the child with respiratory dysfunction. In Irwin S, Tecklin JS: Cardiopulmonary Physical Therapy, pp 334–366. St Louis, CV Mosby, 1985

Fishkind M, Haley SM: Independent sitting development and the emergence of associated motor components. Phys Ther 66:1509, 1986 (Examines the relationship between motor components and a developmental milestone.)

Folio MR, Fewell RR: Peabody Developmental Motor Scales and Activity Cards (Manual), pp 6–12. Allen, TX, DLM Teaching Resources, 1983

Forssberg H, Nashner L: Ontogenetic development of postural control in man: Adaptation to altered support and visual conditions during stance. J Neurosci 2:545, 1982 (Discusses the development of upright postural responses in children and the context-dependent use of various sensory input.)

Gallahue DL: Understanding Motor Development in Children. New York, John Wiley & Sons, 1982

Gilfoyle EM, Grady AP, Moore JC: Children Adapt, pp 47–77. Thorofare, NJ Charles B Slack, 1981

Haley Stephen M: Sequential analyses of postural reactions in non-handicapped infants. Phys Ther 66:531, 1986

Holt KS: How and Why Children Move. In Holt KS (ed): Movement and Child Development, pp 1–7. Clinics in Developmental Medicine 55. Philadelphia, JB Lippincott, 1975

Kelso JAS, Clark JE (ed): The Development of Motor Control and Coordination. New York, John Wiley & Sons, 1982

Keogh J, Sugden D: Movement Skill Development. New York, Macmillan, 1985 (Comprehensive view of motor development; combines information from the biological, psychological, and neurological sciences. A compilation of psychology, physiology, physical education, and motor control literature.)

Leveau BF, Bernhardt DB: Developmental biomechanics: Effect of forces on the growth, development, and maintenance of the human body. Phys Ther 64:1874, 1984 (Definition and review of the effect of forces on the growth and development of the spine and lower extremities.)

Milani-Comparetti A: The neurophysiological and clinical implications of studies on fetal motor behavior. Semin Perinatol 5:183, 1981

Prechtl HFR (ed): Continuity of Neural Functions from Prenatal to Postnatal Life, pp 1–45; 115–125; 144–178. Philadelphia, JB Lippincott, 1984 (Discusses the theoretical explanations for the changes in neural and sensory functions that occur in the species transition from prenatal to postnatal life. Specific developmental changes in wakefulness and vision are addressed.)

Shumway-Cook A, Woollacott MH: The growth of stability: Postural control from a developmental perspective. J Motor Behav 17:131, 1985 (The stage-like development of the ankle strategy of postural control in children aged 15 months to 10 years.)

Slaton D: Muscle fiber types and their development in the human fetus. Phys Occup Ther Pediatr 1:47, 1981

Slaton D: Gait Cycle Duration in Three Year Old Children. Phys Ther 65:17, 1985

Stengel TJ, Attermeier SM, Bly L et al: Evaluation of sensorimotor dysfunction. In Cambell SK (ed): Pediatric Neurologic Physical Therapy, pp 13–88. New York, Churchill Livingstone, 1984

Stratton P: Rhythmic function in the newborn. In Stratton P (ed): Psychobiology of the Human Newborn, pp 119–145. New York, Wiley-Interscience, 1982

Sutherland DH et al: The development of mature gait. J Bone Joint Surg [Am] 62:336, 1980

Tepper RS et al: Physiologic growth and development of the lungs during the first year of life. Am Rev Respir Dis 134:513, 1986

Thelen E: Rhythmical stereotypies in normal human infants. Anim Behav 27:699, 1979 (Developmental description and discussion of stereotypic movement patterns generated by the nervous system during infancy.)

Thelen E, Bradshaw G, Ward JA: Spontaneous kicking in month old infants: Manifestation of a human central locomotor program. Behav Neutral Biol 32:45, 1981

Thelen E, Heriza CB: Development of early motor control. Presented at Combined Sections Meeting, Anaheim, CA, Feb 1986

Touwen B: Neurological Development in Infancy. Clinics in Developmental Medicine 56. Philadelphia, JB Lippincott, 1976

Valadian I, Porter D: Physical Growth and Development: From conception to maturity. Boston, Little, Brown & Co, 1977

VanSant AF: Concepts of neural organization and movement. In Connolly BH, Montgomery PC: Therapeutic Exercise in Developmental Disabilities, pp 1–8. Chattanooga, Chattanooga Corp, 1987 (Overview of the current models of motor control and their implications for assessment and treatment.)

Walker JM: Development and maturation of the hip joint: Significance for physical therapy. Presented at Combined Sections Meeting, Houston, TX, Feb 1984

Wolff PH: Theoretical issues in development of motor skills. In Lewis M, Taft LT (eds): Developmental Disabilities: Theory, Assessment and Intervention, pp 117–134. New York, Spectrum Publications 1982

Wyke B: The neurological basis for movement: A developmental review. In Holt KS (ed): Movement and Child Development, pp. 19–33. Clinics in Developmental Medicine 55. Philadelphia, JB Lippincott, 1975

7 Normal Development of Movement and Function: Child and Adolescent

REBECCA E. PORTER

Remarkable changes occur as the normal developmental process transforms the 2-year-old preschooler, just beginning to master walking and running, to the physically mature post-adolescent. The process spans a period of 16 to 18 years. In discussing the changes that occur, we must consider not only the physiological and anatomical aspects of the developmental process, but also the changes in motor development and motor learning. Understanding of the topic of movement would not be complete without examining the psychosocial influences on the development and expression of movement patterns, particularly the area of differences in movement patterns between males and females.

For physical therapists, knowledge of the normal development of movement underlies the assessment of movement dysfunction and directs the interventions selected to correct or modify the problems. Therapists working with persons with neurological deficits examine the normal developmental process to gain understanding of the acquisition or reacquisition of motor control. Therapists treating clients with orthopedic dysfunctions must understand the normal growth process to correctly design protocols that meet the individual's needs, rather than arbitrarily conform to adult standards. Clients with cardiac or respiratory dysfunctions need to have programs implemented that consider the developmental norms for the age and growth of the individual. Knowledge of the biological, kinesiological, and social influences on human movement and function provide the foundation for physical therapy interventions.

DEFINITION OF TERMS

A common terminology is necessary before discussing normal development. Although some discrepancies exist among authorities on the age ranges to be assigned to different terms, the timelines presented by Valadian and Porter (1977) represent the most frequently used definitions, and will be used for this chapter.

The time span covered in this chapter can be divided into two major categories: childhood and adolescence. Childhood spans the ages of 2 to 10 years for girls and 2 to 12 years for boys. The difference in the cessation of childhood for girls and boys represents the differences in the average age of onset for the changes signaling the start of puberty. Childhood can be divided into the preschool and school-aged periods. A preschooler is considered to be between the ages of 2 and 6 years (both boys and girls). School-aged refers to girls from 6 to 10 years and boys from 6 to 12 years.

Adolescence spans an eight-year period for both sexes, but has different ages of onset and cessation (girls, 10 to 18; boys, 12 to 20). Adolescence is divided into three subunits. Prepubescence covers the two-year prelude to the onset of puberty and the adolescent growth spurt. Pubescence is the two-year period during which the adolescent growth spurt reaches its peak. Marshall and Tanner (1986) refer to puberty as a collective term for the totality of morphological and physiological changes that occur in the growing individual as the gonads change to their adult form and function. The final portion of adolescence, postpubescence, represents the final growth toward the mature individual—the adult. The ages for each of these periods are presented in Table 7-1.

The chronological definitions of developmental periods are less confusing at the younger ages than at the older end of the spectrum. Because children in America traditionally begin first grade at the age of 6 years, the term "preschooler" is generally descriptive. When terms are applied to describe the periods covered by the general term "adolescent," the definitions become more complex. The differences in the age of onset and completion of physical maturity between the sexes contribute to the complexity. Also adding to the confusion are the socioeconomic and cultural influences on the definition of achieving adulthood or terminating adolescence. For example, some authors include in the definition of the termination of puberty not only the physical capability to conceive but also the concept of successfully rearing the children. The point at which one can successfully rear children is determined by the values of the culture or individual and, therefore, adds confusion to the point when one leaves adolescence and enters adulthood.

It is important to differentiate among three terms that will appear throughout this chapter: growth, maturation, and development. Growth is the increase or decrease of some measurable quantity. It is an ongoing process throughout the life of the organism. Growth can be positive (as when a preschooler gains height), negative (as when an aging adult losses overall height), or in a state of equilibrium. Maturation and development have been used as overlapping terms by different authors. In this discussion, maturation will refer to the morphological and physiological changes that occur as various systems of the body reach adult form and function. Development will be used as the more general term, which is the summation of growth, maturation, learning, and the influences of the environment.

PHYSIOLOGICAL AND ANATOMICAL GROWTH AND MATURATION

SKELETAL SYSTEM

The changes in the skeletal system provide the most frequently used indicator of growth and maturation from childhood through the end of adolescence. The infant has a relatively large head, long trunk, short arms, and short legs. As the child grows, the proportions change so that the limbs become relatively longer, the shoulders broader, and the pelvis narrower (Fig. 7-1). Skeletal growth defines the changes in the length and width of bones as the result of the formation of new osseous tissue. Skeletal maturation occurs throughout childhood and adolescence as changes occur in the relative amount of ossified tissue and progress is made in the fusion of the primary and secondary ossification centers. Comparison of the amount of ossification revealed in an x-ray film with normal standards is a method of assessing the physical maturity of the skeletal system. This information is sometimes used as an overall indicator of physical maturity. Establishing the degree of skeletal maturity is important in the correct timing of some types of orthopedic sur-

Table 7-1. Chronological Correlates for Developmental Terms

	GIRLS (YR)	BOYS (YR)
Childhood	2–10	2–12
Preschool age	2–6	2–6
School age	6–10	6–12
Adolescence	10–18	12–20
Prepubescence	10–12	12–14
Pubescence	12–14	14–16
Postpubescence	14–18	16–20

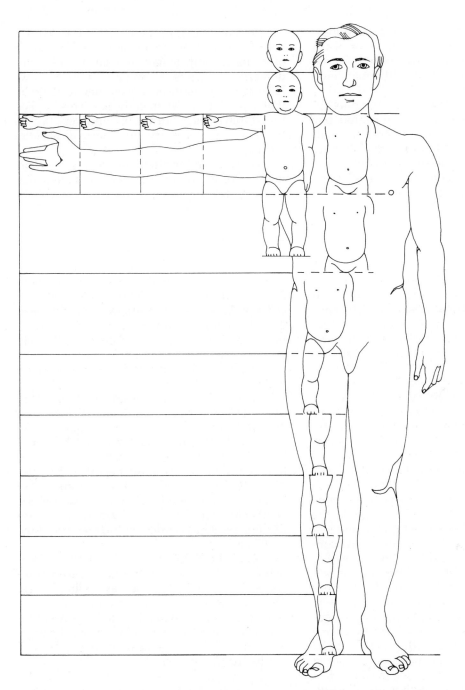

Figure 7-1. Changes in body proportions occur at varying rates in different body segments. Between birth and maturity, the length of the head increases by a factor of 2, the trunk by a factor of 3, the upper extremities by a factor of 4, and the lower extremities by a factor of 5. (Reproduced by permission from Valadian I, Porter D: Physical Growth and Development, p. 30. Boston, Little, Brown & Co, 1977)

gery, such as surgeries to correct a scoliosis. Skeletal growth should be complete, or nearly complete, so that further bone growth following surgery does not result in additional deformities.

Tables have been developed regarding the time of appearance of ossification centers and fusion of epiphyses. These were primarily based on information obtained from well-nourished children and adolescents of white European or American origin. No clear evidence indicates a racially based variation in the order of ossification events. Variations in the timing of ossification are affected by differences in nutritional standards for individuals and populations. Metabolic influences such as the availability of calcium, phosphorus, vitamins A, C, and D, and secretions of the hypophysis, thyroid, parathyroid, adrenal glands, and gonads affect the bone growth at all stages. Girls have an earlier appearance of the centers of ossification and fusion of the epiphyses, which accounts for their earlier cessation of growth relative to boys. Generally, most bones have ossified by the age of 20 years.

Growing bone has different characteristics from adult bone, and therefore responds differently to stresses. Young bone is less dense and more porous than adult bone, with the haversian canals occupying a greater proportion of the bone. The more porous nature of the young bone results in it failing under stresses of both compression and tension, whereas adult bone fails only in tension. The periosteum of the child's bone is much thicker, stronger, and less readily torn than adult bone. Because the continuity of the periosteum determines whether or not a fracture is displaced, the child is less likely to have a displaced fracture. If a fracture does occur, the normal growth process will provide the basis for a greater degree of remodeling than is possible in the adult. As a bone grows in length and girth, asymmetrical growth of the physis and periosteum correct the deformity produced by the healing of a fracture. Damage to the growth plate can result in cessation of bone growth in that area, resulting in shortening and frequently a progressive angulation deformity.

Before the epiphyses are closed, increased use of muscles appears to augment the growth of bones in both length and girth. This phenomenon, which is an example of Wolff's law, is seen in the reduced development of limbs that are paralyzed at an early age. This implies that the stresses of normal use and muscle contraction are necessary for normal skeletal growth.

The data on the effects of greater than normal use of limbs (such as occurs in intensive training activities) on the development of bones in the growing human are limited. Unilateral extremity use, such as pitching a baseball, seems to increase the bone mineral content of the dominant arm. In general, the pressure effects of physical activity may stimulate epiphyseal growth. Excessive pressure may retard linear growth. Unfortunately, the concept of excessive pressure has not been quantified for growing children. Studies reported by Bailey and co-workers (1986) of elite young athletes indicate that they grow as well as nonathletes. Further studies in this area are needed.

Tanner (1978) presents information on the prediction of a child's adult height based on present height, considering the variables of age and sex. For example, a 2-year-old boy is at 49.4% of his adult height; a girl is at 52.7%. A boy is at 62% of his adult height at 5 years, 77.6% at 10 years, and 95.4% at 15 years. A girl is at 66.4% of her adult height at 5 years, 84.5% at 10 years, and 99.1% at 15 years. These predictions are 95% accurate within an error range of ±7 cm.

Skeletal development is the summation of heredity, hormones, nutrition, environment, and stresses applied to the developing bones. These influences account for the variations in stature among individuals. These same influences will result in variations in the development of the other systems of the body, but will not be further discussed.

MUSCULAR SYSTEM

The ratio of skeletal muscle mass to body weight increases throughout development. At birth, skeletal muscle mass is approximately 25% of the total body weight. At age 5 years, skeletal muscle mass accounts for 35% of the body weight as compared to approximately 40% at maturity. The percentage may be higher in males. Between the ages of 5 and 18 years, muscle mass in boys increases more than five times; in girls, more than four times. The growth curve for the addition of muscle mass relative to body weight demonstrates an acceleration in its upward slope between the ages of 1.5 and 5 years and a second acceleration during adolescence. Adult muscle diameter is reached between 12 and 15 years of age.

The amount of muscle per unit height is similar in both sexes until the male adolescent growth spurt begins. During the adolescent growth spurts, proportionately more muscle tissue is deposited per unit height gained in the boy than in the girl. The boy doubles his muscle mass between the ages of 11 and 17 years; the girl, between the ages of 9 and 15 years. The girl is adding only small increments of muscle mass between the ages of 13 and 18 years, while the boy continues his growth. In girls, the peak in muscle growth is reached 6 months after peak height velocity. In boys, the peak velocity of muscle growth and peak height velocity occur simultaneously. Following the termination of growth, factors such as physical exercise, metabolism, nutrition, age, and sex will affect muscle mass.

Muscular strength increases linearly with age from early childhood until adolescence, demonstrating a growth curve similar to that for height and weight gains. In girls, the linear relationship of strength and age continues through age 15 years, with the tendency of strength gains to level off after that point. The peak rate of strength growth appears to occur shortly before menarche. Boys are stronger than girls at all ages. Boys demonstrate a marked acceleration of strength development between the ages of 13 and 20 years. This acceleration in strength development increases the male-female strength differences. The adolescent peak in strength development in both boys and girls occurs about 9 to 12 months after the peak weight and height gain. In general, muscle tissue increases first in mass, and then in strength.

NERVOUS SYSTEM

At birth, the brain is approximately 25% of its adult weight. In terms of total weight, the brain is the organ that is nearest its adult value at birth. By the age of 3 to 4 years, the brain is approximately 75% of its adult size. By the age of 5 to 6 years, the brain weight is approximately 90% of its final weight, although the body weight is less than one third of its mature amount.

The rapid rate of myelination that occurred until the age of 2 years slows during the preschool and school-aged periods. The process of myelination is nearly complete by the age of 10 years, although the myelination of some structures continues into the twenties (reticular formation) and thirties (association areas of the cerebral cortex).

The appearance of function is closely related to the maturation of the structures of the brain. The development of the connections between the cerebellum and the cerebral cortex, which are essential to the development of fine motor control, illustrate this concept. The myelination of the connecting fibers begins after birth and continues until age 4 years. During the third year, as myelination of the fibers is terminating, the child begins the initial exploration of fine motor skills like manipulating a crayon to color. The reticular formation, which is involved in the maintenance of consciousness and attention, continues myelination beyond puberty. Tanner (1978) speculates that the stages of mental functioning described by Piaget and others reflect the development of the brain and other body structures, and that the emergence of one stage after another is dependent upon the progressive maturation and organization of the cerebral cortex.

Studies of the development of cortical thickness demonstrate that each hemisphere and each cortical lobe has its own rate of development. Areas within specific lobes may develop at different rates. Rabinowicz (1986) indicates a relationship between the functional development of the cerebral cortex and changes in the thickness or density of the cerebral cortex or its component layers. Critical periods in the maturation of the cortex appear between 15 and 24 months, 6 and 8 years, 10 and 12 years, and around 18 years.

The wave patterns recorded on an electroencephalograph show that rhythms of low frequency (few waves per second) predominate in the early years of childhood, according to Valadian and Porter (1977). These rhythms are gradually replaced by higher-frequency rhythms during childhood. The mature pattern is established around the ages of 10 to 13 years.

CARDIORESPIRATORY SYSTEM

The heart and lungs increase in weight along the lines of the general growth curve of the individual, including a period of accelerated growth during the adolescent growth spurt. (According to Marshall and Tanner [1986], all abdominal viscera follow this same pattern, although evidence is limited.) The heart increases in weight from approximately 2/3 oz at birth to 7 oz at age 15 to 16 years. The rate of contraction of the heart decreases with increasing size. The average rate of contraction decreases from 120 bpm at birth to an average of 70 to 80 bpm in adulthood. The higher rate, in part, is a compensation for the smaller stroke volume, particularly under conditions of exercise stress. Until the age of 10 years, the average rate of contraction is similar in both sexes. After the 10th year, the average rate of contraction in girls is slightly higher than in boys. The rate of contraction begins to stabilize around the adult values during the 16th year. Blood pressure remains relatively constant during the second to fifth years. The blood pressure gradually begins to rise in the sixth year, and continues until adult values are reached at the end of adolescence.

The heart changes its position in the chest cavity during the growing years. During early childhood, the heart lies in an almost horizontal position. As the child grows and the chest lengthens, the apex (lower end) of the heart shifts downward, causing the heart to assume a more vertical position as well as a position lower in the chest.

The pattern of respiration changes as the child develops. Until the end of the preschool years, the work of respiration is accomplished primarily through the movement of the diaphragm. During the ages of 5 to 7 years, the transition is made to the thoracic muscles as the source of movement for quiet respiration (Valadian and Porter, 1977). The efficiency of respiratory exchange is similar in both sexes through childhood. At puberty, boys become markedly more efficient than girls in respiratory exchange (Valadian and Porter, 1977).

The index of maximum aerobic power is "the maximum volume of oxygen taken up per unit of time under maximal exertion conditions and is generally accepted as the best available measure of the efficiency of the oxygen transport system" (Bailey and co-workers, 1986). Values for both sexes increase with age and have approximately the same absolute values until the age of 12 years. Factors contributing to the differences in values during adolescence may be in part physiological (increase in adipose tissue to lean body mass ratio in girls) and in part cultural (decreased participation of girls in vigorous physical exercise).

Studies of children's physiological response to exercise must deal with problems that make the research design extremely difficult. The normal physiological changes seen in adults with exercise conditioning are also the physiological changes that occur in normal growth. Conclusive studies have not yet differentiated the effects of conditioning from the effects of normal growth.

Bailey and co-workers (1986) report a number of differences between adults and children in physiological responses to exercise. Children have a poorer ventilation efficiency than adults during submaximal and maximal effort, and have a higher respiratory frequency than that of adults performing the same task. Although quantitative differences exist in pulmonary response to exercise, the patterns are similar in children and adults.

Cardiac output (stroke volume multiplied by heart rate) is lower than adults at all levels of exercise. Bar-Or (1983) states that the higher arteriovenous oxygen differences in children compensate during submaximal exercise. Mechanical inefficiency may contribute to the high oxygen cost of activities in children. The influence of aerobic training on children has not been conclusively determined.

ADIPOSE TISSUE

Anthropometry includes tools to measure the growth of adipose tissue during human growth. Given society's concern with the problems of obesity, information is included here to provide the physical therapist with knowledge of the normal parameters for development of adipose tissue.

Most children demonstrate a steady increase in the amount of white adipose tissue from age 8 years until adolescence. The rate of increase of the subcutaneous fat layer slows as the growth of the skeleton and muscle mass begins to accelerate in the adolescent growth spurt. During the adolescent growth spurt, girls continue to add adipose tissue, although at a slower rate than before or after the growth spurt. Boys demonstrate a negative rate of gain of adipose tissue during the adolescent spurt, and so are actually becoming leaner during this period.

Studies of the growth in size and number of adipocytes (fat cells) are not in full agreement on the process. Growth in the number of fat cells increases slowly between age 2 years and puberty, while the size of the cells may increase slightly or remain the same. The rate of increase of the number of fat cells accelerates during puberty (Faust, 1986). By adolescence, the markedly obese person has a greater number of fat cells than the person of normal weight; however, studies are not conclusive on the influence of dietary habits in infancy or patterns of exercise in childhood.

GROWTH IN EACH AGE GROUP

PRESCHOOL AGE (2 TO 6 YEARS)

The preschool period is a time of steady growth for children, with both sexes gaining height at about the same rate. The velocity of growth has decelerated from the sharp upward slope in infancy. Between the second and third years, children may add 10.2 cm to their height.* Height gains continue at a rate of 5.1 to 7.6 cm/yr until the adolescent growth spurt. Birth length has doubled by age 4. By the age of 6 years, the child has reached approximately two thirds of the adult height. These figures represent average changes in large sample populations; however, the amount of variability in growth within a sample, between samples, and within the individual is large.

Weight gains during the preschool years average 2.0 kg/yr.† A child born at the average birth weight of 3.4 kg will quadruple that weight at the age of 2.5 years. At 5 years of age, the child will have doubled the weight at 1 year. Graphs that demonstrate height and weight as a variable of age and sex allow the determination of an individual's percentile status (Figs. 7-2 and 7-3).

The chunky physique of the newborn and toddler elongates during the preschool years. By age 2 years, the lengths of the upper and lower extremities have increased 60% to 75% over the lengths at birth. The posture of a 2-year-old child is characterized by a mild lordosis and protuberant abdomen. By about age 4 years, these features have usually disappeared and the shoulders have become broader. The head and neck have continued to decrease in proportion to the rest of the body.

During the first four years, the rate of growth of the muscular system is proportional to the rate of growth of the whole body. After age 4, muscular development accelerates. Development and motor control of larger muscles exceeds that of small muscles. This is reflected in the motor tasks that are characteristic of this period.

SCHOOL AGE (GIRLS 6 TO 10 YEARS, BOYS 6 TO 12 YEARS)

Physical growth continues with a steady pattern during the school-aged years for both boys and girls, although the rate of growth is declining during this period. The average gain in

*1 in = 2.54 cm.
†1 lb = 0.45 kg.

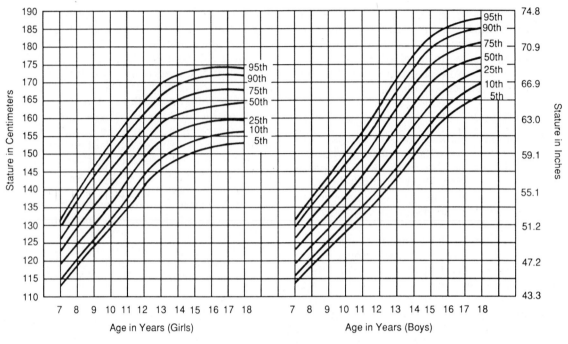

Figure 7-2. Height gain by percentiles for girls and boys. (Adapted from National Center of Health Statistics, Department of Health, Education and Welfare, Vital Health Statistics. Washington, DC, US Government Printing Office, 1977. Reproduced by permission from Ingersoll GM: Adolescents in School and Society, p 32. Lexington, MA, DC Heath, 1981)

height is approximately 6 cm (5.1 to 7.6 cm) per year for both sexes. However, the rate of growth is not proportional throughout the body. A greater increase in length occurs in the limbs than in the trunk, resulting in further changes in the body proportions. The shoulder width to pelvic breadth relationship remains the same in both sexes. The individual's center of gravity is moving caudally during this growth period.

Weight increases about 2.7 kg/yr from ages 6 to 9 years. During the 10th year, 4.1 kg are added. At 10 years of age the child's weight should be 10 times the birth weight. An alternate guideline is that the child's yearly weight gain between the ages of 5 and 10 years should equal the birth weight.

A wide range of heights falls within one standard deviation of the average height and weight for children during the school-aged period. As an indicator of deviations from normal growth, determination of the rate of growth is more important than actual size measurements.

Particularly in the later stages of childhood, girls may be more mature in physical development than boys, although boys tend to be slightly taller and heavier until the girls enter the prepubescent stage growth spurt at 10 years of age. Muscle mass is approximately equivalent in boys and girls during the school-aged period. Muscle mass accounts for an increasing percentage of the total body weight between 5 years of age and adolescence. Increases in strength are usually greater in boys, especially as they begin puberty.

ADOLESCENCE (GIRLS 10 TO 18 YEARS, BOYS 12 TO 20 YEARS)

Adams (1980) describes adolescence in western society as a biological, sociocultural, and cogni-

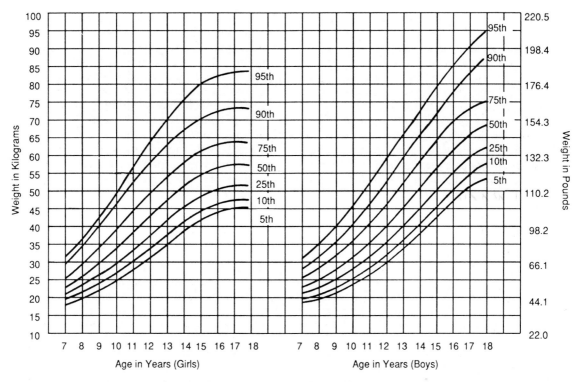

Figure 7-3. Weight gain by percentiles for girls and boys. (Adapted from National Center of Health Statistics, Department of Health, Education and Welfare, Vital Health Statistics. Washington, DC, US Government Printing Office, 1977. Reproduced by permission from Ingersoll GM: Adolescents in School and Society, p 31. Lexington, MA, DC Heath, 1981)

tive or psychological phenomenon. The following summary describes the somatic changes that occur during this period.

Many body parts, such as the skeleton, muscles, and viscera, undergo an increase in the rate or velocity of growth, referred to as the adolescent growth spurt. Not all body parts accelerate at the same time or to the same extent, which results in changes in the body composition or the percentage relationships among muscle, fat, and bone. The average age of onset of the adolescent growth spurt differs in boys and girls, although a wide range occurs in the onset within each sex. In addition, the rate of increase is different between the sexes, which results in sex-specific differences in body composition. The reproductive system matures and secondary sexual characteristics

develop during this period.

The onset of the adolescent growth spurt and puberty is influenced by genetic factors, which are modified by environmental factors. The adolescent growth spurt is variable in onset, intensity, magnitude, and duration among individuals within a population and between populations. The onset of the spurt begins in girls around 10.5 years and in boys around 12.5 years of age. In the six months preceding and following the peak velocity of growth in height, girls grow an average of 6 to 11 cm and gain 3.6 to 4.5 kg, while boys grow 7 to 12 cm and gain 5.4 to 6.3 kg. The peak velocity of height growth usually occurs in girls during the 12th year and in boys during the 14th year. Generally, birth length has usually tripled by the age of 13 years. Girls reach adult stature at age 17 to 18 years, and boys at age 18 to 21 years.

During the adolescent growth spurt, different body parts grow at different rates. Although the legs grow faster than the trunk during childhood, the reverse is true in adolescence. Rapid growth in the size of the foot is one of the first indicators of the onset of the adolescent growth spurt, and the foot probably attains its maximum size before any other region (with the possible exception of the cranium). The brain grows only slightly during adolescence in relation to the growth of other organs. The amount of adipose tissue as a percentage of body weight decreases in boys, who actually lose fat during the period of peak height velocity. Girls do not lose fat during adolescence, but a slowing of its accumulation occurs.

Girls reach the maximum muscle growth in the 12th year, with subsequent slowing of growth. The maximum muscle growth in boys occurs at age 14 years. In both sexes, the maximum muscle growth coincides with the peak height velocity. The combination of muscle growth and the cardiorespiratory changes occurring in adolescence result in a stronger person who has increased endurance.

MOTOR DEVELOPMENT

The topic of motor development is too broad to be covered in detail in this chapter, but trends and generalizations in children and adolescents will be presented to provide a background to understand the topic. The following sections include the sequence of acquisition of motor skills; changes in motor performance as related to age, sex, and maturity; and some of the factors affecting physical fitness and strength.

ACQUISITION OF MOTOR SKILLS

Zaichkowsky and co-workers (1980) divide the development of motor skills into four age-related stages: infancy, early childhood, late childhood, and adolescence. The infant builds on reflexive responses to develop rudimentary movement abilities. In early childhood, general fundamental skills (such as the ability to run, jump, balance, and throw) are developed. These skills are common to all children, and provide the necessary foundation for advanced movement skills. The quality of performance of both the fundamental and advanced movement skills will show large variations within a population. The fundamental movement skills have a general order of appearance that is common to most individuals. Only the rate of appearance is a variable.

In late childhood, the general fundamental movement skills are refined to specific movement skills. As the skills are applied to sport performances, more emphasis is placed on form, accuracy, and adaptability. Movements become more fluid and automatic. During adolescence, specialized skills relating to practiced movement responses may develop. However, specialized skills do not appear universally because they depend upon the amount of practice invested in their development.

Beyond these general descriptions, certain changes are specific to each age group. They are presented below.

Preschool Age

During the preschool years, the gross motor developmental milestones that are most frequently recorded are related to the addition of locomotor skills and the refinement of the throwing pattern. During the second year, the child develops the ability to walk backward, walk up and down stairs without using a support, and hop on one foot. The neuromuscular control for the balance necessary for higher-level activities is beginning to develop.

In the third year, the child makes the transition from a fast walk to a true running pattern with the toe touching the ground first. A horizontal component is added to the vertical component of a hop, so that the child begins to hop forward for several repetitions. The refinement of balance permits the child to display the beginnings of one-foot standing balance. The child can catch a bounced ball and can execute an overhand throw of a ball with directionality.

In the fourth year, the child develops the balance to stand on one foot for four to eight seconds and to walk on tiptoe with control. The 4-year-old child can catch a thrown small ball using outstretched arms, and can throw the ball overhand for some distance. The child is beginning to learn an underhand throw.

During the sixth year, the child can balance on the preferred foot for eight or more seconds and on the nonpreferred foot for five or more seconds. The child is developing a rhythmicity to movements, as demonstrated in the ability to march well in time to music and the ability to skip with alternating feet. A small ball can be caught using the hands more than the arms. The child is beginning to master alternate forms of progression, such as roller skating and riding a bicycle with training wheels. During the previous four years, the child has mastered all the fundamental gross motor skills needed to function successfully as an adult. The remainder of gross motor development is a refinement of those skills.

Fine motor skills also make remarkable advancements during the preschool years. During the second year, the child learns to build a tower of blocks. Following a demonstration of building a bridge with three cubes, the child can execute its construction. A cross and a square can be traced with a crayon. The child has sufficient control of fine grasp and release to place 10 small pellets in a bottle in 10 seconds.

In the third year, the child can copy a picture of a square and a circle, can imitate the drawing of a cross, and can cut a straight line with scissors. In the fourth year, the child can copy a picture of a triangle and imitate the drawing of a diamond, activities that both require the ability to make a diagonal line. The child is developing the ability to color within the outline of a picture. In addition, the child can copy the letters of simple words with reasonable accuracy.

In the fifth and sixth years, gross motor control will be more advanced than fine motor control. Concentration on fine motor tasks may result in associated movements or reactions (overflow movements), which are involuntary movements in resting musculature when another body part is performing a voluntary motor task. Given the development of the fine motor skills described above, the child is prepared to meet the fine motor demands of school. (The motor skills completed at each age were selected from Denhoff and Hyman [1974].)

School Age

During the school years, significant improvement in the levels of coordination allows the child to accomplish increasingly complex motor tasks. Although the individual child possesses vast motor skills, the most common assessments of the level of motor development focus on running, jumping, and throwing. Explanation of the standards applied to various tasks is beyond the scope of this chapter, because the standards may involve distance measurements (how far one jumps), time measurements (how fast one runs a set distance), or determining how closely one's performance conforms to adult form. For example, Ulrich's Test of Gross Motor Development (1985) describes three criteria for the performance of a leap: (1) the child should take off on one foot and land on the opposite foot; (2) at some point, both feet should be off the ground for a period longer than in running; and (3) the arm opposite the lead foot should reach forward. At age 8 years, 80% of the children demonstrate the proper foot positions, but only 60% demonstrate the proper arm position. At age 10 years, 80% of the children demonstrate the proper arm position.

As a general guideline, between 6 and 10 years of age, a child will master the adult forms of running, throwing, and catching. The skill patterns may or may not be further refined during adolescence. Refinement of skill patterns will depend on the amount of practice and instruction invested in improving the movements. Additional information will be presented in the discussion of changes in motor performance in adolescence.

CHANGES IN MOTOR PERFORMANCE

Motor performance steadily improves with age. In boys, the level of performance continues to improve until at least 17 to 18 years of age. After the age of 18 years, studies of performance levels tend to be restricted to college populations. This information indicates that motor performances in boys and men may continue to improve into the early twenties. Performance continues to improve in the general population of girls until the age of approximately 14 years (Bailey and co-workers, 1986). The cessation of improvement may reflect sociocultural influences on the level of physical activity of girls during late adolescence.

Sex differences are evident throughout childhood and adolescence. After the age of 2.5 years, the average boy performs at a higher level than the average girl on a variety of gross motor tasks. Throwing patterns are better for boys than girls at age 5 years (Singer, 1975). Girls are usually better at fine motor tasks than boys in the fifth and sixth years. Throughout childhood, boys outperform girls in running, jumping, and throwing. Variables such as sociocultural influences may also contribute to some of the differences previously attributed to male-female differences. Differences in the levels of motor performance become more marked in adolescence.

The age of onset of puberty appears to influence the level of performance in boys: Those who mature earlier perform at superior levels compared with those who mature later. Boys who mature earlier also have the advantage in size, strength, and endurance. This advantage will disappear over time. The level of performance of girls does not appear to be related to the age of onset of puberty.

In their review of the available literature, Bailey and co-workers (1986) report that the pattern of adaptation of muscle to exercise appears to be the same in children as in adults. Endurance training in adolescents produces the same types of changes in aerobic and anaerobic glycolysis as in adults, but with a different magnitude. Physical training (a regular, systematic practice of physical activities) appears to be an important component in modifying the muscle metabolism of children.

Measures of the level of physical fitness show little difference between the sexes for the initial six to seven years. During childhood, boys test at slightly higher levels. At the beginning of adolescence, boys demonstrate a marked increase in the level of physical fitness while girls level off or decline (Zaichkowsky and co-workers, 1980). As mentioned previously, the differences in sociocultural expectations of boys and girls must be considered in interpreting data about male-female differences.

Multiple factors affect the development of strength. The size of muscles and therefore their potential strength increases with age in both sexes. Because the size of muscles is related to strength, heredity will influence strength development. Children who mature earlier are stronger than those who mature later until both complete the adolescent period. In boys, the apex of the adolescent strength spurt occurs after the height and weight spurts. In girls, the apex of the strength spurt occurs after the adolescent height spurt and before menarche. Boys are stronger than girls at all ages, but the difference is magnified during the adolescent spurt of strength development in boys. The cardiorespiratory system changes that occur in adolescence also contribute to the strength and endurance gained in this period.

MOTOR LEARNING

Cratty (1986) has developed a paradigm to describe the changes that occur in the processes contributing to motor learning and skill acquisition. Three basic tendencies underlay motor learning: seeking information, seeking novel experiences, and development of the ability to move. From infancy, the individual seeks information. Initially the information seeking is confined to a single sensory modality. The maturing individual develops a multisensory, cross-modal approach to information gathering. Movement behaviors are both a source of information to be stored and compared with past experiences, and a means to gather additional information. Infants and preschoolers spend considerable amounts of time using and expanding their capacities for movement. Movements are made, repeated, and expanded because it is fun to do so.

Motor learning is also influenced by the inherent need to prevent boredom by seeking novel experiences. Information gathering, novelty seeking, and the development of the capacity for movement lead to high levels of motor activity in both the infant and preschool child.

As the child develops language, another factor is added to the capacity for motor learning. The expansion of language capacities in middle and late childhood allow the child to use internal language as a form of self-instruction. Although the infant may formulate movement rules based upon simple associations, the older child can formulate increasingly complex rules about movement and movement learning. In late childhood and adolescence, the individual can combine self-instruction with formal instruction from others to produce more complex and more skilled movement patterns.

In the progression through childhood and into adolescence, along with increasing levels of cognitive development, the individual becomes better at planning movement strategies. At the same time, the child is becoming more sophisticated in the ability to formulate or plan movement strategies. The child uses internal talk to analyze the tasks to be accomplished, order the tasks to be accomplished, and assess the outcome of each component and the overall outcome of the strategy. This process improves as the child matures and becomes more intellectually able.

Cognitive development and neuromuscular maturation interact with a third component, maturation and integration of sensory system input, to influence motor learning in the developing child. The infant progresses through stages to integrate visual input and movement abilities. During the second year, the child begins to develop the ability to separate components of the perceptual and motor systems. The child progresses from the linkage of the visual and motor systems to an integration of the visual and motor systems to the highest level of performance, which is the flexibility to be visual, motor, or visual-motor as the situation requires.

The transition in the manner in which a developing individual learns motor tasks is not well defined by age guidelines. Many factors, including movement experiences, have the potential to influence the transition to the mature characteristics of motor learning.

The development of upper extremity control illustrates the progression through the process of motor learning. As the infant seeks information about his surroundings, the presence of an object in his visual field increases his random motor activity. The chance swiping of the object leads to attempts to recreate the event as he seeks to repeat the novel experience. As he develops better separation of eye movements from head movements, and is better able to act upon incoming sensory information, the infant becomes more successful in recreating the movement. The toddler builds upon this knowledge to increase his skill in reaching for and grasping food, initially using his fingers and gradually refining the skill to include using a utensil. The preschooler uses these skills to learn to manipulate a crayon; the school-aged child refines his skills in learning to write. As the individual progresses from adolescence to maturity, the movement patterns acquired through the developmental stages contribute to the increasingly complex upper extremity tasks he must learn.

PSYCHOSOCIAL INFLUENCES ON DEVELOPMENT

PRESCHOOL AGE

The preschool child spends a considerable portion of each day engaged in gross and fine motor activities. The 2-year-old child is beginning to be involved more in peer play situations. Play at this stage tends to be more parallel than interactive, but the child is receiving stimulation from the playmates. Play tends to be more vigorous with a familiar playmate than without a playmate.

Parental influences strongly affect the movement experiences that are available to and appropriate for the child. The parents control the amount of vigorous movement experiences available to the preschooler. Sex-related role expectations influence the child's movement experiences through parental toy selection and peer play situations. Similar behaviors may receive different reactions depending on whether the child is a boy or a girl. The differences in motor skills apparent in the preschooler (boys better at throwing and jumping; girls better at hopping, skipping, and small muscle coordination) may be due to skeletal differences or may reflect societal attitudes on appropriate behavior for each sex.

SCHOOL AGE

The impact of the difference in societal expectations on the motor behaviors of girls and boys was demonstrated in a study by Hayes and co-workers (1981). Children were rated on sexual mannerisms in sitting, standing, and walking. Differences between the sexes were noted as early as kindergarten. By second grade, the sitting patterns of girls and boys were clearly different. Differences in standing developed by the fourth grade. The ability to modify sex-related motor behaviors was apparent in the kindergarten child and increased steadily with age, indicating that at least a portion of the behavior was learned, rather than an inherent difference between the sexes (Hayes and co-workers, 1981).

The school years mark a transition from the cooperative play of the late preschool years to demonstrations of competitiveness among peers. Status in the peer group is influenced by ability to play the games of interest to the peer group. The level of one's skill becomes increasingly important with age. Boys in particular may find that their index of social acceptance in the peer group is directly related to their athletic skills.

Although preschool children are rarely frustrated by their lack of success at physical activities, school-aged children may be easily frustrated if they cannot master a new motor skill. Observation by peers or by an adult may limit the child's willingness to try new activities, because children at this age are sensitive to any signs that they interpret as disapproval.

ADOLESCENCE

As noted in the discussion of motor performance, boys continue to improve through adolescence; however, girls tend to peak at age 13 to 14 years, after which performance stays the same or declines. These changes in performance seem to have less to do with the process of physical maturation than with the influence of society. In the past, the beginning of adolescence marked the time for girls to stop acting like tomboys and start acting like ladies. Changes in society's valuing of physical fitness may change the performance of future generations.

The physical growth and changes associated with the adolescent growth spurt can have an important effect on the individual's status in the peer group and evaluation of self. For boys, size, strength, and endurance will influence their status in sports and peer groups. Marshall (1986) states that it may be advisable to warn early-maturing athletic boys that their advantage in size and strength may only be temporary. Late-maturing boys can benefit from reassurances that they will not always be smaller and weaker than their peers.

Research data has been somewhat conflicting on the differences between early- and late-maturing girls. Adolescents of both sexes are extremely concerned about physical appearance and being "normal." For example, early development of breasts may cause some girls to hide the development and other girls to wear clothing to accentuate the development. Girls with an early height growth spurt may attempt to minimize their tallness by assuming deviant postures, such as slouching. Fears of being different from the norm may interfere with the development of feelings of self-worth in both sexes.

Adolescent behavior may include many examples of risk-taking behaviors, with a focus on the present and a denial of the consequences. Risk-taking behavior and denial of consequences may help explain adolescent sexual behaviors and experimentation with substance abuse; furthermore, it also influences behavior in athletic endeavors. Zito (1985) cites a list of special problems unique to the adolescent athlete developed by the American Academy of Pediatrics. Three of the items relate to physical characteristics of the adolescent: strength disproportionate to size, flexible ligaments and open epiphyses, and unrecognized congenital problems. Four of the items are related to risk-taking behaviors: indifference to restrictions, decreased motivation to work hard, indifference to equipment needs, and inadequate supervision. The tendency toward risk-taking behavior may contribute to the athletic injuries seen in adolescents.

CONCLUSION

Understanding the normal development of movement and function in the child and adolescent is essential to help the physical therapist recognize and understand developmental processes that deviate from normal standards. This information can also provide a basis for building an understanding of the reacquisition of motor skills. This chapter is only an overview of the material available on each topic. The sources listed in the annotated bibliography represent expanded overviews suitable as introductions to the topics. These texts should be consulted for more detailed information.

ANNOTATED BIBLIOGRAPHY

Adams W: Adolescence. In Gabel S, Erickson MT (eds): Child Development and Developmental Disabilities, pp 59–81. Boston, Little, Brown & Co, 1980 (Covers the major physical, motor, sensory, perceptual, cognitive, and social developmental milestones for adolescents. Also presents the diagnostic evaluation of developmental disorders and some of the typical problems associated with developmental disorders.)

Bailey DA, Malina RM, Mirwald RL: Physical activity and growth of the child. In Falkner F, Tanner JM (eds): Human Growth: A Comprehensive Treatise, Vol 2, 2nd ed, pp 147–170. New York, Plenum, 1986 (The authors have reviewed and summarized the literature to provide an concise presentation of the topic. The entire book is recommended as a source of information on the postnatal growth of humans.)

Bar-Or O: Pediatric Sports Medicine for Practitioners. New York, Springer-Verlag, 1983 (Presents information on the normal physiological changes that occur with exercise in childhood. Includes chapters on the effects of various disease processes on the characteristics of the individual's exercise physiology.)

Cratty BJ: Perceptual and Motor Development in Infants and Children, 3rd ed. Englewood Cliffs, NJ, Prentice-Hall, 1986 (Summarizes information on motor development, motor performance, and motor learning relating to gross, fine, and perceptual motor areas.)

Denhoff E, Hyman I: Parent programs for developmental management. Tjossem TD (ed): Intervention Strategies for High Risk Infants and Young Children, pp 381–466. Baltimore, University Park Press, 1974 (The appendix to this chapter contains a detailed developmental assessment of typical behaviors described at various developmental ages.)

Faust IM: Adipose tissue growth and obesity. In Falkner F, Tanner JM (eds): Human Growth: A Comprehensive Treatise, Vol 2, 2nd ed, pp 61–77. New York, Plenum, 1986 (Reviews the literature on the growth of adipose tissue in the developing human.)

Hayes SC, Nelson RO, Steele DL et al: The development of the display and knowledge of sex related motor behavior in children. Child Behav Ther 3(4):1, 1981 (Discusses a study conducted to demonstrate the development on "male" and "female" behaviors in standing, sitting, and walking in children.)

Ingersoll GM: Adolescents in School and Society. Lexington, MA, DC Heath & Co, 1982 (An overview of basic information on adolescent development.)

Marshall WM, Tanner JM: Puberty. In Falkner F, Tanner JM (eds): Human Growth: A Comprehensive Treatise, Vol 2, 2nd ed, pp 171–200. New York, Plenum, 1986 (Describes the changes that occur during puberty. Based on the studies of Tanner and others.)

Rabinowicz T: The differentiated maturation of the cerebral cortex. In Falkner F, Tanner JM (eds): Human Growth: A Comprehensive Treatise, Vol 2, 2nd ed, pp 385–410. New York, Plenum, 1986 (Summarizes the research on the development and maturation of the cerebral cortex.)

Singer RN: Motor Learning and Human Performance, 2nd ed. New York, Macmillan, 1975 (Presents detailed information covering various aspects of motor learning.)

Tanner JM: Foetus into Man: Physical Growth from Conception to Maturity. Cambridge, MA, Harvard University Press, 1978 (Tanner is a noted researcher in the area of growth. This small text summarizes information on a number of topics on growth.)

Ulrich DA: Test of Gross Motor Development. Austin, TX, Pro-Ed, 1985 (This gross motor test is typical of the tools used to assess motor development.)

Valadian I, Porter D: Physical Growth and Development: From Conception to Maturity. Boston, Little, Brown & Co, 1977 (Introductory information on physical growth and development presented by body system in a programmed textbook.)

Zaichkowsky LD, Zaichkowsky LB, Martinek TJ: Growth and Development: The Child and Physical Activity. St. Louis, CV Mosby, 1980 (An introduction to concepts of psychomotor, cognitive, and social-psychological development and their implications for physical education.)

Zito M: The Adolescent Athlete: A Musculoskeletal Update. In Gould JA, Davies GJ (eds): Orthopaedic and Sports Physical Therapy, pp 643–652. St Louis, CV Mosby, 1985 (Summarizes some of the unique problems of the adolescent athlete.)

8 Normal Development of Movement and Function: Older Adult

MARYBETH BROWN

By the time you begin practicing as a physical therapist, 12% of the population will be over the age of 65 years. Most of the patients treated at your facility will be older adults, and you will be working with a unique, challenging, and wonderful group.

So that you may better understand why the older person often is a complex and challenging patient, I will describe some of the age-related changes that occur as we grow older. Most of the changes you are aware of (eg, need for glasses, slower movements), but you may not realize the variability, the magnitude, or the implications of the changes. I hope that after reading this chapter you will be more comfortable, confident, and capable of working with older patients.

Primary physical effects of aging, such as decreased strength, flexibility, and balance, can be evaluated readily by a physical therapist. Translating those findings to functional performance expectations poses a major challenge. Relating secondary changes, such as decreased vision and hearing, to treatment goals requires much of the therapist's art and skill. In addition to identifying and coping with primary and secondary problems, often it is necessary to integrate medical problems with primary and secondary age-related changes. Successfully balancing medical and aging changes requires the ultimate in physical therapy capability. Designing realistic goals and treatment plans for an 83-year-old man who was in bed for four weeks with the flu, who has a fractured hip, congestive heart failure, poor vision, and who lives alone on a five-acre farm is an example of the challenge we face daily.

Muscular atrophy is one type of aging change that occurs directly within the tissue; such tissue change affects function. Other changes in function take place, in part, because of the increased stiffness of the connective tissue present within all organs. Still other changes in performance may be secondary to a failure of the cardiovascular system to deliver fuel and oxygen, or a lack of necessary hormones. All body systems are inextricably tied together; thus, aging change in one system affects all others. The whole aging process is complex.

One of the most difficult elements to grasp about aging is the variability of age-related change. You all have had the experience of seeing two older men or women of the same chronological age who are light years apart in function. On his 70th birthday fitness expert Jack LaLanne held a rope in his teeth and towed 24 rowboats filled with people for two miles. However, I would not consider him typical. At the other end of the spectrum is the wheelchair-bound 70-year-old man with diabetes, an amputation, kidney failure, and heart disease, but this person also is not typical. Variability is the norm, and necessitates individualizing treatment plans and goals for all older clients.

Age-related change can begin in almost any system at almost any time after 20 years of age. It is not uncommon to see gray hair on a 25-year-old person; however, in that same individual, changes in maximal oxygen consumption ($\dot{V}O_{2 \text{ max}}$) may not begin until the age of 40 years. Conversely, a decrease in $\dot{V}O_{2 \text{ max}}$ may begin in the third decade, particularly in a sedentary person. However, that person may show little overt evidence of aging, such as graying hair or wrinkling skin. Decrements in kidney, lung, and heart function can begin at different times even within the same person, or around the same time. In addition, the rate of aging change may be quite variable. Aging is a highly individual process that must be taken into consideration for each older person in physical therapy.

Age-related change occurs in all systems of the human body: skin, cardiovascular, musculoskeletal, respiratory, endocrine, nervous, genitourinary, gastrointestinal, and sensory. We as physical therapists don't work directly with all of these systems, although they affect those systems we do work with. Therefore, this discussion of age-related change will concentrate on those systems that directly affect physical and functional capability.

CHANGES IN PRIMARY SYSTEMS

MUSCULOSKELETAL SYSTEM

Muscle mass decreases with age as a result of fiber atrophy, particularly among type II fibers, and probably as a result of fiber loss. Other changes within skeletal muscle may include disorganization of the myofibril, infiltration of fat and connective tissue, evidence of denervation, and alterations of the neuromuscular junction and sarcoplasmic reticulum. Electrophysiological studies indicate that fewer motor units function in older persons, and that nerve conduction velocity tends to decrease.

Larsson (1978) found that the ratio of type II to type I fiber area in the vastus lateralis muscle of men between the ages of 20 and 29 years was 1.33, but decreased to 0.99 in men between the ages of 60 and 65 years. Interestingly, Larsson (1984) later observed a reversal of type II fiber atrophy in the same 60- to 65-year-old subjects after a four-month program of calisthenics and strength training. This result suggests that much of the skeletal muscle atrophy associated with aging is due to disuse. Even after restoration of fiber size, knee extension torque values for the older subjects were well below those of the 20- to 29-year-old subjects, indicating that other factors in addition to atrophy are responsible for the decline in strength seen with aging.

As expected, skeletal muscle fiber atrophy in subjects aged 75 years and older was found to be of greater magnitude than that found by Larsson (1978) in subjects aged 56 to 65 years (Aniansson and co-workers, 1986; Grimby and co-workers, 1982). It is unclear when atrophy begins to occur in the life span. Larsson's study (1978) suggests that atrophic change does not become apparent until the fifth decade. Yet, life span studies of performance, such as grip strength and elbow flexion torque, indicate that some decrement in strength is noticeable by the end of the thirties. Even if we do not know precisely when age-related change begins to occur in skeletal muscle, it is obvious that we do not suddenly awaken at the age of 65 years to find our muscles atrophied.

Several investigators have reported that the lower extremities are more affected by atrophy than the upper extremities (Serratrice and co-workers, 1968). This suggests that the upper extremities are used to a greater extent than the lower extremities, and that age-related atrophy may be retarded with exercise or activity. The general trend toward a decrease in muscular activity, associated with a more sedentary lifestyle with aging, is a probable cause for age-related muscle fiber atrophy.

Inokuchi and colleagues (1975) removed rectus abdominus muscles from 45 men, from 45 women who had never had children, and from 45 women who had given birth at least once, and counted the number of fibers in cross section. Subjects ranged in age from 20 to over 80 years. Men in their twenties had an average of 150,000 fibers, while men in the ninth decade had less than 35,000. Even though the methods employed in this study are fraught with error, there is no denying that something happened to the fibers within this muscle. Decreases in fiber number were even greater for women, particularly those who had had children.

Lexell and colleagues (1983) removed entire quadriceps muscles at autopsy from 12 men, six between the ages of 19 and 37 years and six between the ages of 70 and 73 years, and counted the number of fibers in cross section. The results again suggested that fiber loss had occurred, because fiber numbers for the men in the eighth decade were one third less than those for the younger men.

Change within skeletal muscle may be due in part to disuse, but other factors also are responsible. A muscle is not an isolated entity. It functions optimally given the following conditions: adequate circulation, intact innervation, sufficient quantity of circulating hormones, and appropriate nutrition. Alterations in the nervous system, circulation, endocrine system, and nutrition frequently occur with aging, which obviously makes muscle less efficient and perhaps contributes to cell death.

A progressive loss of bone mass is a normal consequence of aging. Osteoporosis is not normal. Bone loss has been shown to occur with age in all populations studied so far, including primitive humans. The loss begins earlier and is greater in women than in men, which is related in part to menopause. Women generally achieve their maximum bone mass between the ages of 20 and 30 years. Thereafter, bone loss occurs gradually until the first five years after menopause, when demineralization occurs rapidly. Men also achieve maximum bone mass between 20 and 30 years of age, and then lose bone slowly at a rate of approximately 1% per year. After the accelerated change associated with menopause, bone loss in women approaches the 1% rate.

Whether bone loss reaches a critical state at which fracture is likely to occur depends largely on the amount of bone stock to begin with. Those with more bone stock at the time of skeletal maturity are less likely to develop symptomatic osteoporosis. Hence, the importance of good nutrition during the bone formation years.

A clear relationship between bone mass and degree of physical activity has been established. Increased stress on bone stimulates new bone formation, and lack of stress results in decreased formation and increased resorption. Tennis players, for example, have denser bones in the playing arm than in the nonplaying arm. Bone mass generally is higher in men who have an active occupation such as manual labor or farming, whereas sedentary workers have accelerated bone loss by comparison. Persons confined to bed because of flu, fracture, or other illness begin to lose bone within 24 hours of immobility.

Some of the most exciting research results to emerge within the last few years relates to exercise effects on bone mass in older women. Several studies have shown that bone stock can be increased with physical activity (reversal of loss and increase in bone production), particularly if calcium supplementation is occurring simultaneously. Smith (1982) observed an almost 3% increase in bone in women with an average age of 81 years after a program of relatively mild exercise. Dalsky (1986) has reported increases of up to 7% in postmenopausal women involved in vigorous exercise such as stair climbing and jogging. Findings such as these have enormous implications for physical therapy.

Articular cartilage also sustains age-related change, including a decrease in chondroitin sulfate, decreased resilience, and an increased liability for degenerative change. Cartilage defects are common in the joints of the elderly, and may affect movement either because pain is present or the coefficient of friction between the two joint surfaces has increased significantly. Arthritis may be very debilitating.

Bennett and colleagues (1942) examined knee joints after death in 63 subjects ranging in age from one month to 90 years. Joints were examined roentgenologically and macroscopically. The degree of change in joints for each decade was estimated as maximal, minimal, or average. His findings indicate that some degenerative change of the knee joint was present in every subject over the age of 15 years. Thus, osteoarthrosis is not a phenomenon associated only with advanced age.

NERVOUS SYSTEM

Age-related change within the nervous system has tremendously wide-ranging effects given the diversity of target organs and the fact that the nervous system coordinates the activities of all the other organ systems of the body. Unquestionably, nervous system deterioration is responsible for some of the loss of muscle mass, but nervous system alterations also may affect hormone regulation, temperature adjustment, blood pressure, heart and respiration rate, touch sensitivity, and many other functions. Age-related changes in the nervous system are vast; this section can do little more than highlight certain areas.

During one's lifetime, a pigment called lipofuscin accumulates in the brain and spinal cord, but whether it interferes with function is not known. The brain and spinal cord atrophy as the number of cells within them decreases with advancing age. Peripheral nerves show axonal fallout and alterations of the myelin sheath and motor end plate. These changes probably are related to the increase in central processing time, decreased nerve conduction velocity, and slower reflex responses seen in older adults.

Aging skeletal muscle shows signs of denervation. This denervation process may be secondary to a loss of large efferent nerve fibers and, possibly, anterior horn cells. Studies of the spinal cord and peripheral nerves in humans and animals show a decline in number of myelinated nerve fibers (Rexed, 1944; Swallow, 1966). In humans and rats, the loss of entire motor units with age has been correlated with the loss of axons in the innervating nerve trunks. Rexed (1944) observed a shift toward smaller diameters of ventral and dorsal root fibers with aging in humans, which suggests that selective atrophy and degeneration of the larger, faster conducting nerver fibers occurred. Cotrell (1940) also found a similar loss of the largest myelinated fibers in peripheral nerves. Type II muscle fibers typically are innervated by the large and fast conducting nerve fibers. The selective type II muscle fiber atrophy and type-grouping seen with age may be due in part to a gradual loss of alpha motoneurons innervating type II fibers.

One aspect of brain aging that terrifies people is memory loss and associated loss of intellectual functioning. Alzheimer's disease is not a natural consequence of aging, nor are the other forms of dementia. Memory changes are apparent, but a decline in intellectual capacity is neither universal nor inevitable.

Memory has been divided theoretically into primary and secondary forms. Primary memory is designated as a limited capacity store in which information is still "in mind." Secondary memory is an unlimited, permanent storehouse. In general, findings indicate that primary memory is unaffected by age but processing and response times are increased. Tests of secondary memory indicate loss with age. Older adults acquire new knowledge at slower rates and tend to have difficulty retrieving new knowledge at a later time. Secondary memory failures include forgetting names, faces, objects, appointments, locations, routines, phone numbers, and addresses. Memory failures may occur at any age when the person is faced with an unfamiliar situation such as hospitalization. Your older patient may not report a reliable medical history, particularly in the unfamiliar environment of a hospital. In general, those who maintain a high level of intellectual functioning tend to show less memory loss with aging. This is another example of the principle of "use it or lose it."

It is not known when nervous system change begins to occur, but again, judging by performance decrements in activities like running, which require speed, alterations are apparent by the mid-thirties. Most men and women in their forties and fifties will admit needing more time to learn new material and experiencing lapses in memory, particularly recalling names. The problem of memory intensifies with each passing decade.

RESPIRATORY SYSTEM

Pulmonary function certainly is related to the condition of the lungs and associated air passageways. Equally important to function are the chest wall, diaphragm, circulation, and muscles of inspiration and expiration. Although aging changes occur within the respiratory tree, changes in the chest wall, circulation, and muscles may have a greater impact on function. Abnormalities of the chest wall are common among the elderly, with kyphosis being a primary cause. Calcification of the costal cartilages may occur, which contributes to an increase in chest wall rigidity. If the rib cage becomes less mobile, the diaphragm and abdominal muscles become more important in effecting ventilation. If the muscles are atrophic and have fewer fibers, contraction capability is diminished. The result of all these possible changes is altered pulmonary capacity.

Within the lungs several phenomena occur with advancing age: a loss of alveolar surface area and an increase in lung distensibility. Alveolar surface has been estimated to fall 4% per decade after the age of 30 years. Alveoli tend to become flattened and more shallow, while ducts are enlarged; the alveolar wall is thinner and contains fewer capillaries. With increasing age, elastic recoil of the lungs gradually decreases, contributing to altered lung compliance.

Pulmonary measures for older adults demonstrate variability similar to that found for measures of strength or range of motion. Although variability among the older population is present, pulmonary function tests indicate an overall decrease with age in forced vital capacity (FVC), FEV_1, and an increase in residual gas volume (dead air). These decreases are seen particularly when the patient has respiratory disease, smokes, or is routinely exposed to pollutants. The arterial-venous oxygen difference ($A-\dot{V}O_2$) increases progressively with age, indicating less oxygen extraction by the tissues.

In the elderly person, some of the smaller air passages tend to collapse during expiration, particularly in the lower lobes. The lung volume at which small airways start to close (closing volume) increases with age. Therefore, on expiration, older persons reach the closing volume sooner. This distorts the balance of perfusion and ventilation, particularly during exercise when respiration rate is increased.

Given a more rigid chest wall and altered lung compliance with age, an older person will have a higher respiratory work load for a given external effort, particularly if lung disease is present. In severe emphysema, the energy cost for breathing may be increased 10 to 20 times more than normal. If $\dot{V}O_2$ max is already low, as is typical in a debilitated person, breathing may be virtually the only activity the individual has the energy to accomplish.

Age-associated pulmonary disease is common, particularly among smokers and those regularly exposed to air pollution. The incidence of emphysema, lung cancer, chronic bronchitis, "black lung," infection (particularly pneumonia), and tuberculosis increases linearly with age and accounts for an estimated 15% of all hospitalizations among persons over 70 years of age (Davies, 1985). Age-related change in pulmonary function capacity, coupled with the increased likelihood of lung disease, are likely to result in compromise of other organsand tissues that depend upon oxygen for maximum efficiency.

CARDIOVASCULAR SYSTEM

Anatomical changes in the heart (atrophy, lipofuscin accumulation, increased fat and connective tissue) do occur with age, but they do not explain the declines in function that have been observed. Peak heart rate, maximum cardiac output, and cardiac contractility decrease with aging, which certainly affects the intensity and duration of physical activity that an older person can tolerate. A debilitated 80-year-old patient may reach maximum heart rate with a trip to the bathroom. A 65-year-old man develops almost the same cardiac output as a young adult who is working at a comparable rate, but the 65-year-old man will reach his peak cardiac output at a substantially lower work load.

The elasticity of the major blood vessels declines with age secondary to an atrophy of the elastic lamellae and an increase in collagen in the vessel walls. More rigid arteries accept the cardiac stroke volume less readily. Thus, resting pulse pressure and systolic blood pressure increase with advancing age.

Probably the most significant decline with advancing age is that of maximum working capacity, or $\dot{V}O_{2\ max}$. For a specific intensity of effort each element of the cardiac and respiratory system must operate closer to its maximum value. If the maximum value is low to begin with, a patient's margin of reserve is negligible. For example, if a person's $\dot{V}O_{2\ max}$ is 40 mL O_2/kg/min, walking is an easy task, requiring perhaps 40% of maximum capacity. If $\dot{V}O_{2\ max}$ has declined to 12 mL O_2/kg/min, a very high proportion of that capacity will be used for walking and any other physical task. Thus, the duration the task can be continued will be very short.

When the physical work capacity of a sedentary but healthy older adult is assessed, huge differences are apparent. For example, $\dot{V}O_{2\ max}$ values for a group of 60- to 70-year-old subjects (n = 60) tested at Washington University ranged from 17 to 40 mL O_2/kg/min. $\dot{V}O_{2\ max}$ values obtained for master athletes typically are higher than 40 ml O_2. Recently, I tested a 69-year-old master athlete ($\dot{V}O_{2\ max}$ = 57 ml O_2/kg/min) who had just completed a double marathon, 26 miles of which included the Appalachian Trail! I also have worked with other 69-year-old patients who became exhausted walking 50 ft. Successful program planning for the older adult should be based on an assessment of physical work capacity, taking into consideration what is realistic for the individual client. You also should take into account that maximum working capacity usually can be improved with aerobic exercise.

Working capacity values decrease in almost linear fashion after the age of 30 years, if the person is sedentary (Shepherd, 1978). If a young man or woman maintains a high level of physical activity, capacity changes do not become apparent until the person is closer to 40 years of age. The higher the value to begin with and the longer the value is maintained, the greater the margin of safety for physical function in older age.

The incidence of age-related cardiovascular disease increases dramatically with age, and ranks as the number one cause of death worldwide. Ischemic heart disease, hypertension, and cardiac arrhythmias are common, affecting an estimated 40% of the population over 70 years of age. Cardiac disease may further limit physical activity tolerance and capability.

SENSORY SYSTEMS

Vision

Loss of visual acuity is virtually a universal aging phenomenon. Rarely can a person older than the age of 50 years see the newspaper or detailed objects without glasses. This inability of the eye to accommodate for close vision is called presbyopia.

Remembering the prevalence of presbyopia is important when treating the older adult. You will have far greater success teaching diabetic Mr. Smith how to check his feet if he is wearing glasses and can see what you are trying to point out. Mrs. Jones may catch on to her home exercise program more quickly if she can see the exercises you are teaching her while you are doing the instruction. Patients who wear their glasses in therapy can be treated more effectively and comply more readily.

Another visual change accompanying presbyopia is an increased threshold to light stimulation, or the need for more light to see adequately. For an older person to function optimally at home or in the physical therapy clinic, higher intensity light bulbs should be used. Light-colored walls enhance the illumination of a room and reduce the possibility of patients losing items in dark areas or tripping over an object that does not stand out.

As people reach the eighth decade, the inability to adapt to darkness becomes apparent. Fear of driving at night is well founded because the eyes of an older driver do not readily adjust to the dark. The incidence of nighttime accidents is significantly increased among drivers over 65 years of age. Falling or tripping in dark or dimly lighted areas is more prevalent among the elderly, especially when walking to the bathroom in the middle of the night. Recommendations we can make to our older clients include using night-lights throughout the house, increasing outdoor lighting (especially around patios, porches, or entryways), and pausing for a moment before entering a dark room.

The converse, light adaptation, also slows with aging. When emerging from a movie theater most older people can see very little for several moments. Be tolerant of their slow egress and watchful of anyone likely to miss a step or ramp. Cautioning your older clients to pause for a moment after brightly illuminating a room may prevent a fall.

Strategic use of color in the physical therapy clinic can assist an older person to gain confidence in walking in an unfamiliar environment. A sharp color contrast between the walls and floor makes it obvious where one ends and the other begins. Changes in the color of flooring between a room and the hallway may be perceived as a raised or lowered area. The resulting tendency to stop and "step up" or "down" into the next room will be eliminated if the carpeting or tile is the same color in the rooms and the corridor. However, stairs should be a color different from the corridor, to signal that a break in flat terrain is ahead.

Unfortunately, vision may diminish with advancing age because of a number of other common conditions. Cataracts result in cloudy, dim vision; fortunately, however, cataracts usually can be removed surgically once they have "ripened." Macular degeneration (which increases the area of the blind spot), glaucoma, and diabetic retinopathy may severely compromise vision, diminishing quality of life and ability to function.

Vision is an integral component of balance. For example, I found the average one-legged standing balance time for a group of 60 men and women between the ages of 60 and 70 years was 45 seconds. When asked to stand on one leg with eyes closed, the average standing time was five seconds! The balance of older persons is compromised when they are in the dark and when their sight is markedly diminished.

Hearing

Hearing sensitivity diminishes with advancing age primarily because of a loss of hair cells and

neurons of the auditory pathway. With aging there is a gradual, but usually modest, loss in hearing (presbycusis) along the entire audible sound spectrum. Hearing loss frequently results in functional problems: impaired sound localization, reduced sound sensitivity, disturbed loudness perception, and reduced sound discrimination. Hearing loss rarely proceeds on an even basis, and affects different sound frequencies to differing degrees. Usually, lower frequencies are more readily heard than others. This means that our clients may have difficulty discriminating consonants, which are generally of a higher frequency than vowels. Thus, speech may be audible but incomprehensible.

The degree of hearing loss in later years is related directly to noise bombardment at earlier ages. Persons who live next to freeways or airports, listen to extremely loud rock music, or work in a noisy factory have detectable hearing losses long before middle or old age. A rather extensive survey by Wilkins (1949) revealed that, when questioned, 27% of all those older than 74 years admitted to having a hearing loss. An even higher incidence of inability to hear all the words of a conversation has been reported by others (Pathy, 1985). Being sensitive to a possible hearing loss among our older patients may contribute to more successful rehabilitation.

Touch Sensitivity

A common complaint of older persons is an inability to discriminate fine detail when handling small objects, such as screws. Touch sensitivity, temperature sensitivity, and sharp-dull perception all tend to diminish. Objects are dropped more often, and work requiring fine dexterity and exquisite sensitivity, such as watchmaking, may become impossible. Recognizing reduced sensitivity is important; diabetics must be especially aware of the need to reduce the risk of trauma and subsequent skin breakdown. Simple testing for diminished touch pressure and sharp-dull perception may reveal the need for protective footwear or consideration of safety factors at home or at the workplace.

SKIN

With increasing age, the collagen per unit area of skin decreases, reducing the thickness of the dermis. Remaining collagen within the dermis may undergo some degeneration, decreasing skin strength and elasticity. Older skin is more subject to breakdown, particularly pressure sores. Cells in the basal or germ layer of the epidermis divide at a slower rate as we age, which prolongs healing time after an injury or surgery. Sweat production is diminished with aging, which affects the ability to dissipate heat. Exercise time may be quite limited on very warm days.

ENDOCRINE SYSTEM

Hormones contribute to the regulation of body fluids and cardiovascular performance, the mobilization of fuel for exercise, and the synthesis of new protein. Therefore, a weakening of hormonal control reduces the body's ability to adjust to stress, such as exercise or an increase in temperature. Age-related deterioration of the pancreas, thyroid, adrenal cortex, and pituitary gland has been demonstrated, but it is unclear whether hormone production remains adequate in later years. With aging, there is a definite increase in endocrine disorders such as diabetes and thyroid disease. However, other factors (including obesity, autonomic nervous system dysfunction, circulation, and available receptor sites on target organs) also affect endocrine function. Therefore, one cannot implicate the endocrine system alone if disorders are present.

GENITOURINARY SYSTEM

The number of functioning nephrons and glomeruli decreases with age, and the filtering surface of each glomerulus is diminished. Renal plasma flow is reduced. The major consequence of these changes is a progressive decline in glomerular filtration rate after maturity.

Many older adults are on medications for elevated blood pressure, a chronic age-related disease such as diabetes, or similar problems.

One of the major routes of drug elimination is the kidney, but with diminished kidney function, renal clearance of a drug is slowed. A drug like diazepam (Valium), which normally is cleared from the blood in eight hours, may not clear before 16 hours in an older person. If the patient is given two to three doses of diazepam per day, the drug will accumulate in the system, causing a previously alert and vital person to become dull and somnolent. Watch for rapid personality changes in your older clients. You may suspect a drug overdose in many cases of confusion, especially when a family member reports that grandfather was fine before coming into the hospital. Report your findings to the nursing staff or directly to the physician.

Bladder function also undergoes age-related changes, including an increase in the frequency of urination and in the residual volume of urine remaining in the bladder after voiding. The incidence of incontinence and accidents increases. If present, this is a major source of worry for our older clients. If a patient is likely to have an accident, physical therapy may well provoke it. Active exercise or a change from the supine to standing position, with gravity acting on the bladder, tends to stimulate urine flow. Using a bedpan, commode, or the bathroom before exercising and walking may prevent an accident; voiding before therapy may give the patient enough peace of mind to do a lot better during treatment. Try to be sensitive to bowel and bladder needs, because people are often reluctant to mention such matters.

GASTROINTESTINAL SYSTEM

Age-related changes may involve the entire gastrointestinal (GI) system. If teeth are missing, mastication may be poor, or the patient may choose a diet lacking bulk. Peristaltic movements of the esophagus slow with age, so that the time taken for food to move from the pharynx to the stomach is prolonged. The incidence of gastritis and various ulcers increases with age. The rate of intestinal absorption diminishes. Among older persons common diseases and problems of the GI tract include diverticulitis, GI bleeding, cancer, colitis, bowel obstruction, and constipation.

Constipation is typically due to the combined effects of decreased intake of fluid and lack of dietary bulk. Constipation also may be caused by atrophy of the muscle layer of the bowel and decreased physical activity among sedentary persons. A vigorous session of PT may stimulate bowel evacuation, and you will find that having a bathroom nearby is most convenient for the patient.

The liver functions less efficiently with age because of a number of changes. It is possible that the aging liver is less able to metabolize and detoxify drugs, so that toxic levels may accumulate in the blood. A loss of beta cells occurs in the pancreas, which results in decreasing levels of insulin secretion with advancing age; glucose tolerance is reduced.

CHANGES IN PERFORMANCE

Nothing exemplifies the variety of aging change more than performance characteristics. Identifying a "normal" older man or woman becomes difficult because the range of values for any activity is so great. For example, CAA climbed the Matterhorn and Mont Blanc several times between the ages of 65 and 70 years and still, at age 73, averages 15 to 20 miles of hiking per day on rugged terrain. Conversely, CGG, who is 68 years old, walks to and from his car but prefers not to visit shopping centers because the walking required is too great. Which one is more "normal"? Both are, which is why working with older adults is so challenging. In no other age category are functional or performance goals more varied or difficult to set.

SPEED OF REACTION

The trend toward a slowing of reaction speed with age (after the third decade) is well documented. Movement time, reaction time, and the time to accomplish other movement tasks such as card sorting or shirt buttoning is increased when older adults are compared with younger adults.

Does slowing with age really have to happen? Anyone who has observed Vladimir Horowitz's fingers flying over the piano keyboard has to wonder about the effects of practice. However, Salthouse and Somberg (1982) tested eight young and eight older adults before and after 50 hours of practice (hand skill) and found that, although both groups improved dramatically, perceptual motor performance deficits still were apparent among the older group. Our tests of master athletes, men who have been vigorously active all their lives, indicate that some slowing does occur but that age effects are greatly attenuated or seemingly not present yet. Master athletes cannot run the 100-yd dash as rapidly as an Olympic competitor, regardless of their stage of training. However, values for master athletes' walking velocity, finger tapping, and time to peak torque are comparable with those of 20- to 29-year-old athletes. Unquestionably, physical activity has a modifying effect on the slowing of movement that occurs with age. Kroll and Clarkson (1978) also found physically active older adults (mean age, 63 years) to have faster reaction times than their age-matched but sedentary counterparts.

When speed of behavior is examined in greater detail, it has been found that all of the components of a task take longer to execute. For example, if a 75-year-old person is asked to react to a light stimulus, there will be a delay in perception of the turned-on light, an increase in central processing time, and a delay in the execution of the task to be performed (eg, applying the brakes of the car). This delay between input and output will be even greater if more than one task is assigned simultaneously and if the complexity of the task is increased. So, our chances of success with a patient are increased if we reduce tasks to their simplest form. If working on dressing with Mr. Jones, the activity will probably go faster if he is sitting (thus not having to balance simultaneously), if he is wearing his glasses, and if the lighting is adequate.

WALKING

Walking velocity decreases with advancing age, with a significant decline noted by the seventh decade. It is highly unlikely that people suddenly slow down at the age of 65 years; rather, a gradual slowing occurs over several decades. This slowing becomes statistically noticeable only when comparisons are made between young adults (20 to 29 years) and older adults (over 60 years). Although the trend is toward reduced walking speeds, the range of values for older adults is enormous. I have recorded walking velocities for 60 men and women between the ages of 60 and 70 years, and have values ranging from a low of 49 m/min to a high of 95 m/min. The mean walking velocity for the group (66 m/min) is lower than the velocity of 80 m/min recorded for young adults 20 to 29 years of age (Blessey and colleagues, 1976). These older adults are "normal" because they are without orthopedic complaints or diseases that would affect their ability to ambulate. Thus, their degree of variability also is normal. Walking speeds recorded in our laboratory for men and women between 80 and 90 years of age range from 14 to 44 m/min (n = 13).

BALANCE

Standing balance times also decrease with advancing age, but individual differences are amazing. I have asked the same 60 older adults mentioned in the previous section to stand on one foot for one minute; values range from two seconds to over 60 seconds. One man with a balance time of six seconds sustained a hamstring strain trying to maintain the upright position, whereas others of the same age (66 years) barely swayed or used their arms. None of the 30 control subjects between the ages of 20 and 30 years lost their balance during the 60-second period. Single-limb stance times with the eyes closed are even more interesting. Twelve of the 60 older adults were unable or unwilling to balance on one foot with eyes closed; the average balance time was 5.3 seconds (range, 0.5 to 20.5 seconds). Single-legged balance times with eyes closed for the young adults ranged from 5 to 60 seconds (maximum required) with an average balance time of 43 seconds. These data indicate the critical role vision plays in balancing, and underline the importance of creating a safe environment for our older patients (eg, night-lights in hallways and bedrooms).

In my experience, many of my older patients have a particularly difficult time balancing on soft and uneven surfaces. Thus, for safety's sake, and to improve their chances of success at home, I have clients practice walking on soft carpeting, grass, sand, and mud (if appropriate). Balance on the straightaway may be adequate, but a cane, walking stick, or rail may be required for balance on more challenging terrain.

Balance times are easy to assess, and the process takes but a few moments. Whether we can affect balancing as the result of our treatments is not known. Regardless, taking balance times into consideration for treatment and discharge planning is only prudent.

ISOMETRIC STRENGTH

Decreases in isometric strength with age have been well documented in both cross-sectional and longitudinal studies. Although not all muscle groups have been examined, the downward trend with age is similar for all muscles that have been studied. Burke (1953) assessed hand grip among 311 males between the ages of 11 and 73 years. He found grip strength declined slightly between the late twenties and early sixties, and showed a dramatic decrease thereafter. Asmussen and co-workers (1975) tested grip strength of a group of men and women over a 40-year span. Between the first test when subjects were in their twenties and the last test when subjects were in their sixties, grip strength decreased 37% in women and 28% in men. In one of the few studies of subjects older than 70 years, Aniansson and colleagues (1983, 1986) collected knee extension torque data on the same 73- to 83-year-old subjects in 1975 and again in 1983. As expected, isometric strength values for the older subjects were markedly less than those of young controls 20 to 29 years of age. Also observed was an additional decline in strength of 10% to 22% during that period.

These studies are very important for documenting trends with aging and for providing some normative data that can be used for comparison. However, what does not stand out in any of these publications is the variability in degree of change among persons at different ages or even the same ages. I have studied 60 men and women between the ages of 60 and 70 years, and have found knee extension torque values for the men to range from 78 to 178 ft·lb. The average isometric torque value for young (20 to 29 years) men was 147 ft·lb. Thus, some of the older men had more torque capability than men 40 years younger. This variability is normal and points out that it may be difficult to determine how much of a strength increase to strive for in our older clients. Comparing isometric strength values of an uninvolved to an involved extremity (if possible) is particularly useful. Comparing manual muscle test grades and torque output also helps, because the former takes into consideration the weight of the body part. Keep in mind that a "fair" grade on a muscle test typically reflects a 40% to 50% reduction in strength, and that a patient with this grade has a long way to go before becoming "normal" (Beasley, 1961). Although strength decreases with aging, this finding should not deter physical therapists from prescribing active or resistance exercise for older clients. Some rather exciting preliminary findings indicate that strength gains for aging adults are of a magnitude comparable with those of young adults. Strength increases of 10% to 20% are not uncommon following a strengthening program. Muscular endurance also can increase. One noticeable difference related to strengthening exercise with the older patient as compared to young clients is that strength increases come more slowly. Programs need to be modified on the average of every 10 to 14 days instead of weekly.

DYNAMIC STRENGTH

Concentric strength has not been assessed systematically for very many older persons. This is particularly true for women and those older than 70 years of age. No values exist for eccentric strength. The existing data suggest that losses in dynamic strength are apparent, and of a magnitude similar to that seen for isometric testing. One aspect of interest regarding dynamic strength testing is that some older persons lose the ability to generate torque at the faster rates of speed. I have observed an inability of some older persons (women in particular) to move a Cybex arm into knee flexion and extension at 300°/sec and into plantar and dorsiflexion at 180°/sec. Considering that knee flexion during gait normally is in excess of 300°/sec, this finding represents a marked slowing. After a three-month exercise class, however, all the people who had zero torque readings at high speed with Cybex testing could produce some measure of torque again. This suggests that some of the slowing with age can be reversed.

Interestingly, with the older clients who had difficulty moving quickly, strength increases at faster speeds were disproportionately large following exercises that were not done rapidly. After three months of exercise, improvements in torque of 50% to 100% occurred, which could not be reflective of an actual 50% to 100% increase in contractile prolein. Rather, this finding suggests a "rediscovery" of muscles that had not been used for years or altered patterns of muscle fiber recruitment.

ENDURANCE

Muscle endurance seems to be little affected by age as long as the task can be done aerobically and is matched to the person's strength capability. Grip strength endurance, which is the time that 50% of maximum grip strength can be maintained, is comparable at all ages. I have found that the time it takes to decline to 50% maximum voluntary contraction with continuous active knee extension in Cybex testing is comparable at all ages of clients tested up to 84 years of age. However, initial torque values for older adults are lower than those for younger subjects.

SUMMARY

You may have noticed that information in this text related to onset, rate, and magnitude of age-related change is rather sparse. Unfortunately, for most elements of performance relevant to physical therapists, there is no information. We do not have data that would indicate the normal course of change across the decades in muscular, physiological, and neurological systems. Data for onset, rate, and magnitude of age-related change are needed, and it is hoped that some of you will rise to the challenge of providing this information in the future.

Other significant voids in our physical therapy body of knowledge are performance norms, beginning in the third decade. Often, the physical performance capacity of our clients, regardless of age, is compared with that of the 20- to 29-year-old college student. College students are readily available to investigators, and data from these samples of convenience are being used to represent all 20- to 29-year-old persons. Whether data for college students truly reflect what is normal for others in that age group is uncertain. Data for persons 20 to 29 years old do not provide us with definitive guidelines for what can be expected for persons 30 to 39 years old, 40 to 49 years old, and so forth. Norms for all decades would greatly enhance our abilities to judge impairments in strength, range of motion, posture, activities of daily living, endurance, gait, and other components of function.

OTHER ASPECTS OF AGING

Some people breeze into old age taking each new challenge and change in stride, but others find aging oppressive and depressing. Attitudes toward aging are as varied as the individual biological responses. These attitudes certainly affect expected outcome of rehabilitation. Aging also may bring burdens such as financial worries, loss of friends, loss of spouse, moving from the family home, illness, loss of status, loneliness, loss of independence, and feelings of insignificance. Any one of these burdens may so overwhelm the individual that it is difficult for the physical therapist to break

through the barrier of illness or worry. If Mr. Jones has lost his leg secondary to cancer, he may not hear what you're saying about how to use his new prosthesis because he is so worried about his bedridden wife for whom he is the sole caretaker. Mrs. Smith will never get rid of her neck spasms and headaches while wondering where the next meal is coming from or how to pay the rent.

With advancing age, chronic disease may interfere to such an extent that the expected outcome of rehabilitation is not attainable. Taking disease and its impact into consideration is difficult, and it is easy for a physical therapist to err on the side of optimism. Attaining selected goals may not be possible, particularly if disease such as emphysema, congestive heart failure, or diabetes is present. Adjusting treatment and goals accordingly may be necessary, although embarrassing. However, it is better to be embarrassed than to delude the family or patient into believing he can do the impossible. Maybe the patient is physically capable of dressing, but it takes two hours or is so exhausting that he cannot do anything else the rest of the day. Thus, assistance in dressing would be a better choice than independence.

An additional complication of dealing with older clients is that sometimes the treatment appropriate for a younger patient becomes contraindicated in an older client because of disease. If edema is present in the legs of a 28-year-old patient, she usually is advised to lie in bed with the feet elevated higher than the head. If this same procedure is followed for a 78-year-old woman with congestive heart failure, chances are the lungs will fill with fluid and the patient will be more ill following the treatment than she was before. When gait training a 20-year-old patient who has been in bed for a few days, sitting on the edge of the bed for several moments usually is sufficient to overcome dizziness before starting out on crutches. For an older person, the same practice may result in fainting, if orthostatic hypotension is a problem. A tilt table may be required. Learning safe PT practices comes from experience, but following prudent procedures routinely (eg, monitoring blood pressure, heart rate, and respiration rate, and noting color) will eliminate guesswork and enhance the chances of success. Be very observant.

On occasion, the success of rehabilitation may be foiled by factors that are not physical in nature. If Mrs. Jones has no one to go home to and is enjoying the company and meals provided by the hospital setting, she may not want to become independent. If Mr. Smith is going home to a family that does not want him, he may become incontinent or fail to grasp basic care needs. The fear of going home or losing independence may be overwhelming. These factors must be dealt with if rehabilitation is to be successful.

Variability is the norm for older adults. This variability in function should be kept in mind to ensure that each older client is evaluated properly and that goals appropriate for that individual are made. Under no circumstances should two clients who are 50, 60, or 70 years of age or older be considered "the same."

The data presented in this chapter were obtained primarily from persons who were considered "healthy elderly," not compromised in function by disease or disability. Although the relatively healthy older group constitutes a portion of our patient population, it does not represent the majority of those we see. Most of our patients have some age-related disease such as diabetes, coronary artery disease, or emphysema. The presence of one or more diseases contributes to the potential for even more variability in functional capability. Although age-related disease is common among older persons, not all people have disease, nor does everyone have the same collection of diseases.

Another contributing factor to variability among the elderly is medication. It is not uncommon to find a patient with Parkinson's disease barely able to move at 8 AM, but after medication is in the system, dressing independently by 10 AM. Unfortunately, it is also not uncommon to watch the transformation of a happy, animated, and fully capable person into one who is barely oriented taking diazepam.

Finally, additional variability will be present as a result of the time and the setting in which the patient is seen. The person you respond to in the hospital two days after total hip replacement will be entirely different six weeks later when functioning at home. The same patient seen in an outpatient clinic three months after surgery will be at another level of capability as well.

CONCLUSION

Although the changes that may occur with aging have been presented on a system-by-system basis, I hope that you realize how a change in one system can have pronounced effects on other systems as well. To emphasize this point, I will use Barney Clark, the first recipient of an artificial heart, as an example. Barney Clark went through years of progressive heart failure. As a consequence of his heart failure, coupled with aging change, other systems also began to fail. After he received his heart, he suddenly had blood circulating at pressures so much higher than they had been for years that his blood vessels failed and he had multiple strokes. Even though the heart was fine, too much age-related change and damage were present in other systems. He died because of liver, kidney, and other forms of failure. Another lesson to be learned from the Barney Clark episode is that correcting aging change and disease in one system does not compensate for change that occurs elsewhere. The human body is a magnificent organism, but, like an automobile, it does not run on isolated parts.

Older clients are fascinating and above all challenging to work with. It is fun and exciting to ferret out problems that are age related and those that are associated with disease, and to find treatment procedures appropriate for both. Even more exciting is seeing the progress that can be made with older clients when your treatment is well designed. The rewards are enormous.

ANNOTATED BIBLIOGRAPHY

The following textbooks cover the topic of aging in detail and would serve as a good starting point for anyone interested in developing a broader base of knowledge. Typically, chapters are written by experts who nicely synthesize available literature in their respective fields.

Birren JE, Schaie KW (eds): Handbook of the Psychology of Aging, 2nd ed. New York, Van Nostrand Reinhold, 1985

Brocklehurst JC (ed): Textbook of Geriatric Medicine and Gerontology, 3rd ed. New York, Churchill Livingstone, 1985

Finch CE, Schneider EL (eds): Handbook of the Biology of Aging, 2nd ed. New York, Van Nostrand Reinhold, 1985

Lewis CB (ed): Aging: The Health Care Challenge. Philadelphia, FA Davis, 1985

Pathy MSJ (ed): Principles and Practice of Geriatric Medicine. New York, John Wiley & Sons, 1985

Shock NW et al: Normal Human Aging: The Baltimore Longitudinal Study of Aging. US Dept of Health and Human Services publication No. 84-2450. Bethesda, MD, Public Health Service, NIH, 1984

SKELETAL MUSCLE

Aniansson A et al: Muscle morphology, enzymatic activity, and muscle strength in elderly men: A follow-up study. Muscle Nerve 9:585, 1986

Beasley WC: Quantitative muscle testing: Principles and applications to research and clinical services. Arch Phys Med 42:398, 1961

Grimby G et al: Morphology and enzymatic capacity in arm and leg muscles in 78–81 year old men and women. Acta Physiol Scand 115:125, 1982

Inokuchi S et al: Age-related changes in the histochemical composition of the rectus abdominus muscle of the adult human. Hum Biol 47:231, 1975

Larsson L: Morphological and functional characteristics of the aging skeletal muscle in man. Acta Physiol Scand Suppl 457, 1978 (One of the most extensive studies performed to date.)

Lexell J et al: Distribution of different fiber types in human skeletal muscles: Effects of aging studied in whole muscle cross sections. Muscle Nerve, 6:588, 1983

Serratrice G, Roux H, Aquaron R: Proximal muscle weakness in elderly subjects. J Neurol Sci 7:275, 1968

BONE AND CARTILAGE

Bennett GA, Waine H, Bauer W: Changes in the Knee Joint at Various Ages. New York, The Commonwealth Fund. 1942

Dalsky GP, Birge SS, Kleinheider KS: The effect of endurance training on lumbar bone mass in postmenopausal women. Med Sci Sports Exerc 18(2):520, 1986

Smith EL, Reddan W, Smith PE: Physical activity and calcium modalities for bone mineral increase in aged women. Med Sci Sports Exerc 13:60, 1981

NERVOUS SYSTEM

Cotrell L: Histologic variations with age in apparently normal nerve trunks of limbs. Arch Neurol Psychiatry 43:1138, 1940

Rexed B: Fiber size in the peripheral nervous system of adults and old persons. In Contribution to the Knowledge of the Postnatal Development of the Peripheral Nervous System in Man. Acta Psychiatr Neurol [Suppl] 33:164, 1944

Swallow M: Fiber size and content of the anterior tibial nerve of the foot. J Neurol Neurosurg Psychiatry 29:205, 1966

CARDIOVASCULAR SYSTEM

Shepard RJ: Physical Activity and Aging, pp 63–114. London, Croom Helm, 1978 (The author's vast knowledge and expertise in this field make the book an excellent resource and interesting reading.)

RESPIRATORY SYSTEM

Davies B: The respiratory system. In Pathy MJS (ed): Principles and Practice of Geriatric Medicine, pp 515–536. New York, John Wiley & Sons, 1985

PERFORMANCE CHANGES

Aniansson A et al: Muscle function in 75-year-old women: A longitudinal study. Scand J Rehabil Med [Suppl] 9:92, 1983

Asmussen E, Freunsgaard K, Norgaard S: A follow-up longitudinal study of selected physiologic functions in former physical education students: After forty years. J Am Geriatr Soc 23:442, 1975

Blessey RL et al: Metabolic energy cost of unrestrained walking. Phys Ther 56:1019, 1976

Burke WE et al: The relation of grip strength and grip-strength endurance to age. J Appl Physiol 5:628, 1953

Kroll W, Clarkson P: Age isometric knee extension strength and fractionated response time. Exp Aging Res 4:389, 1978

Larsson L: Physical training effects on muscle morphology in sedentary males at different ages. Med Sci Sports Exerc 14:203, 1984

Moritani T, deVries H: Potential for gross muscle hypertrophy in older men. J Gerontol 35:672, 1980

Salthouse TA: Speed of behavior and its implications for cognition. In Birren JE, Schaie KW (eds): Handbook of the Psychology of Aging, 2n ed, pp 400–426. New York, Van Nostrand Reinhold, 1985

HEARING

Wilkins LT: The prevalence of deafness in a population of England, Scotland, and Wales. Central Office of Information, London, 1949

9 Communication Through Human Movement

KATHERINE F. SHEPARD

The elderly woman with bent posture and thin gnarled hands moved her grocery cart down the aisle. The woman's son, following closely behind her, sadly thought, "I hate to see Mom in so much pain. I wish there was something I could do." A child spied the old woman and exclaimed, "Oh Mommy, she looks just like the witch in my storybook!" The young physical therapy student passed the old woman and mused, "There is a person with advanced rheumatoid arthritis. She walks as if she has had a total hip replacement." Young people moved impatiently around the old woman, considering her an obstacle. Older people patiently waited for her to pass, silently grateful that they were not so impaired. The old woman, aware of the many looks and hesitancies around her, had a strong urge to shout out, "I didn't always look like this—I was once a professional dancer!" Instead, she kept her eyes downcast on her grocery cart and painfully moved on, trying to be as inconspicuous as possible.

It is impossible to discuss human movement and function without considering what movement and function communicate about who we are as human beings. What we communicate through our physical appearance and our way of moving ourselves through space has a powerful influence on our self-image as well as the image of the self we convey to others. Physical appearance and movement include postures, facial expressions, gestures, gaits, the clothes we wear, and the presence or absence of ambulatory aids such as crutches and wheelchairs.

Our perceived self-image influences our thoughts, feelings, and beliefs about our human worth (Fig. 9-1). The self as portrayed by our physical appearance and movement is the single most important factor in eliciting first impressions and setting the framework for subsequent interactions with others.

The primary purpose of this chapter is to explore briefly how a person's physical appearance and movement, which change through the life span, are central to the health care concerns of the physical therapist. A secondary purpose of this chapter is to stimulate your awareness of how nonverbal behaviors can be used in the evaluation and treatment of patients and families.

PHYSICAL APPEARANCE RELATED TO COMMUNICATION

I often show my students a series of photographs of people to underscore how important physical appearance and physical environment are to the perceptions and judgments they hold about others. Upon seeing each photo briefly, students are asked to write down two or three adjectives to describe what they see. A picture of a smiling blonde, blue-eyed girl standing in a flower garden evokes a predictable narrow range of responses such as pretty, sweet, and innocent. A picture of an old woman sitting in

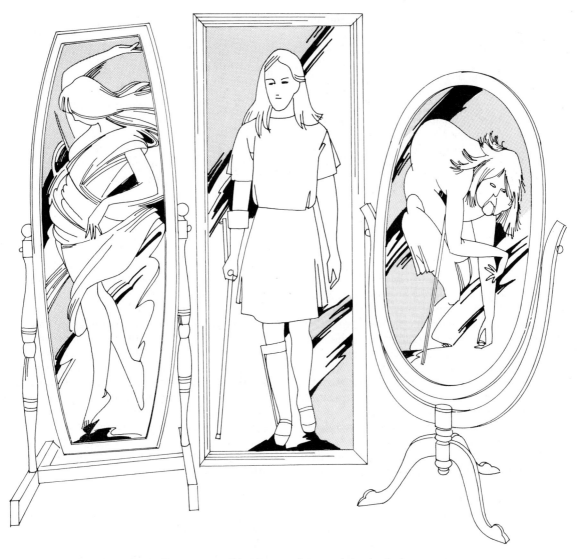

Figure 9-1. Representation of how one's self-image can change when physical appearance changes. (Purtilo R: Health Professional/Patient Interaction, 3rd ed, p 45. Philadelphia, WB Saunders, 1984)

a rocking chair, knitting, with a faraway look in her eyes provokes a more mixed set of reactions, from sad and lonely to loving and grandmotherly. A third picture of a black couple with intense expressions evokes an even greater array of reactions, from defiant and angry (often responses from white students) to proud and beautiful (more likely responses from black students).

Responses to these pictures are more similar when the content is simple, the context (situation) is familiar, and all the elements in the picture are congruent, such as the calendar-like photograph of the smiling young girl in the spring flower garden. As the pictures become more complex (by adding background features, a second person, or cultural or ethnic distinctions with which students are less familiar), responses become increasingly varied.

Students learn through this demonstration that how they immediately react to what they see comes directly from their personal experiences. They can no more ignore these early experiences and the feelings, judgments, and stereotypes that accompany them than they can change the color of their eyes.

However, being *aware* of what stereotypes or ethnocentric reactions you have, and recalling how you acquired them, is the beginning of being able to modify your initial impressions and to see quickly beyond old information to the unique person you are communicating with. Clearly, the more significant contact experiences you have with people who are different from you (eg, in age, culture, or belief system), the more open you are to differences. The more open to differences, the less likely you are to perceive and react within narrow growth-inhibiting frameworks when communicating with others.

The overwhelming importance that physical appearance has in first impressions is especially notable in everyday clinical practice. When our patients put on orthotic devices, or use a cane, or propel themselves in a wheelchair, they are often shocked at how differently people react to them than when they physically looked and moved much like everyone else. They are bewildered when longtime friends avoid them, and when store clerks and waitresses talk to them as if they were small children or, worse, ignore them altogether. They are stunned by the discomfort and embarrassment of immediate family members, especially when in public places. They plaintively tell us, "But I'm the same person I was." Perhaps cognitively and emotionally they are the same. However, in physical appearance they are not, and it is physical appearance that sets the stage for our interactions as human beings.

From the time we are old enough to listen to fairy tales and to see movies, we are made aware of the power of physical appearance. As Thurer wrote, "The physically disabled have bad literary press. Physical deformity, chronic illness, and any outer defect have come to symbolize an inner defect" (Thurer, 1980). Thus, the evil Captain Hook is an amputee; plotting witches are arthritic, kyphotic, and near-sighted; and as Pinocchio tells lies, his nose becomes progressively deformed.

The primary focus of the powerful movie "Mask" is how people responded to the brilliant, sensitive Rocky Dennis as though he were retarded because of his facial deformity. Persons who accepted and loved Rocky for the unique human being he was fell into one of two categories: those who had disabilities of their own (a stuttering motorcyclist and a blind girlfriend), or those without disabilities who were able to see beyond his physical appearance to the person inside.

Goffman has written of this acceptance of individuals who are "different" as acceptance by "the Own and the Wise." The Own empathize with the personal trials of those who are considered different because they are also different. The Wise live or work closely with those who suffer being different, and thus have gained a profound understanding of the individual person. Goffman writes, "Wise persons are marginal men before whom the individual with a fault need feel no shame nor exert self control, knowing that in spite of his failing he will be seen as an ordinary other" (Goffman, 1963). Witness a Special Olympics performance to see a powerful public display of acceptance by the Own and the Wise. We as physical therapists have superb opportunities to become one of the Wise and to demonstrate to patients, families, and the public how to see beyond physical disabilities.

ATTRACTION AND REPULSION

Many researchers who have studied the reactions of the nonhandicapped to the handicapped have noted that physical deviance, or difference, initially dominates the attention of the nonhandicapped. That is, when nonhandicapped people see a handicapped person for the first time they feel "engulfed by deviance." Notice the reactions of strangers (including yourself) to a multiply handicapped child in a wheelchair in a public place. Other children often stop and stare, only to be grabbed by a parent (who has been covertly staring) and told in a loud whisper, "It's not nice to stare."

Actually, staring may be the first step in eliminating social barriers imposed between the disabled and nondisabled because of physical appearance. Donaldson (1980), in summarizing techniques that may be used to change attitudes toward the disabled, has avocated the practice of "sanctioned staring." Sanctioned staring is staring at someone either unobserved or with explicit or implicit permission to stare. Entertainers and other public figures who have physical disabilities allow the phenomenon of sanctioned staring to occur. This sanctioned staring decreases the novelty of one's physical appearance, and thus decreases avoidance of that person because of physical differences.

In a "Bloom County" cartoon, Berke Breathed humorously portrayed the barrier of fear and avoidance that occurs before one is able to get past physical appearance differences (Fig. 9-2). Fortunately, once these physical differences (as well as similarities) are carefully noted, the nonhandicapped person can move beyond the feeling of being engulfed by devi-

ance and begin to respond to the person as a "normal," that is, nondeviant, human being.

IMPORTANCE OF FACE

Facial expressions of basic human emotions are universal. Eckman (1975) used photos of people expressing six different emotions (happiness, fear, surprise, anger, disgust-contempt, and sadness) to do research into the universality of human emotions. People from 13 literate cultures, such as in the countries of Brazil, England, and Africa, as well as two preliterate cultures in New Guinea were shown photos of people expressing these six emotions. They agreed on the emotions expressed approximately 75% or more of the time. Muscle actions of the forehead, eyebrows, and mouth as well as the amount of eye opening that typify each emotion appear to be biologically determined for the human species. Thus, angry people across the globe knit their eyebrows, project a harsh eye stare, and either press their lips tightly together or open them into a square shape.

Morris (1977) notes that children who are born both blind and deaf smile and frown appropriately even though they have never seen another person's facial expressions. Apparently the universality of facial expressions to convey emotions originates far back in our

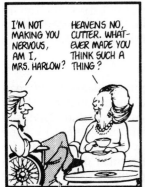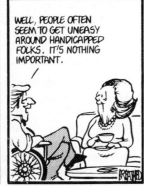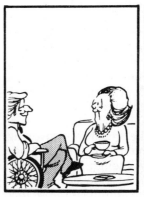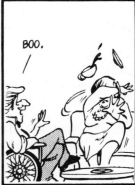

Figure 9-2. Cartoon portrayal of physical appearance that forms an initial barrier and interferes with expected social interactions. (© 1983, BLOOM COUNTY, by Berke Breathed. Washington Post Writers Group, reprinted with permission.)

evolutionary past, and allows us as a species to know who is friendly and who is not, as well as who is sad, fearful, or disgusted.

As physical therapists, we constantly use this innate ability to identify emotions portrayed in facial expressions in patient care. We see and respond to the fear of a patient who is being readied for a hubbard tank treatment for the first time, or the pain in someone's eyes as we move inflamed joints. At the same time, we find it difficult to communicate with a person whose face we cannot see because of bandages. We find similar difficulty in communicating with patients whose facial expressions we cannot "read" because of movement limitations imposed by burn scars, or those whose facial movements are distorted because of nasal-oral cancer surgery. When working with these patients we focus intensely on their eyes, and seek cues from other body movements to assess their comprehension and feeling states.

Our patients and their families also read our faces intently. Thus, they respond with grins to our facial expressions of joy with their hard-won success. Conversely, they feel acute discomfort and withdraw from our unconscious expressions of disgust at the sight and smell of their open wounds. In health care settings, both healers and patients seem particularly attuned to thoughts and feelings through the medium of the human face.

In an interesting series of experiments, Mehrabian (1981) attempted to discover which component of communication had the most powerful effect on conveying an attitude: What someone said (the verbal component), how someone said it (the vocal component), or what someone looked like when saying it (the facial component). The results of his studies showed that the facial component carried over half the weight (55%) and the vocal component (tone of voice) carried 38% of the weight of conveying an attitude. The content of the message counted for only 7%. Although it is probable that these exact percentages do not hold for conveying all situational attitudes, the *relative* weight of each component probably does hold true. Test it yourself. Just say, "Have a nice day" to someone harshly with a frown on your

face and your lips curled up, and see what the response is. Does the person respond to what you said, or to your tone of voice and what you looked like when you said it? When you greet your patient with "Hi, how are you?" are you conveying interest and concern, or harried brusqueness and preoccupation?

Remember, when verbal, vocal, and facial messages are contradictory, it is your face and tone of voice, not your words, that will determine the message you deliver. In addition, unconscious facial expressions may be combined with other body postures and gestures to give forceful (and sometimes unwanted) messages to patients. As Purtilo (1984) notes, "The health professional must be aware that nonverbal communication is as powerful as verbal communication. When a person's response is not what the health professional expects, the health professional's actions are probably speaking louder than his or her words."

BODY MOVEMENT RELATED TO COMMUNICATION

Besides facial expressions, our partial body movements (gestures) and full body movements (postures and gait), as well as movements within our own unconsciously designated personal space give others an enormous amount of information about us. This information conveys elements of our experiences and portrays present moods and expectations about our illness and wellness states.

GESTURES

The most important point in learning to read nonverbal aspects of communication is to learn to read the nonverbal cues *in context*. That is, a single gesture or postural movement by itself conveys little meaning. Movements must be interpreted within the context of the person's entire behavior and the situation in which the behavior is expressed. For example, standing with your arms folded across your chest is a component that could be part of a relaxed posture used while standing and talking to a friend. Conversely, arms folded across your chest could be a component of a defensive body stance if you also hold your trunk rigid, stand with your legs and feet spread apart and have a look of serious intent upon your face. Is the elderly person sitting in the wheelchair with his head lowered, tugging at the end of his short gown embarrassed, cold, frightened, or simply not aware of his surroundings? Skillful therapists move quickly to respond to these nonverbal cues with nonverbal gestures of their own: putting a blanket over the person's lap, touching for reassurance, or lifting the person's head to orient him to his immediate surroundings.

BODY POSTURES AND GAIT

Total body postures and gait reflect generalized moods. As you watch a child walk down the street, can you tell if she is feeling excited and on her way to a birthday party or reluctant and on her way to school? Of course! The position of her head, the amount of arm motion, the style and speed of her gait, and facial expression give you an enormous amount of information about her mood and her expectations for the immediate future. Try it yourself. Walk with determination, and then with sorrow. What is the difference? What message does your body give as you stride down a busy hospital corridor toward the room of your next patient? How does it differ from the message conveyed when you saunter down the street on a Saturday night on the town?

Your ability to receive and react to the psycho-emotional meaning of postural components of human movement will greatly enhance your abilities as a physical therapist. What if you see your patient approaching in a wheelchair with lowered head, slumped shoulders, and a generally "withdrawn" posture. Would you set him up for a vigorous exercise routine he physically "should" be able to perform independently? Or would you stay with him, using physical guidance and reassuring touch to orient him away from despondency and toward productive activity? Does the mother of a multiply handicapped child hold her child close to her with comfort, or away from her body like an object? Along with treating this child, what teaching must you do with this child's parents? Does your patient with low back pain ambulate with greater or less endurance when his family members are present? What is happening? How can you use this information in formulating your treatment goals?

PERSONAL SPACE

Every person has an invisible comfortable boundary around her body. Similar to animals who defend their territories, human beings have similar invisible "territories" that we claim and defend against intrusion. In the classic work, *The Silent Language* (1959), Hall points out that the size of this territory or space that surrounds the body, and to which we lay personal claim, varies considerably across cultures. A person from one culture may feel decidedly uncomfortable with the personal space alloted to him by a person from another culture. To quote Hall:

> In Latin America the interaction distance is much less than it is in the United States. Indeed, people cannot talk comfortably with one another unless they are very close to the distance that evokes either sexual or hostile feelings in the North American. The result is that when they move close, we withdraw and back away. As a consequence, they think we are distant or cold, withdrawn and unfriendly. We on the other hand, are constantly accusing them of breathing down our necks, crowding us, and spraying our faces.

Define your own personal space by having an acquaintance slowly approach you from the front, back, and either side. Tell the person to stop the moment you begin to feel uncomfortable with her closeness. For many of us, our personal space is an oval. We feel more comfortable with public closeness on either side of us rather than in front of us. This may be related to ancient feelings of personal defense during face-to-face contact with unknown animals or other humans.

Neutral conversation space is considered from 2 to 5 ft from the other person. If closer than 2 ft in our culture, you begin to intrude upon personal space that ordinarily is considered comfortable for intimate conversation. Watch your patient's body movements to determine his comfort zone with your closeness during conversation. If he flinches and withdraws physically or turns his head away, try backing up until he relaxes and resumes eye contact with you.

How you stand within your personal space can also feel more or less vulnerable. Try standing with your arms across your chest, then down at your sides, and finally out away from your body with your palms forward. In which position do you feel most vulnerable, and in which do you feel least vulnerable? Think of how you can use this information in caring for your patients. Where might you position yourself to talk closely and quietly with a frightened patient? Is the unsteadiness in training a patient to balance with a new prosthesis the result of physical instability, or a sudden feeling of vulnerability because of a body position with arms away? The more aware you are of intuitive comfort associated with your own body within your personal space, the greater skill you will have in working with patients.

NONVERBAL COMMUNICATION IN PATIENT CARE

There are many nonverbal communication techniques we can use to facilitate our ability to work swiftly and effectively in patient care. Use of nonverbal forms of language to communicate specific concepts, active listening skills, pacing, eye contact, and touch can be used with people from all cultural backgrounds, of all ages, in varying degrees of wellness states. Our knowledge of these psychosociomotor skills is as important to our function as skilled health professionals as is our understanding of biological and physical components of movement.

NONVERBAL LANGUAGE

There are two basic ways of communicating, or coding and transmitting information between two or more people. One form of communication is known as analogic and the other is referred to as digital.

Analogic codification uses a symbol similar to the thing or idea for which the symbol stands. For example, a drawing of a house, two adults, three children, and a dog is an analogic codification of someone's family. Gestures are also a form of analogic codification, as when you point in the direction one is to go, or shake your head vigorously from side to side to indicate "no." Digital codification uses symbols that are not similar to the object. Use of letters (alpha) and numbers (numeric) are the two types of digital codification systems with which we are most familiar.

Analogic codification is the more ancient communication system. It is speculated to have preceded digital communication systems by thousands of years. Primitive people drew pictures of hunting expeditions on cave walls to be read and interpreted by all who passed by. We are each aware that when people have difficulty communicating by use of digital codification, they revert to the use of an analogic system. Thus, while giving directions to someone who is unfamiliar with the English language, we use pantomime and exaggerated facial expressions along with single words to indicate drive, turn right, bridge, turn left, church, and stop. Those who have traveled in foreign countries laughingly remember rubbing their stomachs to indicate hunger when trying to ask directions to a local restaurant. When people are not listening to the words we are saying (digital communication), our use of gestures becomes more frequent and pronounced. Witness an animated conversation between two people, each of whom is trying to communicate verbally a different point and neither of whom is listening to the words of the other.

Deaf sign language codes, especially the American Sign Language Code, are extensively used in the United States. However, Skelly (1979) notes a common problem with most sign language codes: They are 90% symbolic (that is, they employ digital codification), and must be learned as one would learn a foreign language. Thus, these forms of sign language may be ineffective for use with persons who have an impaired cortex, such as patients with head trauma, or those who have endured cerebrovascular accidents affecting language and memory centers, or those with mental retardation. Equally important, digital-based sign language systems are not effective for use with patients and families who use a different digital codification system than one based on the English alphabet.

Skelly makes a strong case for the use of American Indian Hand Talk, which is based on an analogic codification system and uses pantomime. This system was developed for communication among people who did not share a similar linguistic background. For example, Figure 9-3 illustrates how to communicate the word "breathing." Two or more basic pantomime gestures may be combined to communicate a more complex word or feeling. Figure 9-4 illustrates the combination of two words that could be interpreted to indicate "hospital." It takes some practice to use this hand language skillfully, but physical therapists should find many of the gestures in Skelly's book *Amer-Ind Gestural Code Based on Universal American Indian Hand Talk* very useful in their clinical practice.

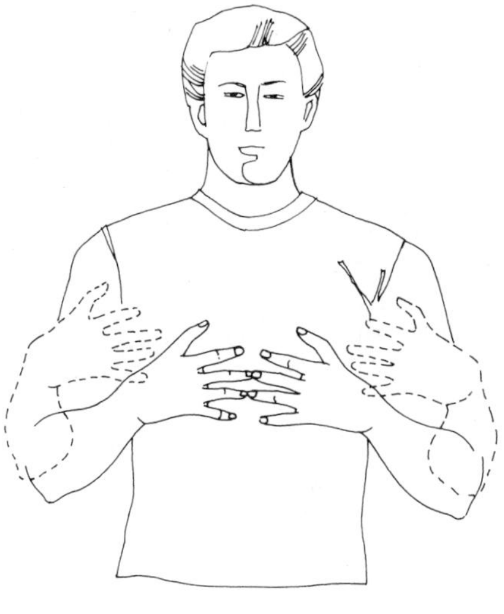

ACTIVE LISTENING

As physical therapists we hold valuable information on how the human body functions and what can be done to prevent and alleviate problems associated with movement dysfunction. Upon entering our first days of clinical practice, many of us rushed eagerly to pour out to our patients our knowledge and opinions about their illnesses. How confident we were that this information would be gratefully received! In time we learned that we often "missed" with our information, giving too much too soon, or in too much detail, or to the wrong family member at the wrong time. Gradually we be-

Breathe
(repetitive)

Breath
Breathing
Exhalation
Inhalation
Lungs
Respiration
Respirator

Both hands rest lightly on chest, palms against body, fingers spread. Hands are moved forward and upward from chest about one inch, then back to chest. Repeat three times.

Figure 9-3. American Indian Hand Talk for the word *breathing*. (Reprinted by permission of the publisher from Skelly M: Amer-Ind Gestural Code Based on Universal American Indian Hand Talk, p 239. Copyright 1979 by Elsevier Science Publishing Co., Inc.)

gan to ask more questions and listen more carefully to what the patient was telling us about his state of health. We learned that patients or family members often had concerns or defined physical functioning in ways that were quite opposite from what we as physical therapists could objectively observe, measure, and make pronouncements about. A beginning physical therapist quickly learns the importance of the subjective examination—the gaining of information about the cause and course of dysfunction from the patient's perspective.

What skills do you need to gather health care information completely and accurately? You must be able to listen, and to coach the patient into sharing with you her experience of illness. Moreover, you must do so without interjecting your thoughts and opinions.

Try this exercise. Find a person who is willing to spend 15 minutes with you in an active

Pain (static)

Ache
Agony
Distress
Hurt
Ill
Nauseated
Sick
Sore
Suffer
Throb
Unhealthy
Unwell
Upset

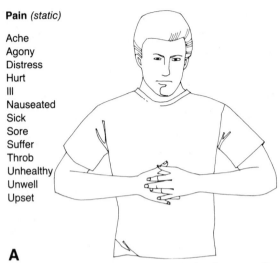

A

Right palm is pressed to abdomen. Left palm covers fingers of right and presses inward. (Signal is clarified if torso leans forward.)

Shelter (static)

Build
Building
Dwell
Home
House
Residence
Roof

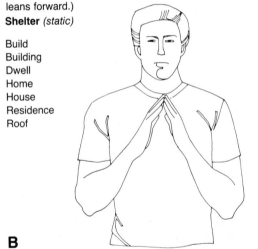

B

Hands are brought together, chest high, palms facing, tips of middle fingers touching. Wrists are about five inches apart, forming a gable roof line. (The signal can be executed with one hand by forming the gable at the finger-base knuckles or at the wrist. It can be clarified, if necessary, by placing it over the head.)

Figure 9-4. *(A, B)* American Indian Hand Talk for the word *hospital* is a combination of two words, *pain* and *shelter*. (Reprinted by permission of the publisher from Skelly M: Amer-Ind Gestural Code Based on Universal American Hand Talk, pp 358, 388. Copyright 1979 by Elsevier Science Publishing Co., Inc.)

listening exercise. This person becomes the problem owner and thinks up a problem she wants to solve. The problem can be very specific (like overeating) or elusive (like procrastination). You as the listener must follow three rules of active listening: no advice, use of probe questions, and empathic support.

The first rule is *not* to give any advice. Along with giving no advice, be careful not to say that you know *exactly* how your partner feels because you have had the same problem! Remember the uniqueness of each human being. No two people have exactly the same set of circumstances surrounding a given problem, and no two people will ever solve even a similar problem in exactly the same way. Your role as an active listener is to create an atmosphere where the problem owner can gain increased insight into a problem and begin to solve it from her own unique perspective.

The second rule of active listening is to question the problem owner, either by paraphrasing and returning information given to you (to clarify what was said) or by using open-ended probe questions. Examples of open-ended probe questions are "Can you say more about it?", "Can you give an example?", "Why is this a problem for you?", and "In what ways have you thought about change?"

The third rule of active listening is to give sympathetic verbal and nonverbal support. Verbal support responses are short, such as, "I see" or "Uh-huh." Nonverbal support responses include empathic body postures such as leaning forward, direct eye contact, and nodding your head in agreement.

After six or seven minutes, switch roles so that you also have a chance to experience talking to a problem solver who is engaged in active listening. When you finish this active listening exercise, talk with each other about the experience. Did the problem (and perhaps potential solutions) become clearer to you as you were supported in talking through your problem? How did you feel about the person who was listening to you in a calm, supportive way? How did you feel as the problem solver who was not engaged in a customary role of giving advice? How did you help the problem owner by *not* giving advice for a few minutes?

The primarily nonverbal communication skill of active listening is a superb technique to use with patients, families, and professional colleagues. Being listened to, *really* listened to, is a rare phenomenon in our bustling health care settings where personnel rely predominantly on invasive diagnostic procedures, laboratory and radiographic tests, and pharmaceutical or surgical interventions to restore health.

For the physical therapist who uses primarily noninvasive manual skills for evaluation and treatment, and who depends upon patient-demonstrated and patient-reported physical performance as a guide to treatment planning, active listening skills are vital. The atmosphere created by consciously engaging in active listening is one of interest, and calm and helpful support. Given such an atmosphere, patients often respond with openness and trust, and the information you seek for evaluation and treatment comes quickly and definitively.

Active listening can also be an extremely powerful and efficient tool to use with people who are having difficulty taking active responsibility in working toward their physical recovery. It is easy to become a passive patient when one is asked questions that demand only "yes" or "no" responses. It is much more difficult to be passive when asked "Please describe. . ." and someone waits quietly and patiently until a response is given. As your patients describe facts, reason, and question out loud, and are supported by you in verbal and nonverbal ways, they unknowingly begin to assume accountability. They move from passive responding to active engagement in their physical and psychological recovery.

Finally, active listening can be a useful technique in working with an anxious or agitated person who needs to calm himself so he can be receptive to information he may need from you. By assuming an active listening stance, you support the person in "talking through" his agitation until he can reach a point where he is ready for input. At this time, the patient will ask questions to elicit the information you are waiting to give.

PACING

Another effective form of nonverbal communication that we can use in patient care comes from the field of neurolinguistic programming. The key to this form of communication is to pace your input to another person's reality. This can be done verbally or nonverbally. King and co-workers (1983) give an excellent example of verbal pacing.

> Thus if a child has just abraded a knee from a fall, a few appropriate statements such as the following could be immediately offered: "I bet that hurts terribly," "It's even starting to bleed a little," "No wonder you're crying, I'd be screaming, too." Phrases such as these, spoken congruently with the appropriate expression and feeling, but not in any particular order, would usually establish an adequate pace for the child at that moment. Inserting a lead statement such as, "And I bet that will continue to really hurt terribly, maybe for a whole minute or two" usually results in the desired outcome—the cessation of pain in a minute or two. Contrast this approach with a more typical approach one might almost instinctively take with such a child; that is, to say "It doesn't hurt that much" (almost trying to convince the child that his or her experience of pain is not valid). Since there is no congruence between your verbalized expression and the child's experience, you have not set up the conditions necessary to lead the child out of the pain.

Nonverbal pacing includes mirroring the patient's body with your own. You might assume the other person's posture, breathing rate, position of hands or feet, and even the tone of voice. Not all of these body aspects need to be mirrored at once; one or two are effective. It is important that this pacing is below the person's consciousness level, and it usually is because we are so often unaware of what our own bodies are doing. Try nonverbal pacing with your friends and see if you don't quickly "connect" with them.

Most effective, of course, is the combined use of verbal and nonverbal pacing that some very effective communicators use naturally. One more example from King (1983) illustrates this.

> A patient had stationed himself inside a room, screaming, cursing, and disrupting the furniture. Initial efforts by the staff could not stop him. The (occupational) therapist, who was passing by, walked in yelling in a loud, frantic voice, "YOU ARE REALLY UPSET!" After a two-second pause the therapist continued in a slow, soft, soothing tone, with relaxed body accompaniment, "Weren't you"? The patient answered in a clear, calm voice as if the event had occurred the day before, that indeed he had been upset, and started to discuss the situation matter-of-factly with this staff member. In only a few moments this professional communicator was able to pace the patient's emotional state and lead him to an alternative state, thereby beginning the therapeutic process.

EYE CONTACT

Another area of nonverbal communication in patient care is eye contact. For skilled therapists more information is conveyed more quickly through the patient's eyes than any other body part. We continually seek eye contact to assess emotional and physical states. How many times have you seen a therapist talking to a patient who is hunched over in a wheelchair? More than likely the therapist is kneeling with her head in an awkward position trying to make face-to-face contact, and more specifically, eye contact with the patient. It is very difficult to talk to a patient who has his eyes averted or closed.

When students are in the process of acquiring their professional skills, they use little eye contact at first. They are watching what position their hands are in, while thinking about what position they should move their hands to next. Students who look at a limb and tell the limb to relax will find, as their skills increase, that their eyes shift from their hands and the patient's limb to the patient's eyes. It then becomes possible to let their increasingly

skilled hands search for muscle tension while their eye contact exchanges information with the patient as to what the patient is feeling. There is basic human connectedness as well as a powerful communication flow in eye contact between two people, which we search for and use in reestablishing health.

Eye contact can also be used to help calm a crying patient. Certainly there are many good reasons why someone may need to cry. Crying helps release the tremendous amount of physical and emotional tension that accrues with loss and despair. At other times crying may have obscure emotional antecedents. Sometimes patients cry because of lack of central nervous system control, or because crying will allow them escape from a new and fearful situation. One technique you can use with these patients is to ask them to look at you while you speak slowly and quietly to them. Because it is physically impossible to look someone in the eye and cry at the same time, this technique can have a calming effect on the patient and may allow both of you to focus on the next important step in the patient's treatment regime.

TOUCH

Perhaps the most basic and powerful form of nonverbal communication between the patient and you is touch. The skin is the largest sensory organ in the body, and tactile sensitivity is probably the first sensory process to be activated when human life begins.

Touch is basic to survival and growth for all high-level mammals, including humans. Montague (1986) writes:

> During the nineteenth century more than half the infants in their first year of life regularly died from a disease called marasmus, a Greek word meaning "wasting away." The disease was also known as infantile atrophy or debility. As late as the second decade of the twentieth century the death rate for infants under one year of age in various foundling institutions throughout the United States was nearly 100 percent.

This high mortality rate was eventually traced directly to the fact that with so many infants and so few nursemaids, only physical care such as feeding, diapering, and bathing was given to infants in foundling institutions. There was no time available for cuddling, rocking, or individual physical bonding with another human being. In fact, not until after World War II, when research was conducted to find the cause of marasmus, was physical touch even identified as a human need that was basic to life.

Today children who are apathetic, have delayed motor abilities, and are well below normal for their birth weight because of lack of physical and social human contact are identified as abused children. Much of the subsequent therapy with these children includes gentle and prolonged physical contact. To assist with normal child development and encourage parent-child bonding, physical therapists are often in a position to teach parents how to touch through infant massage. One particularly good videotape for teaching parents infant massage is "Babystrokes" (Edwards, 1987).

Touch is no less important for older children, adolescents, and young, middle-aged, or older adults. A problem in our society is that beyond earliest childhood, touch is often confused with sexuality. Huss (1977) reports, "We equate touch with sex unless it is perfectly clear there is no connection. Thus we use touch sparingly to express warmth, affection, understanding, and acceptance." Many writers have examined the phenomenon of touch and the cultural consequences of the lack of touch. Everything from eager participation in rough and tumble sport to sex crimes has been attributed to lack of early and ongoing simple, caring touch.

It is virtually impossible for physical therapists to treat patients without using touch. If your touch feels safe to the recipient (shoulder, arm, and hand are generally safe places to touch first-time patients), touch can facilitate immediate rapport between you and your patient. Touch implies that you are interested in and trust the other person. Patients appear to comply with requests more frequently when they are touched than when they are not touched. Touch also implies that the other person has something important to give to you: information, acknowledgment, and return

trust. Verbal exchanges with patients can proceed more quickly and are often more self-revealing when touch is used. Beyond communication, the use of touch by physical therapists to evaluate and treat is self-evident.

In our rapidly changing, highly industrialized society, lack of touch appears to be an increasingly obvious problem. John Naisbitt in his book *Megatrends* wrote of a high tech-high touch society. He suggested that the more people are in contact with high-tech machines in their work, the more they seek high-touch situations. This phenomenon, he contends, explains the rapid rise of birthing centers, hospices, and wellness centers that include "de-stressing" massages. First-person accounts of illness and disability almost always include tender and poignant remembrances of the few health care personnel who touched in a caring way.

We in physical therapy would do well to heed these concerns and ensure that our health care practices continue to carry a strong component of laying on of hands along with our use of the latest high-frequency electrical stimulation equipment. Our hands heal by guiding and stimulating movement and decreasing musculoskeletal pain, as well as calming, reassuring, and comforting people in great physical and emotional stress. When massaging or mobilizing a patient brings forth an unanticipated emotional and cognitive self-disclosure, we are also aware of the intimate relationship between the mind and body. Those of us who know and use ancient acupressure points to induce tranquility and decrease pain are also dramatically made aware of the power of human touch. In fact, we touch people physically so often that we frequently forget the meaning this has for our patients until we become a patient and are touched by someone else.

CONCLUSION

Our awareness of the nonverbal aspects of human movement is as important to our skill as therapists as our basic knowledge of the chemical, biological, and physical basis of human structure and function. Physical therapists have the opportunity to become particularly skilled in nonverbal communication because, from the beginning of our professional education, we train our eyes to interpret movement. Information derived from our patient's facial expressions and postures, our use of active listening skills, and our sensitivity to personal space is absolutely essential to the process of patient evaluation. Our use of nonverbal communication is at least equally as important as any other intervention strategy in the process of healing another human being. You should proceed with the following chapters on evaluation and treatment thoroughly grounded in all the theoretical and applied foundations of human movement: structural, biobehavioral, and sociobehavioral.

ANNOTATED BIBLIOGRAPHY

Donaldson J: Changing attitudes towards handicapped persons: A review and analysis of research. Except Child 46:504, 1980 (Compilation of research data resulting in the identification of specific techniques to induce more favorable attitudes towards people with physical handicaps. Includes ideas for change specific to movement experiences and nonverbal communication.)

Druckman D, Rozelle R, Baxter J: Nonverbal Communication: Survey, Theory and Research. Beverly Hills, CA, Sage Publications, 1982 (Synthesis of a wide range of theories and empirical findings in the field of nonverbal communication research. Includes a reference list of over 240 articles.)

Eckman P: Face muscles talk every language. Psychology Today, Sept 1975, p 35 (Popular account of Dr. Eckman's crosscultural work with facial expressions and emotions.)

Edwards C: The Lifestrokes Library: Babystrokes. (Videotape.) Burlingame, CA, Mentor Publishing, 1987 (Easy-to-learn instructions for joyful infant massage to increase infant physical and emotional health and to bond child with family members.)

Goffman E: Stigma: Notes on the Management of Spoiled Identity. New York, Simon and Schuster, 1963. Reprint, 1986 (Fascinating sociological analysis of how people who are prohibited from full social acceptance in our culture by virtue of physical, mental, or social differences survive. As timely reading today as when the work was first published in 1963.)

Hall E: The Silent Language. New York, Doubleday, 1959 (Delightfully written classic on cultural differences in unspoken aspects of life such as use of time and space. In the author's words, "If this book has a message it is that we must learn to understand the 'out-of-awareness' aspects of communication. We must never assume that we are fully aware of what we communicate to someone else.")

Huss A: Touch with care or a caring touch? Am J Occup Ther 31:11, 1977 (Humanistically written overview of touch as it relates to communication and healing in health care settings.)

King M, Novik L, Citrenbaum C: Irrestible Communication: Creative Skills for the Health Professional. Philadelphia, WB Saunders, 1983 (Intriguing book filled with specific health care examples of direct and indirect communication skills that have been successfully used by creative psychotherapists.)

Mehrabian A: Silent Messages: Implicit Communication of Emotions and Attitudes, 2nd ed. Belmont, CA, Wadsworth Publishing, 1981 (One of the pioneer psychologists in the field of nonverbal communication presents findings from 442 reference sources in this informal and very readable paperback book.)

Montague A: Touching: The Human Significance of the Skin, 3rd ed. New York, Harper & Row, 1986 (First published in 1971, this book was the ground-breaking work on the documented role of touch in human development, especially as it relates to physical and mental health.)

Morris D: Manwatching: A Field Guide to Human Behavior. New York, Harry N Abrams, 1977 (Heavily illustrated with photographs and drawings, this oversized book is a compendium of crosscultural nonverbal behavior in a wide variety of playful and serious situations.)

Purtilo R: Health Professional/Patient Interaction, 3rd ed. Philadelphia, WB Saunders, 1984 (Dr. Purtilo has turned philosophical, psychological, and sociological theories on illness, health, and effective helping behaviors into practical advice for health care givers. The theme of effective interpersonal interactions, including nonverbal communication skills, is sensitively portrayed throughout.

Skelly M: Amer-Ind Gestural Code Based on Universal American Indian Hand Talk. New York, Elsevier North-Holland, 1979 (Well-written, clearly illustrated book presents an analogic codification system useful with a wide variety of patients and families in any health care setting.)

Thurer S: Disability and monstrosity: A look at literary distortions of handicapping conditions, Rehabil Lit 41:12, 1980 (Dr. Thurer explores and attempts to explain the stereotyping of literary and dramatic characters with physical disabilities as being endowed with inherently good or bad traits.)

PART III

Causes of Movement Dysfunction and Physical Disability

10 Musculoskeletal Causes

MARY MOFFROID
NANCY ZIMNY

Potential sources of musculoskeletal dysfunction include structural imbalance, surgical alterations, birth defects, pain, edema, weakness, fatigue, changes in central nervous system control, and tissue degeneration. In this chapter we examine each of these factors from the perspective of its effects on the tissues of the musculoskeletal system, and the subsequent ramifications for the functional unit (the physiologic joint). The specific tissues addressed here include muscle and connective tissue (bone, articular cartilage, fibrocartilage, ligament, fascia, tendon, muscle sheaths, and fat).

Figure 10-1 illustrates the structural relationships of the components of the functional unit, the physiologic joint. Note the continuity of the periosteum with the joint capsule's two layers. The muscle, tendon, and osseotendinous attachment are intimately related and interdependent with each other, as well as with the joint capsule. Intracapsular structures include synovium, articular cartilage, and sometimes fibrocartilage. Although the contributions of blood vessels and nervous tissue to musculoskeletal function and dysfunction are not specifically addressed here, they are also essential components of the physiologic joint. Ideal functioning of the physiologic joint depends on the interaction of all its parts.

STRUCTURAL IMBALANCE

The body appears symmetrical, and the untrained eye expects this to be so. Normal function rests on the assumption that the right and left halves will work together and share equally in movement tasks. Typically, this right-left symmetry includes the expectations that leg lengths are equal; that arm lengths are equal; that the force potential of the right and left erector spinae muscles is the same; and that the right and left hip joints demonstrate equal amounts of active and passive movement.

However, on closer examination, the right and left halves are not symmetrical. This is apparent visually if you juxtapose the right side of the face with its mirror image, and then compare the composite to a face constructed from the left side coupled with its mirror image. The two composite faces are different, demonstrating the lack of symmetry in structure and expression. Figure 10-2 illustrates a full image of an intact face, the two right sides, and the two left sides.

Although not as easily demonstrated, other right-left asymmetries are also present. Functionally, physical therapists are concerned with the balance of the musculoskeletal components of the body, which implies that limb lengths, joint flexibility, ligamentous integrity, and right-left muscle forces are in balance. If some asymmetry is normal, what are the expected ranges of asymmetry that we accept as within normal limits?

Muscle force, which connotes strength, must be assessed with factors of joint position, velocity, acceleration, and lever length in mind. Torque, work, or power are the common means of expressing muscle strength. Muscle

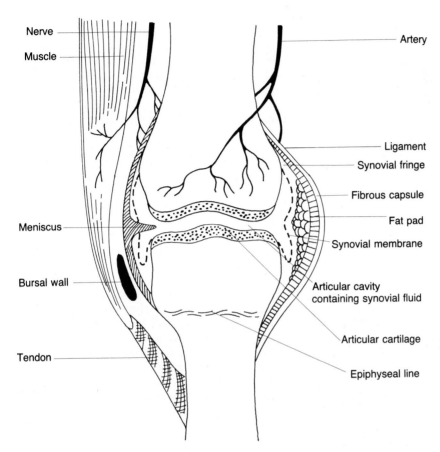

Nerve

Muscle

Artery

Ligament

Synovial fringe

Fibrous capsule

Fat pad

Meniscus

Synovial membrane

Bursal wall

Articular cavity
containing synovial fluid

Tendon

Articular cartilage

Epiphyseal line

Figure 10-1.   Physiologic joint. (Wright V, Dowsen D, Kerr J: Structure of joints. Int Rev Connect Tissue Res 6:106, 1973)

strength of the right and left sides is more similar in the proximal muscles, whereas we accept a 10% to 15% difference in strength of the distal muscles. In the upper extremities, the right distal muscles tend to be stronger regardless of dominance, whereas the differences in the distal muscles of the lower extremities are less predictable, partly because determination of dominance in the lower extremities is less certain.

With joint flexibility, we accept a 5% difference between goniometric measurements of the right and left sides. The difference reflects posture and use habits, which in turn affect muscle length and joint capsule laxity, and produce other connective tissue discrepancies. Circumference of limbs may also differ be-

tween the right and left sides, particularly in persons who engage in unilateral sports, such as tennis or baseball.

Therefore, more than 10% to 15% difference in strength of distal muscles, or more than 5% difference in flexibility between the right and left sides, suggests that an imbalance needs to be addressed. Conclusions about the trunk present a much more difficult problem because there is no right-left basis for comparison. Furthermore, comparison with age- and sex-related values requires norms that currently do not exist.

In addition to right-left balance, physical therapists are concerned with the balance between synergists and their antagonists. For ex-

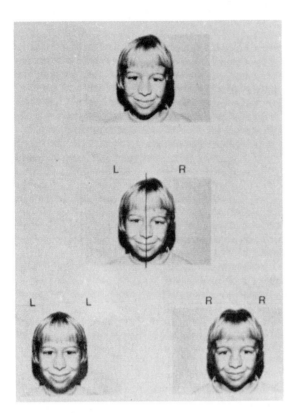

Figure 10-2. Asymmetry of facial expression: *(top, middle)* the intact face; *(bottom left)* composite of the two left sides; *(bottom right)* composite of the two right sides. (Bryden MP: Laterality: Functional Asymmetry in the Intact Brain, p 131. New York, Academic Press, 1982)

ample, the flexors and extensors about a joint need not be equal in contractile force, but it is believed that there is an optimal balance or ratio of agonist to antagonist muscle forces about each joint.

Physical therapists are concerned with musculoskeletal imbalances and recognize that these imbalances can lead to injury or dysfunction or both. However, we must be careful not to identify an imbalance where none truly exists, or where an apparent imbalance masks a problem that has arisen from another source. Correcting an apparent imbalance that is not creating any dysfunction can be as disruptive as failing to identify a musculoskeletal imbalance that is truly disruptive.

The body has the ability to adapt to some degree of imbalance of the musculoskeletal system. The threshold for when an asymmetry will become symptomatic or problematic is unknown, and probably varies from one person to another. Therefore, planning intervention for musculoskeletal imbalances is a clinical judgment. However, if the therapist knows normal variances and expected use situations, rational decisions can be made. For example, comparatively less quadriceps torque at high speeds in the right limb (compared with the left) of an older, sedentary person may not present a problem, whereas a young football player with this inequality may encounter a serious injury. In the latter case, intervention would be prudent, whereas in the former, it would not be. Right-left comparisons to evaluate symmetry are necessary, but alone are not sufficient to determine the appropriateness of intervention. Age- and sex-related norms and individual needs are also important.

Inequalities or imbalances that do not occur in isolation and that produce pain are cause for concern. The body compensates for many imbalances, and these compensations lead to further malalignment and eventual pathologic conditions. Compensatory mechanisms occur in both closed and open kinematic chains. The lower extremity in weight-bearing situations is a good example of a closed kinematic chain. The distal lever (the foot) is fixed on the floor during stance and the positions of the proximal joints are directly determined by what happens at the foot-ankle complex.

Figure 10-3 illustrates the chain of events in a closed kinematic chain with one abnormal link (a short heel cord) at the beginning. If the heel cord is short, prohibiting any dorsiflexion, the tibia cannot advance forward over the fixed foot. If the tibia cannot advance forward, then the body's center of gravity will be further behind the ankle, creating a greater torque and greater work load. To avoid this inefficiency, the knee may hyperextend, permitting the body's center of gravity to be closer to the fulcrum. Hyperextension of the knee does not usually occur in isolation. Short hip flexors may cause the pelvis to tilt anteriorly, inclining the body forward. This new inclined position is

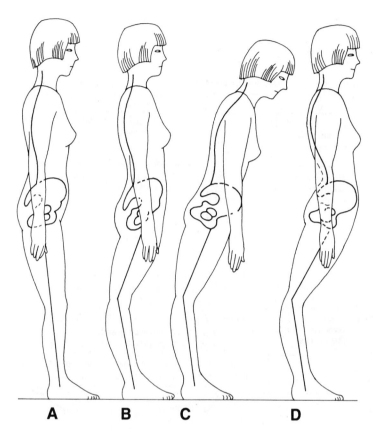

A   B   C   D

Figure 10-3. Postural changes as a compensation for shortened heel cord. *(A)* Center of gravity is behind the base of support. *(B)* Knee hyperextension compensates for the altered center of gravity. *(C)* The body is inclined forward and the head is facing down. *(D)* Increased lumbar lordosis and thoracic kyphosis with continued knee hyperextension compensate for the alterations in center of gravity and head position.

not consistent with our righting mechanisms, which act to maintain horizontal gaze and erect head position. Therefore, additional compensations of increased lumbar lordosis and thoracic kyphosis occur to permit the head to be upright. From the neck up, this person looks fine; however, from the neck down, these postural changes are sufficient over time to evoke damaging structural changes.

A structural limitation, such as a short heel cord, will cause different compensations if analyzed in an open kinematic chain, as in the swing phase of normal gait. In this instance, the ankle may not reach the desired neutral position from plantarflexion. Possible compensations may include extension of the toes or circumduction of the entire lower extremity for the foot to clear the floor.

In the upper half of the body, the interrelationship and interdependence of musculo-skeletal structures are also apparent. Figure 10-4 diagrams the potential results of having a forward head posture.

Not all imbalances arise from compensations for musculoskeletal inequalities. One theory for some types of scoliosis is based on alterations in the vestibular and righting mechanisms. If awareness of body alignment is not accurate, incorrect adjustments occur to achieve a perceived balance. If the spine deviates laterally with accompanying rotation of the vertebrae, then scapular and pelvic relations will be altered, affecting shoulder and hip function. Altered shoulder and hip function will necessarily determine different parameters for hand and foot movement.

Understanding the etiology of imbalances and the resulting compensatory changes are everyday challenges to analyzing and solving problems within the musculoskeletal system.

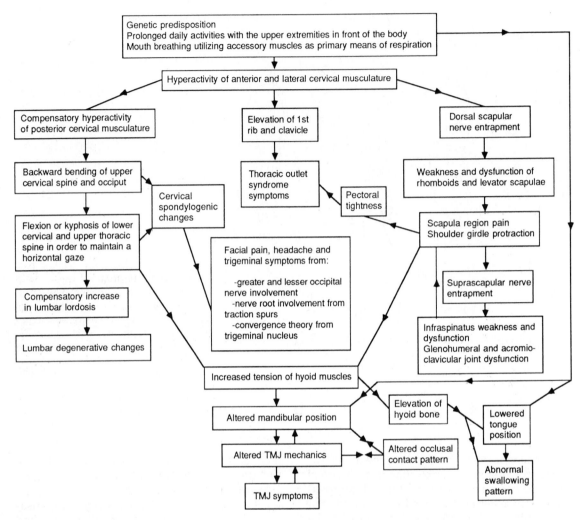

Figure 10-4. Chronology of events for forward head posture. (Darnell M: A proposed chronology of events for forward head posture. Journal of Craniomandibular Practice 1(4):53, © by Chroma, Inc, 1983)

The remainder of this section on musculoskeletal imbalances will consider problems originating in connective tissue and in muscle.

CONNECTIVE TISSUE: BONE

Bone is a dynamic tissue that is constantly being remodeled. The human skeleton replaces 2% to 3% of its organic and inorganic matrices every year. The rate and shape of remodeling is affected by mechanical, physiologic, and pathologic stimuli. The physical therapist is aware of the need for bone to develop and maintain itself so that sufficient support is provided and a balance exists within the entire musculoskeletal system. Failure to achieve these needs results in dysfunctions such as postural faults and pain from uneven leg lengths; ligamentous avulsions from weakened osseoligamentous junctions; unprecipitated fractures from decreases in the gel-like ground substance of bone; and postural changes and pain from compression of cancellous bone in osteoporosis.

Some of the mechanical, physiologic, and pathologic factors affecting bone maintenance are addressed below. In the following discussion, we will look more closely at changes in bone metabolism that eventually result in observable changes in musculoskeletal balance and function. Physical therapists hope that tissue imbalances can be reduced or even avoided, so that the resulting dysfunction from musculoskeletal imbalances can be minimized or prevented.

Mechanical Factors

If bone is excessively bowed, the convex surface (that being stressed) becomes osteoclastic. That is, osteoclasts (cells specializing in bone resorption) work to resorb the bone on the convex surface. The concave surface (that being abnormally compressed) becomes osteoblastic, or bone forming. Because bracing is used frequently to supplement the role of bones as support structures, the bracing must be adequate to maintain the intended shapes of bones. Weight bearing too early in development, or with inadequate support, places stresses on bones that can result in abnormal remodeling. Bone is a viscoelastic substance, with some potential for recovery from positional deformities; thus, time can be a detriment. Sustained periods of excessive stress on bone produce more changes than short periods of stress with intermittent rests. Exercise is considered a stress, and differences in cross-sectional areas between the right humerus and the left humerus have been reported in professional tennis players. In contrast, excessive and unrelenting stresses can actually decrease the amount of bone substance.

Fractures result from excessive bone deformation, either stress or strain. Because bone is a viscoelastic tissue, the occurrence of a fracture depends on the rate of stress as well as on the amount of force. A rapid rate of stress is less likely to cause a fracture. However, soft tissue damage is the unpleasant sequel to the rapid impact. Fractures present short-term and long-term challenges to musculoskeletal balance. Short-term concerns relate to casting, pain, and weakness. The recovery process, in which there may be atrophy, limited flexibility, and structural alterations of the bone, lead to gross imbalances in the musculoskeletal system. If these imbalances are not resolved, posture, patterns of use, alignment, and efficiency of movement will be affected. Even with resolution, long-term problems may still arise because old fracture sites are more vulnerable to arthritic changes.

Physiologic Factors

Bone responds to internal as well as external stresses. *Muscular forces* can remodel the skeleton and cause structural changes. For example, muscle contractions place a stress on bone at the insertion; if the stress is frequent and forceful enough, it will lead to bone hypertrophy at the insertion. Respective sizes of tubercles and tuberosities on skeletal remains provide clues to physical anthropologists about the relative strength and some of the functional activities of the individual.

Circulatory compromise in bony tissue leads to ischemia and collapse of the bony structure. Bone is highly dependent on circulation for development, growth, maintenance, and repair. Without the presence of adequate circulation, bone undergoes necrosis. Obvious structural imbalances result, such as unequal leg lengths due to necrosis of the femoral head. Ground reaction forces during gait have different effects on limbs of different lengths. The asymmetrical forces at weight acceptance are translated differently to more proximal structures, so that hip and lumbosacral activity differs on the two sides. Some clinicians believe that the sacroiliac joints, when unequally stressed, create pelvic obliquities that can lead to low back pain. However, the degree to which the sacroiliac joint is mobile in persons past the fifth decade of life is frequently challenged.

Growth of bone is a complex process. *Uneven growth rates* of long bones can result from a variety of causes, including positional restraints, epiphyseal fractures, and genetic disturbances. Whatever the cause (or causes), uneven lengths of bones or disproportioned bones can dramatically affect musculoskeletal function. Having short upper arms in relation to torso length has been cited as a contributing factor to low back dysfunction. Uneven growth rates of ribs has been suggested as a precipitating cause of scoliosis. Theories abound, but all have a common denominator: normal alignment and proportion are essential ingredients for smooth and efficient function. Balanced alignment with normal opportunity for movement is essential in utero, just as it is during the rest of the life span.

Pathologic Factors

Bone is susceptible to neoplasms, to infections, to changes in the body's regulatory system, and to many other injuries. Any of these insults can precipitate change (either proliferation or resorption) in bone tissue. Because not all bones are affected similarly, imbalances occur, and the results may be postural asymmetries as described above. Other results of changes in bony structure include overall weakness, fatigue, and pain. Bones form movable links and are important for support, shock absorption, muscle attachments, momentum, and metabolic homeostasis. One weak link is usually discernable because of compensatory changes, such as substitutions, limps, malalignment, or inability to perform a movement in a normal fashion.

OTHER FORMS OF CONNECTIVE TISSUE

Connective tissue, apart from bone, provides a network of flexible support. Nerve fibers, muscle fibers, blood vessels, and internal organs are covered with connective tissues that provide support (eg, the patellar retinaculum); provide attachment for functional actions (eg, insertion of the patellar tendon); facilitate movement (eg, the patellar bursae, which reduce friction); and limit movement (eg, the collateral ligaments of the knee, which restrict abnormal movement in the coronal plane). Connective tissue may be firm and unyielding,

like the linea alba of the abdominal muscles; or it may be flexible and supple, like the fascia separating the pectoralis major muscle from the underlying pectoralis minor muscle. Yielding facia allows one muscle to move on another without generating friction, so one muscle can contract without the other necessarily having to shorten.

Normally, the enormous range of connective tissue resilience complements the numerous simultaneous demands of the musculoskeletal system. However, because connective tissue demonstrates the ability to be dense and rigid, or to be scant and forgiving, the potential for error in its composition and effect is great. Furthermore, connective tissue is reasonably plastic. That is, it responds readily to various stimuli, including loading, stretching, inactivity, aging, and disease. Some potential responses are an increased amount of collagen, increased capillary permeability, rupture, elongation, cell proliferation, or cell death.

More specific examples of how changes in connective tissues affect the balance of the musculoskeletal system are considered below. Changes in cells, fibers, and the composite are discussed separately. Finally, the joint is discussed as a complex integration of many forms of connective tissue, including capsules, synovium, ligaments, and articular cartilage.

Cell Changes

Connective tissues are varied, but all are composed of cells, fibers, and ground substance. The cells are the active elements. When stimulated, they may proliferate, although not all proliferation leads to musculoskeletal imbalance, of course. Proliferation is intended to meet a demand for more cells in the matrix. One example of dysfunctional proliferation of connective tissue is an excess production of adipose (fat) cells. It is not known why fat cells are predisposed to accumulate in specific regions of the body, but some of the musculoskeletal imbalances caused by these accumulations are known. For example, when fat accumulates in the abdominal area, the center of gravity is displaced anteriorly. The trunk extensors must then work harder to maintain the erect position, because the body's center of gravity is now further from the fulcrum.

Failure of cells to proliferate adequately, given the necessary stimulus, can also lead to dysfunction. Cartilage, to some extent, repairs itself when stressed. However, if the stress is too frequent or too severe, the cells cannot reproduce enough to keep up with the destruction, and loss of articular surface area results.

Death of connective tissue cells results in a release of histamine. As a result, membrane permeability increases, which in turn leads to swelling and further dysfunction.

Fiber Changes

The cells and fibers make up the matrices of connective tissue. The fibers, whether collagen, elastin, or fibrin, are manufactured by the resident cells. Fiber proliferation increases density and tensile strength of the connective tissue, but the tissue's functional usefulness depends on the internal organization of the fibers. Normal use patterns influence tissue organization and reorganization. Rehabilitation of a repaired bicipital aponeurosis, for example, would require movement of the forearm through supination-pronation, as well as through flexion-extension. Otherwise, the fiber arrangement of the aponeurosis would become too parallel, and would not permit adequate rotation.

The fibers of connective tissue structures can become shortened if their normal excursions are not frequently used. Shortening, tightening, or binding down of connective tissue fibers all result in a structural imbalance leading to limited range of movement, pain, and dysfunction. The structures most affected by shortening of fibers in their connective tissues are joint capsules, ligaments, tendons, fascial sheaths, aponeuroses, the perimysium and epimysium around muscle fibers and fascicles, and the perineurium and epineurium surrounding nerve fibers.

Scarring produces fiber shortening, irregularly arranged fibers, increased density of the connective tissue, and resulting limitation of movement. Scarring may be in deep tissues or may be superficial, as in skin trauma. However, even with superficial scarring, movement restrictions are evident in the skin, the underlying soft tissues, and secondarily in muscle fibers and joint structures. The structural changes then produce an imbalance in the musculoskeletal system, which causes further dysfunction. For example, the weekend athlete who plays a hard game of tennis overstresses the internal rotators of the right shoulder while serving. Fibers of the subscapularis muscle become irritated and inflamed; with improper treatment, they may become scarred and inflexible. With limited external rotation, something as simple as reaching over from the driver's seat in a car to open the passenger door is impossible. The role of the thorax, trunk, and pelvis in simple movements becomes exaggerated, and energy expenditure and body mechanics are inefficient, portending dysfunction of the extensor muscles of the trunk.

Fiber laxity can also lead to a musculoskeletal imbalance. The anterior cruciate ligament of the knee normally guards against hyperextension of the knee. If the ligament is lax because of some prior stretch injury, the quadriceps muscle can act unopposed and drive the femur too far posteriorly on the tibia during forceful knee extension. Knee hyperextension is the primary result, but compensatory changes in the ankle and hip lead to secondary causes of abnormal alignment. The altered biomechanics add stress to the muscles and ligaments active in posture and movement, and further dysfunction ensues.

Composite Changes

The intrinsic balance of cells, fibers, and ground substance provides the necessary degrees of support and flexibility in the normal person. With palpation and kneading of soft tissues beneath the skin, one can determine symmetry, balance, and appropriate tension in the underlying connective tissues. Over the paravertebral region, for example, one should be able to pick up and work the soft tissues that lie superficial to the muscle layers. This type of skin rolling can indicate sites of underlying dysfunction by identifying isolated soft tissue areas that are reluctant to be moved, are bound down, or are otherwise restricted.

Synovial Joints

Synovial joint motion is a product of the joint's surface geometry as well as its surrounding soft tissue constraints. Under normal circumstances, three major types of surface or arthrokinematic movements can occur: spin, roll, and glide (Fig. 10-5).

The type of surface movement that predominates at any one joint depends in part on the congruency of the articular surfaces. For

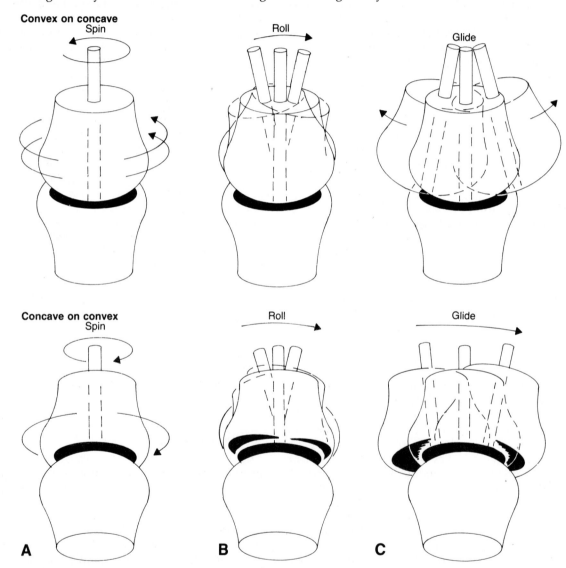

Figure 10-5. Three major types of surface or arthrokinematic movements: *(A)* spin, *(B)* roll, and *(C)* glide. (Reproduced by permission from Gould J, Davies G (eds): Orthopedics and Sports Physical Therapy, p 218. St Louis, CV Mosby, 1985)

example, more congruent surfaces, such as those that are relatively planar in shape, demonstrate greater amounts of glide and lesser amounts of roll. In contrast, joint surfaces that are less congruent, such as concave-convex surfaces, demonstrate more roll and less glide. In reality, glide and roll often occur in combination with each other and with the third type of surface motion—spin or rotation about the longitudinal axis of the bone. The knee joint is a good example of how the surface motions of roll, glide, and spin occur in varying amounts during the performance of physiologic movements such as flexion and extension (Fig. 10-6). Soft tissue constraints such as the joint capsule, surrounding ligamentous tissue, and intracapsular fat help to guide and produce these surface movements.

Physical therapists generally think of the degrees of freedom of a joint as related to the number of axes about which active movement occurs. For example, the wrist has two degrees of freedom because voluntary muscle actions can move the joint in the physiologic motions of flexion-extension and abduction-adduction.

The hip has three degrees of freedom because its muscles can move the joint in physiologic flexion-extension, abduction-adduction, or internal-external rotation. However, surface motions are an equally important part of normal joint mechanics; without surface motions, normal physiologic motions cannot occur. These motions are considered component or accessory elements of physiologic movement, and cannot be produced actively in an isolated manner. They occur about the same axes as physiologic motion, but usually in the form of translations (Fig. 10-7). Therefore, the degrees of freedom in various directions at a synovial joint should include the linear and the angular displacements about movement axes to describe joint motion accurately.

Capsuloligamentous adhesions that prevent these normal arthrokinematic or accessory motions from occurring may change the center of rotation of the joint, upset joint mechanics and lubrication mechanisms, and result in painful or limited gross physiologic movement. Physical therapists use a variety of manual techniques (generically labeled *joint mobilization*

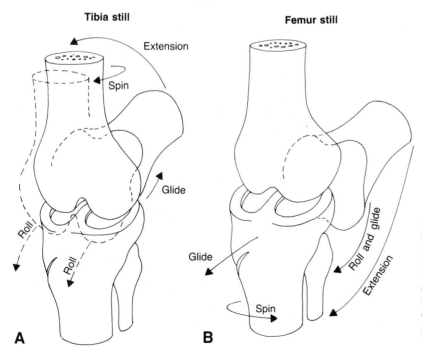

Figure 10-6. Combination of surface motions and physiologic movement: *(A)* convex moving on concave; *(B)* concave moving on convex. (Reproduced by permission from Gould J, Davies G: Orthopedics and Sports Physical Therapy, p 220. St Louis, CV Mosby, 1985)

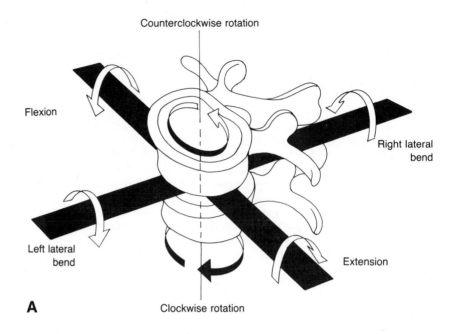

Counterclockwise rotation

Flexion

Right lateral bend

Left lateral bend

Extension

A

Clockwise rotation

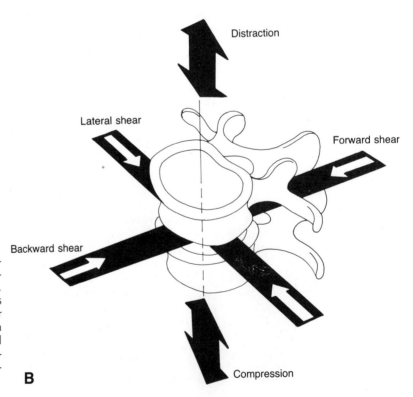

Distraction

Lateral shear

Forward shear

Backward shear

Figure 10-7. Angular (A, physiologic motions) and linear (B, accessory motions) displacements. Joints may have up to six degrees of freedom. (Stokes IAF: Biplanar radiography of the spine. In Grieve G [ed]: Modern Manual Therapy of the Vertebral Column, p 581. Edinburgh, Churchill-Livingstone, 1986)

B

Compression

procedures) to identify the loss of accessory movements and to restore them therapeutically.

The synovial joint illustrates the functional integration of loose connective tissues (synovium, bursae) and dense connective tissues (capsule, ligament, articular cartilage, and disks). Imbalance of these elements will lead to macroscopic imbalances in the musculoskeletal system. Some of the joint tissues are richly innervated, and trauma can disrupt transmission of proprioceptive cues about joint position and joint motion. Therefore, despite the fact that motion of muscles and tendons produces proprioceptive information, gait disturbances have been reported from loss of peripheral nerve branches supplying joint innervation in the lower extremities.

MUSCLE

Muscle as a tissue can be a primary or a secondary cause of musculoskeletal imbalance. Muscle can produce force, create motion, maintain posture, provide direction, and respond to a demand for action within a specified period of time. Although the central nervous system produces the required signals, the muscle must be capable of responding appropriately. If muscle becomes tight, weak, fatigued, stretched, or painful, the responses to central nervous system activation will be partial or inadequate and dysfunction will result.

Physiologic Factors

Muscular force depends on the following five properties of muscle fibers: (1) quantity (more fibers, more force); (2) size (larger fibers generate more force); (3) arrangement (pennate and bipennate arrangements allow more fibers per unit of cross-sectional area); (4) length (in vivo range near rest length is most advantageous); and (5) type (type II or fast-oxidative fibers are capable of generating more force per fiber than type I or fatigue-resistant fibers). Of all these factors, length is the most easily varied.

A muscle lengthened beyond its normal functioning range in vivo may be weak and more easily fatigued during normal use. The gluteus medius muscle has been documented as being prone to unilateral stretch weakness because of the habit of standing in postural adduction on one side. Right-handed persons tend to stand in right postural adduction, thereby stretching the right gluteus medius muscle. This results in a lax joint capsule, hypermobility of the right hip joint, increased contact areas at the articular sites between femur and acetabulum, and eventual development of osteoarthritic spurs. Gait deviations, such as a trunk lean or a positive Trendelenburg, may also result.

Under normal conditions, fiber quantity does not change in mature skeletal muscle, and fiber arrangement is fixed. Thus, fiber type and size are the only other factors that can be altered, and that can create an imbalance in the musculoskeletal system. Fiber size changes with exercise. Adequate exercise produces hypertrophy, and disuse leads to atrophy. The resulting weakness that occurs with disuse atrophy has profound effects on the balance of the musculoskeletal system. (Disuse atrophy is discussed more thoroughly in the section on Weakness later in this chapter.)

Fiber type appears to change under some conditions. An increase in the number of fast-twitch (type II) fibers (which can occur with immobilization of muscle) increases the fatigability of muscle. This situation is usually temporary, and can be modified with functional electrical stimulation, and reversed with resumption of normal activity. A decrease in the number of fast-twitch fibers (which occurs with aging) increases the response time of muscle. For example, if the quadriceps muscle contracts too late at weight acceptance, more momentum must be overcome, so more force is required, with higher loading on the knee joint. The joint is stressed, and the body is at greater risk of falling. Reaction time is also a factor in safety. During normal gait, the quadriceps muscle must contract eccentrically at weight acceptance to counteract the flexion moment at the knee. Because this portion of the gait cycle is single-support phase, failure of the quadriceps to contract within a few hundred milliseconds can be catastrophic. Persons who lack this capability compensate by keeping the center of gravity ahead of the knee, by taking short steps to reduce the time in single limb support, and by walking slowly to minimize the ground reaction forces, or by using a cane or other assistive device.

Mechanical Factors

The angle at which a muscle inserts into a bone determines how much effective torque will be available to rotate the skeletal lever. Given maximal effort of total muscle force, (M), Figure 10-8 illustrates that the closer the angle of insertion is to 90 degrees, the more torque will be produced with which to rotate the limb. This is because torque is the product of the rotary component (Fy) times the distance from the axis to the muscle's insertion. Because distance between bony points is constant, the determinant of torque that varies is the rotary component of the muscle's force. The rotary force varies as the angle of insertion varies throughout a range of motion. This variation, and the changes in muscle length, account for the normal torque variations through a range of motion, and thus for the shape of the normal torque curve.

Although different muscle groups have distinctive torque curves, any one muscle group has the same configuration (but not the same magnitude) in different persons. This is because humans are built proportionately, and taller persons have longer muscles, which insert farther from the joint. Surgery, poorly healed fractures, and postural changes can all change normal angles of insertion. Patellec-

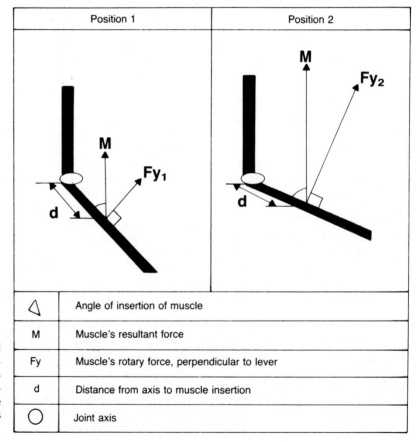

	Position 1	Position 2
△	Angle of insertion of muscle	
M	Muscle's resultant force	
Fy	Muscle's rotary force, perpendicular to lever	
d	Distance from axis to muscle insertion	
○	Joint axis	

Figure 10-8. Given maximal voluntary effort and considering that the only effect on muscle tension is the angle of insertion, the torque increases as the angle of insertion approaches 90 degrees (torque = $Fy \times d$).

tomy reduces the angle at which the quadriceps inserts into the tibia, and results in reductions of quadriceps torque on the order of 30%. Fractures or avulsions at osseotendinous junctions change angles of insertion. Postural changes can also alter angles of insertion. For example, excessively pronating the feet when standing encourages compensatory adjustments of calcaneal eversion, tibial internal rotation, and genu valgum. The quadriceps tendon, although still on the tibial tubercle, is now more medial because of the tibia's internal rotation. The patellar tendon rides over the medial aspect of the patella, and therefore the ability of the patella to increase the angle of insertion of the quadriceps is reduced. Changing angles of insertion reduces the efficiency of the body's system, requires more work, and results in more stress.

Range of motion limitations produce predictable alterations in the balance of the musculoskeletal system. Muscles and their investing connective tissues degenerate during immobilization or disuse. Connective tissue deteriorates more slowly than muscle tissue, and the perimysium and epimysium around the fascicles become thicker, as does the whole muscle. Flexibility is lost and function is altered. Although a single muscle over a single joint may be the only presenting pathology, the body's compensations to the change may be devastating. For example, knee extension may be limited by 15 degrees. With the distal lever free, as in sitting, the person may be inconvenienced and unable to sit comfortably for long periods. But with the distal lever fixed, as in rising from a chair, the situation becomes far worse. The person is not able to place his foot beneath the chair to get up. He has to lean very far forward to get his body over his base of support to push up from the chair. Once upright, he has difficulty standing because one limb is shorter. During ambulation, the quadriceps muscle works twice as forcefully as normal because the flexion moment is increased at weight acceptance as a result of the center of gravity falling farther behind the joint axis.

The body makes its own compensations, but these are never as efficient as the patterns they are replacing. A person with tight hip flexors cannot keep her spine normally contoured *and* stand upright. Instead, she tilts the pelvis anteriorly and increases the lumbar lordosis. Resulting compensations include an increased thoracic kyphosis and a cervical lordosis with a forward head. In this stance, her head is still oriented normally to the world. However, most points on the trunk have moved farther from a line projected through the center of gravity, so the torque required to maintain alignment of the various segments is greater. Finally, in addition to the hip flexors being tight (the starting point in this degenerative story), other muscles become tight, such as the sternomastoids from the forward head position, and the lumbar erector spinae muscle from the increased lordosis.

Moving Origins and Moving Fulcrums

Muscle, by its attachments through tendons and ligaments to bones, can produce complex actions. Muscle has reverse actions, and can contract from a fixed origin (proximal attachment) or from a fixed insertion (distal attachment). However, if the origin and insertion are both moving, the muscle has no stable base from which to exert meaningful forces, and the effort is not productive. For example, the teres major muscle and the latissimus dorsi muscle both extend, adduct, and internally rotate the humerus. The latissimus dorsi is a dynamic muscle and the teres major is a static muscle. In other words, if the scapula is fixed, the teres major muscle works to its best advantage, but if the scapula is moving through downward rotation (as when the latissimus dorsi is contracting) the teres major muscle has a minor role. The teres major muscle cannot develop adequate torque if both of its attachments are moving. The latissimus dorsi muscle serves better in this situation because of its origin from the stable iliac crest. The one exception to the moving attachment problem is the group of lumbrical muscles. These four muscles, which originate from the tendons of the long digital flexors, act on the phalanges from a moving base of attachment, whether the fingers (or toes) are flexing or extending. In this situation, the moving origin of the lumbricals is muscular, but it provides the capability of continuous adjustment in length as a substitute for a fixed origin.

The moving fulcrum is another common biomechanical situation. The axis of motion, or the instant center of rotation, of any joint in the body changes during motion. The amount of movement depends on joint geometry, soft tissue constraints, range of excursion, participating muscles, and torque produced. In normal function, there are adaptations to the moving fulcrum through subtle translatory movements of the bones and through complex patterns of muscle recruitment. For example, the shoulder axis moves dramatically (upward) during flexion or abduction. The sophistication of muscular interplay and joint translations permit smooth motion. You are barely conscious of glenohumeral rotation, depression of the humeral head, elevation and rotation of the clavicle and scapula, or thoracic extension when you raise an arm overhead. Yet, problems become apparent if any alterations prevent normal movement of the fulcrum. Failure to recruit the proper muscles in the appropriate sequences with requisite force, speed, and direction produces significant changes in joint biomechanics because of the potential influences that these factors have on a joint's center of rotation.

In addition to the effect of muscle action on center of rotation, an abnormal joint structure may permit abnormal movement of the fulcrum, resulting in decreased stability of the joint and apparent muscle weakness. The congenitally shallow acetabulum is an example of this, with its resultant chronically dislocating hip and apparent abductor muscle weakness. On the other hand, a structure that does not permit a sufficiently movable fulcrum can also produce changes in biomechanics and lead to altered function. Joint prostheses exemplify this situation because of their fixed centers of rotation.

Muscle as a tissue is critical in achieving and maintaining the balance of the musculoskeletal system, but muscle force is not the only concern. Equally important to efficient overall function are specific characteristics of muscle (such as speed of contraction, response time, recruitment order, and relaxation ability) as well as joint structure and function. Any aberration in these characteristics will alter normal balance of the musculoskeletal system and lead to dysfunction. A variety of factors can cause these aberrations, and they are explored further in the section on Weakness.

PAIN

Pain is now acknowledged as a complex psychophysiologic phenomenon that may be influenced by cultural, racial, and environmental factors. A great deal of information about the anatomical basis for pain was established in the past 50 years. More recently, the information has been revised, updated, and expanded as interest in clinical pain syndromes, the character of pain and pain states, and the importance of learning and perception has increased. Nationally, the proliferation of chronic pain centers reflects a heightened awareness of the need to manage clinical pain more effectively. Certainly, many of the patients seeking treatment in pain centers and similar rehabilitative units have complaints related primarily to the musculoskeletal system.

Even if intense and uncomfortable, pain of brief duration can be considered helpful because it warns of impending tissue damage and is a stimulus to withdraw the body part at risk. Common examples are stepping on a tack or touching a hot stove. In a more general sense, pain can produce self-limited behavior in activity and mobility after an injury. This behavior also could be classified as a protective function, because it results in prevention of further damage to already traumatized tissue.

Besides playing an important role in protection from tissue damage, pain is also a helpful indicator of dysfunction because it encourages persons to seek medical attention to analyze the cause of the discomfort and helps the diagnostician locate the possible source of the dysfunction.

MECHANISMS OF PAIN PRODUCTION

Tissue injury—whether from mechanical, physiologic, or chemical sources—results in a chain of events that produces pain as a by-product. Mechanical stimuli in the form of both macrotrauma and microtrauma is probably one of the most common methods of inducing pain in musculoskeletal tissue. Macrotrauma to bone, induced by compression, axial loading, torsion, or bending moments that exceed the tissue's capability to sustain them, can result in significant bone fractures and secondary disruption of soft tissue structures such as muscle, fascia, ligament, and joint capsule. Primary disruption of soft tissue alone (ligament and tendon tears and ruptures) can also occur when these tissues are subjected to excessive external or internal forces. Ironically, however, the severity of injury cannot always be related to the degree of pain. For example, a total ligamentous rupture may be less painful than a sprain, because in a rupture no fibers are left intact to transmit pain messages. Chronic pain-free anterior cruciate ligament (ACL) ruptures with no known history of trauma are sometimes found during routine knee examinations.

Pain from trauma is the direct result of a tissue injury that produces local biochemical changes acting on chemoreceptive nociceptors to generate A delta and C fiber transmission to the spinal cord and higher CNS levels. At the same time, acute injuries may activate segmental reflexes that stimulate somatomotor cells to increase skeletal motor activity in the same geographic region as the original tissue insult. Muscle splinting around the site of an acute injury is an example of this activity.

Microtraumatic events may follow a similar scenario, though to a lesser degree or intensity. In microtrauma, there is no particular history of a given traumatic event. However, repetitive stresses over time may have cumulative effects that result in low-grade inflammatory tissue responses with the same or similar consequences of pain production as in macrotrauma. In both macrotraumatic and microtraumatic events, certain parts of the inflammation and repair process play a role in pain production.

Initially, edema forms as intracellular fluids leak from damaged cells into the intercellular space. This process is compounded by the increase in permeability of cell walls and the fact that colloids which bind fluids now lie outside of the cell walls and draw more fluid into the extracellular space. The result is a distention of tissue, which alone may be a further mechanical stimulus to pain production. In addition, scarring, which occurs during the maturation phase of healing and which may develop as disorganized and dense connective tissue, may produce sufficient mechanical strain on tissue to deform and subsequently fire local nociceptors during movement that is otherwise normal in range and direction.

An understanding of the sensory receptors, peripheral and central nervous system pathways, and connections that result in the perception of pain is important but is beyond the scope of this chapter. When assuming that the source of pain is within the musculoskeletal system, it is important to consider which tissues within the musculoskeletal system are capable of producing a pain sensation. In general, highly innervated tissues can do so, while those that are considered aneural cannot. The periosteum of bone contains many nerve fiber endings that can produce pain. In contrast, cartilage, which is largely avascular and aneural, is not capable of producing pain sensations. However, if cartilage impinges or encroaches on adjacent pain-sensitive tissue, the result can be pain whose origin is in cartilaginous dysfunction. Other tissue components of the musculoskeletal system have varying levels of inherent sensitivity to pain. Ligaments, tendinous–periosteal junctions, and fibrous capsules can produce pain when their sensory receptors are adequately stimulated, whereas muscle is relatively insensitive to mechanically induced pain. However, pain has long been associated with spasm of muscle, especially in spinal disorders in which the concept of the pain-spasm-pain cycle has been clinically popular.

Physiologists believe that muscle spasm may initiate pain by stimulating mechanical pain receptors, causing ischemia and stimulating chemosensitive pain receptors, or by compressing blood vessels and decreasing blood flow while at the same time increasing the rate of muscle metabolism so that relative ischemia is even greater and pain-inducing substances are released. The concept of muscle spasm, despite its clinical popularity, has been neither fully studied nor adequately defined. Clinicians generally regard it as a reversible state of sustained, involuntary contraction in which there is shortening of the muscle and associated changes in the muscle's electrical activity. However, this definition alone leaves many questions unanswered. Some studies have shown no electrical activity in the muscles surrounding a fracture site, despite their appearance of sustained involuntary contraction. The patient with acute low back pain who demonstrates an involuntary scoliosis also shows no electrical activity of the muscles on the supposedly painful contracted concave side of the curve. This raises the possibility of a chemical, rather than an electrical, basis for the contracted state of the muscle. In addition, the flattening of the lumbar and cervical lordotic curves, which can be radiographically confirmed in acute cases of lumbar and cervical spine pain and which is ascribed to muscle spasm, is not logically supported by the shortening of the lumbar or cervical extensor muscle groups. If shortened, these muscles would tend to increase, not decrease, the lordotic tendency. Without further study, clinical muscle spasm in the patient with musculoskeletal problems remains enigmatic and variously defined.

In persons with an otherwise normal musculoskeletal system and no obvious trauma, muscle pain can develop one to two days after unaccustomed activity. Although most persons are familiar with this event, the exact mechanism for the latent pain is not clear and various theories have been proposed to explain it. One explanation is that the cause is metabolic in nature, because the delayed onset of pain seems to coincide with latent rises in the levels of various enzymes related to intense muscle activity. As further support of the metabolic theory, normal persons who engage in

training exercise programs have been shown to have lowered enzyme levels along with reduced subjective pain complaints. Another possible explanation for postexercise pain is that the muscle pain is mechanically induced from torn muscle fibers. Repetitive eccentric muscle contractions cause higher levels of pain than concentric contractions. This is because in eccentric contractions, greater tension development per muscle fiber predisposes the fibers to greater risk of physical damage. Tearing or damage to the connective tissue within and surrounding the muscle, rather than damage to the muscle fibers themselves, is also proposed as another mechanism for latent muscle pain. Whatever the exact cause of latent muscle pain in normal persons, its existence underscores the need for therapists to consider the type of muscle contraction employed and a paced resumption of former activity levels in both conditioning and rehabilitation programs to avoid iatrogenically induced tissue trauma and pain.

Evaluation of Pain

Clinicians who manage patients with musculoskeletal dysfunction evaluate a patient's pain complaints to guide further evaluation and subsequent management. Although the general categories of pain investigation are straightforward (location, nature, severity, and behavior) the implications of answers to these questions may not be, for several reasons.

Location

If superficial tissue, such as the skin, is mechanically deformed and sensation is intact, the patient can usually localize pain to the site of insult. However, deeper tissues, such as the ligaments, joint capsules, or nerve roots, may give rise to local pain complaints and may produce patterns of pain perception in areas distant from the injured tissue itself. Referred pain may be produced in different ways. Direct irritation of a nerve root at the spinal segmental level produces dermatomal pain, which the patient reports in the skin area supplied by the nerve root. Dermatomal charts have been mapped out for the human body and are available in most neurology texts, although there are differences between texts. These differences are due to natural variation among individuals, to differences in experimental protocols, to a dearth of subjects used for obtaining data, and to the extensive overlapping of dermatomal distributions from adjacent segmental nerve roots.

Dermatomal referred pain is the most commonly recognized referred pain phenomenon, but two other sources that may produce pain perception at sites remote from the original stimulus are sclerotomal referred patterns and myofascial pain patterns. Sclerotomes are de-

fined as deep somatic tissues innervated by one segmental nerve root (Fig. 10-9).

Embryologically, although limb tissue develops from tissue in the limb buds, which are distinct from the mesodermal somites, the limb tissues still share common innervation with their segmental axial counterparts throughout the developmental process. Therefore, during life, if one part of a sclerotome is damaged, the potential exists for pain to be perceived in any or all parts of that same sclerotome. One of the most common clinically accepted examples of the sclerotomal referral process is the young male teenager with knee pain. Upon further

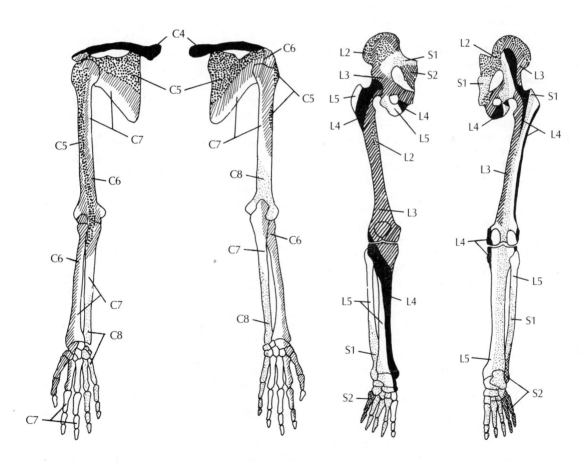

Figure 10-9. Sclerotomes chart. (Kessler RM, Hertling D: Management of Common Musculoskeletal Disorders, p 53. New York, Harper & Row, 1983)

investigation, no intrinsic pathologic problem can be found. Instead, the source is discovered in the hip joint in the form of avascular necrosis of the femoral head (Legg-Perthes disease). This example of a hip joint problem giving rise to a perception of pain in the knee would be familiar to most clinicians, but applying the concept of sclerotomal referred pain to other pathologic problems arising in the facet joint capsules of vertebral segments and referring pain into either the upper or lower extremities is less well-accepted and recognized. However, the fact remains that patient complaints of limb pain cannot always be accounted for by localized dysfunction at the painful site or by implication of nerve root pressure causing dermatomal referral. Sclerotomal referral pain may be one viable explanation for seemingly nonclassical referral patterns of pain into the limbs.

Another alternative mechanism that may account for atypical patterns of pain referral throughout the body is the phenomenon of myofascial referred pain. Travell and Simons have investigated and popularized the concept of trigger points in muscle or fascia, which may serve as intrinsic sources of local pain and pain at sites distant to the muscle in which the trigger point is found. Neither the exact pathology nor the specific mechanism by which the myofascial trigger point gives rise to referred pain has been extensively studied. Consequently, skepticism about the scientific basis of myofascial pain remains. Nevertheless, trigger point charts based on the clinical study of hundreds of patients have been compiled and demonstrate certain typical patterns of both local and referred pain for all the muscles in the body.

Nature

Patients are asked the nature of their pain complaints because the particular characteristics of pain may give clues to its tissue of origin. Pain that arises from deep somatic tissues such as the ligaments or joint capsule is often described as deep and aching, and may be classified as sclerotomal pain. Pain from more superficial tissues may be described as sharp or electric, and classified as dermatomal in nature. Differences in the perceived nature of pain may be derived from the type of tissue that is stimulated and the type of nerve fiber transmission that ensues. Dermatomal pain, which is sharper and more delineated, is carried mostly by myelinated A delta fibers of 1 to 6 μm in width. Pain of sclerotomal origin, which is described as deep and achy, is related more to C fibers of much smaller diameter with little myelin covering. Second-order neurons may also differ for the two types of pain, with the fast pain transmitted in a direct spinal-thalamic route and the dull, diffuse pain routed by numerous short, interconnecting neurons to the medulla and midbrain.

Severity

Severity of a patient's pain complaints can be rather vaguely recorded as mild, moderate, or severe, or it may be more objectively defined by having the patient assess the pain on various types of pain scales. A common method of pain rating is the visual analogue scale. The scale generally consists of a line of a predetermined length, at the poles of which are the extremes of no pain and intense pain. To indicate perception of the severity of pain, the patient marks the line at the appropriate point between the two extremes. More detailed, objective, and reliable assessment of pain may be accomplished by using pain questionnaires, such as the McGill system; however, they are cumbersome and not suited to the efficiency needs of most clinical departments. Some scales, such as the one developed by Harris, attempt to relate activity levels to perception of pain severity. These scales may be particularly helpful in determining the impact the patient's pain has on activities of daily living.

Behavior

How the patient's pain behaves in response to certain types of stimulation can also help differentiate the origin of pain. When patients have musculoskeletal problems, the physical therapist's primary concern is to recognize pain that is not purely musculoskeletal, but instead has a serious pathologic source (eg, neoplasm or disease), so that appropriate treatment is not delayed. The task may be difficult, especially if a serious pathologic problem is in its early stages and is mimicking mechanical pain symptoms. In addition, viscero-somatic reflexes allow dysfunction in an organ to be reflected as skin hyperalgesia or deep somatic tissue pain. Some of the more common examples are cardiac dysfunction reflected as left shoulder pain, kidney or gynecologic dysfunction felt as low back pain, or diaphragmatic irritation represented by shoulder discomfort. A thorough medical history as well as attention to patient reports of a general decline in overall health or weight loss is helpful, but not infallible, in establishing pain related to nonmechanical sources.

Paying attention to how the patient's pain behaves with respect to the time of day, type of static positions used, or dynamic activities engaged in can give clues about whether the pain is of mechanical or chemical origin. Chemical pain or pain of inflammatory origin is described as constant and generally unrelated to the time of day, differences in static positions, or changes in dynamic activities. In contrast, pain of mechanical origin is variable in intensity, usually decreasing with rest and increasing with movement, and can be worsened or lessened by specific positional changes and dynamic activities.

When pain can no longer be identified as serving a protective function, or when it continues despite negative diagnostic results indicating any dysfunction of the musculoskeletal system, it can itself precipitate dysfunction. In general, pain usually results in a decreased willingness to move, with the ensuing attendant effects of immobility and their negative consequences for the musculoskeletal system. These include joint contracture and muscle shortening, venous stasis, and poor nutritional support, especially to tissues that rely upon movement as a mechanism for obtaining nutrients. Pain has also been shown to decrease force development capability in muscle, both for voluntary muscle contraction and in response to electrical stimulation.

The effects of acute compared with chronic pain on the musculoskeletal system may differ. Only recently have persons with chronic pain been subjected to intensive exercise programs in an attempt to raise their thresholds for functional physical activity. Through a combination of work hardening and lifting tasks, resistive exercise, flexibility routines, and aerobic activities, the patient with chronic pain is taught to move again. Little to no emphasis is placed on subjective pain complaints. How these patients' general fitness levels may change, and the subsequent effects on their musculoskeletal systems, have not yet been clarified. However, initial results seem to support an ability at least to push thresholds higher before pain causes a cessation of activity. Thus, higher tolerances for functional activity are achieved.

EDEMA

Under normal circumstances, a constant exchange occurs between the plasma in the capillary networks and the fluid in the interstitial spaces. Starling first discovered the hydrostatic and osmotic pressure differentials between capillary membranes and interstitial spaces, which account for both the rate and direction of fluid exchange. When functioning properly, fluid leaks out of the arterial end of capillaries and is reabsorbed at the venous end. However, this exchange is not perfectly balanced, and a small but significant net filtration of fluid into interstitial spaces occurs. The lymphatic system is responsible for draining this excess fluid from the interstitium and returning it by means of its extensive vessel network into the general circulation.

In general, edema results when the normal process fails, and fluid accumulates in the interstitial spaces. Different factors may initiate and perpetuate edema formation, but they usually originate from one or more of four basic physiologic events: (1) an increase in capillary pressure; (2) a decrease in osmotic pressure; (3) an obstruction in the lymphatic system; or (4) an increase in capillary permeability.

Edema is often associated with trauma to the musculoskeletal system. At the time of injury, trauma is a direct cause of fluid leakage into intercellular spaces because of disrupted tissue and torn vessels. After injury, trauma causes leakage indirectly through the action of various chemicals released in the inflammatory process. Histamine, bradykinin, and serotonin can act on the permeability of capillary membranes to allow colloids that are usually restricted to the plasma within capillaries to leak into the interstitial spaces. Because colloids attract and bind water, their presence outside the capillary walls further encourages fluid migration into the intercellular space, enhancing edema. Posttraumatic edema formation may continue for several days after an injury before stabilizing.

Other factors also combine to extend the edematous process. During the inflammatory period after injury, fibrin clots form in the interstitium and further restrict one of the avenues of fluid reabsorption. Lymphatic system activity may be dampened by the lack of muscle pumping action, and a dependent extremity may have increased capillary pressures, further forcing fluid out into interstitial spaces.

The inflammatory response to injury, which includes edema formation as part of the process, can occur in any musculoskeletal tissue. In muscle, direct trauma from external forces or from excessive internal contraction or stretch can result in edema and extravasation of blood in the form of hematomas. Muscle fiber destruction is possible by means of pressure and subsequent ischemia. In addition, the endomysial tubes (the connective tissue elements that encase muscle fibers) may develop fibrous tissue proliferation after injury, causing an eventual loss of muscle extensibility. Edema as a cause of muscle fiber destruction is dramatically demonstrated by clinical compartment syndromes, such as the anterior tibial syndrome. The etiology of compartment syndromes is unknown, but they seem to occur in deconditioned persons who participate in unusually high levels of physical activity. Compartment syndrome tends to occur where muscle is tightly contained by bony or fascial surroundings, as in the anterior tibial compartment. The exact trigger mechanism for edema formation within the muscles is unclear, but may be related to excessive metabolite buildup. Once the edematous process is initiated, a chain of events occurs wherein lymphatic

drainage channels and venous return become further compromised, trapping fluid in the contained area. Pressure builds, and unless it can be relieved, results in severe muscle destruction.

Joints may also be perceived as contained units, with the joint capsule being the outer covering. When edema forms within a joint, fluid volume increases. Depending on the extent of fluid accumulation and whether the location of the joint is superficial or deep, the joint may appear visibly distended. The degree and progression of edema is often measured clinically through circumferential or volumetric measurements. However, whichever method of measurement is preferred, it is important to remember that muscle atrophy can accompany edema, and you should not confuse atrophic muscle changes with edema reduction.

The fluid within acute posttraumatic edematous joints is considered an inflammatory exudate that represents events occurring in the synovial membrane. Joint effusion following simple injury usually develops within 12 to 24 hours, and may be accompanied by a physical sensation of tightness as the edema changes the intra-articular pressure from a normal negative value to a positive one. Clinicians should be aware that a sudden joint effusion occurring within two hours after injury may denote bleeding into the joint or serious injury to bony or intra-articular structures. In this event, further medical evaluation is required.

Long-standing joint effusions probably relate less to the initiating traumatic episode of long ago than they do to the abnormal alterations in the synovial tissue that have developed since the original tissue insult. These alterations consist of a generalized thickening and gradual fibrosis of synovial tissue that eventually can produce significant intra-articular adhesions that substantially interfere with joint function. Without proper joint movement, newly synthesized collagen fibrils laid down during the repair process are unable to orient themselves appropriately to the planes of imposed stress, and further restrict movement or provide less than adequate stability.

Although edema formation after a traumatic injury is a normal part of the body's inflammatory and repair process, it should also be recognized as having the potential to unnecessarily extend the original injury and, in and of itself, contribute to tissue necrosis. This is especially true if the edematous period is prolonged. When a fluid volume imbalance that favors interstitial accumulation exists, cells are surrounded by a larger than normal space between themselves and their capillary networks; therefore, nutritional exchange must take place over greater diffusion distances. Tissues can also become chronically overstretched by edema of prolonged duration, resulting in pressure-volume changes that actually make it easier for subsequent fluid increases of smaller volume to have edematous results. Aging tissue is particularly vulnerable to edema because of its decreased elasticity and subsequent pressure-volume changes. Besides tissue dysfunction, other effects on the musculoskeletal system include (1) pain from damaged nerve fibers and stimulation of joint nociceptors from distended joint capsules; (2) interference with proper healing of ligaments and subsequent reduced tensile strength capabilities; (3) restriction of active and passive range of motion because of joint fluid accumulation and pain; (4) eventual disuse atrophy and weakness of muscles; and (5) potential joint contracture and adhesions from excessive connective tissue proliferation in muscle and joint cavities.

Immediate physical therapy management of edema is directed at minimizing negative secondary effects and thereby providing an optimal environment in which the normal tissue healing process can occur. Various clinical methods are employed to accomplish this task. Ice is applied to decrease pain and muscle splinting around the injured site. The edematous part is elevated to decrease local capillary pressures and use gravity to aid in lymphatic drainage. External compression in the form of elastic bandages or stockings is provided to counteract forces causing fluid outflow from capillaries. Gentle, controlled muscle activity is used to hasten the rate of lymph flow and subsequent fluid removal. On a long-term basis, restoration of optimal joint and muscle func-

tion may be achieved through a progressive program of range-of-motion, strengthening, and functional retraining, both to rehabilitate fully the original injury and to condition against future occurrences.

Although edema formation affecting the musculoskeletal system is usually associated with trauma from physical injury, the physical therapist should also remember that excess fluid accumulates in extremities as a result of various diseases as well as from specific surgical and medical interventions. Surgical procedures themselves are a form of physical trauma, and a common practice in the immediate postoperative period is to apply compressive dressings over and around the incision to promote healing. Gentle, early active and active-assisted range-of-motion exercises performed within the constraints of the surgical procedure also serve the same goal. Some surgical procedures directly interfere with the fluid absorpion process by removing parts of the lymphatic system. This is the case in some mastectomy patients whose axillary lymph nodes are removed. Such patients therefore demonstrate postoperative edema and a long-term deficit in fluid reabsorption capabilities. Certain medications may also change venous and arterial pressures or fluid retention levels, and contribute to short- or long-term edema formation in the limbs. Certain diseases, especially those with a primary effect on synovial joints (such as rheumatoid arthritis), often produce edema in affected segments.

Edema of surgical, pharmaceutical, or disease origin may not respond in the same time frame or to the same extent that a "simple" posttraumatic injury does. This is because in the patient with a simple posttraumatic injury who is otherwise healthy, the initiating event for the inflammatory process has a finite duration. Once the trauma has occurred, physiologic processes move into the inflammatory and repair phase until pre-injury status is regained. However, if the initiating event for inflammation or edema is a chronic disease, a medication, or a permanent alteration in fluid dynamics, the stimulus for inflammation and excess fluid accumulation continues over time, and normal healing or fluid removal cannot proceed. In this case, physical therapy management of edema is an adjunct to medical management of its underlying cause and is directed at maximizing whatever fluid removal is possible within the constraints of the problem while minimizing functional disability resulting from an edematous limb or body segment. Physical therapy management may consist of long-term use of compressive wraps, exercise programs stressing maximal restoration of joint motion and strength, or splinting devices for joint protection.

WEAKNESS

Weakness creates significant dysfunction, but can often be corrected with physical therapy. The musculoskeletal tissues with which we are concerned in this section are muscle and connective tissue (including bone, cartilage, ligaments, fascia, and joint capsules—in other words, the dense connective tissues).

MUSCLE

When is muscle considered weak? Weakness in an extremity is judged in comparison with muscles of the other limb; in comparison with muscles of the same limb, as in agonist-antagonist ratios; and in comparison with muscles of other persons of the same sex and comparable body weight. Muscles of the trunk are more difficult to assess, and physical therapists rely on evaluating performance of specific tasks, such as trunk curling or leg lowering. More recently, dynamometers have been developed to assess isometric and isokinetic torque of the trunk flexors and extensors, but age-related norms are needed to determine the presence of real weakness.

Muscle is the only voluntary support for joint structure. Although the supporting function of muscle is mostly through involuntary and unconscious control, therapists remain fascinated with muscle support because we can do something to change muscle force. Much has been written about the balance of forces of agonist-antagonist muscles about some joints, especially the knee. Presumably, if the quadriceps do not produce a torque ratio of at least 3:2 against the hamstrings at slow speeds of isokinetic testing, the articular supports (capsule and ligaments) of the knee are vulnerable. This means that if the peak torque of the hamstrings is 60 ft·lb, then the peak torque of the quadriceps should be 90 ft·lb when tested at a slow isokinetic speed, such as 60°/sec. Articular injury at the knee caused by an imbalance in muscular torque is believed to occur because the opposing muscles will not be able to maintain or control the amount of translatory movement between the tibia and femur in the event of sudden impact. At the knee, damaging impact to the extremity generally occurs as an impact to the limb while the foot is fixed on the ground, leaving the knee joint to be the next movable (and destructible) link in the chain.

Similarly, the balance of torque between the flexor and extensor muscles of the trunk is believed to be relevant to low back pain. Authors disagree whether weak muscles predispose one to low back pain, or whether the muscles become weak as a result of chronic low back pain. Furthermore, they disagree whether it is the flexors or the extensors (or both) that are predominantly weak. Testing of patients is confounded by pain, and testing of normal persons is confounded by variables such as axis of rotation, age, sex, speed of testing, and body position. Without controls on these variables, meaningful norms cannot be obtained.

Muscle weakness can affect bone, as well as the joint that the muscle crosses. Bones are subject to compressive forces through weight bearing. These compressive forces are somewhat diffused by muscular contractions, which create tension at the muscle's insertion. A weak muscle is unable to produce adequate tension, and the bone in question becomes subject to excessive compressive forces. For example, the tibial shaft is compressed during weight bearing. The hamstrings (semitendinosus muscle and long head of biceps femoris muscle) act on the hip to generate a hip extension torque at weight acceptance, pulling from a fixed attachment (the proximal tibia). Thus, the tension created by the hamstrings diffuses some of the compressive forces on the tibia at weight acceptance. If the hamstrings are weak and unable to generate adequate torque, the tibia will be subjected to higher compressive forces. Gradually, this will lead to degenerative changes and functional losses. Macroscopically, some compensatory gait adjustments are made because of the weak hip extensors (such as backward leaning to keep the center of gravity posterior to the hip joint). As with any other compensatory adjustment, effort is increased and additional structures are stressed, further compounding the dysfunction.

Muscle is capable of isometric, eccentric, and concentric contractions. Developmentally, the ability for isometric and concentric contractions is functionally present before the ability to control eccentric contraction. Although not confirmed in the literature, our personal clinical impression is that eccentric control decreases in the aging process and may be one of the reasons that older persons fall. Eccentric contractions require less energy, less metabolic work, and fewer motor units than do concentric contractions of the same torque level. For these reasons, eccentric contractions are more efficient, and more total work can be accomplished. The passive resistance to elongation offered by the connective tissues that pervade muscle is the usual explanation for the increased efficiency of the eccentric contraction. Because of the participation of the relatively inert connective tissue, which is capable of absorbing energy, potential damage to the muscle fibers may occur with heavy eccentric loading. Disruptions of the Z bands in skeletal muscle have been demonstrated by electron microscopy after heavy eccentric training. To what extent specific exercises affect isometric, concentric, or eccentric capability remains to be seen. One investigator working with cats on a treadmill reported that the motor units recruited in sartorius muscles during swing phase (concentric contraction) were different from those recruited in the same muscle during stance phase (eccentric contraction). Research of this type raises questions regarding specificity of recruitment and specificity of training.

The potential for measuring eccentric contractions in humans has just become available, and current research may shed light on many pressing questions.

General factors that can produce muscle weakness are considered below. Selected internal factors are physiologic, pathologic, and psychologic in nature, and external factors are mechanical in nature.

Physiologic Factors

Aging

The aging process affects the force potential of muscle fibers. Throughout fetal development, myoblasts participate in the formation of new muscle fibers. After birth, satellite cells, which reside in the basement membrane layer of muscle cells, produce additional myofibrils, the contractile units of muscle. In later years, satellite cells, which are present in fewer numbers, continue to attempt to generate new myofibrils or new muscle cells (especially in the presence of disease), but these attempts are not fruitful.

Inhibition of muscle activity is an important aspect of sensorimotor development. Infants and young children gradually acquire this capability. Without normal inhibition, muscle activity is excessive and lacks coordination. The emergence of inhibitory patterns results from a combination of (1) the maturation of the central nervous system, (2) the opportunities for repetitive practice, and (3) the structure of the synapses. The facilitory and inhibitory synapses are structurally different, and the latter appear later in development.

The later development of eccentric control has already been mentioned, and is another factor to consider when evaluating movement patterns. The 18-month-old baby is expected to drop into his toddler's chair, but the 3-year-old child is expected to lower his body slowly into the chair. Failure to achieve this by the age of 3 years is an indication of weakness or lack of motor control.

In adolescence, hormonal changes stimulate protein synthesis and more actin and myosin filaments result, leading to increased fiber diameter and increased force potential. These hormonal changes are related to changes around puberty and have predictable effects on muscle, especially in boys. However, the purposeful ingestion of androgenic anabolic steroids for increasing muscle capacity has less clear results. Studies are contradictory, and most of the studies that were blinded fail to show significant effects on muscle torque as a result of taking these steroids.

The aging process alters the recruitment patterns of motor units. Muscle increases its voluntary output by recruiting more motor units, or by increasing the rate at which active ones are firing, or both. DeLuca has recorded evidence that a proximal muscle (such as the deltoid muscle) increases its force primarily by recruitment, whereas a distal muscle (such as the first dorsal interosseus muscle) increases its force primarily by increasing the firing rate of its motor units. In the aging person, recruitment strategies are altered, fewer motor units are present, and firing rates are decreased. The cumulative result is less force being produced in the muscle. Strength decreases up to 20% to 40% in the elderly, but this decrease can be minimized with activity.

Gender-Based Differences
Gender is not a basis for weakness in the musculoskeletal system. Muscle force reflects training and use patterns. Generally, untrained men exhibit more force than untrained women of comparable age. However, muscle groups vary, and the differences are more pronounced in the upper body. These differences narrow when one relates strength to lean body mass, suggesting that the potential for force development is similar in the two sexes. Because of gender-based differences in patterns of fat deposits, which result in differences in lean body mass, the actual force development in men is usually greater.

Length-Related Changes During Immobilization
Immobilization of tissue produces profound changes in a short period of time—days, in fact. The ultrastructure of muscle is altered when the muscle tissue is kept immobile by a cast, or by long-term positioning. The length at which muscle is immobilized influences the type of changes occurring, as does the age of the patient. Some research indicates that in the adult, immobilization in a lengthened position produces more sarcomeres, with the new rest length showing an increase in tension. On the other hand, the very young do not demonstrate additional sarcomeres, and the very old actually demonstrate necrosis of muscle cells from long-term immobilization in a lengthened position. If the muscle is immobilized at a shortened length, the number of sarcomeres decreases, although the remaining ones become longer. Some slow-oxidative (type I) fibers decrease or degenerate, and overall peak tension decreases. In addition, contractures may result. These changes are reversible when movement is permitted, but the reversal may take months.

Nutrition
Appropriate quality and quantity of food is vital to normal muscle function. Overall starvation produces atrophy of type II muscle fibers and profound weakness. Rate of contraction is also reduced. Vitamin deficiencies (especially of vitamin E and vitamin B_{12}) have been linked to weakness. However, in healthy persons, vitamin deficiencies are rare. Excess vitamins do not increase muscle force or endurance; in fact, vitamin loading can be harmful.

Insulin deficiency can result in muscle fiber atrophy because muscle cells rely on insulin as a determinant of protein (actin and myosin) synthesis. If plasma levels of insulin are insufficient, muscle fibers (as well as other cells) cannot use glucose, and muscle fibers begin to rely on their own proteins for metabolism. Because exercise stimulates a cell's ability to use insulin for glucose transport, insulin sensitivity can possibly be increased in the diabetic patient who exercises, with less resultant muscle deterioration.

Temporary changes in muscle performance are presumed to occur with many dietary habits, many of which have become fads and most of which are useless. If not overdone, carbohydrate loading before an athletic event is the one nutritional practice that results in increased performance. The glycogen content of muscle can be significantly increased, resulting in increased endurance. Misuse of this practice results in an overload of glycogen in muscle (cardiac as well as skeletal muscle); therefore, caution is advised. Electrocardiograph abnormalities have been reported as a result of excess glycogen and water deposits in cardiac muscle.

Environment

Temperature affects performance of muscle. Superficial applications of heat or cold in therapeutic doses do not affect the core temperature, and hence do not affect muscle temperature. However, studies of prolonged local cooling show that when muscle temperatures drop from around 35°C to about 25°C, the effect of the cold produces a significant increase in maximal voluntary muscle tension. Some have reported that cold of such intensity also increases local muscular endurance. However, general cardiovascular endurance is decreased if the cold application is of sufficient intensity.

Less intense local cooling, such as that obtained with cold packs, does not affect voluntary muscular effort. The desired response of relaxation occurs because of the heightened threshold of afferent nerve fibers. Therefore, we tend to use cold therapeutically to obtain relaxation. Using cold packs makes sense when the application is of short enough duration to reduce the firing rate of the cutaneous receptors. In the absence of transmission of pain signals, muscle is more likely to relax.

Heat is reported to bring about relaxation of muscle, provided the core temperature can be affected. Deep heat or prolonged heat is required to change muscle temperature. Muscle relaxation results because of a general depression of the central nervous system. Superficial warming may also induce muscle relaxation, either because of the psychologic effects of warmth, or because of the theorized interruption of the pain-spasm cycle.

Environmental hazards pose a threat to neuromuscular function. Lead poisoning and mercury poisoning are common causes of neuropathy and muscle weakness. Lead-based paints present a danger because children may eat chips of paint that have flaked off surfaces. Mercury poisoning is experienced by some persons who react to dental amalgams, especially if they have a mixture of metals in multiple fillings.

Time of Day

Voluntary muscle tension demonstrates a diurnal effect. Most persons are capable of significantly higher isometric tension levels in the afternoon than in the morning. Possibly the slight increase in body temperature a few hours after waking is enough to prepare the system for optimal performance. The temperature change is much less than what was discussed previously, which explains why a little warming can increase performance, whereas excessive warming decreases tension. The increased body temperature after waking is associated with increased blood flow. Warm-ups before a workout provide the same priming of the system, which improves performance and reduces incidence of injury.

Pathologic Factors

Muscle diseases can affect the myofibrils, the reticulum, the plasma membrane, the mitochondria, or the nuclei. The motor units appear fractured in an electromyogram tracing (Fig. 10-10). The normally smooth asynchronous recruitment of fibers in each motor unit is fragmented because some diseased fibers have dropped out. The EMG demonstrates motor units that are polyphasic and of short duration. Some repair or replacement of muscle fibers is attempted by the satellite cells located in the basement membrane of the muscle fibers. However, results are not functional, and fatty infiltration and connective tissue proliferation predominate. Muscular dystrophy, an inherited disease, may be arrested in our lifetime because the genetic code that alters the plasma membrane of skeletal muscle has recently been identified.

Tumors in many different organs and tissues produce muscle weakness. Often the pat-

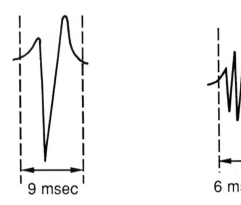

Figure 10-10. Schematic of typical short-duration, low-amplitude polyphasic potential seen in primary muscle disease *(right)*, compared with a representation of a triphasic normal motor unit potential *(left)*. (Goodgold J, Eberstein A: Electrodiagnosis of Neuromuscular Diseases, 3rd ed, p 158. Baltimore, Williams & Wilkins, 1983)

tern is proximal weakness, with the phasic (type II) fibers being more affected. Muscles exhibit weakness and slowed contraction time from atrophy of type II fibers. Physical therapists should be aware that the presence of proximal weakness with no known cause may reflect an undiagnosed tumor.

Metabolic diseases result in muscle weakness as well. The mechanisms are varied, but include high body temperatures and alterations in electrolyte balance. Exercise for patients who are weak due to a metabolic disorder can be painful, possibly because electrolyte balance is abnormal.

Pharmacologic Effects

Drug-induced weakness is a common condition that can be reversed if correctly observed, reported, and relieved. Severe alcohol ingestion acts on the calcium-binding mechanism of muscle. Alcoholic myopathies are characterized by cellular changes and profound weakness. Exercising myopathic muscles of the alcoholic patient is painful and can exacerbate the inflammation and microtrauma occurring in the muscle cells. Rest appears to reverse the soreness in a short time.

Corticosteroids (catabolic) are widely used in the management of many diseases. Essentially the prednisonelike steroids result in a reversible fast-twitch (type II) fiber atrophy in proximal muscles bilaterally. Synthetic steroids, particularly the fluorinated ones, have a more pervasive atrophic effect on all forms of muscle fiber. Withdrawal of steroid therapy might reverse the atrophy, but is often not practical because steroids are effective in managing many diseases. Exercise can retard and diminish the occurrence of muscle weakness that results from steroid ingestion. However, because steroids also cause alterations in bone, and because muscle exerts tension directly on bone, the patient and therapist must strive to avoid pathologic fractures from development of too much muscle tension on a weakened bone.

Medications can cause muscle weakness by affecting peripheral nerves. Vincristine, used to manage some forms of cancer, causes temporary peripheral neuropathy. Patients demonstrate paresthesias and weakness, particularly in the distal muscles.

Other medications also lead to muscle weakness. The pattern is usually bilateral, symmetrical, and most noted in the proximal muscles, with the muscles innervated by cranial nerves being spared. Medications used to control mood swings often result in lethargy, resulting in apparent general weakness because of a lack of desire to exert effort. Physical therapists do not prescribe medications, but do need to be alert to side-effects and drug interactions.

Mechanical Factors

Gravity is the "weak force" to nuclear physicists. To physical therapists (and all others), gravity is a significant force that we actively combat with muscle contraction. When gravitational forces diminish (as on the moon), our muscles cease combat. Atrophy ensues, just as when muscles become inactive through disuse. At this writing, there is minimal physical therapy in space, but NASA studies demonstrate the need for physical exercise in gravity-free environments. When in space, the muscles atrophy within a week because the stimulus of gravity, which normally elicits muscle contractions, has been removed. The converse is that gravity on earth is a potent force that requires muscle contractions to maintain upright posture. As a result of normal upright activity, muscles (especially the antigravity ones) are able to maintain their tone.

Length changes alter the mechanics of the contractile mechanisms of muscle, and hence the force capability of the fibers. A normal muscle's length-tension curve accounts for the active and passive elements of muscle tension, and dictates that optimal tension is developed at one point known as rest length (Fig. 10-11).

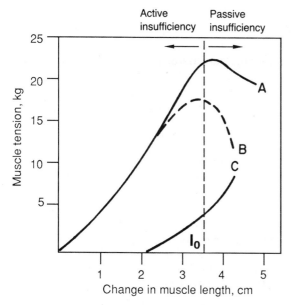

Figure 10-11. Isometric length-tension curve for human triceps muscle. Muscle length tension changes are taken from the length at which total muscle tension is zero. The curves are a summary of many results. *(A)* Most probable total tension curve. *(C)* Most probable passive tension curve with range indicated. *(B)* Net voluntary tension curve obtained by subtracting C from A. Shaded areas indicate range of results; l_0 is rest length or optimal length where voluntary tension is maximal. (Ruch TC, Patton HD: Physiology and Biophysics, 19th ed, p 129. Philadelphia, WB Saunders, 1965. After University of California: Fundamental Studies of Human Locomotion and Other Information Relating to Design of Artificial Limbs, vol 2, 1947)

The entire spectrum of any muscle's length is never available in vivo. In fact, rest length in one-joint muscles is near the muscle's lengthened position.

A muscle stretched past its normal in vivo length is believed to be weak, because conventional muscle testing in the shortened test position produces less torque in this stretched muscle. However, Gossman suggests that a stretched muscle may demonstrate normal peak torque at its new rest length, which may be missed because of test protocols. Therefore, the notion of stretch weakness may be erroneous. However, the concept remains that each muscle has a point in its range where peak torque is normally developed. The point in the range where peak torque occurs is a function of muscle length, and of the angle of insertion of the muscle into the bone.

The *angle of insertion* is a mechanical variable. Resultant muscle force (R) can be represented by two vectors: a stabilizing component (X) and a rotary component (Y). The rotary component is the only component that physical therapists evaluate regularly. The force in this vector becomes proportionately greater as the angle of insertion approaches 90 degrees, and thus more torque can be developed. The stabilizing force does not contribute to the torque, but does contribute significantly to the stability of the joint (Fig. 10-12). Changes in joint position, structural differences, or surgical alterations affect the angle of insertion, which will necessarily alter the tension in each of the components.

Muscle force is closely related to *speed of contraction*. Decreased force (and hence decreased torque) in an athlete means decreased acceleration capacity. Recall that force is the product of mass and acceleration. Decreased force in muscle also means decreased response time to a given stimulus, such as falling. Ordinarily the human muscle can develop maximal voluntary force levels within 200 to 400 msec. Weak muscle often takes longer, and then does so with less than optimal tension. In the gait cycle, inadequate rate of force development of the quadriceps produces instability at weight acceptance.

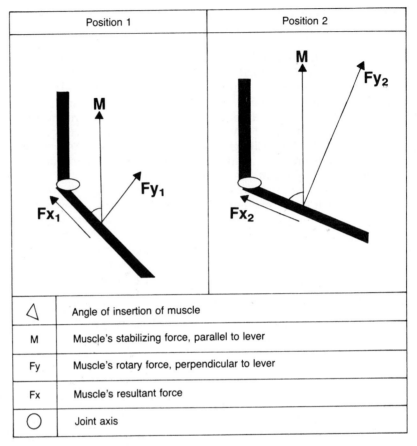

| | Position 1 | Position 2 |

△	Angle of insertion of muscle
M	Muscle's stabilizing force, parallel to lever
Fy	Muscle's rotary force, perpendicular to lever
Fx	Muscle's resultant force
◯	Joint axis

Figure 10-12. Given the same total muscle force *(M)*, as the muscle's angle of insertion increases (position 2), the rotary force *(Fy)* increases and the stabilizing force *(Fx)* decreases (torque = Fy × distance from insertion to joint).

The degree to which potential muscle force (actually, torque is the quantity measured) declines depends on the muscle group being tested. Agonists and antagonists behave differently. Preliminary findings suggest that some antigravity muscles (eg, knee extensors and ankle plantar flexors) are less capable of maintaining previously attained concentric torque levels when the speeds of movement are increased, than are the opposing flexor muscles. With muscle weakness, torque capability during a few slow maximal efforts may appear normal. But when the muscle is made to contract faster, excessive torque decrements with increasing speeds of movement provide clear evidence of muscle weakness. Inability to generate concentric torque at higher speeds may be linked to selective weakness of the fast-twitch fibers, alterations in neural control, or pain.

In studies of flexor muscles of cats, the velocities where torque loads approximate one third of maximal isometric capability are the velocities that produce optimal power output, and thus optimal training effects. Research suggests this optimal point in the velocity spectrum is about 200°/sec. Research of this sort is necessary on humans because generalizations from animal studies may be invalid. However, right-left comparisons with voluntary maximal effort can be made, and the relationship of isokinetic torque at a reasonable velocity to isometric torque measured at the same joint angle as the isokinetic peak torque is certainly a measure of interest. As stated previously, absolute torque is less interesting and less important than the rate at which torque can be produced.

Daily events do not require herculean forces; they do require precision timing.

In eccentric contractions, the force potential of muscle increases with increasing speeds of contraction. Comparison of a concentric and an eccentric contraction at equal levels of torque shows many fewer motor units active in the eccentric contraction. Joint forces in these two types of contraction will be the same, provided the rates and patterns of movement are the same. Little is currently known about the relationship between muscle weakness, joint mechanics, and comparable performance in concentric or eccentric muscle contractions. For example, clinical observation suggests that some patients with pathologic conditions of the knee are able to perform more work concentrically than eccentrically.

Psychologic Factors

Motivation and interest cannot be measured, but they are vital to producing and maintaining muscle tension. You need only to look at the posture of a depressed person to recognize that the trapezius muscle and the erector spinae muscle have let gravity get the upper hand. Lack of motivation and interest are also contaminating factors in the measurement of voluntary maximal effort, and they may mask normal strength in testing. Worse, lack of motivation and interest can ultimately lead to true muscle weakness. The mind-body association cannot be separated. Each aspect is an essential component of the other. In discussions of musculoskeletal dysfunction, physical therapists tend to concentrate on the physical entities. However, the entire discussion is invalid without taking into account the enormously important role that the emotional and cognitive factors have in musculoskeletal function.

CONNECTIVE TISSUE: BONE

Connective tissues serve many important functions, including support. Weakness in bones, ligaments, tendons or joint capsules brings about significant changes in function. Increased flexibility or compressibility alters normal internal forces, which then promote de-generation, pain, and dysfunction. Underlying causes are numerous.

What is meant by weak, flexible, compressible, porous, or brittle bone? All are examples of pathologic conditions in which the bone is unable to withstand normal stress. Factors that give rise to these pathologic states should be viewed in light of bone's composition. Bone is a connective tissue, and has the same three structural components as all other connective tissues: cells, fibers, and ground substance. In addition, bone has an inorganic matrix of minerals, which provides stiffness and rigidity. Bone provides attachment sites for muscles, levers for movement, structures for support, and cushions for shock absorption. The varying composition and arrangement of the cells, fibers, ground substance, and minerals within specific bones conform to the needs these bones normally serve. For example, the weight-bearing metatarsals have a higher density than the metacarpals of the hand. Various factors influence the degree to which bone succeeds in withstanding normal stresses and strains. Other functions of bone relating to homeostasis of electrolytes and formation of red blood cells during development are not addressed here.

Physiologic Factors

Development

Development during the life span affects bone's characteristics. The fetal skeleton is cartilage and, of course, is flexible and unable to support weight. Bone development is a dynamic process. During the growth periods of the long bones, the compact layers have not attained the density characteristics of maturity and are more prone to greenstick fractures. Some epiphyseal centers do not form synostoses until the late teens, and fractures at these sites before the child achieves full stature may result in stunted growth. Avulsion fractures, such as separation of the lesser trochanter from the femur, can occur in young persons. Aging bone also demonstrates compact layers, which are less dense. In addition, because of concomitant reduction in the ground substance with aging, bone is less resilient, and is brittle and less able to withstand compressive or tensile forces.

Disuse

Use and disuse patterns affect all tissues, and bone is no exception. Heavy dynamic exercise can cause hypertrophy, just as immobilization can produce atrophy. The apparent mechanism for bone hypertrophy is that exercise promotes more capillary beds. A richer environment increases cell activity. The responding cells are the osteoblasts, located in the membranous (inside) layer of the periosteum and endosteum. Normal daily activity suffices to keep osteoblasts active in the ongoing remodeling of bone (provided other nutritional conditions are met). Before the fifth decade of life, bone production matches the rate of bone absorption. Disuse dramatically decreases normal stimuli, and the rate of bone absorption exceeds the rate of bone production, with atrophy resulting. This condition of bone absorption is osteoporosis. Bones become more easily compressed because the internal bony architecture softens. Trabecular (or cancellous) bone is more affected by osteoporosis than is cortical (or compact) bone.

Trabecular bone is better suited to handle compressive forces than is cortical bone. Furthermore, trabecular bone is found predominantly in strategic places where compressive forces occur, such as in the vertebral column. Thus, when trabecular bone demineralizes and softens in osteoporosis, the result is the inability to maintain an erect, standard posture. Later, the person becomes unable to achieve an erect posture.

Research on osteoporosis is active at this time. Reports suggest that some bones are more susceptible than others. Reasons for this may be the differing proportions of cancellous to compact bone, or the different loading characteristics of the bone in question. The more a bone is loaded (used), the less notable is the degenerative change.

Nutrition

Nutrition affects bone as well as other tissues. The roles of calcium and vitamins C and D have been recognized for a long time. Other elements such as manganese and zinc are also important. A normal diet supplies adequate amounts of vitamins to maintain bone's inherent and optimal structure, but the same is not true of minerals. Mineral deficiencies lead to osteoporosis, partly because cancellous bone releases minerals to the body's demands more readily than compact bone. For some reason, small-boned women of northern European descent are more prone to osteoporosis in their later years. Current practice is to begin diet supplementation before menopause.

Mechanical Factors

Bone responds to external forces. Long-term bracing or any type of *static positioning* affects the way in which bone remodels itself. Bilateral genu varum (bowed legs) from years of horseback riding is a mild example. Stunted phalanges from the ancient Chinese practice of binding women's feet is a more extreme example. The forward head position from failure to keep gravity at bay is a common clinical example. The forward head, as with any other postural deviation, is accompanied by other compensatory changes, some of which are bony. Because bone becomes less dense with aging (or with fewer demands placed on it), gravitational forces gain an advantage and are more able to dominate the remodeling of the cervical and thoracic vertebrae. Because vascularity is compromised, either through altered forces or through aging or disuse, the internal mechanisms for remodeling bone and balancing the gravitational forces are inadequate. Accompanying compensatory changes in this example may include increased head or neck extension, low cervical and high thoracic spine flexion, and shortened sternomastoid muscles. The reversability of such changes depends on the degree of structural alteration, the duration of the postural change, and the characteristics of the tissues involved.

Implants, such as screws or plates surgically placed within fractured bones, can themselves cause weakness. Living tissues react to the presence of implants by both osteoblastic and osteoclastic activity. An implant alters the manner in which forces are transmitted, and may lead to bone resorption. After implant removal, activity levels must be reduced to allow time for bone tissue to reorganize. Bone resorption without concomitant bone replacement leads to weakness, and finally to total dysfunction.

Healed *fractures* do not present a problem. Often the bone is more dense at the fracture site as a result of repair efforts. Incomplete healing of fractures results in permanently weakened bone structure. Because of the piezoelectric charges of bone, the positive polarity of the convex surface tends toward being osteoclastic (resorptive), whereas the negative polarity of the concave surface tends toward being osteoblastic (regenerative). Excessive bone may be laid down within the concave area, while inadequate repair may occur over the convex area. Strategically implanted electrical stimulation devices have proven helpful in supplementing the repair process in poorly healing fractures.

Diseases

Bone is susceptible to neoplasms, which can affect any of the three substrates (cells, fibers, and ground substance) and lead to changes in dynamic function. If a sarcoma pervades the organic substance, bone becomes less distensible, more stiff, and prone to fracture. If a fibroma proliferates, the fibrous substance increases, with resulting increased tensile strength but decreased flexibility. If the ground substance is affected, bone responds with increased flexibility and decreased strength.

Bone can also become infected or inflamed. Any mechanism, whether parasitic, viral, or bacterial, will destroy bone tissue and lead to weakness and dysfunction. Bone degeneration occurs as a sequela to some diseases. In this instance, the resorption of bone outdistances the regenerative attempts. The recessed mandible and the short extremities of children who have had severe juvenile rheumatoid arthritis are examples of the effects of disease on bone in children.

Some medications used in the management of disease, particularly neoplasms, have bone resorption as a side-effect. Weakened bone is more prone to compression stresses.

Hyperstimulation of growth hormone, which results from abnormal levels of ACTH, will produce abnormal growth in bone. Increased density of bone does not make the bone more weak; but, because it is less flexible, the bone becomes vulnerable to tension stresses and shear forces.

OTHER CONNECTIVE TISSUES AND JOINTS

The tendons, ligaments, capsules, and muscle and nerve sheaths are all examples of connective tissues whose functional role is dependent on normal abilities to withstand stresses and strains. Weakness is the inability to withstand internal and external forces, and it may result from being too flexible or too rigid. The clinical indications of connective tissue abnormalities can be increased flexibility, decreased flexibility, altered patterns of movement, altered rates of movement, frank ruptures, subluxations, or pain.

All connective tissues (like bone) have three major components: the cells and the fibers that together make up the cellular matrix, and the ground substance that forms the extracellular matrix. The cells synthesize the fibers, which lend tensile strength to the material. The ground substance, composed of amorphous glycosaminoglycans, is made up in part by cellular secretions, and lends compressive strength and flexibility to the tissue. Altering these components by a variety of factors will change the balance of the tissue, and hence its functional role.

Stiffness and laxity are measures that indicate relative degrees of stability and flexibility. Stiffness is the rate of change in length with a known change in load. Laxity is the change in length with a known change in load, and has a negative correlation with strength and body weight. Most clinical measures for stiffness and laxity rely on subjective judgments derived from history taking, palpations, passive testing (range-of-motion and accessory movement testing), and subjective end-feel and observation of joint movement. Physical therapists become familiar with what is considered normal for a person of a certain age, sex, and lifestyle.

Then, therapists consider factors that can affect the normal behavior of connective tissue, and arrive at a better understanding of whether or not the tissue is dysfunctional, and what can be done to improve the situation. Factors that may affect the stiffness or laxity of connective tissues are discussed below.

Physiologic Factors

Certain changes occur in all connective tissue as a result of aging, regardless of use patterns. The arterial supply gradually becomes occluded and the tissues rely more on diffusion and less on internal blood supply for nutrition. The central arteries located in tendons atrophy by the third decade of life. The blood supply to the intervertebral disks is also compromised by the third decade, and the structures then rely on imbibition for maintenance. Decreased nutrition affects repair and replacement, and tissues become less supple. Some connective tissue, such as cartilage, has no internal blood supply and has always had to rely on diffusion. However, as cartilage becomes more compressed with aging, the diffusion process becomes less adequate.

Posture alters the arrangement of connective tissue (see discussion of bone). For example, as structures become compressed by a stooping posture, they become more dense. Diffusion becomes more of a challenge and the tissues become less well nourished. Normally cartilage is a metabolically active tissue whose cells participate in regeneration. With increased compression and decreased nutrition, repair is inadequate and the ability to resist compressive forces is compromised. In addition, collagen fibers, normally oriented in parallel to resist stresses, become less well oriented and the elasticity of the tissue is reduced. Shorter periods of stress now result in irreversible changes because the tissue loses its ability to regain pre-stretched or pre-compressed states.

Use patterns affect the organization of connective tissue fibers. Optimal arrangements result from normal physiologic use. Without the proper stimulus of normal movement and normal stress, the normal ongoing repair or replacement process changes, and the connective tissue structure is altered. Sometimes normal movement and normal stress cannot be tolerated. In these situations, fibers become oriented in nonphysiologic arrangements, overall length is inadequate, and ground substance is compressed. The clinical picture is reduced flexibility, altered movement, and, usually, pain.

Exercise

Exercise has an effect on connective tissues. Warming up before exercise is believed to increase the circulation and enhance flexibility, thereby reducing the likelihood of an overstretched tendon or ligament. Intensive, dynamic exercise of several months' duration increases the tensile strength of connective tissue fibers. The increased stiffness is believed to result from the additional collagen fibrils, which increase the diameter of the fibers. However, exercise that is too vigorous can lead to tissue breakdown. Excessive forces create tissue trauma, and excessive durations lead to fatigue and increased laxity. For example, responses to cyclic loading of knee specimens demonstrate that there is an increase in measured ligamentous laxity, which supports the observation that ligamentous injuries in skiing often occur late in the afternoon after a full day of skiing. Protective mechanisms of muscle also become deficient from fatigue by the end of a day's activities, and probably contribute to the injury rate.

Gender-based differences may be apparent in ligamentous composition and capability. Common belief holds that women's ligaments are more lax than men's, but some studies suggest that when mass and strength are factored out, the sexes are comparable in ligamentous laxity, except during pregnancy.

Pharmacologic and Hormonal Influences

Some connective tissues are known to be altered with hormonal changes and with some medications. Pregnancy promotes increased flexibility of some connective tissues. This may be due, in part, to an increased amount of ground substance (proteoglycans and glycoproteins). The incidence of compartment syndromes, such as carpal tunnel syndrome, is reportedly increased during some pregnancies. With an increase in some of the connective tissue components, structures in tight spaces are compressed, producing compartment syndromes with their reversible sensory and motor changes.

Drugs appear to influence connective tissues indirectly. Muscle relaxants, which reduce tension in muscle, will reduce guarding during ligamentous testing and produce more apparent flexibility. For example, when testing for a posterior cruciate ligament abnormality, the therapist determines the relative amount of posterior displacement of the tibia on the femur. If the quadriceps is tensed, the full amount of displacement available will not be exhibited; but if the quadriceps is relaxed, a greater range of tibial displacement would be expected. Drugs that suppress inflammation, such as the corticosteroids, will result in more measurable flexibility because swelling, guarding, and pain are reduced.

Mechanical Factors

Connective tissue is plastic and responds dynamically to stresses placed upon it. Mechanical factors that weaken connective tissue include stretch, compression, and shear.

Stretch, if sufficient in intensity and duration, can elongate or rupture connective tissues. Connective tissue stretches through slow, constant loading and through rapid, forceful movement. Forceful movement is traumatic, and is exemplified by tendon tears, as well as avulsion fractures. Slow, constant loading causes microtrauma, and has a more insidious onset. Both are common and both are preventable. Postural stretches that occur to connective tissues can be from muscle weakness, as in the subluxed shoulder of the patient with hemiplegia and atrophy of the supraspinatus muscles. More often, postural stretches result from poor habits acquired over a lifetime. The situation is compounded when dynamic activity is reduced, so that nothing adequately counteracts gravity's constant presence. Dynamic activity may be exercise, but it

can also be something as simple as frequent changes of position. Capsular laxity can produce impingement syndromes whereby a snip of loose tissue (such as a synovial fold) gets pinched at a specific point in the joint's range, producing a repeatable painful arc of movement. Once a capsule has become lax, repeated trauma is likely. A familiar example is the unstable ankle joint with the overstretched anterior talofibular ligament from previous sprains. A less familiar example, and one more difficult to confirm, is the segmental instability of the vertebral column that is due to overstretched connective tissue components at one or more of the articulations.

"Double joints" do not exist. Excessive or abnormal mobility is simply a result of overstretched ligaments and joint capsules. Because connective tissue is more supple in younger persons, prolonged stretching leads to greater laxity in children than in adults. Early and excessive gymnastic stretching is not advised for children because of the resulting instability in later years.

Lack of movement produces lengthening of some aspects of joint capsules and ligaments, but the concurrent shortening of other aspects is just as detrimental. Shortened fibers restrict range, and are more prone to rupture (either totally or microscopically) at their attachments. Shortened capsular fibers produce capsular patterns that are proportional limitations in a joint's passive range of motion. Sometimes the tightness causes other loose connective tissues, such as bursae near the joint, to become impinged during movement, resulting in a painful arc of movement despite the range of motion being within normal limits.

Compression can also weaken connective tissues. Cartilage is the most susceptible tissue to compressive forces. Ground substance diminishes and the lacunae that house the chondrocytes (cartilage cells) become compressed. Shock absorption capability is reduced. Repeated stresses on neighboring tissues, like the synovial layer of the joint capsule, promote other changes in the cartilage. Decreased production of synovial fluid increases the surface tension and thus increases friction during movement. The chondroblasts, which normally attempt to make new cartilage cells, now behave like fibroblasts or osteoblasts and lay down more densely arranged fibers. Osteophytes at joint surfaces result, as in osteoarthritis.

Mechanical alignment of bones and joints is a complex, but critical, factor in normal function. Intracapsular fat pads increase joint congruency, and their functional necessity is evidenced by their sustained presence, even during starvation. The interactions of adjoining segments influence all structures, and the forces and their effects on the connective tissues must be understood before they can be analyzed and managed.

Trauma has primary and secondary effects on the connective tissues. The primary ones of overstretch, rupture, and avulsion fracture have been mentioned. Secondary effects are more insidious. Blood within a joint capsule destroys hyaline cartilage. Overproduction of synovial fluid in response to trauma can lead to joint swelling and possibly to the formation of ganglionic tissue. Menisci or articular disks may become loose after joint inflammation and interfere with joint mechanics.

Disease

Connective tissues are subject to diseases and neoplasms, although not uniformly. Neoplasms arise in the synovium and in fatty tissues, but not in ligaments, hyaline cartilage, or menisci. Metabolic diseases form an enormous category, and include rheumatoid arthritis and lupus erythematosus. Discussion of connective tissue diseases is well beyond the scope of this chapter, but you are encouraged to apply information about the roles of cells, fibers, and ground substance in all types of connective tissue to understand better the processes of disease and theories of intervention. Keep in mind that the connective tissues embrace bone, cartilage, synovium, ligament, fat, fascia, aponeurosis, joint capsule, bursa, labrum, sheaths of muscle fibers and nerve fibers, and coverings of organs and blood vessels.

FATIGUE

Fatigue implies a decrease over time in the ability of a tissue to perform the purpose for which it is designed. Bone fatigue (with subsequent fracture) results in the inability of bone to sustain and transmit loads. Cartilage fatigue (with subsequent fissuring and erosion) results in a decreased ability of cartilage to distribute and transmit forces at joints. Muscle fatigue (with subsequent decreased force output) results in decreased motor function ability. Fatigue is a natural phenomenon in the sense that all tissues demonstrate an upper limit of tolerance to repeated loading; beyond that upper limit, signs of fatigue and possible breakdown may occur. Normal, healthy connective tissue elements of the musculoskeletal system respond to the demands of repetitive loading with a constant tissue turnover that allows tissue breakdown and repair to occur in a balanced way. However, if upper limits are exceeded, an imbalance develops and tissue breakdown with pain and inflammation occurs. Muscle responds to repeated loading that goes beyond its upper limits of tolerance by ceasing to function, or at least by functioning with a limited force output that does not endanger its basic integrity. In a general sense, then, fatigue may either protect against injury (as it seems to do in muscle), or initiate dysfunction (as it does in bone, tendon, and cartilage). In the musculoskeletal system, the consequences of fatigue are unique to the special contribution each tissue makes to the stability and mobility of the body.

CONNECTIVE TISSUE

Connective tissues such as bone, cartilage, ligament, and tendon have been studied under extreme single-load applications, and under repetitive low-loading and time-dependent situations. Fatigue as the human body's response to physical activity is perhaps best represented experimentally by the repetitive low-loading or time-dependent situations. However, the response of connective tissue to extreme single-load application illustrates the destructive influence of excessively high forces, the consequences of which may make the connective tissue reach fatigue limits sooner. This response is reviewed below.

Response to Single High-Load Application

Stress-strain curves for connective tissues developed under extreme single-load application all demonstrate characteristic shapes and an upper limit of tolerance to mechanical stress, which, if exceeded, threatens the structural integrity of the tissue. The shapes and upper limits of these curves vary for each tissue, depending on relative amount, organization, and orientation of collagen fibers and other composite materials.

Bone possesses a calcified matrix, and therefore has a hard and rigid structure that is well designed for its role of support. Normal healthy bone will deform under moderate loads, but will return to its original position and geometry once the loads have been removed. If loads are increased, deformation increases until the forces overcome the bone's capability to restore itself, and the bone reaches its failure point and fractures. Different physical characteristics of bone (size, shape, organization) as well as variables related to the type of imposed load (tension, compression, bending, shear, torsion) determine a bone's exact response to loading. In addition, bone, like most connective tissue elements, is anisotropic, that is, it exhibits different mechanical properties depending on the direction of loading. The ultimate dysfunction is the fracture, which destroys the bone's structural integrity and no longer allows it to function as a supportive structure (eg, fractures of the long bones). In addition, other bones that primarily protect internal organs may no longer be able to serve this purpose, and by the nature of the injury may actually damage the structure they were designed to protect (eg, lung punctures from fractured ribs). Physically disabling systemic effects of bone fractures may also develop, with the potential for circulatory, respiratory, and neurologic complications, from fat emboli released from fractures that involve the bone marrow.

Cartilage has a semisolid matrix and a high percentage of glycosaminoglycans interwoven with its constituent collagen and elastin fibers. This physical makeup results in relatively little stiffness, but a large water-binding capacity that is well adapted to cartilage's role of spreading loads over a joint surface and allowing motion between joint surfaces while minimizing friction and potential wear. Because cartilage is avascular, it depends upon motion and pressure changes for its nutritional health by means of imbibition. Impact loads are particularly harmful to cartilage, because they put high stress on the collagen fibers and proteoglycan matrix. Once the integrity of the microstructure of cartilage has been disrupted, further mechanical stress, although of normal magnitude and frequency, may compound the problem by adding to a negative cycle of increased wear, fatigue, and tissue failure.

Ligament, capsule, and tendon are also subject to stress and potential failure. Normally, tendons and ligaments are particularly well suited to resist the tensile stresses imposed by either muscle contraction or external loads because a high percentage of their collagen fibers are arranged longitudinally in the direction of imposed stresses. On the other hand, joint capsules are well adapted to movement in multiple planes because of the multidirectional nature of their collagen fiber arrangement. Soft tissues in general, unlike hard bone tissue, possess a high water content. The degree of stiffness or elasticity of connective tissue depends on whether collagen or elastin fibers predominate. Collagen and elastin behave differently under loading; therefore, the stress-strain curves for tissues of higher collagen composition differ from curves for tissues of higher elastin composition. When compared with cortical bone tested in tension, collagen fibers tolerate about one-half and elastin fibers about one-tenth the amount of stress that cortical bone does before tissue failure occurs in single-load application.

Response to Sustained Repetitive Low-Load Application

In general, connective tissue responds to and tolerates loads applied for certain durations of time by a phenomenon called creep. Creep is a property of viscoelastic biologic materials that results in a slow deformation of the tissue over time. Although most deformation occurs when the load is imposed, creep that results in elongation of soft tissue may continue at low rates over many months. Most of the static stretching techniques used in physical therapy to elongate muscle or stretch tight joints probably take advantage of the creep phenomenon. The exact amount or duration of load that is optimal for achieving clinical success in stretching programs is not known, and may be influenced by many factors, such as the patient's age, genetic predisposition to tissue laxity, changes in hormonal levels, or the severity of injury or the type of disease process that initiated the contracture.

Bone depends on a certain amount of "normal" mechanical stress for its healthy state, as is evidenced by the bone loss apparent during prolonged periods of immobilization. However, when the mechanical stress on bone is of such a repetitive and sustained nature that microdamage to bone tissue overcomes the bone's inherent ability for repair, fatigue fractures may occur. Because these fractures begin as microdamage to the bone, they are often not visible initially on roentgenograms and it is only when subperiosteal and endosteal new bone appears that a fatigue fracture is confirmed. Because fatigue fractures of bone often occur in deconditioned persons or during sustained and vigorous activity, muscle fatigue has been suggested as one possible cause. Fatigued muscles are believed to fail in their role as energy absorbers; therefore, bone becomes subject to abnormally high stresses with the potential for subsequent fatigue fractures.

Cartilage will also respond to repetitive loading by tissue failure if an imbalance occurs between the normal breakdown and repair process. This is demonstrated clinically by the fact that persons in certain occupations and sports that produce high repetitive joint load-ing effects suffer from cartilage degeneration. The cartilage that lines joints is particularly susceptible to fatigue from repetitive loading because joints normally function in repetitive modes in all activities of daily living. It has been hypothesized that fatigue failure results from disruption in the collagen fibers themselves, a breakdown in the proteoglycan macromolecular system, or problems at the interface between fibers and the interfibrillar matrix.

The mechanical properties of the soft tissues have been reported to vary considerably. It is unclear if this is due to inherent variability, or to the difficulties in studying these tissues using classical experimental methods and in vivo methods. Nevertheless, soft tissues such as cartilage, tendon, ligament, and capsule follow a bonelike pattern of response to repetitive loading; however, they show a higher tolerance to strain and develop fatigue more slowly than bones, probably because soft tissues are more viscoelastic than bones. Ligaments pushed beyond their fatigue limits develop excessive laxity and can contribute to joint instability. Once fatigue thresholds in cartilage are reached, it is at a higher risk than other soft tissue for tissue degradation because it is avascular and its capacity for self-repair is limited. Clinically, the terms *tendonitis* and *tenosynovitis* refer to an inflammatory process of either the tendon or (as occurs in some locations in the body) the synovial lining of the sheath that surrounds the tendon. These conditions are often referred to as "overuse syndromes," indicating the repetitive or sustained nature of the precipitating event.

Clinical Relevance

Physical therapists are interested in the differing fatigue and failure characteristics of soft and hard tissue in response to immobilization and enforced exercise. Many of our patients are seen after prolonged periods of immobilization; moreover, exercise is a common mode of rehabilitation after an injury and in conditioning regimens for otherwise normal persons. Prolonged immobility is known to result in periosteal and subperiosteal bone resorption along with a decrease in bone strength and stiffness. Joints that are immobilized can develop periarticular and intra-articular adhesions, and the strength and stiffness of tendons, ligaments, and related musculature significantly decrease. Knowing these negative effects of immobility, the clinician should devise a rehabilitation plan with graduated programs of exercise and weight bearing to avoid tissue failure and inflammatory pain responses.

Based on animal research that has demonstrated the negative effects of immobility and the positive effects of remobilization, clinicians and researchers have developed technology that encourages and promotes early controlled movement after injury or surgical repair. Continuous passive motion machines are used to foster repair of articular cartilage defects and to stress ligaments and tendons to improve their response to tensile loading. In addition, electrical stimulators are used to promote muscle activity and engender more normal and prolonged bone stress during imposed immobility periods. However, the intensity of the early mobilization efforts must be geared to avoid overstretching and injury to newly repaired tissue, and use of electrical stimulators for muscle contraction must be monitored because the mechanism of electrically induced muscle contraction differs from physiologic contraction and high fatigue levels can be reached prematurely.

MUSCLE

Muscle, which has a different structural makeup than the primarily connective tissue elements of the musculoskeletal system, has been studied somewhat differently with respect to fatigue. Muscle fatigue is a complex mix of objective and subjective sensations. As such, it can be and has been studied from various viewpoints, including the psychological origins of weariness or perceived tiredness, and the biochemical substrate or circulatory system components necessary for sustained motor activity.

The cardiovascular system plays an important role in allowing muscle activity to continue over a sustained period. Under experimental conditions, muscle force declines rapidly from loss of its nutrient base, especially oxygen. The critical role of vascular support is demonstrated clinically by the marked inability of patients with intermittent claudication syndromes or severe peripheral vascular disease to sustain muscular effort. In addition, patients with heart or lung disease or dysfunction who are unable to supply or transport nutrients or eliminate waste products will also suffer from generalized fatigue during motor activities.

Sources of energy for muscle contraction originate from the ingestion of carbohydrates, fats, and proteins. Therefore, inadequate nutrition can be a source of profound muscle fatigue. These chemical compounds (mostly carbohydrates and fats; protein is used only in starvation) are metabolized by the body to produce the energy needed for muscle contraction. To sustain muscular effort and avoid muscle fatigue, a continuous supply of the energy compound adenosine triphosphate (ATP) is needed. ATP can be produced anaerobically through the process of glycolysis; however, the energy gain is less than in aerobic metabolism and glycolytic by-products such as lactic acid form, which further interfere with muscle contraction ability. Aerobic pathways use glycogen or free fatty acids, and in the process yield high ATP levels as well as non-noxious by-products. Therefore, aerobic pathways are better suited to delaying muscle fatigue.

Specific types of muscle contraction may selectively use anaerobic rather than aerobic methods of energy production, and therefore the ability to sustain effort within that particular mode of contraction is affected. For example, muscle activity that is dynamic, though repetitive, may be sustained for long periods provided the work rate does not exceed either the muscle's glycogen supply or the body's ability to aerobically resynthesize ATP from glycogen or free fatty acid stores. In contrast, the duration of static and sustained efforts, such as isometric muscle contractions, will be limited by the finite supply of energy located within the muscle itself, the relative ischemia caused by the sustained contraction, and the lactic acid buildup from anaerobic metabolism.

Efforts to push the thresholds of fatigue higher in normal persons are well documented in endurance training, where overloading oxygen delivery and utilization systems seems to result in greater capillary densities in muscles, improved aerobic enzyme systems, and more and larger mitochondria in muscle cells. However, an upper limit to endurance exists, dictated in part by the inherited ratio of muscle fiber types. Olympic athletes who compete in endurance events tend to show a higher ratio of slow-twitch versus fast-twitch fibers; the reverse is true for athletes who compete primarily in sprint events. Because there is no clear evidence that, under nonexperimental conditions, fiber type can change from slow to fast or vice versa, conditioning programs are generally directed at maximizing the potential and extending the capabilities of the extant system. Similarly, in rehabilitation programs, resistance to muscle fatigue is improved through graduated and progressive exercises that increase the frequency, duration, and intensity of muscle activity.

Muscle fatigue may be a positive feedback mechanism to shut down motor activity when the muscle's metabolic limits have been reached. The accumulation of metabolic end products signals fatigue and discomfort when the circulation is unable to keep up with the metabolic demands being made, and the patient stops the activity. However, in some patients this positive feedback mechanism may not be operative. For example, in patients with only partially innervated muscle, the ratio of blood supply to remaining active muscle fibers is greater than normal. This means that the buildup of metabolites either does not occur or occurs less readily, and therefore no signal to stop is received. These patients may be in danger of developing overuse syndromes. However, fatigue limits and fatigue mechanisms have not been identified in specific patient populations. Therefore, the advisability and the intensity of exercise in patients with certain disease processes remains a clinical judgment.

Multiple sites of failure have been incriminated when a decline in muscle force output occurs secondary to fatigue. Experimentally, it is possible to discern central and peripheral fatigue. Motor nerve stimulation will still be able to elicit a muscle contraction in central fatigue, but it cannot do so in peripheral fatigue. However, in clinical situations the origin of fatigue may not be as easily discerned. Motivation and cognitive effort play a large role in sustained motor activity, and persons can push themselves or voluntarily decline to do so, modifying the total time to fatigue. Specific sites of failure have been identified in some muscle diseases. Transient muscle fatigue during lower extremity exercise in patients with multiple sclerosis may be related to inadequate nerve transmission across sites of plaque formation in the nerve itself. In myasthenia gravis, neurotransmitter function at the neuromuscular junction has been found to be deficient, and in other rare diseases, mitochondrial defects have been recognized. However, in most normal muscle, fatigue is related to glycogen depletion and intracellular acidosis. Although little is known about fatigue mechanisms in atrophied muscle, it is also believed to be a function of these muscles working at or near their metabolic limits.

The concept of the physiologic joint includes all the elements that contribute to the normal functioning of the musculoskeletal system. The body uses the muscular system, which is driven by neurologic elements and sustained through cardiorespiratory factors, to move joints whose own structures are nourished, strengthened, and protected by such movement. A breakdown in any one element in this complex, interrelated system has serious consequences for the remainder, and the result can be significant physical disability and dysfunction.

LOSS OR CHANGE IN CENTRAL CONTROL

Deficits or changes in the neurologic system can be manifested clinically through changes in musculoskeletal structure and function. Even though the primary lesion is in the central nervous system, a change is brought about in how the structures of the musculoskeletal system behave and relate to each other. In other words, some of the basic rules of maintaining healthy structure and integrated functioning of the parts of the musculoskeletal system may break down if central control mechanisms deviate from normal or are lost.

PARALYSIS OR PARESIS

One of the most obvious problems associated with CNS damage is paralysis. The loss of active control of muscle function and the subsequent immobility that it produces have serious implications for many of the tissues in the musculoskeletal system. In general, during immobility, bone becomes demineralized, muscle tends to atrophy, and joint structures develop contractures.

Much of the understanding of the negative effects of immobility has been derived from studies of immobilized but otherwise normal persons. Differences between the type and severity of the effects of immobility resulting from a damaged central nervous system and the effects of immobility that is imposed on a person with an intact CNS have not been studied in depth. However, one might assume that the effects are at least similar, if not further compounded, in the patient with a damaged CNS.

Bone formation and absorption is dictated in part by weight-bearing stress and muscle contraction activity. In the neurologically normal person, demineralization that occurs during imposed immobility reverses when weight-bearing activities are resumed. However, demineralization that occurs because of immobility caused by muscle paralysis does not seem to reverse as readily, or to the same extent. The implication is that weight bearing alone is not enough to retard the demineralization process in the neurologically damaged patient, and that muscle contraction or certain other neurologic mechanisms may be a critical missing link. A good example is the patient with an injured spinal cord who, despite standing activities, suffers extensive bone demineralization effects below the level of the cord lesion. During attempts to substitute for the loss of muscle function, as in the use of electrical stimulation for standing activity, the therapist should observe caution because these patients lack bone tolerance.

Loss of joint mobility and muscle atrophy following immobilization is well documented in the neurologically normal population. Similar effects occur in the presence of muscle paresis secondary to CNS damage. Muscle atrophy occurs, but in the patient with a damaged CNS, the bias is towards atrophy of the type II muscle fibers. In the neurologically intact, but immobilized person, the bias is towards atrophy of the type I fibers. Joint contractures in the presence of muscle paralysis or paresis compound the patient's difficulties with movement. In addition, in some neurologically damaged patients with muscle paralysis, calcific deposits form in the soft tissues surrounding joints, which results in pain, swelling, and a loss of joint range of motion. The mechanism for this ectopic ossification is unknown. Although not limited to persons with neurologic damage, it can and does occur when muscle paralysis is secondary to a spinal cord injury.

Muscle paralysis can also result in changes in extremity functional use patterns. Depending on the extent and pattern of involvement, the normal physiologic rhythm can be seriously disrupted. Aberrant movement patterns may produce impingement syndromes as force couples can no longer operate either because of ineffective force production, or a change in the timing or onset of muscle activity in one of the partners or synergists of the movement. Paralysis may also dictate that alternate patterns of movements and extreme joint positions be used to accomplish functional tasks. Over time, this may result in capsuloligamentous laxity and joint hypermobility with attendant pain and the potential for changes in joint wear patterns, lubrication mechanisms, and destructive effects on cartilage.

CHANGES IN CHARACTER

Normal muscle at rest has some resistance to passive lengthening, and if severed in vivo, will retract because of the resilience of the tissue. Muscle in the neurologically damaged person demonstrates alterations of this characteristic, historically referred to as *tone*, which, in combination with patterns of muscle weakness, will interfere with normal movement. Increased resistance to passive lengthening and poor active muscle control combine to hold joints rigidly immobile in positions that favor contracture formation. Depending on the particular combination of increased resting turgor and decreased voluntary movement of specific muscle groups, preferential contracture patterns may develop in the trunk or extremities. For example, the patient with Parkinson's disease tends to develop a forward flexed spine, and the hemiplegic patient is at high risk for an adduction-internal rotation contracture at the shoulder.

Changes that result in a decreased amount of resistance to passive elongation (flaccidity) also have an effect on musculoskeletal tissue. Flaccidity accompanied by lack of active muscle control results in a general vascular and fluid stasis in the affected area, predisposing the segment to edema formation, subsequent connective tissue proliferation, and eventual contracture development. Joints also become predisposed to instability, excessive stress, and, over time, stretched capsuloligamentous support so that articular surface relationships change. The subluxed shoulder of the hemiplegic patient is a good example of the effects of lack of resting muscular turgor on joint alignment. Scapula positioning is altered because of reduced voluntary and involuntary tension of the shoulder girdle musculature, and the glenoid fossa becomes excessively angulated in an inferior direction. The weight of the dependent extremity further acts to separate joint surfaces. This, along with the lack of resting tension in the supraspinatus muscle, results in an overstretch of the superior joint capsule and the supraspinatus tendon, which normally maintain joint integrity.

In a lower extremity joint that must tolerate the high stresses of weight-bearing forces, further damage to musculoskeletal structures may occur if precautions are not taken. For example, the patient who lacks muscular support and sufficient muscle activity to stabilize the knee may "lock" the knee into a hyperextended position to attain a stable limb for walking. Over time, the posterior capsule of the knee may overstretch, tibiofemoral and patellofemoral relationships may change, joint stability may be compromised, and soft tissue damage and pain syndromes may develop.

SENSORY CHANGES

Sensory loss secondary to CNS involvement may be another way in which joint damage is produced. Even in the presence of voluntary muscle control, a loss of proprioceptive sensation from joints may interfere with the reflex activation of protective muscle activity, and therefore make the joint vulnerable to unnecessary and damaging extremes of movement. Everyday trauma that the joint is normally protected against then becomes a potential source of serious injury to musculoskeletal structures.

Finally, visual, cognitive, or balance reaction deficits that are not compensated may predispose the patient with CNS damage to falls and subsequent gross trauma to the musculoskeletal system. These injuries may be neither as adequately nor as efficiently resolved as in the neurologically normal person because of the aforementioned problems.

DEGENERATION

All tissues degenerate. Part of our biologic program includes degeneration, and this aspect is present from conception. The rate of degeneration is never noticed, however, until it surpasses the rate of tissue generation or regeneration. Then we become aware of a change. Degeneration is a normal process, but when it advances too rapidly, it becomes a pathologic process. When it advances slowly but reversibly, it is a disuse phenomenon; when it advances slowly but irreversibly, it is aging. Sometimes these processes happen concurrently.

PATHOLOGIC DEGENERATION

Muscle

Muscle degenerates in primary muscle diseases (myopathies). Numerous structures of the muscle cell can be affected, including the mitochondria, the sarcoplasmic reticulum, the plasma membrane, and the nuclei. Functional changes include decreased endurance and decreased force capability from fatty infiltration and reduction of myofibril synthesis. Attempts at self-repair produce connective tissue, not muscle tissue. In humans, different muscle fiber types seem to be affected about equally in the myopathies.

Neuropathies may result in muscle degeneration if they are prolonged or severe enough. Muscle depends on innervation for its maintenance. If innervation is lost, the muscle will atrophy and change to fat and scar tissue in a matter of months. If innervation is altered, as in nerve transplants, the muscle characteristics will reflect those of the newly transplanted nerve (ie, fast twitch or slow twitch).

Trauma obviously creates pathologic conditions in muscle. Overstretching and overworking are the two primary types of trauma. Overstretching can cause tears of the connective tissue sleeves of the muscle fibers, tears at the myotendinous junction, or tears within the muscle fiber itself. Overworking causes fatigue of the muscle. The attachments of the muscle to periosteum become irritated. Membrane permeability increases, and edema occurs. In tight compartments bound by dense fascia, a small amount of edema creates distention and pressure. Sensory nerve endings in the fascia signal pain, which is one possible explanation for the discomfort of shin splints. Some clinicians have postulated that the same mechanism may contribute to the discomfort of low back pain.

Often we overstretch or overwork such small portions of our muscles that we are not aware of the pathologic effects. This microtrauma builds up over time, and one day becomes a frank symptom with no known precipitating cause. These overuse syndromes are common, but are avoidable with proper patient education.

Connective Tissue

The connective tissues, including bone, cartilage, ligaments, tendons, and fascia also degenerate in disease processes and in trauma. Their demise is less rapid than that of muscle. Affected components of connective tissue include cells, fibers, ground substance, and, in the case of bone, mineralization. If the cells (fibroblasts) were affected, a functional change would be altered fiber synthesis. Neoplasms increase fiber synthesis, whereas degenerative diseases reduce fiber synthesis. Changes in the number of fibers and their arrangement alter the structural properties of the tissue (density, stiffness, and flexibility). Changes in the content and amount of ground substance affect the tissue's distensibility and compressibility. Articular cartilage, for example, provides shock absorption and diffusion for a load. If the cells (chondrocytes) fail to produce adequate proteoglycans for the ground substance, the cells will be closer together and less able to absorb the forces produced in weight bearing. If membrane permeability changes and plasma enters the tissue, degeneration is predictable because cartilage does not survive in the presence of blood. Recalling endochondral bone formation, the presence of blood is the necessary stimulus for cartilage resorption and production of osseous material.

DISUSE

All tissues within the musculoskeletal system are negatively affected by disuse. The mechanisms may differ from those discussed above, but the results are predictably those discussed in the section on Weakness. The changes are reversible, but they do take time and effort. Degeneration from disuse can often be avoided. Attention to positioning, exercise, rest, nutrition, and well-being is required. Because posture reflects mental outlook, and because posture is not a conscious attribute, a positive self-image is vital to a healthy posture. And a healthy posture is vital to provide normal and adequate use of structures in the musculoskeletal system.

AGING

At some point the degenerative processes in humans exceed the restorative process in all tissues. The point when this happens and the degree to which it happens vary with individuals, and depend somewhat on lifestyle. "Use it or lose it" is a worthwhile axiom, provided we understand that it really means "Use it more and lose less of it."

The aging process can be slowed, but it cannot be reversed. As the human life span increases with biomedical improvements, clinicians will have to learn more about the musculoskeletal systems of the aging population to improve the quality of life for those living longer. Some of these tissue changes are discussed below.

The pattern of muscle degeneration with disuse and aging is to atrophy. The fast-twitch motor units are affected first. Exercises and activities are needed to maintain all fibers, but the predilection of aging for the fast-twitch variety implies that exercise programs should include anaerobic activities with reasonable resistance. To accomplish this, the tolerance of the cardiovascular system will also have to be maintained or improved.

Osteoporosis currently is the focus of most studies on aging bone. Bone stores 90% of the body's calcium, so naturally bone is depleted when the body demands calcium. Cancellous bone gives up calcium more readily than compact bone, so bones that have more cancellous matrix are demineralized earlier. Thus, the femur shows more osteoporosis in aging than the tibia, and the cervical vertebrae show more than the lumbar vertebrae. Proper nutrition can prevent osteoporosis, but calcium is not the only required element. Zinc, manganese, and some hormone supplements are also suggested. Exercise and weight bearing are also

necessary to maintain electrolyte balance and associated mineralization in the bones.

Bone resorption is a different process from demineralization. In bone resorption, the rate of osteoclastic activity exceeds the rate of osteoblastic activity. The bone now has reduced numbers of osteocytes and fewer fibers, hence a reduced matrix. Changes in facial structure, including mandibular recession and enlarged tooth sockets, attest to the passage of time. Because fibrocartilage does not recede as bone does, the ears and nose become proportionately more prominent with aging. In addition, the buccal fat pads (which are also connective tissue) shrink, producing hollow cheeks.

The synovial layer of the joint capsule degenerates with time, producing less synovial fluid. The stratum synoviale of the capsule is not equally distributed throughout the capsule. Changes in joint surface configuration may lead to alterations in the synovial layer and its function. Decreased levels of lubrication increase friction in the joint, create pain, stimulate changes in the cartilaginous end zones of the joint surfaces, and produce musculoskeletal dysfunction on a macroscopic level.

Other connective tissue changes from aging appear to be secondary to changes in circulation, to changes in use patterns caused by changes in muscle, or simply to decreased use. All of these are fully discussed elsewhere in this chapter.

Aging changes of the musculoskeletal tissues cannot be stopped, but some can be slowed and others can be prevented. At this time, physical therapy is active in slowing some of the aging changes through exercise and education. Health professionals are becoming involved in retarding some aging changes through education, nutritional counseling, prophylaxis, and community activities. Orthopedic surgery is providing artificial joints when preventive and rehabilitative efforts are either too little or too late.

Philosophically, physical therapy will age with the rest of the population. As physical therapists become more knowledgeable about tissue maintenance and repair today, the tissues with which we are working will require more maintenance and repair tomorrow. The history of this profession suggests that it will not stop at this point and wait for artificial muscles or bones to be perfected. Physical therapists have barely begun to explore the health and maintenance of the musculoskeletal system.

ANNOTATED BILIOGRAPHY

DeLuca CJ, Le Fever RS, McCue MP et al: Control scheme governing concurrently active motor units during voluntary contractions. J Physiol 329:129, 1982

Gossman MR, Sahraman SA, Rose SJ: Review of length-associated changes in muscle: Experimental evidence and clinical implications. Phys Ther 62(12):1799, 1982

Guyton AC: Textbook of Medical Physiology, 7th ed. Philadelphia, WB Saunders, 1986 (A detailed text that explains physiology of human body systems of relevance to physical therapists from a viewpoint of cellular and macroscopic structure in both normal and abnormal function.)

Harris WH: Traumatic arthritis of the hip after dislocation of acetabular fractures: Treatment by mold arthroplasty. J Bone Joint Surg 51A:737, June 1969 (An end-result study using a new method of results evaluation.)

Junqueria LC, Carneiro J, Long JA: Basic Histology, 5th ed. Los Altos, CA, Lange Medical Publications, 1986 (Chapters 5–8 provide an in-depth study of the varieties of connective tissue and their intrinsic properties. Electron micrographs are clear and support the text, which is detailed and well-organized.)

Kendall HO, Kendall FP, Boynton DA: Posture and Pain, Chap 10. Huntington, NY, Robert E. Frieger Publishing, 1977 (Analyzes the compensations the body makes to varying stresses. Many examples of children and adults give practice to the reader in analyzing musculoskeletal imbalances.)

LeVeau B: Williams and Lissner's Biomechanics of Human Motion, 2nd ed. Philadelphia, WB Saunders, 1977 (A good basic text that graphically presents concepts of muscle and joint forces and torque. The analysis of static systems is clearly diagramed, and sample problems with solutions assist in understanding the material.)

Mannheimer JS, Lampe GN: Clinical Transcutaneous Electrical Nerve Stimulation. Philadelphia, FA Davis, 1984 (Chapters throughout this text address the structural, physiologic, and behavioral aspects of clinical pain. Written by physical therapists, the chapters are heavily referenced and provide an informative blend of scientific support with clinical experience.)

Melzak R: The McGill Pain Questionnaire: Major properties and scoring methods. Pain 1:277, 1975

Nahum AM, Melvin J (eds): Biomechanics of Trauma. Norwalk, CT, Appleton-Century-Crofts, 1985 (Specifically addresses the biomechanics of accidental trauma and includes both basic science issues and clinical aspects of injury. Although an advanced text, it provides important information on the scientific basis for the mechanisms and management of musculoskeletal trauma commonly seen by the physical therapist.)

Phys Ther 62(12):1754–1830, 1982 (The entire December issue of this journal addresses muscle. Several articles by physical therapists Rose S, Gossman M, Rothstein J, and Speilholz N are pertinent to this chapter, and are relevant to physical therapy intervention. Numerous citations are referenced.)

Shipman P, Walkman A, Bichell D: The Human Skeleton. Cambridge, MA, Harvard University Press, 1985 (Provides information that is basic, yet applicable to clinical practice. Some of the more pertinent chapters address bone healing, bone aging, and bone tolerance to various stresses.)

Steinberg FU: The Immobilized Patient: Functional Pathology and Management. New York, Plenum, 1980 (Written by a clinician, this short text examines the musculoskeletal system from the perspective of a functional problem well known to physical therapists: immobility. The author summarizes the effects of immobility on human function, based on previous human and animal research. Numerous references are provided.)

Travell JG, Simons DG: Myofascial Pain and Dysfunction: The Trigger Point Manual. Baltimore, Williams & Wilkins, 1983

11 Neuromuscular Causes

CAROLYN A. CRUTCHFIELD

In this chapter we will examine the potential sources of physical disability and movement dysfunction that arise in the neuromuscular system. Therefore, we must review selected neurophysiologic bases or theories of action that will affect movement and our understanding of it. Much of the information concerning the muscular system has been presented in Chapter 10; this chapter should be considered a companion to that one.

The functional unit of the neuromuscular system is the motor unit. Although most of the activity of the nervous system takes place elsewhere, the motor unit is the final common pathway for the expression of movement. The emphasis of this chapter is to foster understanding of how a disorder affects the motor unit to produce the resultant movement dysfunction.

It is difficult not to be exuberant and poetic about the brain, perhaps because the brain not only controls the entire body but may be considered to do so for its own purposes—to perceive, feel, think, and exist. The brain provides the expression in movement experienced daily by human beings. The dancer, baseball player, pianist, and painter fill us with wonder at their creative perceptions and movements, but the commonplace motor acts of dressing, fixing breakfast, walking, and hugging someone are just as wondrous even though they are usually taken for granted. There is nothing simple about their elaboration, and the world is indeed changed forever when these capacities are lost.

How human movement is produced is a question for which we have been seeking answers for most of this century. How close have we come in that time? Investigations of some of the theories of motor control should be pertinent to physical therapists. The theories we choose to accept, either consciously or unconsciously, have profound effects upon the choice and administration of treatment.

Other questions arise. Does the brain function as if it were two relatively independent organs? Does the popular view of "right brain-left brain" provide some implications for physical therapy rehabilitation programs? What changes take place in the aging brain? Could they be altered?

Physical therapists are naturally interested in the disease processes that afflict the nervous system because the information tells us what to expect from the patient so affected and provides a framework for suggesting treatment intervention. The processes involving the nervous system are much the same as those that occur elsewhere in the body; however, there are special features of the nervous system that modify the expression of disease. These special features include the presence of unique cell types, the correlation between function and location in the nervous system, and the snug encasement of the brain by the skull. All three profoundly influence the response of the nervous system to a host of diseases and disorders.

The understanding of spasticity and other "disorders of tone" has been a constant quest by physical therapists since the earliest days of our profession. How much closer is that goal? It seems relevant to investigate the current knowledge concerning one of the greatest problems physical therapists face in treating patients with neurologic deficits. Some insight into these questions will be presented in this chapter in association with neurophysiologic foundations for suggested answers.

THE MOTOR UNIT

The motor unit is composed of (1) the motor neuron, which consists of the cell body, and its axon and terminal branches; (2) the neuromuscular junctions; and (3) all the muscle fibers (cells) that the neuron innervates (Fig. 11-1). It is the elementary unit of behavior in the neuromuscular system. This unit is the final common pathway for the expression of sensory input. Nervous system activity converges on this final pathway to produce a single event— muscle contraction. The entire unit responds in an "all or none" fashion.

The anterior horn cell receives input from the other nerve cells including interneurons in the spinal cord, from afferent axons, both direct and indirect through interneurons from the periphery, the cortex, and from other higher centers of the central nervous system. This input determines the excitability level of the motor neuron (Fig. 11-2).

Like muscle fibers, motor units may be classified by type. Naturally, the motor unit name is the same as that of the muscle fibers that it contains, thus, a type I motor unit contains type I muscle fibers. Additionally, the characteristics of the motor neuron match or complement the muscle fibers it innervates. For example, type I muscle fibers are innervated by the smallest motor neurons. The type I motor units usually contain fewer numbers of muscle fibers per unit than the other types do. Because the total tension developed in the motor unit depends upon the type and number of muscle fibers it contains, the type I motor units will develop the least amount of peak twitch tension of all the motor unit types available (Fig. 11-3). The total tension developed in a given muscle is determined by number of motor units activated and the tension produced by each muscle fiber in those motor units.

The proper functioning of the motor unit as a whole depends upon the appropriate contributions of all the components. Each component has its own characteristics and functions within the unit. Diseases and disorders may affect different parts of the motor unit as well as the inputs the unit receives.

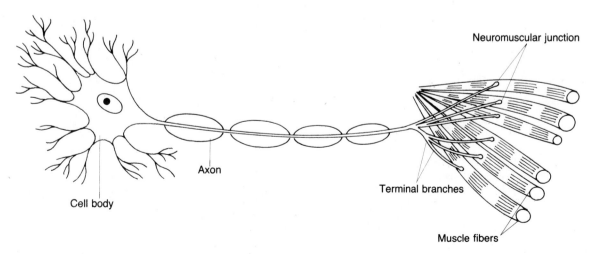

Figure 11-1. Components of the motor unit.

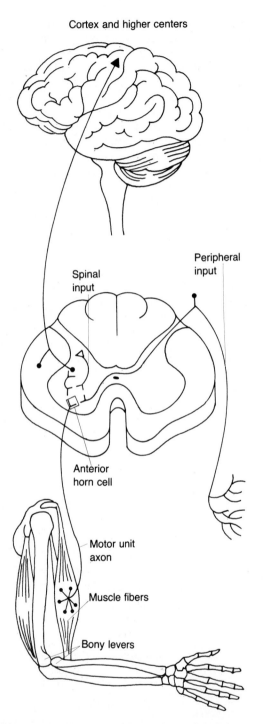

Cortex and higher centers

Peripheral input

Spinal input

Anterior horn cell

Motor unit axon

Muscle fibers

Bony levers

Figure 11-2. Input from areas of the central nervous system and the periphery determine the level of excitability of the motor neuron that activates muscle.

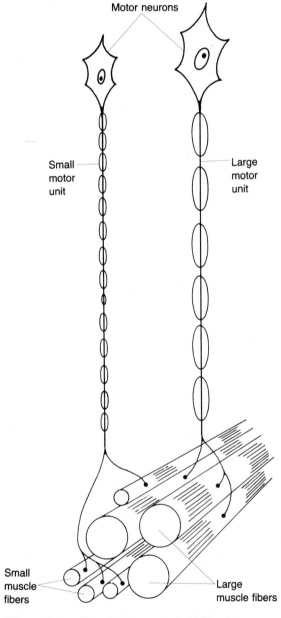

Motor neurons

Small motor unit

Large motor unit

Small muscle fibers

Large muscle fibers

Figure 11-3. The arrangement of neighboring motor units. Note the intermingling of different types of motor units and their muscle fibers.

THE MOTOR NEURON

The cell bodies of the motor neurons lie within the ventral horn of the spinal cord. The cell bodies of all the neurons that innervate a single muscle are referred to as the *motor neuron pool* (Fig. 11-4). The motor neuron pool is designed for the single purpose of producing precise mechanical effects in its muscle. To produce these effects and to operate under a wide variety of conditions the motor neuron pool must produce perfectly timed contractions of various numbers and types of its motor units. The organization of the motor neuron pool must be understood if one is to understand some of the basic concepts of motor control.

There are various sizes of cell bodies in a motor neuron pool. The largest motor neurons generally innervate the greatest number of muscle fibers and the largest muscle fibers. Therefore, these components constitute the largest motor units. The cell bodies of the motor neurons have a number of characteristics that are strongly correlated with size. One of these is the size principle of activation.

According to the size principle, there is a critical firing level for each cell body, and this level is related strongly to size. Thus, the smallest motor neurons are most likely to be activated first and the very largest ones last. Even preprogrammed circuitry for certain movements appears to include recruitment of neurons according to the principle of their size. Other characteristics of the small motor neurons are that they are the least susceptible to inhibition, have the slowest maximum firing rate, and have the longest afterhyperpolarization, which prevents rapid reactivation. The largest motor neurons have the opposite characteristics.

AXONS AND NEUROMUSCULAR JUNCTIONS

The largest motor neurons have the largest axons. These axons have the heaviest myelin sheaths, which contribute to the fast conduction velocities of the large motor neurons. The largest axons are the most susceptible to temperature changes and ischemia, and are the most resistant to local anesthetics. Action potentials propagated along the axon will be

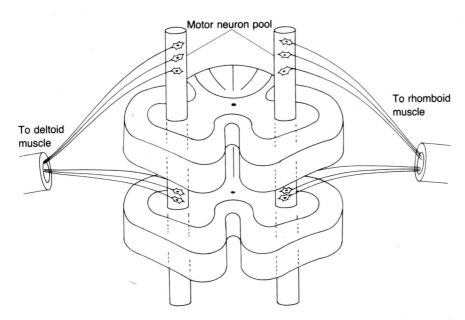

Figure 11-4. The intersegmental arrangment of motor neuron pools within the spinal cord.

faithfully reproduced in all the collaterals and terminal branches.

Each terminal branch ends in a neuromuscular junction complex formed with the muscle fiber it innervates. The distinct types of neuromuscular junctional complexes are related to the types of muscle fibers, and thus contribute specific characteristics to each type of motor unit (Fig. 11-5).

MUSCLE FIBERS

The muscle fibers, the last component of the motor unit, have characteristics that also differ from type to type. Type I muscle fibers are the smallest, have the slowest speed of contraction, produce the lowest maximal tension, and fatigue the least. These fibers have an oxidative metabolic system and thus have an aerobic capacity. Type IIB fibers have opposite characteristics, and are anaerobic in nature. Type IIA fibers are intermediate and have various qualities of one or the other or both muscle fibers.

It is apparent that the various components of the motor unit are matched up: that is, the large, high-threshold cells have large, fast-conducting axons that innervate large, fast-contracting muscle fibers. These combinations result in a high-threshold, rapidly contracting, high-tension output, but produce rapidly fatiguing movements.

Putting all of this together to produce a specific movement among the many possible movements that might occur would seem to be a formidable task. We used to believe that the central nervous system could pick and choose from a wide variety of motor units in many different combinations to achieve the desired total outputs. The possible combination of active units in a single motor pool of 300 neurons would be on the order of 10^{90}. Selective activation, then, would require tremendous circuitry and an eternity for the necessary calculation to be accomplished.

Therefore, it would appear that a pool of cells activated by a simple rule "such as by size" would decrease the demand on the CNS. Much research on animal and human subjects shows that type I motor units are activated first in any type of movement and that the order of recruitment is relatively fixed. As you might expect, there are also research results suggesting that the size principle most likely is not the only mechanism available for motor neuron activation.

In addition, the organization of motor pools within the cord assists in patterns of activation. The motor neuron pools to the proximal muscles are located medially in the cord, whereas the pools that innervate the extremities are in a lateral position. The pools can also be grouped dorsally and ventrally, the former innervating flexors and the latter extensors. These arrangements permit logical and convenient groupings for functional activation (Fig. 11-6).

PERIPHERAL SENSORY MECHANISMS

Although the sensory system is not part of the motor unit, incoming sensory input must be considered for complete understanding of the

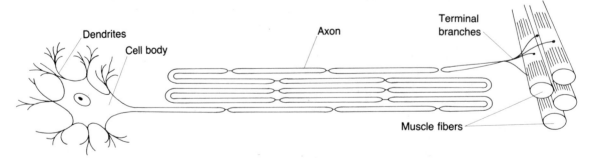

Figure 11-5. The parts of a motor unit.

neuromuscular system. The peripheral sensory system will be considered here because its components are often in close proximity to the motor components. Certain dysfunctions and disorders will affect the sensory system selectively or in association with the motor system. Alterations in the sensory system, in and of themselves, will affect the motor system.

The peripheral sensory system consists of sensory receptors, which pick up stimuli, and axons, which enter the dorsal root ganglion to bring sensory impulses into the spinal cord. The receptor behaves as a transducer and converts various environmental energies into a generator potential. Once the threshold value is achieved, an action potential is generated along the axon and into the central nervous system (Fig. 11-7). At this point numerous possibilities arise for the interaction and continuation of sensory input. The neuron may synapse at various points within the dorsal horn to interact at segmental levels with other sensory-motor information. Some branches will ascend to higher centers in the brain and brain stem. Some branches will come directly or indirectly to the ventral horn to influence motor neurons.

A sensory nerve cell consists of (1) a specialized segment that is receptive to a specific stimulus, (2) an axon or conductive segment, and (3) a transmissive segment, the central terminus that contains the secretory vesicles (Fig. 11-8). Sensory receptors behave as transducers by reacting to one form of energy (such as

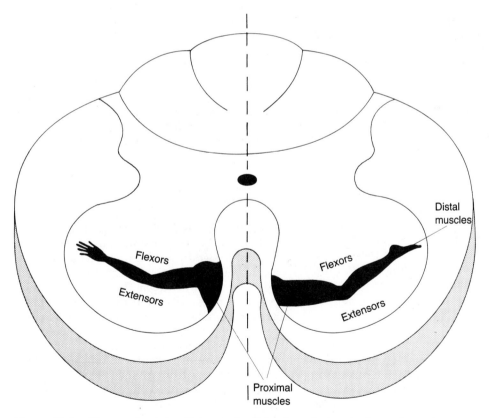

Figure 11-6. The proximal (medial group), distal (lateral group), flexor (posterior group), and extensor (anterior group) groupings of motor neuron pools within the ventral gray horn of the spinal cord.

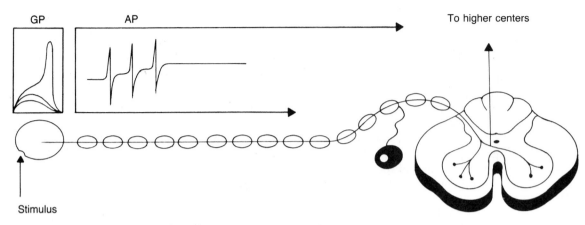

Figure 11-7. The sequence of activity in response to stimulating a sensory receptor (GP, generator potential; AP, action potential).

mechanical energy) and triggering action potentials (electrical energy) in the axons. Thus, all forms of energy can be transduced or "translated" into electrical energy, the "language" of the nervous system.

One mechanism for the coding of stimulus intensity is the frequency of action potentials conducted along the axon. The frequency of action potentials is determined by the amplitude of the generator potential, which is directly related to the stimulus intensity. How sensation is perceived is a combination of the specific receptors activated, the frequency of impulses, and the pattern of receptor activation.

Sensory receptors may be generally classified as rapidly adapting or slowly adapting. Clinically, the former would be stimulated through repetitive application of the stimulus. The latter would continue to respond as long as the stimulus is maintained.

DISEASES AND DISORDERS OF THE MOTOR UNIT

Because the motor unit is the avenue through which movement is expressed, it should be apparent that influences affecting the motor unit or the peripheral sensory system will have an impact or effect on movement. Some disorders affect each component of the motor unit, whereas some result from combined influences. These disorders can be classified further as resulting from structural imbalances, inflammatory processes, degenerative processes, and chemical imbalances.

The Anterior Horn Cell

Diseases of the anterior horn cell are usually referred to as *motor neuron diseases,* and include structural imbalances from trauma or mechanical disruption, infections, degeneration, chemical imbalances, and disorders of unknown etiology.

Structural imbalances resulting from mechanical disruption include the avulsion of the ventral root from the cord. This may occur from traumatic circumstances in which violent stretching forces have been applied to the peripheral nerves. For instance, a collision with a tree while sledding at high speed may produce a brachial plexus lesion in which ventral or dorsal roots are torn from the spinal cord. The prognosis for recovery through peripheral regeneration when root avulsions are present is poor.

Inflammatory diseases of the anterior horn cell may be represented by poliomyelitis. Poliomyelitis results from a viral infection affecting motor neurons in the ventral horn of the spinal cord. The bulbar form affects the motor neurons in the brain stem (the "bulb"). This disease results in an acute and usually severe motor dysfunction. The more motor neurons

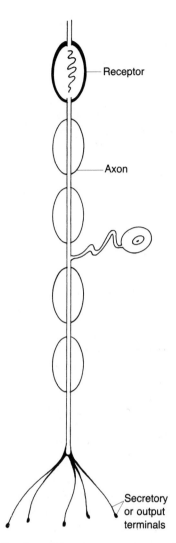

Figure 11-8. A peripheral sensory nerve cell.

ing functional activities, and preventing contractures.

If poliomyelitis involved the muscles of respiration and respiratory support was inadequate, the disease was fatal. Because the cells were injured, but not dead, some recovery through axonal regeneration usually occurred. For instance, very few patients who survived had to remain on the "iron lung." The amount of recovery varied from patient to patient, but most had some residual loss of function, which may have been limited to one muscle or one extremity or may have involved all extremities.

Degenerative disorders include some motor neuron diseases that affect the pyramidal tract cells as well as those in the anterior horn. Amyotrophic lateral sclerosis is a disease in which both are affected. Spinal muscular atrophy and progressive bulbar palsy are also progressive motor neuron diseases. The pathogenesis of these diseases is unknown. Their onset is usually in early middle age. All lead to death within a few years. The bulbar form is particularly lethal because it interferes with swallowing and breathing and easily leads to aspiration pneumonia. In these cases, physical therapy is directed at relieving discomforts such as pain, stiffness, and pressure sores, and maintaining function as long as possible through exercise.

Werdnig-Hoffmann disease is a congenital motor neuron disorder in which the affected infants are born "floppy" or flaccid. The condition progresses until death, usually by 2 years of age.

Axonal Diseases

Diseases that affect the peripheral axons primarily fall into two categories. One is segmental demyelination in which Schwann cells die, resulting in loss of myelin at the segments of the axon they covered. When this occurs the axon itself is intact and for the most part may continue to conduct action potentials. However, when segments of myelin are missing, the conduction can no longer be through saltatory means, by jumping from one node of Ranvier to another. Thus, the conduction velocity will be slowed in the involved axons (Fig. 11-9).

involved, the greater the weakness or paralysis. Because only the motor unit is affected, the patient has no sensory disturbances. Although the disease has been effectively eradicated in the United States through vaccination, it is still prevalent in many other countries. In the late 1940s and 1950s the largest group of patients receiving physical therapy were probably those afflicted with polio. Rehabilitation was directed at strengthening the remaining muscles, train-

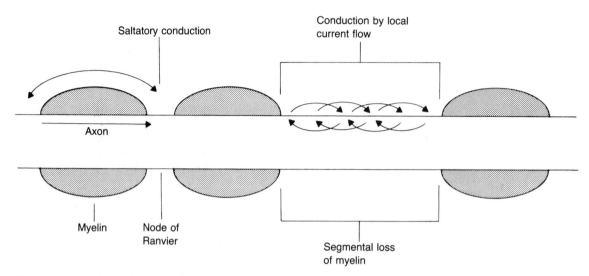

Figure 11-9. When Schwann cells are destroyed, myelin is lost in a segmental fashion, resulting in a change in the type of current propagation in the affected areas of the axon.

Timing is critically important in the nervous system. A delay of 5 msec, as is found in the synapse, is imperceptible to our senses. When compared to the fastest conducting axons, however, this delay is 1 million times as slow. Reflexes and other coordinated functions rely on critical rapid timing. Thus, segmental demyelination that results in slowing of the conduction velocity may produce marked effects in function.

Structural imbalances that result in segmental demyelination include entrapment syndromes and herniated disks in which the nuclear material compresses an area of the axon in the dorsal roots. Entrapment syndromes such as carpal tunnel syndrome or Saturday night palsy result when outside pressures or connective tissue constrictions compromise the axon at vulnerable points. Crossing the legs constricts the blood flow to the nerves as well as compresses the peroneal nerve as it courses around the head of the fibula. This action results in a temporary conduction block of the axons involved. If such conditions are continued for a long period of time or are repeated sufficiently, actual degeneration may occur and more permanent disability will result.

Severe forms of this demyelination may be seen in inflammatory diseases such as Guillain-Barré syndrome, which may result in total paralysis. In this disease the onset of paralysis is rapid and often follows an upper respiratory tract infection. Complete or near complete recovery, however, usually occurs within a few months to a year.

Milder polyneuropathies may result from certain hereditary degenerative conditions, such as Charcot-Marie-Tooth disease. Although victims may be confined to a wheelchair by their later years, symptoms do not usually appear before the teens and disability during young and middle adult years is minimal. Chemical imbalances such as those resulting from metabolic toxins (diabetes), and environmental toxins (lead and arsenic poisoning) usually produce mild polyneuropathies that may be slowly progressive if conditions persist or the disease is not controlled. There may be some muscular weakness, as well as pain and sensory loss.

The presence of the sensory symptoms indicates that more than the motor unit axons are involved. The sensory and motor axons are usually encased in the same nerve from the point where they join just outside the vertebral foramina to make the spinal nerve until close to their termination. Therefore, peripheral neuropathies in which the major lesion is segmental demyelination involve the sensory axons as well as the motor axons.

The other category of axonal lesion involves both the axon and the myelin. In traumatic lesions the axon is compromised and usually is disrupted. This results in wallerian degeneration, in which the entire axon distal to the lesion degenerates along with the myelin sheath (Fig. 11-10). Because most nerves are mixed with both motor and sensory fibers, sensation and motor functions are lost. For example, a transection of the radial nerve will produce paralysis of the wrist extensors and loss of sensation over the thumb and the dorsolateral surface of the hand.

Neuromuscular Junction Diseases

In the healthy person, the impulses reaching the muscle through the terminal axons of the motor neuron are faithfully propagated throughout the muscle fibers of the motor unit. This process perpetuates the "all-or-none" character of the motor unit activity. Impulses arriving at the nerve terminus expel quanta of acetylcholine, which binds with the postsynaptic muscle cell, permitting specific changes in ionic flow, resulting in the muscle action potential.

All diseases of the neuromuscular junction could probably be classified under the heading of chemical imbalances. Diseases may affect the various components of the neuromuscular complex. Each vesicle contains a normal amount of acetylcholine, referred to as a *quantum*. Packaging defects or other such abnormalities will result in a decreased amount of neurotransmitter in each vesicle.

Various substances may also compete with acetylcholine for the membrane receptor site. This occurs when curare extracts or succinylcholine are administered during surgery to prevent unwanted muscular contractions. In botulism, the toxins prevent the release of acetylcholine from the nerve terminus. Obviously, the person will have muscular paralysis commensurate with the amount of substances or toxins involved. In these circumstances, death occurs from respiratory failure. Thus, early respiratory support is necessary until the substances are rendered ineffective.

Abnormalities of the receptor site will also underlay muscular weakness. This occurs in myasthenia gravis and is believed to be caused by autoimmune mechanisms. In this case, the muscular weakness is of a fluctuating nature. Drugs that slow the breakdown of acetylcholine are effective in correcting this weakness. Unfortunately, most of these have very short-term effects and are useful only for testing. Currently, anti-inflammatory and anti-immune drugs, such as cortisone, are used with some success.

Muscle Diseases

Muscle is often secondarily involved in many diseases and disorders of almost all parts of the

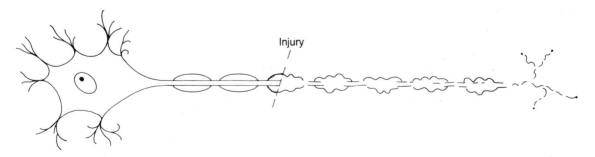

Injury

Figure 11-10. Wallerian degeneration in which both the axon and myelin degenerate back to the first node of Ranvier proximal to the lesion.

body. Age, gender, immobilization, nutrition, environment, and time of day are physiologic factors that affect the function of muscle. Mechanical factors such as effects of gravity, length of muscle, angle of insertion, and velocity of contraction also have influence.

Primary muscle diseases are those in which pathologic changes affect the muscle tissue first during the disease process. These diseases are most often of an inflammatory or degenerative nature. Inflammatory disease of muscle (myositis) may be an acute condition caused by infectious agents. Its more devastating form occurs with diseases such as polymyositis or dermatomyositis, in which the inflammation does not result from an invading organism, and the victim experiences insidious and progressive weakness with swelling and tenderness of the muscles. Myositis has been treated with such anti-inflammatory drugs as cortisone with some success.

The most well-known primary muscle diseases are the muscular dystrophies. These are genetic disorders in which the muscular tissue degenerates and is replaced with noncontractile tissue, such as fat. In almost all cases the weakness first affects the proximal muscles. Thus, patients lack the stability to climb stairs or get up from the floor. Scapular stability needed for hand placement for upper extremity activities is affected. Weakness in the respiratory muscles predisposes the victims to respiratory infections.

There are several forms of muscular dystrophy. The most familiar is the Duchenne form, in which the symptoms appear in male children about 4 years of age and the victim dies in his late teens or early twenties. Other forms have an older age of onset, and the prognosis is less grave. In addition, other forms may have a different genetic pattern of transmission, in which women are affected at the same ratio as men.

LOWER MOTOR NEURON SYNDROME

The peripheral nervous system has been referred to as the *lower motor neuron system*. This label probably occurred because the anterior horn neurons are "lower" in relation to the brain and brain stem structures, which are "higher." (At least, this is so when we stand up.) These labels have often been used to imply level of control as well. It is easy to visualize that the cortex has control over everything below it or "lower" than it. As will be discussed later, however, this hierarchical view can be misleading.

Irrespective of its value, the term "lower motor neuron" persists in medical jargon and refers to some very important concepts. Involvement of the peripheral nervous system produces signs and symptoms that are very different from those encountered when the central nervous system, or "upper motor neuron," is involved. The classic signs of the lower motor neuron lesion are flaccid paralysis, decreased deep tendon reflexes, and muscle atrophy. To these signs could also be added the specific local effects, and the loss or alteration of sensation in predictable patterns consistent with the nerves or disease process involved.

The presence of lower motor neuron signs is an aid in the diagnosis of the problem. The signs indicate that the disease or disorder is limited to the motor unit or the peripheral nerves. Knowledge of the anatomy, physiology, and pathology that causes such signs is essential for developing the proper treatment for the condition and provides insight into the prognosis for recovering movement.

Flaccid Paralysis

When the peripheral nerves that supply the muscles are disrupted by injury or disease, a very specific type of muscle weakness occurs. The muscle feels flabby, and if the loss of the nerve is complete, a nonresistive, flaccid paralysis occurs. Such a weakness or paralysis is limited to muscles supplied directly by the nerves or motor neurons involved. If the radial nerve is cut about the elbow, for example, all muscles innervated by this nerve below the elbow will undergo flaccid paralysis. The triceps muscle and others innervated by the radial nerve above the elbow will be unaffected. Thus, when peripheral nerves are affected, very localized effects occur.

Anterior horn cell or motor neuron disease affects muscles in the same manner as peripheral nerve injuries, and produces flaccid paralysis. Because the motor neuron pools to several muscles are at the same spinal level and each pool spans more than one level, the effects are not so localized. Depending upon the extent and locus of the disease, very mild and spotty or severe and total paralysis may occur. It is possible for only one extremity to be affected, or even one side of the body.

Diseases of the nerves in which nervous tissue is the prime target are referred to as neuropathies. In neuropathies weakness is usually first noted in the distal musculature. This distribution is in direct contrast with the proximal weakness noted in myopathies or primary muscle diseases.

Loss of the motor nerve supply to the muscle produces very distinctive changes in the muscle. Besides the degenerative changes that will ultimately occur, alterations develop at the neuromuscular junction. The neurotransmitter receptor proteins are usually confined to the synaptic cleft area. With denervation, receptor proteins are spread along the muscle membrane. This changes the permeability of the membrane and results in spontaneous rhythmic contractions of the single denervated muscle fibers, which are referred to as *fibrillations.* As long as viable contractile tissue remains in the denervated muscle cell, it will fibrillate. Once fatty degeneration and fibrous replacement occur, the fibrillations will cease and the muscle cannot be restored by reinnervation.

In spotty diseases such as anterior horn cell disease, the single denervated cells may be reinnervated by sprouting of axons of nearby intact motor units. This results in units that have more than their original number of muscle fibers. During needle electromyogram, the motor unit potentials from such motor units can be observed and are referred to as *large* or *giant units.* Obviously, the larger unit loses some of its fine control, but the overall strength of the remaining unit is increased.

In anterior horn cell diseases, as peripheral nerve fibers die, spontaneous impulses are generated, which result in the activation of the entire motor unit or groups of units. This phenomenon is referred to as *fasciculation.* These larger spontaneous contractions can be seen by an observer and felt by the patient. Fasciculations also occur commonly in normal persons and are sometimes referred to as "tics." The mechanism probably comes from irritation phenomena. Substances such as caffeine, and stress and fatigue often result in fasciculations.

Regeneration of the peripheral nervous system components is a functional reality. If the cell body remains alive, the axon may be regenerated. Damaged axons will die back to the first node of Ranvier proximal to the lesion, and then begin the reparative process. The distal axon and myelin sheath will degenerate, fractionate, and be absorbed. New axon buds grow from the stump outward at the rate of approximately 1 mm per day or 1 inch per month.

The functional outcome of this regeneration depends upon several conditions. If a nerve has been completely transected, the two ends must be opposed in order for the sprouting axon to be guided back to its original position. Microsurgical techniques that allow the matching of fascicles within the nerve have resulted in even better return to the denervated muscles. The distance the nerve must grow is also significant. Axons regenerating from the sacral plexus and growing to the muscles of the foot have lesser success rates than lesions involving shorter distances, such as in Bell's palsy. The complexity of the pathway is also important. For example, injuries to a plexus produce a relatively poor prognosis for functional recovery. Although physical therapy probably will do little to speed the rate of regeneration, much effort is made to keep the muscle, connective tissue, and joint in as good a condition as possible to accept any reinnervation effectively. Such techniques include electrical stimulation, splinting, and passive and assistive range of motion.

Decrease in Deep Tendon Reflexes

It is interesting that by definition the lower *motor* neuron does not include sensory structures, but when signs and symptoms are described sensory mechanisms cannot be ignored. This becomes obvious when deep tendon reflexes are encountered.

The simplest reflex, the monosynaptic myotatic reflex, involves the interaction of two neurons from the periphery—one sensory and one motor—and is basically a peripheral reflex. It is true that there are synapses on the motor neuron itself, which come from CNS structures. These inputs may certainly affect the motor neuron such that the result of an activated monosynaptic reflex can be modified.

Nonetheless, if the only abnormality is in the peripheral system, the reflex will be diminished or absent. If anterior horn cells have died, they cannot be activated. If axons are severed, muscle fibers cannot be activated. If the sensory fibers are disrupted, the exciting stimulus cannot be activated. Remember that demyelination may occur rather than axonal disruption. The timing defects and functional blocks that occur also produce weakness and loss of or alteration in sensation.

Localized Sensory Loss

Although localized sensory loss is not generally described as a lower motor neuron finding, sensory changes do occur as previously noted. Sensory changes found in peripheral nerve involvement differ from those that are found in central nervous system deficits. There are no sensory changes at all in motor neuron disease. If a mixed nerve is cut or damaged, very specific sensory loss will occur. In the case of generalized peripheral neuropathies, a "dying back" phenomenon occurs in which the fine distal portions of the nerves degenerate first as the process proceeds proximally. This distal involvement produces a distinctive "glove and stocking" anesthesia. This pattern of anesthesia obviously does not follow a dermatomal distribution as would be present in a nerve root lesion, nor does it follow the pattern expected if a particular nerve were disrupted (Fig. 11-11).

Muscle Atrophy

A classic lower motor neuron sign is muscle atrophy. When the motor supply to the muscle cell is disrupted, myofibrils and sarcoplasm are lost. The muscle cell becomes smaller and is referred to as *atrophic*. The distribution of the atrophy depends upon the pattern of involvement of the nerves.

CENTRAL LOCALIZATION OF BEHAVIOR

All behavior is a reflection of brain function. This includes not only such common motor acts as walking or smiling but also elaborate affective and cognitive functions such as feeling, thinking, and perceiving. The motor unit described previously serves the will of the brain. Of course, automatic circuits and reflex connections exist at all levels of the nervous system and work together to produce behavior.

CELLS AND STRUCTURE

The brain is made up of individual, elaborately organized units—the nerve and glial cells. Nerve cells, the signaling component, have considerable variation in their shape and the extent of their processes. Figure 11-12 shows a typical cell with four distinct parts or functional regions: input (dendrites); integrative (cell body); conductive (axon); and transmissive or output (secretory vesicles and terminals).

Glial cells, the other type of brain cell, outnumber the neurons in the central nervous system 9 to 1. These cells are very small and generally lack axons. In large part they provide the supporting network for the nervous system, much as the connective tissue elements support the musculoskeletal system. Glial cells surround and separate groups of neurons and provide nutritive functions. The oligodendroglia are responsible for producing the myelin in the central nervous system. One glial cell type, the microglia, behaves as a scavenger much like the monocytes in the connective tissues. The astrocytes, with their glial foot processes that attach to capillaries, provide one portion of the blood-brain barrier (Fig. 11-13).

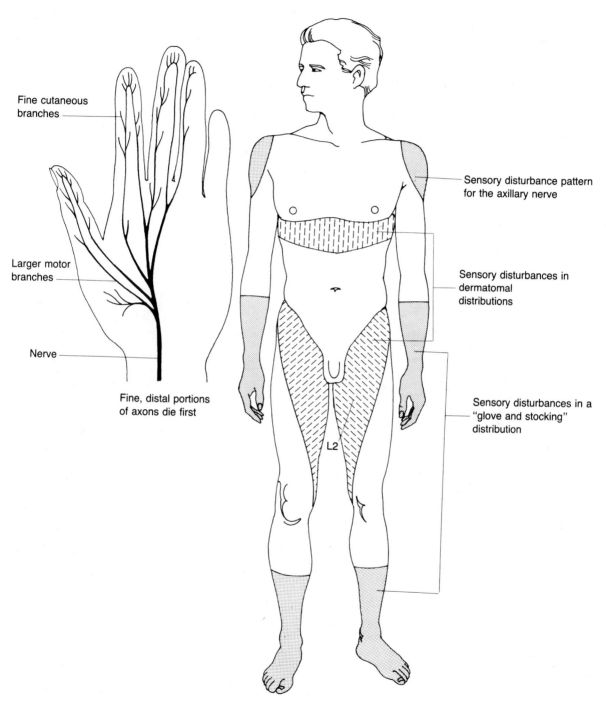

Fine cutaneous branches

Larger motor branches

Nerve

Fine, distal portions of axons die first

Sensory disturbance pattern for the axillary nerve

Sensory disturbances in dermatomal distributions

Sensory disturbances in a "glove and stocking" distribution

L2

Figure 11-11. The "glove and stocking" distribution of sensory disturbances resulting from the dying-back phenomenon compared with the dermatomal distribution found in segmental lesions and nerve pattern distributions present when a particular nerve is involved.

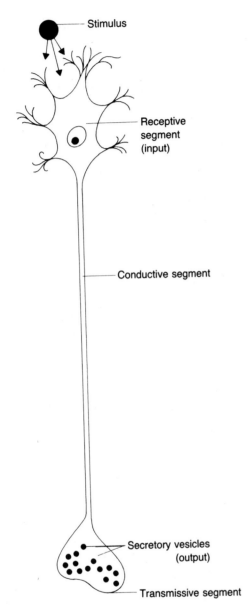

Figure 11-12. The functional components of a typical nerve cell.

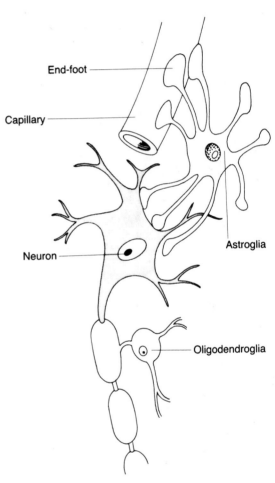

Figure 11-13. Two types of glial cells.

ORGANIZATION OF THE CENTRAL NERVOUS SYSTEM

Most of the cytoarchitectural maps of the central nervous system have been developed by electrically stimulating the various areas of the brain and observing the responses. It is un-likely that all areas have a known function and it is possible that subtle activities occur that have escaped the attention of neural cartographers. Some studies also suggest that areas of the brain may become reorganized in response to certain circumstances, such as the removal of a body part. Nonetheless, many of these areas are well documented and provide a guideline for understanding brain function and for clinical localization of lesions.

Cortex

The most well-known name associated with mapping functional areas of the cortex is Brodmann, who in 1909 described 52 fields. Later researchers subdivided the cortex into as many as 200 fields, and more division is likely as our knowledge and techniques advance. Most of us are familiar with such terms as Brodmann's area 4 (the motor strip) or areas 1, 2, and 3 (the primary sensory areas). Broca's areas 44 and 45 are familiar as the motor speech areas, and so forth. The more the clinician knows about brain arrangement, the better able she is to localize a lesion that involves those areas.

A general idea of the function of various areas of the cortex is presented in Figure 11-14. Most areas have complex functions and certainly interact with other areas through associational connections. Speech functions, for instance, occur in at least seven areas. Some are concerned with perception of auditory impulses, whereas others are essential for the interpretation and appreciation of intricate sounds. Still others synthesize data into a sensory language pattern. Other connections are responsible for turning the head to follow sound.

Brodmann also described a further organization of some areas in a somatotopic fashion. The most familiar is the representation of the areas of the body within area 4 (the motor strip) and areas 1, 2, and 3 (the sensory cortex) (Fig. 11-15). Thus, it is possible to localize cortical activity governing the knee to the top of the cortex in the center of the brain at area 4.

Of what interest is this information, other than satisfying the curiosity of those who would wish to know it? It allows the clinician to observe the symptoms and assess the signs from a patient with a neurological insult to the cortex and pinpoint the lesion. Further, the ability to map out the lesion assists in determining its cause. Such information is useful to the physical therapist in determining prognosis, understanding the patient's signs and symptoms, and planning types of intervention.

For example, if the patient experiences loss of motor and sensory functions primarily to the head, trunk, and arms, the one place that these functions are distributed together is on the lateral surface of the cortex. This area is supplied by the middle cerebral artery. Thus, the thera-

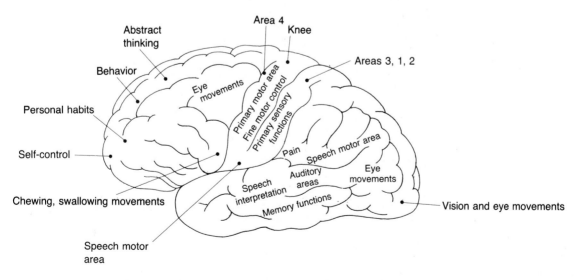

Figure 11-14. Some functions localized to particular areas of the cerebral cortex.

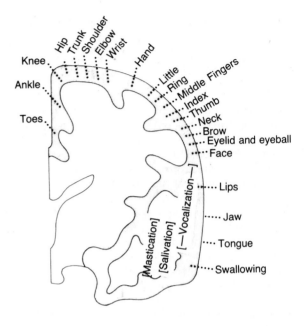

A

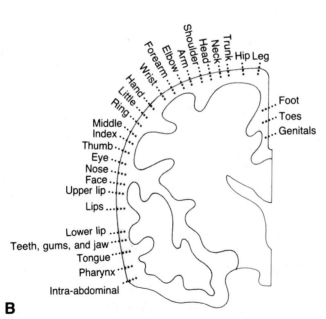

B

Figure 11-15. *(A)* Body areas represented along the primary motor area (area 4). *(B)* Body areas represented along the primary sensory area of the cortex (areas 1, 2, 3).

pist may conclude that involvement of this artery at the point specified could be the cause of patient's symptoms (Fig. 11-16).

No matter what the type of lesion, if it is located in this area the same signs and symptoms will appear. So, in areas 1, 2, 3, and 4, traumatic laceration, vascular compromise, demyelination, or cellular aberrations will affect the same general area of the body. Because certain types of lesions occur in particular patterns in the cortex, the type of lesion may be identified by the pattern. An example is a vascular lesion. A particular artery supplies a known area of the cortex. As a result, if it is occluded the functions served by that area will be compromised. Therefore, it can be concluded that the pattern of signs and symptoms results from involvement of that particular artery.

Deep Brain Structures and the Brain Stem

From the cell bodies in the motor cortex, the axons travel through various deep brain areas, through the brain stem, and into the spinal cord. These pathways are also arranged in a very orderly fashion just as is the cortex itself. The first major structure through which the

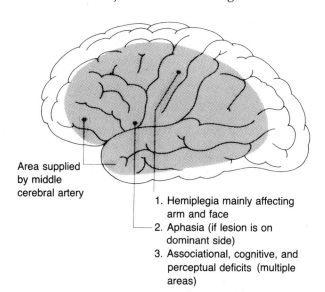

Area supplied by middle cerebral artery

1. Hemiplegia mainly affecting arm and face
2. Aphasia (if lesion is on dominant side)
3. Associational, cognitive, and perceptual deficits (multiple areas)

Figure 11-16. Functions that are disturbed by damage to the areas of the cerebral cortex supplied by the middle cerebral artery.

cerebrospinal fibers pass is the internal capsule.

If we were to look at a horizontal section through the internal capsule, the organization would be apparent. The fibers are arranged in an orderly fashion beginning in the genu of the capsule with the fibers to the face (Fig. 11-17). The order of fibers from the genu through the posterior limb of the capsule is the arm, the trunk, and then the lower extremity. Sensory fibers are grouped near the motor fibers to the leg with visual and auditory information passing at the extreme posterior of the capsule.

It should be obvious that a lesion involving all of the posterior portion of the internal capsule would affect sensory and motor functions on one entire side of the body. A very discrete lesion here, however, may affect only one specific area of the body. In addition, some functions such as vision and audition may have dual connections from both sides of the brain. If so, those functions will not be as clearly affected by a one-sided lesion as will functions that have only unilateral representation.

The deep brain structures and the brain stem also enjoy orderly arrangements. For instance, the thalamus serves as a relay station for sensory information from the periphery to the cortex. Closely associated with the thalamus are the nuclei that make up the basal ganglia. The basal ganglia form a broad, collaborative system of connections between the cerebral cortex and the thalamus, thus providing for ease and flexibility of movement. The anterior limb of the internal capsule carries the reciprocal fibers connecting these structures. Lesions in these areas produce profound alterations in movement.

In addition to the sensory and motor fibers that ascend and descend through the brain stem, there are specific areas of function located within the brain stem. Lesions involving these areas will result in alterations of the functions served. Examples of such lesions are presented in Figure 11-18.

Spinal Cord

The neurons and tracts in the spinal cord are also organized into specific patterns. The as-

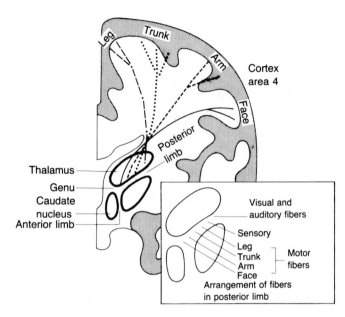

Figure 11-17. Somatotopic arrangement of fibers from the primary motor area as they pass through the internal capsule.

cending and descending axons found in the white matter of the spinal cord are located in very specific areas of the ventral, lateral, or dorsal funiculi (Fig. 11-19). The senses of two-point discrimination and vibration are carried in the dorsal columns or funiculi of the cord. A lesion at this point thus results in alteration or loss of these senses. In fact, tabes dorsalis, a lesion caused by syphilis, involves the dorsal columns and results in the loss of these very important proprioceptive senses.

There is also a cytoarchitecture to the gray matter of the spinal cord. As mentioned earlier, the organization of the ventral horn assists in the activation of related neurons. The gray matter has been systematically subdivided into ten laminae. The neurons in a lamina share related functions (Fig. 11-20). For instance, laminae II and III comprise the substantia gelatinosa, which is believed to play a role in regulating afferent input to the spinal cord. Laminae VII, VIII, and IX contain neurons involved in motor control as well as neurons that project to the motor regions of the brain. The neurons of lamina VII are particularly related to lamina

IX and participate in motor movements of the extremities. Lamina VIII is particularly related to IX_m, which controls the muscles of the neck and trunk.

The organization of the central nervous system at all levels is apparent. Structures such as the cerebellum, which have not been enumerated here, also have cytoarchitectural and somatotopic organization. Such an organization is a valuable underpinning for efficient control of functions. Nervous system organization helps simplify neuron selection as does the size principle of neuron activation. This organization helps the clinician localize a lesion in the nervous system and may suggest the probable cause for the abnormality.

DISEASES AND DISORDERS OF THE CENTRAL NERVOUS SYSTEM

Almost all diseases or disorders of the central nervous system result in some alteration in motor control or sensory perception, or both. Most often the location of the lesion is as important, if not more important, than the particular nature of the disease itself.

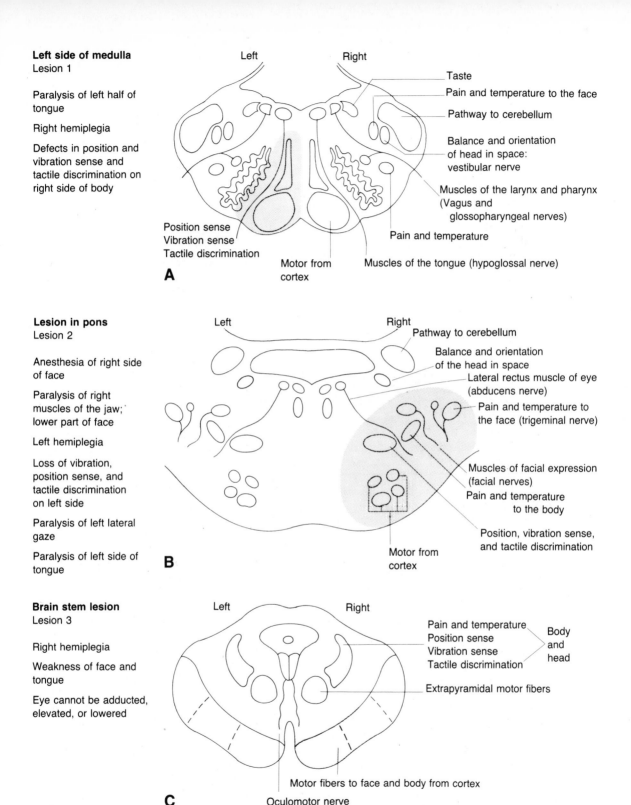

Left side of medulla
Lesion 1

Paralysis of left half of tongue

Right hemiplegia

Defects in position and vibration sense and tactile discrimination on right side of body

Left

Right

Taste

Pain and temperature to the face

Pathway to cerebellum

Balance and orientation of head in space: vestibular nerve

Muscles of the larynx and pharynx (Vagus and glossopharyngeal nerves)

Pain and temperature

Position sense
Vibration sense
Tactile discrimination

Motor from cortex

Muscles of the tongue (hypoglossal nerve)

A

Lesion in pons
Lesion 2

Anesthesia of right side of face

Paralysis of right muscles of the jaw; lower part of face

Left hemiplegia

Loss of vibration, position sense, and tactile discrimination on left side

Paralysis of left lateral gaze

Paralysis of left side of tongue

Left

Right

Pathway to cerebellum

Balance and orientation of the head in space

Lateral rectus muscle of eye (abducens nerve)

Pain and temperature to the face (trigeminal nerve)

Muscles of facial expression (facial nerves)

Pain and temperature to the body

Position, vibration sense, and tactile discrimination

Motor from cortex

B

Brain stem lesion
Lesion 3

Right hemiplegia

Weakness of face and tongue

Eye cannot be adducted, elevated, or lowered

Left

Right

Pain and temperature
Position sense
Vibration sense
Tactile discrimination

Body and head

Extrapyramidal motor fibers

Motor fibers to face and body from cortex

C

Oculomotor nerve

Figure 11-18. Functional alterations resulting from lesions at various levels are listed for each lesion of the brain stem: *(A)* lesion in the medulla, *(B)* lesion in the pons, and *(C)* lesion in the midbrain.

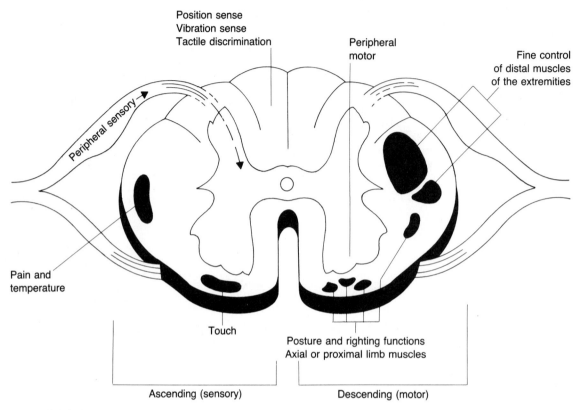

Figure 11-19. Some functions localized to particular areas of the spinal cord. Ascending or sensory functions are illustrated on the left, and motor functions on the right.

Structural Imbalances

Edema, Hydrocephalus, and Increased Intracranial Pressure

No other organ is as rigidly encased as the brain. Such an arrangement may provide great protection against injury, but it becomes detrimental when the brain expands. This expansion may result from space-occupying lesions, such as hematomas and tumors. Edema is a major cause of expansion of tissues. Hydrocephalus, the accumulation of excess cerebrospinal fluid in the ventricles, also enlarges the brain. The fact that the tissues need to expand but are prevented in doing so by the skull has serious implications for the patient.

Edema is not a specific disorder. Intracranial pressure from expanding tissue occurs as a response to a host of insults. The tissue becomes heavy and boggy. The gyri are flattened and the sulci are obliterated. The increased fluid content is principally intracellular in cytotoxic forms of edema and extracellular in vasogenic edema.

Hydrocephalus results from several types of problems. If there is an overproduction or an under-resorption of cerebrospinal fluid, an accumulation of the excess occurs. Congenital malformations can interfere with the flow of CSF. Additionally, scarring from diseases such as meningitis or pressure from tumors may encroach upon the circulating pathway of the CSF (Fig. 11-21).

Edema, hydrocephalus, and many other disorders such as tumors, hemorrhage, toxic problems, and trauma all produce intracranial

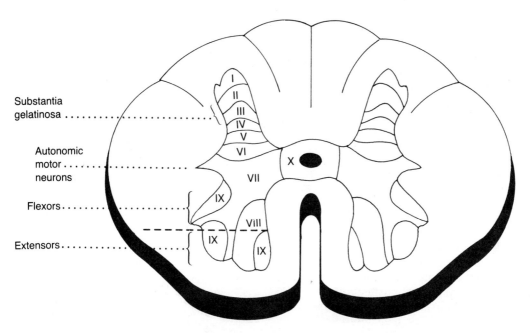

Substantia gelatinosa

Autonomic motor neurons

Flexors

Extensors

Figure 11-20. Rexed's laminae, which indicate functional grouping of cells within the gray matter of the spinal cord.

pressure. Such pressure squeezes and compromises various neurons and nervous centers resulting in headache and vomiting followed by drowsiness, seizure, and perhaps coma.

Vascular Diseases

A stroke or cerebrovascular accident (CVA) is probably the best known neurologic disorder. Vascular diseases do not result from primary neurologic disease. The nervous system is damaged when the oxygen system is compromised by a thrombus, embolus, or hemorrhage. Interruption of the oxygen supply for more than three to four minutes results in widespread damage and death to nerve cells. Direct destruction of the nervous tissue may also result from the escape of blood into the tissues when a vessel ruptures.

The major etiologic factors in CVAs include atherosclerosis of the cerebral arteries. Sudden arterial occlusion often results from cardiac emboli. Vascular malformations such as aneurysms and arteriovenous (AV) malformations result in cerebral damage through encroach-

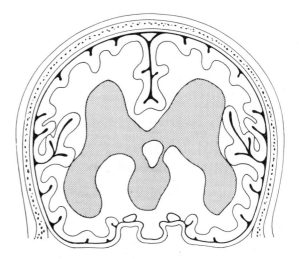

Figure 11-21. The marked dilatation of the ventricles in hydrocephalus compresses and encroaches upon the substance of the brain.

ment of the tissues by a space-occupying aneurysm, or through rupture of one.

The exact symptoms the patient exhibits are determined by which structures have been compromised. The blood supply to the cortex and deep structures of the brain comes from two sets of arteries. These are the internal carotid artery, which arises from the aorta, and the vertebral-basilar system, which arises from the subclavian arteries. These arteries meet at the base of the brain to form the circle of Willis.

Cerebral hemorrhage usually results from a weakness in an arterial wall. Arteries have gaps in their smooth muscle coat at the points where branching occurs. Given the many branches off the circle of Willis, there are many points of inherent weakness in the vascular wall. Congenital weaknesses particularly involve the circle of Willis, where berry aneurysms are quite common. The weakened walls allow the artery to bubble out like a small balloon. These aneurysms are often visualized as small bumps or "berries," thus the name "berry aneurysm" (Fig. 11-22). The weakened walls may rupture, producing cerebral hemorrhage. Such hemorrhage tends to occur in persons who have hypertension. Vascular walls may also be weakened by the invasion of an atherosclerotic plaque. Vascular lesions of the spinal cord are relatively rare. However, the spinal vessels may be involved in another disease process, such as pressure on an artery from a spinal tumor.

Trauma

Head trauma is a common cause of movement dysfunction. The skull and vertebral column provide excellent protection for the vulnerable tissues of the brain and spinal cord. As a result, a relatively severe injury is usually necessary to damage the neural tissues.

However, the brain may be bruised (contusion) and lacerated without fracturing the skull. Skull fractures, especially depressed fractures, are likely to damage nervous tissue. If either an artery or vein is pierced or torn, an epidural or subdural hematoma will likely form, which can damage nervous tissue by

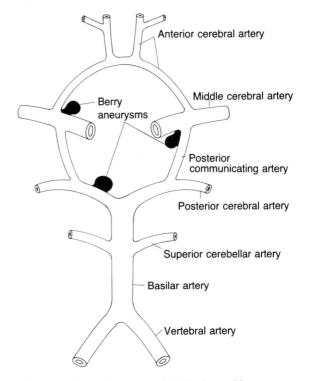

Figure 11-22. The circle of Willis formed by anastamosing arteries supplying the brain. Berry-shaped aneurysms balloon from the arterial walls at areas of weakness, such as bifurcations.

direct destruction from escaping blood. A hemorrhage also becomes a space-occupying mass as the blood collects, producing an increase in intracranial pressure and causing further swelling (Fig. 11-23). The greatest danger from a swelling brain is that part of the cerebrum will herniate through the connective tissue tentorium that separates it from the cerebellum and brain stem. If herniation occurs, the cerebral tissue will encroach upon the brain stem or its blood supply. Because the brain stem contains the reticular formation or arousal system and other vital centers such as the respiratory center, death usually results.

If the trauma involves the motor areas of the brain, some paralysis may occur. In most cases it occurs on the contralateral side of the body and is referred to as *traumatic hemiplegia*.

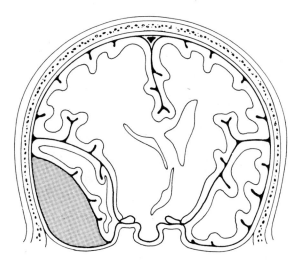

Figure 11-23. An extradural hematoma encroaches upon brain tissue and produces an increase in intracranial pressure.

Areas of the brain that are healed, with resultant scar tissue, may be prone to developing posttraumatic epilepsy.

Perhaps the greatest problems encountered with brain trauma are the personality changes and cognitive deficits that accompany such injury. Because the pathways from the reticular formation in the brain stem may be damaged, a change in consciousness occurs. The change may range from drowsiness to stupor to frank coma. Some victims may never regain consciousness even if they survive other medical aspects of the injury. Those who do regain consciousness may find that cognitive tasks are beyond them. They will have short attention spans and will be unable to concentrate. The biggest roadblock in their rehabilitation is more likely to be cognitive than physical.

Spinal Cord Trauma

Traumatic injuries to the spinal column usually result from the fracture and displacement of the vertebrae. When this occcurs the spinal cord may be crushed, overstretched, or partially or completely transected. The resulting movement disorder is usually termed *paraplegia* or *quadriplegia*. Because the cord is organized into segments, the level of the transection can be determined by observing what neurological functions have been compromised and which muscles retain their function.

Respiratory functions provide insight into the level of the lesion in the cervical portion of the cord. "High" quadriplegics who have injuries between C1 and C4 rarely survive because of respiratory depression. The innervation to the accessory muscles of respiration, the anterior neck "strap" muscles, and the diaphragm comes from C3-C5. The intercostal muscles receive innervation from T1-T12. So a "rocking horse" breathing pattern, which occurs when intercostal muscles are not used, indicates to the physical therapist that the damage is to the high thoracic or low cervical portion of the cord (Fig. 11-24).

Obviously, the farther down the cord the lesion occurs, the more functions remain. Lower cord damage below S1 results primarily in bowel and bladder incontinence and sexual impotence. Partial lesions will show peculiar distributions of motor and sensory impairment depending upon the level of the injury and the amount and portion of the cord involved.

Initially, the victim experiences "spinal shock" in which a flaccid paralysis occurs. As the shock dissipates, the residual paralysis often becomes spastic. In most cases of neurologic disease, including traumatic injury and CVAs, many cells are only temporarily involved and are not destroyed. As recovery takes place, the cell will once again function and some "return" occurs. It is impossible to predict with complete accuracy how much function will return or at what point the return will begin or cease. Nonetheless, most of the return in function usually occurs within the first 18 months following the insult.

Tumors

The symptoms and signs of an intracranial tumor are due mainly to two factors: the local destructive effects of the tumor and increasing intracranial pressure. The cranium is able to accommodate a comparatively large mass if it

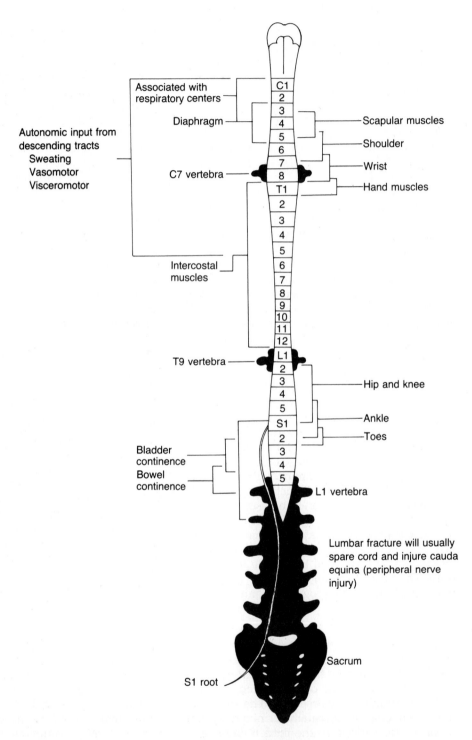

Figure 11-24. Muscles innervated from various levels of the spinal cord.

grows slowly and does not obstruct the CSF from the ventricular system. The location of the tumor is of prime importance. A tumor of the frontal lobe can be relatively silent for a long time. In contrast, brain stem tumors rapidly encroach upon vital areas and give rise to symptoms early.

Benign tumors may be just as serious as malignant ones because they may be located in vital areas that cannot be reached surgically. The types of tumors are classified according to the cells of origin. Tumors arising from glial cells are called gliomas, all of which are malignant. Benign tumors include the meningiomas and pituitary tumors. The brain is also a favored site for secondary neoplasms that have metastasized from elsewhere.

Tumors that arise in, infiltrate, or press upon the sensory-motor regions of the brain give rise to motor or sensory seizures, contralateral weakness, and sensory impairment. The exact location, of course, determines the distribution of findings. Parasagittal tumors of this area are apt to involve both legs, thereby giving rise to asymmetrical spastic weakness and sphincter disturbances.

Spinal cord tumors are less common than intracranial neoplasms. Primary intraspinal (intramedullary) tumors occur in the same varieties as those found in the cranial vault. Extramedullary tumors are the most common, and the most common of these are the meningiomas and neurofibromas. The spinal cord is smaller than its protective canal, so at the beginning there is room for the tumor to expand.

The extramedullary tumors disturb function by displacing the cord against the bony canal or by producing local pressure upon the cord. Blood supply to the cord may also be compromised and nerve roots may be compressed. Intramedullary tumors are often accompanied by cavitation of the cord and dilation of the central canal.

Onset of symptoms is usually slow. Paresthesias may take the form of pins and needles, numbness, tightness, or coldness. The first symptoms may be pain, paresthesias, weakness, or sphincter dysfunction. When treating patients for back pain, a major red flag should

be pain that is constantly present and is not altered by position changes or rest.

Congenital and Developmental Disorders

There are many congenital and developmental disorders of the nervous system. They may range from severe malformations, such as total lack of brain development (which is incompatible with life), to spina bifida occulta in which no functional abnormalities usually occur. Three of these disorders that are quite familiar to physical therapists and involve distinctly different processes will be presented here: cerebral palsy, syringomyelia, and spina bifida.

Cerebral Palsy

The term "cerebral palsy" is neither specific to one disorder nor particularly descriptive. Some of the newer terms, such as "infantile encephalopathy," are not much better. These terms refer to a heterogeneous group of syndromes that are dominated by disorders of movement and posture. The lesion may result from a number of causes, such as maternal illness, birth injury, and asphyxia. The lesion is situated in the brain and the damage occurs during fetal life, during birth, or in the neonatal period. The condition is permanent and nonprogressive. The results may be mild and referred to as "minimal brain dysfunction." This classification includes the clumsy child and those often referred to as having developmental delays. The most severe forms include spastic quadriplegia or severe athetosis accompanied by mental retardation.

The more common forms of cerebral palsy are spastic diplegia (in which the lower extremities are more involved than the upper), spastic quadriplegia, hemiplegia, and athetosis. The pathologic features vary from patient to patient and types often overlap, so that a child may have both spasticity and athetosis. The clinical features may be apparent soon after birth, or the child may be regarded as normal for the first few months. Then, someone may notice that he fails to hold up his head, and his limb movements may be rigid, spastic, or clumsy. As time progresses, the familiar motor milestones such as rolling over, sitting up, and creeping do not appear. There may be a tendency for the lower extremities to cross over one another in a scissor gait pattern.

In the case of athetosis the child has involuntary movements and abnormal postures. Athetoid movements invade the face, neck, arms, and legs, interfering with all voluntary movements, including speech and swallowing. The movements are not present at rest, but as soon as a muscle is activated the child is handicapped by athetoid movements and a background of fluctuating muscle activity.

It is common for mental retardation to be associated with the physical abnormalities. However, it is necessary to be extremely cautious in assuming the child to be retarded. As technology permits us a deeper understanding and ability to communicate with such persons, it has become apparent that many of them are not retarded or at least not as severely as once thought, but are simply unable to communicate appropriately. Providing a rich environment of experience and support is necessary because physical and psychosocial deprivation can lead to or increase the severity of mental retardation.

Syringomyelia
Syringomyelia is characterized by gliosis and cavitation (syrinx) of the upper portion of the spinal cord or the medulla. It is believed to be a congenital abnormality and is often associated with other congenital abnormalities such as cervical rib, kyphoscoliosis, and spina bifida. Possibly, it may result from abnormalities that obstruct the foramen of Magendie, thereby raising the pressure in the central canal of the spinal cord.

The cavity usually extends transversely across the cord into the dorsal areas. As the cavity increases in size, it often invades the ventral horns, and may be either unilateral or involve both sides of the cord. It most often involves the spinothalamic decussation, the spinothalamic and pyramidal tracts, the dorsal columns, the anterior horn cells, and the posterior horns (Fig. 11-25).

Symptoms usually have their onset be-

tween 20 and 40 years of age, but can be seen in childhood or later life. Early symptoms are usually segmental in nature, with loss of pain and temperature sensation at the level of the lesion and intact sensation above and below it. The first sign of the disease usually occurs when the patient burns or cuts his hand and fails to notice it. As the cavity spreads to involve motor cells, the hands and arms become atrophic and weak. In later stages spasticity may appear as the lateral tracts become involved.

Myelomeningocele (Spina Bifida)
Spina bifida results from the defective closure of the neural tube and the vertebral canal in early fetal life. It leads to one of a graduated series of abnormalities of the spine, spinal cord, and cauda equina. The spinal cord may be involved in varying degrees of severity. In spina bifida occulta, for example, the site is marked with a dimple, nevus, or tuft of hair and is seldom associated with neurologic symptoms.

Other forms include the association with a meningocele, which is a sac on the back containing the meninges, but no involvement of the spinal cord. Forms of this disorder that result in sensory and motor disturbances involve the spinal cord itself. In these meningomyeloceles, the sac contains both the meninges

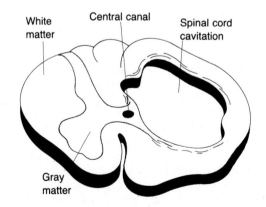

Figure 11-25. Cavitation of the spinal cord in syringomyelia, damaging both white and gray areas of the cord.

and the spinal cord or the cauda equina (Fig. 11-26).

When the defect is at the cervical level, the cord is herniated into the sac. As you might expect, the arms and legs are spastic and there may be symmetrical loss of pain and temperature sensations in the cervical dermatomes. The lumbar form of this disorder involves the cauda equina. Because the cauda equina are actually ventral roots that are outside the spinal cord, any injury to them would be considered a lower motor neuron lesion. The muscles atrophy and are afflicted with flaccid paralysis, but sensory loss is usually mild.

Demyelinating Diseases

Myelin is primarily a lipid substance laid down in multiple layers around the axon. This substance behaves as an insulator, which prevents the flow or loss of ions and speeds the rate of conduction from five- to sevenfold over non-myelinated fibers. The speed of conduction is directly related to the cross-sectional area of the axon and its myelin sheath.

Several diseases of the nervous system can cause demyelination. Any injury or disease of nervous tissue usually will involve the myelin as well; however, there are diseases in which the degeneration of myelin is the key factor. They occur in the central nervous system just as they do in the peripheral system. These diseases can have devastating effects on the control of behavior, because they alter the temporal relationships between neurons or between neurons and effectors.

If the axon is not involved in the disease process, but only the myelin, the possibility that it can be repaired is significant. Repair or regeneration becomes less likely if the axon is also involved. Although axons do regenerate in the central nervous system, the regeneration is not likely to be functional as it is in the peripheral nervous system. One reason for this failure is that the glial cells that react to the injury produce a glial scar, which is not conducive to allowing neurons to recommunicate with one another.

The most important disease in this category is multiple sclerosis. Its cause is not known, but the disease results in widespread patches of demyelination within the CNS. The clinical picture is highly variable, as would be expected with the widespread anatomic distribution of the lesions. The most common symptoms are visual disturbances, ataxia, weakness, and paresthesias. Because the plaque will most likely undergo some repair and regeneration of myelin, the patient experiences periods of recovery of function with a remission of the symptoms. Exacerbations occur when a demye-

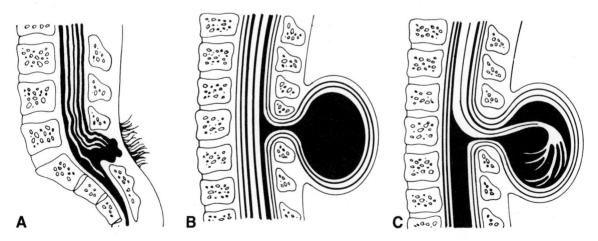

Figure 11-26. Various forms of spina bifida: *(A)* spina bifida occulta, *(B)* meningocele, and *(C)* meningomyelocele.

lination process again occurs at the same or another site.

The disorder may manifest itself by disturbances of mind, mood, speech, cranial nerve function, motor control, sensation, and sphincter performance. These patients usually have a progressive course and may become bedridden in middle age. The disease progresses rapidly in some patients, and they are disabled very quickly; others may experience a complete remission. The main object of physical therapy is to maintain function as long as possible, particularly by avoiding continued immobilization following an exacerbation.

Another demyelinating disease that results in movement dysfunction is Schilder's disease, which has no remissions and tends to affect children. The disease usually begins with paresthesias of the hands and feet. Subacute combined degeneration of the spinal cord accompanies pernicious anemia. Because the lesions are found in the dorsal and lateral columns of the spinal cord, the patient loses vibration sense as well as proprioception, and becomes ataxic. Lateral tract involvement results in spastic paralysis.

Degenerative Diseases

Degeneration is a relatively broad and nondescriptive term. The degenerative diseases are no less heterogeneous. "Degeneration" refers to situations in which the cells and fibers cease to function and gradually degenerate and disappear. To be classified as a degenerative disease, the cells must undergo these changes in the absence of specific vascular lesions, toxic poisoning, or other known causes of nervous system dysfunction.

One degenerative disease that is becoming more familiar through exposure in the media is Alzhemer's disease. Like most of the degenerative diseases, the symptoms usually occur relatively late in adult life. The degenerative processes involve the cerebral cortex and primarily result in dementia.

Parkinson's disease, on the other hand, is one of the more familiar diseases involving degeneration of subcortical areas of the brain. The major lesion is in the black pigmented cells of the substantia nigra in the midbrain, which is part of the basal ganglia. These cells produce the neurotransmitter dopamine. This area of the CNS is responsible for integrated movement.

The patient experiences muscular rigidity and a resulting paucity of movement. The face is unexpressive and mask-like. Movements are very stereotyped and the patient has a "pill-rolling" tremor at rest. The gait is shuffling, and once started the patient has difficulty stopping.

Unlike the cortical degenerative diseases, the mind is not affected in Parkinson's disease. Physical therapy is usually directed at maintaining function at the highest level for as long as possible. If drug or surgical treatments are effective, the patient will need help in learning to move again.

Huntington's chorea is a familial disease that involves both the cortex and subcortical structures, particularly the basal ganglia. The patient experiences involuntary movements, such as chorea or athetosis. Because the cortex is involved the patient experiences mental deterioration as well as memory failure and difficulty concentrating. Disorders of mood are prominent. The disease is slowly progressive, and death usually occurs within 15 years of onset.

Inflammatory Diseases of the Nervous System

Infections of the nervous system may occur through blood-borne infectious agents or through direct extension from infected structures in near proximity such as the middle ear, mastoid bone, and nasal sinuses. Additionally, organisms may be introduced directly into the skull or spine as a result of penetrating wounds or compound fractures. Organisms may enter the subarachnoid space by spinal tap, and by injections of spinal anesthetics and contrast media.

The areas of the brain or brain structures involved in the inflammatory process are readily apparent from the name: meningitis, encephalitis (brain substance proper), myelitis (spinal cord), and so forth. There is an almost unending list of bacterial and viral organisms that participate in these processes. In any event, this entire class of disorders constitutes a medical emergency such that the prime objective is to identify the culprit rapidly enough to limit the damage. This task is not easy and the victim may die before treatment can be effected.

Physical therapists generally encounter the survivors of these infectious processes. Unfortunately, the sequelae to these diseases often result in neurological abnormalities and movement dysfunction. Patients may suffer hydrocephalus, blindness, deafness, cranial nerve palsies, seizures, mental retardation, and weakness. The weakness may be spastic or flaccid depending upon the locus of the infection. Rigidity may occur. In poliomyelitis, a lower motor neuron disease, the paralysis is flaccid.

In syphilis, the victim may experience atrophy of the entire brain or specifically of the posterior columns and dorsal roots of the spinal cord. The movement disorder that results from the latter is quite distinctive. The patient has pain, paresthesias, sensory impairment, and loss of tendon reflexes. Ataxia is caused by loss of sensory information from the proprioceptors, which pass through the posterior columns. During gait, the feet are raised too high and put down too forcibly because of diminished feedback from sensory involvement.

UPPER MOTOR NEURON SYNDROME

The upper motor neuron syndrome refers generally to involvement of the nervous system "above" the anterior horn cell. It reflects involvement of the central nervous system. In some cases the term specifically refers to the pyramidal tract or the corticospinal tract. This is the long tract from the cortex to the motor neurons in the anterior horn of the spinal cord. A lesion in the corticospinal tract leaves the peripheral reflex arcs and cells intact.

Spastic Paralysis

The classic sign of upper motor neuron disease is spasticity, which usually is slow in developing. The initial motor response to an acute lesion is most often flaccidity. Spasticity is manifested through increased deep tendon reflexes and resistance to passive stretch, particularly quick stretch, as exhibited by the patient with CNS disease. Putting the two terms "spastic" and "paralysis" together has probably caused many of the misconceptions about upper motor neuron disease. The paralysis is, in fact, a weakness or paralysis of muscular ability. The appearance of hyperactivity associated with spasticity is misleading. The hyperactivity exists only in response to quick stretch. The posturing and mass pattern activity apparent in patients with upper motor neuron lesions is not hyperactivity, but instead is uncoordinated or inappropriate muscle activity that occurs when voluntary contractions are attempted. These phenomena are thoroughly discussed later in this chapter. Thus, the two conditions, spasticity and paralysis, have no functional relationship to each other.

Increased Deep Tendon Reflexes

The patient with upper motor neuron lesions shows hyperreflexia upon examination. A defect in the central mechanisms results in hyperactivity of the anterior horn cells. When the tendon is tapped, the stimulus adds excitement to an already excited pool of neurons. The resulting response is an exaggerated jerk. In the case of the upper motor neuron lesion, the peripheral wiring mechanisms are intact, allowing the reflex arc activity to take place. In contrast, the lower motor neuron lesion disrupts some portion of the reflex arc, and the deep tendon reflexes are diminished or absent.

No Muscular Atrophy

As noted previously, muscular atrophy occurs primarily from the loss of the motor neurons to the muscle. Because the motor neuron remains intact in corticospinal tract involvement, the muscles do not atrophy as they do in lower motor neuron disease. There may be some wasting from prolonged disuse of the muscles in some cases, but the frank atrophy of denervation is not present.

Other Central Nervous System Symptoms

Symptoms also occur in upper motor neuron syndrome from involvement of tracts in the central nervous system that do not come from the motor strip. These tracts involve fibers from the cortex, thalamus, basal ganglia, reticular formation, and other areas of the brain stem. Lesions in these areas may produce rigidity, tremor, chorea, athetosis, nystagmus, and autonomic nervous system dysfunction. Dysfunction of the cerebellum results in unsteadiness of motor performance such as ataxia, asynergy, past pointing, and tremor.

Sensory Systems

The sensory changes that occur with nervous system disease are useful in identifying the area of the lesion. There are differences in the pattern and quality of sensory loss produced by lesions of the peripheral nerves, sensory roots, spinal cord, thalamus, and parietal cortex.

The notion that a sensory stimulus evokes potentials that travel unhindered along well-defined pathways to the thalamus and then to the cortex ignores the tremendous interactions and modulations that occur with sensation. It is believed that sensory input can be modulated by the cortex and subcortical structures, and incoming volleys may be inhibited at the level of the spinal cord.

The sensory interactions are very complex. Lesions of the central nervous system invariably involve sensation to some degree. Because of the complexity, the lesion rarely involves anesthesia as it does in the peripheral system or in the ascending tracts in the spinal cord. Rather, paresthesias are usually present, although they may also be present in peripheral lesions. Complex sensory perceptions are altered. Perceptual alteration is much more global and subtle in its effects than is localized loss of sensation.

Of the many diseases and disorders of the nervous system, some are relatively common and others are exotic and extremely rare. Whatever the nature of the disease, its signs and symptoms invariably relate to the area of the nervous system that is involved and the extent of that involvement. Because the nervous system is cytoarchitecturally arranged, the lesion can be located by observing the neurological signs. Conversely, when the site and extension of the lesion are known, one should be able to predict the resulting signs and symptoms. Clinical neurology is truly the arena of applied neuroanatomy.

For the most part, physical therapy cannot alleviate the neurological disorder. However, it can assist the patient to regain lost function or sustain current function as long as possible. Neuromuscular reeducation involves a very complex but promising avenue for treating these patients.

HEMISPHERIC SPECIALIZATION

GENERAL PRINCIPLES OF SPECIALIZATION

In the nineteenth century, Broca and others established that the left hemisphere was dominant for language and for hand usage in right-handed persons. Since that time, much work has been done to document the asymmetrical organization of the brain. "Right brain-left brain" theories have come and gone and come again in the popular press and in the scientific laboratory.

These studies imply that the two hemispheres have unique and distinctive cognitive styles. The right hemisphere is nonverbal, holistic, intuitive, and appositional. The left hemisphere does best at being verbal, analytical, logical, and propositional. The left hemisphere is suspected of organizing information in temporal sequences in contrast to the right, which may be more apt to be spatial and relational. The popular press informed the public that humans had, in a figurative sense, the luxury of two minds. One was conscious and rational and the other was mute, unconscious, and mystical.

Before the 1960s, however, people interested in the differing roles of the left and right hemispheres depended almost entirely on evidence drawn from animal research, from studies of neurological patients with one-sided brain damage, or from patients who had the corpus callosum surgically severed. A method of studying hemispheric processing in normal populations was needed.

Neurophysiologists believe that sensory input to one side of the body is relayed to and processed in the contralateral side of the brain. Based on this principle, methods for studying brain function in normal subjects were developed. The subject was asked to listen to two different words coming to the two ears at the same time. It was assumed the subject would report the sounds most often associated with the hemisphere that was dominant for that function. When several word pairs were given in a row, subjects were unable to report them all. Right-handed subjects and most left-handed subjects tended to report the words presented to the right ear most accurately. This would suggest that sound stimuli from the right ear, although sent to both hemispheres, are preferentially sent to the left hemisphere, which controls speech (Fig. 11-27).

Each technique was designed to promote perceptual rivalry between the hemispheres. Using these processes, visual stimuli and tactual-spatial stimuli were presented. The results of the studies produced data from which the dominance for the function was inferred. The major contribution of these studies is confirmation that the cerebral hemispheres have a normal functional dominance in a pattern consistent with that reported in pathological cases.

The brain is not as simply organized as these descriptions of hemispheric dominance may suggest. Some individuals depart from the general pattern. For instance, in some subjects the right hemisphere is dominant for words presented in the auditory experiments. In contrast to the right ear-left hemisphere dominance for auditory speech, other auditory signals such as music are processed in the right hemisphere. This leads to the observation that dividing a specific stimulus into some functional components can be confusing and misleading.

Further complications arise with the discovery that there are differences in right and left brain function between men and women.

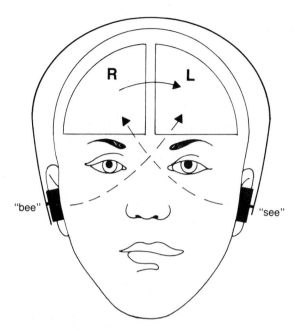

Figure 11-27. Sounds entering either the left or right ear are carried to both hemispheres and are reported accurately when tested individually. When two syllables, "bee" and "see," are given simultaneously, only the sound going to the dominant hemisphere for speech should be heard. Therefore, "bee" is more often accurately reported than "see."

In producing speech the function is said to be localized to the left hemisphere in both sexes, but women show a more focal location to the front of the hemisphere. In vocabulary skills and defining words men have a localization to the left hemisphere, but women are more diffusely organized and both hemispheres are used. In some other verbal tests men and women are the same. Hand movements for motor skill are also more focal for women because they appear to be localized to the front of the left hemisphere.

There is reason to believe that brain organization varies widely from person to person. For example, when persons of above average reasoning ability were given spatial tests, left-handed men showed poorer performance than right-handed men. However, left-handed women were better at these tasks than right-handed women. When persons with below average reasoning ability were tested, just the opposite occurred.

These observations suggest that problem-solving abilities are related not only to gender and hand preference but also to overall intelligence. Therefore, it is most likely that there are not one or two types of brain organization, but several types. Very little can be predicted about an individual's mental abilities based on his or her gender. However, it is clear that the brain is, indeed, organized in some way even if it differs from person to person, between sexes, or even within the same person at different times. It is likely that the brain is not as organized as the popular press would have us believe. Some organization appears to be developmental in that certain dominance patterns develop at a later age than others.

A simple task in the past was to determine the handedness of an individual. The investigator either asked which hand the individual preferred or observed which hand was used. Actually, a whole battery of tests are needed to determine handedness. The handedness an individual expresses will be somewhere on a continuum in which "pure" right-handedness is on one end and "pure" left-handedness on the other. In between, it is apparent that an individual will use one hand for a particular task and another for a different task. Cultural differences must be taken into account as well. For instance, in some societies, eating with the left hand is taboo. Irrespective of cerebral dominance, training will alter the expected observational outcome.

DIFFERENCES IN RIGHT-LEFT HEMIPLEGIA FOLLOWING A CEREBROVASCULAR ACCIDENT

Even if some of the finer aspects of the localization of brain function are not as clear as we would like, some general observations may be useful in assessing and treating the patient with one-sided brain injury, such as the stroke victim. The patient with a left hemiplegia has had an insult to the right side of the brain. The most obvious result is the motor paralysis on the left side of the body. But, as noted earlier, many different functions and interactions involve the areas of the brain that undergo such an insult.

One of the first problems a therapist must face with a hemiplegic patient is that many bilateral and associational functions are altered because of changes in communication between hemispheres. Therefore, there is no such thing as true left or right hemiplegic. Many problems will be encountered on the contralateral side as well, although they may be more subtle than the frank paralysis of the "involved" side. For instance, research has shown that similar abnormalities in muscle activation patterns of the lower extremities during gait will be found on the contralateral side. Thus, it is important to consider both sides when assessing the patient and developing rehabilitation programs.

Patients with left hemiplegia (right hemisphere CVA) generally have impairment in visual, spatial, and perceptual operations involving the discrimination and appreciation of form, distance, position, and movement. Right-sided damage seems to involve integration of sensory modalities that contribute to the development of body scheme and body awareness. As a result, the patient ignores or denies having a left side. The patient thus becomes disoriented in space because he does not relate to people and objects on the left side. Such deficits permit a distortion of internal and external circumstances. Patients often have a particular visual disturbance called heteronymous hemianopia in which the left visual field is obliterated. This condition is also often denied. The patient with left hemiplegia usually has little verbal impairment. Because of his tendency to cover deficits, he may be overconfident and often unsafe alone because he moves too quickly and impulsively with disturbed judgment in speed and time. Therefore, he may be accident prone.

Closer examination may show subtle difficulties with such tasks as discriminating positions of objects, disorientation in a familiar environment, and deficits in understanding and using words indicating direction such as up, down, and beside. There is impairment in sequential ordering of numbers and a loss of the ability to discern the meanings of symbols. For instance, the subject may not recognize that a "+" means "positive" or "to add."

Further visual-spatial deficits may be in figure-ground relationships. Figure-ground is most easily demonstrated in the visual illusion so constructed that when looking at the picture the first time a vase may be seen and the next time two faces appear. In this case the illusion is so well constructed that the eye, or rather the brain, vacillates about which portion of the illustration constitutes the figure and which the background. The result is that two objects are perceived in alternating fashion. The ability to focus on relevant aspects and maintain attention to the situation are flawed in the patient with left hemiplegia.

All or most hemiplegic patients demonstrate such behaviors as irritability, confusion, and fatigue. These patients may perseverate, that is, repeat the same motor act or verbal phrase over and over. There is often a lability of mood with exaggerated mood swings or inappropriate responses, such as weeping for no apparent reason. Patients are easily distracted.

Those patients with right hemiplegia resulting from a left CVA have a greater impairment in language than those with left hemiplegia, as might be expected. They are likely to suffer receptive or expressive aphasia, or both. In the former, the patient cannot process the spoken word and so does not comprehend what he hears. In the latter, the patient may understand what he is told but cannot form appropriate words. There is often an impairment in the sequential ordering of steps necessary to accomplish an activity. As a result the performance is slow and the patient may forget some of the steps. The patient may have a body scheme disturbance with right-side neglect, but this neglect is more common in patients with left hemiplegia.

IMPLICATIONS FOR TREATMENT

In this section we have tried to identify some of the many subtle and not so subtle alterations and deficits that may occur when the brain is damaged. In fact, the motor deficit itself ultimately may be less a deterrent to functional performance than are the other problems. It is also clear that no particular problem is invariable or that those who suffer right-sided insults will never experience any of the deficits that are more likely to accompany left-sided insults, and vice versa. Nonetheless, this information is likely to provide some insights into the numerous problems experienced by persons with brain injury and possibly to suggest some considerations that may make rehabilitation easier or more effective. Siev and co-workers (1986) provide many practical insights into the evaluation and treatment of perceptual and cognitive disorders in stroke patients.

When approaching the patient with left hemiplegia, make sure that objects of importance are in the right visual field. However, activities must include the left side of the body and the left portion of the environment to help minimize denial. Because verbal language is intact, the emphasis should be on verbal cues as a teaching technique. The rehabilitation potential for those with left hemiplegia, which involves so many perceptual deficits coupled with an underestimation of disability and lack of motivation, is often not as secure as for those with right hemiplegia.

The major deficits in patients with right hemiplegia are in communication. Although this makes it difficult to get them to follow instructions, they probably have more potential for functional rehabilitation. When teaching these patients it is necessary to simplify directions. Give visual instructions or demonstrations rather than verbal cues. Use pictures rather than words. When giving positive feedback, do it by gesturing your approval, smiling, clapping your hands, or shaking their hands. Divide tasks to be performed into simple steps.

Innervation to the more proximal muscles, including the trunk, appears to be more bilateral and contains more synaptic opportunities than that to distal muscles. The pyramidal tract provides much direct monosynaptic input to the distal muscles. As a result, the distal areas such as the hands will be the most severely involved and fine motor skills will be affected. Because the pathways are unilateral and relatively direct, recovery of function is usually more difficult and less effective for fine motor skills.

Patients with left hemiplegia usually have greater deficits in kinesthesia than those with right-sided involvement. They also tend to have what may be termed motor impersistence. That is, they lack the ability to keep the motor activity going and to maintain the muscle contraction. Some therapists have tried the "forced use" programs for the involved side. Such programs restrict the use of the less involved side and require that the task be accomplished by the more involved extremity.

Future research will no doubt provide more insight into any possible differences in right and left brain function. Knowledge of these differences should be of great assistance in developing programs for patients with brain damage, particularly unilateral brain damage such as that sustained by stroke victims.

CHANGES THAT OCCUR IN THE NERVOUS SYSTEM WITH AGING

Some gerontologists consider aging to be a pathologic process in itself. However, it does not seem reasonable that changes occurring over time to most, if not all, persons should be labeled pathologic. Pathology refers to abnormalities that do not occur naturally but rather are associated with some state of disease. It might be more useful to consider aging as a developmental process like birth, growth, and the achievement of adulthood.

"Normal" aging of the nervous system includes changes that occur in persons who do not have actual neurologic disease. These changes are characterized by slow changes in specific functions. For instance, there is little change with age in the ability to store information. However, there is a continual loss in speed functions such as learning time and reaction time to stimuli.

Peripheral and central nervous system changes may occur with increasing age. Specific anatomic alterations in the peripheral nerves and muscles appear to relate to some expected physiologic changes. Central nervous system phenomena are much more difficult to identify, from either an anatomic or physiologic standpoint, than are the peripheral ones. Determining alterations in central processing, for instance, requires much more complex yet less exacting studies than does determining conduction velocities in the peripheral nerves.

CENTRAL NERVOUS SYSTEM

Identifying the mechanisms responsible for aging is necessary before any procedure, device, or substance can be developed that might retard its progress. Undoubtedly, aging begins at the subcellular level just as does disease. Improved technology will be required to identify and understand these molecular alterations. Before delving into cellular and subcellular alterations that have been identified, however, some gross observations may be useful.

Gross Changes

Most of the studies on aging tissues have been done on animals. Such findings are often difficult to extrapolate to humans. When human analysis is performed, we often do not know if "aging" caused the problem or whether some pathologic condition produced the findings that have been labeled as resulting from aging. Biopsies and autopsies provide most tissue material and the circumstances necessitating the tissue removal often make it difficult to know whether some disease process is already present. Identifying a "normal" brain at the time of death is not an easy task.

Certainly, neurons are lost, but the popular view that we loose 1 million cells a day is not accurate and is overstated. Some areas of the brain are affected more than others. The frontal gyrus is one area that is clearly affected; however, the loss of cells within this area occurs more in the fifth decade than at any other time in the life span. Any estimate of daily loss is neither useful nor justifiable.

Lord Byron's brain, one of the largest ever

weighed, was reputed to weigh 3000 g. Another highly intelligent person, Anatole France, had a brain which weighed 1200 g. From these two cases it would appear that intelligence does not relate to brain size or weight; however, standardization of brain-weighing techniques had not occurred. Studies using computed tomography have confirmed that age does affect the size of the brain. Brain weight studies, which are necessarily cross-sectional studies performed at autopsy, suggest that the average weight ranges from 930 to 1100 g.

The peak brain weight occurs between 20 and 25 years of age, and by about 70 to 80 years of age the brain weighs approximately 100 g less. It might be expected that the heavier and larger body of a 20-year-old person would need more brain tissue to support it. There appears to be a distinct relationship between brain weight, muscle weight, muscle strength, and age.

Cell counts within the nervous system are more difficult to perform than gross weight or size studies. Again, relatively few such studies have been done and they are of necessity cross-sectional studies. Those that have been completed suggest that a decrease in cell number occurs with aging in specific cortical areas to varying degrees. The precentral, superior temporal, and superior frontal gyri are the most clearly affected. Purkinje cells in the cerebellum may decrease in number, but not until the sixth decade of life. Most brain stem nuclei do not show loss of cells in association with age.

Microscopic Changes

Almost every known cytoplasmic organelle has been shown to exhibit subtle transformations as the neuron ages. The Golgi complex may fragment into globules and loose its characteristic distribution within the cell. Mitochondria have shown abnormal swelling, vacuolation, and disruption of the cristae. A decrease in number of mitochondria also may occur. A decrease in the amount of Nissl substance in older animals and humans strongly suggests that age-dependent changes take place in the endoplasmic reticulum. The loss of the nucleolus, a decrease in nuclear chromatin, and infolding of the nuclear membrane indicate alterations in genetic material, and a resulting deviation of instructions to the cell machinery could be expected. Lipofuscin, the "aging pigment," is definitely more prevalent within cells as age increases. However, it is not known whether the substance is cytotoxic.

These changes in organelles suggest that some fundamental transformation in cellular functions may occur. The most conspicuous alterations would most likely be in producing and packaging cellular substances. Some of the most important of these cellular secretions are the neurotransmitters.

Modification of neurotransmitters includes a decrease in dopamine. Animal studies also have shown decreases in acetylcholine synthesis, norepinephrine content, and serotonin concentration. There appears to be a marked loss of cells within the monoamine oxidase systems that regulate the autonomic nervous system. Again, assays of these substances in humans are usually accomplished through biopsy of brain tissue, a process not likely to occur in normal, healthy persons.

Microscopic observations suggest that there may be a loss of dendritic arbor. The loss of dendritic spines results in a loss of synapses. Loss of dendrites is associated with shrinkage and distortion of affected cell bodies. The richness of synaptic connections that differentiates the immature fetal brain from the adult brain undoubtedly has a great correlation with physical, emotional, and intellectual capacity and flexibility of function. Synaptic loss must provide some "hardwiring" changes in these capabilities.

Changes in Function

General intellectual performance peaks between the ages of 20 and 30 years. Intellectual function as measured by tests of verbal abilities in vocabulary, information, and comprehension is maintained until at least the mid-seventies. Other cognitive functions requiring speed, such as performance on timed tests, peak at about 20 years of age and decline slowly throughout life. Almost everyone notes this change by 70 years of age. Slowing occurs in simple motor tasks such as running or finger tapping. Slowing of sensory perceptual responses monitored by reaction time also occurs. Slowing is one of the most significant changes in function of the nervous system of normal aging persons.

The cognitive skills requiring central processing show steady decline. Reaction time is slower, but choice reaction time that interposes a decision in the process of reacting is increased to an even greater degree in older persons. It appears that practice can enhance skills requiring speed at any age; however, there is little transfer effect. This means that improvement in the skill under consideration, such as the speed of copying words, will not improve other timed skills (Katzman and Terry, 1983).

Learning and memory are complex processes that are of interest to those studying the aging process. One of the most frequent complaints of the elderly is forgetfulness. Studies show that most persons develop some degree of impairment in learning and memory, especially after age 70 years. New learning is more difficult for the aging person. Short-term learning and memory are the most likely to show some impairment, and these changes may be related to the longer processing time required by the elderly.

In terms of postural functions, the elderly appear to rely heavily on vision for balance. This may be a result of the dysfunction and alteration of somatosensory receptors. Additionally, the vestibular neurons undergo degenerative changes, as do other peripheral neurons. When intersensory conflicts are presented, such as standing on a soft and yielding surface that fails to provide accurate information to the somatosensory system, postural instability results. Alterations in somatosensory, visual, and vestibular senses in concert with the slowing and dysfunction of central processing may account for the inability to resolve intersensory conflicts. Falls are likely to occur under circumstances of diminished sensation or intersensory conflicts, such as the diminution of vision in the dark or inaccurate somatosensory input that may result from support surface alterations.

Changes in the central motor system resulting from normal aging are difficult to differentiate from those that are secondary to age-related disorders such as cardiovascular disease. Many of the biochemical and microscopic changes noted earlier, such as the degeneration of neuronal systems involving the monoamine oxidase neurotransmitters and the pathways involving the basal ganglia (corpus striatum), are also characteristic of Parkinson's disease although the alterations are much more dramatic in the latter. Many of the clinical signs of Parkinson's disease, however, are characteristic of old age.

A progressive decrease in dopamine within the striatum has been observed in aging persons. In addition, other substances and cofactors such as tyrosine hydroxylase are decreased and may compound the changes from the diminishing monoamine systems. Acetylcholine also decreases, but to a lesser extent than dopamine. The net result of such a condition is a relative overactivity of acetylcholine. The changes in neurotransmitters may compound the alterations produced by the loss of neurons and synaptic communications. These central changes, in association with peripheral nervous system degenerations described later such as segmental demyelinization, may produce the senescent signs that resemble an extrapyramidal syndrome. Extrapyramidal-like signs include a decrease in movement, weak voice, slow or shuffling walk, flexed posture, muscular rigidity, and often a tremor. It appears that some loss of central inhibition occurs. Impairment in balance, postural tremor, and unsteady hand movements may be related to degenerative changes in the cerebellum, the vestibular system, or their connections (Katzman and Terry, 1983).

PERIPHERAL NERVOUS SYSTEM

Two types of structural changes in aging nerve fibers have been well documented, especially in sensory fibers. One type is associated with myelin regression, in particular segmental demyelinization. The largest axons suffer the greatest demyelinative processes. Segmental demyelinization of both sensory and motor axons decreases conduction velocity along the axons. The second change in peripheral nerves involves degeneration of the axon itself. This usually begins in the most distal areas and regresses proximally. The most significant axonal finding is the loss of neuronal fibers or axons, which may result from the loss of neuron cell bodies.

The neuromuscular end plate of the motor fibers exhibits some swelling and regressive changes. Motor nerve endings in distal muscles may have spherical axonic swellings in addition to elaborate and multiple motor end plates, as opposed to the single motor end plate in each muscle fiber, as is the usual case in the normal younger person. Some of the motor problems are undoubtedly associated with the loss of motor neurons. There is evidence of denervation and reinnervation of muscle, which indicates that neurons have degenerated and regenerated over time. These findings are similar to those found in patients with motor neuron disease such as poliomyelitis. The loss of muscle fibers in old age may relate to this pattern of degeneration of neurons in which the type II motor units are possibly the most affected.

Sensory receptors in the skin undergo a variety of alterations. The pacinian corpuscle increases in size, and remodeled endings have been noted or new ones have been formed on the axons of obsolete corpuscles. Merkel's corpuscles decrease in number, as do Meissner's corpuscles. The latter also shows coiled and lobulated nerve endings within the capsule, which differs from their normal state. Free nerve endings undergo the least changes. The most affected aspects of cutaneous sensation would be, therefore, the very specific and localizing information carried by the larger fibers such as light touch, deep pressure, and two-point discrimination. The changes in pacinian corpuscles may cause the diminished vibratory perception in the lower extremities seen by the seventh decade. Ultimately, most sensory modalities are diminished in the distal portions of the extremities.

Some of the compromise in cutaneous sensation may be related to the changes in the skin itself, such as increasing collagen and loss of skin elasticity. Blood vessels supplying the neural tissues may be thickened, and the endoneurial connective tissue is likely to be increased.

As far as proprioceptors are concerned, some researchers indicate that there may be up to a 50% loss of joint receptors. Muscle spindles may have increased capsular thickness, a decrease in the intrafusal fibers as well as changes consistent with denervation, and end plate abnormalities. The diminished deep tendon reflexes that occur in normal aging thus may result from conduction slowing and impaired activity of the muscle spindles. Muscle fiber atrophy, joint stiffness, and changes in elastic connective tissue undoubtedly make some contribution to the suppression of reflexes.

It is difficult to determine the extent to which these changes are the result of biologic aging per se or repeated trauma, ischemia, local nerve entrapment, and poor regenerative capacity.

AUTONOMIC NERVOUS SYSTEM

Diminished competence of the autonomic nervous system is common in old age. A vast number of functions are affected. The most prevalent changes include disorders of pupillary, cardiovascular, thermal, and secretory functions. Some of these changes may result from deterioration of the peripheral system, others from dysfunction of the CNS control centers of the autonomic nervous system. A portion of the dysfunction undoubtedly results from deterioration of the non-neural tissues as well. The more serious autonomic changes include the compromise of body temperature regulation, and dysfunction of the baroreceptor reflex, which results in an increase in blood pressure.

The health of the nervous system depends upon the health of other systems as well, especially the cardiovascular system. Habits of lifestyle, such as smoking and diet, that increase the chances of arterial disease will profoundly affect the nervous system. A cerebrovascular accident or stroke that results in motor and sensory abnormalities is not a nervous system disease, but a cerebrovascular disease.

Exposure to some substances directly affects the nervous system. Excessive intake of alcohol and exposure to arsenic and heavy metals all produce generalized peripheral neuropathies, which may result in decreased sensory acuity and impaired motor function. Many drugs administered for other conditions, such as cancer therapy, may produce neuropathies as a side-effect. Nutritional deficits and vitamin deficiencies may affect both the peripheral and central nervous systems.

THE GOOD NEWS

Whether the aging phenomena of the nervous system can be altered or delayed is an extremely important and relevant question. Much of the decline in motor performance can be related more to the physical inactivity usually associated with aging than to actual senescent alterations. Physical training appears to improve such phenomena as reaction time and work capacity. Such training also has a general effect on the body including improvement in heart rate, blood pressure, and joint mobility. These improvements should also affect general longevity and prevent the compromise of the nervous system from the involvement of other systems.

Some forms of drug and nutritional therapy may prove to be useful in the future. The administration of dopaminergic agents appears to influence some aging phenomena in animals. Such substances may also affect humans. Additionally, the presence of dietary precursor substances may be critical. Often the elderly persons's diet is deficient in one or more nutrients. A good, well-balanced diet, possibly including an increase in certain nutritional elements, certainly can do no harm and may be beneficial in retarding some of the dire effects of aging.

Some of the oldest adages appear to have significant meaning for all of us who are destined to join the world's largest minority. "Use it or lose it," "practice makes perfect," and "you are what you eat" are but a few. Although immortality may not be achievable greater longevity most likely will be. The most important aspect of this, however, is the maintenance of the quality of life during the later years. To live and work, to be productive, happy, and healthy are far more important than to exist for 90 or 100 years or beyond.

THEORIES OF MOTOR CONTROL

Insight into the neurophysiologic substrata of motor acts is of paramount importance in developing treatment strategies aimed at correcting or overcoming abnormalities in motor control. Motor control deficits and resulting movement dysfunction plague all patients who have suffered nervous system insults.

When a physical therapist treats a neurologically involved patient, the treatment is based upon the therapist's conscious or unconscious model of motor control. Associated with the model the therapist has chosen to accept are certain assumptions. For example, you might espouse what is considered to be a mostly outmoded view that cerebral spasticity results from a hyperactive muscle spindle system. In this case, it is likely you will assume that the patient with brain damage who demonstrates resistance to passive stretch has a short and sensitive muscle spindle. Treatment will thus be aimed incorrectly at desensitizing the muscle spindle and gaining control over the system by gradually increasing the length the muscle can attain before resistance appears. If our model is incorrect, our assumptions will lead us astray, and the treatment procedures that are devised will most likely be incorrect. Even if the treatment technique is useful, it may be applied for the wrong reason or with inappropriate expectations of the result.

The question of how movement is generated to produce complex motor patterns of behavior has been a subject of research for the past 80 years. Although the technology necessary to obtain neurologic data has increased or improved by quantum leaps, it is likely that only the first layers of understanding have been reached. How much understanding is necessary to generate consistently effective treatment interventions is unknown. No universally acceptable theory of motor control has been articulated. In addition, those theories that are available often give an extremely divergent view of the controlling system. For some theorists the controlling mechanisms are specific neural structures that may involve reflexes or pattern generators. For others, activities of the controller are minimized and understanding the process does not require the identification of specific complex neural substrata. A completely different notion of control is present in theories in which movement results from self-organizing processes.

Several of these theories will be discussed in this chapter with the intent to identify some of the assumptions that are likely to accompany them. Also of concern is how the theories may relate to understanding the patient with movement dysfunction and the treatment approaches that may be needed.

REFLEX HIERARCHY THEORIES

Ever since Sherrington's clever experiments early in this century, neurophysiologists and motor control theorists have attempted to reduce complex human behavior to certain reflex reactions or combinations of reflex behaviors. A reflex requires a stimulus and a response. A reflex may be considered as that response which occurs with great probability when a particular stimulus or stimuli are presented. The simplest example of such a reflex is the deep tendon reflex, or monosynaptic spinal reflex, which is mediated by the muscle spindle. In this case a tap on the tendon exciting the stretch receptors results in a synchronized contraction of the muscle stretched, and in response a "jerk" or movement of the joint occurs.

Other early researchers, such as Magnus and de Kleijn, using cats whose nervous systems had been surgically transected at increasingly higher and higher levels, observed more complex reflexive behaviors. Further patterns of complex activity have been described from observing newborn humans and patients with central nervous system insults as well as animal experimentation and observation. Proponents of reflex-based behavior have attempted to explain complex motor behavior as resulting from the "chaining" of simple reflexes into combined patterns of activity (Delong, 1971). Thus, the basic unit of movement in this theory is the reflex (Easton, 1972).

Reflex responses result in specific spatial and temporal activation of the muscle groups involved in elaborating the pattern. Because this activation is relatively invariant a readily identifiable movement is observed. The reflex responses are associated with specific sensory stimuli that are believed to be necessary to elicit the motor response. Examples of what are or were believed to be primitive reflex behaviors that can be elicited in normal neonates and young infants are the flexor withdrawal, automatic walking, asymmetric tonic neck, tonic labyrinthine, and Moro reflexes.

Attempts have also been made to categorize these reflex patterns into a specific hierarchy of neural organization. In order to do this, it is necessary to assume that some area of the nervous system is responsible for generating or controlling the reflex. Through ablation experiments, it was concluded that the lowest level reflexes are generated in the spinal cord. Next up the hierarchy are the brain stem and midbrain reflexes, and finally the cortically governed reflexes. However, the fact that a reflex does not manifest itself after section or destruction of a particular level of the CNS can have several interpretations, only one of which is that the region is responsible for generating or controlling the reflex.

Although primitive and more mature reflexes are often presented in this manner, some distinct problems are associated with such attempts. For instance, the Moro reflex, one of the most primitive reflexes, is apparently generated or controlled in the medulla. Spontaneous stepping has been assumed to be an intrinsic reflex property of the spinal cord. In humans, however, because stepping is relatively uncommon in those with spinal cord injuries, it has been hypothesized that the reflex is controlled from the brain stem and possibly the diencephalon (Brooks, 1986). What quickly becomes apparent is that the assumed hierarchy does not always hold true, at least for centers of possible generation. This theory of hierarchical reflex organization, which rests so heavily on animal studies of the early 1900s, has dominated our view of motor control for so long that it still probably provides the most prevalent underpinnings of therapeutic intervention.

In the hierarchical approach, the higher-order reactions are those that develop after birth and are usually present throughout life. These are the righting and equilibrium reactions. Assumptions made in accepting the reflex-hierarchical model of motor control are that the "higher"-level reflexes will inhibit the "lower" ones, or that the primitive reflexes prevent the development of the righting and equilibrium reactions. It is also assumed that the primitive reflexes interfere with the development of normal movement or the elaboration of normal movement. Because these stereotyped movement patterns can also be elicited in adults who experience neurological insult, it is assumed that the higher systems of organization have been damaged and have released their control over the primitive system.

Treatment approaches based on these theories involve the assumptions that a specific stimulus is required to elicit the response and that sensation is necessary for movement. Therapists are likely to assume that higher centers dominate movement and that lower centers never dominate unless some pathologic condition arises. In the latter case the movements are primitive and stereotyped. Treatment will be directed at attempting to decrease the dominant effects of the primitive patterns first, and then at eliciting the equilibrium and righting reactions. The assumption is that the primitive reflexes prevent the elaboration of the higher reactions, and that the latter assist in the integration of the former. Treatment programs in this case are highly organized around specific reflexes. The patient in many respects becomes the passive recipient of therapy.

SERVOMECHANISTIC THEORIES ("LOOP" THEORIES)

Advances in control systems theory have also influenced models of motor control. In computer programming, sequences are developed that circle or "loop," allowing for the repetition of certain functions. Neurophysiologists have used the loop concept to explain rhythmic and repetitive motor behaviors such as the gait cycle.

Closed Loop

Closed loop models have been dominant with motor control theorists for years. The origins of this view grew out of the engineering sciences and servomechanistic approaches. In a closed loop model, the executive controller needs to be given the result of the response to any activation. The neurons are arranged in a circular fashion or in loops in which the neurons influence one another, providing feedback with further activation (Fig. 11-28). Such theories require an internal reference with which to compare such feedback and thus determine if modification of the response is necessary.

Much evidence has been interpreted as to support this theory. For example, one experiment often cited showed that if a subject's muscle was vibrated, the vibration produced an illusion of movement (Goodwin and co-workers, 1972). Some muscle receptors are responsive to vibration. Apparently the activation of the sensory receptors is sufficient to induce the perception that movement has occurred when it has not. In this case, the higher centers were overridden by the stimulation of a peripheral receptor. Such circumstances might favor a closed-loop control. This data suggests that sensory input, especially muscle sensory input, contributes to the perception of movement but does not necessarily, of itself, support a closed-loop theory of motor control.

This is an error-centered theory in which error detection, error correction, and knowledge of results are the major requirements. The theory requires two memories: the memory trace and the perceptual trace (Adams, 1976). The memory trace is a learned capability for the

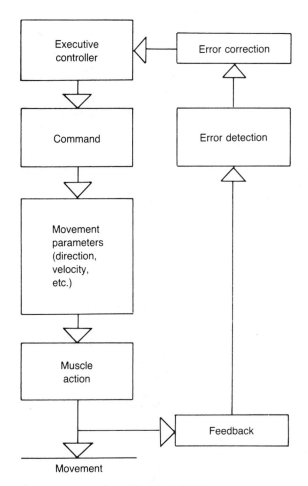

Figure 11-28. Closed-loop model of motor control.

late movements. Thus, both fast ballistic movements and slow movements requiring feedback could be elaborated (Stelmach; see Kelso, 1982).

Hypotheses that have been developed to explain the function of the muscle spindle have evolved through various theories of motor control. Muscle spindle function has been explained through hypotheses based on closed-loop theories. For instance, an early hypothesis was called the length-servo hypothesis. In this hypothesis, the misalignment between intended muscle length and actual muscle length would be determined by activity of the fusimotor system. That is, if the systems were activated by a certain load requirement and the load was increased, the gamma output would increase. Thus a feedback system was present that controlled the constancy of activity. We will see that other hypotheses of muscle spindle physiology have evolved that relate to other theories of motor control.

There is also considerable experimental evidence that has been interpreted as being in opposition to closed-loop theories. Such theories require the subject to have the knowledge of the results of previous trials to learn the task. There is evidence that this knowledge is not always necessary and learning may take place without knowledge of results. Kelso (1982), for example, removed the sensory input from the digits by using constricting cuffs that impeded the blood supply and abolished sensation. He found that subjects were just as accurate in reproducing positions of the finger without the sensory feedback as they were with it. On the other hand, subjects could not reproduce distance accurately. Thus, the perceptual trace may not exist, or at least it may not always function as earlier described.

Closed-loop theories may adequately describe a small portion of human motor behavior, but they appear to be inadequate for a far greater percentage. Aspects of this approach will resurface, however, within other theories.

In a closed-loop view the motor learner is an active participant in controlling, manipulat-

selection and initiation of a desired response and behaves in an "open" loop fashion, that is, no feedback is required. The perceptual trace is a structure for evaluating the correctness of the response as executed by the memory trace. The perceptual trace determines the extent of movement but not the choice of movement. It is not a single entity, but rather is a complex distribution of traces produced over many practice trials. To address the variety of movements that can be elaborated, the open-loop structure might be used to generate movements and the closed-loop system would regu-

ing, and generating behavior. The environment, or the therapist, is not expected to precipitate or generate the activity. When the nervous system is considered to be an active agent in controlling movement outcomes, treatment approaches are geared differently than when the patient is considered to be a passive recipient of external stimuli. In a closed-loop view, the patient will be expected to be an active agent experiencing and exploring the environment. Spontaneous and voluntary movements should be observed and encouraged within a varied context of environmental constraints.

Open Loop

One model of motor control involves the concept of an open loop. In an open loop system the motor "command" contains all the information necessary to produce the movement. The neurons are activated in one direction, so no feedback loops return to neurons within this system (Fig. 11-29). The movement is completed without any alteration of parameters. This type of central control theory has been out of date as an exclusive theory of motor control for some time. However, the observation that motor acts may be programmed in advance has received considerable support and resurrects at least some aspects of this theory. Fast movements that occur too rapidly for feedback to modify them would be the most likely candidates to be under open-loop control.

In following the earlier example of explaining the muscle spindle, further evolution can be seen. Later research concerning the muscle spindle showed that gamma or fusimotor activity did not precede the alpha activity, but that alpha and gamma motoneurons are co-activated. Therefore, primary muscle activation occurs in an open-loop fashion. Spindle discharge strength increases as the extrafusal muscle contraction rises, which accounts for the name "servo-assist" hypothesis. Spindle bias through gamma motor neurons allows for sensitivity to changes in muscle length, providing for feedback. When it was discovered that muscles working against a load produced a significant discharge of the muscle spindle and

unloaded movements did not, the hypothesis was modified as the "load-dependent servo-assistance" hypotheses. Both forms of this hypothesis combine open- and closed-loop mechanisms.

By observing patient treatment it could be concluded that physical therapists have often viewed the nervous system as operating in an open-loop fashion. If the idea is that the therapist can trigger the desired movement by manipulating input to the patient, the treatment is

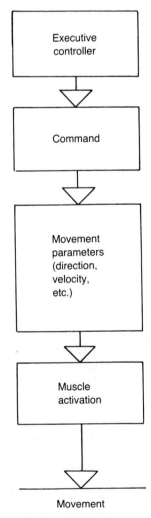

Figure 11-29. Open-loop model of motor control.

then oriented in a passive manner with the patient being the mere recipient.

COGNITIVE THEORIES

When analyzing highly skilled and rapid movements some theorists have suggested that primary components enter into skill: a decision component and an action component. People are assumed to assess a situation, make a decision, select a movement or some other action, and then execute that action. Duration of the decision component can be assessed by reaction time and duration of the action component can be assessed by movement time.

Movement time reflects the primary component of skill called the action component. The efficiency of skilled performance typically depends on either speed or precision of the movement, or more often a combination of the two (Keele; see Kelso, 1982). Fitts's law combines distance and precision into a single formula: $MT = A/W$ (movement time equals the ratio between distance to the target and width of the target). The faster the movement to be made to a target at a given distance, the greater the force that must be imparted to start a movement and the greater the opposing force to stop movement as the target is neared. Fitts's law makes it clear that there is a trade-off of speed for accuracy. Part of the trade-off is the result of increasing force in order to increase speed because greater force results in less precision.

When a large motor unit is activated a relatively large force results by combining the force output of all the muscle fibers contained in that unit. In reverse, to produce a large force, the large type II motor units must be activated. Therefore, it would seem impossible to make fine gradations in motion when using large forces. Thus, if one needs precision, moving slowly and minimizing the force required should result in a more precise movement without feedback.

Reaction time reflects the primary component of skill called the decision component. It has been observed that the more a skill is practiced, the more it improves. Improvement over the years show that world records are broken all the time. Some of this may be due to better equipment and technology but some is undoubtedly due to refining the movement technique. Bernstein (1967) showed that motion in the body parts of a world-class runner were more complex than those of ordinary runners, implying that technique, not just conditioning, improves.

Others suggest that the information being picked up becomes more and more subtle and precise, which leads to skill development. The skilled performer resonates to the information and becomes attuned to it over time (Kelso, 1982). Information is always available, and thus there is no need to access stored knowledge structures for the purposes of prediction and anticipation.

Certain variables, for example, compatibility and the probability of expected events, have well-known effects on the time it takes to make decisions. Reaction time is often slow when the situation calls for movements or reactions that are not natural or easily linked together. Sometimes this results from having too many choices to make within a certain time. More often reaction time is prolonged because the actions are not compatible. For instance, touch a person's finger and ask him to press the finger that is touched. The reaction time should be very fast. On the contrary, if the person is asked to move the same finger on the right hand that you have touched on the left hand his reaction time should increase markedly. The response is not compatible with what is natural to do.

Keele (see Kelso, 1982) applied these variables to sports skills and suggested a number of interesting applications of these concepts. He suggests that knowing ahead of time what stimulus is about to appear vastly reduces decision time, and in theory, the skilled basketball player or boxer could use such cues to anticipate what might happen next. According to Keele, a highly skilled behavior may be as much cognitive as it is perceptual or motor.

Cognitive theories would suggest to physical therapists that the acquisition of movement requires concentration and practice. Although these tools may be useful in therapy, it may not be appropriate to equate basic posture and movement underlaying average everyday activities with highly skilled athletic or artistic acts. Most neurologic patients lack these fundamental movements, which are likely to be much less cognitive in nature than are movements involving high levels of skill.

PATTERN GENERATOR THEORIES

The existence of predeveloped patterns of activity would be an additional mechanism for simplifying motor activity. With patterns of movement, muscles are activated in certain spatially and temporally organized relationships. For instance, under a specific circumstance the plantar flexor, hamstring, and paraspinal muscles may be linked together in that order with very specific timing to produce a particular movement. Those who espouse the theories of pattern generation suggest that perhaps the most classic movement that could result from a pattern generator is gait and locomotion. According to Brooks (1986), we know that locomotor patterns are programmed because neural control signals associated with locomotion are recorded even in animals who have been paralyzed with curare or some other such agent.

In human infants the patterns of spontaneous kicking, flexor withdrawal, crossed extension reflexes, and automatic stepping are quite similar. Rather than being "primitive reflexes" these movements may reflect the activity of a pattern generator involved in locomotion. As will be discussed later, many maturational influences may produce the particular part of the pattern that is seen and labeled a primitive reflex.

Nashner (Nashner and Woollacott, 1979) developed some elegant human experiments that identified specific patterns of activity elaborated under certain circumstances. When a subject is standing on a platform that provides forward or backward perturbations, reliable movement patterns occur in response to the disturbances in balance produced by the moving platform. These patterns may be called the hip and ankle synergies. If the perturbation is

small the control of the center of gravity is achieved by "postural sway," a pendulum motion controlled from the ankles. The pattern of muscular activity is very specifically timed and organized. If the perturbation is such that the platform under the feet is jerked backward, it causes a forward displacement of the body. As a result the gastrocnemius, hamstring, and lumbar paraspinal muscles contract in that order to return the center of gravity to a more stable position (Fig. 11-30). A forward perturbation resulting in a backward displacement of the body produces an activation of the opposite muscles, the anterior tibialis, quadriceps, and abdominals.

If the center of gravity is perturbed too far for the ankle synergy to correct it, or if the ankle synergy cannot be effective in a given environmental context, a more proximal strategy is elicited. This is called the hip synergy, and the hamstrings and paraspinal muscles or the quadriceps and abdominal muscles are activated with little or no activity from the ankle musculature. This synergy results in a much wider excursion of the body in an attempt to return the center of gravity to a stable position.

According to Nashner (Nashner and Woollacott, 1979) these synergy patterns of muscular activation occur too quickly to be voluntary and are too slow to be considered reflexive. At least, they are too slow to result from a basic monosynaptic reflex as would be elicited simply from stretch on the involved muscles during perturbation. However, the suggestion is that these movements are preprogrammed linkages of specific muscles constrained to act together in particular patterns. These patterns are thus activated under certain conditions of the destabilization of the center of gravity.

How many patterns are there? Where do they come from? Do all our movements consist of predictable patterns of muscular activity? These are all questions that remain to be answered by those investigating the mysteries of motor control.

Evidence suggests that at least some of these patterns are genetically determined and communications are established in the system before birth. Milani-Comparetti (1981) has observed the spontaneous activity of fetuses using ultrasonography. Very competent and complex movements have been documented. Reaching, grasping, thumb sucking, and changing positions are a few. Because no stimuli could be identified to elicit many of these behaviors, Milani-Comparetti concluded that

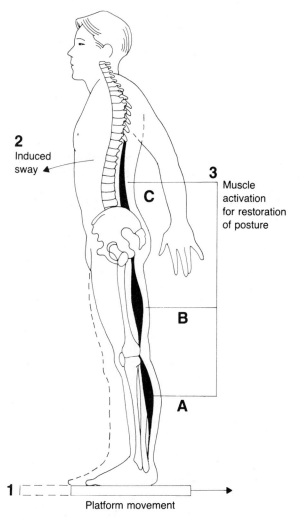

2
Induced sway ◄

3
Muscle activation for restoration of posture

C

B

A

1

Platform movement

Figure 11-30. Posterior platform perturbation induces a forward sway of the body, which is counteracted by a specific sequence of muscle contractions: (A) gastrocnemius, (B) hamstring, and (C) paraspinal muscles.

motor actions result from pattern generators. These generators would then form the underlying neural basis for such spontaneous movement. It should be noted, of course, that other interpretations may be placed on this information.

It is likely that the failure of the neonate to demonstrate many of these movements competently at birth relate to the environmental states that occur before and after birth. Before birth the fetus is floating in a fluid medium in which the antigravity effects could provide a most suitable environment for expressing such movements. Once the child is born the effects of gravity completely alter the environment in which movements are to be made. In some cases the infant is undoubtedly too weak to produce the pattern against gravity. Learning and maturation are undoubtedly needed to perform in this new set of circumstances. Other mechanical or developmental factors may influence the expression of motor behavior. Further weight gain and maturation will continue to alter the expected pattern and the child's ability to produce it.

In opposition to the pattern theories, some theorists would suggest that the elaboration, disappearance, and reappearance of certain motor acts raises serious questions about the interpretation of the pattern as being caused by a pattern generator. If the pattern was indeed present, then it should be encountered in some manner. EMG records could show underlying patterns even if sufficient strength was not present to produce joint movement. Such research projects could clarify these assumptions about patterns that are present during neonatal life but not expressed at birth.

Because neurons are highly differentiated cells, they are not capable of cell division and multiplication once the differentiation has taken place. Therefore, at the time of birth all the neurons the child will ever have are present. However, much of the communication between neurons has not been completed. One clear difference between the nervous tissue of neonates and more adult animals is the connections or synapses that are completed and activated. The processes of learning and maturation apparently have strong influences on the development of synaptic connections and the activation of synapses present. So the basic structure for some program generators that are not expressed at birth or in utero may be present at birth, but connections are not yet complete.

Myelination is also an important process of maturation. Myelination is not completed in the newborn and continues for some years after birth. The critical timing factors noted at the beginning of this chapter may have an impact on the accessibility of any given pattern or system of activation.

It has been postulated that the generator may be accessed from peripheral stimulation of sensory receptors. Early studies of locomotion using animal subjects showed that even if the sensory input was eliminated by cutting the sensory roots, a locomotor pattern could still be generated. The question arises then, how is the pattern accessed? Some theorists have proposed that the pattern is expressed from within the central nervous system itself. Combination theories suggest that the spinal and supraspinal centers function together with the interaction of continuous sensory input and cortical refinement to modify motor pattern activity.

If the first elaboration of motor patterns is spontaneous and occurs without sensory input, the role or value of such input may be questioned. Reflex models of motor control clearly indicate that sensory mechanisms are active by definition, and cannot be separated from the motor response. In Milani-Comparetti's view, even though movement is initially spontaneous, later in prenatal development the link between sensory input and motor output is observed. Even if specific stimuli are not necessary to elicit a movement, they may be of value for feedback to the central nervous system for motor learning. This feedback would bring into the central mechanisms knowledge of the movement and its results. The results of the act can be used to make the next movement more refined or better suited to the purpose.

Fatigue studies in humans have supported the theory that some learned human move-

ments may be stored as motor patterns. If an act is repeated until the subject is fatigued, the question arises: What is fatigued—the arm or the pattern or the program? Measurements showed that greater fatigue occurs in the same pattern in the other arm than when a different act is performed. That is, if a pattern of activity is performed by the left arm until it is fatigued and then the pattern is repeated by the right arm, the right arm will be more easily fatigued performing that particular activity than if a completely different activity is attempted (Brooks, 1986).

Experiments with handwriting showed that the trajectory shape of the writing was similar whether written with the right hand, the right hand with enlarged letters, the left hand, the foot, or with the pen in the mouth. Thus, the writer's style was recognizable no matter how the writing was produced. This observation suggests that the same program is drawn on by diverse muscle systems.

According to Brooks (1986) motor acts consist of postures, which are made up of "hold" programs, and transitions from one posture to another, which consist of "move" programs. Complex actions are produced by overall plans that are composed of several programs. The programs themselves are further composed of smaller subroutines or subprograms. Subprograms contain the code for actual muscle activity and also initiate other subroutines, which execute patterns of muscle contractions and so forth. This hierarchy of plans, programs, and subprograms ultimately converges on neurons executing nonlearned automatic or reflex adjustments, which we might call patterns. Movements are learned when successful combinations occur and the entire sequence of action is planned thereafter as a single unit.

This process suggests that continued practice is essential to learning new motor tasks. In addition, synaptic strength is reduced when the pattern is unused. So the old adage "use it or lose it" makes sense.

The motivation or desire to move is another important aspect of generating movement. The limbic portions of the brain are involved with the emotional aspects of motor control, such as the need or wish to move. The motivation to accomplish a motor learning task thus originates in the limbic system.

According to Brooks (1986), the sensorimotor areas of the brain are concerned with sensations and motor programs. The brain directs the elaboration of movement in a command hierarchy that may be thought of as occurring on three levels. The highest level is the association cortex. At this level the overall plans and perceptions are elaborated. The middle level, which consists of the sensorimotor cortex, the cerebellum, the basal ganglia, and the brain stem, convert the plans into programs and packages. The lowest level, the spinal cord, executes the programs. Brooks states that this hierarchy is not to be thought of as a rigid vertical line of command. Levels interact through internal feedback loops to correlate ascending and descending messages.

Two kinds of errors may occur with programs when attempting to achieve an environmental goal (Schmidt; see Kelso 1982). These are errors in either selection or execution. In selection errors the subject will choose the wrong program. For example, a batter who expects a fast ball sets the spatiotemporal program that will allow him to hit it effectively. He is thrown a slow curve instead. The bat swing that he executes is inappropriate and he is not successful.

Errors in execution occur when the program is correct but is not executed correctly. The muscles do not do what they were intended to do. If muscles are fatigued, for example, the variation in timing that results from fatigue will alter the execution of the pattern. Errors in selection are thought to involve the central mechanisms, whereas those in execution may involve spinal or cerebellar mechanisms. Attention or cognitive awareness is probably necessary to correct selection errors. It takes much longer to initiate a correction with selection errors than with execution errors (Schmidt; see Kelso, 1982).

Therapists who espouse the view that there are pattern generators within the nervous system would be expected to incorporate them into treatment programs. The assumption is that a movement package or at least part of it is available if it could be accessed. The first step would be to identify patterns in normal persons with an attempt to observe how they are altered or whether they even exist in patients afflicted with nervous system disorders.

Anyone who has treated patients with neurological deficits knows that the motor organization and adaptability of the normal person are not apparent. The patient may demonstrate consistent movement patterns or synergies, but these synergies are dominant and nonadaptable, and the patient has a limited repertoire of movements.

Closer analysis of the muscular activation patterns found in response to perturbations noted earlier showed differences between those with nervous system disease and normal persons. In some cases the order of muscular activation was altered. As might be expected, such alteration in sequence would result in the elaboration of a different motor act or movement than that produced with the normal sequence.

From a clinical perspective, it would seem logical that when treating patients one approach might be to attempt to change the patterns that are demonstrated if they are abnormal. Undoubtedly our understanding of the mechanisms of movement is ahead of clinical methods of intervention. There is no proof that it is possible to access a new synergy or to correct an abnormal one. Nonetheless, it appears more prudent to attempt such a feat with logical reasoning based on available knowledge than to persist in treatments based on clearly outmoded concepts. So be creative!

Perhaps the wrong sequence or synergy is used in the activity. Possibly the synergy itself is abnormal with alterations in the activation sequences of the muscles. The direction of treatment, then, would be to foster the elaboration of the correct pattern or synergy for the appropriate task and the diminution of the improper one. These objectives might be accomplished in any number of ways. Biofeedback, electrical stimulation, or cutaneous stimuli might be used to trigger the appropriate order of muscle activation. Situations may be contrived, such as using a balance beam or a soft support surface to force the elaboration of a specific pattern. Allowing the person to move and providing useful guidance and support through handling might be a good approach.

MOTOR SCHEMA

Schmidt (1982) has described problems with the concept of patterns and programs. Many questions arise: How many programs are there? Does changing the speed of a throw require a new pattern generator? Is there a pattern generator for every possible combination of new throws? If a pattern was required for every one of the infinite variations of throwing, hundreds or thousands of pattern generators and programs would be necessary. This will present a major problem for storage of such programs. Another problem with programs is the novelty problem. How does one make a movement never made before? We are quite capable of executing movements for which no evolutionary purpose could be construed. It has been observed that repeated movements may be similar but are never identical.

Schmidt suggests that rather than consisting of specific pattern generators, movements result from more generalized programs. If the controllers are supplied with informational parameters such as in computer programs, the program could be run off in a variety of ways depending on the goal. This would eliminate the massive storage required for individual patterns. He indicates four kinds of information that might be stored: (1) parameters such as duration, force, spatial relationships, movement size, and so forth; (2) movement outcome—what happened? (3) sensory consequences—what did it "feel" like? and (4) initial conditions—weight and size of objects that will be manipulated, the initial state of the body, and so forth. In the course of running a given program, after each response the subject briefly stores these four pieces of information. The brain then abstracts the relationships among the stored bits of information and generates or updates any rules that describe the relationship

between them. Thus, a motor schema or general plan is stored rather than vast numbers of individual patterns.

SYSTEMS OR DISTRIBUTED CONTROL THEORIES OF MOTOR CONTROL

The idea of a systems or distributed control approach to motor control probably has many roots. Underlying a system view of control is the concept that the whole is greater than the sum of the parts and the control does not reside within one area but is broadly distributed. There are properties and behaviors that are exhibited which cannot be determined by investigating or by limiting the investigation to the component parts. For example, the elements sodium and chloride can be studied through many avenues—electrochemically, in solution, and so forth. But combined into sodium chloride, or table salt, they exhibit properties that could not be ascertained from studying only the elements themselves. In the systems view of motor control the common thread is that all of the parts are interrelated to all the other parts and recording the behavior of an isolated circuit or unit fails to explain the functioning organism as a whole. Although there are many areas of basic agreement and common research foundations, various researchers have viewed the systems approach somewhat differently.

Biomechanical Models

Aside from formal theories of motor control that focus on central nervous system action, some investigators have proposed less ambitious models of specific motor behaviors that include or consider the importance of biomechanical factors as well as nervous factors. These models are not totally inconsistent with other aspects of systems theory or even such concepts as central pattern generators or motor programs, and are often incorporated into those models or hypotheses.

In movement there is what has been termed the degrees of freedom problem. Each joint in the body may have up to three degrees of freedom. The degrees from each joint then may be combined because most movements involve a multisegmental or multijoint action. Such combinations produce a very large, if not infinite, number of possible joint positions. How to control all of those possibilities becomes a problem for the nervous system.

There are additional components involved in defining the degrees of freedom. Each muscle has to be controlled. Further, each motor unit within the muscle is controlled. Given that there are different types of motor units, something must provide the proper selection of each type. The number of items a controlling system has to manage exponentially expands to mind-boggling proportions. Some solutions were presented earlier in the chapter when the size principle of motor unit activation was described. Selection according to the size principle would decrease some of the tremendous demands for activating specific motor units. Also, the existence of pattern generators would greatly reduce the degrees of freedom that would burden an executive controller.

Bernstein (1967), a Russian physiologist, was probably the first to address the problem of degrees of freedom. He defined three major sources of variability that are conditioned by the context in which they occur. The first is the variability that results from anatomical factors. For example, the pectoralis major muscle will either flex or extend the shoulder, depending upon the position of the arm in relation to the trunk in horizontal adduction. The muscle, therefore, changes its role based on the biomechanical function of its angle of pull.

The second source of variability is mechanical. Depending upon the condition of the limb, a given amount of muscular contraction of a specific muscle will have different movement consequences. This means that there are many nonmuscular forces at work, such as gravity and changes in moments, that determine the context of the movement. The relationship between the state of contraction of a muscle and the movement consequence is variable. The result depends upon the context in which the muscle is activated and the relationship between one link and another. When one link is controlled, the others necessarily change.

The third source of context variability is physiological variability. The supraspinal or "higher" mechanisms do not dominate the spinal ones. The interneurons in the spinal cord change the descending information, not just relay it. This concept is similar to Brooks's statement that the command hierarchy should not be pictured as a rigid vertical pipeline from cortex to muscle.

Bernstein implied that the highly skilled athlete discovered ways of reducing the degrees of freedom involved in the movement under consideration. When one is just beginning to learn a skill, the first approach is to eliminate some of the degrees of freedom by making the body relatively rigid. As improvement occurs some of the degrees of freedom are released. As skill increases, the developing child learns to work with the reactive forces and releases a ban on the degrees of freedom. When a batter swings at a ball and the hips rotate, a certain rotation in the upper part of the body will occur (Fig. 11-31). The batter can exploit the reactive forces to regulate rotational degrees of freedom and does not actually have to control the entire trunk through every part of the movement. The process of acquiring skill primarily involves two processes. One is finding ways of controlling the degrees of freedom. The other is to make use of the forces provided by the context in which they occur (Turvey and co-workers; see Kelso, 1982).

The fundamental problem is how to regulate systematically the many degrees of freedom of the body within a wide variety of contexts. A further goal is to involve an intelligent executive system as little as possible. Bernstein suggested that this could at least in part be solved by what is termed a muscle linkage or coordinative structure (functional synergy). A coordinative structure consists of a group of muscles constrained to act as a single functional unit. These muscles often span several joints. Thus, when performing a task such as aiming a gun, the joints are linked through the

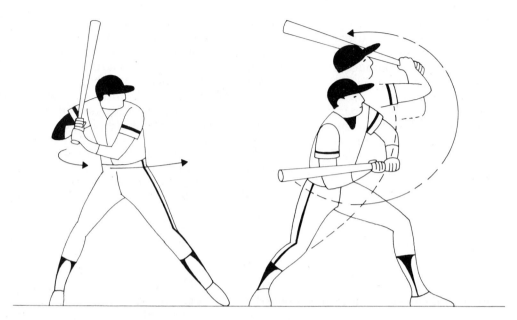

Figure 11-31. When hitting a baseball, the player's shoulders follow the movements imparted by the hips and pelvis.

muscles and act together. When the shoulder moves in one direction the wrist moves in another, which keeps the aim on target. Skill is developed by learning to activate such constraints.

A mechanical example of constrained activity occurs with an automobile. There are four wheels on the car. To simplify successful guiding of the vehicle the designers built in some very specific relationships. Mechanisms were designed to link the two front wheels together. If the steering wheel is turned to the right, both of the wheels turn to the right. Independent control over each wheel is not possible. The rear wheels are set in concert with the front wheels, with a much simpler and less flexible linkage than that between the two front wheels. Thus the multiple problems of controlling all four wheels have been simplified to one control, the steering wheel, which permits only the rotation of the steering device to provide full control over the direction of the vehicle.

In the body, when the abdominals contract to rotate the pelvis into posterior tilt, the gluteal muscles can usually be felt to contract as well. This would imply that there are functional linkages between various muscles.

A fundamental question to be asked is where do these constraints come from? Nervous system activation and muscle contraction certainly provide the ultimate expression of these linkages. Perhaps there is some relationship to programs or pattern generation. Obviously, there are multiple possibilities but only certain responses manifest themselves, depending upon the biomechanical context.

If you reach for a large and close target with your hand, you will accomplish the task faster than if you reach for a little target that is further away. If both targets are reached for at the same time, you would expect the hand aiming at the large close target to get there first. If the distance and target width ratio hold true for one hand, it would be expected that it would also hold true when two hands are used. In fact, both hands get to their respective targets at the same time. In this case, Kelso (1982) attempted to apply Fitts's law to two-handed movements. This result challenges Fitts's law under the conditions of a two-handed activity.

Some other lawful relationship has been in effect in which both of the upper extremities have been linked together, putting constraints on the activity and simplifying the control.

When independent muscles are constrained to act together, a self-regulatory system is created. When locomotion in the horse is analyzed it becomes apparent that the different phases of gait such as a walk, trot, rack, and gallop are very similar to the walking phase. The positional relationships of the joints of the limbs change very little. As the speed increases and the horse changes to a gallop, the time required to go from flexion to extension and the time from extension to landing on the hoof do not change. The only change that occurs is a decrease in the duration from landing on the hoof to the next flexion of the extremity. Therefore, the transfer time is not altered, only the support time changes (Tuller and co-workers; see Kelso, 1982) (Fig. 11-32).

The differences in the gait patterns result from what might be called nesting constraints. That is, larger constraints govern smaller linkages. For instance, there are linkages for the forelimbs and the hindlimbs. There must also be linkages over the pelvic and scapular girdles. Thus, the synchronization differences noted in the trot, rack, and gallop depend upon what girdles and what limbs are in phase with each other. When two limbs are moving, the position of the one in relation to the other is described by the term *phase*. This relationship can be expressed in degrees. For instance, when the two limbs are doing exactly the same thing they are in phase or at 0 degrees. When they are in totally opposite positions, the limbs are 180 degrees out of phase with each other.

In the trot gait pattern of the horse, the right forelimb and left hindlimb are in phase (Fig. 11-33). The right forelimb and right hindlimb are in phase in the rack gait (Fig. 11-34). In the gallop both the right and left forelimbs are in phase with each other as are both hindlimbs (Fig. 11-35). In the walking or alternate-step gait, any limb is one-half cycle out of phase with the other limb of the same girdle (Tuller and co-workers; see Kelso, 1982) (Fig. 11-36).

Another aspect of constraint is a process

called *entrainment*. Many oscillating systems become mutually synchronizing. For instance, if two clocks are hung on the same backboard they will eventually run at the same speed. The phenomenon of entrainment appears to happen in movement as well. In this case coordi-

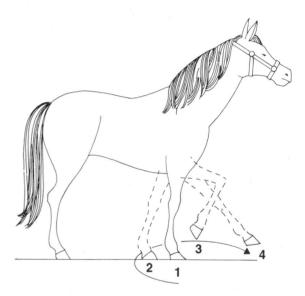

Figure 11-32. A complete step cycle of the horse proceeds from 1 to 4, in which 4 represents the support phase. As velocity increases, only the duration of the support phase is decreased. Flexion and extension phases are changed very little or not at all.

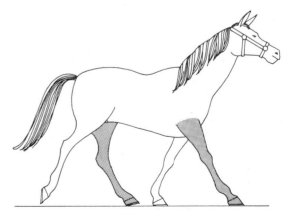

Figure 11-33. Opposite limbs of the shoulder and pelvic girdles are synchronized in the trot gait.

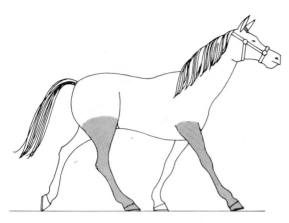

Figure 11-34. Limbs of the same side of the shoulder and pelvic girdles are synchronized in the rack gait.

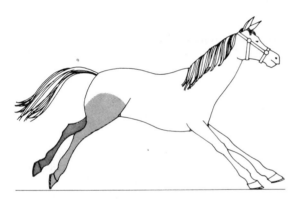

Figure 11-35. Both limbs of the same girdle are in phase with each other in the gallop.

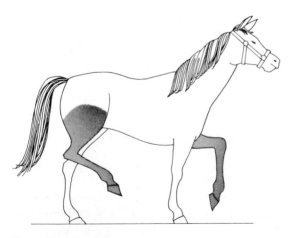

Figure 11-36. Alternate-step gait.

nation among various limbs would be maintained without the need for executive control. The nature of the entrainment, especially in living organisms, and the action of the neural components involved are all conditions awaiting clarification.

Another hypothesis that addresses constraints is the mass-spring model. According to Bernstein and others the mass-spring is a simple mechanical device in which elements of the motor apparatus are linked by equations of constraint. The muscular system can be modeled as a spring that is attached to a fixed support at one end with a mass suspended at the other. No matter what the elongation or compression of the spring, it always returns to the same length (Fig. 11-37). In such oscillatory systems no error correction is necessary be-

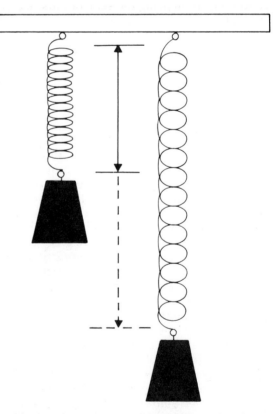

Figure 11-37. A mass-spring system. After being stretched, the spring always returns to the same position.

cause the position of the mass-spring is law-fully specified by the relation between the spring's stiffness and resting length, and the magnitude of the mass. No executive controller is necessary to direct it. Experiments by Kelso described earlier, which showed that movement is accurate even when sensory input from joints and muscles is removed, support the mass-spring model for movement in living systems.

Fel'dman (1986) further developed the mass-spring model into what he calls the equilibrium point model of motor control. He maintains that joint stiffness and position are regulated by the length-tension characteristics of the agonist and antagonist muscles. He describes a set of invariant characteristics for each muscle, which is an abstract concept that represents the viscoelastic, mechanical, and neural conditions influencing the state of muscle contraction and stiffness. The equilibrium point is where the plots of length-tension curves (selected invariant characteristics) of the agonist and antagonist intersect. In the equilibrium point hypothesis the limb position can be changed by selecting a new invariant characteristic for the contributing muscles. Muscle stiffness is regulated through the stretch reflex, which represents regulation from many avenues including descending tracts in the nervous system.

Fel'dman's hypothesis also presents a dynamic alternative to the requirement for monitoring proprioceptive information continually and comparing it with some internal memory of the movement. The mass-spring concept allows the limb to assume a specified position even without feedback. He argues that the nervous system "sets" the desired position by adjusting the length-tension relationships of the muscles involved. The "spring" will always reach a final or equilibrium point depending upon the system's dynamic parameters, such as mass and stiffness. Muscles have only to be adjusted by those parameters and the desired behavior, including the trajectory of the limb, is closely approximated by mechanical principles. No constant feedback is necessary unless the resulting equilibrium point does not match the desired end point because some unwanted mechanical disturbance occurs that is more than transient in nature.

In motor control, the multitude of sensory perceptual processes are no less demanding on the controller than are the modes of motor output or muscular expression. In terms of sensory perception, the job of dealing with all possible combinations of perceptual states is as overwhelming as coordinating all possible muscle responses.

From a biomechanical or physical perspective, sensory information may be considered to be of three types. The first relays information about the environment—exteroceptive. The second relays information about the relationship of body parts—proprioceptive. The last relays information about the environment in relation to the observer—exproprioceptive.

Actually the exteroceptive and proprioceptive work together in the exproprioceptive type. For instance, consider the optical information you receive when standing in a room. What happens if the walls suddenly move toward you? Lee (1978) discovered that you will respond by falling backward. One compensates for the perceived difference in "time-to-contact" with the wall. Hitting a tennis ball or other such athletic event is regulated by this lawful relationship between optic flow and time-to-contact. Visual exproprioceptive information may bias reflexes underlying motor activities as seen in the moving room experiments. Sound and tactile information will produce the same results. That is, there may be many different sources of information that alter the muscular responses but they are also constrained to some reference system. Apparently they all convey the information in the same "language" (Fitch and co-workers; see Kelso, 1982). There are numerous sources of information that will affect the tuning or activity of the muscle.

The human body has a posture-preserving system and a movement system. All theorists have attempted to show how these are or could be integrated within the framework of their hypotheses. The first system is involved with keeping the body upright. Superimposed on these postural movements are movements of the body or parts of the body with respect to the environment. All activities are performed in terms of these two classes of movements. Every movement acts to disturb the upright posture, so it is necessary to be sensitive to what can be done and still remain upright. One must in some way be aware that there is a region of reversibility. Within this region any movement that disturbs balance may be counteracted by another movement that restores balance. Given a system engineered to preserve upright posture, an individual must choose movements that will not go beyond this region in which the balance can be restored.

The posture-preserving system is tailored to all movements. Before a movement occurs, the rest of the body makes adjustments in anticipation of the movement. Different movements are preceded by different postural adjustments. Thus, the movement and postural systems constrain each other. This is accomplished cooperatively, not by one dominating the other. Much of skill acquisition focuses on discovering the relationship between these two systems.

Neurological Models of Motor Control

A systems or distributed model of motor control revolves around a network of neural connections that are not vertically oriented, as some of the previous hierarchical models would suggest. Rather, the entire nervous system can be considered to consist of complex systems and subsystems that interact in a flexible manner rather than in a strict hierarchial fashion. The various systems and subsystems would share information and work together to control movement.

In this approach the area or unit responsible for being the controller in motor control will vary from circumstance to circumstance. The subsystem with the most accurate information relative to the demands of the environment and the state of the individual would have the greatest effect on the resulting actions.

If the somatosensory system is correctly registering the condition of the supporting surface, it should have major influence on the motor outcome. This is especially true if some other system such as the visual system is registering inaccurate information. Some other system or subsystem will determine which information is accurate and select the appropriate response.

With a distributed control view of motor control, some of the closed-loop aspects of neural organization become apparent. In such a system feedback is part of the loop. When feedback is present a system of comparison arises that is postulated to be active in motor learning. A feedback mechanism provides knowledge of results to the motor control system. When such knowledge of results is present, the result can be compared with the intention and the next movement can be modified accordingly. This aspect of systems theory has little difference in principle from Schmidt's schema theory presented earlier.

The role of the environment is critical in the systems view of motor control. The neurological approach considers that all movements are done within the context and constraints of the environment. Patients must then be exposed to a variety of conditions and requirements when rehabilitation is attempted.

In motor learning do we have to learn all of the subsystems down to the smallest muscle twitches? At least to some extent the final coordination of different muscles is already built into the organism. What the learner does is learn particular goals at an abstract level. At lower levels some part of those goals are automatically translated into action. The human body has many more ways to move than it actually uses, because body movements are partly constrained by patterns already built into the organism. We have already suggested this is true of locomotion patterns in animals and of specific patterns of activity that result when anterior-posterior balance is disturbed.

For instance, consider the asymmetric tonic neck reflex (ATNR). The ATNR is present in young infants and is also exhibited by children with CNS dysfunction. Normal adults do not exhibit this reflex in such stereotyped fashion. However, studies have shown that under conditions of fatigue or need for greater strength, the normal adult will turn the head away from the arm producing extension movements and toward the hand that is producing flexion movements. When movements combine with the reflex activity, additional strength is conferred. This illustration is highly suggestive of the notion that much final selection of movement is based on already existing motor patterns.

This reflex pattern as well as others appear in movement patterns in sports and dances. Given certain circumstances, the effects of one reflex such as the labyrinthine reflexes may overrule the tonic neck, and the pattern is altered. Some consider that a motor program itself is a hierarchical representation of action. The action begins with determining general goals and proceeds to the selection of specific muscles. Much of the learning may take place at higher levels, which plan the general sequence of action. Final details may be woven into the movement by innate reflex patterns. Reflex and voluntary performance blend into one another gradually. They are connected by activities that may be automatic in nature but may also be modified by cognitive actions.

Self-Organizing Models of Motor Control

Theorists attempting to understand the neurologic determinations of motor control have discovered that the requirements for identifying even one pattern generator is a task almost beyond comprehension at the present time. The pattern generator, no matter how it is viewed, is a theoretic concept that may or may not be valid. This is true of all theories of motor control. Adding to the confusion is the fact that the same research results often can be interpreted in such a manner as to support or refute a given theory.

Because the greatest problem is establishing the link between the neural levels and behavioral levels in motor control, the dynamic or self-organizing theories suggest that it might be more profitable to study motor control from a completely different perspective. Perhaps it is more useful to identify principles of organization underlying motor behavior.

Physicists have known for centuries that there are basic laws governing the universe. Identifying and applying these laws has provided a much simpler base for understanding the universe and ultimately enabled us to make headway in conquering it. It is through the application of these laws that space travel and much of our scientific technology has developed.

In this systems approach it is necessary to define the total system and interactions of the parts of the system. Of basic interest is the change of motion in a system and the flow of energy within it. For example, consider a pot of water. Just sitting on the stove it would contain a quiet, smooth volume of consistent, even fluid. If heat is added, the water boils and is no longer quiet. The relationship of the parts or molecules to one another has changed. If heat is continually applied, the water turns to steam. Now the parts are again in a different relationship. There is no mechanism in the pot of water that made an executive decision to start boiling. It simply followed basic laws of physics. Therefore, there may be basic laws that govern living systems and result in the spontaneous self-organization of parts into different relationships.

The question arises whether there are laws or principles that transcend the biological properties of the system and will help us to understand the complex patterns of movement. Some theorists suggest that principles of self-organization can be discovered, which do not limit us to the anatomy or physiology of the organism. If so, it might be expected that those principles would be applicable to such diverse biological organisms as the centipede, cockroach, cat, horse, and human.

In the early 1900s some extraordinary experiments were conceived and implemented by von Holst. Working with a centipede, he systematically removed pairs of legs until six legs (three pairs) remained. The animal immediately assumed the gait of a six-legged animal. If another pair was removed, the animal demonstrated a quadruped gait. Thus, the original gait in which each leg was one seventh out of phase with every other leg completely changed to a new organization.

Research on animals and human infants has been done with a split-belt treadmill. On such a treadmill each belt can be run independently. When locomotion is occurring and the belts are made to run at different speeds, complex interlimb patterns emerge. Infants shortened the stance on the slow belt and increased the stance on the fast belt to maintain regularly alternating steps (Thelen and co-workers, 1987). This was an instantaneous change in the pattern of activity to meet demands resulting from changes in the environment.

Both the centipede experiments and the split-treadmill experiments cast doubt on the presence of central pattern generators for locomotion. It does not seem reasonable that the centipede has hardwired programs available just in case it loses certain pairs of legs. The same conclusion is reached about walking on split treadmill. Such activity would not be expected for any species. These experiments suggest there must be more all-encompassing principles or laws that govern, or at least play a crucial role in governing, the activity of living organisms.

Other examples of instantaneous changes in patterns of activity were encountered earlier in this section about the different gaits found in horses. Similar studies on humans suggest that when certain parameters are changed the pattern of activity changes. For instance, if the wrists are alternately flexed and extended, they may do so either in phase or out of phase. That is, both may flex and both extend or one may flex while the other extends (Fig. 11-38). When a parameter change is imposed, such as requiring an increased frequency of movement, subjects shift to an in-phase pattern. An out-of-phase pattern cannot be sustained (Kelso and Scholz, 1985). Horses walk until the speed increases to the point where the gait is no longer energy efficient and the gait pattern changes. The frequency of an activity may determine the pattern that is used. The principle may be one of energy efficiency or conservation of energy.

When walking, for example, a lot of movements happen just by momentum. Elastic energy is stored in the muscles and the tendons through stretch and potential energy is changed to kinetic energy as movement takes place. Perhaps some elaborate program is not necessary to produce a gait sequence. Studies of horses show that there is a specific gait that is most energy efficient for a particular speed or range of speeds. The horse will walk until a certain speed is reached, and then the gait pattern is changed. The pattern will persist at a higher speed until it is more energy efficient to change the organization of movement and switch to a trot.

Perhaps rather than elaborate neural switching of programs, the system reorganizes itself when the energy requirements reach a certain level. Just as with the pot of water, there is a reorganization of the system that is going to be more efficient. Try walking fast as opposed to jogging. You will discover how

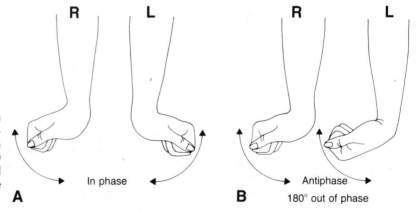

Figure 11-38. *(A)* When both the left and right wrists are extending or flexing, the pattern is considered to be in phase. *(B)* When one wrist is flexing and the other is extending, they are in an out-of-phase pattern.

much more difficult and energy consuming it is to maintain the speed of a fast walk than to change to a jog.

Studies covering the past 50 years on a wide variety of animals such as the cockroach, cat, dog, and stick insects have shown some striking results. Studies indicate that the initiation of swing phase in gait depends upon reflexes that appear to be identical in all the species studied. Swing phase is initiated when the support leg is unloaded. Some pathway signals the decrease in load at the end of stance, which triggers the initiation of swing on the opposite limb.

A second mechanism is the position of the hip joint at the transition point, which causes a switch from stance to swing. Movements in 7-month-old infants who performed little or no stepping patterns were studied by supporting them over a treadmill. The infants immediately produced alternating stepping movements that closely resembled mature walking. It is possible that providing the full extension stretch to the stance leg together with unloading the ankle and producing a weight shift supplies the passive energy required to overcome gravity and swing the leg forward (Thelen, 1986). Past concepts that maturation of the executive control system is required to allow stepping in a developing child do not appear to be valid. Certainly the underlying mechanisms have not "disappeared" with the failure to elicit further the automatic stepping of the newborn.

If full extension and limb unloading are important events in triggering swing phase, consider this: How many stroke patients or patients with cerebral palsy ever achieve full hip extension and appropriate unloading of the limb during gait? It may be that these studies allow us to begin to identify some of the critical factors that cause the system to reorganize itself. If the patient can be helped to establish that critical factor, perhaps that human organism can spontaneously reorganize itself.

Many of the biomechanical principles or observations made about motor control such as muscle constraints, mass-spring models, and limit cycle oscillators contribute to self-organizing models of motor control. These factors de-

scribe lawful relationships and behaviors concerning some aspects of living systems. In this approach the environment becomes a crucial element in the elaboration of movement and may play a role as important as that of the nervous system.

The task to be addressed by the dynamic systems or self-organizing theorists is to identify the principles at work that may govern biological movement. At this juncture it is apparent that altering the speed, velocity, or frequency of an activity would be important in clinical evaluation and treatment.

The question arises as to just what happens in the case of a stroke victim. If the system self organizes, what organizational change occurs that results in the readily identifiable gait and posturing of the patient with such a neurologic deficit? The first understanding that must occur is to recognize that the dynamic systems theorists are not denying that the nervous system has a role in movement. It is viewed, rather, that areas of the nervous system participate or produce the self-organizing behavior and that strict neural circuits that are destined to become pattern generators and so forth may not exist. Some studies with monkeys, for instance, have shown that an area of the sensory cortex that is activated upon stimulation of the hand is no longer responsive when nerves carrying afferent input are removed from the hand. The area reorganizes itself to participate in other sensory activities. If the afferentation is restored the cortex reorganizes itself, and once again that area responds to hand stimulation. The brain itself may be a self-organizing system that is even more dynamic than we suspected.

SUMMARY OF MOTOR CONTROL THEORIES

From this relatively short exploration it is apparent that much is yet to be discovered before a full understanding of motor control is possible. Only the major or most familiar theories have been presented here. There are numerous other aspects or approaches to motor control that have not been mentioned. Some theorists of motor control have approached it by attempting to identify the areas or specific structures of the brain that appear to be responsible for variations in movement. Brooks (1986) probably best represents the neurophysiologist who can integrate the anatomy and physiology of the brain into a story of movement. Much of the work on integrated systems has been postulated by Nashner (1979) and colleagues.

Other theorists have approached the problem of motor control from the perspective of identifying general laws and principles that may govern movement. They suspect that biologic systems are governed by natural laws just as there are lawful relationships governing the universe. Bernstein (1967) and Feldman (1986) have contributed biomechanical models to a dynamic self-organizing systems approach to movement, which is probably best explained by Kelso and Scholz (1985) and their colleagues.

Information presented from these theorists leads us to expect that more of these laws and principles will be discovered. The knowledge of such laws and principles will provide guidance for understanding movement deficits and developing rehabilitation procedures for intervention. These principles may ultimately prove to be the most valuable to the practicing clinician because they may provide the clearest suggestions about which parameters may be altered for rehabilitation. In the clinic, it is quite possible to vary such parameters as velocity, speed, and frequency. Identification of prerequisite acts, such as full hip extension for the triggering of swing phase in gait, will provide eloquent guidance as to the choice of activities within a rehabilitation program.

Even if we do come to know exactly what part of the brain contains a program (if programs exist), this knowledge in and of itself may not likely be very helpful in selecting treatment protocols in physical therapy. The same is not true for those in medicine who may discover drug or surgical treatments for such disorders. Of course, careful clinical observation of the patterns of movement that result may give us clues about the normal and abnormal nature of such a pattern and guide us to find methods of altering undesirable patterns.

The mechanical issues of movement have been ignored for too long. Although those theories do not really explain what the CNS is doing, it may not be critical to understanding movement or correcting movement disorders. Perhaps no one area must be in control. Possibly all of the parts of the system are equally important in causing a reorganization. In terms of abnormal motor control, perhaps when any part is atypical the entire system is going to reorganize itself around that.

From a nervous system perspective, you can be fairly certain that influences can be made on the anterior horn cells. I am pretty sure I can influence the anterior horn cells. But the more synapses and reflexes and loops and structures that can be identified and might be influenced, the less confident one becomes about what is actually being manipulated or changed. But in some sense the concept of self-organizing systems and biomechanical principles provides better access to treatment. It is very possible, for instance, to observe and change the amount of hip extension a child has.

It is an exciting and frustrating time to be involved in clinical physical therapy because the complete understanding of motor control is still ahead. Even further in the future is the understanding of abnormal motor control. The exact approach to take with a patient eludes us, but many new thoughts, experiments, and theories are providing new insights into treatment and evaluation. Clinical application necessarily lags behind the discovery of facts, laws, and principles; however, by keeping up to date and approaching the problems with flexibility, more appropriate clinical applications will be made.

TONE

The term *tone* has been used in physical therapy to refer to a variety of conditions or states. In fact, it conveys a whole constellation of data and the information is reinterpreted by the receiver in terms of the perceptions he has developed to accommodate such concepts. As such, it is of little value as a descriptive term. The purposes of this section are to examine the variety of descriptions for the term muscle tone; explore the nature of the conditions that have fostered such descriptions; and suggest alternatives in both understanding the underlying mechanisms of dysfunction and the terminology used to describe them.

Attempts to define clearly or measure quantitatively muscle tone have met with little success. In various contexts muscle tone has been described as (1) normal tissue firmness; (2) tension in resting muscles; (3) the response to passive stretch; (4) variations in the ability of the muscle to fully elongate; and (5) the state of muscle activity. The latter includes the notion that motor neuron activity to the muscle may be either too high (hypertonicity) or too low (hypotonicity). None of these descriptions have led to clear objective criteria for measurement or even categorization of what might be observed.

Physical therapists who use "tone" to describe tissue firmness mean how the muscle feels to the touch. The normal muscle has a particular turgor or firmness to it when palpated. Atrophied or diseased muscle has a different "feel." The muscle may feel pasty, or stringy, or soft and boggy. All of these adjectives notwithstanding, no objective, reliable way to measure this feel has been developed. The descriptive terms, on the other hand, convey a multitude of meanings and implications dependent upon the bias and field of experience of the reader or listener.

MECHANICAL ASPECTS OF TONE

Those who most often use the term muscle "tone" to refer to how the muscle looks or feels are usually orthopedically oriented or are referring to patients who have orthopedic conditions. Attempts at objective evaluation have included such observations as girth measures. There are two problems with this method of assessment. First, it is difficult to take a girth measurement of a single muscle. For instance, a measurement of the upper arm usually includes biceps, triceps, and other muscles depending upon which portion of the arm is measured. Nonetheless, if one side is measured and compared to the other side of the same individual, some conclusions can be drawn about the atrophic or hypertrophic state of the muscle or muscles. Secondly, one assumption behind this method of assessment is that the larger the muscle, the more powerful that muscle may be. However, no studies have been done showing that a girth measure is correlated with any kind of firmness measure or provides any proven physiologic or functional measure. Thus, there has been no success in either objectively measuring this meaning of tone, or of accurately predicting function based upon its assessment.

No studies have been reported correlating histopathologic changes with changes in the "feel" of muscle. Therefore, the elements that make up this tissue firmness are not always agreed upon. Nervous input undoubtedly affects the health and state of muscle tissue and, therefore, how it feels. However, even a denervated muscle does not droop and fall off the bone, and changes in texture are slow and progressive as degeneration proceeds. In addition to innervation states and dynamic changes in actomyosin attraction, the sarcoplasm and connective tissue elements provide additional mechanical support, structure, and their own viscoelastic properties to the look, feel, and function of the muscle.

Tardieu and colleagues (1982a) coined the term "hypoextensibility" to refer to the resistance to passive stretch and loss of elongation in a noncontracting muscle that results from the loss of sarcomeres. They showed that this lack of range is related to both loss of sarcomeres in series and to loss of extensibility of the parallel elastic elements. Their studies demonstrate a correlation between these structural changes and loss of elongation of muscle. The changes in the connective tissue also provide a basis for explaining some changes in the texture of these adaptively shortened muscles. No studies have been done, however, to determine whether those logically anticipated changes in texture can in fact be reliably detected.

Muscle tone has also been described as the tension in resting muscles. It was at one time believed that tension in resting muscle resulted from some state of active contraction. However, electromyographic examination shows that if a resting muscle is supported and relaxed, it does not generate action potentials. Thus, the resting texture of muscle cannot be the result of some minimal state of active contraction.

Evidence suggests that some contractions do take place in the absence of an action potential. Such a contraction would likely be chemically based and not dependent upon ionic charges. Older research by Gasser (1930) showed a type of shortening or tension development characterized by a mechanical change that did not produce a wave-like electrical response and was not propagated. The resistance to elongation that results has sometimes been called a physiologic contracture. This term is used to differentiate it from a myostatic contracture, in which lack of elongation results from the loss of sarcomeres, or a contracture resulting from changes in the soft tissue such as adhesions or connective tissue scarring.

Physiologic contractures without action potentials are not the result of any injury to the contractile mechanism. Certain states of fatigue might cause such contracture. Clinical situations in which physiologic contracture exists would clearly affect muscle texture, its ability to elongate fully, and its resistance to passive motion, all of which have been described as "changes in tone."

Cummings (1984) designed an experiment to investigate which tissues limit normal joint range at the elbow. The range of joint motion in the normal relaxed person could be limited by ligaments, capsule, muscle, or skin. Extension of the elbow joint approaches a "close-pack" position of the joint, which indicates that the ligaments and joint capsule should limit extension. Elbow extension in the relaxed subject, as determined by EMG biofeedback, was compared with the extension available when the subject was paralyzed by a myoneural blocking agent. The clearly significant results show that additional range is available when muscles are totally inactivated. This study not only reveals that muscle rather than ligament or capsule is the limiting factor in elbow extension in normal persons, it also shows that, even when the muscle is completely voluntarily relaxed, more muscle elongation is available.

No action potentials were elicited during the phase in which relaxation was taking place to account for the failure to achieve full elongation. It could be hypothesized that the lack of full elongation may have resulted from low levels of the same phenomena as occurs in physiologic contracture. Simple observations of paralyzed patients confirm such a conclusion and show that joints crossed by paralyzed muscles allow a much greater range than normal.

This phenomenon of physiologic contracture or a residual state of contraction that does not involve the generation of action potentials might be referred to as "residual stiffness." A possible mechanism by which this type or state of contraction occurs is the availability of adenosine triphosphate (ATP) during regular active muscle contraction. When the ATP is used up, the muscle remains in a contracted state until new ATP is available. The muscle rigidity seen in rigor mortis, for instance, relates to this chemical condition. Thus, in a state in which the muscle is relatively relaxed, there may be residual cross-bridging of actin and myosin filaments resulting in some form of muscle contraction. This cross-bridging may be physically broken by muscle elongation, or changed by a new active contraction.

This physiologic contracture may change with the gradual availability of new ATP, which causes separation of the cross-bridges. A muscle may show greater elongation following an active contraction. The postcontraction relaxation of a muscle probably relates to the infusion of new ATP from the latest contraction. The efficacy of the clinical technique of "contract-relax" may be explained on this basis. It is a common experience for therapists who use the hold-relax and contract-relax techniques to observe the changes in muscle stiffness. When these techniques are applied to any muscle at virtually any joint it is clear that marked, transient increases in muscle length occur.

Additionally, factors affecting the contractile state of smooth muscle such as local tissue factors or circulating hormones may also have an effect on skeletal muscle. Some local tissue factors that may affect the contractile state of muscle are lack of oxygen, the presence of lactic acid, increased potassium ions, and diminished calcium ions.

Other conditions under which muscle may be contracting, either in association with action potentials or without them, include "trigger points," "spasms," "cramps," and muscle "splinting." Trigger points, which can be palpated as a localized lump or thickening in a muscle, suggest that that portion of the muscle is contracting. Researchers and clinicians have noted that the range of motion decreases in the presence of trigger points. However, when electrodes are inserted into the trigger point prolonged insertional activity is present but no action potentials are recorded on EMG. In contrast, cramps usually produce considerable active EMG activity. Muscle spasm is another term that suggests the muscle is in some state of contraction. Although in most cases a spasm is clearly an active contraction, the term is widely used as a clinical descriptor without strict criteria. It is possible that either the active type of contraction, which produces action potentials, or the residual stiffness type of contraction could be present depending upon the conditions. Muscle splinting or guarding is often used synonymously with spasm and probably involves both types of contraction as well.

In summary, the mechanical aspects of muscle tone include the various mechanisms that contribute to the look and feel of a muscle. The viscoelastic properties of the muscle cell are derived from the sarcoplasm and the parallel elastic components. The texture of the muscle can be influenced by pathologic states such as denervation. Variations in the ability of the muscle to elongate fully might result from myostatic contracture in which the muscle is shortened from loss of sarcomeres or physiologic contracture (residual stiffness). These also will influence the texture of the muscle. Regardless of the mechanism involved, reliable measures do not exist for most of the problems encountered. When evaluating and communicating the condition of a muscle or muscle group, it should be most effective to report that a muscle has a normal texture and appearance rather than remark on the tone of the muscle. Abnormalities in texture or appearance could simply be described as fully as possible. Techniques do exist in the literature (Tardieu and co-workers, 1982a) for reliable measures of extensibility.

HYPERTONIA AND TYPES OF SPASTICITY

Still another description of "tone" relates to the resistance offered by muscles to either brief or continuous stretch. In deeply relaxed normal subjects, resistance to joint displacement is moderate at all speeds of movement. This moderate resistance has been postulated to be solely dependent upon the viscoelastic properties of the muscle and the joint. Sahrmann and Norton (1977), however, have shown that active EMG potentials are recorded during passive movement during both lengthening and shortening phases.

The reaction to stretch becomes stronger when stretch reflexes are reinforced, such as when the subject is concentrating or performing a Jendrassik's maneuver. In contrast, highly tense and nervous subjects cannot suppress the stretch reflexes. The arousal system influences the state of muscle activity through the descending supraspinal systems. Such descending input has significant control over the activity of the anterior horn motor neurons. Thus, tense individuals may already have such a low threshold to activity that responses from the stretch receptors produce motor neuron activation and result in obvious muscle contraction. Low-keyed individuals with a higher spinal level threshold may not respond to stretch reflex activity with noticeable muscle contraction.

Joint rotation that is more prolonged than a tendon tap produces a sustained muscle stretch. The resulting stretch reflex is called a *tonic stretch reflex* and consists of two parts. The initial "phasic" part is relatively intense. The "tonic" component is sustained but less powerful. The tonic stretch reflex is likely to be modulated by supraspinal influences because it would involve multisynaptic pathways. The tendon jerk or phasic stretch reflex is monosynaptic in nature; therefore, it is not subject to other influences. The motor neuron is subject to descending influences, and if the neuron is in an already heightened state, as when the subject is concentrating or performing a Jendrassik's maneuver, the monosynaptic responses may be exaggerated.

Neurologic patients are often classified by physical therapists as having normal or abnormal tone. The abnormal characteristics are most often referred to as *hypertonicity* or *hypotonicity*. Those patients with increased tone, or hypertonicity, might be described as stiff because the clinician feels resistance to passive movement of the limbs. The patient may also show various posturing of the extremities such as holding the upper extremity in shoulder, elbow, and wrist flexion with fisting of the hand when making an effort to move (Fig. 11-39). Physical therapists have identified such posturing as being characteristic of hypertonia. Under such circumstances, when the term hypertonicity is used it indicates that the patient has spasticity.

HYPOTONIA

Other clinical entities have been described using the term *hypotonia* to mean less than adequate muscle contractions. Hypotonia would be defined physiologically in those cases as a state of decreased motor neuron excitability. Patients such as those with Down syndrome are often described as being hypotonic. They experience developmental delays in the acquisition of motor control. There is joint hypermobility, persistence of primitive reflexes, and no exaggerated response to passive stretch.

Shumway-Cook and Woollacott (1985) have shown, however, that the motor neuron pool excitation and stretch reflex mechanisms in children with Down syndrome are no different from those in the normal child. The children showed delayed onset of muscular con-

tractions when their balance was disturbed by perturbations. The children could not adapt responses to changing forms of perturbation. The deficits appear to be within higher-level postural mechanisms rather than hypotonia.

Davis and Sinning (1987) found that mentally handicapped subjects, including those with Down syndrome, produce significantly less torque with an isometric muscle contraction. Thus, what separated the normal from the mentally handicapped subjects was the degree to which they could voluntarily increase the level of stiffness in a muscle rather than the resting level of stiffness. It was postulated that some central deficiency is responsible for the deficit.

Thus, the child with Down syndrome does not have hypotonia as physiologically defined, and treatment of the hypotonia in those patients may be less than effective. Drugs and therapeutic procedures designed to alter the

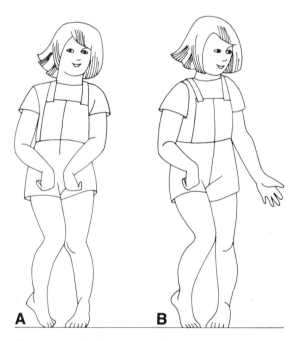

Figure 11-39. Typical muscle patterns or "posturing" in children with cerebral palsy: *(A)* spastic quadriplegic; *(B)* hemiplegic.

muscle tone show little functional gain in terms of acquiring developmental skills.

Cerebellar lesions have been postulated to result in hypotonia. In experimental cerebellar lesions, the hypotonia produced results from decreased gamma bias. It is not likely that this mechanism works in humans. The hypotonia in cerebellar lesions may result from the dysfunction, or loss, of motor programs. With program dysfunction there may be deficient premovement tensing of muscles. Cooke (1980) has shown that simple movements can be modeled by plotting the limb velocity and amplitude of the movement. A linear relationship exists, which results in a line with a given slope when plotted (Fig. 11-40). Any change in the resting stiffness of the muscle will alter the slope of the line (Fig. 11-41). When the amplitude and velocity of the movement is plotted for patients with cerebellar disease, there is a decrease in the slope of the line. Thus, it may

be concluded that patients with cerebellar disease have a resting stiffness that is lower than normal, which may explain the presence of hypotonia. Cooke also suggests that the hypermetria exhibited by cerebellar patients may be explained by a decrease in resting stiffness. If the movement is learned in terms of the final stiffness level, getting to such a level when starting at a lower than usual level will result in an increase in the amplitude of the movement. As a result, the limb overshoots the target, producing hypermetria.

MECHANISMS IN SPASTICITY

A clear definition of spasticity eludes us despite the fact that therapists can invariably recognize its various states. Perhaps more useful than a specific definition is a list that characterizes some of the motor signs of spasticity, including active resistance or involuntary con-

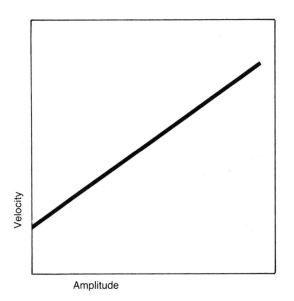

Figure 11-40. A line representing the relationship between velocity and amplitude in modeling a movement. (Modified and reprinted with permission from Cooke JD: The organization of simple, skilled movements. In Stelmach GE, Requin J (eds): Tutorials in Motor Behavior. Amsterdam, North Holland Publishing, 1980)

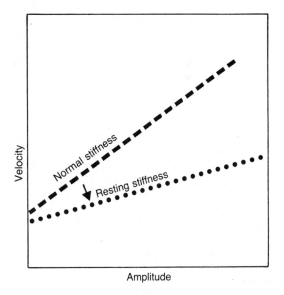

Figure 11-41. Two different slopes result when velocity and amplitude are plotted from different levels of resting stiffness. (Modified and reprinted with permission from Cooke JD: The organization of simple, skilled movements. In Stelmach GE, Requin J (eds): Tutorials in Motor Behavior. Amsterdam, North Holland Publishing, 1980)

traction in response to passive stretch, clonus, spread of contraction to include synergists, and a lower threshold of the stretch reflex. Alterations in the stretch reflexes do occur in disorders of tone; however, the deficit is not in the stretch reflex system itself, as will be discussed shortly.

The characteristics of spasticity differ depending upon the area of the nervous system involved. For instance, spinal spasticity follows transection of the spinal cord. The tendon reflexes are exaggerated and can become oscillatory by re-excitation, which produces clonus. Flexor spasms or contractions are common in spinal spasticity. The descending modulation from the reticular and vestibular systems is removed in spinal lesions, which leads to exaggerated flexor facilitation and extensor inhibition when the flexor reflex afferents are stimulated. These changes trigger the clasp-knife phenomenon, in which stretched extensors collapse at a certain point in the stretch.

The tonic vibration reflex may be clinically useful in evaluating some patients with spasticity. This reflex is elicited by placing a vibrator firmly into the muscle belly. In most normal persons, a slowly building tonic muscle contraction will occur in response to the vibration. The contraction will be sustained as long as the vibration is present. This reflex involves the stretch reflex system, but is not solely monosynaptic in nature and requires support from higher centers. Obviously, no tonic vibration reflex should be elicited if the spinal cord is completely transected, cutting off higher center support. However, the tonic vibration reflex may be present if the lesion is incomplete. The muscle contraction begins abruptly and the spastic patient cannot enhance or suppress the reflex voluntarily, as can the normal person.

Cerebral spasticity is caused by lesions above the brain stem. This condition exhibits less manifestation of the clasp-knife reflex and fewer flexion spasms. In this situation the dorsal lateral reticulospinal tract is uninterrupted and functions normally because it is not under direct cortical control. In contrast, the lateral vestibulospinal tract is disinhibited, which favors physiologic extension. Therefore, in the human hemiplegic the effects are most severe in leg extensors and arm flexors. The tonic vibration reflex is usually suppressed in patients with cerebral lesions.

Rigidity in the patient with Parkinson's disease is characterized by hypertonia that is not dependent on the velocity of muscle stretch. The rigidity is of a "cog-wheel" or "lead pipe" variety and is distributed mostly in the flexors of the upper and lower extremities. The lesion involves the basal ganglia, and animal studies show that the gains of many long-loop responses are regulated by the basal ganglia. Tonic reflexes are elevated. Phasic stretch reflexes are normal, but tonic reflexes have a lower threshold. Tonic vibration reflexes may be hyperactive.

Research in the field of neurobiology has failed to tell us just what spasticity is in humans. However, we have some ideas as to what it is *not*. An ever increasing body of research results refutes our old view that spasticity is the result of a hyperactive fusimotor system with resultant hypersensitivity of the muscle spindle afferents. Stretch reflexes may be exaggerated in spasticity, but the mechanism for such activity is most likely the lack of central modulation. It is not from a hypersensitive or "biased" muscle spindle. Crutchfield and Barnes (1984) have presented an extensive review of these mechanisms.

The biggest problem with effectively evaluating persons who have motor deficits has been to demonstrate a connection between what can be evaluated and the actual sensorimotor deficit within the CNS. For example, if a patient shows an increased resistance to elongating a muscle group, we decide the patient has spasticity. The same conclusion is reached if the patient demonstrates clonus. Our assumption usually is that hypertonus interferes with the patient's ability to produce normal movement. However, it has been noted that when the perceived excessive activity in the muscle has been decreased through handling or drugs, the movements produced have changed relatively little.

Hughlings Jackson long ago categorized the symptoms of neurologic dysfunction into two groups: negative symptoms and positive symptoms. The negative symptoms are by definition the deficits in the patient. Such deficits would include weakness or lack of mobility. The positive symptoms were defined as release phenomena. Spasticity and abnormal reflexes and possibly stereotypic movement synergies would be positive symptoms. It is postulated that the two types of signs result from different mechanisms. The presence of increased resistance to passive stretch cannot be given a causal relationship to the patient's weakness.

Sarhmann and Norton (1977) completed a classic research project that proved the movement dysfunction in patients with upper motor neuron lesions was not the result of increased antagonistic stretch reflexes. Most interestingly, they showed that the inability of a patient with spastic hemiplegia to flex and extend the elbow joint rapidly could be related to three abnormalities.

The first abnormality was that the onset latencies of muscle activity were delayed. This observation is in agreement with the observation that there is delayed onset of muscle activation during gait and in defective preparatory postural sets in hemiplegics.

The second abnormality noted was that the muscle contraction was of insufficient magnitude for a movement. We have come to believe that spastic contractions are actually hyperactive or excessively strong. Failure to generate an adequate tension may be considered to be a disorder of gain. The hypertonus or what is perceived as excessive muscle activity may be the result of inadequate gain, and the patient recruits everything possible to help with the movement. In effect, it is possible that hypertonus is the effect of movement dysfunction rather than the cause of it.

The third abnormality noted was that muscles failed to "shut-off" at the appropriate time. In normal persons, the biceps muscles ceased activity long before the triceps muscles came in to reverse the motion at the elbow. In hemiplegic patients, rapidly extending the elbow was made difficult by inappropriate but not excessive activity in the elbow flexors. This becomes a state of excessive co-contraction, which inter-

feres with the rapid activation and suppression of antagonists that occurs in the normal person. Figures 11-42 and 11-43 show the muscle patterns in a normal person and a hemiparetic person.

Spasticity is often defined as a velocity-dependent resistance to high-velocity passive stretch. This passive stretch is the quick stretch test that physicians do to patients, and conclude that the patient has increased tone. This response bears no resemblance to what happens when someone attempts a voluntary movement that results in abnormal movements. The response of a spastic muscle to stretch is not the same during active motion as during passive motion. The disorders may in fact be due to abnormalities in programming

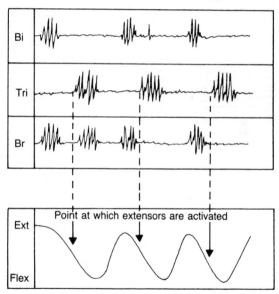

Normal isotonic elbow flexion and extension performed as rapidly as possible

Figure 11-42. EMG tracings of three elbow muscles during normal isotonic elbow flexion and extension performed as rapidly as possible. Note that the flexors cease to be active and the extensors become active before the peak of flexion is achieved. (Modified and reprinted with permission from Sahrmann SA, Norton BJ: The relationship of voluntary movement to spasticity in the upper motor neuron syndrome. Ann Neurol 2:460, 1977)

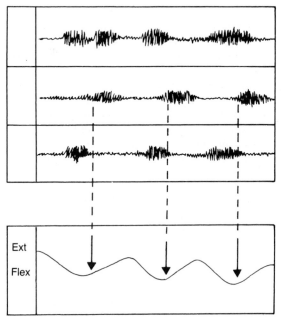

Isotonic elbow flexion and extension performed as rapidly as possible by a hemiparetic patient

Figure 11-43. EMG tracings of a hemiparetic patient while performing isotonic elbow flexion and extension as rapidly as possible. Note that (1) the triceps are activated later at the beginning of extension; (2) the biceps are active during the extension phase; and (3) the movements are slower and smaller than in the normal person. (Modified and reprinted with permission from Sahrmann SA, Norton BJ: The relationship of voluntary movement to spasticity in the upper motor neuron syndrome. Ann Neurol 2:460, 1977)

and regulating the motor neuron pool. Motor control disturbances may result from disorders of reciprocal innervation, which will increase the resistance to voluntary movement.

The symptoms and complaints of the patient with an upper motor neuron lesion are generally more important than hypertonia. Movement may be significantly restrained by co-contraction or by a dyssynergic pattern of muscle contraction. Some patients have exaggerated or spontaneous involuntary flexor spasms. Paresis or loss of dexterity are important aspects of the patient's inability to function (Davidoff, 1984). Davidoff suggests that just as

there are several forms of spasticity depending on the location of the lesion and the extent of the damage to the central nervous system, there is no reason to expect that all patients will have the same pathophysiologic abnormality or respond equally to therapeutic agents.

Some of the pathophysiologic alterations found in the presence of spasticity include alteration in the contol of neurotransmitter release affecting the efficacy of presynaptic inhibition. Other changes include sprouting of unaffected axons, denervation hypersensitivity, transsynaptic degeneration, and activation of normally ineffective synapses. Any of these alterations may contribute to plastic changes that could modify existing circuits and pathways. These changes develop over time with some occurring within hours or days of the insult and others over weeks and months. The fact that such plasticity exists suggests avenues by which both short-term and long-term effects may be produced through therapeutic intervention.

A research project completed over 35 years ago by Hirschberg and Nathanson (1952) showed that abnormalities in the gait cycle of patients with spastic hemiplegia were due to late onset of contractions, weak contractions, and inappropriate contractions. When an obturator neurectomy was performed on the innervation to the adductor muscles, the EMG activity was markedly reduced, as might be expected. However, none of the other muscle patterns changed, which indicates that removal of the "tonus" from one muscle does not alter others. Most important, strikingly similar findings of muscle patterns were found in the nonparetic extremity. The marked decrease in muscle activity in the paretic limb was contrasted with marked increase in amplitude of muscle activity in the nonparetic limb. Undoubtedly this imbalance was in part the result of requiring the nonparetic limb to do most of the work.

These researchers also showed that the use of braces and canes, and the application of resistive exercises did not alter the pattern of muscle activity, although in some instances functional improvement was shown. Most likely, such improvement was the result of mechanical support provided by such devices, or perhaps a greater control over the amount of effort expended in the activity.

In a recent research project patients with hemiplegia were asked to produce a maximal voluntary contraction of two wrist muscles, and the amplitudes of the motor unit potentials were recorded by EMG (Nutter and co-workers, 1987). The amplitudes of the maximal voluntary recruitment were significantly greater in normal control subjects than in either the paretic or nonparetic sides of the hemiplegic subjects. This difference was postulated to result from reduced numbers of superimposed action potentials, thus a lack in recruitment in general, as well as difficulty in recruiting large, high-threshold motor units. This research provides further insight into the weak and slow movements experienced by spastic patients.

Tardieu and colleagues (1982b) studied the hypoextensibility in children with different types of cerebral palsy who had increased resistance in the triceps surae muscles when they were not contracting. Full relaxation and the greatest muscle length of the triceps surae muscles was obtained by abolishing the ankle reflex through ischemia. Subjects were put into one of two groups depending on whether they had what was described as persistent plantarflexor hyperactivity resulting in an imbalance between the triceps surae muscles and the dorsiflexors producing actual muscle shortening. The other group consisted of children who had primary defective trophic regulation in which the growth of the muscle does not keep up with the growth of the bone. The steepness of passive torque curves produced by passive dorsiflexion of the ankle were studied before and after treatment.

Children in the group with defective trophic regulation had excessive muscle shortness with a lack of sarcomeres. The condition is often associated with an abnormally long tendon. These circumstances result in resistance to passive elongation and the inability to generate maximal active contraction at full plantarflexion. Passive range of motion or immobilization from casting the ankle may only lengthen the tendon further, which will result in the inability to generate adequate tension in a physiologically useful position.

Children with imbalance in muscle activity responded to casting, although measures had to be taken to maintain the increase in passive range of motion. Surgery was also initially successful, but showed that the condition would likely recur as the muscle imbalance persists.

Nashner and co-workers (1983) examined postural movement patterns in children with spastic cerebral palsy using EMGs and a platform perturbation protocol. With the rotating platform the subject may receive an unexpected perturbation by rotating the ankles into dorsiflexion. Results from platform studies were not consistent with what might be expected from the clinical examination of the children. A common assumption among many clinicians is that passive stretch to the triceps surae muscles in patients with extensor spasticity will produce increased resistance, signifying a hyperexcitable output.

EMG analysis of postural movement patterns showed that, contrary to expectation, so-called spastic muscles were delayed in their onset and produced less force, not more, than nonspastic muscles. These studies support those by both Sahrmann and Hirshberg and confirm that the patient with neurologic deficit suffers from an inability to generate an adequate force and excessive co-contraction occurs, blocking effective movements. However, hyperactivity of stretch reflexes, is not the cause of functional disability.

Additionally, children showed a reversal in the sequence of muscles that are usually activated as the ankle synergy. Proximal musculature was activated before distal musculature. This disassociation of the synergy results in excessive excursions of the proximal joints, often mistaken for proximal instability by clinicians.

A recent communication in a newsletter (Ploeger and Yamada, 1987) indicated that some spasticity in children with cerebral palsy is being treated by dorsal rhizotomy in which the sensory nerve rootlets are cut. Of course, the expression of spasticity will be modified because incoming information, particularly the stretch reflex input, will be abolished and will no longer be an exciting factor. Naturally, the lower extremities can be easily taken through the range of motion.

However, it is interesting to note, that following rhizotomy the child presents with a stiff back and the hip fixed in flexion and the back in extension. The therapists note that the child now has very little movement and insufficient strength. Patients ambulated with a very similar gait pattern preoperatively and postoperatively. The therapy is now directed toward developing normal movement patterns as the child relearns how to move and control his body. Most likely this should have been the appropriate approach in the first place. The therapists have assumed that spasticity is causing the abnormal patterns, so therapeutic intervention has often been aimed at decreasing the spasticity. It is further stated that sufficient strength must be developed or the child will revert to "fixing" in abnormal patterns, thus suggesting that the "spastic" pattern may not be the result of spasticity.

MUSCLE TONE: SOME BETTER DESCRIPTORS

Because "tone" has come to mean how a muscle looks and feels, the state of stretch reflexes, and a whole constellation of characteristics of movement and posture, it is best to dispense with the term. It is better to describe the movement carefully so that another clinician can picture it than to call it "abnormal tone." Perhaps the best descriptor of the resistance to passive joint movement is simply to indicate the presence of spasticity.

The tension generated during active motion could be equated with muscle "stiffness." Thus, a patient could be described as having normal muscle compliance, or being too compliant or too stiff. Excessive muscle stiffness would reflect the state of co-contraction that occurs during movements attempted by those afflicted with spasticity. The terms "muscle activity" or "muscle contraction" also make good substitutes for certain meanings currently held for tone. "Inappropriate muscle activity" is a phrase signaling the actual physiologic response that occurs during movement dysfunction in the presence of cerebral insult, which is primarily one of co-contraction.

In summary, the movement dysfunction that is apparent in patients with upper motor neuron lesions may be the result of the following: inadequate recruitment of motoneurons such that the resulting movement is weak; incorrect timing of contractions, particularly those of late onset, which results in functional weakness; and the persistence of muscle contractions beyond the time they should cease, which produces an ineffective co-contraction. In addition, muscles are not activated in the appropriate order or sequence within the normal prepackaged and programmed synergies that have been identified. Also, there may be an inability to access the appropriate synergy.

Certain physical or biomechanical prerequisites may not be present, resulting in inadequate movement. An example is the failure of most patients with neurologic deficit to achieve full extension at the hip, along with unloading the ankle and appropriate weight shifts. Perhaps key movements can be facilitated that will allow the system to reorganize itself and produce more normal movement.

The most important concept to conquer is that the passive measures of spasticity (ie, the resistance to passive stretch or increased stretch reflex responses) have nothing to do with the conditions occurring when active contractions are generated. By knowing that patients who experience brain injury have specific types of deficits such as delayed onset of muscle response as opposed to "increased tone," it becomes possible to devise more appropriate evaluation procedures to assist in preparing more effective treatment programs. If it is clear that the deficit is not in the muscle spindle system itself, the response to a reflex stretch or an attempt to isolate a joint action need no longer lead us astray. The tonic vibration reflex may be a useful tool for evaluating the various characteristics of spasticity in different types of nervous system lesions.

It is most important to realize that some of the standard tests of spasticity, such as increased resistance to passive stretch and exaggerated deep tendon reflexes, represent the positive signs of upper motor neuron dysfunction. These signs have no functional or causal relationship with the weakness and movement deficits present in such patients. Treatment will not likely alter stretch reflex responses and even if it does, the change will not affect the movement dysfunction present.

Treatment programs should address the deficits identified. Many treatment tools traditionally used will not have to be altered. It is still possible, for example, to use quick stretch, vibration, or proprioceptive neuromuscular facilitation. Most importantly, they will be applied from a new perspective, with a different intermediate objective, ultimately to accomplish the same goals of improved function that this profession has always held dear.

ANNOTATED BIBLIOGRAPHY

Adams JA: Issues for a closed-loop theory of motor learning. In Stelmach GE (ed): Motor Control: Issues and Trends. New York, Academic Press, 1976

Bernstein NA: The Co-ordination and Regulation of Movements. Oxford, Pergamon Press, 1967 (A classic work that presents the foundations of several present theories or models of motor control.)

Brooks VB: The Neural Basis of Motor Control. New York, Oxford University Press, 1986 (A very detailed but readable text in which the various levels of the nervous system are described as they relate to movement.)

Cooke JD: The organization of simple, skilled movements. In Stelmach GE, Requin J (eds): Tutorials in Motor Behavior. New York, Elsevier North-Holland, 1980

Crutchfield CA, Barnes MR: The Neurophysiologic Basis of Patient Treatment, Vol III, The Peripheral Components of Motor Control. Atlanta, Stokesville Publishing, 1984 (Extensive review of muscle spindle physiology and the mechanisms in spasticity.)

Cummings GS: Comparison of muscle to other soft tissue in limiting elbow extension. Journal of Orthopaedic and Sports Physical Therapy 5:170, 1984 (Study showed that muscle limits elbow extension and that additional range of motion is available when muscle is paralyzed as compared to voluntarily relaxed.)

Davidoff RA: Antispasticity drugs: Mechanisms of action. Ann Neurol 17(2):107, 1985 (Excellent review of drug action and mechanisms in spasticity.)

Davis WE, Sinning WE: Muscle stiffness in Down syndrome and other mentally handicapped subjects: A research note. Journal of Motor Behavior 19(1):130, 1987 (Research report showed that subjects with mental handicaps cannot generate the same level of muscle stiffness that normal subjects can.)

Delong M: Central patterning of movement. Neurosciences Research Program Bulletin 9:10, 1971

Easton TA: On the normal use of reflexes. Am Sci 60:591, 1972

Fel'dman AG: Once more on the equilibrium-point hypothesis for motor control. Journal of Motor Behavior 18:17, 1986 (This discussion of the author's hypothesis for motor control is very difficult to read but is a thorough review of his thesis.)

Goodwin GM, McCloskey DI, Matthews PBC: The contribution of muscle afferents to kinesthesia shown by vibration induced illusions of movement and by the effects of paralyzing joint afferents. Brain 95:705, 1972

Hirshberg GG, Nathanson M: Electromyographic recording of muscular activity in normal and spastic gaits. Arch Phys Med April, 1952, 217 (Study showed abnormal muscle patterns during gait in patients with spasticity that are not altered by surgery, bracing, or exercise.)

Katzman R, Terry RD: The Neurology of Aging. Philadelphia, FA Davis, 1983 (Very thorough discussion of the effects of aging on the nervous system.)

Kelso JAS (ed): Human Motor Behavior: An Introduction. Hillsdale, NJ, Lawrence Erlbaum Associates, 1982 (Excellent and readable discussions of various models and theories of motor control.)

Kelso JAS, Scholz JP: Cooperative phenomena in biological motion. In Haken H (ed): Complex Systems: Operational Approaches in Neurobiology, Physical Systems, and Computers. Berlin, Springer-Verlag, 1985 (Discusses the self-organizing models of motor control.)

Lee DN: On the functions of vision. In Pick H, Saltzman E (eds): Modes of Perceiving. Hillsdale, NJ, Lawrence Erlbaum Associates,

1978

Milani-Comparetti A: The neurophysiologic and clinical implications of studies on fetal motor behavior. Semin Perinatol 5:183, 1981

Nashner LM, Woollacott M: The organization of rapid postural adjustments of standing humans: An experimental conceptual model. In Talbot RE, Humphrey DR (eds): Posture and Movement: Perspectives for Integrating Neurophysiological Research on Sensormotor Systems, pp 243–257. New York, Raven Press, 1979 (The typical synergies produced as a response to surface perturbations are described.)

Nashner LM, Shumway-Cook A, Marin O: Stance posture control in select groups of children with cerebral palsy: Deficits in sensory organization and muscular coordination. Exp Brain Res 49:393, 1983 (Research study indicates that children with spastic cerebral palsy fail to generate as much tension on the involved side as the less involved side as a result of stretch and have derangements within the synergies, which are normally elicited when perturbated.)

Nutter PB, Fitts SS, Hammond MC et al: Maximal Voluntary Recruitment Amplitudes in Upper Motor Neuron Paralysis. Presented at the AAEE Annual Meeting, San Antonio, TX, 1987 (Unpublished study showed that the amplitude of motor unit recruitment was significantly less in patients with hemiplegia.)

Pearson KG, Duysens J: Function of segmental reflexes in the control of stepping in cockroaches and cats. In Herman RM, Grillner S, Stein PSG et al (eds): Neural Control of Locomotion. New York, Plenum Press, 1976 (Gait research shows that some components of the gait cycle are controlled by identical mechanisms in diverse animal species. This suggests that mechanisms other than nervous system pattern generators produce locomotion.)

Ploeger DN, Yamada SJ: Spasticity eliminated; Now what? Physical Therapy Forum 6(40):1, 1987 (Treatment suggestions for patients who have undergone dorsal rhizotomies to eliminate spasticity.)

Sahrmann SA, Norton BJ: The relationship of voluntary movement to spasticity in the upper motor neuron syndrome. Ann Neurol 2:460, 1977 (Classic study by physical therapists indicates that the deficits in spasticity do not relate to hyperactive stretch reflexes.)

Schmidt, RA: Motor Control and Learning: A Behavioral Emphasis. Champaign, IL, Human Kinetics Press, 1982 (Presents several aspects of motor control including schema models.)

Shumway-Cook A, Woollacott MH: Dynamics of postural control in the child with Down syndrome. Phys Ther 65(9):1315, 1985 (Experimental work suggests that hypotonia is not the deficit present in children with Down syndrome.)

Siev E, Freishtat B, Zoltan B: Perceptual and Cognitive Dysfunction in the Adult Stroke Patient. Charles B Slack, Thorofare, NJ, 1986 (Excellent resource for evaluating perceptual problems in stroke patients and suggestions for treatment procedures.)

Tardieu C, Huet de la Tour E, Bret MD et al: Muscle hypoextensibility in children with cerebral palsy: I. Clinical and experimental observations. Arch Phys Med Rehabil 63:97, 1982 (Classic work shows that the inability to lengthen a noncontracting muscle has multiple causes.)

Tardieu C, Tardieu P, Colbeau-Justin A et al: Muscle hypoextensibility in children with cerebral palsy: II. Therapeutic implications. Arch Phys Med Rehabil 63:103, 1982 (Classic work in which children with different mechanisms producing hypoextensibility were treated with either serial casting or surgery to reduce shortened plantarflexors. Results show that the treatment success depends upon the condition present. All children with cerebral palsy are not afflicted in the same manner.)

Thelen, E: Treadmill-elicited stepping in seven-month-old infants. Child Dev 57:1498, 1986 (Infants who did not voluntarily produce stepping movments did so when placed on a treadmill.)

Thelen E, Ulrich BD, Niles D: Bilateral coordination of human infants: Stepping on a split-belt treadmill. J Exp Psychol 13(3):405, 1987 (Work on seven-month-old infants who did not produce stepping movements until placed on the treadmill. Stance was altered to maintain regularly alternating steps even when the belts were run at different speeds.)

12 Cardiovascular Causes

CLAIRE P. KISPERT

The cardiovascular system consists of the heart and blood vessels. Its status is an important determinant of ability to perform physical tasks. The heart is a muscle that contracts and relaxes continuously throughout life to pump blood through the body. The vascular system is a series of vessels, varying in size, that allow blood to flow to all regions of the body. The cardiovascular system delivers oxygen to the body in response to metabolic needs. The amount of blood delivered per minute, or cardiac output, is determined by the strength and rate of contraction of the heart. The amount of blood delivered to specific areas of the body is determined primarily by the size of the vessels leading to that area. The system is dynamic, a characteristic that is reflected by rapid changes in heart rate, myocardial contractility, and regional blood flow, which occur in response to changes in physical, mental, and emotional states.

Cardiovascular reserve is defined as the ability to increase function in response to needs. Specifically, the amount of reserve is the difference in cardiac output from rest to maximal levels of exercise. Persons with large reserves will have high capacities for performing exercise. Factors that influence the amount of reserve include age, sex, and level of cardiopulmonary fitness. The presence of a pathological condition decreases the reserve, thus impairing physical abilities.

Abnormalities of the heart and vascular system can produce pain, decrease muscular strength and endurance, and decrease ability to perform activities of daily living. The nature and severity of the abnormality determine the clinical manifestations. As cardiovascular reserve decreases, capacity for maximal exercise decreases. Relative exercise intensity is defined as submaximal exercise and is expressed as a percentage of maximal exercise. The value increases in the presence of a pathological condition for the same amount of work. Because relative exercise intensity directly correlates with cardiac workload, there is an increase in cardiac stress for a comparable level of exertion.

Abnormalities of the cardiovascular system that produce physical disability can be categorized as resulting from abnormal cardiac muscle function, structural abnormalities of the heart and vascular system, abnormal control of the cardiac impulse, or changes in cardiovascular structures resulting from aging. This chapter will define specific problems included in each category of abnormality, describe the mechanisms producing abnormal function, and discuss the clinical manifestations that result. Pictured in Figure 12-1 is a diagram of the heart showing the major vessels in which many abnormal functions occur.

ABNORMAL CARDIAC MUSCLE FUNCTION

Heart failure occurs when the heart is unable to contract sufficiently to satisfy the metabolic needs of the body. The condition can result from a variety of causes, including hyperten-

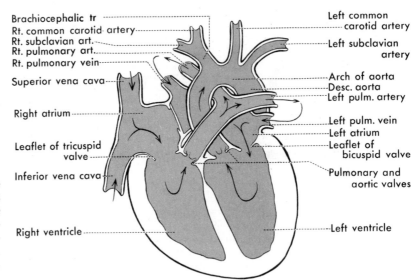

Figure 12-1. Diagram of the heart and the major arteries and veins. Arrows indicate the direction of blood flow. (Hollinshead WH, Rosse C: Textbook of Anatomy, 4th ed, p 78. Philadelphia, JB Lippincott, 1985)

sion, anatomical and valvular abnormalities, cardiomyopathies, and arrhythmias. Even though causes differ, the signs and symptoms are similar.

INADEQUATE CARDIAC OUTPUT

Heart Failure

Heart failure results when an increase in diastolic filling volume does not produce the normal increase in stroke volume (Fig. 12-2). There is a decrease in intrinsic myocardial contractility, or the strength of the contraction of the heart. The mechanism producing reduced contractility is not known, but may be an abnormality in the function of the contractile proteins. Alpert (1984) documented the existence of low levels of the enzyme adenosine triphosphatase (ATPase) and abnormal regulation of intracellular calcium in the myocardium of hearts that have failed to function.

Initially, when cardiac output is inadequate, the body attempts to compensate in several ways. One mechanism is an increase in sodium and water retention, which increases blood volume. This results in an increased end-diastolic volume and pressure, and consequently an increased stroke volume. Ultimately this leads to an enlarged, dilated left ventricle.

A second compensating mechanism is increased activity of the sympathetic nervous system, which produces increased levels of circulating norepinephrine. This results in an increase in myocardial contractility and peripheral vascular constriction. The increased peripheral vasoconstriction results in an increased afterload, or the force that the heart muscle must contract against to eject blood from the left ventricle. Hypertrophy of the cardiac muscle ultimately occurs, which helps to maintain output but also produces increased myocardial work and decreased myocardial compliance. Thus, the compensatory mechanisms function to increase output, but they also have detrimental effects.

Left Ventricular Failure

When the primary problem is failure of the left ventricle, the term *congestive heart failure* is used. If the defect is mild, cardiac output may be normal, with an increase in left ventricular end-diastolic pressure. As the condition worsens, cardiac output decreases and atrial pressure increases. The sequence of events is shown in Figure 12-3. The increased pressure is transmitted upstream to the pulmonary vessels, increasing pulmonary blood volume. The result is a decreased compliance of the lungs,

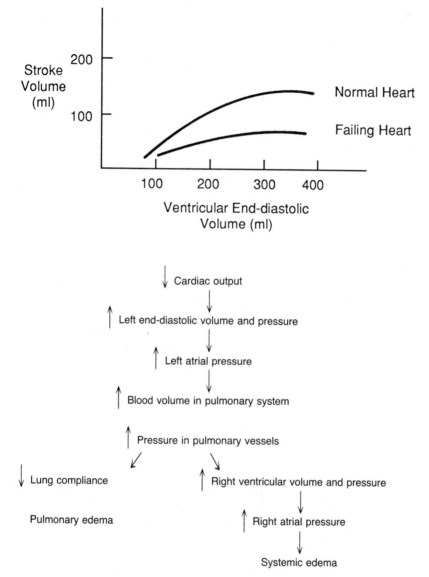

Figure 12-2. Relationship between ventricular end-diastolic volume and stroke volume for normal and failing hearts. (Vander AJ, Sherman JH, Luciano DS: Human Physiology, 4th ed, p 370. St Louis, McGraw-Hill, 1985. Used with permission.)

Figure 12-3. Sequence of events in left ventricular failure, progressing to right ventricular failure.

or increased lung tissue stiffness. The amount of air that can be exchanged is decreased, producing the symptom of dyspnea. The increase in pulmonary blood volume causes fluid to move from the pulmonary capillaries to the interstitial spaces and alveoli. The result is pulmonary edema, further decreasing lung compliance and air exchange. As pressure backs up further, cardiac output from the right ventricle decreases, resulting in right-sided heart failure.

Right Ventricular Failure

Failure of the right ventricle, occurring as a result of pulmonary disease, is referred to as *cor pulmonale.* In this situation right ventricular output is decreased, and right ventricular end-diastolic pressure is increased. As the condition worsens, right atrial pressure and jugular venous pressure increase. Distention of the jugular vein is a sign of right-sided heart failure. The increase in right atrial pressure contributes to the retention of sodium and water by the kidneys. Fluid increase in the intravascular and interstitial spaces produces edema in the dependent areas of the body. Because of the increase in blood returning to the heart and lungs when moving from the upright to the supine position, the pulmonary congestion worsens when supine. The term *orthopnea* describes difficulty with breathing that worsens with positional changes.

Responses to Exercise

During exercise, the metabolic needs of the body increase, and cardiac output must increase to support this need. Signs and symptoms of heart failure often occur during physical activity before being noted to occur at rest. Exercise testing can be used to identify persons in the early stages of heart failure when symptoms are not present at rest (Kaltenbach, 1976). Such individuals experience dyspnea at relatively low levels of work, and the heart rate response may be exaggerated. The excessive increase in heart rate occurs because of the inability to increase stroke volume. Blood flow to active skeletal muscles may not increase normally, leading to early dependence on anaerobic metabolism and signs of fatigue (Braunwald and co-workers, 1982). For persons with signs and symptoms of heart failure at rest, attempting to increase cardiac output with exercise increases the severity of the symptoms. For these persons, exercise is contraindicated until the condition has been medically controlled.

CARDIOMYOPATHIES

Cardiomyopathies are diseases of heart muscle that can result in abnormal systolic or diastolic function, or in cardiac arrhythmias. A "primary" cardiomyopathy is one that affects only the heart muscle, whereas a "secondary" cardiomyopathy occurs as a result of a known disease that affects other parts of the body.

Common causes of secondary cardiomyopathies include alcoholism, nutritional deficiencies, collagen diseases, and myocarditis. Cardiomyopathy is also associated with the neuromuscular disorders of Duchenne muscular dystrophy and Friedreich's ataxia.

Depending on the anatomical and physical abnormalities, cardiomyopathies can be classified into four major types: hypertrophic, congestive, restrictive, and obliterative.

Hypertrophic Cardiomyopathies

The primary defect in hypertrophic cardiomyopathy is abnormal myocardial hypertrophy. The condition can be inherited as an autosomal dominant trait (Hampton, 1984). Alpert (1984) noted the formation of zones of abnormal cardiac cells that work in opposition to each other rather than together. The abnormal process can involve the septum, the free wall of the ventricle, or both structures. The hypertrophied ventricle is noncompliant, or stiff, resulting in increased diastolic pressure. The increased pressure is transmitted backwards to the left atrium and pulmonary vessels, producing symptoms of dyspnea and signs of congestive heart failure.

Hypertrophic cardiomyopathies can be nonobstructive or obstructive in nature. In the nonobstructive form, ejection fractions are normal or above normal. The ejection fraction is the ratio of the volume of blood ejected from the left ventricle with each contraction, or stroke volume, to the diastolic filling volume. In the obstructive form, left ventricular outflow is impeded, possibly from an enlarged septum, or abnormal motion of the mitral valve (Roskamm, 1982). Because of the obstruction, ventricular volume and pressure are increased, also contributing to pulmonary congestion. Systolic function is usually preserved until the later stages of the disease, when ventricular dilation often develops. Mild hypertrophic cardiomyopathies are often asymptomatic. In more severe cases, symptoms of heart failure, angina, or syncope may be present. Heart failure occurs when cardiac output is insufficient to meet the needs of the tissues. The angina probably results from an increase in myocardial oxygen demand that is not met by the coronary blood flow. Syncope occurs because of inadequate cerebral blood flow, usually resulting from ventricular arrhythmias.

Congestive Cardiomyopathies

In congestive cardiomyopathy, left ventricular contractility decreases, producing a decrease in cardiac output. In response to this abnormality, the blood volume increases, producing an increase in end-diastolic volume. The result is a large, dilated heart with approximately normal wall thickness. The process usually involves both the right and left ventricles. Enlargement of the ventricles also produces abnormal function of the papillary muscles, and atrioventricular valve regurgitation. Both low cardiac output and abnormal valve function produce pulmonary congestion and edema, and symptoms of dyspnea and fatigue.

Restrictive Cardiomyopathies

The primary abnormality of restrictive cardiomyopathy is decreased compliance of the cardiac muscle. This results in abnormal diastolic function. The ventricle is not adequately able to fill with blood during diastole, producing an increase in diastolic pressure, and consequently elevated pulmonary and venous pressures. Symptoms include dyspnea, and swelling of the ankles and abdomen. A decrease in cardiac output may also be present.

Obliterative Cardiomyopathies

In obliterative cardiomyopathy, the ventricular cavities are obliterated by disease of the endocardium. The disease is rare in North America, and occurs mainly in Africa (Alpert, 1984). There is fibrosis and scarring in one or both ventricles leading to left- or right-sided heart failure. Decreased ventricular compliance leads to increased diastolic pressures. Systolic function may also decrease.

STRUCTURAL ABNORMALITIES OF THE HEART AND VASCULAR SYSTEM

Structural abnormalities of the heart include deformities of the valves, the walls of the chambers, and the major vessels connecting the heart to the lungs and systemic circulation. The result is an abnormal path of blood flow through the heart and lungs. These abnormalities can occur during the development of the heart in the fetus, or they can be acquired later in life. Structural abnormalities of the vascular system include narrowing of vessels (usually from an atherosclerotic process), occlusion of vessels from emboli or thrombosis, and weakening with possible rupture of vessel walls.

ABNORMAL CARDIAC VALVES

The cardiac valves open and close in response to changes in the pressures between the chambers of the heart. This allows blood to flow in an orderly manner from the right side of the heart to the lungs, and then to the left side of the heart and the systemic circulation. Stenosis is a narrowing of the valve opening, which limits the forward movement of blood. An incompetent valve is a valve that does not close completely, allowing blood to flow in the opposite direction from normal. Incompetent valves produce a leaking or regurgitation of blood. A valve that is severely damaged can result in both stenosis and regurgitation such that not enough blood flows forward and some blood actually flows backward. The consequences of an abnormal valve depend on the specific valve involved, and the nature and severity of the abnormality.

Pulmonary and Aortic Valve Stenosis

Stenosis of the pulmonary or aortic valve produces an increased resistance to flow of blood from the right or left ventricle, respectively. Pulmonary valve stenosis often occurs congenitally. The narrowing results either from an abnormality in the area of the pulmonary artery adjacent to the valve, or from an abnormal valve. The increased resistance to flow will cause the right ventricle to hypertrophy, and may produce right-sided heart failure.

In aortic stenosis, there is an increased pressure gradient between the left ventricle and the aorta. Aortic valve stenosis results in left ventricular hypertrophy and, if severe, produces left ventricular failure. During exercise, stroke volume and cardiac output cannot increase adequately. An increase in intraventricular pressure occurs, which increases ventricular wall tension and the oxygen requirements of the myocardium. The oxygen delivered to the heart may be decreased because the obstruction occurs proximal to the origin of the coronary arteries. Clinical symptoms during exertion may include chest pain, dyspnea, and lightheadedness. Sudden death during strenuous exercise can occur in aortic valve stenosis, and has been attributed to ventricular fibrillation (Hampton, 1984). Consequently, exercise stress testing to maximal levels and high-intensity competitive activities are contraindicated in persons with aortic valve stenosis.

Mitral Valve Stenosis

In mitral valve stenosis, increased pressure in the left atrium is transmitted backwards, causing an increase in pressure in the pulmonary capillaries, the pulmonary artery, and the right ventricle. An increase in blood flow to the lungs and right ventricular hypertrophy result. If the defect is severe, fluid will move from the pulmonary capillaries to the alveoli, causing pulmonary edema.

Aortic and Mitral Valve Incompetence

With an incompetent aortic valve, blood moves backwards from the aorta into the ventricle during diastole. The increase in left ventricular volume produces an increased stroke volume, and left ventricular hypertrophy. With mitral valve incompetence, blood moves backwards from the left ventricle to the left atrium during systole. The result is a decrease in both stroke volume and cardiac output.

Tricuspid Valve Stenosis and Incompetence

Isolated abnormalities of the tricuspid valve are rare. Tricuspid stenosis occasionally occurs in combination with a mitral valve disorder in rheumatic heart disease, but is usually not the dominant problem (Downie, 1982). Tricuspid regurgitation may also occur with rheumatic heart disease, or because of dilation of the valve ring occurring secondary to right-sided heart failure.

Heart Murmurs

Valvular defects produce heart murmurs, which vary in timing (systole versus diastole) depending on the location, nature, and severity of the defect (Table 12-1). Because pulmonary and aortic valve stenosis increase resistance to the outflow of blood, these conditions produce murmurs during systole, when blood is ejected from the heart. Stenosis of the tricuspid or mitral valves produces an increased resistance to flow from the atria to the ventricles. Consequently, these conditions produce diastolic murmurs. The backflow of blood resulting from incompetent aortic or pulmonary valves occurs during diastole, producing diastolic murmurs. The backflow of blood resulting from incompetent mitral or tricuspid valves occurs during systole, producing systolic murmurs. The location on the chest wall where the intensity of the murmur is loudest is used to assist in determining the specific valve that is not functioning correctly.

ABNORMAL CARDIAC CHAMBERS AND MAJOR VESSELS

Abnormal development of the heart during the fetal period or failure of normal changes to occur during the early neonatal period result in malformations of the cardiac chambers or major vessels. If the defect is severe, signs of cardiac failure and cyanosis may be present at birth. These infants often have difficulty feeding, and may become fatigued quickly during feeding. Minor defects may not be detected until later in life, when the individual has a routine physical examination. Abnormalities are functionally classified as either "left-to-right" shunts or "right-to-left" shunts, depending on the direction of the abnormal flow of blood (Table 12-2).

Left-to-Right Shunts

In left-to-right shunts, blood moves from the left side of the heart to the right side. Causes include ventricular and atrial septal defects. In these conditions, there is an opening between the left and right ventricles, or between the left and right atria. Because the pressure is higher in the chambers on the left side of the heart, blood moves from the left side to the right side. The result is an increase in blood flow through the pulmonary circulation in comparison to the systemic circulation. If the defect is between the ventricles, the infant may develop left-sided heart failure. Both defects result in an increased risk of developing pulmonary vascular disease (Hampton, 1984).

Failure of the ductus arteriosus to close after birth also results in a left-to-right shunt. The ductus arteriosus connects the pulmonary artery to the aorta, allowing blood to bypass the lungs in the fetal circulation. Because the pressure is higher in the aorta, blood moves from the aorta to the pulmonary artery. A large defect will result in heart failure and an increased risk for developing pulmonary vascular disease.

Right-to-Left Shunts

In a right-to-left shunt, blood moves from the right side of the heart directly to the left side of the heart, without going through the lungs to receive oxygen. Cyanosis occurs because of the excess of deoxygenated hemoglobin. Tetralogy of Fallot is a condition of four abnormalities that results in a right-to-left shunt. The four abnormalities include a ventricular septal defect, pulmonary valve stenosis, an abnormal position of the aorta, and right ventricular hypertrophy. Because the pulmonary stenosis obstructs blood flow from the right ventricle to the lungs, blood moves through the ventricular septal defect to the left ventricle. The result is cyanosis, which becomes worse with an increase in activity.

Another condition that often produces a right-to-left shunt is coarctation or narrowing of the aorta, occurring distal to the branching of the subclavian artery. In one type, the ductus arteriosus remains open, connecting the right ventricle to a point on the aorta distal to the narrowing. Because the pressure is low distal to the narrowing, a right-to-left shunt results, producing cyanosis.

A second type of coarctation of the aorta has no shunt because the ductus arteriosus closes. Because the narrowing occurs distal to the branching of the major arteries to the upper extremities, the result is high blood pressures in the upper extremities and low pressures in the lower extremities. Femoral pulses are weak or absent, and ventricular hypertrophy results.

Table 12-1. Valvular Abnormalities and Associated Heart Murmurs

VALVE	ABNORMALITY	TIME OF MURMUR
Aortic, pulmonary	Stenosis	Systolic
	Regurgitation	Diastolic
Mitral, tricuspid	Stenosis	Diastolic
	Regurgitation	Systolic

Table 12-2. Functional Consequences of Anatomical Abnormalities

FUNCTIONAL EVENT	ABNORMALITIES	POSSIBLE CLINICAL CONSEQUENCES
Left-to-right shunt	Atrial septal defect Ventricular septal defect Patent ductus arteriosus	Pulmonary vascular disease Heart failure
Right-to-left shunt	Tetralogy of Fallot Coarctation of aorta with patent ductus arteriosus	Cyanosis

ABNORMALITIES OF THE VASCULAR SYSTEM

Structural abnormalities of blood vessels include narrowing or a decrease in size of the lumen of vessels, occlusion of vessels, and enlargement of a section of vessel wall. Permanent vessel narrowing usually results from atherosclerosis; reversible narrowing occurs from smooth muscle spasm of vessel walls. Occlusion of a vessel results from formation of a blood clot, or thrombus, within a vessel. A dislodged clot, or embolus, travels through the circulation and terminates in vessels of a size that impede movement. Aneurysms are enlargements of vessel walls. The walls become weak and thin, and are at high risk for rupture and hemorrhage.

Atherosclerosis

Atherosclerosis is the formation of fibrous plaques in the intima of vessels. The plaques occupy space in the interior of vessels, resulting in a decrease in blood flow. The plaques consist of smooth muscle cells that have migrated from the media to the intima of the vessel. The smooth muscle cells proliferate, stimulate the formation of connective tissue, and serve as an area for the accumulation of lipid. The clinical manifestations of atherosclerosis depend on the anatomical location of the vessels involved. Atherosclerosis of peripheral vessels, peripheral vascular disease, and atherosclerosis of the coronary vessels are discussed in this chapter.

Peripheral vascular disease is a term describing the presence of atherosclerosis in the lower aorta or the blood vessels supplying the lower extremities. In the early stage of the disease, the delivery of oxygen is inadequate only during activities when oxygen needs are increased. The increased activity, such as walking, may cause intermittent claudication and pain. As the disease progresses, the distance that the person can walk decreases and the person may experience pain at rest. Clinical signs of inadequate circulation include an absence of peripheral pulses or the presence of bruits. Bruits are sounds heard over peripheral vessels, usually indicating turbulent blood flow.

The skin of the affected extremity is dry, scaly, hairless, and may feel cold. Consequences of peripheral vascular disease include poor wound healing and cardiopulmonary and muscular deconditioning, because activity is decreased secondary to pain.

Atherosclerosis of the coronary arteries produces a condition where blood flow to the heart is compromised. Normally, increased myocardial demand is met by an increase in flow, rather than by an increase in the amount of oxygen extracted from the blood. Blood flow may be adequate for myocardial activity at rest, but inadequate as oxygen demands increase with physical activity or emotional stress. Clinical manifestations include angina and myocardial infarction.

Angina is described as pain in the chest, often radiating to the arm, neck, or jaw. The onset of classical angina is associated with physical exertion or emotional stress. This type of angina is referred to as *exertional angina,* and is relieved by discontinuing activity and by taking medication. Other types include variant or Prinzmetal's angina and unstable angina. Variant angina often occurs at rest, and is thought to result from a coronary artery spasm. Unstable angina is characterized by a changing pattern of frequency, duration, and severity, may occur at rest, and may not be relieved with medication (Van der Werf, 1980).

Angina is thought to result from an imbalance between myocardial oxygen demands and myocardial oxygen supply. Myocardial oxygen needs are determined primarily by heart rate, myocardial contractility, and ventricular wall tension. Both heart rate and contractility increase in response to increased catecholamines in the blood, which occurs with exercise and stress. Ventricular wall tension is determined by intraventricular pressure and volume. Increases in systolic and diastolic blood pressures increase wall tension. Myocardial oxygen supply is determined by the blood flow through the coronary arteries. The amount of flow is determined by the diameter of the vessels, the diastolic blood pressure, and the duration of diastole. The primary cause of inadequate flow is reduced size of the vessel lumen from atherosclerosis, coronary artery spasm, or a combination of both abnormalities. Angina results in cardiopulmonary and muscular deconditioning, because physical activity is avoided secondary to pain.

Myocardial infarction occurs when heart muscle becomes necrotic because of inadequate oxygen. Events can result from a prolonged increase in myocardial oxygen demands, causing damage to the subendocardial areas, or from a sudden occlusion of a vessel from the formation of a thrombus or the rupture of an atherosclerotic plaque. Symptoms include chest pain, excessive sweating, and nausea. Emergency medical care is essential to avoid sudden death, which usually occurs because of abnormal cardiac rhythms.

The damaged heart muscle is progressively replaced by a fibrous scar. The healing process involves the formation of collagen fibers, and begins in the third week after the event (Hampton, 1984). By the end of the second month, a fairly strong matrix of collagen fibers is formed. The amount of tissue replaced by scar and the location of the scar determine the amount of loss of cardiovascular reserve. During systole, an ischemic area will not contract, but will bulge outward. If a significant portion of the ventricle is ischemic, there will be an increased end-systolic volume, and a decrease in stroke volume. During diastole, the scarred area is noncompliant, causing an increase in end-diastolic pressure. Small myocardial infarctions (less than 8% of the area of the left ventricle) have minimal effects on stroke volume (Wenger, 1984). These investigators state that if the area is greater than 10%, stroke volume will be decreased during activities; if the area is greater than 15%, diastolic pressure will also be elevated, and if the area is 23% or greater, clinical symptoms of heart failure will be present.

Damage to an area of the heart responsible for generation or conduction of the cardiac impulse results in cardiac arrhythmias. Bradyarrhythmias, or arrhythmias associated with a slow heart rate, may result from damage to the sinoatrial (SA) node, atrioventricular (AV) node, bundle of His, or conducting fibers. Atrial and ventricular ectopic beats, flutter, and fibrillation may result from damage to either atrial or ventricular muscle. The nature and frequency of the arrhythmia determine the clinical signs.

Damage to the papillary muscles affects the functions of the atrioventricular valves. Damage to the mitral valve is fairly common, occurring in 25% to 33% of patients sustaining a myocardial infarction (Brand and co-workers, 1969). The result is an incompetent mitral valve; the severity of the defect depends on the specific lesion. A complete rupture will produce signs and symptoms of acute heart failure.

Thrombotic Disease

Deep vein thrombosis is the formation of a blood clot, usually in the veins of the calf or thigh muscles. Causes of thrombosis include abnormal blood flow and abnormalities of blood components. With immobility, the rate of blood flow is decreased, allowing the chemicals in the blood that are responsible for blood clotting to build up and support a growing clot. An increase in platelets or fibrinogen in the blood also increases the probability of clot formation. The risk of developing a clot increases with age, obesity, the presence of cancer, a history of deep vein thrombosis, the presence of varicose veins, and the use of estrogens. Clinical symptoms include pain and swelling in the affected extremity, increased skin temperature, and dilation of superficial veins. Immediate treatment is necessary to prevent the clot from dislodging and traveling to the lungs.

Aneurysm

An aneurysm is a localized swelling of the wall of an artery. The wall weakens, and thinning of all layers occurs. The aorta and popliteal arteries are most commonly affected (Downie, 1982). Aneurysms may be asymptomatic, especially if the abnormality extends over a long distance of vessel. Symptoms occur if the swelling is large enough to apply pressure to surrounding tissues. Pressure on adjacent veins can obstruct blood flow, leading to venous stasis and thrombosis. Pressure on bone can lead to erosion of the bone, and pressure on nerves can produce pain and muscular weakness. Preventing excessive increases in blood pressure is important until surgery can be performed to correct the abnormality.

ABNORMAL CONTROL OF THE CARDIAC IMPULSE

The cells of the SA node, which lie under the epicardium close to the junction of the superior vena cava and the left atrium, are responsible for generating the cardiac action potential. The impulse travels through the atria to the AV node, where there is a slight delay, providing time for the ventricles to complete the filling process. The impulse continues through the intraventricular conduction system, moving rapidly to allow simultaneous contraction of the ventricles. Abnormalities result if the impulse originates at a site other than the SA node, or if the impulse is blocked at any point along the path of conduction. Abnormal beats that occur only occasionally and do not produce symptoms are often observed but not treated. Symptoms may develop, depending on the nature of the abnormality. Slow ventricular rates often produce hypotension, lightheadedness, or fainting from inadequate blood perfusion to the brain. Fast ventricular rates produce "palpitations," or sensations that the heart is beating fast and irregularly.

Causes of abnormal impulse generation or conduction include defects occurring within the heart itself, abnormalities in the neural control of the heart, abnormalities in the composition of the blood, or a combination of the three. Myocardial abnormalities that can affect the cardiac impulse include local areas of ischemia, and the presence of small calcified plaques placing pressure on muscle cells. Neural control of the heart involves afferent information from various areas of the body, and efferent output through the parasympathetic and sympathetic nerves. Diseases that affect either peripheral nerves or the central nervous system can produce inappropriate efferent signals, resulting in abnormalities in rate and rhythm. Blood-borne substances such as nicotine and

caffeine influence the cardiac impulse. Abnormal electrolyte concentrations, especially potassium, can also produce significant alterations in cardiac rhythm.

DISORDERS OF IMPULSE FORMATION

Excessive Stimulation

The formation of the impulse can be altered by excessive parasympathetic or sympathetic stimulation, or by irritable foci within the heart. Stimulation by the vagus nerve of the parasympathetic nervous system slows the rate of impulse generation at the SA node and the conduction velocity through the AV node. Excessive stimulation may produce symptoms of dizziness and lightheadedness. If the conduction time through the AV node is too long, the impulse is not propagated. Unless the AV node or ventricles take over, the heart is in asystole, or standstill. Stimulation by the sympathetic nervous system speeds up the heart rate. Symptoms of palpitations may occur. Disadvantages of a rapid rate include a shortening of the diastolic time period, which limits ventricular filling, and shortening of the time available for blood flow through the coronary arteries.

Premature Contraction

Premature contractions, also referred to as extrasystoles or ectopic contractions, are contractions of a part of the heart that occur prior to the normal time for contraction of that area of the heart. Premature atrial contractions originate at a location in the atria other than the SA node. The impulse travels through the atria, stimulating the SA node and then the AV node. The resulting ventricular contraction occurs slightly early, compromising ventricular filling and producing a decrease in stroke volume. Therefore, peripheral pulses may be absent or weak. The next contraction will be slightly delayed because of the time needed for the SA node to recover before it can initiate the next beat. The stroke volume in this instance may be greater than normal, producing a strong pulse.

Premature contractions can also originate

in the AV node, bundle of His, or ventricular muscle. A beat originating in the AV node travels backward to the atria and forward to the ventricles at the same time. The result is simultaneous contraction of both atria and ventricles, slightly decreasing ventricular filling. Premature ventricular contractions, depending on the precise timing, may result in inadequate stroke volume because of inadequate time for ventricular filling. The presence of early ventricular contractions is a more serious situation than early atrial or nodal contractions, because there is an increased chance of developing ventricular tachycardia and fibrillation.

Abnormal generation of the cardiac impulse may also result from a rapid rhythmic discharge of impulses from a localized area called a *focus*. This focus becomes the pacemaker of the heart. If the irritable area is in the atria or AV node, the abnormality is referred to as atrial or nodal paroxysmal tachycardia. The onset and the termination of this arrhythmia is usually sudden, with the rhythm lasting from minutes to days. This type of tachycardia usually occurs in young, healthy persons, does not produce serious symptoms, and is not life threatening. However, a rapidly discharging focus located in the ventricles results in ventricular tachycardia, which is a considerably more serious arrhythmia. This abnormality occurs when the ventricles are seriously damaged, and may lead to ventricular fibrillation.

Fibrillation

With fibrillation, many small depolarization waves spread in different directions in an unorganized manner. The result is lack of an organized contraction, which is necessary to move blood through the heart. Atrial fibrillation produces irregular ventricular beats because impulses arrive at and fire the AV node randomly. Cardiac output may be depressed because of an inadequate time period for ventricular filling. In ventricular fibrillation, there is no organized contraction of the ventricles and consequently no cardiac output. Immediate electroshock is necessary to restore organized ventricular contractions.

DISORDERS OF IMPULSE CONDUCTION

Blocks

The impulse can be blocked at any point in its path through the heart. Blocks can result from areas of ischemia, inflammation, or scarring, or from excessive vagal stimulation. In a sinoatrial block, conduction is blocked between the SA node and the atrial muscle. The AV node usually takes over initiating impulses, producing bradycardia because of the lower intrinsic rate.

Several types of blocks can occur at the AV node. The term *incomplete heart block* is used to describe a prolonged conduction time through the AV node. In a second degree heart block, some beats are conducted and others are not, depending on the strength of the impulse. In this situation the atria may beat two or three times for each ventricular contraction. In complete or third degree heart block, the atria and ventricles beat independently of each other. Because the intrinsic rate of ventricular contraction is slow, symptoms of lightheadedness or fainting are often present. Blocks may also occur in the right or left bundle branches, or in peripheral parts of the conduction system. The result is asynchronous beating of the ventricles.

CHANGES RESULTING FROM AGING

Certain changes occur normally in the cardiovascular system as a person becomes older. The decrease in activity level as a person ages and the increased incidence of disease are two factors making the distinction of "true" aging changes difficult. Performing longitudinal studies of healthy persons has facilitated the identification of changes resulting primarily from aging. In general, the changes produce a limitation in performance at moderate and high levels of work.

Age-related changes in the heart and vascular system have been documented by Weisfeldt (1980), and include prolonged contraction and relaxation of cardiac muscle, decreased responsiveness to sympathetic stimulation, decreased ventricular compliance, and increased resistance to ventricular ejection. A longer time for myocardial relaxation produces a shorter period for diastole, and may result in increased ventricular pressures during diastole. The time period for diastole is important to assure coronary blood flow to the left ventricle, and to allow the ventricles to fill with blood prior to ejection.

A specific decrease in responsiveness of the older heart and vascular system to catecholamines is evident as decreased inotropic and chronotropic responses. *Inotropic* refers to the strength of the cardiac contraction, and *chronotropic* refers to the timing of the contraction. This alteration may be at least partially responsible for the decrease in maximal exercise heart rate. A decreased responsiveness to catecholamines that produce peripheral vasodilation limits the decrease in total peripheral resistance that normally occurs with exercise, and may explain the higher systolic blood pressures in older persons compared with younger persons.

A decrease in ventricular compliance primarily affects diastolic function. This alteration could cause problems under conditions when left ventricular diastolic volume is increased, which occurs during exercise. The resulting increase in diastolic pressure may cause dyspnea. This increased stiffness might be responsible for an earlier onset of dyspnea during exercise in older persons. The decreased compliance may also limit the increases in stroke volume that occur with progressive exercise. A lower stroke volume for the same level of oxygen consumption occurs in older persons in comparison with younger persons (Wenger, 1984).

The increased resistance to ventricular ejection results from changes that occur in the peripheral vessels. Changes in elastin and collagen occur, making the vessel walls less extensible (Weisfeldt, 1980). The decreased compliance increases the load that the ventricle must overcome to eject blood. To compensate, there is an age-associated myocardial hypertrophy (Weisfeldt, 1980). This alteration is probably responsible for the increased systolic and diastolic blood pressures both at rest and during exercise in older persons.

Cardiac output, stroke volume, heart rate, and oxygen consumption are all lower for maximal exercise for older persons compared with younger persons. If age-related changes occur in isolation, they produce functional limitations during high-intensity exercise. If these changes occur in combination with changes resulting from disease or inactivity, the functional limitations are greater, often occurring at low levels of activity or even at rest.

CONCLUSION

The condition of the cardiovascular system is a major determinant of ability to perform work because of the system's role in the delivery of oxygen. Changes in the cardiovascular system that limit the delivery of oxygen include abnormal cardiac muscle function, anatomical defects, an abnormal sequence of cardiac muscle stimulation, and age-related structural and functional changes. These alterations are analogous to changes in the musculoskeletal system that include muscle weakness, inadequate joint motion, and incoordination of movement.

The changes in the cardiovascular system are not as easily detected by the physical therapist as changes in the musculoskeletal system. Abnormalities often occur in combinations, such as coronary artery disease and abnormal cardiac rhythms, or abnormal function of a valve and congestive heart failure. With careful monitoring of vital signs, observation of patients, and listening to and documenting subjective information, the clinician can identify possible cardiovascular abnormalities, and make the appropriate referrals for further evaluation. It is important for the clinician to measure and document vital signs routinely because cardiovascular disease often occurs in combination with neurological or musculoskeletal abnormalities. This practice becomes important because physical therapy usually includes physical stresses. Understanding the possible causes and the clinical signs and symptoms related to these causes will help the therapist prevent life-threatening cardiovascular events.

ANNOTATED BIBLIOGRAPHY

Alpert JS: Physiopathology of the Cardiovascular System. Boston, Little, Brown & Co, 1984 (This text provides a comprehensive review of heart failure, including the specific cardiac abnormalities that can produce heart failure, and the associated renal and respiratory system responses.)

Brand FR, Brown AL, Berge KG: Histology of papillary muscle of the left ventricle. Am Heart J 77:26, 1969

Braunwald E, Mock MB, Watson JT (eds): Congestive Heart Failure. New York, Grune & Stratton, 1982 (The proposed mechanisms for the development of congestive heart failure are reviewed, followed by a discussion of clinical evaluation procedures and medical and surgical strategies for intervention. Selection by Zelis and Flaim is relevant.)

Downie PA (ed): Cash's Textbook of Chest, Heart, and Vascular Disorders for Physiotherapists. Philadelphia, JB Lippincott, 1982 (The pathology, medical management, and physical therapy management of cardiac and pulmonary disorders are discussed. A description of the information obtained from radiographs, electrocardiographs, and pulmonary function tests is included. Chapters by Fowler and by Pickering and Bourne are of interest.)

Hampton JR (ed): Cardiovascular Disease. Chicago, Year Book Medical Publishers, 1984 (The structural, functional, and cellular adaptations that occur with cardiovascular disease are presented, with application to specific clinical problems. See chapters by Bailey and co-workers; Fentem and Hampton; and Morris.)

Kaltenbach M: Exercise Testing of Cardiac Patients, pp 87–99. Baltimore, Williams & Wilkins, 1976

Roskamm H, Csapo G (eds): Disorders of Cardiac Function. New York, Marcel Dekker, 1982 (The pathology and management of abnormalities of the generation and conduction of the cardiac impulse are presented. Discussions of ventricular function at rest and during activity in individuals with cardiovascular dysfunction are included. Selection by Bertrand is relevant here.)

Van der Werf T: Cardiovascular Pathophysiology. New York, Oxford University Press, 1980 (Abnormal function of the heart resulting from cardiovascular pathology is discussed with reference to normal cardiac physiology. Included are conditions that result in volume or pressure overload on the heart, a decrease in myocardial contractility, cardiac arrhythmias, and hypertension.)

Weisfeldt ML (ed): The Aging Heart, Vol 12, Aging. New York, Raven Press, 1980 (This text reviews current research on the effect of aging on the structure and function of the heart, the coronary vasculature, and the neural control of the heart. Information is included on the response to exercise in the aging heart. Chapters by Weisfeldt and Yin are of interest.)

Wenger NK, Hellerstein HK (eds): Rehabilitation of the Coronary Patient, 2nd ed. New York, John Wiley & Sons, 1984 (This book presents a multidisciplinary approach to the long-term management of individuals with cardiovascular disease. Programs designed for postcoronary bypass surgery patients, postmyocardial infarction patients, and patients with other conditions affecting cardiac function are presented. See especially chapters by Tommaso and co-workers, and Wenger.)

13 Respiratory Causes

PEGGY CLOUGH

The ability to move and interact with the environment is usually thought of as the primary function of the musculoskeletal system mediated through impulses and reflexes in the central and peripheral nervous systems. However, the physical ability to move or exercise is based on the capacity of the pulmonary and circulatory systems to deliver oxygen (O_2) and nutrients to the exercising muscles. Without sufficient O_2, the muscles would be unable to produce energy for muscle fiber contraction. Fatigue would result and the person would be unable to continue the exercise or activity. The central nervous system (CNS) is very sensitive to decreased O_2 levels. Without sufficient O_2 to the brain and other parts of the nervous system, motor function is impaired with loss of motor planning, balance, and coordination. In addition, hypoxemia can produce confusion, headache, restlessness, impaired judgment, delirium, and ultimately coma.

It is the primary function of the respiratory system to deliver sufficient O_2 and remove carbon dioxide (CO_2) at the cellular level for all body systems; therefore, the respiratory system is closely interrelated with each body system. This interrelatedness means that pathology or stress in the respiratory system usually has some effect on other body systems. Conversely, pathology in other body systems often has some component that affects the respiratory system. The discussion in this chapter will focus on primary and secondary pulmonary pathology, and how this pathology may affect the patient's ability to move and interact with the environment.

PULMONARY SYSTEM

The pulmonary system is made up of many interactive parts and functions. The airways, lung parenchyma, pulmonary circulation, gas transport, control of respiration, and the respiratory musculature will be discussed briefly.

AIRWAYS

The airways serve several functions within the pulmonary system. They are the route for inhaled and exhaled gases. With each inspiration, air passes through the nose or mouth, pharynx, larynx, trachea, mainstem bronchi, and then lobar, segmental, and smaller bronchi and bronchioles. The conducting airways end with the terminal bronchiole leading to the alveolus, where gas exchange takes place (Fig. 13-1). Within the airways, particularly the nose, each inhaled breath is warmed and humidified. The airways also have the ability to move, which alters airway resistance and can move secretions upward for easier expectoration. With each inspiration, the bronchi elongate and their internal diameters increase. Both of these motions are reversed on exhalation.

Within the walls of the trachea and bronchi are located two body defense mechanisms. The first defense mechanism is made up of the cilia

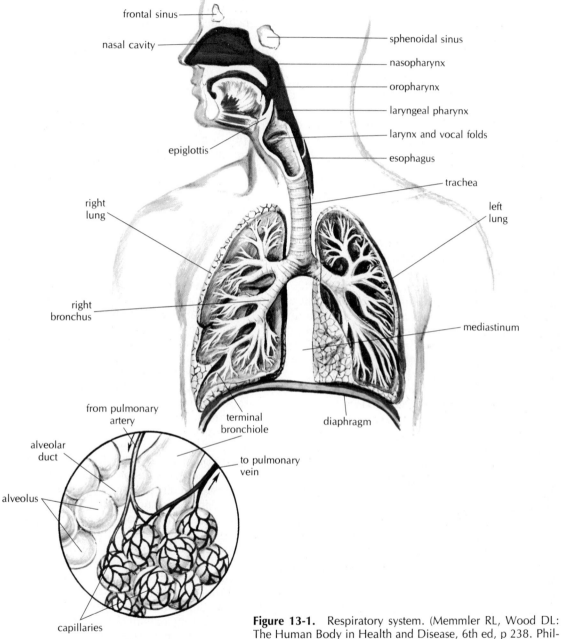

frontal sinus

nasal cavity

epiglottis

right lung

right bronchus

sphenoidal sinus

nasopharynx

oropharynx

laryngeal pharynx

larynx and vocal folds

esophagus

trachea

left lung

mediastinum

terminal bronchiole

diaphragm

from pulmonary artery

alveolar duct

to pulmonary vein

alveolus

capillaries

section of lung enlarged

Figure 13-1. Respiratory system. (Memmler RL, Wood DL: The Human Body in Health and Disease, 6th ed, p 238. Philadelphia, JB Lippincott, 1987)

and goblet cells, which work together to eliminate inhaled small particulate matter. The ciliated epithelial cells contain up to 200 cilia each, which beat in a rhythmic upward motion 12 to 25 times per second. The cilia move particulate matter toward the mouth at a rate of 3 mm/min, so that 90% of deposited particles are cleared within two hours.

The irritant receptors are the second defense mechanism, and are responsible for the cough reflex. The cough reflex is triggered by the irritant receptors located in the larynx, trachea, bronchi, pleura, and diaphragm. These irritant receptors are particularly concentrated at the carina. The afferent impulses from these receptors travel by means of the vagus, trigeminal, glossopharyngeal, and phrenic nerves to a poorly defined cough center in the medulla. Efferent signals are then carried by the recurrent laryngeal nerve, which controls the glottis, and by the phrenic and spinal nerves, which innervate the diaphragm and abdominal and thoracic wall musculature. A vigorous cough can produce intrathoracic pressures up to 300 mm Hg, which then is used to force air out at the speed of sound. This high-velocity airflow also moves mucus within the lungs so that excess mucus can be expectorated.

These irritant receptors can also cause bronchoconstriction, which increases airway resistance and the work of breathing. The increased airway resistance reflexly causes a decrease in the respiratory rate in an effort to decrease the work of breathing. Small changes in airway resistance can mean significant increases in the work of breathing. Over 50% of the total airway resistance occurs in the nose; about 20% in the mouth, pharynx, larynx, and trachea combined; about 20% in the bronchi; and only 10% in the smaller bronchioles (<2 mm^2). With increased flow rates or exercise, airway resistance is significantly increased. When exercising, one compensatory mechanism used to decrease airway resistance is to inhale through the mouth rather than the nose. This change is often made automatically without conscious decision. Airway resistance is also affected by body position. It increases in the supine position and decreases when the person is upright. Because the small peripheral bronchioles contribute so little to total airway resistance, diagnosis of small airway disease is difficult until the disease is well advanced.

LUNG PARENCHYMA

The lung parenchyma is made up of the 300 million alveoli present in the adult lung. Gas distribution to the alveoli, sensory innervation of the lung parenchyma, and defense mechanisms within the lung parenchyma contribute to the function of this part of the pulmonary system. The millions of alveoli that make up the lung parenchyma have a total surface area of 50 to 100 m or an area approximately 50 times the total surface area of the body. It is over this surface area that the essential lung function of gas exchange takes place. Even at rest, the amount of air and blood passing in and out of the lungs to participate in gas exchange is about 5 L per minute.

The normal lung is very elastic and easy to distend. To take a normal tidal volume of 500 mL requires an inspiratory mouth pressure of -3 cm of water (H_2O). To accomplish the same volume change in a child's balloon might require 300 cm H_2O pressure. The reason that the alveoli are so much easier to distend is due to the presence of surfactant. Surfactant lowers the surface tension of the alveoli and increases lung compliance. It promotes the stability of the alveoli so that smaller alveoli do not empty into larger alveoli, causing atelectasis. Surfactant prevents transudation of fluid from the capillaries into the alveoli. Even though surfactant is present throughout the lung, the alveoli are not uniformly ventilated. Because of hydrostatic pressure, unequal pleural space pressures (more negative at the apex and less negative at the base), and the weight of the lung itself, the dependent lung tissue is best ventilated. In sitting or standing, the apex of the lung would have a larger resting volume but poorer ventilation (volume change per unit resting volume) than the base. The bases would be relatively poorly expanded but better ventilated than the apex. This regionalization of ventilation is also true with the patient supine, prone, or sidelying. The uppermost part of the lung is better expanded and the dependent part of the lung is better ventilated.

This concept takes on importance with a variety of pathological processes that promote ventilation/perfusion ($\dot{V}/\dot{Q}$) mismatching. The sensory innervation of the lung parenchyma can account for some of the changes noted in specific pulmonary pathologies. Basically, the lung parenchyma contains specific sensory nerve endings that are activated by volume changes, the rate of lung volume change, and irritants such as smoke or chemicals. The lung also contains J receptors, which respond to increased pulmonary congestion. The impulses from the lung's sensory receptors travel to the medulla by means of the vagus nerve and can change the rate, pattern, and depth of ventilation as well as protect the lung from overinflation. The lung tissue itself contains no sensory nerve endings for pain. However, the parietal pleura contains numerous pain receptors. The lung tissue contains two defense mechanisms to protect itself from particulate matter not cleared by the mucociliary escalator. Alveolar macrophages destroy and eliminate inhaled particles reaching the alveoli. Lymphohematogenous drainage also can clear particles from deep within the lung through lymphatic channels, but this mechanism takes months or years to accomplish.

PULMONARY CIRCULATION

The pulmonary circulation is a high flow/low pressure system capable of altering the distribution of blood flow in the lungs in response to changes in body position, ventilation, or activity. Like ventilation, pulmonary blood flow is not equal throughout the lungs. Because of gravity and the weight of the lungs, perfusion is greatest at the base of the lungs when the body is in an upright position. Conversely, blood flow through the pulmonary capillaries in the apices of the lungs is diminished in the upright position. Therefore, regionalization of blood flow is dependent on body position, with the dependent lung segments always bet-

ter perfused. With any changes in the distribution of inspired gases, vasoconstriction and vasodilation within the pulmonary capillary bed can alter pulmonary circulation. For example, if a portion of the lung was not being ventilated, the pulmonary capillaries in that area would undergo vasoconstriction because of alveolar hypoxia. Normally the entire cardiac output flows through the pulmonary circulation, making blood flow to the lung higher than that of any other organ. However, at rest only about 100 ml of blood is in the pulmonary capillary system, and it remains at the capillary level for only 0.8 second. With exercise pulmonary vascular resistance (which is low to begin with) decreases and pulmonary blood flow increases, thus increasing the amount of blood in the lungs. The speed with which the blood flows through the lungs is also increased, which decreases the amount of time it remains at the capillary level. The distribution of blood flow is also changed with activity. Exercise in the upright position increases pulmonary pressures so that blood flow to the apices improves and perfusion throughout the lung becomes more uniform than at rest.

GAS TRANSPORT

The primary reason for having a pulmonary system is to oxygenate the blood so that O_2 can be carried to all body cells. Normal oxygen transport is dependent on many factors within the pulmonary and circulatory systems and at the tissue level (Table 13-1). Gas diffusion is a passive process in which the O_2 and CO_2 levels in the alveoli and capillary blood seek to equalize. Gas transport occurs at the alveolar-capillary interface, which measures approximately 70 m^2 of membranous surface area only 0.5 μm thick. Normally it takes only a quarter of a second for the capillary blood to give up excess CO_2 and replenish its supply of O_2. Oxygenation of the blood can be impaired in a variety of ways. Any pathology that thickens the alveolar-capillary membrane, causes increased physiological dead space, enhances ventilation/perfusion mismatching, impairs ventilation, or limits blood flow or the O_2-carrying

Table 13-1. Oxygen Transport*

Gas Phase

Room air	Adequate inspired O_2 concentration
Airways	Unobstructed Normal resistance to flow
Lungs	Normal volumes/capacities Normal compliance
Alveoli	Normal PaO_2 Normal ventilation/perfusion matching Normal diffusing capacity

Blood Phase

Pulmonary capillaries	Normal volume and flow Normal ventilation/perfusion matching Normal diffusing capacity
Blood	Normal PaO_2 Normal pH Normal electrolytes
Red blood cell	Normal hemoglobin content Normal binding to O_2
Heart	Normal cardiac output Appropriate distribution

Tissue Phase

Tissue capillaries	Normal membrane permeability
Tissues	Normal metabolism

*Normal oxygen transport depends upon several factors being normal in a variety of locations.

capability of the blood can affect gas transport and impair oxygenation of the blood. Decreased oxygenation of the blood causes hypoxemia, which is a leading cause of tissue hypoxia.

CONTROL OF RESPIRATION

Respiration is controlled by the interrelationship of a myriad of automatic and voluntary influences. It is not clear exactly how the clusters of cells that make up the respiratory control center in the medulla, the apneustic center in the lower pons, and the pneumotaxic center in the upper pons work to generate the respiratory rhythm. Current evidence seems to support a theory of a reverberating neural circuit being responsible for the basic rhythmic respiratory pattern. The two groups of respiratory neurons found in the medulla are surrounded by the reticular formation, which influences wakefulness and arousal. These two groups of respiratory neurons are self re-exciting, and the groups are mutually inhibitory. Impulses from the respiratory control center descend through the reticular spinal fibers in the lateral and ventral columns of the spinal cord. Whereas the medulla is thought to be responsible for the normal rhythmicity of the respiratory cycle, the pons is thought to be responsible for the smooth, regular characteristics evident in normal breathing. The outflow from these centers is influenced by a number of peripheral, somatic, and visceral receptors relaying information on changes in skin temperature, movement of peripheral joints, pain, exercise, emotions, and information on other changes in the internal or external environment, all of which can then affect respiration. In addition, the voluntary control of respiration located in the somatomotor and limbic forebrain structures allows us to speak, sing, or play a wind instrument. This voluntary control is mediated through two pathways, one to the reticular formation through the corticobulbar fibers and the other to the spinal cord through the corticospinal fibers of the dorsolateral column.

Respiration is also controlled by central and peripheral chemoreceptors. The central chemoreceptors, located on the ventral surface of the medulla in the area of the ninth and tenth cranial nerves, are sensitive to changes in the hydrogen ion (H+) concentration in the cerebrospinal fluid, which is affected by the CO_2 level in the blood. The central chemoreceptors are the primary receptors responsible for the minute-to-minute control of ventilation. The peripheral chemoreceptors are located in the carotid and aortic bodies. Those receptors in the aortic bodies are sensitive to the increased partial pressure of carbon dioxide in the arterial blood ($PaCO_2$) and the decreased partial pressure of oxygen in the arterial blood (PaO_2). Chemoreceptors in the carotid bodies are sensitive to increased $PaCO_2$, decreased pH, and decreased PaO_2. The hypoxic ventilatory drive mediated through the peripheral chemoreceptors is considered secondary because the central chemoreceptors are much more sensitive to changes in pH and $PaCO_2$.

However, the hypoxic drive can become very important in cases such as chronic obstructive pulmonary disease (COPD) where there is chronic CO_2 retention and therefore decreased sensitivity to changes in $PaCO_2$ by the central chemoreceptors. The peripheral chemoreceptors also seem to become more sensitive to changes in $PaCO_2$ during periods of exercise.

MUSCLES OF RESPIRATION

The major function of the respiratory muscles is to inflate the lungs by increasing the volume of the thoracic cage, and thereby decreasing the pleural space pressure. The major muscle of respiration is the diaphragm. The diaphragm's motor innervation is from C3-C5 by means of the phrenic nerve. The sensory innervation of the diaphragm is sparse. It has few proprioceptors with relatively more tendon organs than muscle spindles. The diaphragm is also not well supplied with pacinian corpuscles or free nerve endings, which discern pressure and pain sensations. Therefore, diaphragmatic pain is often indistinct and perceived as pain in the shoulder area.

The action of the diaphragm contributes two thirds of the tidal volume (TV) in the sitting or standing position and three fourths of the TV in the supine position. The average diaphragmatic movement for tidal volume in the upright position is 1.5 cm and in supine is 1.7 cm. During a forced vital capacity (FVC) maneuver the diaphragm contributes two thirds of the total volume and its excursion averages 9.5 cm. The diaphragm in the normal adult contains 55% high-oxidative slow-twitch muscle fibers, 21% high-oxidative fast-twitch muscle fibers, and only 24% low-oxidative fast-twitch muscle fibers. The predominance of high-oxidative slow-twitch muscle fibers makes the diaphragm resistant to fatigue.

The diaphragm is a pancake-shaped domed muscle that forms a movable boundary between the chest and abdominal cavities. Although the diaphragm has long been accepted as the major inspiratory muscle, more recently it has become clear that its efficiency is dependent on the action of the scalenus and abdominal muscles, the resting lung volume, and to some degree body position. The scalenus muscles elevate and fix the first two ribs, which stabilize the thorax so that it is not pulled inferiorly with diaphragmatic contraction. This stabilization of the upper thorax allows the diaphragm to increase the vertical diameter of the thorax more effectively. The abdominal muscles are known to be the major muscles of expiration and are particularly necessary to generate an explosive, expulsive expiratory effort in coughing. However, in the upright position, the abdominal muscles are active during inspiration. These muscles provide postural tone in the abdominal wall, which exerts pressure on the underlying abdominal contents and places the diaphragm higher in the thorax, and therefore at a better mechanical advantage for the next diaphragmatic contraction. With larger lung volumes the diaphragm is forced to a lower resting position, which is less efficient. The upright position versus the supine position also favors a lower diaphragmatic resting position, and therefore the length-tension relationship of the muscle fibers is less efficient.

The external intercostal muscles are active on inspiration and the internal intercostals are active during expiration. Both muscle groups are innervated by the intercostal nerves from T1-T12. The external intercostals are responsible for enlarging the thorax in both the sagittal and anteroposterior planes. These muscles also change the configuration of the chest wall, making it more elliptical during inspiration and more circular during expiration. The circumference of the rib cage increases by approximately 8 cm during a vital capacity maneuver. The intercostal muscles have a much better supply of muscle spindles, tendon organs, pacinian corpuscles, and free nerve endings. Together with the mechanoreceptors in the costovertebral joints, these sensory endings are thought to contribute to a person's perception of tightness in the chest during labored breathing and to the sensation of dyspnea.

The scalenus and sternocleidomastoid muscles are the major accessory inspiratory muscles. The scalenus muscles are innervated by ventral rami from levels C4-C7. The sternocleidomastoid muscles' motor innervation is from levels C2-C3 by means of the spinal accessory nerve. The scalenus muscles, although considered accessory muscles of respiration, are active even during quiet inspiration to stabilize the upper thorax. With deep breathing at larger lung volumes, the scalenus muscles become more active. Unlike the scalenus muscles, the sternocleidomastoid muscles are quiet during normal breathing. They contract towards the end of a maximum inspiration, elevating the sternum and increasing the AP diameter of the chest.

The abdominals, primarily the external and internal oblique muscles and rectus abdominis muscle, are innervated by the intercostal, subcostal, iliohypogastric, and ilioinguinal nerves from T5 to L1. Within the pulmonary system these muscles are used primarily for forceful exhalation, and can exert 300 to 400 cm H_2O pressure on the abdominal contents. Average flow rates during a vigorous cough approach the speed of sound. In the upright position, the abdominals are also active during inspiration to enhance diaphragmatic contraction. In supine, the abdominals are quiet during inspiration.

WORK OF BREATHING AND EXERCISE

A decreasing level of activity tolerance is frequently the most prominent symptom in patients with pulmonary problems. Changes in how the pulmonary system functions, both from pulmonary pathology and extrasystem causes, often affect the patient's mobility and ability to exercise. Before we can discuss the impact of pulmonary dysfunction on the musculoskeletal system, we must review briefly the work of breathing and how exercise and ventilation are related.

The pulmonary system very capably makes continuous minor adjustments in the ventilation pattern and rate to minimize the work of breathing. For any given alveolar ventilation, there is an optimum respiratory rate and tidal volume to keep the total mechanical work of breathing minimal. This balances the work needed to overcome the elastic recoil of the

lung against the work needed to overcome airway resistance and wasteful ventilation of the anatomic dead space. During quiet breathing the body uses 200 to 300 mL O_2/min, of which less than 5% or 3 to 14 mL O_2/min is used to support the work of breathing. Anything that increases airway resistance increases the work of breathing. For example, lying supine instead of standing upright, decreased lung volumes, increased flow rates, bronchial constriction, or bronchoendothelial hyperplasia can all cause a significant increase in the work of breathing. Anything that decreases the compliance of the lung or chest wall also increases the work of breathing.

Exercise increases the minute ventilation by increasing the respiratory rate and tidal volume. This increases the work of breathing so that the O_2 consumption of the respiratory musculature can reach 25% to 30% of total body O_2 consumption. During exercise, total body O_2 consumption is also increasing significantly. During mild to moderate exercise there is a linear relationship between minute ventilation and O_2 consumption. However, as exercise becomes vigorous and O_2 consumption reaches 50% to 75% of maximum, the minute ventilation rises out of proportion to the O_2 consumption. The work of breathing increases disproportionately so that the respiratory muscles take a larger and larger percentage of the total O_2 uptake. Several events occur to meet the increasing O_2 demand brought on by exercise: (1) cardiac output is increased with a tenfold increase in pulmonary blood flow to the bases of the lungs; (2) ventilation is increased with the total volume increasing in a linear relationship as exercise increases, until TV is approximately 50% FVC—after that, respiratory rate increases to a limit of about 50 breaths/min in young healthy adults; (3) ventilation/perfusion relationships are improved because of more uniform distribution of gas and blood within the lungs; and (4) tissue cells become more efficient in extracting O_2 from the circulating blood. With exercise, receptors in muscles and joints are activated so that even passive movement of the extremities causes hyperventilation. The increased pulmonary blood flow increases the pulmonary capillary pressure, which stimulates the J receptors. Activation of the J receptors triggers hyperventilation and produces reflex inhibition of the limb muscles. Even before exercise is begun, when it is only anticipated, learned responses from higher brain centers and cortical factors accelerate ventilation in an effort to meet expected metabolic demands from the muscles. During exercise the main chemical stimulus for hyperventilation is the increased concentration of H^+ ions, but this stimulus to ventilation takes longer than the neural changes. The peripheral chemoreceptors become more sensitive to PaO_2 levels during exercise so that the O_2 concentration is maintained at normal levels. Most often in normal subjects, the $PaCO_2$ is normal or slightly decreased during exercise because of the hyperventilation. With ongoing exercise the body temperature may increase 1 to 2 degrees, and this stimulates further hyperventilation.

Strenuous exercise may result in an O_2 consumption of 4 L/min and a total ventilation of up to 120 L/min, or 20 times the resting level of ventilation. When aerobic metabolism can no longer meet the energy demands of the exercising muscles, exercise becomes anaerobic. $PaCO_2$ usually drops slightly, the PaO_2 begins to fall, and the pH falls because of the production of lactic acid. Anaerobic metabolism is very inefficient, using approximately 19 times the glucose to generate the same amount of energy when compared with aerobic metabolism. The anaerobic threshold is usually exceeded due to circulatory factors rather than ventilatory factors. However, ventilatory impairment caused by any or all of the following can limit exercise tolerance: (1) gas exchange abnormalities leading to inadequate oxygenation of the blood; (2) decreased ventilatory response to exercise driving the alveolar and arteriolar O_2 down and the alveolar and arteriolar CO_2 up; (3) severe ventilation/perfusion mismatching creating an increased alveolar-arteriolar difference in O_2 tension; or (4) cor pulmonale, which would result in decreased cardiac output and decreased mixed venous O_2 content.

PULMONARY DYSFUNCTION

We have discussed briefly pulmonary physiology, particularly as it relates to mobility and exercise. We are now ready to discuss 10 factors that can influence mobility and the person's ability to interact with the environment. For each factor, possible respiratory and nonrespiratory causes will be explored to show how different pathologies result in pulmonary dysfunction. The symptoms and signs of this pulmonary dysfunction are detailed in Tables 13-2 to 13-5, which also show how a variety of symptoms and signs, caused by both pulmonary and nonpulmonary diseases, interrelate to cause the pulmonary dysfunction. It then becomes clear how impairment of the pulmonary system can alter a person's mobility.

PAIN

Pain anywhere in the body can have a striking effect on ventilation, usually increasing the ventilatory drive and causing hyperventilation. The pulmonary pathology most commonly associated with pain is lung cancer. However, there is no lung pain with lung cancer because the lung tissue itself has no sensory nerve endings specific for pain. This is unfortunate, because lung cancer is often advanced or metastasized before symptoms such as cough, weight loss, or shortness of breath are significant enough to cause the patient to seek medical attention. Once diagnosed, lung cancer often has a painful and fatal prognosis with only a 10% five-year survival rate. This statistic has not changed appreciably in the past three decades. Pain from lung cancer is experienced as the cancer invades the mediastinum, pleura, or chest wall or metastasizes to other structures such as the brain and bone. Because bone metastases are present in 25% of all lung cancer patients, the patient may experience a boring type of bone pain, pathological fractures, hy-

Table 13-2. Symptoms of Respiratory Dysfunction in Pulmonary Disease

DISEASE	DYSPNEA	COUGH	SPUTUM
Lung cancer	Possible	Productive	Purulent, minimal
Pulmonary edema	+, acute or gradual onset	Dry or productive	Pink, frothy
Cystic fibrosis	+	Productive	Mucoid/purulent, ↑ viscosity, copious
Asthma	+, acute onset	Dry or productive	Tenacious with mucus plugs
Chronic bronchitis	+, on exertion	Productive	Mucoid, purulent
Pneumonia	Occasionally	Productive	Purulent
Diffuse interstitial fibrosis	+, insidious onset	Dry	−
Pneumoconiosis	+, insidious onset	−	−
Emphysema	+, insidious onset	− or productive	Mucoid
Pulmonary emboli	+	Dry or productive	Mucoid
Lung abscess	−	Productive	Purulent, foul-smelling, copious
Croup (laryngotracheobronchitis)	+	Barking	↑ viscosity

Key: +, present; −, not present; ↑, increased.

pertrophic osteoarthropathy, and joint pain. Intercranial metastases can result in movement dysfunction (similar to hemiplegia), epilepsy, personality changes, speech defects, and confusion. Pain, joint changes, and pathological fractures all combine to decrease the patient's mobility. If the pleura are involved, breathing and coughing will be very painful and the patient will try to minimize chest wall expansion and limit tidal volume. The involvement of the lung tissue can cause consolidation, blockage of airways, and atelectasis resulting in increased ventilation/perfusion mismatching, decreased oxygenation of the blood, and decreased exercise tolerance. The problem of decreased exercise tolerance is often compounded by inadequate nutrition and weight loss, which cause muscular weakness and wasting.

Although the lung itself is not a source of pain, other parts of the pulmonary system do contain sensory nerve endings specific for pain. The pleura and chest wall are particularly rich in pain receptors. Therefore, pathologies such as pleurisy, fractured ribs, or burns and incisions on the chest wall cause severe localized pain that diminishes the person's ability to breathe deeply, cough, rotate the thorax, stoop, or lift. Pain from rib fractures will decrease markedly over the first 10 days, although coughing may cause pain for six months. Pain generated by the standard posterolateral thoracotomy incision markedly decreases FVC and maximum minute ventilation

HEMOPTYSIS	CHEST PAIN	CNS CHANGES	APPETITE
Possible	Possible, pleuritic	Metastasis to brain may cause changes	Depressed, weight loss
Streaking	—	—	Depressed
Streaking	—	—	Depressed, malabsorption, weight loss
—	—	Anxious	—
Streaking	—	Morning headaches	—
—	Pleuritic with some pneumonias	Headaches	Depressed
—	Possible, pleuritic	—	Weight loss
—	—	—	Weight loss
—	—	—	Depressed, weight loss
Streaking	Pleuritic, substernal	Headache, apprehension, agitation	—
Streaking	Possible, pleuritic	Headache	Depressed, nausea
—	—	Restless, irritable	Depressed

(MMV) and causes ipsilateral shoulder movement to be painful and weak. Following any painful chest trauma, chest wall excursion and ventilation are reduced nonuniformly, ventilation/perfusion mismatching increases, and there is often a drop in PaO_2. This can result in tissue hypoxia and a diminished exercise tolerance.

Pain outside the pulmonary system almost always causes ventilatory changes, which may then result in movement dysfunction. For example, following an abdominal incision, the vital capacity and expiratory flow rates are significantly reduced. This can lead to decreased PaO_2, secretion retention, fever, weakness, malaise, and decreased activity tolerance, all present because of the effect of pain on the pulmonary system. The patient would also have guarded movement of the trunk as a direct result of the incisional pain in the abdominal muscles.

EDEMA

Edema within the lungs can be caused by intrinsic pulmonary pathology, by secondary effects from pathology of other organ systems, or by environmental factors, any of which will result in similar pulmonary dysfunction. Pulmonary edema is caused by damage to the pulmonary capillary bed, which increases the permeability of these capillaries. This leads to engorgement of the peribronchial and perivascular spaces known as interstitial edema. At a

Table 13-3. Signs of Respiratory Dysfunction in Pulmonary Disease

DISEASE	TACHYPNEA	BREATH SOUNDS	CHEST EXPANSION	CHEST PERCUSSION
Lung cancer	Possible	Wheezing, friction rubs	Normal	Dull
Pulmonary edema	+	Rales	Normal, ↓ lung compliance	Dull
Cystic fibrosis	+	Rales, rhonchi, bronchial breath sounds	↓ lateral excursion	Normal or dull
Asthma	+	Wheezing	Normal	Normal or hyperresonant
Chronic bronchitis	+	Rales, rhonchi	Normal	Normal
Pneumonia	+	Rales, rhonchi, bronchial breath sounds	↓, asymmetrical	Dull
Diffuse interstitial fibrosis	+, insidious onset	Dry rales, friction rub, ↓ breath sounds	↓, ↓ lung compliance	Dull
Pneumoconiosis	Possible	Dry rales, rhonchi	↓, ↓ lung compliance	Dull
Emphysema	+	↓ breath sounds	↓, en bloc	Hyperresonant
Pulmonary emboli	+	Rales, wheezing, friction rub, ↓ breath sounds	↓ same side	Dull
Lung abscess	−	Rales, rhonchi, bronchial breath sounds, ↓ breath sounds	Normal	Dull
Croup (laryngotracheobronchitis)	+	Stridor	Substernal/intercostal retractions	Normal

Key: PFTs, pulmonary function tests; ABGs, arterial blood gases; +, present; −, not present; ↑, increased; ↓, decreased; PaO₂, partial pressure of oxygen in arterial blood; PaCO₂, partial pressure of carbon dioxide in arterial blood; VC, vital capacity; FRC, functional reserve capacity; RV, residual volume; TV, tidal volume; AP, anteroposterior; NA, not applicable.

later stage fluid crosses into the alveoli and they become unventilated, so that oxygenation of the blood cannot occur. Damage to the pulmonary capillaries can be caused by lung contusion, left ventricular failure, hypoxia, hypercapnea, uremia, acute renal failure, or increased intracranial pressure.

Environmental factors that may result in pulmonary edema are near drowning, smoke inhalation, inhalation of chemical fumes, radi-

PFTs	ABGs	FEVER	CYANOSIS	CLUBBING	MUSCULOSKELETAL CHANGES
Normal or ↓ volumes, normal flows	↓ PaO_2, ↓ $PaCO_2$	+, low grade	Possible, central	+	Myalgias, painful swollen joints, bone pain, sensory/motor neuropathy
Normal or ↓ volumes, normal flows	↓ PaO_2, $PaCO_2$ (↓ early and ↑ late) ↓ PaO_2, ↑ $PaCO_2$	Possible with sepsis	+, central and peripheral	–	Labored breathing, use of accessory muscles
↓ VC, ↑ FRC and RV, ↓ flows	↓ PaO_2, ↑ $PaCO_2$	+	+, central	+, early	↑ AP diameter of chest, kyphosis, flat diaphragm, general muscle weakness
Normal or ↑ volumes, ↓ flows	↓ PaO_2, ↓ $PaCO_2$	–	+, central	–	Labored breathing, use of accessory muscles
↓ VC, ↑ FRC and RV, ↓ flows	↓ PaO_2, ↑ $PaCO_2$	+ with exacerbations	+, central	+, late	Use of accessory muscles
Normal volumes, normal flows	↓ PaO_2, normal $PaCO_2$	+	+, central	–	Myalgias, use of accessory muscles
↓ volumes, normal flows	Normal or ↓ PaO_2, normal or ↓ $PaCO_2$	–	+, central	+	Labored breathing, use of accessory muscles
↓ volumes, normal flows	↓ PaO_2, normal $PaCO_2$	–	+, central	–	Muscle weakness, muscle wasting
↓ VC and TV, ↑ FRC and RV, ↓ flows	↓ PaO_2, ↑ $PaCO_2$ (late)	–	+, peripheral	+, late	Barrel chest, flat diaphragm, use of accessory muscles, muscle wasting
↓ VC, normal TV, FRC, RV, normal flows	↓ PaO_2, ↓ $PaCO_2$	+, low grade	+, central	–	Use of accessory muscles
Normal volumes, normal flows	↓ PaO_2, normal $PaCO_2$	+, spiking	+, central	+	Use of accessory muscles, muscle weakness
NA (infants)	↓ PaO_2, ↓ $PaCO_2$	+, low grade	+, central	–	Labored breathing, use of accessory muscles

ation exposure of the chest, heroin overdose, severe burns, or high altitudes. The resulting pulmonary dysfunction includes pulmonary congestion, dyspnea, cough, production of frothy sputum, cyanosis, increased $PaCO_2$, decreased PaO_2, decreased lung compliance, increased work of breathing, hypoventilation, increased ventilation/perfusion mismatching, and an increased alveolar-arterial O_2 difference. The outcome is that more of the O_2 con-

Table 13-4. Symptoms of Respiratory Dysfunction in Nonpulmonary Disease

DISEASE	DYSPNEA	COUGH	SPUTUM	HEMOPTYSIS
Fractured Ribs	+, acute onset	Painful	−	Possible
Kyphoscoliosis	−	−	−	−
Ankylosing spondylitis	−	−	−	−
Obesity	+	−	−	−
Aspiration of foreign body	+, acute onset	Barking	−	−
Poliomyelitis	+, gradual, progressive	Weak	−	−
Guillain-Barré syndrome	+, gradual, worsening	Weak	−	−
Amyotrophic lateral sclerosis	+, gradual, worsening	Weak	−	−
Myasthenia gravis	+	Weak	−	−
Multiple sclerosis	−	−	−	−
Muscular dystrophy	+ on exertion	Weak	−	−
Parkinson's disease	−	−	−	−
Stroke	−	↓ cough reflex	Possible ↑ production	−
Quadriplegia	Possible	Weak	−	−
Smoke inhalation	+, acute or gradual onset	Productive	Sooty	Possible
Systemic lupus erythematosus	+	Dry	−	Possible
Scleroderma	+ on exertion	−	−	−
Rheumatoid arthritis	−	−	−	−

Key: +, present; −, not present; ↑, increased; ↓, decreased.

sumption is used to aerate stiff, wet lungs. This decreases the amount of O_2 available to the muscles for activity. Tissues may become hypoxic, the anaerobic threshold is lowered, exercise becomes inefficient, and activity tolerance can be severely impaired.

INFLAMMATION

Inflammation within the pulmonary system can be caused by a number of pathologies or environmental factors. The pathologies may be primary to the pulmonary system or may arise in other body systems with secondary effects causing inflammation within the lungs. A few pathologies will be discussed briefly to show you how the pathology or environmental factor causes respiratory dysfunction, which then compromises how a person moves or exercises.

Sudden infant death syndrome (SIDS) is a

CHEST PAIN	CNS CHANGES	APPETITE
Sharp, localized	—	—
Anterior chest pain	—	Possible weight loss
—	—	—
—	—	Increased weight gain
—	—	—
—	—	—
—	Disorientation, ↑ fatigue	—
—	—	Weight loss
—	↑ fatigue	—
—	Emotionally labile	—
—	—	Weight loss
—	↑ fatigue	—
—	Headache, ↓ consciousness, emotionally labile, ↓ mental acuity, poor judgment	—
—	—	—
—	Headache, confusion, irritability, ↓ vision, ↓ judgment, hallucinations, convulsions, coma	Nausea
Possible pleuritic	Psychoses, convulsions	Depressed, weight loss
—	—	—
Possible pleuritic	↑ fatigue	Weight loss

pulmonary syndrome of unknown cause affecting infants of low birth weight, particularly premature infants. Although the cause is unknown, one of the manifestations of this syndrome is mild to moderate inflammation of the upper respiratory tract with pulmonary edema and congestion. These pathological changes then lead to chronic hypoventilation and hypoxemia. This decreases the amount of O_2 available to the muscles for movement, includ-

ing respiratory movement. Often these babies are described as quiet: They do not cry loudly, wave their arms, or kick their feet.

Cystic fibrosis (CF) is the most common genetically transmitted fatal disease of childhood. The disease is transmitted by an autosomal recessive trait and involves the exocrine glands, particularly of the lungs and pancreas. Although the disease is fatal, life expectancy has been significantly increased over the past

Table 13-5. Signs of Respiratory Dysfunction in Nonpulmonary Disease

DISEASE	TACHYPNEA	BREATH SOUNDS	CHEST EXPANSION	CHEST PERCUSSION
Fractured ribs	+	↓ breath sounds	↓ same side, paradoxical, asymmetrical	Normal
Kyphoscoliosis	−	Possible bronchial breath sounds, ↓ breath sounds	Asymmetrical	Normal
Ankylosing spondylitis	−	Possible ↓ breath sounds	↓ , fixed chest cage	Normal
Obesity	Possible	↓ breath sounds	↓	Normal or dull
Aspiration of foreign body	+	Stridor, wheezing, rhonchi, absent breath sounds	↓ same side, asymmetrical	Normal or dull
Poliomyelitis	−	Normal	↓ , asymmetrical	Normal
Guillain-Barré syndrome	−	↓ breath sounds	↓ , possible asymmetrical	Normal
Amyotrophic lateral sclerosis	+	Rales, ↓ breath sounds	↓	Normal
Myasthenia gravis	+	↓ breath sounds	↓ , asymmetrical	Normal
Multiple sclerosis	−	Rales, ↓ breath sounds	↓	Normal
Muscular dystrophy	−	Rales, ↓ breath sounds	↓	Normal
Parkinson's disease	−	↓ breath sounds	↓	Normal
Stroke	−	Possible wheezing, ↓ breath sounds hemiplegic side	↓ hemiplegic side, asymmetrical	Normal
Quadriplegia	Possible	Rales, ↓ breath sounds	Paradoxical, ↓	Normal

Key: PFTs, pulmonary function tests; ABGs, arterial blood gases; +, present; −, not present; ↑, increased; ↓, decreased; VC, vital capacity; FRC, functional reserve capacity; RV, residual volume; TLC, total lung capacity; TV, tidal volume; PaO_2, partial pressure of oxygen in arterial blood; $PaCO_2$, partial pressure of carbon dioxide in arterial blood; CO, carbon monoxide.

PFTs	ABGs	FEVER	CYANOSIS	CLUBBING	MUSCULOSKELETAL CHANGES
↓ VC and TV, normal FRC and RV, normal flows	Normal PaO_2, normal $PaCO_2$	−	−	−	Use of accessory muscles
↓ VC and TLC, normal TV and RV, normal flows	↓ PaO_2, normal or ↑ $PaCO_2$	−	−	−	−
↓ VC, ↑ FRC and RV, normal flows	↓ PaO_2, normal or ↑ $PaCO_2$	−	−	−	−
↓ VC and FRC, normal TV and RV, normal flows	↓ PaO_2, ↑ $PaCO_2$	−	Possible	−	↓ muscle efficiency, ↓ exercise tolerance
Normal volumes, normal or ↓ flows	↓ PaO_2, ↑ $PaCO_2$	−	Possible, central	−	Labored breathing, use of accessory muscles
Normal or ↓ volumes, ↓ flows	↓ PaO_2, ↑ $PaCO_2$	+	−	−	Respiratory muscle weakness, ↓ exercise tolerance
↓ VC, normal FRC and RV, ↓ flows	↓ PaO_2, normal or ↑ $PaCO_2$	−	Possible with respiratory muscle weakness	−	Respiratory muscle weakness, ↓ exercise tolerance
↓ volumes, ↓ flows	↓ PaO_2, ↑ $PaCO_2$	Possible with aspiration	−	−	Respiratory muscle weakness, use of accessory muscles, muscle wasting, ↓ exercise tolerance
↓ VC, normal FRC and RV, ↓ flows	↓ PaO_2, ↑ $PaCO_2$ (late)	Possible with aspiration	Possible late	−	Respiratory muscle weakness, ↓ exercise tolerance
↓ volumes, ↓ flows	↓ PaO_2, ↑ $PaCO_2$	−	−	−	↓ exercise tolerance
↓ volumes, ↓ flows	↓ PaO_2, ↑ $PaCO_2$	−	−	−	Muscle wasting, ↓ exercise tolerance
↓ volumes, ↓ flows	↓ PaO_2, normal or ↑ $PaCO_2$	−	−	−	↓ exercise tolerance
Normal volumes, normal flows	↓ PaO_2, normal $PaCO_2$	−	Possible	−	−
↓ volumes, normal or ↓ flows	↓ PaO_2, normal or ↑ $PaCO_2$	−	−	−	Use of accessory muscles, ↓ exercise tolerance

continued

Table 13-5. (continued)

DISEASE	TACHYPNEA	BREATH SOUNDS	CHEST EXPANSION	CHEST PERCUSSION
Smoke inhalation	Possible	Rales, wheezing, rhonchi	Normal, ↓ lung compliance	Normal or dull
Systemic lupus erythematosus	Possible	Rales, friction rub, ↓ breath sounds	Normal, ↓ lung compliance	Normal
Scleroderma	—	Normal	Normal, ↓ lung compliance	Normal
Rheumatoid arthritis	—	Unilateral friction rub	↓	Normal or dull

Key: PFTs, pulmonary function tests; ABGs, arterial blood gases; +, present; −, not present; ↑, increased; ↓, decreased; VC, vital capacity; FRC, functional reserve capacity; RV, residual volume; TLC, total lung capacity; TV, tidal volume; PaO_2, partial pressure of oxygen in arterial blood; $PaCO_2$, partial pressure of carbon dioxide in arterial blood; CO, carbon monoxide.

50 years. When CF was first described in the 1930s, 80% of affected children died during the first year of life. Currently, 75% of children with CF survive to adolescence or adulthood. Within the lung, the disease is manifested by increased abnormal mucus production. These tenacious secretions cause obstruction, infection, inflammation, and areas of parenchymal damage. These chronic pulmonary changes lead to increased work of breathing, increased ventilation/perfusion mismatching, air trapping, increased AP diameter of the chest with a low flat diaphragm decreasing diaphragmatic excursion, hypoxia, and hypercapnea. This means exercise tolerance may be severely limited with impaired motor planning, coordination, and balance. These patients also experience significant gastrointestinal absorption defects, which compromise their nutritional status. Because of these problems, they often have a wasted appearance, short stature, and delayed maturation. These children often do not participate in physical activities because they are awkward, have decreased stamina, and look different from their peers. Yet exercise is good for them, because it increases their physical capacity, aids in mucus clearance, and increases ventilation.

Asthma is a pulmonary disease characterized by periodic attacks of bronchospasm caused by an allergic reaction to dust, pollen, animal dander, aerosols, smoke, or upper respiratory tract infection. Children and adults with asthma are usually free of symptoms between attacks. However, during an asthmatic attack there can be severe bronchospasm, inflammation of the bronchial mucosa with thickening of the basement membrane, production of sticky opalescent mucus with mucus casts, air trapping with hyperinflated lungs, and increased ventilation/perfusion mismatching. This complex of pathological changes dramatically increases the work of breathing; because of the hyperinflation, all of the muscles of respiration are at a mechanical disadvantage to carry out this increased work load. Because the supine position increases airway resistance, these patients are usually sitting straight up in bed and gasping for air through the mouth. During an attack all other movement is kept to a minimum to conserve energy for the work of moving the chest wall. If asthma is severe in childhood, it can limit activity, which then contributes to decreased strength and endurance and increased weight gain. If a child is taking corticosteroids for the asthma, the drugs can cause growth depression and enhance weight gain. Some children and adult asthmatics have a hypersensitivity to exercise so that airway resistance rises significantly after only a few minutes of exercise. These persons require careful counseling in the importance of warm-

PFTs	ABGs	FEVER	CYANOSIS	CLUBBING	MUSCULOSKELETAL CHANGES
Normal volumes, ↓ flows	↓ PaO$_2$, normal PaCO$_2$	–	Possible cherry red skin color with CO poisoning	–	–
↓ volumes, normal flows	↓ PaO$_2$ normal or ↓ PaCO$_2$	+	–	–	Muscle weakness, ↓ exercise tolerance
↓ volumes, normal flows	↓ PaO$_2$, normal PaCO$_2$	–	–	–	↓ exercise tolerance
↓ volumes, normal flows	↓ PaO$_2$, normal PaCO$_2$	+, low grade	–	–	Muscle weakness, ↓ exercise tolerance

up and cool-down periods, types of exercise to use, regularity of exercise, and the selection of safe exercise environments.

Chronic bronchitis is a diagnosis given to a clinical symptom complex in which the person has a productive cough for at least three months of the year for two or more years. Cigarette smoking is the principal cause of chronic bronchitis. The incidence of chronic bronchitis increases in areas of high pollution or in workers exposed to chemical fumes or high dust concentrations. These irritating factors cause inflammation with hypertrophy of mucus glands. There is also an increased number of mucus glands to serous glands in the bronchial mucosa, which leads to increased mucus production. Over time this causes a slow rise in PaCO$_2$ and a drop in PaO$_2$, which means less O$_2$ is available to the tissues for movement and exercise. The fact that many patients with chronic bronchitis continue to smoke also brings into effect all the negative factors of smoking (which will be discussed later in this chapter). Chronic bronchitis is worsened by the aging process, prolonged bed rest, pregnancy, obesity, and increased left atrial pressure (mitral stenosis). Many of these factors in themselves cause pulmonary dysfunction, which results in changes in the person's ability to move and exercise. When these factors are combined with chronic bronchitis, the limits

set on the patient's exercise tolerance will be even more severe.

Pneumonia is a term used to describe a pulmonary symptom complex usually associated with bacterial infection (pneumococcal, staphylococcal, klebsiella). It is also used to denote aspiration, postoperative, postanesthesia, immunosuppressive, or radiation problems that secondarily affect the pulmonary system (aspiration pneumonia, pneumocystis carinii pneumonia, radiation pneumonitis). This symptom complex includes fever, increased respiratory rate, decreased FVC, decreased functional reserve capacity (FRC), increased sputum production, cough, chest pain, shortness of breath, decreased lung compliance, increased ventilation/perfusion mismatching, decreased O$_2$ uptake, weakness, and muscular aches. In addition, depending on the causative agent, other specific pulmonary pathology may occur. Aspiration pneumonia may include hemorrhage into the alveoli with transient consolidation. Pneumocystis carinii pneumonia, most commonly associated with acquired immune deficiency syndrome (AIDS), damages parenchymal cells and alters the alveolar-capillary permeability. Infections (such as pneumonia) that raise body temperature increase the metabolic rate and therefore the body's demand for O$_2$. The O$_2$ uptake, however, is decreased because ventilation is decreased and ventilation/

perfusion mismatching is increased. The work of breathing is increased due to mucus obstructing the airways and decreased lung compliance. Gas transport is affected by the presence of secretions, consolidation, and ventilation/perfusion mismatching. The resulting respiratory dysfunction is that of increased work for decreased oxygenation of the blood, and therefore decreased O_2 available to the tissues. This hypoxemia along with myalgias common with pneumonia cause the patient to limit movement and decrease activity tolerance.

Diffuse interstitial fibrosis (DIF) is a progressive restrictive pulmonary disease characterized by an increase in connective tissue within the lung. DIF may occur secondary to chronic bronchitis, viral pneumonia, drug reactions, chemical vapors, radiation exposure, or connective tissue disorders. Once diagnosed it has an average survival time of under four years. The most prominent symptom is shortness of breath. Other pathological changes include hyperventilation, cough, decreased lung compliance, impaired gas transport, ventilation/perfusion mismatching, decreased lung volumes, and hypoxemia. These factors significantly increase the work of breathing and decrease exercise tolerance. With DIF it is quite common for the PaO_2 to fall with exercise. It is interesting that patients with DIF have a high incidence of rheumatoid factor in their serum, whether or not they have joint problems. Conversely, patients with rheumatoid arthritis (RA) can have lung involvement in one of four ways: DIF, discrete nodules, Caplan's syndrome, or pleurisy. Rheumatoid patients with a high titer of rheumatoid factor are particularly likely to develop DIF with the same pathological changes outlined above.

Pneumoconiosis is a disease caused by the inhalation of organic (bacteria, viruses, fungal spores) or inorganic (industrial exhaust, dusts, smoke, fumes) agents. The organic agents cause more acute illness, whereas the inorganic agents cause chronic progressive debilitating illness. Table 13-6 is a list of some of the organic and inorganic substances that can cause pneumoconioses. These substances cause inflammation, edema, and diffuse fibrosis within the

Table 13-6. Causative Agents of Specific Pneumoconioses

CAUSATIVE AGENT	PNEUMOCONIOSIS
Organic Substances	
Coffee bean dust	Coffee worker's lung
Moldy cork dust	Suberosis
Cotton dust	Byssinosis
Moldy hay	Farmer's lung
Moldy redwood sawdust	Sequoiosis
Moldy sugarcane fiber	Bagassosis
Inorganic Substances	
Asbestos	Asbestosis
Beryllium dust	Berylliosis
Coal dust	Coalworker's pneumoconiosis
Iron dust	Siderosis
Silica	Silicosis
Tin	Stannosis

lung. This results in ventilation/perfusion mismatching, decreased lung compliance, increased residual volume (RV) caused by premature small airway closure, decreased diffusing capacity in some patients, inflammation of the airways, bronchospasm, shortness of breath, increased secretion production, decreased maximum breathing capacity (MBC), and hypoxemia. Because of the respiratory dysfunction, pulmonary reserve is severely limited and the work of breathing and O_2 demand of the respiratory muscles is significantly increased. This leads to decreased exercise tolerance, weakness, muscle wasting, and weight loss. Besides the general pulmonary picture, a specific type of pneumoconiosis may have other manifestations that can also affect movement. For example, silicosis can lead to an increased incidence of connective tissue disorders, particularly scleroderma and rheumatoid arthritis, both of which would limit movement.

Another environmental cause of inflammation in the pulmonary system is cigarette smoking. A single inhalation of cigarette smoke causes a 200% to 300% increase in airway resistance. Cigarette smoke damages the cilia, rendering ineffective this lung defense mechanism. Cigarette smoking also slows bacterial clearance by the macrophages, hindering a second lung defense mechanism. This results in a higher incidence of respiratory infections in smokers. One study of approximately 200 males showed the incidence of significant respiratory infection was nine times greater in smokers than in nonsmokers. Smoking also causes mucous gland hypertrophy and increased mucus production. Smoking also changes the composition of the bronchial mucus. Cigarette smoking impairs gas distribution and enhances ventilation/perfusion mismatching. Smokers also have a higher level of carbon monoxide (CO) in their lungs, which combines with hemoglobin to form carboxyhemoglobin. This means that 4% to 7% of the smoker's hemoglobin may be combined with CO, and therefore is unavailable to carry O_2 to the tissues. This decreases the person's work capacity by decreasing the O_2 content of the blood and the available O_2 at the tissue level. These are the more immediate pathological changes caused by smoking. They result in the increased work of breathing, decreased O_2 carrying capability of the blood, and increased incidence of possible repeated respiratory infection. Because of the large pulmonary reserve, these changes may result in no appreciable change in the normal person's ability to move and exercise. However, cigarette smoking also has long-term effects. Cigarette smoking is the most significant cause of lung cancer. Cigarette smokers have 10 to 20 times the risk of dying of lung cancer compared with nonsmokers. Cigarette smoking is the principal cause of chronic bronchitis. In addition, cigarette smoking is linked with emphysema, coronary artery disease, peripheral vascular disease, hypertension, stroke, low birth weights in infants, and small airway disease. All these long-term effects individually and collectively affect the person's ability to move and to exercise; many are discussed in this chapter. The information now available on secondhand smoke shows that these same pathological changes can be seen in nonsmokers who work or spend time in smoke-filled environments.

STRUCTURAL IMBALANCE

Structural integrity of the pulmonary system can be affected by pathologies that cause intrinsic structural changes in the lung tissue and those that cause imbalance in the thoracic wall. Emphysema is the primary example of a disease that actually destroys the internal structure of the lung parenchyma. Structural changes that affect the thoracic wall include kyphoscoliosis, ankylosing spondylitis, sternal abnormalities, and obesity. Related to obesity, but not directly causing changes in the chest wall, is pregnancy.

Emphysema is an irreversible pulmonary disease in which there is destruction of the acinus. Both alveolar walls and the surrounding capillary beds are destroyed. This leads to the formation of bullae. The elastic recoil of the lung is diminished and there is increased air trapping. The surface area available for gas exchange is decreased due to the destruction of the alveolar walls and capillary beds. The position of the diaphragm is low and flat and the AP diameter of the thorax is increased, both of which are due to the increased air trapping. The residual volume and functional reserve capacity are both increased and the vital capacity is decreased. These pathological changes lead to increased work of breathing because all the respiratory muscles must work in shortened ranges, and decreased oxygenation of the blood because of the decreased surface area for gas diffusion. Because the capillary beds are also destroyed, these patients exhibit pulmonary hypertension, which can progress to cor pulmonale. These changes in the respiratory system lead to insidious but progressive decreases in the patient's activity tolerance. In an effort to avoid shortness of breath, the patient does less and less physical work. Using the arms in over-the-head activities, vigorous recreation, and stair climbing are some of the first activities to be eliminated. With end-stage emphysema the patient is so short of breath with any activity, that dressing and eating may be impaired. These patients may become anorexic, and there is often muscle wasting and severe generalized weakness.

Kyphoscoliosis denotes abnormal curvature of the spine, specifically kyphotic changes in the thoracic region with lateral curvature in the cervical, thoracic, and lumbar regions. Kyphoscoliosis may be idiopathic, or it may be caused by neuromuscular weakness or disease such as poliomyelitis or quadriplegia. With kyphoscoliosis the lung tissue itself is normal; however, the respiratory mechanics are affected in proportion to the degree of abnormal angulation. These changes in the dynamics of the thorax could cause decreased total lung capacity (TLC), decreased FVC, increased RV, irregular distribution of inspired gas between the lungs and within the lungs, decreased chest wall compliance, increased ventilation/perfusion mismatching, and decreased MBC. These pulmonary changes result in increasing the work of breathing, cause dyspnea on exertion (DOE), and over time may cause alveolar hypoventilation, hypercapnea, hypoxemia, pulmonary hypertension, and cor pulmonale. With severe spinal deformity, the dynamics of the chest wall musculature will be impaired and O_2 demand will be increased. Because the body is out of alignment, other movement and exercise may also require increased O_2 and energy expenditure. As the lung ages and these structural changes cause alveolar hypoventilation, less O_2 will be available to the tissues, and mobility and exercise will be diminished.

Ankylosing spondylitis is a chronic inflammatory disease affecting the joints of the spine and the sacroiliac joints. Approximately 8% of patients with ankylosing spondylitis have pulmonary involvement. Involvement of the pulmonary system can take the form of patchy infiltrates in the upper lobes, pulmonary nodules with cavitation, pleural thickening, colonization by fungus, or interstitial fibrosis. Most patients with ankylosing spondylitis have a rigid thorax so that the dynamics of breathing depend upon the diaphragm. The amount of respiratory dysfunction depends upon the type and degree of pulmonary involvement. In most cases there are few significant respiratory symptoms, and the increased work of breathing is well tolerated unless other pulmonary pathology becomes evident. Because of the stiffness of the spine and sacroiliac joints, posture is affected and movement may be painful; however, these changes are a direct result of the ankylosing spondylitis and are not mediated through the pulmonary system.

Sternal deformities, such as pectus excavatum or pectus carinatum, cause no respiratory symptoms or significant changes in the mechanics of breathing. They are essentially only cosmetic deformities. Pectus carinatum may be associated with childhood asthma. These deformities have no impact on the person's ability to move or exercise.

Obesity denotes an increase over ideal body weight of 20% or more of ideal body weight. This extra weight represents a gross increase in body mass, which requires increased O_2 consumption and CO_2 production. The excess weight on the chest wall decreases chest wall compliance and increases the work of breathing four fold. The increased soft tissue in the abdominal area exerts pressure on the abdominal contents, forcing the diaphragm up into a higher resting position. This results in decreased expansion and ventilation of the lungs, especially at the bases, and leads to early small airway closure in the dependent lung regions. The bases of the lungs are hypoventilated, increasing ventilation/perfusion mismatching. Obesity acts as a restrictive impairment on the lungs. Expiratory reserve volume (ERV) and inspiratory reserve volume (IRV) are especially diminished, but all lung volumes and capacities are decreased, except residual volume, which is unchanged. In an effort to maintain minute ventilation, the respiratory rate is increased, adding to the work of breathing. In very obese patients, alveolar hypoventilation results in decreased PaO_2 and in some patients causes chronic, increased $PaCO_2$, which blunts the responsiveness of the central chemoreceptor area in the medulla. The work of breathing is further increased because of the abnormal length-tension relationships of the respiratory muscles. With long-standing obesity, the hypoventilation leads to chronic hypoxia, causing pulmonary hypertension and right ventricular hypertrophy. Therefore, the respiratory dysfunction caused by obesity increases the work of breathing. Even when this increased work load is met, alveolar ventilation is impaired. The obese patient is hypoxemic and yet has increased O_2 needs to support this extra soft tissue. This makes less O_2 available to the muscles for movement or exercise. Because of the extra weight, the skeletal muscles are required to work harder to move a body part through space or to exercise. Functionally, exercise tolerance is reduced and patients are more prone to DOE.

Pregnancy in the third trimester has some of the same effects as obesity on the pulmonary system. It impairs ventilation to the dependent lung regions, which results in early small airway closure and increased ventilation/perfusion mismatching. Pregnancy also decreases the voluntary lung volumes, particularly ERV, and increases respiratory rate. These changes increase the work of breathing, and make the woman feel as if she is unable to take a deep breath. To counteract some of these negative pulmonary changes, the increased level of progesterone in the pregnant woman increases her ventilatory drive so that normal PaO_2 levels can be maintained.

AMPUTATIONS

Amputations within the pulmonary system can occur physiologically or mechanically as a result of pulmonary pathology or trauma. Amputations can occur in both the pulmonary ventilatory system or the pulmonary circulatory system. Because of the degree of pulmonary reserve, the amputation has to be of significant magnitude before any respiratory dysfunction will be evident.

Pulmonary embolism is the primary example of a physiological amputation in the pulmonary circulatory system. Pulmonary embolism is the most common acute pulmonary disease among hospitalized patients and accounts for 50,000 to 100,000 deaths annually in the United States. The most common causes of pulmonary emboli are detached thrombi from the veins of the calf following orthopedic surgery or prolonged bed rest. If the pulmonary embolism is large and blocks over 65% of the pulmonary

circulation, acute right ventricular failure occurs, resulting in death within minutes. More commonly, the emboli lodge in smaller pulmonary vessels, blocking the pulmonary circulation. This results in pulmonary hypertension and increased right ventricular work. There is increased alveolar dead space, pneumoconstriction, possibly a pleural friction rub with pain on deep breathing, fever, hemoptysis, and, over time, loss of alveolar surfactant (which promotes atelectasis). Some pulmonary emboli can result in infarction of a portion of the lung. The degree of dyspnea, ventilation/perfusion mismatching, and hypoxemia are directly related to how much of the pulmonary circulation is affected by the emboli. The resultant degree of tissue hypoxia will determine how movement is affected in a given patient. If hypoxemia is significant, then motor function will be impaired.

Pneumonectomy or lobectomy are the primary examples of mechanical amputations of the pulmonary ventilatory and circulatory systems caused by pulmonary pathology. Because of the degree of pulmonary reserve, these amputations or resections are well tolerated. Following pneumonectomy, the volume of the remaining lung increases. The PaO_2 and $PaCO_2$ levels remain within the normal limits and gas diffusion remains normal. The patient's maximum breathing capacity is reduced and the patient may experience dyspnea on exertion with moderate to vigorous levels of exercise. Lung resections are usually performed through a posterolateral thoracotomy incision, which initially would cause pain and might limit movement of the hemithorax and the ipsilateral shoulder. Approximately 4 to 6 weeks following lung resection, there should be no discernible effect on the patient's movement. With a pneumonectomy the patient's exercise tolerance will be decreased due to the decrease in ventilatory reserve and maximum breathing capacity, which results in the patient's anaerobic threshold being reached more quickly.

Lobar consolidation resulting from pneumonia is an example of a physiological amputation in the pulmonary ventilatory system due to pulmonary pathology. The resulting respiratory dysfunction would be similar to a lobectomy. However, this dysfunction would be reversible as the consolidation cleared.

Aspiration of a foreign body is an example of a physiological amputation in the pulmonary ventilatory system caused by trauma. Depending on where the foreign body lodged, the resulting respiratory dysfunction would be similar to a lobectomy or pneumonectomy until the foreign body could be removed.

Traumatic pneumothorax is an example of a physiological amputation involving both the pulmonary ventilatory and circulatory systems as a result of trauma. If the trauma causes a tension pneumothorax, the patient is in a life-threatening situation due to the continually rising intrathoracic pressure, which collapses the lung and decreases venous return and cardiac output. If the trauma causes a simple pneumothorax, then the resulting respiratory dysfunction would be similar to a pneumonectomy except that it would be completely reversible when the lung was reinflated.

WEAKNESS AND ENDURANCE

Weakness of the respiratory muscles may result from pulmonary pathology, neuromuscular diseases, musculoskeletal changes in the configuration of the thorax, or any debilitating condition that decreases the patient's energy stores or requires protracted bed rest.

Chronic obstructive pulmonary disease (COPD) is a prime example of a pulmonary pathology that affects the efficiency of the respiratory pump and decreases the endurance of the respiratory musculature. With COPD the residual volume becomes very large, and because of air trapping the lungs are hyperinflated. This increase in lung volume moves the diaphragm caudally to a low, flattened position, increases the AP diameter of the rib cage, causes anterior bowing of the sternum, and can contribute to kyphosis of the thoracic spine. These changes in the configuration of the thorax change the length-tension relationships of the respiratory muscles, putting them in their shortened ranges and thereby making them less efficient. The work of breathing is in-

creased, and yet the volume of gas these muscles are able to move in and out of the lungs (breathing efficiency) is decreased. To counteract the decreased efficiency of the respiratory pump, the accessory muscles of respiration become more active, which further increases the work of breathing and the O_2 consumption of the respiratory muscles.

COPD also destroys lung parenchyma and significantly decreases the elastic recoil of the lung. These changes result in the air trapping already noted, but also make exhalation an active respiratory phase. Because the passive recoil of the lung is diminished and the thorax is rigid in a hyperinflated posture, contraction of the abdominal muscles and internal intercostal muscles is needed to move air out of the chest. Changing exhalation from a passive to an active process significantly increases the work of breathing. Airway resistance in COPD is also increased due to bronchospasm, increased secretions in the airways, and inflammation. This airway resistance may be as much as six times the normal airway resistance, which markedly increases the work of breathing. COPD patients often experience dyspnea, and over time progressively reduce their activity to avoid this unpleasant sensation, which further decreases the endurance of the respiratory muscles.

End-stage COPD usually has the patient gasping for breath so that even eating is problematic. These patients often lack the pulmonary reserve to prepare or eat nourishing meals. This lack of proper nutrition means the energy stores in the muscles are not replaced, which further weakens the muscles and limits the patient's ability to exercise, move, or breathe. These factors mean that even at rest, the COPD patient's cost of breathing (O_2 consumption), is 4 to 10 times that of a normal person. Because so much of the O_2 must be directed to the respiratory muscles, these patients become short of breath at progressively lower levels of activity. They routinely continue to limit their activity, until finally they are having difficulty with the simple activities of daily living.

A number of neuromuscular conditions can significantly affect respiratory muscle function and cause pulmonary dysfunction. These conditions include poliomyelitis, Guillain-Barré syndrome, amyotrophic lateral sclerosis (ALS), multiple sclerosis (MS), cerebral palsy (CP), parkinsonism, and hemiplegia. Although the specific mechanism for pathological changes may vary, the resulting respiratory dysfunction has many common elements. A few of these conditions will be briefly discussed, and the common overall pulmonary changes caused by these conditions will be explained.

Poliomyelitis is a viral disease that attacks the motor nerve cells in the spinal cord and brain stem. Both the diaphragm and intercostal muscles can be weakened or paralyzed in this disease. Guillain-Barré syndrome is of unknown etiology, but often follows a viral illness and may be related to the immune system. This syndrome is characterized by ascending symmetrical motor paralysis followed by sensory changes such as burning, tingling, and numbness of the extremities. Both the intercostal muscles and diaphragm may be involved. Paralysis usually reaches its peak in 7 to 10 days, and is usually slowly reversible, taking weeks to months for recovery. Both poliomyelitis and Guillain-Barré syndrome can acutely change the patient's ability to use muscular activity to ventilate the lungs or interact with the environment. In addition to the common changes seen in the pulmonary system, neuromuscular conditions often require bed rest, intubation, and mechanical ventilation, which also affect respiratory function.

Other neuromuscular conditions, such as ALS and myasthenia gravis, change the patient's ability to use muscular activity to breathe or move; however, this occurs in a slowly progressive pattern over a period of years. ALS is a degenerative disease that involves both upper and lower motor neurons. Muscles innervated by both cranial and spinal nerves are usually involved. The disease course is one of progressive muscular weakness and wasting, eventually leading to profound weakness of the respiratory muscles and ultimately death. Myasthenia gravis is a neuromuscular disease of unknown etiology, which

has its primary abnormality at the neuromuscular junction. Transmission of impulses from nerve to muscle is impaired by a decrease in the number of receptors in the muscle for the neurotransmitter substance. This causes weakness and fatigue of voluntary muscles, most frequently those innervated by the cranial nerves. As a result these patients exhibit ptosis, dysphonia, and dysphagia, which can lead to aspiration problems. These chronic neuromuscular diseases profoundly change how a patient is able to move and interact with the environment. Simple activities become more difficult, with increasing levels of energy expenditure required, until even breathing becomes too difficult and respiratory failure occurs.

Neuromuscular diseases commonly exhibit a restrictive ventilatory pattern. Total lung capacity is reduced, with residual volume normal or slightly increased. The major change is decreased vital capacity. With end-stage disease, even tidal volume may be decreased. Although respiratory rate increases, maximum minute ventilation is decreased. The changed breathing pattern is less efficient, resulting in hypoventilation. The abdominal muscles often cannot generate an effective cough, which can lead to retained secretions, areas of atelectasis, and recurrent respiratory tract infections. There is often CO_2 retention, which can depress the ventilatory centers, and hypoxemia may result. With hemiplegia the breathing pattern is asymmetrical. During quiet breathing, upper chest expansion is decreased about 10% on the hemiplegic side while lower chest expansion is symmetrical. During voluntary deep breathing, upper chest expansion is decreased about 15% and lower chest expansion decreased about 10% when the hemiplegic side is compared with the normal side. These common pathological changes in the pulmonary system (like the neuromuscular diseases that cause them) are often progressive, leading to total respiratory collapse, which is often the cause of death in these patients.

DEGENERATION

Chronic obstructive pulmonary disease causes degeneration within the pulmonary system.

Specifically, COPD causes (1) inflammation of the airways, leading to changes in the bronchial mucosa such as mucous gland proliferation and damaged cilia; (2) destruction of alveolar walls with loss of alveolar surface area for gas exchange; and (3) destruction of the pulmonary capillary bed resulting in pulmonary hypertension and cor pulmonale. These three degenerative pulmonary changes common to COPD lead to severe respiratory dysfunction, which then compromises other body systems and leads to muscular weakness (Fig. 13-2).

The normal aging process also causes some degenerative changes within the pulmonary system. With age, the lung loses some of its natural elastic recoil, which results in the early closure of small airways, paticularly in the dependent lung regions. In young, healthy persons airway closure would occur only at low lung volumes, but in the elderly, airway closure will occur at higher lung volumes, possibly at FRC. Cigarette smoking also affects the terminal bronchioles, contributing to early airway closure and atelectasis in the elderly. With age, ventilatory ability declines, the physiological dead space increases because of less uniform ventilation/perfusion matching, and the diffusing capacity decreases. All these changes work together to decrease the PaO_2. Airway resistance does not change with age. Lung volumes within the total lung capacity alter with age; most noticeably, the residual volume increases and the vital capacity decreases, so that at age 70 the vital capacity is about 75% of what it was at age 30. The TLC is usually unchanged. The compliance of the chest wall is decreased, often with increased AP diameter and kyphosis of the thoracic spine. Maximum O_2 uptake is also diminished. These normal changes seen with the aging process are insidious, and because of the degree of pulmonary reserve, they often are not subjectively recognized until the seventh or eighth decade of life. Even before they are recognized, the person has been making slight alterations in activity patterns, exercise, and recreational pursuits.

LOSS OF CENTRAL CONTROL

As already discussed, respiration is controlled by neural, chemical, and voluntary mechanisms. If the pons and medulla were obliterated, respiration would cease. However, there are many lesser pathological or traumatic factors that affect the central nervous system and have an effect on respiratory function. In addition, the CNS is extremely sensitive to changes in the H+ ion concentration in the cerebrospinal fluid, which is affected by the $PaCO_2$. Table 13-7 lists the significant changes that can occur within the CNS as a result of hypercapnea. The CNS also has a higher than average rate of O_2 consumption, and is therefore sensitive to a low PaO_2. Table 13-8 lists the CNS alterations that can occur because of hypoxemia. To show the close relationship between the CNS and the pulmonary system, and how each can affect the other, a few disorders arising from pathology or trauma will be discussed.

Depression of the CNS from any cause (eg, trauma, stroke, ischemia, metabolic alkalosis, alcohol, or the overdose of opiates, barbiturates, or sedatives) will result in depression of the ventilatory centers and hypoventilation.

Table 13-7. CNS Changes Caused by Hypercapnea

Headache
Dizziness
Drowsiness/agitation
Dimness of vision
Flattened affect
Decreased memory
Decreased insight
Clouding of intellect
Decreased ability to concentrate
Decreased motor planning skills
Depression
Apathy
Disorientation
Visual/auditory hallucinations
Unconsciousness
Convulsions
Coma

Table 13-8. CNS Changes Caused by Hypoxemia

Headache
Restlessness/combativeness
Somnolence
Decreased judgment
Sensory disorders
Impaired motor function
Confusion
Delirium
Coma

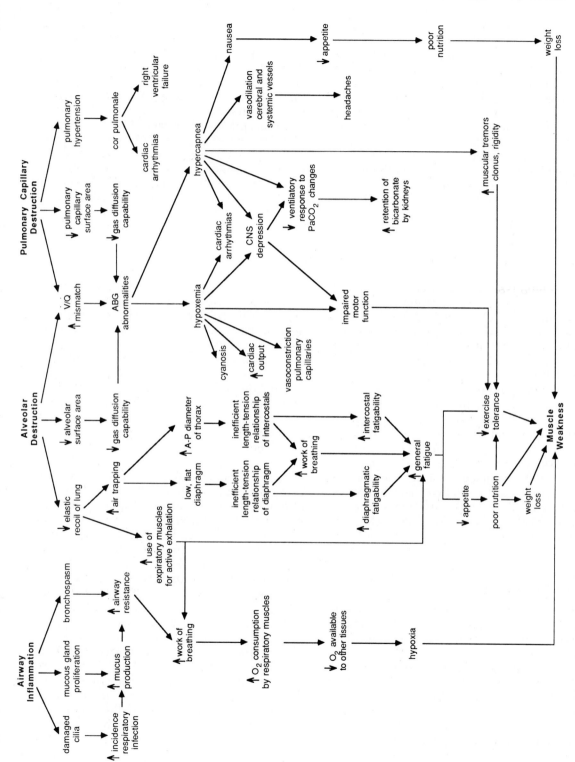

Figure 13-2. Effects of degenerative changes in COPD on the pulmonary system and other body systems. (Peggy Clough, 1989)

Lesions in the respiratory centers in the medulla produce chaotic breathing in which both frequency and depth vary. Lesions in the lower pons can cause apneustic breathing, in which each deep inspiration is followed by a pause, or cluster breathing, wherein three or four breaths are followed by a pause. Lesions in the upper pons or midbrain result in central neurogenic hyperventilation. Cerebellar involvement can decrease ventilation, and the patient may have disordered control of the expiratory muscles. With involvement of the cerebral hemispheres, Cheyne-Stokes respiration may occur. This breathing pattern shows a smooth incremental-decremental change in tidal volume separated by periods of apnea. Encephalopathies can also affect the breathing pattern. The respiratory system itself has profound effects on the CNS and its efferent neurons, as shown in Tables 13-7 and 13-8. Psychological factors such as anxiety or fear can increase the central respiratory drive and ventilation. Pathology in any body system may affect ventilation. For example, increased body temperature increases the central respiratory drive and increases ventilation. Atherosclerosis, involving cerebral arteries, can cause alveolar hypoventilation. Unfortunately, nothing to do with the nervous system is straightforward. The exact location of the lesion, other body systems affected by the pathology, the response of the respiratory system, the activity of all buffer systems to maintain the internal homeostasis, and psychological factors would all interrelate and modify the interaction between the CNS and the pulmonary system.

MUSCLE IMBALANCE

The respiratory musculature normally works synergistically to carry out smooth rhythmic motion of the chest wall, thereby aerating the lung. When any of the respiratory musculature becomes paretic or paralyzed, muscle imbalance results. The activity and function of all the respiratory muscles may be affected, and the respiratory pattern may become very inefficient. The dysfunction is increased if more than one respiratory muscle is involved.

The diaphragm may be weakened or paralyzed. COPD diminishes the effectiveness of the diaphragm by moving its resting position caudally. This position change aligns the muscle fibers of the diaphragm horizontally so that with diaphragmatic contraction the diaphragm constricts the lower rib cage. The diaphragm is therefore working antagonistically against the pull of the external intercostal muscles. The lowered position of the diaphragm also decreases its downward excursion so that the vertical diameter of the chest is not increased as much with each contraction. The air trapping seen with COPD also has the intercostal muscles working in their shortened ranges, making them less efficient in expanding the rib cage. Because of these changes in muscle dynamics, the sternocleidomastoid muscles become much more active, moving the upper rib cage in a cephalic direction and stabilizing the thorax against the pull of the other respiratory muscles.

Diaphragmatic paralysis may result from phrenic nerve invasion by bronchogenic cancer, poliomyelitis, Huntington's chorea, diphtheria, measles, surgical trauma, Guillain-Barré syndrome, or motor neuron trauma or disease. Paralysis of one hemidiaphragm will decrease ventilation in the ipsilateral lung by 25% to 50% and expiratory flow rates may be slightly decreased. Patients usually have no subjective symptoms but may have dyspnea on exertion at lower levels of exercise. Bilateral diaphragmatic paralysis may also be well tolerated if the person is in the upright position, not engaged in heavy exercise, and the other respiratory muscles are intact. However, these patients will have DOE because the vital capacity has been decreased by 25% to 50%. These patients also become severely short of breath if lying supine for even 15 to 20 seconds. This happens because when the patient is supine and the external intercostal muscles contract instead of the rib cage expanding, as it does in the upright position, the diaphragm and abdominal contents are sucked up into the rib cage. The abnormal upward motion of the diaphragm during inspiration is facilitated by gravity in the supine position. This means that the normal intercostal muscles are made less efficient by diaphragmatic paralysis, particularly in the supine position.

Paralysis of the abdominal muscles decreases the efficiency of the diaphragm in the upright position. However, the major effect is the decreased forcefulness of the cough, which can lead to retention of secretions, consolidation, atelectasis, and repeated respiratory infections.

In quadriplegia, all the muscles of respiration may be weakened or paralyzed. If the diaphragm, as well as the intercostal and abdominal musculature, is involved, the effect on ventilation is devastating and these patients must be on mechanical ventilation to sustain a PaO_2 compatible with life. Because of the high level (C3-C5) at which the phrenic nerve exits the spinal cord, many quadriplegic patients may have the diaphragm intact but both the intercostal and abdominal muscles paralyzed. This pattern of paralysis can result in paradoxical breathing. If the chest wall and abdominal wall are flaccid and the diaphragm contracts, creating a negative pleural space pressure, the abdominal wall will move outward and the chest wall inward during inspiration. In patients with paradoxical breathing, chest expansion is expressed as a negative number. In the upright position, because of the lack of abdominal tone, the diaphragm will assume a lowered resting position and therefore be at a mechanical disadvantage. Quadriplegic patients thus usually require abdominal binders to ensure proper diaphragmatic positioning in the upright posture. In the supine position, the effect of gravity on the abdominal contents is sufficient to position the diaphragm for more efficient contraction. The scalenus and sternocleidomastoid muscles are more active in quadriplegic patients. They contract to move the upper chest cephalad and stabilize it against the downward pull of the diaphragm.

Two strategies may be used to overcome respiratory muscle imbalance. If the muscle's nerve supply has been interrupted, resulting in paralysis, then positioning, equipment, and exercises for the remaining respiratory muscles can be used to compensate for the paralyzed muscle. If the respiratory muscle is only paretic, then endurance training can be used to increase the capillary density, mitochondria, and level of oxidative enzymes within the involved musculature. These changes within the muscle, along with adequate nutrition, will increase the oxidative capacity of the muscle and its endurance.

BURNS AND SKIN PROBLEMS

Burn injuries of any significant magnitude always trigger a response in the pulmonary system. The response is particularly severe with an inhalation injury, but can also be dramatic with a purely thermal injury.

Three specific mechanisms cause respiratory dysfunction following smoke inhalation injuries. The first, inhalation of carbon monoxide, is the most life threatening. Carbon monoxide is a colorless, odorless, tasteless, nonirritating gas produced by the burning of carbon-containing substances. This gas has over 200 times the affinity for hemoglobin than does oxygen. Therefore, the CO in the lungs will quickly diffuse into the pulmonary capillaries, enter the red blood cells, and combine with hemoglobin to form carboxyhemoglobin. This decreases the available hemoglobin binding sites for O_2, decreases the O_2-carrying capacity of the blood, and therefore causes hypoxemia, hypoxia, and possibly death.

The second mechanism for respiratory dysfunction is direct injury from inhaling hot, dry air at approximately 300°F and heated particulate matter. Most of the injury from inhalation of hot air occurs in the upper airway because most of the heat can be dissipated in the nasopharynx. Nasal hairs may be scorched, and there may be laryngospasm, edema of the laryngeal and tracheal mucosa, some bronchospasm, and increased mucus production. Most of the particulate matter is filtered in the upper airway, but some may reach the bronchial airways, causing direct damage to the mucosa.

The third mechanism causing respiratory dysfunction is the inhalation of noxious gases produced by the burning of different natural and man-made materials. The degree of pulmonary involvement depends upon the particular noxious gases inhaled and the amount of time exposed to these gases.

The clinical course of patients with smoke inhalation injuries is characterized by acute pulmonary insufficiency, followed by pulmonary edema related to surfactant inactivation or chemical pneumonitis, or both. Somewhat later in the clinical course, these patients are also susceptible to bronchopneumonia, possibly because of damage to the mucociliary clearance mechanism or because of the high incidence of sepsis.

Thermal injuries not involving inhalation injuries may also result in pulmonary edema or bronchopneumonia. The pulmonary edema may result from increased pulmonary vascular permeability and can be exacerbated by more than optimum fluid replacement. Bronchopneumonia may occur because of the impaired immune system and the enforced bed rest following a significant thermal injury. If the thoracic or abdominal walls are involved in the burn, a restrictive ventilatory pattern will be seen. This is particularly true if the burns are circumferential.

Burn injuries can cause serious respiratory dysfunction for weeks to months following the acute injury. During this time ventilation is impaired and gas diffusion may be diminished because of atelectasis, pulmonary edema, and bronchopneumonia, all of which decrease ventilation/perfusion matching. This dysfunction leads to hypoxemia, which impairs motor control and can decrease the O_2 available to the muscles. These patients are often on bed rest, which further weakens the musculoskeletal system. With thermal injuries and eschar formation, mobility can become very limited and painful.

Connective tissue constitutes 25% of the normal adult lung and is composed of collagen, elastin, and proteoglycans. Major connective tissue pathologies include systemic lupus erythematosus (SLE), scleroderma, polymyositis, dermatomyositis, and RA. All these pathologies can include pulmonary system involvement.

Systemic lupus erythematosus is a chronic inflammatory collagen vascular disorder. It usually involves the skin, joints, kidneys, lung, nervous system, and heart. Of all the connective tissue diseases, SLE has the highest rate of pulmonary involvement; 50% to 70% of these patients have pathological changes involving the lung. These pathological changes may include diffuse interstitial fibrosis, pleural effusion, pleurisy with a friction rub and pleural chest pain, pulmonary infiltrates, pneumonitis, uremic pulmonary edema, or atelectasis.

Scleroderma is a systemic inflammatory connective tissue disease that usually affects the skin, small blood vessels, gastrointestinal (GI) tract, kidneys, lungs, joints, and muscles. Raynaud's phenomenon is present in 90% of these patients. GI involvement affects the esophagus, small bowel, and colon. These patients may experience inflammatory joint changes and myopathies of proximal muscles. Approximately 50% of these patients exhibit pulmonary system involvement such as pulmonary fibrosis, pleural thickening, pulmonary edema, or pneumonitis.

Polymyositis is a diffuse inflammatory and degenerative disorder of striated muscle that causes symmetrical weakness and atrophy of proximal muscle groups. This muscular weakness may include the posterior pharyngeal muscles, which can lead to dysphagia and aspiration. This disease can cause weakness in the respiratory muscles, leading to a restrictive ventilatory pattern, hypoventilation, atelectasis, and lower lobe infiltrates. Five percent of these patients also exhibit changes within the lung parenchyma, including pulmonary fibrosis, aspiration pneumonia, or interstitial pneumonitis.

Dermatomyositis is very similar to polymyositis, except that the major dysfunction involves the skin rather than the muscles. Rheumatoid arthritis as a cause of pulmonary dysfunction was discussed earlier in this chapter. As in polymyositis and dermatomyositis, approximately 5% of rheumatoid arthritics have pulmonary system involvement.

Although there may be some differences in the respiratory dysfunction caused by the various connective tissue diseases, the primary pattern is one of restrictive ventilatory impairment. Lung compliance is decreased, all lung volumes are decreased, the diffusing capacity may be decreased, and there is increased ventilation/perfusion mismatching, as well as hypoxemia, DOE, a dry, nonproductive cough, and in some cases hemoptysis.

Movement and the ability to interact with the environment would be affected directly by these diseases through joint inflammation and muscle weakness. However, in some of these patients in which DIF is prominent, pulmonary reserve would be severely limited and the work of breathing increased. These changes would decrease exercise tolerance and contribute to muscular weakness and wasting.

CONCLUSION

Some ways in which the pulmonary system interrelates with other body systems are now clear. The supportive function of the pulmonary system in supplying O_2 to all the tissues makes these close relationships necessary. This means that pathological changes or trauma to the pulmonary system have far-reaching effects, including altering the person's ability to move and interact with the environment. Disease processes in other body systems also affect respiratory function, often to a much greater degree than would sometimes be expected. Again, as soon as the pulmonary system is affected, and there is respiratory dysfunction, the effects can create alterations in other systems. These continued interactions and alterations between the pulmonary system and other body systems can be likened to a never-ending reverberating circuit.

As you continue to study the pulmonary system and how to evaluate respiratory function and treat respiratory dysfunction, its interrelatedness with all the other body systems is an important concept to keep clearly in mind. The evaluative and treatment skills that you will learn are not exclusively for application to pulmonary patients. These are skills that will need to be applied to all the patients you work with as a physical therapist. You will be working with the pulmonary system whenever you are treating patients, for example, when working on head control with a child with cerebral palsy, rolling with a hemiplegic patient, ambulation with a 70-year-old patient with a hip fracture, posture activities with a patient following a radical neck dissection procedure, conditioning exercises with a post-myocardial infarction patient, relaxation imaging with a low back pain patient, gait training with an amputee, or strengthening exercises for a polymyositis patient. In none of these examples would the patient's diagnosis be considered a pulmonary diagnosis. In all of these examples the patient's pulmonary system would be involved. Therefore, your ability to determine your patient's pulmonary status and foster good pulmonary functioning will be a vital part of the care you provide to each of your patients.

ANNOTATED BIBLIOGRAPHY

Bates DV, Macklem PT, Christie RV: Respiratory Function in Disease. Philadelphia, WB Saunders, 1971 (The first three chapters of this book outline the normal anatomy and physiology of the lung; the next twenty are comprehensive discussions of different pulmonary pathologies. The chapter contents are listed at the beginning of each chapter, making it an easy reference to use.)

Cahill M (ed): Signs and Symptoms. Springhouse, PA, Springhouse, 1986 (This alphabetized reference book of clinical signs and symptoms is a handy quick reference. Each sign or symptom is defined and related to a variety of systemic diseases.)

Campbell EJM, Agostini E, Davis JN: The Respiratory Muscles: Mechanics and Neural Control, 2nd ed. London, Lloyd-Luke Medical Books, 1970 (A specialized reference that discusses the kinematics of the chest wall, the neural control of respiration, and the functioning of the respiratory muscles in health and disease.)

Dantzker DR: Cardiopulmonary Critical Care. Orlando, FL, Grune & Stratton, 1986 (This book is divided into three sections on pathophysiology, principles of treatment, and specific pulmonary disorders. Each chapter includes a detailed and up-to-date bibliography. Of particular interest are chapters on respiratory muscle function, mechanical ventilation and weaning, and ethical and legal aspects of caring for the critically ill.)

George RB, Light RW, Matthay RA (eds): Chest Medicine. New York, Churchill Livingstone, 1983 (Divided into three sections, the main topics are pulmonary structure and function, pulmonary evaluation procedures and interpretation, and clinical patterns of lung disease. The last section emphasizes the clinical manifestations and treatment of lung disease.)

Glauser FI: Signs and Symptoms in Pulmonary Medicine. Philadelphia, JB Lippincott, 1983 (This practical guide to the interpretation of a variety of respiratory signs and symptoms is easily readable and uses tables extensively.)

Hiller FC, Wilson FJ Jr, Bone RC (eds): Pulmonary Diseases: Focus on Clinical Diagnosis. New Hyde Park, NY, Medical Examination Publishing, 1983 (This book focuses on diagnostic tools used in the evaluation of the respiratory system and a variety of respiratory diseases. The chapters on interstitial lung disease, pulmonary malignancies, and respiratory control: defects in respiratory drives are particularly interesting.)

Hodgkin JE, Zorn EG, Conners GL (eds): Pulmonary Rehabilitation: Guidelines to Success. Boston, Butterworth, 1984 (This book is a useful adjunct to pathophysiological references because it covers a range of pulmonary rehabilitation topics such as education, patient compliance, sexuality, vocational rehabilitation, cost effectiveness, and marketing strategies. Its focus is on enhancing the pulmonary patient's quality of life, not just improving physiological functioning.)

Irwin S, Tecklin JS (eds): Cardiopulmonary Physical Therapy. St. Louis, CV Mosby, 1985 (This excellent comprehensive reference on pulmonary physical therapy and rehabilitation brings together several skilled clinicians as authors. The chapters on respiratory physiology, respiratory assessment, and respiratory muscles would particularly enhance and deepen the student's understanding of the material presented in this chapter.)

Weinberger SE: Principles of Pulmonary Medicine. Philadelphia, WB Saunders, 1986 (This excellent reference links basic respiratory physiology with pulmonary pathophysiology and clinical pulmonary medicine. Each chapter discusses the etiology, pathology, pathophysiology, clinical features, and diagnostic and therapeutic approaches for a particular pulmonary diagnosis. This text uses a clear style and readable format.)

14 Integumentary Causes

CAROL A. GIULIANI

In this chapter, I will discuss the effects of damage to the integument or skin as they relate to musculoskeletal dysfunction. Injuries to integument may occur from pressure and ischemia (decubitus ulcers), physical trauma (abrasions), or thermal, electric, and chemical agents (burn injury). In all cases the skin is lost or damaged and any or all of its functions may be affected. Consequences of any injury may result in movement dysfunction; however, the sequelae and physical therapy approach to preventing or treating the resultant dysfunction may differ. It is important that the physical therapist understand and be able to identify the causes of movement dysfunction prior to developing a plan of treatment.

FUNCTION AND COMPOSITION

Skin is the largest organ of the human body. Some of its important functions are preventing infection, regulating body temperature, providing sensory information, and contributing to our physical appearance. The skin is composed of two layers, the epidermis and the dermis (Fig. 14-1). The epidermal layer contains (1) a lipid layer (corneum) that acts as a vapor barrier to prevent fluid loss and to protect the underlying tissue from bacterial invasion, and (2) a cell layer (germinativum) that produces new squamous epithelial cells. It is the presence of the epidermis that determines whether a wound will heal in a reasonable period of time or require grafting. The dermal layer contains collagen, cells, and epidermal appendages, such as hair follicles, sebaceous glands, and sweat glands. Nerves, blood vessels, and lymph vessels are also located in the dermal layer. Destruction of the dermal layer results in scar tissue formation and subsequent limitation of joint motion. The epidermal appendages are important to the sequelae of wound healing. These appendages, located in the dermal layer, are lined with squamous epithelial cells, and may be the only source of new skin tissue when the epidermal layer is destroyed (Jacoby).

PATHOPHYSIOLOGY

The results of injury to the skin depend on the specific body area involved, the causative agent, the size or amount of body surface area (BSA) involved, and the extent or depth of injury. Each specific body area injured presents a unique problem for the physical therapist. For example, wounds to the trunk and limbs that do not cross major joints may not result in physical disability, whereas injuries to the hands, feet, and axillae are potentially incapacitating.

The extent may vary from a small superficial abrasion that heals without incident, to a decubitus ulcer that may destroy tissue from superficial epidermal layers to the level of bone and require grafting, or to a major third-degree burn that involves destruction of more than 70% of BSA and may result in death. Extent of

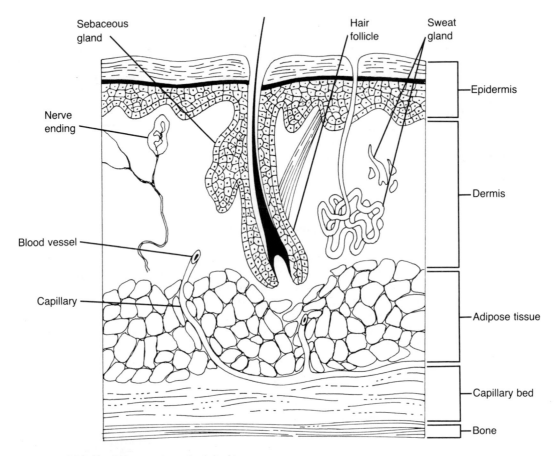

Figure 14-1. Cross section of adult skin.

injury also affects the body's response to injury, which may be localized to the tissue damaged, or may involve many body systems primarily or secondarily. Integumental trauma often affects the function of the cardiovascular, cardipulmonary, renal, metabolic, muscular, nervous, and skeletal systems. Understanding the consequences of disturbing these systems and how that affects movement will increase the efficiency of physical therapy assessment and treatment.

LOCAL TISSUE RESPONSE

Pain

Evidence of the skin as a sensory organ is apparent when it is removed. As most people have experienced, pain from a small blister on the hand or foot may be disabling. Joint dysfunction as a result of pain may occur because the patient does not move the injured area. This immobility may result in capsular and ligamentous stiffness and muscle atrophy. Superficial tissue damage causes more pain than deeper injuries. For example, superficial burns that damage only the epidermal layer are more painful than full-thickness burns that involve damage to the dermal layer because the free nerve endings are not destroyed by the superficial burn. Patients with full-thickness burns may not experience pain within the first few days following injury; however, as nerve endings regenerate and eschar (devitalized tissue) is removed, intense pain may result. Prolonged pain experienced by patients with burn injury is the major deterrent for patient participation in exercise and tolerance for proper positioning to prevent joint dysfunction.

Edema

Histamine release following injury causes capillary leakage of serous fluid into extravascular tissue. Fluid collecting in and about joint spaces limits joint range of motion and may cause tissue destruction by creating local ischemia or tissue strain. A good example of the effects of edema on joint function is seen in the burned hand (Fig. 14-2). The hand assumes a "claw" position, in which the interphalangeal joints are flexed and the metacarpal phalangeal joints are extended. Joints accommodate to a position that allows maximum space for fluid accumulation. This "open" position of the joints tends to distribute the fluid pressure and minimize tissue damage. However, if joint structures are immobilized in this position, hand function may be compromised. Mobility of the metacarpal phalangeal joint is critical for normal hand function. Destruction of the extensor tendon at the proximal interphalangeal

joint may cause the lateral bands to slip anterior to the joint axis, thus producing flexion instead of extension when the finger extensors contract. Maintaining the extensor mechanism is a major goal of physical therapy in patients with burned hands. Physical therapy treatment should be directed at preventing or decreasing edema, maintaining functional joint position, and minimizing periods of immobilization.

Tissue Destruction

Tissue damage may occur as a direct result of external causative agents (eg, heat, chemicals, electricity), and secondarily as a result of ischemia and infection. Continued pressure to the skin, especially over bony structures, creates areas of ischemia that may cause tissue destruction. Decubitus ulcers are the results of tissue damage from ischemia and infection that may involve large areas of skin. The loss of the skin as a bacterial barrier allows organisms easy access to many body systems. Bacterial infection in a second-degree burn may produce a tissue necrosis that converts an original partial thickness injury to full-thickness tissue destruction.

Figure 14-2. Claw hand deformity secondary to edema in a third-degree burn.

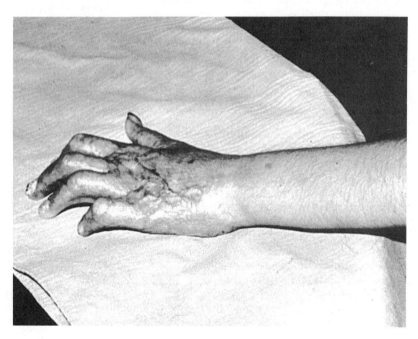

SYSTEMIC RESPONSE

Cardiovascular System

If a large amount of the skin is damaged, as in a major burn injury (greater than 20% BSA), many systems of the body are affected that can limit movement and are of interest to the physical therapist. In patients with major burns, the cardiovascular system may be severely compromised. Edema occurs locally as well as throughout the body. Leaking intravascular substances tend to deplete the circulating cardiovascular volume. If untreated, this hypovolemia will compromise cardiac output, kidney function, and eventually brain function. To prevent the consequences related to decreasing intravascular volume, intravenous fluid replacement is the treatment of choice (Dingeldein). Fluid input and output volumes are monitored closely and treatment is adjusted to maintain an adequate urine output (approximately 30 to 50 cc/hr) (Jacoby). Urine output is an indication of renal function, which may be seriously damaged by hypovolemia. Fluid replacement formulas are based on percent BSA burned and body weight and must be carefully administered to avoid creating cardiopulmonary complications such as pulmonary edema, congestive heart failure, and acute respiratory distress syndromes. The therapist's awareness of the medical treatment, physiological stress on the patient, and potential complications will aid developing a rational plan of treatment.

Metabolic

Thermal injury results in more loss of body mass than any other disease process (Wilmore). High metabolic rates are responsible for the large weight loss in patients with thermal injury and systemic infection. This increase in metabolic activity has been attributed to loss of the skin's ability to regulate body temperature and control evaporation. In addition, increased catecholamine levels reported following thermal injury were identified as major mediators of the hypermetabolic response.

Continued demands on the metabolic system are required for the massive healing process the body must accomplish to close the wound and replace damaged tissue. High caloric and protein supplements are important in these patients to diminish weight loss. Patient weight loss and muscle atrophy are inevitable consequences of major integumentary loss and wound sepsis. Muscle weakness associated with massive weight loss is of prime importance to the physical therapist, whose goals are to maintain and promote the patient's strength and function. However, while attempting to maintain strength and function, the therapist must consider the catabolic state of the patient and develop physical therapy programs that increase strength without increasing metabolic stress. Restoring muscle strength and mass is a formidable task for the physical therapist in burn rehabilitation.

Nervous System

Functions of the central nervous system may be compromised by decreased tissue perfusion from edema or from subsequent hypovolemia. Episodes of confusion, lethargy, disorientation, and irritability are signs of decreased oxygen perfusion to the CNS. Physical therapists must be aware of these signs and consider the effects of an exercise program that may increase peripheral vasodilation and further compromise CNS tissue perfusion. Peripheral motor and sensory nerve function also may be damaged primarily from trauma or secondarily from infection.

Skeletal System

Deep integumentary trauma damaging bone or peripheral circulation may result in amputation. Fingers and toes are amputated most frequently in thermal trauma. Electrical injury may create massive tissue loss at any point between the entry and exit points, depending on the path of the current. Amputation is common in electrical injury, and may be performed shortly after injury to decrease the possibility of infection and preserve healthy tissue (Artz, 1979). Tissue destruction that involves the joint capsule leaves the joint synovium and its articulating surfaces open to sepsis, which may cause additional skeletal system damage.

CONSEQUENCES OF INJURY RESULTING IN MOVEMENT DYSFUNCTION

Although I will primarily address the consequences of burn injury in this section, the same principles may be applied to any skin injury. Physical therapists treat a wide variety of skin injuries and diseases that result in a loss of skin tissue. I intend to show the basic concepts of the acute and chronic processes involved in skin injury that can produce movement dysfunction.

WOUND HEALING

Partial-Thickness Wounds

Injuries limited to the epidermal layer are defined as partial-thickness or second-degree wounds. Histological studies show that wound healing occurs in several stages, provided complications of infection, trauma, or impaired circulation do not intervene. Any of these complications may prolong the healing process and complicate rehabilitation efforts. During the first stage of healing, the inflammatory cells (leukocytes, histiocytes, and macrophages) remove dead tissue. Within 48 hours of the injury, fibroblasts at the wound site begin forming new collagen. New epithelium needed for wound closure is produced from viable tissue at the perimeter of the wound and the epithelial cells lining the epidermal appendages. Epithelialization occurs quite rapidly if it is not impeded by infection, trauma, or impaired circulation. For these reasons it is important to keep the wound clean and protected, and promote circulation.

Healing of second-degree wounds usually takes 10 to 21 days depending on the depth of burn. The more tissue damaged, the longer the healing time. As wound healing proceeds, nerve endings regenerate and the patient may experience considerable pain during wound care and during active and passive movement. Patients are much more comfortable and willing to participate with exercise programs after substantial wound closure occurs. To increase treatment effectiveness during the period of wound healing, the therapist must address the problem of pain and gain the patient's participation in an exercise program.

Full-Thickness Wounds

Full-thickness or third-degree burns cannot reepithelialize. As these wounds heal, fibroblasts and capillaries form a network that fill the burn wound with a red, richly vascularized, moist surface known as granulation tissue. The development of this collagen and capillary network is the beginning of scar tissue formation. Normally, integumentary layers are formed of collagen fibers that are well organized in parallel bundles; however, in the burn wound, collagen synthesis is elevated and its arrangement is disorganized. In hypertrophic scar tissue, whorls or supracoils of collagen are reported. The effects of this formation on joint movement will be explored further in the discussion of scar tissue.

Full-thickness wounds require grafting for timely wound closure and to decrease scar tissue formation. Once the wound is closed, collagen fiber organization tends to regain its typical parallel arrangement, but a normal architectural network is seldom restored (Larson and co-workers).

EFFECTS OF SCAR TISSUE FORMATION

Burn scar formation is a prolonged inflammatory response to trauma that is positively related to the depth of injury. The more of the dermal layer that is disrupted, the greater the inflammatory response and resulting scar tissue. Unfortunately, long after the wound is closed, scar tissue formation continues for approximately one year with maximum activity occurring 2 to 6 months after injury (Baur and co-workers; Larson and co-workers). Scar tissue may cause skin shortening and loss of joint mobility in addition to creating discomfort and disfigurement. When scar tissue is active it appears red, raised, edematous, and usually itches. As scar tissue matures collagen is absorbed, the scar flattens, lightens in color, and blends in with healthy skin.

Scar tissue shortening tightens skin across

joints and limits range of motion. This skin shortening is caused by the formation of collagen whorls. The formation of these whorls is due to the natural helical configuration of the collagen molecule, and is described by Larson as similar to the knots formed when one releases tension upon a twisted and stretched rubber band. Larson suggests that normally the presence of the skin provides sufficient tension for the collagen to form its parallel arrangement. Once this tension is removed, as in a burn injury, the collagen arrangement is haphazard and the collagen bundles tend to form cross links and knot upon themselves. As skin shortens, the tension created by scar tissue may be of sufficient force to cause severe joint dislocation (Larson).

Burn patients and patients with other inflammatory processes and joint edema assume positions of joint flexion because it seems to be a position of comfort. If patients are allowed to remain in this position, the collagen fibers fuse together and produce joint contracture. Even after scar tissue matures and collagen is absorbed, the contracture will persist because the fibers are fused in a shortened position. Joint motion is lost easily in patients with inflammatory processes and scar tissue formation.

Early wound closure by skin grafting will decrease scar tissue formation because the newly grafted skin provides tension to the collagen fibers as they form. Histological studies show a more normal arrangement of collagen fiber in wounds that were grafted early compared with wounds left open and treated less aggressively (Larson and co-workers). If therapists are to be succesesful in maintaining joint function, the effects of patient positioning and scar tissue shortening must be considered.

MUSCLE WEAKNESS

As mentioned earlier, the stress on the metabolic system following a burn causes the patient to lose weight and considerable muscle mass. Once the wounds are closed, however, the patient begins to recover body weight rapidly. The loss of muscle mass and fiber atrophy results in profound weakness, and contributes

to continued edema in distal limbs. Normal muscle tension supports vascular beds and subcutaneous tissue, and muscle contraction helps to pump blood through distal capillary beds and prevent venostasis.

Furthermore, the patient with burns is immobilized for long periods of time for a number of reasons. Frequent skin grafting procedures require immobilization; splinting and pinning joints to prevent joint contracture immobilizes limbs; severity of a patient's medical condition may prevent movement; edema limits motion; and large, bulky dressings make movement difficult, if not impossible. The effects of immobilization on muscle fiber are profound. Muscle fibers shorten by losing sarcomeres, the connective tissue surrounding the fibers shortens, and the muscle becomes more stiff and less compliant. These changes in both active and passive elements of muscle created by immobilization compound the problem of weakness produced by atrophy and contribute to muscle proteolysis.

NEUROLOGIC COMPLICATIONS

Electrical injury frequently affects nerve function. Damage may occur to the brain spinal cord, or peripheral nerves if the current traverses those pathways. The effect of injury may be an immediate onset of neurological deficit, or a deficit may develop later. Neurological deficits of the CNS with late onset may result from vascular thrombosis and associated ischemia. Patients with electrical injury require a careful physical therapy assessment to identify early signs of neurological deficit and a vigorous program to prevent limited range of motion should limb nerve function return (Pruitt).

Peripheral neuropathies with loss of function are frequently associated with burn trauma (Helm, 1984). The initial injury may damage nerves directly by laceration, or by thermal, electrical, and chemical agents. In the patient recovering from skin trauma, decreased range of motion or muscle weakness may be the result of compressed or overstretched nerves (Helm). Many of these nerve lesions are the result of poor positioning or splinting, pressure from bulky dressings over superficial nerves, and overly vigorous stretching (Helm and co-workers, 1982). Scar tissue formation also may cause nerve compression. For example, carpal tunnel syndrome secondary to the proliferation of hypertrophic scar over the anterior wrist surface is a common complication of wrist and hand injury (Fig. 14-3). Neuropathy secondary to multiple intramuscular injections have been reported to injure muscle and nerve tissue (Helm, 1984). Many of these secondary neuropathies may be prevented by increasing the awareness of the medical team to avoid those conditions that may compromise neuromuscular function.

PAIN

As discussed earlier, when the wound is open and nerve endings are exposed, pain limits spontaneous movement and participation in exercise programs. After wounds have healed or been grafted, pain decreases. However, newly healed skin may be exquisitely sensitive. This new skin is dry and fragile, and cracks easily because normal lubrication from sebaceous

glands is diminished. Patients frequently complain of itching and increased cutaneous sensitivity to heat, cold, and touch long after wounds are closed (Giuliani and Perry, 1985). Exercise also may cause pain because the skin stretches across joints and tends to crack. The therapist can avoid pain and skin cracking by lubricating the skin prior to exercise (Helm and co-workers, 1982).

CARDIOVASCULAR DECONDITIONING

General deconditioning of the patient can be attributed to the high metabolic demand for wound healing, vascular incompetence, muscle weakness, and long periods of inactivity. Endurance is decreased and tolerance for activity is compromised further by the patient's inability to dissipate heat during exercise. Sweat glands normally located in the skin are responsible for dissipating heat and regulating core temperature during exercise. The decreased number of sweat glands in the healed or grafted skin of patients with extensive burns make temperature regulation difficult. Caution is urged during exercise of these patients to avoid undue stress on the cardiovascular sys-

Figure 14-3. Proliferation of hypertrophic scar tissue and skin shortening in a third-degree burn, causing a wrist flexion deformity and compression of the median nerve.

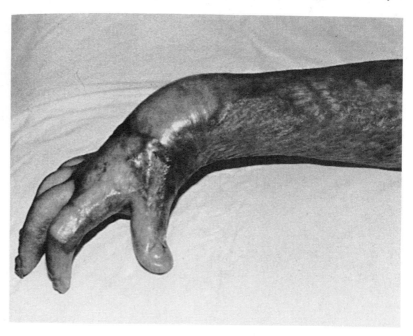

tem. The therapist's goal should include maintaining maximal cardiovascular conditioning throughout the course of treatment and preparing the patient for the demands of activity following discharge.

SKELETAL CHANGES

Osteoporosis was reported by radiographic assessment in 36% of severely burned patients (Shiele). Prolonged periods of immobilization, hyperemia, and increased adrenocortical activity following burn injury may contribute to osteoporosis. Therapists may utilize exercise to minimize osteoporotic changes.

Heterotopic ossification, resulting in limited joint movement and pain, was reported in 23% of severly burned patients (Shiele). Joints in the area of burn injury or remote from the wound area may be involved. Many joints may be the site of heterotopic ossification, but it occurs most frequently at the elbow (Pruitt). The etiology of heterotopic ossification in burn patients is unclear; however, several factors may contribute, including a disturbance of calcium metabolism, overly zealous joint manipulation, immobilization, and infection (Hartford; Varghese). Onset of heterotopic ossification may occur from 3 to 12 weeks after injury. Pain and a sudden loss of joint motion are early symptoms. Bone scans and roentgenograms are useful in diagnosing this condition (Fig. 14-4). Spontaneous resolution occurs in some patients, but if mature cortical bone has formed, surgical excision may be required. Therapists may be the first to detect early signs of heterotopic ossification. In the burn patient, these signs may be hard to detect. The therapist must be aware of the possibility of this complication, be sensitive to daily changes in joint motion, and alter treatment plans accordingly. Because stress to a joint is implicated as a contributing factor to heterotopic ossification, exercise programs must be executed carefully.

ANNOTATED BIBLIOGRAPHY

Artz CP, Moncrief JA, Pruitt BA Jr (eds): Burns: A Team Approach, p. 583. Philadelphia, WB Saunders, 1979 (An excellent anthology covering a broad spectrum of burn care.)

Artz CP: Electrical injury. In Artz CP, Moncrief JA, Pruitt BA Jr (eds): Burns: A Team Approach, pp 351–362. Philadelphia, WB Saun-

Figure 14-4. Heterotopic ossification at the elbow joint eight weeks after burn injury.

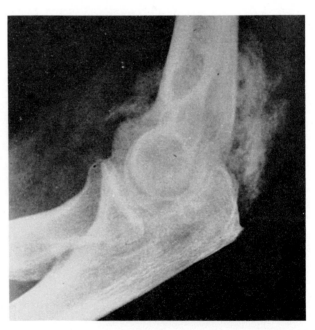

ders, 1979 (Discusses the pathology and treatment of electrical injury.)

Artz CP: Epidemiology, causes, and prognosis. In Artz CP, Moncrief JA, Pruitt BA Jr (eds): Burns: A Team Approach, pp 17–22. Philadelphia, WB Saunders, 1979 (A succinct discussion of epidemiology, cause, and prognosis of burn injury.)

Baur PS, Barratt G, Linares HA: Wound contracture, scar contractures and myofibroblasts: A classical case study. J Trauma 18:8, 1978 (An excellent study on the pathophysiology of burn wound healing and scar tissue formation.)

Davidson SP: Nursing management of emotional reactions of severely burned patients during the acute phase. Heart Lung 2:370, 1973 (Identifies common emotional problems of burned patients and suggests methods of intervention.)

Dimick AR: Pathophysiology. In Fisher SV, Helm PA (eds): Comprehensive Rehabilitation of Burns, pp 16–28. Baltimore, Williams & Wilkins, 1984 (An overview of burn pathophysiology and mechanisms of injury.)

Dingeldein GP: Fluid and electrolyte therapy in the burn patient. In Salisbury RE, Newman NM, Dingeldein GP (eds): Manual of Burn Therapeutics, pp 9–20. Boston, Little, Brown & Co, 1983 (Reviews the need for replacement therapy, various replacement formulas, and medical complications associated with replacement therapy.)

Feller I, Archambeult C: Nursing the Burned Patient, pp 2–13. Ann Arbor, MI, Institute for Burn Medicine, 1973 (Basic information on burn injury and nursing care with many graphic color plates. Not suggested as a reference for rehabilitation.)

Fisher SV, Helm PA (eds): Comprehensive Rehabilitation of Burns. Baltimore, Williams & Wilkins, 1984 (A valuable collection of articles by prominent persons in burn rehabilitation that contains current issues related to physical therapy and rehabilitation of burned patients.)

Giuliani CA, Perry GA: Factors to consider in the rehabilitation aspects of burn care. Phys Ther 65:5, 1985 (Information for physical therapists in assessment and treatment of patients with burns.)

Hartford CE: Surgical management. In Fisher SV, Helm PA (eds): Comprehensive Rehabilitation of Burns, pp 28–64. Baltimore, Williams & Wilkins, 1984 (Information on burn wound care, surgical techniques, scar tissue, and heterotopic bone formation.)

Helm PA: Neuromuscular considerations. In Fisher SV, Helm PA (eds): Comprehensive Rehabilitation of Burns, pp 235–242. Baltimore, Williams & Wilkins, 1984 (Identifies previously overlooked neuromuscular complications in burned patients. Emphasizes complications caused by poor positioning and other medical treatments.)

Helm PA, Kevorkian CG, Lushbaugh M et al: Burn injury: Rehabilitation management in 1982. Arch Phys Med Rehabil 63:6, 1982 (An excellent review of problems in burn rehabilitation and current methods of treatment.)

Jacoby FG: Nursing Care of the Patient With Burns, pp 7–13. St Louis, CV Mosby, 1976 (A basic text of burn care discussing pathology, wound care, medical treatment, and nutrition.)

Larson D, Huang T, Linares H et al: Prevention and treatment of scar contracture. In Artz CP, Moncrief JA, Pruitt BA Jr (eds): Burns: A Team Approach, pp 466–491. Philadelphia, WB Saunders, 1979 (A review of the pathophysiology of scar tissue formation and suggestions for prevention and treatment that are useful to the physical therapist.)

Linare HA, Kischer CW, Dobrokovsky M: On the origin of hypertrophic scar tissue. J Trauma 13:70, 1973 (A classic histological study on the formation of burn scar.)

Marvin JA, Heimback DM: Pain management. In Fisher SV, Helm PA (eds): Comprehensive Rehabilitation of Burns, pp 311–330. Baltimore, Williams & Wilkins, 1984 (Discusses the physiology of pain and suggests methods of intervention. A useful chapter for any therapist dealing with patients in pain.)

Moncrief JA: Topical antibacterial treatment of the burn wound. In Artz CP, Moncrief JA, Pruitt BA Jr (eds): Burns: A Team Approach, pp 250–267. Philadelphia, WB Saunders, 1979 (Discusses burn wound sepsis and major topical agents used to decrease bacterial infection.)

Petro JA, Nicosia JE et al: Hospitalization of burned patients. In Nicosia JE, Petro JA (eds) Manual of Burn Care, pp 15–88. New York,

Raven Press, 1983 (A problem-oriented manual of medical and physical treatment in burn care with little rationale for treatment.)

Pruitt BA Jr: Other complications of burn injury. In Artz CP, Moncrief JA, Pruitt BA Jr (eds): Burns: A Team Approach, pp 523–554. Philadelphia, WB Saunders, 1979 (A review of complications in burns by systems.)

Shiele HP, Hubbard RB, Buick HM: Radiographic changes in burns of the upper extremities. Diagnostic Radiol 104:13, 1972 (A prospective radiographic study of changes in 70 burned patients.)

Varghese G: Musculoskeletal considerations. In Fisher SV, Helm PA (eds): Comprehensive Rehabilitation of Burns, pp 242–249. Balti-more, Williams & Wilkins, 1984 (An overview of prevention and treatment of musculoskeletal complications in burned patients.)

Wilmore DW: Metabolic changes in burns. In Artz CP, Moncrief JA, Pruitt BA Jr (eds): Burns: A Team Approach, pp 120–131. Philadelphia, WB Saunders, 1979 (A discussion of metabolic complications in burned patients and the rationale for treatment.)

Wright PC: Fundamentals of acute burn care and physical therapy management. Phys Ther 64:1217, 1984 (A review of burn injury, local and systemic complications, and physical therapy treatment during the acute phase.)

15 Obstetric and Gynecological Causes

LINDA O'CONNOR
LINDA M. PIPP

An understanding of the pathology and the accompanying signs and symptoms of any dysfunction allows the practitioner to provide more effective care. This is particularly true when treating disorders of the reproductive system, for this system may not be viewed as an obvious source of movement dysfunction. Yet, both natural occurrences and reproductive pathology have far-reaching dysfunctional consequences throughout the body systems. In this chapter, we address structural imbalances (including the pelvis, spine, posture, and gait) and muscular imbalances (including the abdominal muscles, pelvic floor, and uterus). The influence of the reproductive system extends to the neurological, circulatory, and integumentary systems and may disturb the very delicate coordination between reproductive dysfunction and psychological affect. Although the focus of this chapter is on the female through the adolescent years, menstruating and childbearing years, and postmenopausal years, male patients may also clinically exhibit symptoms related to reproductive system dysfunction. Hence, some awareness of associated pathology is both prudent and beneficial for the practitioner.

STRUCTURAL IMBALANCE

PELVIS AND SPINE

The sacroiliac joints have been the focus of increasing interest by practitioners. Once considered immobile, it is now agreed that the sacroiliac joints and, to a lesser degree, the symphysis pubis, may indeed move and cause symptoms of pain, ache, and muscular spasm. During pregnancy, release of the hormone relaxin, which causes relaxation of connective tissue, is responsible for this movement and may result in pelvic obliquity demonstrated by torsion of the ilium on the sacrum or in separation of the pubic rami. Pelvic obliquity may be confused with leg length discrepancy or may be masked by scoliosis. Practitioners need to be aware of these joints as a cause of referred pain to the lumbosacral area, hips, groin, thighs, pubis, pelvic floor, and vulvar region.

POSTURE

Spinal dysfunction may be produced or aggravated by pregnancy as the result of increase in joint laxity. Added fetal weight, which shifts the center of gravity, may exacerbate pre-existing scoliosis or cause faulty posture. Improper posture and improper body mechanics are frequent causes of dysfunction, often accompanied by radicular symptoms or neuropathy. Backache is a common complaint of the general population at any age, but especially during pregnancy. Depending on the patient's physical status prior to pregnancy, backache may be relieved through posture control, body mechanics instruction, or the use of an external support. Other causes of backache include trauma, infection, bone or disk disease, uterine displacement, pull from uterosacral ligamentous structures, and referred pain from pelvic organ dysfunction, hip disease, metastases, or joint relaxation.

Functional backache in pregnant adolescents and women in their early twenties creates the need to focus on posture control and body mechanics. Although documentation in this area is sparse, some practitioners believe that prolonged postural stresses, combined with muscular weakness associated with pregnancy, can precipitate bony changes.

GAIT

Pregnant women may exhibit a characteristic waddling gait with decreased trunk rotation, decreased stride length, and decreased swing phase, which may result from separation of the symphysis pubis. Sacroiliac joint dysfunction, pelvic obliquity, pelvic instability, pelvic discomfort, and coccygodynia due to sacrococcygeal joint sprain may also be responsible for gait abnormalities.

MUSCLE IMBALANCE

ABDOMINAL MUSCLES

A major abdominal muscle dysfunction related to pregnancy is diastasis recti. This dysfunction is characterized by midline separation of the two halves of the rectus abdominis muscle. Some clinicians theorize that diastasis of the rectus abdominis muscle is a passive process in which the muscle is a prisoner of its separating connective tissue sheath. This condition can result from or be aggravated by inherent muscular or connective tissue weakness, hormonal ligamentous softening, obesity, or repeated efforts at straining. The stress on the abdominal muscles caused by pregnancy and delivery can cause diastasis during pregnancy or during the puerperium. Postural instruction, therapeutic exercise, assistive devices, and external supports may provide relief.

The integrity of the abdominal wall may be compromised by pregnancy or abdominal and gynecological surgery, including laparotomy, abdominal hysterectomy, and cesarean childbirth. Incisional pain, postural weakness and guarding, and respiratory difficulties affecting coughing and deep breathing are resultant dysfunctions that need to be addressed by the therapist. Postoperative complications increase with abdominal hysterectomy, because these women usually have more serious pelvic disease than vaginal hysterectomy patients. The abdominal hysterectomy poses a higher risk for infection and injury of the urinary and intestinal tracts. In addition, infection is the major threat of the classical longitudinal cesarean incision, because a broader area is available for organism dispersement compared with the transverse bikini-type incision.

Whether the state of pregnancy concludes in a vaginal or a cesarean delivery, the abdominal wall musculature has been stretched and stressed over a nine-month period. This situation requires physical therapy to correct the weakness and structural imbalances through exercise and postural correction.

PELVIC FLOOR

Three muscular diaphragms and their surrounding fascia form the floor of the bony basin of the pelvis. The pelvic floor supports the urethra, vagina, rectum, bladder, and uterus. The most important of these muscular diaphragms is the levator ani muscle group, consisting of the pubococcygeus, iliococcygeus, and coccygeus muscles. This hammock-like levator sling mechanism between the pubis and the coccyx is vital to support the pelvic contents and for pressure and sphincter control. Any compromise of its integrity through weakness or surgical disruption can cause dysfunction (Fig. 15-1).

During pregnancy, the increase in size and weight of the abdominal and pelvic organs causes pressure and stress on the pelvic floor, often resulting in aching discomfort. Increased vascularity and hormonal tissue softening add to the aching of pelvic congestion and swelling. Childbirth itself may result in stretching of the pudendal nerves that innervate the pelvic floor, compromising its ability to contract. Routine use of episiotomy risks the occurrence of

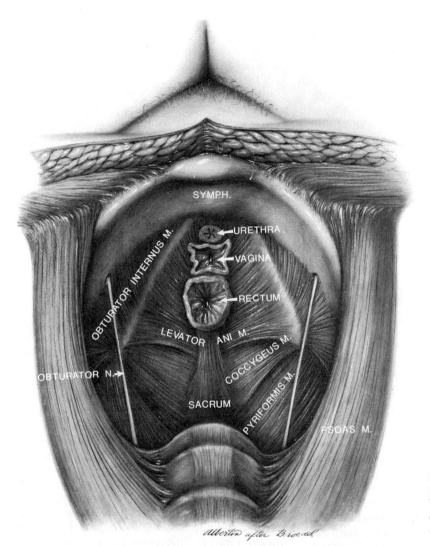

SYMPH.

←URETHRA

←VAGINA

OBTURATOR INTERNUS M.

←RECTUM

LEVATOR   ANI   M.

COCCYGEUS M.

OBTURATOR N.→

PYRIFORMIS. M.

SACRUM

PSOAS M.

Alberton after Brodel

Figure 15-1. Anatomy of the pelvic floor. (Mattingly RF, Thompson JD: Te Linde's Operative Gynecology, 6th ed, p 41. Philadelphia, JB Lippincott, 1985)

pain, edema, dyspareunia, infection, and delayed healing. Surgical disruption of the fascia that acts as a lubricant for the pelvic diaphragm can result in adhesions, loss of tissue mobility, and decreased proprioception for the patient.

Pelvic relaxation, whether congenital or acquired, can lead to structural defects and displacements. These may include cystocele, urethrocele, rectocele, and enterocele. Enterocele is a possible complication of vaginal hysterectomy. Pelvic pain, pressure, sexual dissatisfac-

tion, and urinary incontinence are common complaints.

Pelvic floor exercise is extremely valuable for increasing strength, comfort, and proprioceptive awareness of this area. Electrical stimulation is currently under investigation for pelvic floor muscle re-education.

UTERUS

Laxity of the pelvic floor and supporting ligaments, especially the cardinal ligaments, can contribute to uterine prolapse. This is manifest by the bulging or herniation of the uterus through the vaginal canal. Discomfort can accompany the protruding mass and the urinary tract may be damaged or obstructed. Although these conditions are more common in multiparas as they advance in age, similar symptoms have been documented in pediatric and adolescent patients.

Other structural displacements also produce dysfunction. Uterine retrodisplacement can contribute to pelvic pain, dysmenorrhea, chronic pelvic congestion, and secondary backache. Fistulas are abnormal communications between the genital and urinary areas and can contribute to urinary incontinence. They occur as a consequence of obstetric injury, gynecological surgery, abdominal hysterectomy, and cancer metastasis or radium therapy.

Understanding the etiology of these displacements allows the therapist to choose treatment techniques most beneficial for the problem, including pain relief through exercise and transcutaneous electrical nerve stimulation (TENS).

PAIN

PELVIC ORGAN DYSFUNCTION

Causes of pain from pelvic organ dysfunction can be related to uterine fibroids or to uterine, ovarian, or vaginal neoplasia. In the nonpregnant woman, dysplasia of the reproductive system, endometriosis, and neurologically referred pain can be debilitating and disruptive to sexual function. Women with teratogenic dysplasia, such as that caused by diethylstilbestrol (DES) exposure in utero, have been able to have uncomplicated spontaneous vaginal deliveries. However, theories vary on the effect of cervical scarring or other anomalies on the progress of labor. Severe dysplasia, of course, can cause reproductive and sexual dysfunction.

Vulvar and vaginal infections can cause pain and discomfort or can be asymptomatic. Infection can occur before, during, or after pregnancy. *Candida albicans* is the most commonly treated fungal infection, but bacterial and viral infections also occur.

PELVIC FLOOR TENSION MYALGIA

Pelvic floor tension myalgia can occur in both sexes. In the male, it may be confused with prostatic problems. The patient continually contracts the pelvic floor muscles and the short hip external rotator muscles, possibly secondary to pain and inflammation. This habitual dysfunction may be accompanied by aching, fatigue, and urinary frequency or urgency. Physical therapy awareness of this problem may clarify selection of treatment techniques, including exercise and relaxation.

MENSTRUAL DYSFUNCTION

Some degree of lower abdominal pain and cramping, which radiates to the low back and inner thighs, may accompany normal menstruation. When the discomfort is so severe that activites are limited, this dysfunction is termed dysmenorrhea. Amenorrhea (absence of menstruation) and oligomenorrhea (scanty or infrequent menstrual flow) can occur at any age. Both have been reported in some athletes who train heavily, implicating the role of excessive exercise in menstrual dysfunction. Athletics and trauma in the adolescent, pregnancy and endocrine-related dysfunctions during the active reproductive years, and organic pathology during the perimenopausal cycle can also cause menstrual dysfunction. Regulation of exercise intensity and duration and possible pain relief through TENS are potential physical therapy interventions.

PERIPHERAL NEUROPATHY

Numerous peripheral nerves may be compromised by pressure or stretching injuries as a result of pregnancy, delivery, and surgical positioning. Numbness, paresthesia, pain, and weakness are subsequent dysfunctions. Carpal tunnel syndrome may result from pregnancy-related swelling. Thoracic outlet syndrome is possible due to postural changes such as sagging shoulders and the weight of the breasts impinging at the clavicular-rib area. Brachialgia and vascular symptoms may also result from postural changes. Femoral nerve compression may be the result of impingement caused by anatomical or surgical factors. Numbness of the anteromedial thigh and leg, anterior hip joint pain, instability of the knee during ambulation, and muscle weakness are subsequent dysfunctions. Sciatic nerve injury may result if compression or stretching of the nerve occurs during pregnancy or gynecological procedures. Footdrop and muscle weakness can result. The sacral plexus can be traumatized as a consequence of regional analgesia or anesthesia. Severe buttock and posterior lower extremity pain with ambulation difficulty follows. Physical therapy treatment of peripheral neuropathies involves the use of exercise, assistive devices, orthoses, and pain relief methods.

Treatment of peripheral or central neurological dysfunction, including disk herniation repairs, is restricted during pregnancy. Causes of fetal compromise related to use of physical therapy electrical modalities are undefined at this time, although recordings of electronic fetal monitors have been disturbed by use of TENS. It is unclear whether this is an electrical artifact or indicative of fetal reaction. Because of concern for fetal safety, most obstetrical physical therapists remain conservative on the use of electrical modalities during pregnancy. Use of positioning, superficial heat, and body mechanics and transfer instructions are beneficial.

AGING

MENOPAUSE

Menopause, the completion of the menstrual years, heralds the arrival of some dysfunctions that are also attributable to the aging process. Decreasing estrogen levels are responsible for atrophy and dryness of the genitourinary tissues along with decreased elasticity and support. An increased incidence of pelvic floor weakness, urinary tract infection, and stress incontinence may also occur with aging. Pelvic floor awareness and strengthening are vital.

OSTEOPOROSIS

Osteoporosis may be responsible for midline thoracic and lumbar pain, erector spinae muscle spasm, and kyphosis with associated movement dysfunctions. Fractures of the spine, forearm, and hip are common during the perimenopausal period, with further complications caused by the resultant immobility. Physical therapy plays a preventive role through education and a therapeutic role through muscle strengthening, postural correction, and activity level determination, which provide opportunity for complete care.

CIRCULATION

VARICOSITIES

Varicosities of rectal, vulvar, or scrotal veins can be uncomfortable and painful. Vulvar and rectal varicosities are often exacerbated by increased pelvic congestion that normally occurs during pregnancy. Breasts may become enlarged and veins may be visible through the skin overlying the breasts. Varicosities of the lower extremities are often aggravated by pregnancy, sometimes without spontaneous recovery postpartum. Postural and circulatory exercise, leg elevation, and the use of support garments may help relieve discomfort.

HYPOTENSION AND HYPERTENSION

Other vascular and interstitial complications of pregnancy include hypotension, hypertension, and general swelling with sluggish venous and lymphatic return. Hypotension, especially in the second and third trimesters, may be caused by fetal weight compressing the inferior vena cava when the patient is supine. Physical therapists can provide instruction in positioning, transfers, and comfort techniques.

COMPLICATIONS

During the menstruating years, the dysfunctions of pelvic pain and abnormal uterine bleeding can be the result of ectopic pregnancy, placenta previa, or abruptio placentae. Patients with endometriosis can also present with pelvic pain, bleeding, dyspareunia, and possible infertility. Postpartum hemorrhage resulting from uterine atony, lacerations, hematomas, or rupture can progress to shock if left untreated. Postoperative hemorrhage can also complicate abdominal hysterectomy and extensive pelvic surgery. The occurrence of abnormal bleeding may be accompanied by prolonged immobility, either for the surgical procedure itself or during the immediate postoperative period, allowing venous stasis and possible thrombophlebitis. Breathing exercises following abdominal surgery, TENS for pain relief, and the fitting of support garments are within the scope of physical therapy treatment. Bedside exercise and positioning can diminish the negative effects of immobility.

Air embolus to the heart is a potential danger during pregnancy and during and after delivery. The distensibility of the vagina and the availability of the uterine sinuses may be affected by the introduction of air under pressure. This may occur as a complication of diagnostic or therapeutic procedures or as a consequence of vascular problems during delivery. The knee-chest position has also been implicated in the creation of negative abdominal pressure, which can initiate the cycle of events leading to an air embolus. The physical therapist should advise patients and health team members to avoid improper exercise techniques (eg, speed, lack of control) and positions that may be harmful.

Integument

BREAST

Pregnancy can cause temporary or permanent changes in the skin color, which are related to hormonal stimulation of melanin production. Postpartum persistence of darkened nipples, areolae, face, and abdomen is not unusual. Breasts may remain enlarged, but hypersensitivity often diminishes. Some women experience enlargement and hypersensitivity of breasts premenstrually. Pendulous breasts may cause neck and back symptoms that require additional tissue support, postural instruction, and exercise to decrease pain.

PERINEUM

Pelvic and genitourinary tract infections include salpingo-oophoritis, postpartum endometritis, postoperative pelvic and perineal infections, vaginitis, and cervicitis. Trauma to the perineal area can also result in infections and may be caused by douches, suppositories, tampons, intrauterine devices, and foreign bodies. Localized symptoms of pain, pruritis, burning, edema, and discomfort often accompany a discharge from the perineum, while generalized symptoms include malaise, anorexia, and fever. Skin integrity may be compromised by excoriations and ulcers.

Medications are the treatment of choice, although previously it was thought that heat relieved symptoms of pelvic inflammatory disease. It is now accepted that heat may actually aggravate the infectious process associated with pelvic inflammatory disease. Physical therapists are often the health care provider chosen by the patient to discuss these problems and make recommendations for referral care.

OTHER OBSTETRIC AND GYNECOLOGIC CAUSES

HIGH-RISK OBSTETRIC PATIENTS

Approximately 10% to 30% of obstetric patients can be classified as high risk for perinatal mortality and morbidity. Maternal and fetal abnormalities are often implicated as causative factors; however, large numbers of variables may produce a cumulative effect. Among the most common high-risk cases are those of premature labor and rupture of the membranes and cervical incompetence.

Premature labor refers to labor that occurs

between the 20th and 37th week of pregnancy. The early uterine contractions produce dilation and effacement of the cervix. Premature rupture of the membranes (PROM) involves the loss of amniotic fluid prior to the onset of labor. PROM may accompany preterm labor or precipitate it, and may be a source of ascending infection in the genital tract.

Cervical incompetence is characterized by painless dilation of the cervix during the midtrimester of pregnancy. The membranes usually rupture and the fetus may not survive. Although the cause is obscure, concealed lacerations at the time of a previous delivery or of a surgical procedure, such as a dilation and curettage (D and C) in a young nulliparous girl, may conduce cervical injuries and later incompetence. In providing bedside therapy to high-risk obstetrical patients, a balance must be achieved between conservative care, exercise, and activity levels to obtain optimum maternal functioning and yet maintain fetal health and safety. Consistent monitoring of the patient's vital signs and adaptation to treatment is extremely important.

Bed rest, one of the common treatments in high-risk cases, often causes weakness, loss of mobility, decreased flexibility, and vascular stasis. This creates a dysfunctional state for the patient, which needs to be addressed by the physical therapist.

According to Hellman and Pritchard, "Essentially all diseases that affect a woman when nonpregnant may be contracted during pregnancy. Moreover, the presence of the majority of diseases does not prevent conception." Variations in symptoms, signs, and laboratory values are often influenced by the normal anatomical and physiological changes of pregnancy.

Diabetes mellitus complicates 2% to 3% of pregnancies. Hormones such as cortisol, estrogen, and progesterone interact with the maternal hyperinsulinemia associated with insulin resistance and excessive fetal growth. "Gestational diabetes" refers to the state of impaired glucose tolerance that may be initially noted or accelerated during pregnancy. The balanced roles of diet and exercise are extremely crucial in management of the pregnant diabetic.

CARDIOPULMONARY CHANGES

Cardiopulmonary changes affecting tolerance to exercise occur in the pregnant woman. There is increased sensitivity of the respiratory center, which is possibly related to increasing levels of serum progesterone. The pregnant woman will also experience increased cardiac output, peaking at 20 weeks of pregnancy, and increased stroke volume during the uterine contractions of labor. Plasma expansion without equal increase in red cell volume causes a physiological anemia during pregnancy. Heart rate increases and usually remains elevated.

The enlarging uterus reduces functional lung reserve capacity. Practitioners may see distended neck veins related to hypervolemia, hyperventilation, decreased endurance, and decreased tolerance for exercise as pregnancy progresses. Pulmonary embolism is a significant cause of maternal mortality, and is believed to be reduced by early ambulation postpartum. The physical therapist must recognize the cardiopulmonary status of the patient when prescribing activity levels.

SEXUAL DYSFUNCTIONS

Sexual dysfunctions are most obvious in men, but infertility, frigidity, and hypogonadism can occur in either sex. Male impotence can be hormonal, psychological, or physical. Causes of male infertility can be linked to chromosomal abnormalities, cryptorchidism, decreased semen volume, drug therapy, ductal obstruction, endocrine disorders, ejaculatory disorders, failure of sperm maturation, immunologic reactions, increased heat, increased semen viscosity, infection, or varicocele. Female impotence is usually termed lack of arousal. Both sexes may have orgasmic dysfunction, and some women may be susceptible to vaginismus.

PSYCHOLOGICAL AFFECT

Anxiety accompanies any birth experience or disease or dysfunction process. Vaginal or cesarean childbirth, multiple gestations, and pelvic surgery are times of stress, ranging from eustress to distress. Freeman states that, according to Massler and Devanesan,

The magnitude of the (emotional) response is expected to be proportional to the degree of emotional investment one has in the part of the body being assaulted. Among females, the parts of the body that are most vulnerable to this emotional reaction to assault are the face, hair, breasts, genitalia and perhaps intestine.

Because patients tend to react to current stress in a way similiar to previous crises, a good history is imperative.

CONCLUSION

Musculoskeletal, neurological, vascular, and integumentary symptoms may originate from the reproductive system; thus, a thorough history and physical assessment is necessary. Female patients in the childbearing years must always be considered potential obstetric patients. Their reproductive status must be noted to ensure fetal safety. Care of the obstetric patient always requires care of at least two patients—the mother and her child—and requires appropriate adaptation of treatment techniques. Practitioners are advised to consider wisely the interrelation of systems, because an understanding of the pathology can only enhance treatment.

ANNOTATED BIBLIOGRAPHY

Cherry S, Berkowitz R, Kase N (eds): Rovinsky and Guttmacher's Medical, Surgical and Gynecologic Complications of Pregnancy, 3rd ed. Baltimore, Williams & Wilkins, 1985 (Complete, well-organized text.)

Danforth D, Scott J (eds): Obstetrics and Gynecology, 5th ed. Philadelphia, JB Lippincott, 1986 (Thorough, comprehensive text.)

Freeman MG: Psychological Aspects of Pelvic Surgery. In Mattingly RF, Thompson JD (eds): Te Linde's Operative Gynecology, 6th ed, p 15. Philadelphia, JB Lippincott, 1985 (Excellent resource for operative gynecology.)

Garrey M, Govan A, Hodge C et al: Obstetrics Illustrated, 2nd ed. New York, Churchill-Livingstone, 1974 (Outlined, diagrammed, easily comprehensible text.)

Hellman L, Pritchard J: Williams Obstetrics, 14th ed, p 748. New York, Appleton-Century-Crofts, 1971 (Well-organized, basic text.)

Mattingly RF, Thompson JD: Te Linde's Operative Gynecology, 6th ed. Philadelphia, JB Lippincott, 1985 (Classic text on operative gynecology; originally from Johns Hopkins.)

O'Connor L (ed): Bulletin of the Section on Obstetrics and Gynecology: APTA. Special Issue: TENS 7:3, 1983 (Concise review of the literature on the efficacy and safety of TENS and the pregnant woman.)

O'Connor L (ed): Bulletin of the Section on Obstetrics and Gynecology: APTA. Special Issue: Exercise 8:3, 1984 (Concise reviews of the literature on exercise and pregnancy, including compilation on the knee-chest position.)

Ostergard D (ed): Gynecologic Urology and Urodynamics Theory and Practice. Baltimore, Williams & Wilkins, 1985 (Thorough reference.)

16 Renal Causes

GEORGE A. WOLFE

Kidney disease, in both its acute and chronic forms, is a significant health problem. Over 60,000 persons in the United States are currently being maintained on dialysis or have received kidney transplants. Physical therapists treat many patients whose medical conditions manifest or result in renal failure. Chronic renal failure itself produces systemic changes that result in disorders for which physical therapy is often indicated. Although this chapter is not intended as a pathology reference, it is important to define the nature and major causes of renal failure so the functional impairment necessitating physical therapy involvement can be understood. Understanding the disorders that can arise in renal disease should aid the physical therapist both in selecting appropriate evaluative techniques and in planning effective treatment programs.

RENAL FAILURE

ACUTE RENAL FAILURE

Acute renal failure is defined as a rapid decline in renal function manifested by an elevation in serum urea and creatinine. It is usually accompanied by oliguria, hyperkalemia, and sodium retention. Normally a 50% decline in glomerular filtration rate is necessary before significant signs are noted. The major causes of acute renal failure can be grouped into three classifications: pre-renal, renal, and post-renal. Pre-renal causes include decreased blood flow to the kidneys because of hypovolemia, hypotension, shock, or trauma. Renal causes refer to damage to the functional units of the kidneys (the nephrons) as a result of sepsis, inflammation, ischemia, or drugs. Post-renal causes refer to obstruction of urinary outflow at any point from the tubules to the urethra. Table 16-1 summarizes the causes of renal failure. Treatment of acute renal failure consists of diet, diuretics, intravenous fluids (fluid challenge), and dialysis. Despite intensive medical intervention, the mortality rate can be as high as 50%, usually because of intercurrent infection.

CHRONIC RENAL FAILURE

Chronic renal failure is a persistent, usually progressive decline in function of the kidneys resulting in most cases from glomerular damage. Progression can be relatively rapid or may last for years. Primary signs are edema, hypertension, and uremia. Laboratory findings include proteinuria, hematuria, azotemia, alterations in sodium excretion, and decreased glomerular filtration rate. Many secondary signs of chronic uremia may benefit from physical therapy intervention, and are discussed below.

Chronic renal failure can have many causes. Acute renal failure may become chronic if the precipitating factor is prolonged and the glomeruli are permanently damaged. Hypertensive nephrosclerosis accounts for up to 30%

Table 16-1. Major Causes of Renal Failure

ACUTE	CHRONIC
Pre-renal	Acute renal failure
Hypovolemia	Hypertensive nephrosclerosis
Hypotension	Diabetes mellitus
Trauma	Immune mediated
Renal	Postinfectious
Sepsis	Systemic lupus erythematosus
Inflammation	Goodpasture's syndrome
Ischemia	Polyarteritis nodosa
Drugs	Mixed connective tissue disease
Post-renal	
Obstruction	

of all cases, especially in blacks. Diabetes mellitus results in about 25% of all cases. Immune responses are also a major cause of chronic renal failure. Many patients with collagen vascular diseases such as systemic lupus erythematosus, polyarteritis nodosa, and mixed connective tissue disease ultimately develop chronic renal failure. An immune response to alpha hemolytic streptococcus can also result in chronic glomerulonephritis.

Treatment of chronic renal failure consists of medical management followed by dialysis or transplantation when needed. Protein and sodium-restricted diets, blood pressure control, management of phosphorus intake, and treatment of acidosis are the most common medical interventions. When symptoms of uremia such as anorexia, nausea, and mental confusion occur despite this treatment, or if uremic pericarditis or neuropathy develops, the decision is usually made to begin dialysis or to perform a transplant.

Transplantation has become more successful in recent years, and well-matched recipients have a high probability of long-term graft survival. If a good result is obtained, the uremia is resolved and its symptoms abate. To avoid rejection, patients are required to continue taking drugs that can have undesirable side-effects. Many patients, however, are not candidates for transplantation, have had transplant failures, or do not desire the surgery. These patients must be managed by dialysis.

Dialysis is a process in which the patient's blood is circulated on one side of a semipermeable membrane and a fluid called a dialysate is circulated on the other. By varying the constituents of the dialysate, undesirable amounts of electrolytes and other metabolites can be removed from the blood of the patient by osmosis. Proper electrolyte and fluid balance can thus be obtained. One form of dialysis is peritoneal, in which the dialysate is introduced into the abdominal cavity and the peritoneum serves as the membrane. The other, more common, form is hemodialysis in which blood is removed from the patient, circulated through a dialyzer consisting of a membrane and the dialysate, and then returned to the patient's circulatory system. Both forms, as well as other techniques such as hemofiltration, have advantages and disadvantages. Discussion of them is beyond the scope of this text. It is important to remember that even when dialysis is adequate, patients still manifest signs and symptoms that can limit their function. This is because most dialysis treatments are intermittent instead of continuous. Dialysis is also unable to remove unidentified substances that apparently are deleterious. Trace elements and contaminants such as aluminum and chloramines in the dialysate can also be harmful.

CONSEQUENCES OF RENAL FAILURE

Renal failure, especially in its chronic form, creates multisystem abnormalities. Many of these result in functional impairments that are amenable to some degree to physical therapy. The rest of this chapter presents the disorders resulting from renal failure that can require intervention by the physical therapist (Table 16-2).

PAIN

Patients with chronic renal failure can experience pain attributable to several causes. Over 80% of all patients develop pruritus to some degree. A primary cause of this condition is hypohydrosis of the skin resulting from atrophy of the sweat glands. Increased parathyroid hormone, resulting from derangement of calcium and phosphorus metabolism, can also lead to an increase in mast cells in the skin, which release irritating chemicals. Coupled with this is the deposition of calcium in the form of hydroxyapatite crystals in the subcutaneus tissue. This is termed calciphylaxis and can be a constant source of irritation to the patient. Calcification of small arteries can also lead to ischemia pain. Peripheral neuropathy is another source of skin discomfort.

A second major cause of pain experienced by many patients undergoing hemodialysis is muscle cramping during or following dialysis treatments. During these treatments excess fluid must be removed from the circulation, and this triggers painful muscle cramps in about 60% of all patients. Usually occurring in the legs, the cramps may continue after dialysis and can limit function.

The skeletal system can be the origin of a third type of pain. Skeletal system abnormalities observed in chronic renal disease will be reviewed below. However, one consequence of these disorders can be pathologic fractures. These, as well as bone disease without fracture, can be a source of pain.

Many of the modalities employed by the physical therapist may prove useful in managing the pain associated with renal disease. Unfortunately, objective documentation of the efficacy of these methods is currently lacking. Research remains to be performed to establish which treatments are most useful for the several types of pain experienced by these patients.

EDEMA

Fluid retention in the patient with renal failure is a major problem. Because of the reduced glomerular filtration rate, urine formation in most cases is reduced and body fluids increase. Edema of the distal extremities, especially the legs, is a consequence. Restriction of fluid intake is a very important part of the management of renal failure. Excessive water retention can result in the necessity for removing high amounts of fluid during dialysis, increasing the likelihood of cramping as described previously. Fluid retention may also result in pulmonary edema ("fluid lung"), which can be life threatening.

STRUCTURAL IMBALANCE

The skeletal system can be severely affected by chronic renal disease. As the kidneys fail, the

Table 16-2. Consequences of Renal Failure that May Require Physical Therapy Intervention

Pain
   Pruritus
   Calciphylaxis
   Peripheral neuropathy
   Muscle cramps
   Osteodystrophy

Edema
   Fluid retention

Structural imbalance
   Osteodystrophy

Weakness
   Peripheral neuropathy
   Myopathy

Decreased endurance
   Anemia
   Cardiovascular impairment
   Pulmonary disease
   Deconditioning

Loss of central control
   Autonomic neuropathy

amount of phosphorus excreted decreases. Increased serum phosphorus results in decreased serum ionized calcium, which stimulates production of parathyroid hormone (PTH). Hypertrophy of the parathyroid gland can result. Simultaneously, calcium absorption in the gut is impaired due to a lack of the active form of vitamin D, which is produced by the kidney. In an attempt to increase the serum calcium, PTH mobilizes calcium from the bones. The result is a group of disorders collectively termed renal osteodystrophy. Any of the following types can be seen: osteomalacia, osteoporosis, osteitis fibrosis cystica, osteosclerosis, and subchondral resorption of bone. Pathologic fractures, pain, heterotopic ossification, calciphylaxis, and deformity can result. In children, this commonly leads to severe growth disturbances. Treatment includes reduction of phosphate intake, oral phosphate binders, calcium supplements, and treatment with activated forms of vitamin D.

WEAKNESS

Weakness is a relatively common sequela of renal failure. It occurs secondary to peripheral neuropathy as well as myopathy. It is unclear specifically what causes the peripheral neuropathy of renal disease. Malnutrition as well as unidentified uremic toxins have been implicated. Axonal atrophy and patchy demyelination result in decreased motor nerve conduction velocity. The neuropathy can result in abnormalities in all modes of sensation, paresthesias, weakness, and atrophy. The lower extremities are most commonly involved, with the upper extremities manifesting weakness only after symptoms are severe in the legs. As dialysis techniques have improved, peripheral neuropathy has become less of a problem. However, it remains a significant finding in most patients and is a common reason for referral to physical therapy.

The causes of myopathy in renal disease are also obscure. Malnutrition, increased PTH, decreased vitamin D, disturbance of the microcirculation, and uremic toxins all have been cited. There is elevation of the skeletal muscle fraction of creatinine phosphokinase (CPK). Microscopy reveals streaming of the Z bands and loss of normal arrangement of the actin and myosin filaments. Unlike the weakness of neuropathy, renal myopathy is primarily proximal. Though usually not severe, in some cases myopathy limits function to the point of compromising gait. It may respond favorably to treatment with vitamin D.

DECREASED ENDURANCE

The ability of the patient with renal disease to perform exercise or functional activities can be compromised by decreased endurance. It can affect the patient's ability to comply with a physical therapy program, or it may be an indication for the physical therapist to initiate an endurance training program. Anemia, cardiovascular impairment, pulmonary disease, and deconditioning can play a role in reducing the exercise tolerance of the patient (Table 16-3).

Patients with chronic renal disease are usually anemic, with the average hemoglobin of a patient on hemodialysis varying between 6 and 8 g/dL. This degree of anemia can markedly

Table 16-3. Causes of Decreased Endurance in Renal Disease.

Anemia
  Decreased erythropoietin
  Decreased erythrocyte life span
  Iron deficiency
  Blood loss
  Decreased folic acid
  Hypersplenism
  Chloramine, copper, zinc
Cardiovascular impairment
  Hypertension
  Atherosclerosis
    Hypertension
    Hyperlipidemia
  Cardiomyopathy
  Pericarditis
  Arteriovenous shunts
  Autonomic neuropathy
Pulmonary impairment
  Pulmonary edema
  Calcifications
Deconditioning
  Sedentary life-style

decrease endurance by lowering the oxygen-carrying capacity of the blood. The causes of anemia in this patient group are numerous (see Table 16-3). Chief among them are decreased production of erythropoietin by the kidney and decreased life span of erythrocytes from a normal 115 days to an average of 70 days. This decreased life span is caused by increased PTH and unidentified uremic toxins. Treatment is usually iron supplementation, splenectomy, androgens, and transfusion.

The cardiovascular system of patients with renal disease can be severely impaired because of the elevated incidence of hypertension, atherosclerosis, cardiomyopathy, pericarditis, and the presence of arteriovenous shunts created to allow vascular access for hemodialysis. Hypertension results primarily from fluid retention and excess production of renin. Hyperlipidemia is common in these patients and manifests itself in increased triglycerides and decreased HDL cholesterol. The combination of hyperlipidemia and hypertension leads to an increased risk of coronary artery disease because of atherosclerosis. More than 50% of all deaths of patients with chronic renal disease result from cardiac failure. In addition to ischemic cardiac disease, there is evidence that uremic toxins can cause cardiomyopathy. Of patients with uremia, 25% to 40% have evidence of left ventricular dysfunction. Pericarditis resulting from irritation by toxins and infection is also common, and can result in cardiac tamponade. Combined with the above problems, patients dependent upon hemodialysis have an additional cardiac stressor. Arteriovenous shunts for vascular access typically carry 300 to 400 mL of blood per minute, requiring the cardiac output to be that much higher at any given work load in order to compensate.

The pulmonary system can be impaired. Fluid overload may result in pulmonary edema. Calcium deposits can also form in the lungs. In worst cases, this results in a diffusion block across the alveolar membrane, decreasing oxygen delivery to the blood.

Most patients with chronic renal disease are sedentary. Coupled with the above considerations, this results in deconditioning. De-creased endurance is thus magnified. Many patients, despite what is believed to be adequate maintenance on dialysis, are unable to work on a consistent basis because of fatigue. This produces significant economic stress.

LOSS OF CENTRAL CONTROL

Neuropathy also can affect the autonomic nervous system, decreasing central control of several functions, chief among them heart rate and blood pressure. In patients with autonomic neuropathy, there is decreased heart rate and blood pressure response to a Valsalva maneuver. The blood pressure also fails to rise normally during handgrip tests, and compensation for orthostatic hypotension is decreased, especially in diabetics. This decrement in response may have an effect upon the ability to perform physical work.

ANNOTATED BIBLIOGRAPHY

Bagdade J: Accelerated atherosclerosis in patients on maintenance dialysis. In Hamberger J, Cronier J, Grunfeld J-P et al (eds): Advances in Nephrology from the Necker Hospital, vol 9, p 7. Chicago, Yearbook Medical Publishers, 1980 (A good review of the incidence and causes of atherosclerosis in renal patients.)

Bibra H von, Castro L, Autenrieth G et al: The effects of arteriovenous shunts on cardiac function in renal dialysis patients: An echocardiographic evaluation. Clin Nephrol 9:205, 1978 (Definitive experimental study with good discussion of the problem.)

Conger J, Howard A, Alfrey A et al: Pulmonary calcification in chronic dialysis patients: Clinical and pathological studies. Ann Intern Med 83:330, 1975 (Discussion of incidence and causes as well as experimental results.)

Drueke T, LePailleur C, Zingraff J et al: Uremic cardiomyopathy and pericarditis. In Hamberger J, Cronier J, Grunfeld J-P et al (eds): Advances in Nephrology from the Necker Hospital, Vol 9, p 33. Chicago, Yearbook Medical Publishers, 1980 (Excellent discussion of both problems and their implications.)

Goldberg AP, Hagberg J, Delmez JA et al: The metabolic and psychological effects of exercise training in hemodialysis patients. Am J Clin Nutr 33:1620, 1980 (Except for lack of specific quantification of exercise program, an excellent experimental study and discussion of the limitations of endurance in these patients.)

Henderson RG, Ledingham J, Oliver D et al: Effects of 1,25-dihyroxycholecalciferol on calcium absorption, muscle weakness, and bone disease in chronic renal failure. Lancet 1:379, 1974 (An overview of the effects of activated vitamin D. Describes the myopathy and bone disease nicely.)

Neff M, Kim M, Persoff M et al: Hemodynamics of uremic anemia. Circulation 43:876, 1971 (An old study, but one that describes the cardiovascular stress imposed by the anemia seen in these patients.)

Smith R, Stein G: Myopathy, osteomalacia and hyperparathyroidism. Brain 90:593, 1967 (An early, but good discussion of the relationship of PTH to bone disease and myopathy.)

Tenckhoff HA, Boen E, Jebsen RH et al: Polyneuropathy in renal insufficiency. JAMA 192:1121, 1965 (A valuable overview of signs and symptoms.)

Wiedmann P, Maxwell MH: Hypertension. In Massry SG, Sellars AC (eds): Clinical Aspects of Uremia and Dialysis, p 100. Springfield, IL, Charles C Thomas, 1976 (A thorough discussion of all aspects of this persistent problem.)

17 Psychological Causes

CAROL SCHUNK

A person with a disorder that includes physical and psychological symptoms will usually attempt to find an organic cause by consulting a medical professional. This occurs in part because physical symptoms may dominate the clinical picture, causing the person to believe his illness is physical in origin. This belief determines the pattern of medical consultation. Another reason the initial focus might be on the physical aspect is the availability and social acceptance of seeking medical care over seeking psychological services. Because a medical professional such as a physician or physical therapist is commonly the entry point for health services, it is imperative that practitioners have a background in the psychological complications of or reactions to organic disease as well as the somatic presentation of psychiatric disorders. This chapter will focus on somatic presentations of psychiatric disorders. The physical therapist's understanding of all factors contributing to a movement disorder is essential so that the treatment goals and program may be modified to accommodate the psychiatric influence.

The mind-body dichotomy, once an accepted part of the medical model, no longer is a viable explanation for the complexity of medical conditions. Just as a person cannot be split into two factions, illness does not affect only the body or only the mind. The complexity of the situation is reflected in the controversy surrounding the terminology currently used, particularly the terms *psychogenic* and *psychosomatic*. As explained by Lipowski (1985), the notion of psychogenesis or attributing the origin of an illness to the psyche is incompatible with the prevailing doctrine of multicausality of disease. Although the term psychosomatic is commonly used to describe physical disorders caused or aggravated by psychologic factors, its use may encourage dualism or mind-body orientation to disease. This connotation limits the applicability of a multidimensional approach to diagnosis and treatment. Therefore, the term psychosomatic is used given the absence of a more appropriate term. However, the meaning should refer to the reciprocal relationship between psychosocial and biologic factors in health and disease.

Lloyd (1986), in his review of psychiatric syndromes, indicates that somatization or the appearance of physical symptoms occurs in most psychiatric illnesses. In fact, in the majority of cases the initial presentation of symptoms is physical rather than psychiatric in nature. Unfortunately, the presence of somatic complaints tends to distract the medical professional from the correct diagnosis of a primarily psychiatric disorder. If the possibility of psychiatric contribution to physical symptoms is ignored, mismanagement or misdiagnosis may occur. When a movement disorder is a symptom, a physical therapist frequently is consulted and therefore becomes part of the diagnostic team. If the psychiatric condition is undiagnosed, the physical therapy evaluation will probably include several unusual or unexplained findings. Likewise, the patient will not progress in the expected manner with physical

313

therapy, despite treatment modifications. In such a situation, the physical therapist who is aware of the characteristics of psychiatric conditions will be in a better position to make a positive contribution to the diagnosis and eventual case management.

Physical therapists should be familiar with several specific mental disorders in which somatic symptoms are a primary diagnostic criteria. These disorders are identified by the American Psychiatric Association in the Diagnostic and Statistical Manual of Mental Disorders (DSM III).

DIAGNOSTIC CATEGORIES

The third edition of the Diagnostic and Statistical Manual of Mental Disorders (DSM III) is a glossary of descriptions of the diagnostic categories for mental disorders. For some disorders, somatic symptoms are a primary diagnostic criteria. When discussing movement disorders attributable to a psychological condition, it becomes necessary to refer to the DSM III, because the referring diagnosis is often dependent on criteria stated in the manual. Although it is unlikely that the physical therapist will need to read the DSM III, familiarity with the

disorders will facilitate treatment planning because terminology in psychological reports is usually consistent with DSM III guidelines. The diagnosis made by a psychologist probably will follow DSM III format, because most third party payers reimburse based on DSM III codes. Therefore, the Manual can be a useful reference for the physical therapist involved with patients whose mental condition influences physical functioning.

Each diagnostic category has specific diagnostic criteria related to the characteristics of the presenting physical symptoms. Consideration of the presence or absence of each diagnostic criterion provides the basis for diagnosis. Awareness of these criteria will allow the physical therapist to accurately assess patients who have a psychiatric disorder that involves physical symptoms (Table 17-1).

One main distinguishing characteristic between disorders is the identification of the somatic symptoms as being attributable to a typical pattern of illness. If organicity cannot be demonstrated, then the issue of voluntary control is examined. Identification of voluntary control is controversial. It is recognized in the DSM III as being subjective and only inferred by an outside observer, who may be the physical therapist. Symptoms that appear to be fo-

Table 17-1. Presence or Absence of Diagnostic Criteria for Diagnostic Categories Involving Physical Symptoms

DIAGNOSTIC CRITERIA	DIAGNOSTIC CATEGORY					
	Psychological Factors Affecting Physical Condition	Factitious Disorder	Malingering	Somatization Disorder	Conversion Disorder	Psychogenic Pain Disorder
Organic findings	Yes	No	No	No	No	No
Apparently under voluntary control	No	Yes	Yes	No	No	No
Recognizable goal	No	No	Yes	No	No	No
History of recurrent, multiple symptoms	No	No	No	Yes	No	No
Loss of physical function attributed to psychological factors	No	No	No	No	Yes	No
Limited to pain	No	No	No	No	No	Yes

cused on a situational goal is another criterion for diagnosis, as is the history and presentation of the physical symptoms. Although not characterized by the presence of physical symptoms, depression does influence movement and will be discussed with the other disorders to provide a background for the physical therapist treating a patient with somatic presentation of a psychiatric disorder.

PSYCHOLOGICAL FACTORS AFFECTING PHYSICAL CONDITION

A physical condition may be exacerbated or initiated by the contribution of psychological factors. In such cases, a mental diagnosis of psychological factors affecting physical condition is appropriate. Even though the condition can be attributed to demonstrable organic pathology or a pathophysiological process, the extent to which the symptoms are displayed is not in keeping with the medical diagnosis. An environmental stimulus, such as divorce, may be the psychological factor that can prompt or exaggerate physical symptoms such as migraine headaches or arthritis.

When patients are seen in physical therapy with organic symptoms that occur without physical cause, psychological factors should be considered. Investigation of environmental issues will often contribute more to the resolution of physical symptoms than will traditional therapy.

FACTITIOUS DISORDERS WITH PHYSICAL SYMPTOMS

A factitious disorder with physical symptoms is characterized by symptoms that are voluntarily produced by the individual and that have no organic basis. Although the issue of voluntary control is critical to the diagnosis of a factitious disorder, the DSM III uses the term "apparently under the individual's voluntary control." This acknowledges the necessity of clinical judgment in making the decision whether a symptom is indeed voluntary or involuntary. The display of symptoms is deliberate and purposeful, the objective apparently being to assume the "patient" role. Diagnosed

persons often have a history of multiple hospitalizations and are knowledgeable in medical terminology, procedures, and routine. Behavioral characteristics usually involve noncompliance, arguing with medical personnel, and dramatic presentation of complaints. A chronic factitious disorder has also been called Munchausen syndrome.

MALINGERING

Malingering is differentiated from factitious disorder by the presence of an easily recognizable objective that is achieved by the person's illness behavior. This objective can usually be determined by a knowledge of the patient's environmental situation. Litigation over a workmen's compensation claim is an example of a specific goal that might precipitate voluntary prolonged recovery from a shoulder injury and meet diagnostic criteria for malingering. If the same injury occurred in conjunction with a factitious disorder, the only apparent goal would be to retain the role of a patient. In both cases the patient will complain of symptoms that have no physical origin.

SOMATIZATION DISORDER

Somatization disorders are characterized by recurrent and multiple physical symptoms. To meet diagnostic criteria, the symptoms must have started prior to age 30 and include numerous physical complaints. Complaints may involve several organic systems and are not clinically explained by physical disorder, injury, or the side-effects of medication, drugs, or alcohol. These complaints are often presented in a dramatic, vague, or exaggerated manner. The clinician need not observe the symptom; the patient's report of the existence of a symptom is sufficient to meet diagnostic criteria. However, the patient must report that the symptom was severe enough to have caused him to take medication, see a physician, or alter the life pattern.

The symptomatic presentations that may be observed in patients referred for physical therapy take various forms. Conversion or pseudoneurological symptoms such as varying degrees of muscle weakness and abnormal gait patterns may be exhibited. Cardiopulmonary symptoms and pain are other common complaints of persons with somatization disorders.

CONVERSION DISORDER

Conversion disorder was previously referred to as hysterical neurosis, conversion type. The clinical picture is one of alteration of physical functioning that is an apparent expression of a psychological conflict rather than a physical disorder. Diagnostic criteria include an inability to explain symptoms by a physiologic examination, and determination that the symptom is not under voluntary control. The uniqueness of conversion disorder is reflected in the specific mechanisms to which the disorder is attributed. One mechanism involves a relationship between an environmental stimulus related to psychological conflict and the appearance of the symptom. An example of this mechanism is a lower extremity paralysis following failure in a sports event in which the person's self-image was dependent on the outcome. A second mechanism is based upon secondary gain through avoiding an activity or gaining support from the environment relative to the display of the physical symptom.

Movement implications of conversion disorder include symptoms such as paralysis, weakness, coordination disturbance, sensory changes, dyskinesia, or akinesia. Within a given episode there is usually only one symptom, although variation may occur if the disorder repeats. Clinically, the physical therapist may evaluate an undiagnosed patient and obtain inconclusive or unusual results. For example, the gait pattern of a patient with complaints of lower extremity weakness will appear inconsistent with the motor findings. Paralysis or sensory changes will not follow motor root or dermatomal patterns. When evaluation results in the identification of abnormal movement and function, consideration of a diagnosis of conversion disorder may be appropriately initiated by the physical therapist.

PSYCHOGENIC PAIN DISORDER

The predominant symptom for psychogenic pain disorder is severe and prolonged pain that cannot be attributed to organic pathology or a pathophysiological mechanism. The disorder can also be diagnosed in the case of identifiable organic pathology when the complaint of pain is grossly exaggerated given the physical findings. An additional diagnostic criteria is the involvement of psychological factors similar to the conversion disorder. In this case the pain is enabling the person to avoid a noxious activity or gain support from the environment that is not available without the pain behavior. Or, as seen in some cases, a relationship exists between an environmental stimulus related to psychological conflict and the initiation of the pain.

Psychogenic pain disorder should be differentiated from malingering, which may also involve pain behavior. In malingering, the presentation of symptoms is under voluntary control and is in pursuit of a goal. Although the issue of voluntary control may be difficult to determine, the goal in the case of malingering is usually identifiable upon assessment of the person's environmental circumstances.

Reinforcement of the pain behavior quickly becomes an issue when the patient is referred for physical therapy. If passive modalities are prescribed, the treatment may be counterproductive to diminishing the symptoms. Although movement is often disturbed by the pain symptoms, treatment will usually focus on minimizing the pain behaviors rather than the physical limitations.

DEPRESSION

Depression, or the loss of interest or pleasure in activity, is often characterized by movement dysfunction. One of eight documented symptoms of clinical depression is psychomotor retardation or agitation. The occurrence of such symptoms might initiate a physical therapy referral. Psychomotor retardation can be characterized by slowed body movements or decreased energy level experienced as continuous fatigue despite the lack of physical exertion. Excessive concern with physical health is common. Symptoms must be present nearly every day for a period of two weeks, and may include psychotic features such as delusions or hallucinations. Psychological reaction to a serious illness or disability may also result in a depressed mood and influence physical therapy treatment.

Attempts in physical therapy to enhance activity or increase endurance will often be unsuccessful. Until the factors precipitating the depression are explored and discussed, the physical symptoms may remain unchanged. Recognition of the limitations of treating the physical symptoms may reduce the frustration that often occurs when working with a depressed person.

COMPLIANCE

Although not a psychiatric disorder, compliance is a behavioral issue that can affect the therapeutic outcome. Based on the results from an initial evaluation, a physical therapist establishes treatment goals and designs a treatment plan. As treatment continues, the therapist has certain expectations for progress and the time required to accomplish specific treatment objectives. If movement dysfunction continues without explainable complications, compliance should be considered as a treatment issue. Compliance refers to the exact adherence to a treatment regimen. It is expected by most health professionals despite research estimates showing that noncompliance ranges from 20% to 80% with an average of 50% across studies. If a patient does not follow instructions, the physical limitations or disability may fail to improve or may even get worse. Therefore, although noncompliance does not cause the movement dysfunction in a physiological sense, the behavioral issue will influence the patient's recovery.

Compliance traditionally has referred to undercompliance or the patient doing less than prescribed. The factor of overcompliance or doing more than prescribed has rarely been a consideration in the design of most studies. When a patient does not progress as expected, consideration of overcompliance as a therapeutic variable may be appropriate as a cause of prolonged or unexplained symptoms. Taking too much medication or doing too many exercises may have adverse effects quite different from those related to underutilization of the therapeutic regimen.

The identification of motivational factors likely to influence compliance to a medical regimen is the basis of the Health Belief Model developed by Becker and Maiman (1975). They proposed that the decision to comply or not comply is based upon the patient's belief that

- he is susceptible to the condition,
- the condition has severe consequences,
- the treatment is effective, and
- the cost (financial and personal) will not outweigh the benefits.

Although prediction of noncompliance is difficult, the therapist's awareness of the possibility of noncompliance is important. Self-report can be a valuable tool in identifying the noncompliant patient if administered in a nonthreatening, nonjudgmental manner. This allows the patient to maintain a sense of self-respect when reporting noncompliant behavior. Use of a self-report would allow the therapist to intervene in cases that might otherwise be mishandled on the assumption that the treatment regimen was being followed.

CONCLUSION

Physical therapists have the opportunity to play an important role in the diagnosis and treatment of patients with somatic symptoms related to a psychiatric disorder. The knowledge of normal movement and function is essential to determine if a person is producing symptoms with no physiological origin. Given the physical therapist's educational background, he is in a unique position to assess when a patient being treated for a medical condition may have a movement disorder attributable in part to a psychiatric condition. Awareness of the mental disorders associated with physical symptoms and behavioral issues that influence treatment will prevent mismanagement and facilitate patient recovery.

ANNOTATED BIBLIOGRAPHY

American Psychiatric Association: Diagnostic and Statistical Manual of Mental Disorders, 3rd ed. Washington, DC, American Psychiatric Association, 1980 (Glossary of the descriptions of the diagnostic categories for mental disorders.)

Becker MH, Maiman LA: Social behavioral determinents of compliance with health and medical care recommendations. Med Care 8:1, 1975 (Original development of the Health Belief Model, which continues to be a model for compliance behavior.)

Lipowski ZJ: Psychosomatic Medicine and Liaison Psychiatry: Selected Papers. New York, Plenum, 1985 (Presents a broad overview of psychosomatic medicine. Includes both theoretical and clinical aspects of a biological and psychosocial perspective of illness and disability.)

Lloyd GG: Review article: Psychiatric syndromes with a somatic presentation. Psychosom Res 30:2, 1986 (Reviews the presenting symptoms and diagnostic problems of psychiatric illness with physical symptoms.)

PART IV

Analysis of Movement Dysfunction and Physical Disability

18 The Evaluation Process

JUDITH S. CANFIELD

You will consistently hear that patients must be evaluated before they can be treated. Indeed, how could you treat a patient without first knowing what conditions existed? In order for a therapeutic program to prevent certain pathological conditions from occurring or for a treatment regimen to alleviate dysfunction, the intervention must be directed toward some specific goals. Specific goals cannot be established unless the practitioner is fully cognizant of the capabilities, limitations, and potential of the client. Such factors can only be determined on the basis of a thorough collection and interpretation of patient information.

Evaluation techniques are not used solely to design and initiate treatment programs. These techniques are just as useful in determining the extent of patient progress. Such reevaluation may formally take place on a weekly or monthly basis, and informal reevaluations are an integral part of treatment. Most physical therapists compare a client's signs and symptoms as they appear with those noted on the previous visit and alter the treatment accordingly. If the client requires an assistive device, results of evaluations are used to select the specific features to be included on the device. Evaluation techniques are also used to determine the status of a patient at the time of discharge from physical therapy and the type of follow-up plan or continued care to be recommended.

The collection and interpretation of patient information is also known as evaluation, examination, screen, and assessment. The primary difference between the terms appears to be a function of the breadth of focus of each collection and interpretation process. *Evaluation* seems to be the broadest term, referring to the consideration of the physical and mental state of a patient or of a healthy person. The term *examination,* although broad, refers to the inspection of the body's systems specifically to determine the absence or presence of disease. *Screen* is the most focused of these terms because it refers to systematic inspection directed towards determining the presence of a specific disease or characteristic. *Assessment* is the assignment of a value to or the determination of the quantity and quality of a characteristic, sign, or symptom.

Regardless of the breadth of focus, some elements are common to these investigative processes. One element is knowledge. A certain level of knowledge in the human biological, behavioral, and medical sciences is necessary. If the practitioner does not know what constitutes normal functioning and normal values, he cannot hope to identify abnormalities or recognize their effect on their own or related systems. A second element is a rational and logical system of data acquisition. Unless the practitioner employs such a scheme, data may not be uncovered or, once uncovered, may not appear relevant. During acquisition, data are examined, sorted, and grouped. A complete picture of the client is developed through this analysis and synthesis of data.

REASONS FOR EVALUATING

Why do we use these investigative processes? There are three traditional reasons. (1) The practitioner needs to determine the current health care status of the client. To do this, the practitioner must identify the problems that potentially and actually exist for the client as well as the present and projected future capabilities. (2) The practitioner must establish the diagnosis and subsequently predict the outcomes of treatment for the client. To design an effective therapeutic intervention, one must first establish treatment goals or outcomes. Only then can appropriate therapeutic techniques be selected. (3) The examination of a client provides a baseline against which future measurement values may be compared. These comparisons or reevaluations are necessary not only to monitor the degree of change in the client's condition but also to determine the effectiveness of the intervention. Such comparative documentation is also required by some third-party reimbursement agencies if continued care is to be provided to the patient.

These traditional reasons for client evaluation are just as valid today as ever. However, as the profession gains greater autonomy of practice, additional compelling evaluation issues arise. In direct access situations where the physical therapist is the entry point for clients into the health care system, several critical issues must be addressed before therapeutic intervention can be initiated. One of these issues is the ethical decision of which client should be treated in a particular setting by which therapist. Among any group of physical therapists, whether in an institutional department or a private practice, there exists only a finite number of clinical skills. The physical therapists in one particular setting may be experts in the treatment of adult patients whose physical dysfunctions are orthopedic in nature. However, those same therapists may have little experience treating pediatric patients who have neurologic dysfunctions. Whether or not a patient with primarily neurologic symptoms should be treated in this particular setting is a significant question. To answer this question, a gross patient evaluation should be done, including a brief history and some description of the behavior of these symptoms. If the resulting information indicates that the client should be treated in this particular setting, a second question arises: Which therapist should further evaluate and treat the client? If the client's dysfunction is common and uncomplicated, the assignment of a therapist may not be critical. However, for the patient with an unusual or complex problem, it would be best to assign the therapist with the greatest expertise. If the client should not be treated in this particular setting, he should be referred.

A second issue related to evaluation and direct access is the issue of referral. Clients may be referred for various reasons. The patient data revealed during an initial evaluation may indicate that a physical therapist is not the appropriate practitioner to treat the type of dysfunction exhibited by the patient. Alternatively, the initial data may suggest that, although a physical therapist is the appropriate practitioner to treat the dysfunction, a physical therapist with the necessary extensive evaluation and treatment skills is not available at the particular setting. On the other hand, the initial evaluation data may result in the decision that the evaluating therapist is the appropriate practitioner but that additional information is needed about the client. The physical therapist may have thoroughly gathered the appropriate patient information, but requires some laboratory values or the results of radiography and other imaging techniques to confirm or clarify the diagnosis. Or, the physical therapist may require a diagnosis by a physician. In each of these instances, the therapist's concern for the quality and effectiveness of patient care can only be addressed through referral of the client to another practitioner.

COLLECTING INFORMATION

Evaluation, examination, screening, and assessment all follow an orderly sequence of collection and interpretation of client information. Most data are collected through replicable, standardized techniques. These techniques are valid in that, when administered properly, they measure what they purport to measure. They are considered to be reliable in that subsequent use of the technique with the same or similar clients will produce similar results. The integrity of the results of tests administered solely through manual intervention are subject to factors internal to the test itself, such as the amount of pressure applied by the practitioner to the anatomical area being examined. External factors such as differences in techniques employed by different practitioners can also affect the results. Although the results of mechanically applied tests have a higher degree of reliability, their integrity can be compromised by factors external to the test such as computer crashes, electrical surges, and inaccurate calibration.

Through the application of standardized evaluation techniques, client data emerge. The practitioner has a preset order for administering the evaluative techniques and collecting the data. Minimally, the collected data are grouped in terms of their representation of normal or abnormal states or conditions (negative or positive findings, respectively). In addition, more discrete groupings may be used. The specificity of the grouping can be a function of the complexity of the dysfunction, the frequency with which the dysfunction occurs in the population, the protocol of the facility where the client is being seen, the purpose of the evaluation, and the professional or agency for whom the evaluation is being completed.

EVALUATION IN THE PRACTICE OF PHYSICAL THERAPY

Because information about the client is frequently available from sources other than the client himself, a physical therapist may begin to formulate ideas about a patient's dysfunction, treatment goals, and therapeutic program before the client is actually seen. If the patient is being seen by a therapist in an institutional setting, information about the client may already exist in the patient's chart or medical record. These sources usually contain admission information, medical histories, evaluations by other health professionals, laboratory findings, surgical and special procedures reports, and discharge summaries for any prior admission. If the client is being seen in a private practice or in his home, such visits are usually the result of a referral. Referrals, for the most part, contain at least a preliminary diagnosis or expected outcomes of the visit. The latter provides less comprehensive information regarding the client's condition.

Physical therapists practicing in home health settings, large academic health care centers, small rural acute care hospitals, and in their own private practices all engage in a similar continual process of collecting and gathering data about their clients. Some of the client data is gathered directly from the client through observation. When the physical therapist greets his client for the first time, he is also noting cues about the client: "Her right shoulder is higher than the left. I wonder if this is secondary to a leg length discrepancy, a pelvic obliquity, or a scoliosis?" Noting abnormalities in size, shape, color, sound, smell, alignment, symmetry, and function demonstrated by a client can provide data indicative of hypertrophic disease, skeletal deformity, compromised circulation, infection, degenerative joint disease, peripheral nerve injury, or central nervous system involvement.

At the same time he is observing the client, the therapist also talks with the person about her problems. The data collected from the client in this history-taking fashion is referred to as subjective data. It is considered subjective because it is dependent on the client's perception of the problem and cannot be externally verified. Subjective data may be elicited by asking questions, such as: "Where is the problem/pain? When did it start? Was it the result of an injury or did it just start? Describe how it feels. Has it spread or gotten smaller since it started? Does anything relieve/aggravate the problem/pain? Have you ever had this before? Have you had any treatment for it? What were the results of the treatment?'' The simultaneous mental processing of cues gathered through observation along with the client's responses to the questions will provide the physical therapist with potential etiologies.

The preliminary identification of etiologies forms the basis on which the physical therapist will select specific evaluative tests to perform with the patient. Physical therapists are knowledgeable about and skillful in applying various replicable and standardized techniques. These techniques allow for the evaluation of the musculoskeletal, neuromuscular, cardiovascular, pulmonary, and integumentary systems. The information gathered through these techniques is referred to as objective data. It is considered objective in that it is quantifiable and verifiable.

As information about the client is collected, the physical therapist will begin to group the findings. The collected data will be filtered through the therapist's knowledge of anatomy, kinesiology, neuroscience, physiology, and pathology as well as his understanding of psychoemotional and cultural responses to pain and dysfunction. The filtering first allows the therapist to determine if the client demonstrates any positive findings. Based on this gross determination, more discrete filtering allows the therapist to begin to identify which systems appear to be functioning within normal limits for the client's age and sex, and which systems show abnormal functioning. Exactly when this analysis of information begins and probable diagnoses or problem identifications are generated is a matter of some uncertainty.

As additional evaluative techniques produce subsequent data, they are correlated with an emerging pattern of dysfunction. This allows the therapist to begin to identify the involved tissues as well as the degree of acuteness of the problem. If a pattern is corroborated, the practitioner will be able to determine the etiology more accurately. If the pattern is not substantiated, additional evaluation and correlation of new data with existing data must be done. Depending on the complexity, novelty, and predictability of the client's problem,

the physical therapist may use one or more clinical reasoning processes. Through these processes, the therapist identifies the patient's problems, determines treatment goals, and selects the therapeutic interventions that will be included in the treatment program.

To elaborate further on evaluation, I will use as examples two techniques—goniometry and manual muscle testing—with which physical therapists can gather and interpret information about their clients. These two evaluative techniques are most commonly associated with the practice of physical therapy.

Goniometry is a method of measuring the amount of motion available at any given joint. The measurement may be of the active or the passive motion of the joint. Active motion refers to the movement achieved by contraction of the muscles around the joint. Passive motion refers to the movement achieved when the joint is moved by a force outside the body, such as a pulley or a therapist. When compared, the gross difference between active and passive motion of the same joint can begin to indicate the nature of the client's problem.

For example, a client stated during the subjective portion of the evaluation that he has a painful shoulder and he cannot move it as far as he used to. This condition started the day after he pitched five innings of softball at the family reunion three weeks ago. He had not pitched since the previous reunion. The physical therapist can filter this subjective information through her knowledge base. Her knowledge of anatomy provides a mental picture of all the structures about the shoulder joint: articular surfaces, joint capsule, ligaments, bursae, tendons, and muscles. Knowledge of kinesiology allows her to distinguish between the types of active motion (active assistive, free active, and active resistive) and passive motion (classical movements and the accessory movements of joint play and components). Kinesiology also provides an understanding of the way in which the shoulder joint should function, as well as its normal ranges of motion. All of this knowledge helps the physical therapist to select the objective tests by which to evaluate the client and determine where the problem is located and what the problem is.

As one evaluation technique, the therapist would select goniometric measurement. She then would take active and passive range of motion measurements to identify any limitations of each shoulder movement, the degree of any limitations, and the point in each motion when any pain occurred. The therapist can group these measurements into abnormal and normal measurements (positive and negative findings). These findings are then compared with patterns of shoulder dysfunction that the therapist has seen in the past. Based on the interpretation of the results of the comparison, a few additional tests might be done before the therapist would be able to identify the client's problem as being in the joint capsule and the nature of the problem as being a subacute inflammation. She now can set treatment goals, select therapeutic interventions, and implement treatment.

The second evaluative technique most frequently associated with physical therapy is manual muscle testing (MMT). As the name implies, manual muscle testing tests muscles, not movements. When a physical therapist uses MMT, he must isolate the muscle being tested from other muscles. Realistically, this cannot be done with many muscles. Therefore, the therapist must differentiate the action of one muscle from the action of others. This is done by carefully considering positioning of the client, fixation and stabilization of the bodily segments involved in the test, the amount of pressure applied to the line of pull of the test muscle, and the potential for substitution of action by other muscles. Information gathered through MMT provides a picture of the functional abilities of the patient, helps to localize weakness, and assists in differential diagnoses by distinguishing between problems of contractile and noncontractile tissue.

Consider for a moment the previous example of the client who pitched five innings at his family reunion. The evaluating physical therapist has determined that active movement in one particular direction is painful for the client, but passive movement in the same direction is not painful. However, passive movement in the opposite direction is painful. The therapist might also discover that resistance applied to an isotonic contraction of the muscle that produced the painful active motion is also painful. The constant selection and analysis of patient information, the interpretation of the findings, and the comparing of patterns of information allows the therapist to arrive at a diagnosis. In this case the problem is tendinitis of the subscapularis muscle. However, if the client did not have any limitations in range, and if the shoulder pain had been much more diffuse and accompanied by night pain in the hand, some weakness in grip strength, and poor cervical and shoulder posture, a very different clinical diagnosis would have been reached. This information, when supported by positive findings from other evaluative tests, might indicate a thoracic outlet syndrome.

Although some techniques may be used to assess the functioning of more than one system of the body, each test is designed to elicit very specific information. It is through the skillful selection, application, and interpretation of these techniques that the physical therapist accurately determines a diagnosis.

ANNOTATED BIBLIOGRAPHY

American Academy of Orthopaedic Surgeons: Joint Motion: Methods of Measuring and Recording. Chicago, American Academy of Orthopaedic Surgeons, 1965 (Thorough overview of techniques for measurement of joint extremity and spinal motions. Compares ranges of motion for most joints from four sources.)

Daniels L, Worthingham C: Muscle Testing: Techniques of Manual Examination, 5th ed. Philadelphia, WB Saunders, 1986 (Discusses manual testing techniques for extremity, trunk, and facial muscles and describes proper testing for grades trace to normal.)

Kendall F, McCreary E: Muscles: Testing and Function, 3rd ed. Baltimore, Williams & Wilkins, 1983 (This discussion of manual testing techniques for extremity, trunk, and facial muscles primarily describes proper testing for grades fair and above. Also discusses posture analysis.)

Kessler R, Hertling D: Management of Common Musculoskeletal Disorders: Physical Therapy Principles and Methods. Philadelphia, JB Lippincott, 1983 (Reviews concepts of joint structure, function, and dysfunction and the application of specific assessment and treatment techniques to each extremity joint.)

Minor M, Minor S: Patient Evaluation Methods of Health Professional. Reston, VA, Reston Publishing, 1985 (Reviews basic evaluative techniques and contains excellent photos.)

Norkin C, White D: Measurement of Joint Motion: A Guide to Goniometry. Philadelphia, FA Davis, 1985 (Thorough discussion, with exceptional photos, of goniometric measurement of extremity, TMJ, and spinal motions.)

19 Musculoskeletal Analysis: Introduction

GAIL M. JENSEN

Why is evaluation of the musculoskeletal system necessary? What should that evaluation include? What information needs to be gathered and how do you interpret that information? These are questions this chapter will address. This chapter will provide a general overview of basic concepts critical to musculoskeletal evaluation. Hopefully, this will facilitate your reading of the specific evaluations of the upper and lower quadrant joints in the chapters that follow. There are many excellent sources that provide a more comprehensive discussion of musculoskeletal evaluation, and you will be referred to these throughout the chapter.

Cyriax is responsible for many of the principles followed in evaluation of the musculoskeletal system. In his extensive writings on orthopaedic medicine he argues for logical treatment and the use of reason, not mere custom, as a basis for treatment. He believes that physical therapists need to apply a systematic evaluation in the treatment of patients with musculoskeletal problems and he states:

> Throughout, the choice of method depends on the diagnosis. Accurate treatment follows as a logical result and requires a high degree of skill. . . . Routine physiotherapy forms no part of the practice of orthopaedic medicine. . . . Consequently she cannot allow herself imprecise measures even if the doctor refers the patient with an inexact request. To this end, she assesses the function in turn of every tissue that could be relevant to the symptoms. She singles out the structure at fault, and which part of it, and selects the

individually correct treatment. This intellectual approach involves thought, a clear concept of applied and functional anatomy and never failing interest and care (Cyriax and Coldham, 1984).

Patients with musculoskeletal problems come to physical therapy from many different routes. Some patients have a medical diagnosis that may be as broad as low back pain or as specific as supraspinatus tendinitis. Other patients may have no medical diagnosis and come to a physical therapist for evaluation, consultation, or treatment. Regardless of how the patient reaches a physical therapist, a thorough evaluation lays the foundation for any intervention. This intervention may include consultation, treatment, or referral to another practitioner. The evaluation includes both quantitative and qualitative data, which provides a guide for the therapist throughout the treatment process.

The evaluation by the physical therapist of a patient with a musculoskeletal problem is built on the therapist's knowledge of kinesiology, applied anatomy, pathology, and behavioral sciences. This chapter will provide an overview of how this knowledge is used in the evaluation of a patient with a musculoskeletal problem.

SUBJECTIVE EXAMINATION

The most common distinction made in evaluating a patient with a musculoskeletal problem is the distinction between the subjective and objective examination. The subjective examination is sometimes referred to as the history; however, it includes more than just a history of the patient's complaint. The subjective examination addresses the present and past medical history and the patient's detailed account of the course and behavior of the symptoms. This examination represents a critical part of the musculoskeletal evaluation and demands skill and patience in extracting appropriate information from the patient. The subjective exam also establishes rapport and trust between the therapist and patient because the therapist demonstrates that she wants to understand the patient's complaint.

There are several approaches to the subjective examination that help the therapist organize the subjective information collected. Maitland (1986) advocates a detailed, methodological system of recording subjective data. His approach is described well in his books, and should be reviewed for further understanding of subjective examination. Here is a brief overview.

PATIENT COMPLAINT

In the first series of questions you ask the patient to help you determine what kind of disorder is present. This is done by asking the patient, "What is your main problem? Why have you come here? What is it you cannot do?" Let the patient describe in his own words why he is seeking treatment. These questions acknowledge the therapist's interest in the patient's problem and allow the patient to describe in his own terms why he is seeking treatment.

The patient's account of his onset of symptoms is critical to the evaluation. In general, a straightforward patient will be able to give a chronological account of the symptoms associated with the present episode. Patients will vary, however, and patients with chronic, nonepisodic problems or patients with unfounded pain may have difficulty presenting the concise chronology of events that led to their disorder. Taking a history is a skill that becomes more refined with increased knowledge and experience. It is important that the therapist not jump to conclusions too early, but use a blend of both open- and closed-ended questions in carefully guiding the patient through the history-taking process. For example, with open-ended questions you allow the patient to describe his symptoms or associated problems, but with closed-ended questions you are looking for a simple one- or two-word response. You may find with some patients that you have to use more closed-ended questions to keep them on track.

PRESENT HISTORY

First, background data on the patient, such as age and occupation, should be recorded. Age is an important factor because many disorders may affect only certain age groups. Next, you should find out the onset and development of the present episode. You will want the patient to describe his onset. If he said gradual, does that mean four days or four hours? If he said the onset was sudden, what was the precipitating event? If it was an outside force, what direction did the force come from? Not all symptoms follow directly after an incident. For example, spinal pain may be the result of activities that a patient did some time in the past that actually set the stage for the current onset of symptoms. A simple activity like a cough or sneeze could bring on back pain but it may have been previous activities that contributed to the episode. Find out what other predisposing factors could have contributed to the patient's problem. Was there postural stress, fatigue, emotional stress, or illness that may have contributed to the patient's symptoms? The onset of the present problem provides the therapist some preliminary data about the musculoskeletal disorder. Some musculoskeletal problems have characteristic histories, but nothing should be concluded at this point.

SITE OF SYMPTOMS

Once you have established how the musculoskeletal problem started, you can begin to shift the patient's focus to his area of symptoms.

Here you want to recreate an accurate map of where the symptoms started and where they spread since the onset. A body chart can be used to record this data (Fig. 19-1).

The therapist applies her knowledge of dermatomes, myotomes, and sclerotomes and must also have some understanding of referred pain. Understanding the mechanisms of referred pain in musculoskeletal problems is necessary for accurate evaluation and safe treatment. Here are some general guidelines regarding mechanisms of referred pain.

1. The reference of pain increases in its extent as the lesion becomes more severe. For example, a minor shoulder problem causes local shoulder pain. However, a more severe arthritis of the shoulder can refer pain down the extent of the C5 dermatome (Cyriax, 1986).
2. The stronger the symptoms, the less accurately a patient can tell where they originate (Cyriax, 1983).
3. The further the lesion is from the trunk, the more clearly the patient can localize the problem (Cyriax, 1983).
4. Referred pain that is well delineated and felt throughout a relevant dermatome suggests pressure on a nerve root (Cyriax, 1983).
5. More diffuse referred pain that is deep and vague may be a sclerotomic or myotomic reference of pain (Kessler and Hertling, 1983; Maitland, 1986).

Figure 19-1. An example of a body chart. Note that different symbols can be used to communicate findings. Check marks (√) indicate that a joint is free of signs and symptoms or has been "cleared."

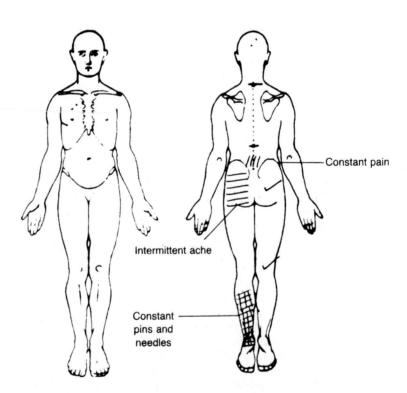

Constant pain

Intermittent ache

Constant pins and needles

6. Diffuse segmental reference of pain may originate from the viscera, somatic structures or a nerve root where the large myelinated fibers are no longer conducting, but C fibers are (Kessler and Hertling, 1983). Cyriax (1983) also suggests that the dura mater and other viscera may cause referred pain outside a segment, or extrasegmental referred pain.

For a better understanding of referred pain, refer to the bibliography at the end of this chapter.

BEHAVIOR OF SYMPTOMS

Not only must the site of the symptoms be described, but the behavior of the symptoms must be recorded as well. Behavior of the symptoms has two components: (1) the character of the symptoms, and (2) how the site and intensity of these symptoms may vary in relation to rest, postural activity, and exertion. The therapist also needs at this point to distinguish between symptoms that are local and symptoms that are referred.

First, have the patient describe the character of these symptoms. Is the pain sharp or stabbing? Does it radiate down an extremity? Is the deep, dull ache constant or intermittent? Is it superficial? Is the area numb or tingling, or does it feel more like pins and needles? The distinction between a patient's subjective complaint of numbness or the presence of pins and needles is often difficult to make. It would have to be confirmed during sensory testing in the objective examination. Does the patient feel weak or are there episodes of giving way? These different qualities of the symptoms can be indicative of certain structures. For example, stabbing pain can be indicative of nerve root involvement, whereas dull, aching pain is often somatic pain (Kessler and Hertling, 1983; Maitland, 1986).

Next, you want to determine how the patient's symptoms respond to rest, posture, or activity. The change in behavior of a patient's pain with different activities also gives the therapist an idea of the severity of the patient's symptoms. Knowing the severity of the pa-

tient's symptoms (ie, how much or how little activity provokes pain) is important to know before proceeding with the objective examination. For example, back pain that comes on immediately upon standing and takes two hours to subside in the supine position is more irritable than back pain that comes on after sitting for three hours and goes away in 10 minutes. Maitland (1986) suggests assessment of a patient's irritability through three criteria: (1) determine the activity that provokes the patient's symptoms; (2) determine the degree and quality of increased symptoms caused by the activity; and (3) determine how long it takes for the increased symptoms to subside.

One of the easiest ways to collect information on the behavior of symptoms is to ask the patient to give an account of what his symptoms are over a 24-hour period. You will want to know what aggravates the symptoms, what eases them, and what his symptoms are like after activity and rest. Here are some general guidelines that may be helpful:

1. Pain that does not change with rest or postural changes may not be the result of a musculoskeletal problem, and the patient may need to be referred to another practitioner.
2. Persistent night pain is unusual for a musculoskeletal problem, except in the case of an acute condition such as nerve root involvement or bursitis. This may be indicative of a more severe pathology such as neoplasm.
3. Patients with degenerative joint disease are more apt to have morning stiffness, and patients with inflammatory processes are more likely to have morning pain.

SPECIAL QUESTIONS

Special questions need to be asked. You will want to ask about the patient's general health, medications, weight loss, or any other information that may help determine what else may have contributed or needs to be considered in treating this patient. In addition, there are special questions specific to each part of the body. (These will be covered in the other musculoskeletal analysis chapters that follow.)

PREVIOUS MEDICAL HISTORY

What about the patient's previous medical history? Is the present episode a recurrence of the same problem? What other kinds of treatment has the patient sought? Does the patient have other joint-related problems? Questions like these give you information about the stability of the lesion, other problems the patient may have, and the amount and kind of treatment the patient has sought.

OCCUPATIONAL AND FAMILY HISTORY

Finally, you need to find out how these symptoms affect the patient's daily life activities and his ability to work. Find out what kind of support the patient has from family or friends. This information gives you a better idea of the nature of the patient's problem, what other factors may be contributing to the symptoms, and how you might want to plan for patient and family education during your course of treatment.

OBJECTIVE EXAMINATION

Once the subjective examination has been completed, the therapist proceeds to the physical or objective examination. Here, numerous tests are performed that help the therapist evaluate the basic musculoskeletal structures. The therapist systematically evaluates joints, muscles, ligaments, nerves, and other soft tissues. The specific testing procedures for each area of the body will be discussed in later chapters. The following overview presents the major parts of the exam and provides definitions of the concepts central to the objective evaluation process.

OBSERVATION

Observation begins the minute the patient walks into the clinic. The therapist should take note of how the patient walks, his posture, and the ease or difficulty with which he moves. The patient's carriage and posture may also give you additional information about how this problem may be affecting his life, as well as information that can be used to look for inconsistencies (eg, the patient may complain of excruciating pain, yet he moves with ease).

EXAMINATION OF JOINT MOVEMENT

Evaluation of joint movement requires an understanding of several key concepts. These concepts are used both in the evaluation and treatment of musculoskeletal problems. Joint movement involves both osteokinematics (the study of bone movement) and arthokinematics (the study of articular movements between two joint surfaces). The book *Muscles and Movement* (MacConaill and Basmajian, 1977) and the chapter on arthrology in the British edition of *Gray's Anatomy* (Warwick and Williams, 1980) are excellent sources for understanding more about joint mechanics. The major concepts relevant to objective examination of joints will be briefly described here.

Physiological and Accessory Joint Movement

Physiological movements are normal movements we perform during our daily activities. These movements can be performed actively by the patient or passively by the therapist. When you examine physiological movements in the objective examination, you first have the patient do the movement actively (eg, shoulder flexion). Then, you apply gentle overpressure, that is, you push the joint passively into more flexion. What you will feel at the end of the range of motion is called the *end-feel* of the joint. It is the sensation imparted to your hands as you push the joint to the end of range. The different types of joint end-feels are discussed later in this section. Physiological movements are also done passively with a patient, and again, gentle overpressure must be applied to assess joint end-feel. Physiological movements can be easily recorded through goniometric measures for evaluation and reassessment. Refer to Maitland (1977, 1986) for a more thorough discussion of physiological movements.

In contrast to these large physiological movements are the relatively small accessory movements. These movements occur between joint surfaces and are involuntary. A patient cannot isolate his accessory joint movements. Remember that accessory movements pertain to the arthrokinematics of the joint. One cannot have normal physiological movement without having normal accessory joint movement. In the objective examination, both physiological movements and accessory movements are assessed.

Accessory movements are small in comparison with physiological movements and difficult to measure. One way to have a similar communication system about joint movement is to use a grading system. An example of the grading system used by Maitland (1986) is shown in Figure 19-2. He uses this classification system for both physiological and accessory joint movement.

Grade I: A small-amplitude movement near the beginning of range.

Grade II: A large-amplitude movement that extends well into the range of movement. This movement occupies any part of the range that is free of stiffness and muscle spasm.

Grade III: A large-amplitude movement that reaches the end of range and does move into stiffness and spasm.

Grade IV: A small-amplitude movement at the end of range, stretching into stiffness or spasm.

Grade V: A high-velocity, small-amplitude range, but still within the anatomical range.

Another critical concept related to accessory joint movement is the understanding of what movements occur between the joint surfaces. Rolling and gliding movements take place between joint surfaces with all active and passive bone movements. Rolling between two joint surfaces is possible only between two surfaces that are incongruent. Gliding occurs between two joint surfaces that are congruent. Human joints are never fully congruent. Therefore, the combination of roll and glide movements takes place between joint surfaces. The gliding movement is the critical component of accessory joint movement. The direction of the gliding movement necessary to restore normal physiological movement follows the concave-convex rule (Kaltenborn, 1980; Warwick and Wilkins, 1980).

Testing of this roll-gliding movement in the joint can also be estimated manually and graded according to the following scale (Kaltenborn, 1980).

0, No movement (ankylo-
   sis)
1, Considerable decrease in }Hypomobility
   movement
2, Slight decrease in movement

3, Normal

4, Slight increase in movement
5, Considerable increase in }Hypermobility
   movement
6, Complete instability

Close-Packed and Loose-Packed Positions

Another concept important in evaluation of joint movement is the difference between close- and loose-packed positions of the joint. The close-packed joint position is where the joint surfaces are in their maximal congruent position. The joint capsule and ligaments are taut and the articular surfaces cannot be sepa-

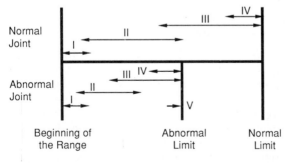

Figure 19-2. Grades of movement can be used to describe both normal and abnormal joints. The abnormal joint still has grades I to IV; however, these grades would change as the range of motion continued to improve.

rated by traction forces. This position cannot be used for testing of accessory joint, joint play movement, or mobilization, but it can be used to stabilize or fixate a joint.

The loose-packed position or resting position of the joint is the position where the joint capsule and ligaments are most relaxed and the greatest amount of joint play is available. This is also the position that allows the maximal amount of space for joint effusion. For example, when a patient has a swollen joint, he would want to keep his joint in the loose-packed position because it is more comfortable. The loose-packed position is important for the testing of accessory joint movement and the best possible position for mobilization. The close- and loose-packed positions of joints are listed in Table 19-1.

Two other concepts necessary for evaluation of joint movement are an understanding of capsular and noncapsular patterns and how to assess joint end-feels.

Capsular and Noncapsular Patterns

Irritation of the joint capsule or synovial membrane of the joint will cause a limitation of passive joint movement in capsular proportions. The term *porportional* means certain physiological movements of the joint are limited in a distinct order. For example, if a patient has a capsular pattern present in his shoulder, you would find shoulder abduction limited most, followed by external rotation, followed by internal rotation. The presence of a capsular pattern indicates joint irritation or arthritis, but does indicate what type of joint irritation is present. Capsular and noncapsular patterns for joints will be discussed in each of the assessment sections. These capsular limitations vary from joint to joint depending on where the laxity is in the joint capsule. The key element in a capsular pattern is not limitation of movements in fixed degrees, but a *fixed proportion* or distinct pattern particular to that joint. The capsular and noncapsular patterns of specific joints are listed in Table 19-2.

A noncapsular pattern reveals that capsular irritation is not present because there is no restriction of movement in that joint's designated proportions. (For example, the capsular pattern in the knee is grossly limited flexion and slightly limited extension.) The noncapsular pattern is just the opposite—extension is limited more than flexion. The presence of a noncapsular pattern means only that irritation of the joint capsule is not contributing to the limitation of physiological movement, and thus it must be something else. Cyriax (1983) classifies these three conditions as possible causes of noncapsular patterns:

1. Ligamentous adhesions: These usually occur after injury when adhesions form. Pain is localized and can be brought on by stretching the ligament.
2. Internal derangement: This occurs in joints where there is the possibility of having an intra-articular fragment of cartilage or bone (eg, the knee or spine). If the loose fragment becomes suddenly displaced within the joint, one or more movements are blocked or painful, or both.
3. Extra-articular limitation: Here, the restricting structure is outside the joint. Often the restriction of physiological movements will be a gross restriction in one direction and full painless range in the other direction. For example, a partial rupture of the gastrocnemius muscle could cause gross limitation of dorsiflexion as the injured muscle is stretched and little restriction of plantarflexion.

Joint End-Feel

When a therapist examines active and passive movement within a joint, a distinctive sensation called end-feel is noted when the end of range is reached. The significance of determining joint end-feel is knowing first what a normal end-feel is for that joint, then knowing how an end-feel may depart from normal. Cyriax (1983) describes six different types of joint end-feels.

1. Bone to bone. This end-feel is normal in elbow extension, but is abnormal when accompanied by a restriction of normal

Table 19-1. Close-Packed and Loose-Packed Positions for Upper and Lower Quadrant Joints

JOINT	CLOSE-PACKED POSITION	LOOSE-PACKED POSITION
Shoulder		
Glenohumeral	Maximal abduction and external rotation	Abduction 55° Horizontal adduction 30°
Elbow		
Humero-ulnar	Full elbow extension/supination	Elbow flexion 70° Supination 10°
Humeroradial	Elbow flexion 90° Supination 5°	Elbow extension Supination
Forearm		
Proximal radioulnar	Mid-pronation/supination (supination 5°)	Supination 10°
Distal radioulnar	Mid-pronation/supination (supination 5°)	Supination 35° Elbow flexion 70°
Hand		
Carpo-metacarpal	Full opposition	Mid-abduction and adduction, flexion and extension
Metacarpophalangeal (II–V)	Full flexion	Semiflexion/slight ulnar flexion
Interphalangeal	Full extension	Slight flexion
Wrist	Full extension with radial extension	Mid flexion and extension, mid ulnar and radial deviation
Hip	Full extension Internal rotation and abduction	Hip flexion to 90° Abduction to 30° and slight external rotation
Knee	Full extension and external rotation	Flexion 25°
Ankle		
Talocrural	Full dorsiflexion	Plantarflexion 10° mid-inversion/eversion
Subtalar } Midtarsal	Supination	Mid-position
Toes		
Metatarsophalangeal	Full extension	Neutral (extension 10°)
Interphalangeal	Full extension	Slight flexion
Vertebral	Maximal extension	Semiflexion
Temporomandibular	Mouth closed	Slight opening

(After MacConaill MA, Basmajian JV: Muscles and Movement. Huntington, NY, Robert E Krieger, 1977; and Kaltenborn F: Mobilization of the Extremity Joints. Oslo, Olaf Norlis Bokhandel Universitetsgaten, 1980)

movement in a joint (eg, degenerative joint disease).

2. Soft tissue approximation. This end-feel is normal. It occurs when a joint cannot be pushed farther because of soft tissue approximation (eg, elbow flexion).

3. Spasm end-feel. Here, the end-feel is an abrupt stop where muscle spasm prevents any further range. It may indicate severe arthritis or other joint pathology.

4. Empty end-feel. The movement causes considerable pain before the end of range is

Table 19-2. Capsular Patterns for Upper and Lower Quadrant Joints

JOINT	PROPORTIONAL LIMITATION
Cervical spine	Equal limitation in all movements except flexion
Shoulder Glenohumeral	Greater limitation of external rotation, followed by abduction and internal rotation
Elbow	Flexion more limited than extension
Wrist	Equal limitation of flexion and extension
Trapeziometacarpal	Limitation of abduction and extension, full flexion
Fingers Metacarpophalangeal and interphalangeal	More limitation of flexion than extension
Thoracic spine	Limitation of extension, side flexion, and rotation with less limitation of flexion
Lumbar spine	Marked and equal limitation of side flexion, limitation of flexion and extension
Hip	Limitation of flexion and internal rotation, some limitation of abduction, no or little limitation of adduction and external rotation
Knee	Flexion grossly limited, slight limitation of extension
Ankle Talocrural	Plantarflexion limited more than dorsiflexion
Talocalcaneal	Increasing limitation of varus, joint fixes in valgus
Midtarsal	Limitation of dorsiflexion, plantarflexion, adduction, and medial rotation
First metatarsophalangeal	Marked limitation of extension, slight limitation of flexion
Metatarsophalangeal (II-V)	Variable; fix in extension with interphalangeal joints flexed

(After Cyriax J: Textbook of Orthopaedic Medicine: Diagnosis of Soft Tissue Lesions, Vol 1, 7th ed. London, Bailliere Tindall, 1983)

reached and the therapist feels no restriction to movement. It is abnormal and can occur in cases such as acute bursitis or severe pathology. This pathology may be joint related or may be another more serious pathology, such as neoplasm or fracture.

5. Capsular end-feel. This is described as the stretching of leather. When it occurs at the end of range, it is normal. When it occurs before the normal full range, it suggests some form of arthritis.
6. Springy block. This end-feel results in a rebound or elastic feeling. The block indicates some form of internal derangement (eg, displaced meniscus in the knee).

Another useful way to consider restricted motion is known as the *barrier concept*. The barrier may be described according to the end-feels previously discussed. Barriers exist at the end of normal active range of motion, where the soft tissues about the joint have reached a degree of tension beyond which the person cannot voluntarily move. This is known as the physiologic barrier. Passively, the joint may be taken beyond its physiologic barrier to the anatomic barrier. Here the soft tissues are on maximum stretch and going farther will either cause failure of the soft tissues or fracture. In a state of dysfunction, a restrictive barrier may occur, causing either a major or minor loss of mobility (Fig. 19-3).

This is an overview of concepts important in evaluating joint movement. The evaluation chapters that follow will apply these principles for each area of the body. The last section of the objective examination is examination of soft tissue.

EXAMINATION OF SOFT TISSUE

Cyriax (1983) has provided us with the most detailed explanations for examination of soft tissue. He divides soft tissue into contractile and noncontractile structures. Contractile structures are those that form part of the muscle, including tendon and bony insertion. Pain can be elicited from these structures by active contraction of the muscle or passive stretching in the opposite direction. Noncontractile or inert structures pertain to tissues that cannot contract or relax, that is, joint capsule, ligaments, fasciae, bursae, dura mater, and dural sheaths of nerve roots. One can distinguish contractile from noncontractile structures by using selective tension tests.

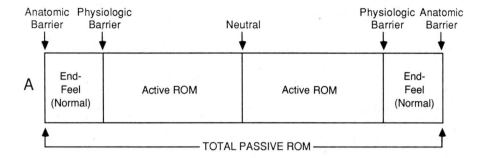

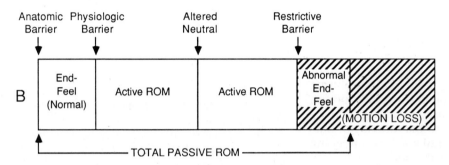

Figure 19-3. Illustration of soft tissue tension development during passive examination procedures. (*A*) Normal mobility and associated barriers. (*B*) Dysfunction and associated restrictive barrier. (Adapted from Kimberly PE: Outline of Osteopathic Manipulative Procedures [manual]. Kirksville College of Osteopathic Medicine, 1980).

Resisted Tests

I have already stated that usually the therapist begins by assessing the patient's active physiological movements. These active movements provide information about the patient's willingness to move, range of motion, and presence or absence of pain. Passive joint movements are then used to assess joint range, pain, end-feel, and presence or absence of a capsular pattern. Passive movements also provide information on the state of inert structures (eg, a bursa may be pinched with passive shoulder abduction or the dural sheath of a nerve root can be stretched with a passive straight leg raise). Resisted movements are used to test contractile structures or muscles and their attachments. These tests give you information on strength and pain. Throughout the entire examination, remember to keep in mind compar-

ing assessment of your patient's muscles and joints bilaterally.

For resisted tests, the patient must contract (isometrically) his muscles against resistance strong enough to provoke a maximal contraction, and all articular movement must be prevented at the involved joint. The joint should be in mid-range or loose-packed position if possible. When resisted tests are done, the possibilities are as follows (Cyriax, 1983):

1. Strong and painful: a minor lesion in some part of the muscle or tendon
2. Weak and painless: a major lesion in muscle or tendon or neurological lesion
3. Weak and painful: a major lesion in muscle or tendon or a gross lesion, such as a fracture or neoplasm
4. All painful: gross lesion or emotional hy-

persensitivity

5. Strong and painless: normal
6. Pain on repetition: If the movement is strong and painless, but hurts after repetition, intermittent claudication is a possibility.

These resisted tests give information on strength and pain, whereas passive movements can be used to assess muscle length and perhaps pain on stretching. Weakness of muscles and potential muscle imbalance problems should be assessed through muscle testing procedures. Further evaluation of muscle weakness can also be done through electrophysiological testing.

Palpation of Soft Tissue

When palpation of soft tissue is done during the objective examination is a matter of preference. Cyriax (1983) advocates waiting until the end of the examination so that one is not misled by finding the "painful spot" before going through a systematic evaluation process. Palpation is used to detect any abnormalities in the skin, soft tissues, and bone. Palpation of joint movement has already taken place during assessment of physiological and accessory joint movement. In examining the soft tissues and bony structures underlying the soft tissue, you should look for localized warmth, edema, the behavior and consistency of the edema, synovial thickening, bony enlargements, relationship of bony parts, sweating, excessive dryness, pulses, and changes in the texture (eg, thickening, resistance, or plasticity) of the soft tissue.

In acute conditions, the skin may feel sweaty and warm, the ligaments exquisitely tender, and the various muscular layers swollen and hypertonic. In chronic cases, the skin may be cold and tight or "bound down" to underlying layers. The ligaments may feel thickened and the muscular layers hardened or even fibrosed. If the therapist is able to discern such palpation findings, it can be valuable in selecting the type and dosage of treatment and in making a prognosis.

NEUROLOGICAL ASSESSMENT

Assessment of neurological function is important for detecting the presence of neurological deficits, and as treatment proceeds, to determine if neurological changes are occurring. A neurological examination should be done in all spinal problems and in peripheral problems if you suspect any neurological involvement.

The assessment includes testing of muscle strength, deep tendon reflexes, mobility of nerve roots (tension signs), sensation, and spinal cord signs (eg, hyperreflexia, gait disturbance, or extensor plantar response). Table 19-3 provides an overview of representative muscles, reflexes, and tension signs that are part of nerve root assessment.

Muscles should be tested against maximal resistance and relative weakness assessed (ie, one side compared to the other). This is the only way to detect muscle weakness, especially in those instances where muscle weakness is minimal (Cyriax, 1983). The presence or absence of a neurological deficit is confirmed by testing a muscle or joint action representative of a given spinal cord level (Grieve, 1981; Maitland, 1986). Deep tendon reflexes are also tested for given nerve root levels. Maitland (1986) and Grieve (1981) advocate doing repeated tapping of a tendon, that is, at least six successive times. They propose that a fading reflex response may indicate developing nerve root signs.

Tension Tests

The mobility of selected nerve roots is tested through passive tests sometimes referred to as *tension tests*. Each nerve root has an external aspect or dural sheath, which moves in relation to other neighboring structures (Cyriax, 1983). Here are the five most common tension tests generally done in the clinic.

1. The straight leg raise is a tension test for lumbosacral roots L4-S2. Pain may be felt in the back or radiating down the lower extremity in a positive test.
2. The prone knee bend is a tension test for

Table 19-3. Examination of Nerve Roots

JOINT ACTION	ROOT LEVEL	REFLEX	TENSION SIGN
Neck rotation	C1		
Shoulder elevation (trapezius)	C2, C3, C4		
Elbow flexion (biceps) Shoulder abduction (supraspinatus, deltoid) Shoulder external rotation (infraspinatus)	C5	Biceps jerk	
Elbow flexion (biceps) Wrist flexion (extensor carpi radialis)	C6	Biceps jerk Brachioradialis jerk	
Elbow extension (triceps) Wrist flexion (flexor carpi radialis)	C7	Triceps jerk	
Thumb adduction (adductor pollicis) Ulnar deviation (flexor carpi ulnaris, extensor carpi ulnaris)	C8		
Finger adduction (interossei)	T1		
Hip flexion (iliopsoas)	L2		
Hip flexion (iliopsoas) Knee extension (quadriceps)	L3	Knee jerk	Prone knee bend
Dorsiflexion (anterior tibialis) Great toe extension (extensor hallucis longus)	L4	Knee jerk	Straight leg raise
Great toe extension Eversion (peronei) Hip abduction (gluteus medius)	L5		Straight leg raise
Eversion (peronei) Plantarflexion (gastrocnemius) Knee flexion (hamstrings)	S1	Ankle jerk	Straight leg raise
Hip extension (gluteus maximus) Knee flexion (hamstrings)	S2	Ankle jerk	Straight leg raise

(After Conesa-Hernandez S, Argote M: A Visual Aid to the Examination of Nerve Roots. London, Bailliere Tindall, 1976)

the femoral nerve and stretches the L3 nerve root. Pain felt in the back and sometimes the anterior thigh is a positive result. Pain felt only in the anterior thigh is not a positive sign.

3. The neck flexion tension test stretches the dura from above because the neck is 3 cm longer in this position. Pain elicited with this test may be a dural sign for thoracic or lumbar problems, depending on where the pain is felt (Cyriax, 1983).

4. Scapular approximation. Cyriax (1983) proposes that scapular approximation stretches the T1 and T2 nerve roots and is a sign for thoracic joint problems.

5. The Elvey test or upper limb tension test is advocated by Elvey (1985) as a tension test for the brachial plexus. The test combines shoulder, elbow, wrist, and neck movements in an attempt to *stretch the brachial plexus and cervical nerve roots.* Maitland (1986) and Elvey (1985) are excellent sources for reading more about this test.

Finally, sensory testing using light touch, pin prick, and vibration may be used to detect any sensory changes in the dermatomes or interference with the cutaneous distribution of pheripheral nerves. Magee (1987) also offers an excellent discussion of the neurological examination for patients with orthopaedic problems.

FUNCTIONAL ASSESSMENT

In addition to the data collected during the subjective examination, the therapist should also determine how the musculoskeletal problem has affected the patient's daily activities and ability to work. What changes has the patient made in his daily routine? What kind of tasks does the patient need to perform for daily work activities?

ANNOTATED BIBLIOGRAPHY

Barak T, Rosen E, Sofer R: Mobility: Passive orthopaedic manual therapy. In Gould J, Davies G: Orthopaedic and Sports Physical Therapy. St Louis, CV Mosby, 1985
(An excellent chapter, it provides more detail on basic concepts such as joint movement, grades of movement, and arthrokinematics. Several of the chapters in this volume also provide a thorough description of musculoskeletal evaluation and treatment.)

Conesa-Hernandez S, Argote M: A Visual Aid to the Examination of Nerve Roots. London, Bailliere Tindall, 1976
(This booklet is an excellent guide for use in the clinic. It contains a page on each nerve root level with a picture of the dermatome, the muscles, and the reflexes one should test for that root level. The introduction also gives a clear, concise overview of referred pain mechanisms.)

Cyriax J: Textbook of Orthopaedic Medicine: Diagnosis of Soft Tissue Lesions, Vol I, 7th ed, pp 1–103. London, Bailliere Tindall, 1983
(Cyriax's Volume I contains all of his theory on orthopaedic medicine. The beginning chapters on referred pain and diagnosis of soft tissue lesions are essential reading for understanding many of the concepts used in orthopaedic physical therapy. The book also

includes detailed chapters on each area of the body. These chapters provide an overview of Cyriax's examination and discuss how he makes a differential diagnosis.)

Cyriax J, Coldham M: Textbook of Orthopaedic Medicine: Treatment by Manipulation, Massage and Injection, Vol II, 11th ed, pp 3–6. London, Bailliere Tindall, 1984
(Volume II has been called Cyriax's "cookbook of treatment." It contains photos and explanations for all of Cyriax's treatment techniques. The introduction also includes a thorough discussion of friction massage. Another Cyriax reference, although not referred to in this chapter is Cyriax J, Cyriax P: Illustrated Manual of Orthopaedic Medicine, Boston, Butterworth, 1983. This book includes both Cyriax's theory and treatment techniques. The charts that summarize his theoretical concepts and evaluation procedures are excellent. The artwork illustrating friction massage and injection sites is well done and would be an excellent reference in the clinic.)

Elvey R: Brachial plexus tension tests and the pathoanatomical origin of arm pain. In Glasgow E, Twomey L et al (eds): Aspects of Manipulative Therapy. New York, Churchill Livingston, 1985
(This short chapter describes in detail Elvey's proposed tension test, and includes several photos illustrating how the test is applied.)

Grieve G: Common Vertebral Joint Problems, pp 69–73, 421. New York, Churchill Livingstone, 1981
(Pertains only to spinal problems, but has an extensive bibliography and contains much detail about spinal pathologies.)

Kaltenborn F: Mobilization of the Extremity Joints, pp 9–25. Oslo, Olaf Norlis Bokhandel Universitetsgaten, 1980
(The first few chapters in this paperback thoroughly describe joint mechanics and how they apply to mobilization. Kaltenborn provides an excellent clinical interpretation of much of MacConaill's work on joint mechanics. The book also has evaluation and selected treatment procedures for the extremities.)

Kessler RM, Hertling D: Management of Common Musculoskeletal Disorders, pp 75–104. Philadelphia, JB Lippincott, 1983
(Contains some excellent chapters on the

basic concepts of musculoskeletal evaluation. Of particular interest are the chapters on friction massage and the use of heat and cold in treating musculoskeletal disorders. Included in the specific treatment chapters are creative exercises you can use in teaching patients self-mobilization techniques.)

MacConaill MA, Basmajian JV: Muscles and Movement, pp 13–44. Huntington NY, Robert E Krieger, 1977

(Provides a thorough description of Mac-Conaill's work on joint mechanics.)

Magee D: Orthopedic Physical Assessment, pp 1–21. Philadelphia, WB Saunders, 1987

(Provides an excellent discussion of the basic concepts and principles of orthopaedic evaluation as well as separate evaluation chapters for each major joint. Many excellent tables and figures are included within a good, easy-to-understand text.)

Maitland GD: Peripheral Manipulation, 2nd ed, pp 7–31. Boston, Butterworths, 1977

(Contains a detailed description of the subjective examination procedure and physiological and accessory movements as they pertain to the extremities.)

Maitland GD: Vertebral Manipulation, 5th ed, pp 43–56, 96–99. Boston, Butterworths, 1986

(Maitland's most recent edition on vertebral evaluation and treatment. It includes much more description and interpretation of both his techniques and philosophy than did his previous edition. The material on subjective examination and interviewing techniques is excellent.)

Warwick R, Williams PL (eds): Gray's Anatomy, 36th ed, pp 420–505. Philadelphia, WB Saunders, 1980

(The chapter of arthrology in British Gray's is a must for anyone wishing to understand thoroughly the basic principles of joint mechanics.)

20 Musculoskeletal Analysis: The Shoulder

LEONARD PARÉ
RUSSELL M. WOODMAN

In order to evaluate soft tissue lesions at the shoulder, the examiner must remember that neck and visceral pathology are capable of referring pain to the upper extremity. Intraspinal space-occupying lesions such as tumors or intervertebral disk lesions can press against either the anterior aspect of the dura mater or the dural sleeve of a nerve root, referring pain to the shoulder. Visceral conditions such as trauma to the diaphragm muscle or coronary heart disease can also refer pain to the upper extremity.

ANATOMICAL OVERVIEW

The examination of any joint requires an indepth knowledge of anatomy and kinesiology. Highlighting some important anatomical idiosyncrasies of the shoulder will be helpful in identifying lesions at the shoulder.

Figure 20-1 illustrates the relationship between the acromioclavicular joint, subdeltoid bursae, supraspinatus, and glenohumeral joint. The deltoid and rotator cuff muscles work synchronously to perform elevation of the shoulder. This synchronous movement helps prevent impingement of the greater tuberosity of the humerus against the acromion process. However, this sophisticated joint arrangement and complementary muscle function is still not enough always to prevent impingement and irritation of the tissues located between the acromion and greater tuberosity.

The subdeltoid bursae, inferior fibers of the acromioclavicular ligament, rotator cuff tendons, and intracapsular portion of the long head of the biceps can become inflamed.

Figure 20-2 shows the location of the subcoracoid bursae and how the subscapularis tendon traverses the proximal medial aspect of the humerus. When one of these tissues is inflamed, passive horizontal adduction is painful because the movement causes the bursae and lower fibers of the tendon to press against the coracoid process.

In Figure 20-3, you can see the location of the musculotendinous junction of the supraspinatus and the body of the infraspinatus tendon. These two structures are located medially, and thus cannot be impinged between the greater tuberosity and acromion process.

Table 20-1 lists the soft tissues of the shoulder and their embryological dermatome derivation. Structures of the same embryological origin can refer pain to part or all of the dermatome. For example, fibers of the diaphragm and acromioclavicular ligament both developed from the C4 mesodermic somite and refer pain to the C4 dermatome at the shoulder.

SUBJECTIVE EXAMINATION

Patients suffering a soft tissue lesion at the shoulder frequently state that elevating the arm or using it repetitively exacerbates the pain. Occasionally, you may encounter a pa-

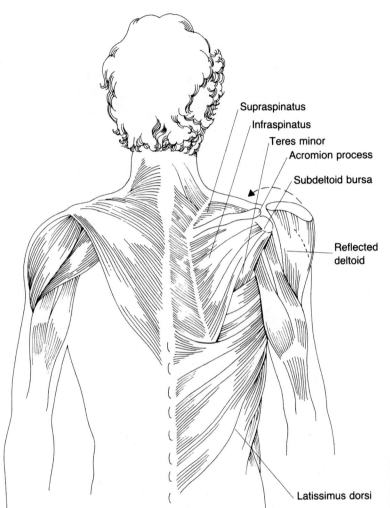

Supraspinatus
Infraspinatus
Teres minor
Acromion process
Subdeltoid bursa
Reflected deltoid
Latissimus dorsi

Figure 20-1. Relationship among acromioclavicular joint, subdeltoid bursa, supraspinatus, and glenohumeral joint.

tient who can describe an injury that precipitated the pain. For example, a middle-aged person who has fallen on his shoulder may develop traumatic arthritis. Some patients, however, are unable to state what activities increase their pain. Asking the following nine questions produces additional important information.

1. Where is your pain?
2. Does your pain ever spread?
3. How long have you had the pain?
4. How old are you?
5. Did you have an injury?

6. Do you have pain during the day even when the arm is at rest?
7. Can you sleep on the shoulder?
8. Are any other joints affected?
9. Have you had any recent surgery?

Questions one and two help assess the severity of the lesion and the likelihood of the acromioclavicular ligament being the only tissue at fault. Remember the acromioclavicular joint is a C4 structure. Therefore, the pain will be only in the C4 dermatome and not spread down the shoulder. A patient whose pain remains in the shoulder, never spreading dis-

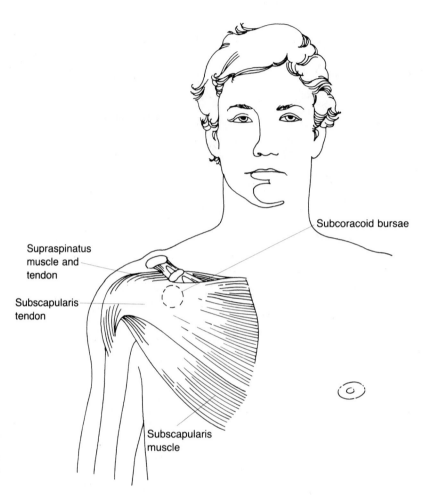

Subcoracoid bursae

Supraspinatus
muscle and
tendon

Subscapularis
tendon

Subscapularis
muscle

Figure 20-2. Location of sub-coracoid bursae and subscapularis tendon.

Table 20-1. Embryological Derivations of Shoulder Tissue

SOFT TISSUES	DERMATOME
Acromioclavicular ligament	C4
Shoulder joint capsule	C5
Subdeltoid bursae	C5
Subcoracoid bursae	C5
Supraspinatous muscle	C5
Infraspinatous muscle	C5 to C6
Subscapularis muscle	C5 to C6
Biceps muscle	C5 to C6
Triceps muscle	C7

tally, is either suffering from an injured acromioclavicular ligament or a minor lesion to another shoulder soft tissue.

Inquiring about the duration of the pain is important because acute bursitis lasts only six weeks, with or without treatment. The pain associated with traumatic arthritis lasts about one year. Most other inflammatory conditions at the shoulder can go on indefinitely.

Age is critical to know because traumatic arthritis rarely occurs before the age of 40 years. Monarticular arthritis occurs between the ages of 45 and 60 years. Osteoarthritis is more common in the elderly.

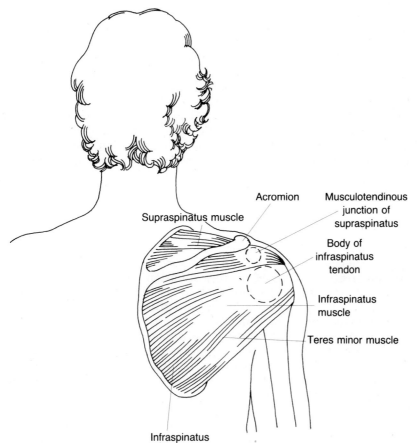

Supraspinatus muscle

Acromion

Musculotendinous junction of supraspinatus

Body of infraspinatus tendon

Infraspinatus muscle

Teres minor muscle

Infraspinatus muscle

Figure 20-3. Location of musculotendinous junction of supraspinatus and body of infraspinatus tendon.

Injuries should be clearly described. Falling on an outstretched arm may rupture a rotator cuff muscle or fracture the clavicle or humerus. A direct fall may rupture a ligament or upwardly sublux the clavicle. On a rare occasion, a severe fall or twisting motion will lead to a shoulder subluxation.

The answers to questions six and seven, along with that of number two, determines the severity of the problems. The more inflamed the tissue is, the more capable it is of referring pain down the arm, causing pain at rest, and preventing the patient from lying on the shoulder at night.

Involvement of other joints can suggest a systemic inflammatory disease such as gout or rheumatoid arthritis.

Inquiring about recent surgery in the shoulder area may serve as a subtle way of finding out about metastasis from breast cancer. You should also inquire about the patient's general health and any unexplained weight loss. With pain in the shoulder area, you must make sure you rule out nonmusculoskeletal causes.

OBJECTIVE EXAMINATION

You begin the objective examination with observation. Inspect the shoulder for visible deformities such as a dislocated shoulder, separated acromioclavicular joint, or displaced sternoclavicular joint. Muscular development or atrophy is noted, making allowances for right-and left-handedness.

PHYSICAL EXAMINATION

Because cervical spine pathology frequently refers pain to the shoulder and upper extremity, you must first rule out cervical problems. Have the patient perform active cervical movements of rotation, lateral flexion, extension, and flexion. Overpressure must be given at the end of range to clear these motions. Then you will proceed with the shoulder examination.

The first movement is active flexion. Is the patient willing and able to complete the motion? Does the test increase the level of pain?

The second movement is passive flexion. Is it limited or painful? What is the end-feel? The normal end-feel at the shoulder is soft, or what we call a capsular end-feel.

The third movement is active abduction. This is a specific test for a painful arc. A painful arc occurs between 70 and 110 degrees of abduction. Sometimes a painful arc may be identified on active or passive flexion.

Movement four is passive glenohumeral abduction. With one hand, the therapist stabilizes the inferior angle of the scapula, while the other passively abducts the humerus. Normally, the humerus can be moved to about 90 degrees before the scapula starts to abduct. If a patient has any restriction in the glenohumeral joint, then the scapula would begin abducting earlier than 90 degrees.

To perform movements four and five, the therapist stands at the patient's side directly next to the arm being evaluated. The arm is held in normal anatomical position with the elbow flexed to 90 degrees. The therapist places one of her arms around the patient's torso for stabilization, and then grasps the forearm of the extremity being tested and externally rotates the shoulder. Normally, the joint can be moved 90 degrees painlessly. Next, the therapist stands behind the patient, holding the patient's humerus in slight adduction. The therapist then gently grasps the forearm and rotates the patient's arm away from his back, moving the shoulder into internal rotation. If the shoulder can be passively moved so that the forearm is behind and slightly away from the patient's back, then the shoulder possesses about 90 degrees of internal rotation. If a capsular pattern was present, you would see a greater limitation of external rotation than internal rotation.

The last six movements assess contractile structures. Movements seven and eight are isometric abduction and adduction. These are performed with the arm held out in about 20 degrees of abduction.

Movements nine through twelve test the remaining muscles most likely to suffer tendinitis. They are isometric shoulder external rotation, internal rotation, and elbow flexion and extension. They are tested by placing the patient's arm in normal anatomical position and in 90 degrees of flexion. The therapist uses her hip and trunk to stabilize the arm against the patient's hip and trunk to minimize muscle substitution.

Passive horizontal adduction compresses the subcoracoid bursae and lower fibers of the subscapularis tendon between the humerus and coracoid process and stretches the acromioclavicular ligament.

Occasionally, isometric extension or horizontal adduction may be used to test the latissimus dorsi or pectoralis major muscles. For example, if your patient has pain upon resisted adduction, you might suspect a lesion in one of these muscles.

ACCESSORY MOVEMENTS

Accessory movements are assessed with the glenohumeral joint in the loose-packed position: slight abduction, flexion, and neutral rotation. These movements include lateral distraction, longitudinal movement in a caudal direction (distraction along the longitudinal axis of the bone), and anterior-posterior and posterior-anterior movements of the humeral head in the frontal plane.

INTERPRETATION OF DATA

The data collected from the objective examination should lead to a shoulder assessment that can be placed in one of five categories.

1. Loss of range of motion in the capsular pattern.
2. Loss of range of motion in the noncapsular pattern.
3. Full passive range of motion with pain on resistive muscle testing.
4. Full passive range of motion with one or more muscles weak.
5. Full passive range of motion; all muscles are strong and painless.

Occasionally, situations arise where two lesions exist at one time. For example, a patient may have a strong and painful muscle indicating tendinitis, but may also be arthritic and have a loss of range of motion in the capsular pattern.

CAPSULAR PATTERN

Capsular pattern usually indicates the presence of an arthritis of some sort. The capsular pattern is a gross loss of external rotation, moderate loss of scapula humeral abduction, and a slight loss of internal rotation. When the loss of range of motion is in the capsular pattern, the therapist must remember a slight possibility exists that the diagnosis is not arthritis. Serious pathologies that can cause a capsular pattern are myeloma and reflex sympathetic dystrophy. Furthermore, if arthritis is present, it is essential to identify the type. For example, cortisone is indicated for the treatment of traumatic arthritis, but contraindicated in the treatment of septic arthritis. If arthritis is present, it is essential to ascertain the extent of inflammation. This information is useful in designing a treatment program for traumatic arthritis and monarticular arthritis. A severely inflamed shoulder in the third stage of capsulitis is more likely to benefit from joint mobilization techniques rather than traditional stretching techniques. The following description of stages can help you determine how irritable the joint capsule is.

Stage One

1. The pain is confined to the shoulder region.
2. The joint is pain free if it is not moved.

3. The patient can lie on the involved shoulder when sleeping.
4. On passive joint movement, the capsular end-feel is reached before the pain is exacerbated.

Stage Two

1. The joint has a mixture of symptoms of both stages one and two (eg, there may be pain below the elbow but the patient can lie on that side at night).
2. On passive movement, pain is exacerbated as the end-feel is reached.

Stage Three

1. The pain has spread to the wrist.
2. There is pain even when the joint is not moved.
3. The patient can no longer sleep on the involved shoulder.
4. On passive movement, the pain increases before the end-feel is reached. The capsular end-feel is less elastic.

NONCAPSULAR PATTERN

Acute subdeltoid bursitis, sprained acromioclavicular ligament, capsular adhesion, pulmonary neoplasm, and psychogenic limitation are examples of lesions that may cause a noncapsular pattern. Remember, a noncapsular pattern means the patient does not have limitations of motion that are proportional in the capsular pattern.

The distinguishing features of acute subdeltoid bursitis are the development of severe pain over a few days' time and usually a gross loss of abduction with little or no loss of both shoulder rotations. The painful bursae is palpable inferior to the lateral lip of the acromion process and also over the head of the humerus when the shoulder is placed in extension.

With an acromioclavicular ligament problem, the ligament can be painfully stressed at or near the extreme end of some or all of the passive joint movements. Passive horizontal adduction is particularly painful when the ligament's posterior fibers are inflamed. A painful arc implicates a lesion in the inferior fibers. Joint laxity occurs if the ligament is overstretched. Because horizontal adduction can become painfully limited, this lesion is classified as noncapsular.

A novice may confuse a sprained acromioclavicular ligament with subcoracoid bursitis because this lesion also causes pain on passive horizontal adduction. You should keep in mind that subcoracoid bursitis is much less common, and unlike a sprained acromioclavicular ligament, the pain can spread down the arm. When in doubt, the two tissues can be palpated for tenderness.

On a rare occasion, trauma to the shoulder injures a portion of the joint capsule, for example, the anterior fibers can be injured when a defensive player grabs a quarterback's arm as he cocks it back to make a forward pass. After the patient's acute pain dissipates, he is left with a chronic ache. On physical examination, the positive findings are full but painful abduction and painfully limited passive external rotation.

As a physical therapist you should also be aware of those painful conditions that require referral to other specialists. It is possible that a patient with shoulder pain may be referred with minimal diagnostic information and a general prescription for treatment. When glenohumeral mobility is normal, but any attempt to lift the arm beyond 90 degrees is agonizing with a spasm end-feel, the therapist should suspect a pulmonary neoplasm. A growth in the lower lung tissue will cause the pectoralis major muscle to go into spasm to protect the underlying pathological tissue. In this case x-ray film of the lower lung field is diagnostic.

The shoulder joint also reflects our emotional state. We eagerly reach out to shake a friend's hand. We hold our arms in adduction and internal rotation when expressing emotional withdrawal. In long-standing psychological disabilities, a patient may progressively lose shoulder abduction. The psychological stress has been converted into a bodily symptom. This is known as a conversion reaction. If the reaction goes undetected, the patient is referred to physical therapy for merely a "stiff shoulder."

Unknown to the patient, even an ankylosed shoulder can be moved into 60 degrees of passive abduction as long as the scapula remains mobile. Therefore, in truly organic lesions passive abduction equals passive glenohumeral range plus 60 degrees. It is likely that a patient is suffering a conversion reaction if the scapula is mobile and the patient exhibits less than 60 degrees of abduction. The phenomenon of conversion reaction can be one cause of myofascial syndrome, an illness sometimes characterized by chronic pain and loss of mobility. Talley's clinical work indicates this syndrome responds well to tricyclic antidepressants, but not analgesics. Myofascial syndrome could be the manifestation of depression cloaked under a socially and psychologically acceptable name to enhance patient acceptance.

TENDINITIS

Tendinitis is a common shoulder problem. Selective tissue testing will identify the painful tissue, providing that the following points are kept in mind.

Double lesions sometimes occur. For example, a patient may have both a tendinitis and a chronic bursitis, or a tendinitis in two muscles. The first problem may be overcome by carefully palpating the bursae or with a diagnostic injection of xylocaine. If more than one isometric muscle test is painful, the therapist can differentiate which test is more painful by testing the patient in the supine rather than the standing position. If in the supine position the patient clearly states that one test is more painful than the other, then a single lesion exists. If both tests are still equally painful, then a double lesion probably exists.

Pain on resistive internal rotation indicates involvement of the subscapularis, latissimus dorsi, or pectoralis major. The latissimus dorsi and pectoralis major muscles are then tested by resistive adduction. If resistive adduction is painless, then the lesion lies in the subscapularis muscle. If resistive adduction is painful, then resistive horizontal adduction and extension are used to test the pectoralis major and latissimus dorsi muscles.

Patients with tendinitis frequently exhibit a painful arc or pain at the extreme end of flexion or abduction. Cyriax hypothesized the painful arc was caused by the rubbing of the acromion arch against a scar located superficially in the tendon. Figure 20-4 illustrates the location of these three scars. Pain elicited at the end of flexion or abduction was caused by the stretching of a deep distal scar. A scar traversing the complete tendon resulted in both a painful arc

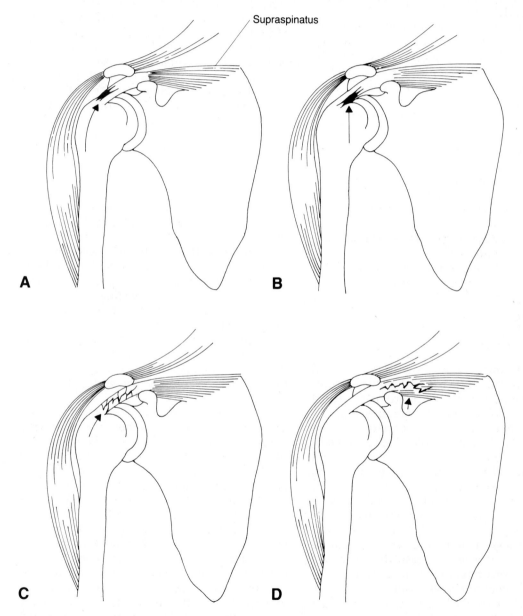

Figure 20-4. Location of scars associated with tendinitis. *(A)* Superficial aspect of supraspinatus tendon. *(B)* Deep aspect of supraspinatus tendon. *(C)* Both superficial and deep aspects of supraspinatus tendon. *(D)* Musculotendinous junction of supraspinatus tendon.

and pain at the extreme end of movement.

The following axioms are helpful in interpreting data from the objective examination.

1. Tendinitis will result in a strong but painful muscle test.
2. Pain elicited at approximately 180 degrees of flexion or abduction indicates the patient may have a sprained acromioclavicular ligament or a scar at the deep distal end of the supraspinatus, infraspinatus, or subscapularis.
3. A painful arc indicates one of the following lesions.

   - Supraspinatus tendinitis—superficial fibers
   - Infraspinatus tendinitis—superficial fibers
   - Subscapularis tendinitis—superficial fibers
   - Acromioclavicular sprain—deep fibers
   - Chronic bursitis
   - Tendinitis of the intracapsular fibers of the long head of the biceps.

NEUROLOGICAL DEFICIT AND MUSCLE BREACHES

A shoulder exhibiting full range of motion with one or more muscles weak and painless brings to mind the possibility of a neurological deficit or a total breach in one or more muscles.

Nerve injury can occur secondary to severe trauma to the shoulder girdle. A fractured surgical neck of the humerus can lacerate the radial nerve, and a dislocated humeral head can compress the axillary nerve.

Virtually all physical therapists learn how to evaluate patients for these obvious peripheral nerve injuries as part of their basic studies. Somewhat less obvious and more difficult is examination for a neurological deficit caused by a disk lesion or neuritis. Remember that you can quickly clear the cervical spine as a part of your shoulder examination. A more detailed examination of the cervical spine has been described in a previous chapter, so our discussion will be limited to neuritis.

The spinal accessory, long thoracic, and suprascapular nerves can develop a neuritis. In these cases, the history may be vague. The patient may state that he suffered a scapular ache that lasted about three weeks. The ache may have been preceded by a stretching type of injury to the shoulder. The inability to elevate the arm normally became apparent to the patient as the scapula ache subsided.

Neuritis may be initially mistaken for a cervical disk lesion because disk problems can also cause a scapula ache eventually leading to muscle weakness. With neuritis, however, the examination reveals that the cervical movements are normal. Of greater significance, the pattern of neurological deficit indicates involvement of a peripheral nerve distal to the nerve root.

Suprascapular neuritis results in painless weakness of the supraspinatus and infraspinatus.

Patients with long thoracic nerve involvement complain of the inability to flex the shoulder more than 45 degrees. Inspection reveals a winged scapula. Muscle testing indicates the serratus anterior muscle is extremely weak.

The spinal accessory nerve innervates the trapezius muscle. The two most obvious clinical findings are a slight loss of active shoulder flexion and projection of the vertebral border of the scapula when testing the middle trapezius muscle.

With neuritis, spontaneous recovery usually commences about six months after the initial onset of the scapula ache. The role of the physical therapist is to assist the physician in reaching a specific diagnosis and to offer the patient a program of strengthening exercises.

A total breach in a muscle or its tendon is caused by trauma or overexertion. Pain is felt immediately and the patient notices a sudden loss of muscle strength. The involved muscle is weak and painless. The examination requires very clear communication between you and the patient. The patient must state accurately whether or not the muscle test increases the amount of pain being suffered. A weak and painful muscle is due to a partial tear or extremely severe tendinitis.

Table 20–2. Common Soft Tissue Lesions at the Shoulder

	AC JOINT SPRAIN SUPERIOR FIBERS	AC JOINT SPRAIN INFERIOR FIBERS	SUPRASPINATUS TENDON TPI Superior Fibers	SUPRASPINATUS TENDON TPI Inferior Fibers	SUPRASPINATUS TENDON Entire TPI	SUPRASPINATUS TENDON Musculotendinous junction	INFRASPINATUS TPI Superior Fibers	INFRASPINATUS TPI Inferior Fibers	INFRASPINATUS Body of Tendon	SUBSCAPULARIS TPI Superior Fibers	SUBSCAPULARIS TPI Inferior Fibers	BICEPS TENSINITIS	CAPSULITIS/ CAPSULAR PATTERN	BURSITIS Acute Subdeltoid Bursitis	BURSITIS Chronic Subdeltoid Bursitis	BURSITIS Subcoracoid Bursitis	Long Thoracic Neuritis	Suprascapular Neuritis	Spinal Accessory Neuritis
Active elevation at shoulder (flexion)	PER	PER	P	P	P		P	P	P	P	P		LP	L			LW	LW	LW
Passive elevation (flexion)	PER	PER		PER	PER			PER			PER		LP						
Painful arc	PA	PA	PA		PA		PA			PA					PA				
Passive abduction (0–90°)													LP	LP					
Passive external rotation (0–90°)	PER	PER											LP						
Passive internal rotation (0–90°)	PER	PER											LP						
Resisted abduction			P	P	P	P											W		
Resisted abduction																			
Resisted external rotation							P	P	P									W	
Resisted internal rotation										P	P								
Resisted flexion of elbow (biceps)												P							
Resisted extension of elbow (triceps)																			
Passive horizontal abduction	LP	LP											LP			P			

Key: P, pain; L, limited; W, weak; PA, painful arc; LP, limited painful; PER, painful extreme range; TPI, tenoperiosteal junction.

NORMAL FINDINGS ON EXAMINATION

Situations arise where the musculoskeletal examination indicates that the shoulder has full painless passive range of motion and, within the confines of the examination as performed, all musculature is strong and painless. The examiner must now look for alternative sources of pain and possibly re-examine the shoulder with greater intensity. As already mentioned, pain at the shoulder can be referred from the diaphragm, heart, or cervical spine. Furthermore, the symptoms may have a psychological origin.

The neck should be examined again and the therapist should refer the patient to other specialists if the pain seems to be caused by something other than a simple musculoskeletal problem.

Patients with minor inflammatory conditions may have no pain at the time of the initial examination. These patients frequently state that it takes numerous repetitions of movement to bring on the pain. In such cases, the physical examination should follow a vigorous session of shoulder exercises.

Lastly, the possibility of a neurovascular syndrome must be considered. Briefly, the absence of pain at rest suggests that the therapist examine the arterial system. Edema, skin tightness, cyanosis, and fatigue suggest a venous problem. Intermittent pain varying with arm position combined with complaints of numbness, tingling, or weakness requires a careful neurological examination.

Table 20-2 synthesizes the information on the various common soft tissue lesions at the shoulder. It may be useful to help the examiner interpret the data collected in the physical examination.

ANNOTATED BIBLIOGRAPHY

Calliet R: Shoulder Pain, 2nd ed, Philadelphia, FA Davis, 1984 (A useful introduction to the functional anatomy of the shoulder with easy-to-understand stick figures. The author emphasizes the proper use of patient history and examination in reaching a diagnosis.)

Lord J, Rosati L: Neurovascular compression syndromes of the upper extremity. Clin Symp 10:35, 1958 (An excellent description of the anatomical relationships of soft tissues at the shoulder to thoracic outlet syndromes. Useful anatomical drawings, clinical photographs, and case studies help explain neurovascular compression syndromes.)

Talley J: Masks of major depression. Medical Aspects of Human Sexuality 20:16, 1986 (An excellent article for physical therapists who wish to gain insight into psychogenic pain.)

21 Musculoskeletal Analysis: The Elbow and Hand

JANET C. COOKSON

ELBOW

ANATOMICAL OVERVIEW

The humeroradial and humeroulnar joints combined with the proximal radioulnar joint make up the elbow. They are all enclosed in the same fibrous capsule, making the structure a compound joint.

The humeroradial and humeroulnar joints function together as a uniaxial hinge joint, enabling the arm to flex and extend. Range of motion (ROM) in extension is limited by the olecranon process of the ulna approximating the olecranon fossa of the humerus. Children and women may have up to 15 degrees of hyperextension available, because the olecranon process is smaller in these groups and can pass deeper into the olecranon fossa during extension. ROM in flexion is limited by approximation of the soft tissue structures in the arm and forearm. In a less muscular person, flexion may be limited by the bone-to-bone block because the coronoid process of the ulna blocks on the coronoid fossa of the humerus.

Supination and pronation at the elbow take place at the proximal radioulnar joint. ROM in pronation is stopped by the approximation of the radius on the ulna, but because of the muscular attachments on these bones the end-feel is leathery. ROM in supination is stopped by the stretch of ligaments.

Component Joints

Humeroradial Joint

In the humeroradial joint the convex-shaped capitulum articulates with the cup-shaped, concave proximal portion of the radial head. It is a triaxial, ball and socket joint. Its arthrokinematic characteristics are:

> Type of joint: ovoid
> Close-packed position: semiflexion and semipronation
> Loose-packed or resting position: extension and supination

The radial collateral ligament passes from the lateral epicondyle of the humerus to the annular ligament, which encircles the radial neck.

Humeroulnar Joint

In the humeroulnar joint, the trochlear notch of the ulna articulates with the trochlea of the distal humerus. Its arthrokinematic characteristics are:

> Type of joint: sellar
> Close-packed position: full extension
> Loose-packed or resting position: semiflexion

Because the trochlea is oriented obliquely with respect to the sagittal plane, the elbow joint demonstrates a valgus carrying angle. This angle may measure from 7 to 20 degrees, and is greater in women than men. The ligamentous support on the ulnar aspect of the elbow is massive compared to the radial side (Tullos and co-workers, 1981). The ulnar collateral ligament fans out from the medial epicondyle along the whole lip of the coronoid process of the ulna.

351

Proximal Radioulnar Joint

The proximal radioulnar joint belongs structurally to the elbow and functionally to the forearm, because its motions of pronation and supination mainly affect the wrist and hand, not the elbow. The convex edge of the radial head articulates with the concave radial notch of the ulna. The arthrokinematic characteristics are:

Type of joint: ovoid

Close-packed position: midway between pronation and supination

Loose-packed or resting position: full pronation or supination

It has one ligament, the quadrate ligament, which passes from the radial notch on the ulna to the medial neck of the radius, and supports the synovial joint capsule.

Nerves

The elbow joint receives articular branches from four different nerves: the musculocutaneous, radial, ulnar, and median nerves. Because many nerves innervate the joint and its surrounding skin and soft tissues, spinal segments C5 through T1 are represented at the elbow. Referred pain from these spinal nerves or any of their structural derivatives can therefore be felt at the elbow. However, unlike other body areas, such as the shoulder, elbow lesions are less likely to refer pain distally.

Muscles

For details on specific muscles producing movement at the elbow, the reader is referred to standard anatomy texts. In evaluating the elbow, remember that some hand and wrist muscles also cross the elbow joint to insert on the humerus. These include the extensors carpi radialis longus and brevis laterally, and medially the muscles making up the common flexor tendon.

Other Soft Tissue Structures

Vessels

The brachial artery traverses the cubital fossa deep to the bicipital aponeurosis and medial to the biceps tendon. The deep lymphatics accompany the brachial artery and may demonstrate some nodes in the cubital region. Medially the cephalic vein and laterally the basilic vein course through the superficial fascia of the elbow.

Bursa

The notable bursa in the elbow region is the olecranon bursa, situated between the skin and the posterior surface of the olecranon process.

SUBJECTIVE EXAMINATION

The subjective examination at the elbow, wrist, and hand identifies the position and behavior of the patient's pain or stiffness, so change can be documented as treatment progresses. Described below are four general areas of inquiry: identifying information, area of pain, history, and behavior of pain. The discussion of the latter three areas is based on Maitland's work (1977).

Identifying Information

The subjective examination begins by noting the patient's identifying information, as follows.

1. Age. Certain lesions in the region have particular ages of onset. These are described in the sections on interpretation.
2. Sex. This is for purposes of identification.
3. Occupation. A habitual sustained posture, a repeated action, or a new activity may be causing or aggravating the pain. At the elbow, look especially for the following habits.

- *Elbow flexion* may aggravate an ulnar nerve compression at the elbow.
- *Leaning on a hyperflexed elbow* may cause an ulnar nerve compression, or an olecranon bursitis.
- *Varus or valgus stress against resistance* may cause lateral or medial epicondylitis.

Correlate any repeated occupational movement with the findings on the objective evaluation.

Area of Pain

Ask the patient, "Where is your pain?" and record its full extent on a body diagram. Be certain to note the following.

1. Define the proximal and distal boundaries of the pain. Include any pain in the fingers. This will identify involvement of a particular cervical segment or peripheral nerve.
2. Label the point of worst pain. Elbow, wrist, and hand pain usually comes from a local cause. The point of worst pain usually overlies the structure that is causing the pain.
3. Diagram reported changes in sensation. Note these in order to compare them with a pinprick test later.

History

Ask the patient, "How and when did this all come about?" Many elbow, wrist, and hand problems have characteristic histories, which are further described in the sections on interpretation. In the history, identify the following.

1. Any causative incident
2. How soon after the incident the symptoms started to occur
3. The order in which the symptoms occurred
4. Any treatment to date and any previous episodes, their treatment, and the results

Behavior of Pain

Ask the patient the following three questions:

1. "How does this feel throughout the day and night?"
2. "What makes it better?"
3. "What makes it worse?"

The answers to these questions will give you an idea of the functional limitation caused by the elbow, wrist, or hand problem. Use the information to design an objective evaluation and treatment plan that will minimize discomfort.

OBJECTIVE EXAMINATION

Observation

Observe the elbow as the patient moves toward the treatment area.

1. Is the patient holding it in a flexed position, or is it in a sling? (There will probably be a loss of ROM on examination.)
2. Is the patient guarding the elbow with the other hand? (The joint may be irritable; handle it gently.)
3. How smooth are the elbow movements? (If they are jerky or guarded, the joint may be irritable, and have a decreased ROM. Alternatively, there may be a neurological problem.)

After the patient exposes the entire upper extremity, place the arm as close to anatomic position (extension and supination) as possible and note the following.

Swelling or Atrophy

Localized swelling indicates a local problem, such as olecranon bursitis. Diffuse swelling usually indicates joint capsule involvement. If there is atrophy, note which muscles are atrophied to determine any pattern of spinal or peripheral nerve involvement.

Carrying Angle/Deformity

Compare the limb to the other side. The elbow may display: (a) cubitus valgus—an increase in carrying angle; (b) cubitus varus—a decrease in carrying angle; or (c) hyperextension because of hypermobility. If any deformity is found, consult the radiographic report. Full ROM may be structurally unavailable.

Skin Condition

Redness indicates inflammation. Hypertrophic changes (shiny, smooth, red skin) indicate an autonomic disturbance in the upper extremity. If there are any scars, note how well they are healed. A burn scar may contract and limit the ROM of an otherwise normal elbow.

Skin Temperature

Although it properly belongs in the examination by palpation, palpate the skin for any increase in temperature at this time. Movement produced later during the objective examination may increase the skin temperature. Palpation for heat at this point avoids this artifact.

Body Type

Is the patient ectomorphic, mesomorphic, or endomorphic? Expect a mesomorphic or endomorphic person to have total ROM of elbow flexion at the lower limit of normal. Palpating the epicondylar area will require deeper pressure in an obese patient.

Joint Movement Assessment

Passive Physiological Movement

There are four physiological motions to examine at the elbow: extension, flexion, supination, and pronation. The patient may be supine, seated, or standing. Stabilize the patient's upper arm, and move the arm to the end of each motion. Apply the pressure at the end of range proximal to the wrist joint, to isolate the stress to the elbow. Range of motion, end-feel, and pain are assessed. The elbow's movement characteristics are:

> Normal ROM: extension, 0 degrees; flexion, 135 or more degrees; supination and pronation, 90 degrees each
>
> Capsular pattern: marked limitation of flexion compared with some limitation in extension. Occasionally there is equal limitation of flexion and extension. If the proximal radioulnar joint becomes involved, there is also a limitation in supination.
>
> Normal end-feel in extension: bone-to-bone
>
> Normal end-feel in flexion: soft tissue approximation
>
> Normal end-feel in pronation and supination: leathery or elastic

Compare ROM and end-feel with that found on the patient's other side. Ask yourself:

1. Is a capsular pattern present? It signifies arthritis: joint capsule involvement.
2. Is the end-feel normal? Arthritis produces a hard end-feel; a soft end-feel in extension

occurs together with a noncapsular pattern when the elbow has a loose intra-articular fragment (loose body).
3. Where in the ROM does pain occur? The relationship between pain and resistance at the end of ROM is discussed below.
4. Is there any crepitus or snapping on movement? Coarse crepitus indicates long-standing osteoarthritis; fine crepitus indicates long-standing rheumatoid disease; and snapping can occur if the ulnar nerve persistently dislocates from the ulnar groove.

Passive Accessory Movement

Distraction of the humeroulnar joint and inferior and superior glides of the superior radioulnar joint may be used to evaluate passive accessory movement at the elbow. Try to assess the degree of motion available in comparison with the normal side. Perception of the amount of passive accessory motion occurring at the elbow requires some practice. It is also helpful to note whether or not the motion produced pain or relief of pain, and whether the pain occurred before, concurrent with, or after resistance or stiffness. If the motion relieved pain, it may be used as a treatment technique. If pain occurs before resistance is felt at the end of the movement, the joint is irritable and requires gentle handling. Pain occurring concurrent with or after resistance is felt means that the joint is not irritable and can tolerate some degree of stretching (Maitland, 1970).

Static Resisted Movement

There are six static resisted motions tested in examining the elbow: elbow extension, flexion, supination, and pronation; wrist flexion and extension. Resisted wrist motions are tested because the wrist extensors and flexors are attached to the lateral and medial epicondyles, respectively, of the elbow. Any pain arising from their dysfunction may present in the cubital area.

All of the motions may be tested with the patient supine, sitting, or standing. Resisted flexion, extension, supination, and pronation are tested with the patient's elbow flexed to 90 degrees. Stabilize the patient's arm with one hand, and apply the appropriate motion-free resistance with your other hand placed proximal to the patient's wrist joint. Wrist flexion and extension are tested with the wrist muscles placed at a mechanical advantage: Test them with the patient's elbow extended.

Assess strength and the presence or absence of pain on contraction. The evaluation of strength will be more accurate if all of the resisted tests are performed on one side and then the other, rather than testing both sides at the same time. If each test is performed bilaterally at the same time, the difference between a muscle grade of 4+ on one side and 5 on the other may not be apparent. If weakness is found, correlate it and any sensation changes with spinal and peripheral nerve distributions. If gross weakness is present in any motion, perform graded muscle tests on the specific muscles in question.

Palpation

At this point in the evaluation, the tissue at fault will be fairly evident, and directed palpation of particular structures can be performed to evaluate pain on pressure, minor swelling and structural abnormalities, and changes in skin sensation.

The olecranon process and the medial and lateral epicondyles are immediately subcutaneous and easy to identify. Palpate anteriorly and deeply on the epicondyles if palpation of the origins of the wrist flexor and extensor tendons is desired. The radial head is located in the depression medial and posterior to the wrist extensors. Rotate the patient's forearm to feel the radial head's motion, verifying the location. Synovial thickening in the elbow joint capsule is best found laterally over the head of the radius. Because the normal feeling of this area is bony, any synovial thickening present will feel like intervening soft tissue over the radial head. A synovial effusion will first bulge into the area posterior to the radial head in the region lateral to the olecranon process. For specifics on palpation of individual muscles, refer to any standard anatomy or muscle testing text.

Other Tests

Sensation testing is performed with the patient's eyes closed. Test pain with a large pin or a sensation wheel, and light touch with a piece of cotton. Test the distributions of spinal segments C5 through T1, and the cutaneous distributions of the ulnar, raidal, and median nerves.

If there is any question about the integrity of forearm circulation, the brachial pulse may be found by palpating deeply in the cubital fossa medial to the biceps tendon. The radial pulse lateral to the flexor carpi radialis tendon at the wrist may also be examined.

Special Tests

Nerve Conduction Velocity
If there is evidence of peripheral nerve compression, it can be confirmed by performing motor and sensory nerve conduction velocity tests on the nerve in question. Consult Goodgold and Eberstein (1972) for an excellent description of these tests.

Tinel Sign
If the ulnar nerve is compressed in the ulnar groove, tapping on it in the groove may cause a tingling sensation radiating down the forearm into the hand in an ulnar distribution. This is a Tinel sign at the elbow.

INTERPRETATION OF FINDINGS

The following section describes the clinical presentation of some common pathologic conditions at the elbow, as described by Cyriax (1975; 1983) unless otherwise noted.

Noncontractile Lesions

Osteoarthritis
Subjective Findings.   Subjective findings in osteoarthritis include nontraumatic, gradual development of osteoarthritic changes in middle-aged patients. The joint is usually not acutely painful, but is uncomfortable when moved to the end of ROM.

Objective Findings.   Objective findings include a capsular pattern, with elbow stiffness and limited ROM. If the condition is long-standing, coarse crepitus may be present. The arthritis is usually present bilaterally.

Rheumatoid Arthritis
Subjective Findings. Pain and loss of ROM occurring in the absence of trauma are subjective findings of rheumatoid arthritis. There may be gross limitation of function in the upper extremity because of the limited ROM and intensity of pain.

Objective Findings. Objective findings are a marked capsular pattern with a hard, spasm end-feel. There may also be warmth, synovial thickening, fine crepitus on movement, synovial effusion, and rheumatoid nodules. Other joints may also be affected. Roentgenograms may demonstrate decalcification and joint cartilage erosion.

Joint Stiffness After Trauma, Fracture, or Surgery
The category of joint stiffness includes sprained collateral ligaments at the elbow. These are so close to the joint capsule that any sprained ligament involves the elbow joint capsule itself.

Subjective Findings. Subjective findings in the patient with joint stiffness will include a history of trauma, such as a bad sprain or a broken bone, with or without surgical repair. The elbow has usually been immobilized with a sling or a cast for a period of time.

Objective Findings. Capsular pattern is the usual objective finding, although surgical repair may alter it. Diffuse swelling may be present.

Internal Derangement
Subjective Findings. In the patient with internal derangement, the joint periodically locks, with full extension or flexion being limited. ROM returns gradually over several days. Frequent occurrences can set up a reactive osteoarthritis, even in adolescents.

Objective Findings. The patient will exhibit a noncapsular pattern: the joint is limited in full extension (soft end-feel) or full flexion (hard end-feel).

Nursemaid's Elbow
Subjective Findings. Nursemaid's elbow occurs when the parent of a child under the age of 8 years pulls upward on the child's extended arm. The child immediately experiences pain and cradles the elbow.

Objective Findings. Noncapsular pattern: the child holds the elbow in 90 degrees flexion, and is reluctant to supinate because of pain.

Olecranon Bursitis
Subjective Findings. The patient with olecranon bursitis may have a history of trauma or repeated irritation to the olecranon, such as habitual leaning on the elbow.

Objective Findings. The usual finding is palpable localized swelling on the tip of the olecranon. If it occurs in conjunction with rheumatoid disease, there may be palpable thickening of the bursa. In an acute case, there may be limited passive flexion because of pain; however, no resistance to movement is felt.

Ulnar Nerve Compression in the Ulnar Groove
Refer to Smorto and Basmajian (1972) for a detailed explanation of ulnar nerve lesions.

Subjective Findings. The patient with ulnar nerve compression may report habitual or prolonged flexion of the elbow, or prolonged leaning on a hyperflexed elbow.

Objective Findings. Painless weakness and possible atrophy in forearm and hand muscles in an ulnar nerve distribution will be noted. There may be sensation changes in an ulnar distribution in the hand. The elbow may demonstrate cubitus valgus or a Tinel sign, or both. The motor nerve conduction velocity of the portion of ulnar nerve that crosses the elbow will be slower than normal. (The practitioner performing the test will have a table of normal values for his own practice.)

Radial Nerve Compression
Subjective Findings. The patient with radial nerve compression usually has a history of an incident where the upper arm was compressed over a sharp edge. Use of an improperly ad-

justed axillary crutch or a mid-shaft fracture of the humerus are alternative histories.

Objective Findings. Painless weakness and sensation changes in a radial nerve distribution will be noted. Weakness in the wrist extensors is especially notable.

Contractile Lesions

Muscle Strain and Tendinitis
Subjective Findings. The patient with muscle strain or tendinitis may report trauma to the elbow, or a history of overuse.

Objective Findings. A static resisted motion is strong, but produces pain when performed. Table 21-1 includes an overview of contractile lesions for various motions at the elbow.

WRIST AND HAND

ANATOMICAL OVERVIEW

The wrist joint is classified as a compound joint, and has three primary synovial joints: the distal radioulnar joint, the radiocarpal joint, and the intercarpal joint. The intercarpal, carpometacarpal, and intermetacarpal joints are structurally related: With the exceptions of the first carpometacarpal (CMC) and pisiform triquetral joints, they share the same synovial joint capsule. The intercarpal joint is therefore the link between the wrist and the hand proper. Joints making up the fingers are functionally linked in series: the intermetacarpal joints, the metacarpophalangeal (MP) joints, and the proximal (PIP) and distal (DIP) interphalangeal joints.

Two transverse arches, concave palmarly, help position the thumb for efficient pinching and grasping. The static, proximal transverse arch is formed by the proximal row of carpals. The deformable, distal arch is located at the level of the metacarpal heads. A third concave palmar arch, the longitudinal arch, is defined by the phalanges and the natural curve of the palmar surface of the metacarpals. If lost, these arches must be restored for normal hand function.

Table 21-1. Contractile Lesions at the Elbow Indicated by Strong, Painful Resisted Motion

JOINT	MOTION	MUSCLE AFFECTED	OTHER OBJECTIVE FINDINGS	OTHER COMMENTS
Elbow	Flexion	Biceps: back of belly	Pain to resisted supination	Palpate by reaching around sides and pinching biceps
		Biceps: lower tenoperiosteal (TP) junction	Increased pain to passive pronation; pain to resisted supination	Refers pain down forearm to wrist
	Extension	Triceps: musculotendinous (MT) or TP junction		If resisted extension is tested with the arm dependent, a pinched subacromial structure could also cause the pain
	Supination	Biceps (see above)	Pain to resisted elbow flexion	
		Supinator		Palpate between upper radius and ulna on posterior forearm
	Pronation	Common flexor tendon: TP junction	Pain to resisted wrist flexion	
		Pronator teres: muscle belly		
Wrist	Flexion	Common flexor tendon: TP junction	May be pain to resisted pronation	History of valgus strain to the elbow: "golfer's elbow"
	Extension	Extensor carpi radialis longus: supracondylar ridge; extensor carpi radialis brevis: TP, MT junctions; muscle belly		History of varus strain to the elbow: "tennis elbow"; pain begins several days after the strain.
				Usually occurs after age 30

Component Joints

Distal Radioulnar Joint

In the distal radioulnar joint, the convex head of the ulna articulates with the concave ulnar notch of the distal radius. These are bound together by the triangular articular disk. It is a uniaxial pivot joint. Its arthrokinematic characteristics are:

> Type of joint: ovoid
>
> Close-packed position: midway between pronation and supination
>
> Loose-packed or resting position: full pronation or supination

Pronation and supination take place at the distal radioulnar joint, with pronation being limited by the approximation of the radius on the ulna, and supination being limited by ligamentous stretch.

Radiocarpal Joint

The radiocarpal joint is composed of the convex surfaces of the scaphoid, lunate, and triquetrum articulating with the concave surface of the radius and the triangular articular disk. It is classified as a biaxial, ellipsoid joint. Its arthrokinematic characteristics are:

> Type of joint: ovoid
>
> Close-packed position: full extension with radial deviation
>
> Loose-packed or resting position: neutral flexion/extension, midway between radial and ulnar deviation

Wrist motions occurring at both the radiocarpal and intercarpal joints include extension, flexion, and radial and ulnar deviation. Range of motion in extension is usually limited by the extensibility of the flexor tendons, but tension may fall on the palmar ligaments during hyperextension trauma. Ulnar deviation (UD) is similarly limited by the extensibility of the antagonistic tendons and additionally by tension in the radial collateral ligament. Wrist flexion is limited by the approximation of the carpals on one another and on the radius; radial deviation (RD) is limited by the bony approximation of the scaphoid on the radius.

The significant ligaments at both the radio-carpal and intercarpal joints are the radial and ulnar collateral ligaments and a number of palmar ligaments. These palmar ligaments are generally thicker and stronger than their counterparts on the dorsum of the wrist.

Intercarpal Joint

At the intercarpal joint, the convex distal scaphoid and the concave trapezium and trapezoid articulate with the convex surface formed by the combined capitate and hamate bones, and the concave surface formed by the scaphoid, lunate, and triquetrum. Although it is structurally a sellar joint, it functions as an ovoid joint (MacConaill and Basmajian, 1977). Its arthrokinematic characteristics, motions, and limitations of motion are the same as the radiocarpal joint.

Carpometacarpal and Intermetacarpal Joints

The joints that join the metacarpals with the triquetrum, capitate, and hamate are plane joints, with only slight gliding possible. The first carpometacarpal joint departs from this pattern and is considered below. Of the joints between the bases of the second through fifth metacarpals, that between the second and the third is immovable because of structural locking with the trapezoid and capitate. The third metacarpal is therefore the least mobile and acts as a fixed point about which the other metacarpals rotate. The metacarpals rotate inwardly towards the axis of the third metacarpal during finger flexion, increasing the cup shape of the palm.

Pisiform Triquetral Joint

The pisiform triquetral joint is a small plane joint, with its own separate synovial capsule. A small amount of pisiform gliding is available. Its two primary ligaments, the pisohamate and piso fifth metacarpal ligaments, are occasionally sprained (Cyriax, 1975).

First Carpometacarpal Joint

The joint between the trapezium and the base of the first metacarpal is more mobile than the other carpometacarpal joints because of its separate synovial capsule and thick, loose fibrous capsule. Its movement characteristics are:

Type of joint: sellar

Close-packed position: full opposition of the thumb

Loose-packed or resting position: slight flexion of the thumb

Mobility at this joint helps to accentuate the distal transverse arch of the hand.

Metacarpophalangeal Joints

The five metacarpophalangeal joints are formed by the convex distal heads of the metacarpals fitting into the shallow concave bases of the proximal phalanges. Their arthrokinematic characteristics are:

Type of joint: ovoid

Close-packed position: full flexion

Loose-packed or resting position: slight flexion

They are classified as triaxial condyloid joints. Extension, flexion, abduction, and adduction occur actively at the MP joints. Extension is limited by the extensibility of tendons and soft tissues on the palmar surface of the hand, and flexion is limited by the approximation of these same tissues. Both abduction and adduction are limited by tension in the collateral ligaments and the soft tissues of the web space. Involuntary, conjunct rotation also occurs at the MP joints, rotating the proximal phalanges inwardly towards the axis of the third digit during finger flexion (MacConaill and Basmajian, 1977).

The separate MP joints are attached to each other by the deep transverse metacarpal ligament. Each MP joint has a collateral ligament on either side, and a thick, volar ligament (volar plate, palmar ligament), which is grooved for the passage of the digital flexor tendons. Figure 21-1 demonstrates these structures.

Proximal and Distal Interphalangeal Joints

In the PIP and DIP joints, the shallow concave bases of the phalanges articulate with the convex heads of the phalanges proximal to them. Arthrokinematic characteristics are:

Type of joint: technically sellar, functionally ovoid

Close-packed position: full extension

Loose-packed or resting position: slight flexion

They are uniaxial hinge joints, with active flexion and extension limited by the tension in the opposing tendons and other soft tissues. These joints also demonstrate slight rotatory conjunct movements, so that with the fingers fully flexed, each digit points in the direction of the scaphoid. They have collateral and palmar ligaments similar to those at the MP joints.

Nerves

Terminal branches of the median, ulnar, and radial nerves all reach the hand through the wrist. Although there is a variable amount of overlap in the areas that these nerves supply, the areas of most distinct supply are:

- Radial nerve: dorsal web space of the hand over the first dorsal interosseus muscle
- Median nerve: palmar side of the terminal phalanx of the index finger
- Ulnar nerve: palmar side of the terminal phalanx of the little finger

Spinal segments C5 through T1 are represented at the wrist and hand, with the distribution of C5 ending on the radial side of the wrist, and that of T1 ending on the ulnar side of the wrist. Segment C6 is distributed to the thumb, C7 to the middle finger, and T1 to the little finger, with some variation in segmental distribution displayed by the index and ring finger. Pain from an injured wrist or hand structure is rarely referred. However, this region is a common recipient of referred pain or paresthesia from the cervical and shoulder region.

Muscles

In general, each physiological motion taking place at the wrist and hand has at least two muscles producing it. Muscles originating outside the hand are labeled extrinsic muscles; muscles originating within the hand itself are labeled intrinsic muscles. For details on specific muscles and the motions they produce, refer to any standard text in anatomy. Notable details

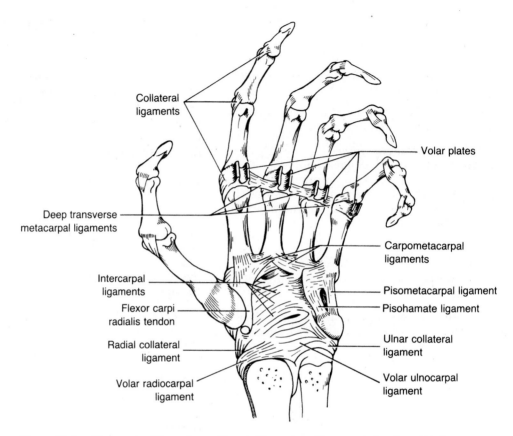

Figure 21-1. Ligaments of the wrist and hand. (Reproduced by permission from Wadsworth CT: The wrist and hand. In Gould JA, Davies GJ (eds): Orthopaedic and Sports Physical Therapy, p 440. St Louis, 1985, The C.V. Mosby Co.)

about special tendon structures in the hand are found on Figures 21-1 and 21-2.

Other Soft Tissue Structures

Retinaculae, Sheaths, and Fascia

The extensor and flexor retinaculae prevent bowstringing of the extensor and flexor tendons at the wrist. As the flexor retinaculum traverses the proximal transverse carpal arch, it encloses the median nerve, digital flexors, and vessels to the hand. This carpal tunnel is a common site for compression of the median nerve. In the hand, bowstringing of the finger flexor tendons is prevented by the attachment of their fibrous digital sheaths to the grooved volar plates of the MP, PIP, and DIP joints (see Fig.

21-1). Bowstringing of the extensor tendons is prevented because the tendons are connected to the volar plates through their extensor hoods, which also attach to the deep transverse metacarpal ligaments. Swan-neck and boutonniere finger deformities can arise from deficiencies in these sheath mechanisms.

All of the extrinsic muscles of the wrist and hand have synovial sheaths in the regions of the retinaculae, palm, and fingers. Both Lampe (1969) and Hollinshead (1982) have excellent diagrams and discussions of these synovial sheaths. In tenosynovitis, these synovial sheaths become irritated. An infection in the sheaths can spread through them throughout the hand.

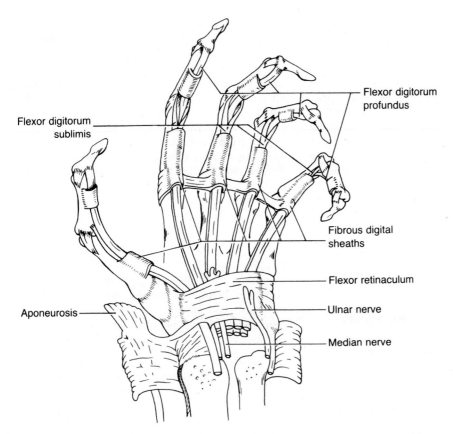

Figure 21-2 Volar soft tissue relationships in the wrist and hand. (Reproduced by permission from Wadsworth CT: The wrist and hand. In Gould JA, Davies GJ (eds): Orthopaedic and Sports Physical Therapy, p 441. St Louis, 1985, The C.V. Mosby Co.)

The deep fascia on the palm is thick and triangular. This palmar aponeurosis binds the skin and flexor retinaculum, and then proceeds distally to attach to the fibrous tendon sheaths of the digital flexors. When the palmar aponeurosis becomes contracted, it limits affected finger extension as in a Dupuytren's contracture.

Vessels

The radial artery passes laterally in the wrist, and then passes deep into the hand at the anatomic snuff box. The ulnar artery crosses the wrist medially, and runs superficial to the flexor retinaculum into the hand.

The superficial and deep veins of the hand drain medially into the cephalic vein, and laterally into the basilic vein. The lymph plexes from the palm and fingers drain to lymph vessels on the dorsum of the hand, which then pass upward in the forearm in association with the cephalic and basilic veins. Because these lymph nodes drain to the dorsum, and the skin is loose and can accommodate, a hand infection will produce swelling on the dorsum.

SUBJECTIVE EXAMINATION

The subjective examination of the wrist and hand is similar to that previously described for the elbow. Habitual motions or positions to be aware of are as follows:

1. *Sustained wrist flexion* may cause median nerve compression in the carpal tunnel, or a subluxed capitate.
2. *Repeated fine finger movements* may also contribute to median nerve compression in the carpal tunnel, cause strained intrinsic hand muscles, or extrinsic flexor tenosynovitis.
3. *Repeated prolonged pressure on the palm by grasping a tool, or striking or pushing an object* can cause median nerve compression, or flexor tendon thickening that could lead to a trigger finger.

OBJECTIVE EXAMINATION

Observation

Note the wrist and hand as the patient enters the treatment area.

1. Does the arm swing normally? If it doesn't, the involved joint is probably irritable.
2. How much is the patient using the hand? Look for things such as the manner in which a woman handles her purse, or if a man uses both hands to undo the buttons on his shirt. Get an initial estimate of the functional limitations posed by the wrist or hand problem.
3. Look for any obvious deformities such as absent digits, or any splints or assistive devices that will need to be noted. Have the patient expose the entire upper extremity, so that it may be examined in full if the pain is found to be referred from a proximal structure. Have the patient place both hands with palms downward on a treatment table and note the following.

Swelling or Atrophy
Common localized swellings are:

1. Heberden's nodes: Hard, sometimes tender nodules at the DIP joints in osteoarthritis
2. Ganglion: A cyst-like swelling in the soft tissues of the wrist or hand, usually over the dorsal carpal area
3. Localized swelling about one particular digit because of local trauma

Synovitis at the wrist will produce diffuse swelling on the dorsum of the wrist. In the fingers, synovitis will produce dorsal edema. In less obvious cases at the MP joints, this can be detected by comparing the patient's clenched fists: The effusion will fill in the normal "valleys" between the metacarpal heads. If the swelling is severe, volumetric measurements may be performed to document the progression of treatment. To assess the effect of diffuse swelling as an extrinsic source of joint limitation in an aseptic hand, use an intermittent compression pump to decrease the swelling prior to re-examination. Examine the contours of the hand for atrophy. Ulnar or median nerve compression may cause hypothenar or thenar atrophy, respectively.

Posture
Compare the hands for symmetrical posture, checking for normal arches and any deviations in length and alignment, such as postfracture deformities. The wrist and hand may display a number of different deformities.

1. Hand posture in rheumatoid arthritis: fixation in wrist flexion with palmar subluxation of the carpals on the radius; finger posture, ulnar deviation
2. PIP hyperextension: swan-neck deformity
3. PIP hyperflexion with DIP extension: boutonniere deformity
4. DIP flexion: mallet finger
5. Fixed thumb adduction: present in first carpometacarpal joint arthritis
6. Fixed finger flexion: present in Dupuytren's contracture and severe trigger finger

Consult x-ray films to determine the extent of the bone and joint involvement if there is a deformity.

Condition of Skin and Nails
Note the color of the hands. Blanched white hands are present in Raynaud's phenomenon. Hands may be red in gout, liver disease, inflammation, or reflex sympathetic dystrophy. In reflex sympathetic dystrophy the skin will also be smooth and shiny. Examine the mobility of any scars on the hand. An immobile scar can extrinsically limit wrist and hand movements.

Skin Temperature

Palpate skin temperature before the objective examination to avoid the artifact of increased temperature because of joint movement. Elevated temperature indicates active inflammation.

Joint Movement Assessment

Passive Physiological Movement

Passively move the various joints through the motions outlined below, recording the ROM, end-feel, presence of pain, and relationship of pain to any resistance felt at the end of the ROM. Be sure that the joint is isolated by your hand placement to avoid inconclusive results caused by testing multiple joints at the same time. As you move the joint, also feel for crepitus. Fine crepitus indicates tenosynovitis, and coarse crepitus indicates advanced rheumatoid arthritis. Passive motions to test and movement characteristics (Cyriax, 1975) for each joint are outlined below.

1. Wrist—distal radioulnar joint

   - Motions to test and their normal ROM: supination (90 degrees), pronation (90 degrees)
   - Capsular pattern: equal limitation of supination and pronation
   - Normal end-feel for supination and pronation: leathery or elastic

2. Wrist—radiocarpal and intercarpal joints

   - Motions to test and their normal ROM: extension (70 degrees), flexion (80 degrees), radial deviation (20 degrees), ulnar deviation (30 degrees)
   - Capsular pattern: equal limitation of extension and flexion, slight limitation of radial and ulnar deviation
   - Normal end-feel for extension and radial deviation: elastic or bone to bone, depending on the elasticity of opposing structures
   - Normal end-feel for flexion and ulnar deviation: elastic

3. Thumb—carpometacarpal, metacarpophalangeal (MP), and interphalangeal (IP) joints

   - Motions to test and their normal ROM: backward movement of thumb in full extension in a screening examination. In a complete examination also examine: CMC abduction (70 degrees), adduction (0 degrees); MP extension (0 degrees), flexion (50 degrees); and IP extension (20 degrees), flexion (90 degrees).
   - Capsular pattern: first CMC joint—limited abduction and extension, developing into fixation of the thumb in adduction; MP, IP joints—equal limitation of extension and flexion
   - Normal end-feel: elastic for all except adduction, which is soft tissue approximation

4. Fingers—MP, PIP, DIP joints

   - Motions to test and their normal ROM: gross extension and flexion in a screening examination. A complete examination would cover: MP flexion (90 degrees), extension (30 to 45 degrees) MP abduction/adduction (20 degrees); PIP extension (0 degrees), flexion (100 degrees); and DIP extension (20 degrees), flexion (90 degrees).
   - Capsular pattern: equal limitation of extension and flexion
   - End-feel: elastic for all motions

Compare any abnormal ROM or end-feel with that found on the patient's other side. Determine whether or not a capsular pattern indicating arthritis is found at any joint.

Passive Accessory Movement

Passive movements that may be assessed at the wrist and hand are listed here and described in more detail in Kaltenborn (1976) and in Kessler and Hertling (1983).

> Distal radioulnar joint: pronatory and supinatory glides
>
> Wrist joint: general distraction, dorsal and volar glides
>
> Fingers: distraction, dorsal and volar glides

Comparing the motions available with those on the contralateral side will demonstrate if any of these motions are abnormal. Record whether or not the motion was limited, and whether pain was relieved or produced during the movement. See comments earlier in this section on passive accessory movement at the elbow regarding the relationship of pain to joint resistance.

Static Resisted Movement

Test maximal contractions, applying motion-free resistance to the following motions:

> Wrist: supination, pronation, extension, flexion, radial deviation, ulnar deviation
>
> Thumb (resist at distal phalanx): extension, flexion, abduction, adduction
>
> Fingers (test all together as a quick test, or individually if a complete test is needed): extension, flexion, abduction, adduction

Stabilize the joint adequately to prevent any motion from occurring. Record strength and note the character and location of any pain produced on contraction. Test one motion at a time, one side at a time for accurate results. If a motion is weak, perform specific graded muscle tests on all of the muscles that perform the motion. Correlate any muscle weakness with sensation changes and compare the pattern with known spinal root or peripheral nerve distributions.

Functional Movement

If a functional assessment seems warranted, evaluate coordination by having the patient button a button, tie a shoe, handle a knife and fork, or perform similar functional activities. Test active and resisted thumb opposition in two ways: thumb pulp to digital pulp, and thumb tip to digital tip.

Palpation

Palpate the distal radioulnar joint by spanning either side of the joint with your thumb and index finger. Synovial thickening at the wrist is most easily detected at the dorsum. With practice, each carpal may be individually palpated for position and tenderness. Hoppenfeld

(1976), as well as Kessler and Hertling (1983), include excellent descriptions of this. Once the carpals are located, the ligaments between the individual carpals on the dorsum of the hand can then be identified. The radial and ulnar collateral ligaments on either side of the wrist can also be palpated.

Palpate the first carpometacarpal joint by pushing through the thenar eminence at the base of the first metacarpal. The metacarpal shafts, phalanges, interposing joints, and collateral ligaments are easily located. Palpate these for deformity, tenderness, and any soft tissue swellings or deformities such as Heberden's nodes.

If a muscle was weak or painful on static resisted contraction, palpate it from origin to insertion for atrophy and the specific location of tenderness. For the location of specific muscles, consult an anatomy or muscle testing text. Also palpate the mobility of any thickened fascia or scar tissue.

Other Tests

Sensation testing is performed as previously described for the elbow. Compare the sensation between the tips of the fingers and their bases, and between medial and lateral sides to identify any peripheral or spinal nerve involvement. Compare any positive findings with sensory nerve and dermatome charts.

If circulation of the hand is in question, the pulses may be palpated. Find the pulse of the radial artery at the wrist lateral to the tendon of the flexor carpi ulnaris. The pulse of the ulnar artery may be found by pressing firmly proximal to the pisiform.

Special Tests

Finklestein Test

The Finkelstein test is a test for deQuervain's syndrome. The patient encloses his thumb within his fist, and ulnarly deviates the wrist. This stretches the abductor pollicis longus and the extensors pollicis, increasing pain.

Tinel Sign

To elicit the Tinel sign, tap on the flexor retinaculum. This will produce a tingling sensation in a median nerve distribution if the nerve is compressed within the carpal tunnel.

Phalen's Test

Another test for carpal tunnel syndrome is Phalen's test. Maintain the wrist in hyperflexion for one minute. The test is positive if any sensation changes are felt in a median nerve distribution.

Nerve Conduction Velocity

Slowed motor and sensory nerve conduction velocities will verify if a peripheral nerve is compressed. Consult Goodgold and Eberstein (1972) for a description of nerve conduction measurements.

Thumb Abduction Stress Test

Thumb abduction is a test for the integrity of the ulnar collateral ligament of the MP joint of the thumb. With the MP joint flexed, apply valgus stress (abduction motion) to the proximal phalanx of the thumb, trying to radially deviate the thumb at the MP joint. The test is positive if it is found to be hypermobile (gamekeeper's thumb) (Green and Rowland, 1984).

INTERPRETATION OF FINDINGS

The following are significant clinical findings for some common pathologic conditions at the wrist and hand, as described by Cyriax (1975; 1983) unless otherwise noted.

Noncontractile Lesions

Osteoarthritis

Subjective Findings. Osteoarthritis is indicated by slow development of stiffness with little associated pain in a middle-aged to elderly person. Alternatively, there may be trauma to the wrist or fingers, with painful stiffness.

Objective Findings. Objective findings include capsular patterns in affected joints. Hands are affected symmetrically with age. The DIP joints are usually involved first, then the PIP joints. Passive thumb hyperextension/abduction will be painful if the first carpometacarpal joint is affected. Fingers may develop a varus deformity, especially at the DIP joints. Heberden's nodes and crepitus may be present.

Rheumatoid Arthritis

Subjective Findings. The patient with rheumatoid arthritis will have painful decreased ROM without history of trauma. Other joints in the body may also be affected. Rheumatoid arthritis may "flare" with increased pain, and then go into painless (but stiff) remission.

Objective Findings. The patient will have a capsular pattern in affected joints. Progression is usually from MP joints, to PIP joints, to wrists. An active case has signs of inflammation. There may be deformity and eventual ankylosis in wrist flexion with palmar subluxation of carpals, and fingers in ulnar deviation. Coarse crepitus is present in motion, with a hard, spasm end-feel.

Fractured Carpal (Usually Scaphoid)

Subjective Findings. Trauma to the wrist, usually a fall, is the typical subjective finding for a fractured carpal.

Objective Findings. The patient will have a capsular pattern at the wrist, pain on passive radial deviation, and a spasm end-feel. The affected carpal is very painful to palpation. The x-ray film may not show the fracture for up to two weeks.

Subluxed Capitate

Subjective Findings. The patient with a subluxed capitate will have a history of trauma or prolonged repetitive wrist flexion.

Objective Findings. The patient will have a noncapsular pattern at the wrist, with limited extension and a hard, spasm end-feel. Other motions may be painful, but not limited. When the wrist is hyperflexed, the capitate is prominent where there is normally a depression on dorsum of the wrist. X-ray films are inconclusive.

Ligament Sprains and Tears

Refer to Kessler and Hertling (1983) and Green and Rowland (1984) for detailed discussions of ligament injuries.

Subjective Findings. A history of trauma to the appropriate ligament will be noted in the patient with a sprain or tear.

Objective Findings. The patient will exhibit a noncapsular pattern. The affected ligament is painful when stretched. Ligaments that may be affected are the radial and ulnar collateral ligaments at the wrist, the palmar radiocarpal ligament, the capitate third metacarpal and capitate lunate ligaments on the dorsum of the hand, and the ulnar collateral ligament at the MP of the thumb (gamekeeper's thumb). Any hypermobility on stretch indicates a ligamentous tear.

Dupuytren's Contracture

Subjective Findings. Dupuytren's contracture exhibits gradual development of painless nodular thickening and contracture of the palmar fascia of the hand. This may occur bilaterally. The typical patient is a 40- to 50-year-old male.

Objective Findings. Palmar aponeurosis is thick and contracted, pulling the affected MP and IP joints into a flexion deformity.

Median Nerve Compression: Carpal Tunnel Syndrome

Refer to Smorto and Basmajian (1972) for an explanation of median nerve compression.

Subjective Findings. The patient with carpal tunnel syndrome reports a history of manual work with the hands, such as prolonged grasping (which puts pressure on the flexor retinaculum). Alternatively, the patient may do prolonged detailed work in wrist flexion. Carpal tunnel syndrome also happens in pregnancy, rheumatoid arthritis, and other collagen diseases.

Objective Findings. Paresthesia or burning in a median distribution in the hand will be noted. In a severe case, there will be atrophy and weakness in thenar muscles innervated by the median nerve distal to the flexor retinaculum. Tinel's and Phalen's tests will be positive. Sensory and motor nerve conduction velocities will be decreased when performed across the carpal tunnel.

Contractile Lesions

Mallet Finger

Mallet finger results from a ruptured extensor insertion at the DIP joint.

Subjective Findings. The patient will have a history of trauma: forced flexion at a DIP joint actively held in extension.

Objective Findings. The patient will be unable to actively extend the DIP joint, with the tip of the finger dropping into flexion in the actively extended finger. Dorsal base of the distal phalanx may be tender and swollen.

Trigger Finger/Thumb

Trigger finger occurs when a thickening on a flexor tendon becomes entrapped within the fibrous flexor sheath at the level of the MP joint in full flexion.

Subjective Findings. Subjective findings may include a history of repetitive trauma to the palm of the hand, or insidious development with no identifiable cause.

Objective Findings. Objective findings may include snapping of a finger as it extends or flexes, or inability of the finger to actively extend after flexion, with a snapping as it is passively extended.

Tenosynovitis

Tenosynovitis is a tendinous irritation within the synovial sheath.

Subjective Findings. The patient will report a history of repetitive use or trauma to the involved tendon.

Objective Findings. See Table 21-2 for specific muscles involved. Resisted motion is strong and painful. Passive stretch in the opposite direction, and movements sliding the tendon back and forth in its sheath also hurt. Fine crepitus may also be present.

Tendinitis and Muscle Strain

Subjective Findings. The patient will report a history of repetitive use or trauma to the involved structure.

Objective Findings. Resisted motion is strong and painful, and the opposite passive motion may also hurt. See Table 21-2 for specific muscles involved.

Table 21-2. Contractile Lesions at the Wrist and Hand Indicated by Strong, Painful Resisted Motion

JOINT	MOTION	MUSCLE AFFECTED	OTHER OBJECTIVE FINDINGS	OTHER COMMENTS
Wrist	Flexion	Flexor carpi radialis: whole tendon	Painful resisted RD	Rule out finger flexors by testing wrist flexion with fingers extended
		Flexor carpi ulnaris: proximal and distal to pisiform	Painful resisted UD	
	Extension	Extensor carpi radialis longus, brevis: TP junctions at metacarpals, distal half of tendons	Painful resisted RD	Rule out finger extensors by testing wrist extension with fingers flexed
		Extensor carpi ulnaris: TP junction, tendon between ulna and triquetrum, tendon in ulnar groove	Painful resisted UD If in ulnar groove, painful passive supination	
Thumb	Flexion	Flexor pollicis longus: whole tendon, insertion into metacarpal	Painful passive extension at end range Possible crepitus	
	Extension/abduction	Extensor pollicis brevis, abductor pollicis longus: metacarpal insertion, level of carpus, radial groove	Possible crepitus Positive Finklestein test	deQuervain's syndrome Radial styloid may be tender
Fingers	Flexion	Flexor digitorum superficialis: tendons in palm, and proximal to wrist	Painful passive finger extension	
	Extension	Extensor indicis: carpal extent	Possible crepitus	Occurrence is rare
		Extensor digitorum	Painful passive finger flexion	
		Extensor digiti minimi		
	Abduction	Abductor digiti minimi: at pisohamate and piso 5th metacarpal ligaments	Painful resisted ulnar flexion (flexor carpi ulnaris lies in series with abductor digiti minimi)	Palpate deeply around pisiform for tender spot
		Dorsal interosseus: insertion at MP joint, distal muscle belly		History of repeated, fine finger movements, such as in a musician
	Adduction	Palmar interosseus		Palpate between metacarpals

CONCLUSION

This chapter has presented an overview of the anatomy, subjective and objective evaluation, and interpretation of findings of the elbow, wrist, and hand. Using a consistent scheme of evaluation combined with knowledge of anatomy and an understanding of the physical presentation of elbow, wrist, and hand lesions will provide a firm basis for treatment planning.

ANNOTATED BIBLIOGRAPHY

Cyriax J: Textbook of Orthopaedic Medicine: Diagnosis of Soft Tissue Lesions, Vol 1, 6th ed. Baltimore, Williams & Wilkins, 1975 (A classic work on evaluation of the musculoskeletal system by selective tension. Chapter 12 on the elbow and Chapter 13 on the wrist and hand provide extensive information on evaluation and treatment of lesions in these regions.)

Cyriax J, Cyriax P: Illustrated Manual of Orthopaedic Medicine. Boston, Butterworths, 1983 (Illustrated with color photographs and drawings, this introductory textbook is a condensation of Cyriax's larger *Textbook of Orthopaedic Medicine,* Volumes I and II. Chapters 4 and 5 cover the elbow, wrist, and hand.)

Goodgold J, Eberstein A: Electrodiagnosis of Neuromuscular Diseases. Baltimore, Williams & Wilkins, 1972 (A clear text on electrodiagnosis. Chapter 7 describes motor and sensory nerve conduction measurements.)

Green DP, Rowland SA: Fractures and dislocations in the hand. In Rockwood CA, Green DP (eds): Fractures in Adults, 2nd ed, pp 388–390. Philadelphia, JB Lippincott, 1984 (In Rockwood and Green's classic work on fractures, these pages describe the anatomy, mechanism of injury, and diagnosis of gamekeeper's thumb.)

Hollinshead HW: Anatomy for Surgeons: Vol 3, The Back and Limbs, 3rd ed. Philadelphia, Harper & Row, 1982 (Chapter 6 presents a detailed account of the anatomy of the wrist and hand.)

Hoppenfeld S: Physical Examination of the Spine and Extremities. New York, Appleton-Century-Crofts, 1976 (Well illustrated with line drawings and succinctly written, Hoppenfeld describes the evaluation of the musculoskeletal system for beginning health practitioners. Chapter 2 covers the physical examination of the elbow, and Chapter 3 that of the wrist and hand.)

Kaltenborn FM: Manual Therapy for the Extremity Joints, 2nd ed. Oslo, Olaf Norlis Bokhandel, 1976 (Covers the arthrokinematic rationale of joint evaluation, the general scheme of joint evaluation, and specific passive accessory movements for each peripheral joint.)

Kessler RH, Hertling D: Management of Common Musculoskeletal Disorders: Physical Therapy Principles and Methods. Philadelphia, JB Lippincott, 1983 (A text covering basic concepts in evaluation, selected treatment techniques, and clinical applications for most peripheral joints. Chapter 13 on the elbow and Chapter 14 on the wrist review relevant anatomy and describe common lesions and their findings on evaluation.)

Lampe EW: Surgical anatomy of the hand. Clin Symp 9:66, 1957 (Anatomy of the hand is described by Lampe and beautifully illustrated by Frank Netter.)

MacConaill MA, Basmajian JV: Muscles and Movements: A Basis for Human Kinesiology, 2nd ed. Huntington, NY, RE Krieger, 1977 (Interspersed throughout technical chapters on the theories of arthrokinematics are examples using the joints of the wrist and fingers. Chapter 12 discusses aspects of kinesiology of the wrist and hand.)

Maitland GD: Peripheral Manipulation. London, Butterworths, 1970 (Illustrated with line drawings, Maitland describes evaluation and treatment procedures for peripheral joints, including how to perform numerous passive physiological and accessory joint movements.)

Maitland GD: The Peripheral Joints: Examination and Recording Guide, 4th ed. Adelaide, Australia, Virgo Press, 1977 (A small and easy-to-use guide outlining the steps necessary to perform a subjective and objective evaluation of each peripheral joint, including many of the component joints of the elbow, wrist, and hand.)

Smorto MP, Basmajian JV: Clinical Electroneurography. Baltimore, Williams & Wilkins, 1972 (Chapters 6 and 7 discuss the anatomy, lesions, and electrodiagnostic measurement techniques of the ulnar and median nerves.)

Tullos HS et al: Factors influencing elbow stability. In Murray DG (ed): Instructional Course Lectures, Vol XXX, pp 185–199. St Louis, CV Mosby, 1981 (Includes a clear anatomical description of the ligaments at the elbow.)

22 Musculoskeletal Analysis: The Hip

THOMAS MOHR

JOINT CAPSULE

The hip joint is a multiaxial ball and socket type of joint with three degrees of freedom. Even though the hip joint allows a great deal of mobility it is a very stable joint. The acetabulum is hemispherical in shape and is surrounded by a labrum, which serves both to deepen the acetabular fossa and provide added stability to the joint. The femoral head is round and forms about two thirds of a sphere. The femoral neck forms an angle of inclination with the shaft of the femur of approximately 125 degrees, and an angle of antetorsion of approximately 15 degrees. The hip joint is a synovial joint with a joint capsule that attaches to the innominate bone medially, and to the base of the femoral neck laterally. The joint capsule is strengthened anteriorly by the *iliofemoral* and *pubofemoral* ligaments, and posteriorly by the *ischiofemoral* ligament. All three of the ligaments become taut in hip extension and relaxed in flexion (Kapandji, 1976). The iliofemoral and pubofemoral ligaments become taut in external rotation, and the ischiofemoral ligament is taut in internal rotation. Hip adduction tightens the iliofemoral ligament, whereas hip abduction tightens the pubofemoral and ischiofemoral ligaments.

During hip extension, the capsular ligaments tighten or "wind up." This "winding" action tends to approximate the femoral head into the acetabulum to stabilize the joint. During relaxed standing, the center of gravity of the head, arms, and trunk falls slightly posterior to the hip joint, "locking" the hip joint in

extension. In patients with hip flexor contractures, the center of gravity falls anterior to the hip joint and acts to "unlock" the joint. When this occurs, both muscle activity around the hip and energy expenditure increase, making standing much more difficult for the patient.

Tension on the hip joint capsule can be altered by changes in position. The position in which the capsule is maximally tensed is called the *close-packed position,* and the position in which the capsule is most relaxed is termed the *loose-packed* or *resting position.* The close-packed position for the hip is with the hip maximally extended, internally rotated, and abducted. The resting position is with the hip in approximately 30 degrees of flexion and abduction, and 20 degrees of external rotation.

The prevalence of degenerative joint disease may, in part, be due to the large compressive forces generated across the femoral head during functional activities. Compressive forces at the hip are about one third of the body weight during two-legged standing, and 2.5 times the body weight during one-legged standing. Forces of 1.3 to 5.8 times body weight have been recorded during walking and running (Singleton, 1975). These large forces are the combined result of body weight, abductor muscle force, and ground reaction forces during gait.

BURSA

The hip joint has three clinically important bursa. The *trochanteric bursa* is located between the tendon of the gluteus maximus and the posterolateral aspect of the greater trochanter. The *iliopectineal* bursa lies between the iliopsoas muscle and the iliopectineal eminence overlying the hip joint capsule. The *ischiogluteal* bursa is located over the ischial tuberosity.

SUBJECTIVE EXAMINATION

Taking a patient's history is a very important aspect of any evaluation process. Although there are many different questions one may ask to gather the history information, the following are examples of some applicable questions regarding evaluation of the hip joint:

1. Ask the patient what the chief complaint or symptom is, and how long the problem has existed. Some conditions such as osteoarthritis can have a long, episodic onset, whereas muscle strains or bursitis may have a relatively sudden onset.
2. If the major complaint is pain, then inquire as to the exact location of the pain and ask for a description of the pain. For instance, it may be described as a pins and needles sensation, or perhaps a dull ache. The patient may be experiencing hypoaesthesia over some area surrounding the hip joint, which might indicate a nerve lesion.
3. With hip problems, the age of the patient is very important. Congenital defects are a common cause of hip dysfunction in infants. Coxa plana (Legg-Calvé-Perthes disease) most commonly occurs in children from 3 to 12 years of age, and slipped femoral capital epiphysis is more common among children 10 to 15 years old (Turek, 1984). Some problems such as trauma, rheumatoid arthritis, and malignancy can occur within any age group, whereas osteoarthritis is more common after 40 years of age.
4. You should inquire about any congential defects or a family history of similar problems.
5. The patient should be asked if he recalls any trauma that may have brought on the problem.
6. The timing of the problem or pain is important. For example, is the pain constant or intermittent? Is there any particular time of day when the problem is better or worse? What types of activity or maneuvers, if any, accentuate the symptoms? What, if anything, relieves the symptoms?
7. If the problem is recurring, you should inquire about any previous treatment and its effectiveness.
8. Find out if the patient is currently receiving any form of treatment. If so, is the treatment effective? For example, the patient may be using heat or ice at home or taking prescribed medication for the problem. The patient also may be taking analgesics, which can obliterate pain and can subsequently alter the patient's response to your objective evaluation.
9. Because surgical procedures to the hip are common, inquire about any past surgeries the patient may have had, either related or unrelated to the present problem. For example, an elderly patient may have had a prior surgical procedure earlier in life, which subsequently caused structural changes in the femur. These changes may have led to secondary problems, such as leg length discrepancies or limitations in range of motion, which would show up in the objective evaluation.

Remember that the purpose of the subjective evaluation is to gain information about the problem from the patient's perspective. Often, by taking a good history, you can save yourself a lot of time with the objective portion of the evaluation. Do not underestimate the importance of a good history, because the patient can often relate to you in minutes what might take you hours to discover or confirm on your own.

OBJECTIVE EXAMINATION

The subjective evaluation generally deals with the symptoms, such as pain, that the patient is experiencing. However, the objective evaluation relates to the definite signs the patient exhibits, such as a leg length discrepancy. In order to minimize pain or discomfort on the patient's part, you should try to minimize positional changes for the patient. However, for ease of discussion the objective tests will be discussed together by topic.

OBSERVATION

Because the hip is a weight-bearing joint, it is important to observe the patient's standing posture and gait pattern. When doing these observations, you should observe the patient from anterior, posterior, and lateral views. When assessing standing posture from an anterior or posterior view, you should note any pelvic obliquity in the frontal plane or any lateral shift in the vertebral column. Changes of this nature could suggest a leg length discrepancy. Note the position in which the patient holds the lower extremity, observing if there is a tendency to rotate the limb internally or externally. This posture might indicate a contracture around the hip joint, or if the hip joint is painful, the patient may tend to hold the hip in the resting position (ie, flexion, abduction, and external rotation).

From the lateral view, changes should be noted in anterior or posterior pelvic tilt along with subsequent changes in the normal lumbar lordotic curve. A flexion contracture at the hip will often cause an increased anterior pelvic tilt with a subsequent increased lumbar lordosis.

A number of hip joint problems are reflected in the patient's gait pattern. Therefore, careful examination of the patient during ambulation is crucial with hip joint problems. If the patient has a shortened leg on one side, the pelvis may drop excessively on the involved side during swing phase in an attempt to "lengthen" the extremity (Tepperman, 1981). In addition, there may be increased flexion of the contralateral lower extremity during its swing phase to clear the floor while moving past the short leg. A contracture, or spasticity, of the hip adductors may cause a "scissoring" of the involved lower extremity during swing phase. A patient with a painful hip joint may exhibit an antalgic gait pattern. With this gait pattern, the patient shortens the time spent in

the stance phase of the involved limb to minimize joint pressure and therefore decrease pain in the hip.

Muscle weakness at the hip may show up in a variety of ways. Uncompensated weakness of the hip extensors would cause a forward bending movement to occur shortly after heel strike on the affected side. To compensate for this, the patient will often "throw" the trunk posteriorly shortly after heel strike to counteract the tendency towards hip flexion. Hip flexor weakness would present itself at the initiation of the swing phase. In an effort to compensate for weak hip flexors, the patient will often "throw" the trunk posteriorly to help move the affected limb through the swing phase of gait. In addition, there may be excessive knee flexion and ankle dorsiflexion to help the affected limb clear the floor during the swing phase.

Hip abductor weakness is quite common and is often seen following hip surgery. With uncompensated hip abductor weakness, the pelvis drops on the contralateral side during stance on the affected limb. This excess pelvic drop in the frontal plane is also referred to as a Trendelenburg gait or a gluteus medius gait pattern. Along with the pelvic drop, the patient will often laterally protrude the pelvis towards the affected side during stance phase of the involved extremity. To compensate for hip abductor weakness, the patient may "throw" the trunk laterally towards the affected hip during stance phase of that hip. If a patient exhibits either a painful hip or abductor weakness, it may be useful to have that patient try ambulating with a cane held in the contralateral hand to see if it reduces the hip pain or alters the gait pattern. Compressive forces at the hip may be reduced by as much as 25% to 30% with the proper use of a cane (Tepperman, 1981). The use of a cane can therefore reduce the patient's pain or aid the weak abductor muscles.

The patient should be checked for any scars that would indicate a history of past trauma or surgery. Look for any obvious deformities or contractures or for areas of skin redness that might indicate an area of inflammation. Also check for the presence of any swelling or edema, although this is not as easily detected at the hip as it is in other joints.

ASSESSMENT OF JOINT MOVEMENT

As with all joint evaluations, you should measure and record the available joint movement. Specific techniques for measuring hip joint movement can be found in standard texts (Daniels, 1986). Normal ranges of motion at the hip are as follows:

- hip flexion—0 to 120 degrees
- hip extension—0 to 30 degrees
- hip abduction—0 to 45 degrees
- hip adduction—0 to 30 degrees
- hip external rotation—0 to 45 degrees
- hip internal rotation—0 to 45 degrees

Accessory motion or "joint play" can also be assessed at the hip. The patient is positioned supine with the involved extremity flexed at both the hip and knee. The patient's knee is positioned over the shoulder of the examiner and the examiner's hands are placed around the proximal thigh (Fig. 22-1). Joint play can be evaluated by applying traction in both distal and lateral directions.

SOFT TISSUE ASSESSMENT

Contractile Tissue

Muscles, tendons, and their points of attachment to bones are considered as contractile tissue (Cyriax, 1983). Contractile tissue is evaluated by resistive movements. If a resisted movement brings on or accentuates the pain the patient is experiencing, then the examiner should suspect the muscle or muscles that accomplish that particular motion. To test the resisted movements, the joint is usually held in mid-range while the patient performs an isometric contraction of the muscle or muscle groups. During the resisted movements, the examiner should be assessing both strength of the muscles and whether or not there is associated pain.

Selected Resisted Movements

Traditional manual muscle testing procedures can be found in standard texts on the subject

(Daniels, 1986). However, a modified approach such as that described here is often more efficient for evaluating hip joint musculature (Cyriax, 1983). Table 22-1 lists the muscles that perform the various hip joint actions.

Although hip muscle strength can be tested in a variety of positions, the most efficient way is with the patient in the supine position. Testing all the muscles in the supine position eliminates repositioning of the patient for each muscle test. To test resisted hip flexion, both the hip and knee are flexed to 90 degrees, the pelvis is stabilized, and resistance is applied to the anterior thigh. For hip extension, the hip is flexed to about 45 degrees and the knee is extended; resistance is then applied to the posterior thigh.

To test knee extension the hip is slightly flexed and the knee is flexed to approximately 45 degrees, the thigh is stabilized, and resistance is applied to the anterior ankle. Knee flexion is tested with the hip slightly flexed and the knee flexed to 90 degrees; the thigh is stabilized and resistance is applied to the posterior ankle.

Resisted hip rotations are done with both the hip and knee flexed to 90 degrees and placed in midposition for internal and external rotation. Resistance is applied to the lower leg with one hand while stabilizing the thigh with your other hand. Resisted abduction and adduction are performed with the lower extremities in midposition for abduction and adduction. For adduction, resistance is applied to the medial thigh; and for abduction resistance is applied to the lateral thigh.

Although resisted motions are usually indicative of a problem in the muscle or muscles performing the action, pain during certain resisted movements may be indicative of bursitis at the hip joint (Cyriax, 1983). Pain during internal and external rotations as well as hip abduction and extension is considered to be an accessory sign in bursitis. With trochanteric bursitis, resisted abduction may be painful; in iliopectineal bursitis, resisted hip flexion may be painful; and in ischiogluteal bursitis, resisted hip extension may be painful (Turek, 1984).

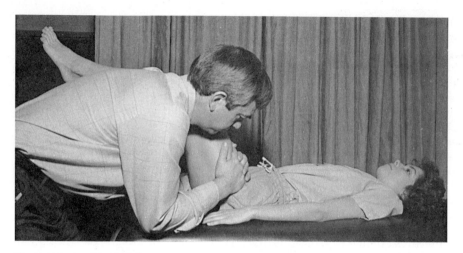

Figure 22-1. Distal glide.

Table 22-1. Prime Mover Muscles Acting on the Hip Joint

HIP MOTION	MUSCLES	INNERVATION	NERVE ROOTS
Flexion	Psoas major	Femoral	L2, L3
	Iliacus	Femoral	L2, L3
	Sartorius	Femoral	L2, L3
	Rectus femoris	Femoral	L2, L3, L4
Extension	Gluteus maximus	Inferior gluteal	L5; S1, S2
	Semitendinosus	Tibial portion sciatic	L5; S1, S2
	Semimembranosus	Tibial portion sciatic	L5; S1, S2
	Biceps femoris (long head)	Tibial portion sciatic	L5; S1, S2
Abduction	Gluteus medius	Superior gluteal	L4, L5; S1
	Gluteus minimus	Superior gluteal	L4, L5; S1
	Tensor fascia latae	Superior gluteal	L4, L5; S1
Adduction	Pectineus	Femoral	L2, L3, L4
	Gracilis	Obturator	L2, L3, L4
	Adductor longus	Obturator	L2, L3, L4
	Adductor brevis	Obturator	L2, L3, L4
	Adductor magnus (anterior portion)	Obturator	L2, L3, L4
	Adductor magnus (posterior portion)	Tibial	L4, L5
Internal rotation	Gluteus minimus	Superior gluteal	L4, L5; S1
	Gluteus medius	Superior gluteal	L4, L5; S1
	Tensor fascia latae	Superior gluteal	L4, L5; S1
External rotation	Obturator externus	Obturator	L2, L3, L4
	Obturator internus	Nerve to obturator internus and superior gemellus	L5; S1, S2
	Superior gemellus		L5; S1, S2
	Quadratus femoris	Nerve to quadratus femoris and inferior gemellus	L4, L5; S1
	Inferior gemellus		L4, L5; S1
	Piriformis	Nerve to piriformis	L5; S1, S2

Noncontractile Tissue

Noncontractile (inert) tissue is not capable of contraction. Examples of noncontractile tissue around the hip are the ligaments, fascia, and bursa. Noncontractile tissue is tested by passive movements that stretch the inert tissues. If a passive movement causes pain, then the examiner should suspect noncontractile tissue involvement. When carrying out the passive movements you are looking for (1) limitation of motion, (2) pain, and (3) end-feel (Cyriax, 1983).

As you carry the extremity through the passive movement, you should also look for a limitation of motion pattern that might be indicative of a capsular pattern. A *capsular pattern* at the hip would present itself by marked limitation of internal rotation followed by some limitation of flexion and abduction. This capsular pattern would indicate a hip joint problem such as one might see with osteoarthritis or rheumatoid arthritis. The normal end-feel at the hip is a capsular or elastic end-feel, although hip flexion and adduction are usually limited by tissue approximation.

Neurological Examination

Because the hip joint is innervated by branches of the femoral, sciatic, and obturator nerves, hip pain may be referred medially, laterally, anteriorly, or posteriorly. Because hip pain can also be referred from the spine, the spine and sacroiliac joints must be "cleared" to rule them out as possible causes of the hip pain. Both the hip and knee joints are innervated by L3. Therefore, hip pain can often be referred to the anterior, medial knee area. If a patient is experiencing knee pain and the knee has been "cleared" as the cause of the pain, the hip joint should be examined to determine if the pain is being referred from the hip to the knee.

If the patient is having pain, you should note the type of pain and the area or dermatome involved. If the patient is experiencing painless weakness in any of the resisted motions, this might be an indication of a nerve lesion and should be noted. Although nerve root impingement problems are common in the lumbar spine, thus referring pain into the hip area, nerve entrapments around the hip joint itself are not very common. Peripheral nerves around the hip are occasionally injured by trauma, hip surgery, and tumors, and in women during pregnancy or childbirth.

Special Tests

Thomas Test

The Thomas test is used to test for hip flexor tightness or contracture. The patient is placed supine with the hips extended. If a hip flexion contracture is present, there may be an accentuated lumbar lordosis when the patient's thighs are resting on the table. To do the test, the extremity contralateral to the affected side is maximally flexed towards the patient's abdomen. The lower extremity is held in this position to posteriorly tilt and stabilize the pelvis, thus flattening the lumbar spine against the table. In a normal individual, the ipsilateral thigh will remain on the table. If a hip flexion contracture is present, the involved thigh will lift up off the table as the pelvis is posteriorly tilted (Fig. 22-2). The angle of hip flexion on the affected side can be measured to determine the amount of contracture present. Because hip flexion contractures are so common, this test should be done routinely in a hip evaluation.

Ober Test

The Ober test is used to test for a contracture of the iliotibial band. The patient is tested sidelying with the involved side up. The examiner flexes the knee to 90 degrees, and then passively abducts and hyperextends the involved hip. The limb is then released and allowed to passively adduct. If normal range of motion is present in the iliotibial band, the limb should adduct and approximate the uninvolved extremity. If an iliotibial band contracture is present, the involved limb will not adduct; instead, it will remain abducted, indicating a positive Ober test (Fig. 22-3). This test can also be performed with the knee extended, which puts the iliotibial band on further stretch.

Rectus Femoris Test

The patient is positioned supine with both knees flexed to 90 degrees and bent over the end of a table. The contralateral hip and knee

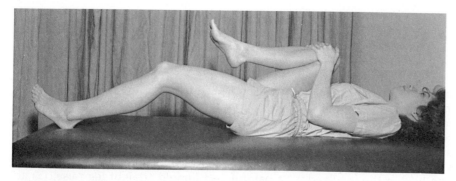

Figure 22-2. Thomas test.

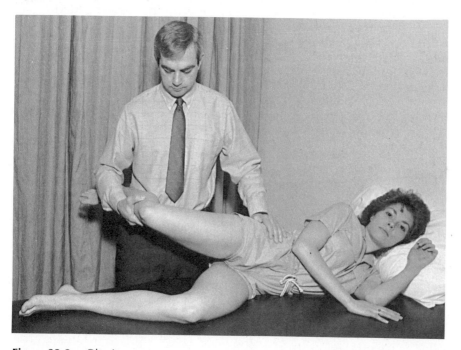

Figure 22-3. Ober's test.

are flexed towards the abdomen as in the Thomas test. If tightness is present in the rectus femoris, the affected knee will extend as the contralateral limb is flexed. If the rectus femoris is normal, the knee will remain in 90 degrees of flexion (Magee, 1987).

Hamstring Test

The patient sits on a table in the long sitting position. Normally, a patient should be able to reach forward and touch his toe with an outstretched arm. An alternate method is to have the patient lying supine with the involved hip and knee flexed to 90 degrees. The thigh is stabilized and the patient is asked to extend his knee through the available range of motion. An angle of 20 degrees from full extension is within normal limits, but a larger angle is considered indicative of hamstring tightness (Saudek, 1985).

Patrick's Test

Patrick's (Faber) test is used to detect an inflammatory disease of the hip joint (Turek, 1984), although the test can also be positive in some sacroiliac joint problems (Magee, 1987). The Faber test is an acronym for the hip movements performed by the examiner during the test: *f,* flexion; *ab,* abduction; and *er,* external rotation. This manuever stretches the anterior hip joint capsule. The patient is positioned supine with the lower extremity on the involved side flexed at the hip and knee. The heel of the involved extremity is placed on top of the contralateral knee. One of the examiner's hands is placed on the contralateral anterior superior iliac spine and the other is placed on the medial side of the knee on the involved side. The examiner then slowly pushes downward on the involved side while gently forcing the hip into maximal abduction and external rotation (Fig. 22-4). A positive test would be indicated by a painful response or a restriction in the range of motion.

Sign of the Buttock

The presence of the sign of the buttock indicates a major lesion. The lesion does not involve the hip joint itself, but instead may indicate a serious condition such as osteomyelitis, septic arthritis, or a neoplasm (Cyriax, 1983). The patient is tested supine. The examiner first does a passive straight leg raise with the patient. Then the examiner passively flexes the hip with the knee flexed. The sign of the buttock is indicated by (1) the presence of both a painful and limited straight leg raise, (2) an even more painful and limited hip flexion, and (3) the absence of a hip capsular pattern.

Leg Length Measurement

There are several methods of measuring leg length using both indirect and direct methods. The most accurate and precise method of determining a leg length discrepancy is the indirect method performed with the patient standing (Woerman, 1984). The examiner palpates the iliac crests to determine if they are level with

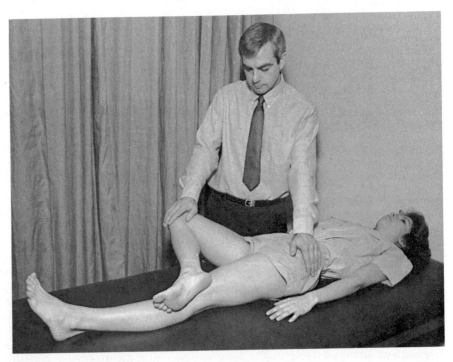

Figure 22-4. Patrick's test.

each other. If the iliac crests are not level, small lift blocks of different thicknesses are placed under the shorter limb until the iliac crests are level. The amount of leg length discrepancy is indicated by the total thickness of the lift blocks used.

To perform the direct leg length measurements, the patient should be supine with the anterior superior iliac spines (ASIS) level with each other. The lower extremities should be positioned perpendicular to an imaginary line drawn between the ASIS, and placed in a neutral position between abduction and adduction. The examiner should first measure real leg length and then apparent leg length, comparing the measurements between the two lower extremities.

Determining real leg length involves a measurement from one of the ASIS to either the lateral or medial malleolus of the same side. The most accurate method of real leg length measurement is to use a tape measure to measure the distance from the ASIS to the lateral malleolus. This method was shown to be more accurate than a measurement to the medial malleolus because differences in thigh girth do not affect this method of measurement as much (Woerman, 1984). Although apparently not as accurate as the previous methods, probably the most common method of measuring real leg length is to perform a measurement from the ASIS to the medial malleolus of the same side.

Common causes for discrepancies in real leg lengths are (1) an abnormal angle of inclination of the femoral neck such as one might see in coxa vara or coxa valgus, (2) differences in the length of the femurs, or (3) differences in the length of the tibias.

After you measure real leg length, you should then measure apparent leg length. Apparent leg length is the measured distance from the umbilicus to the medial malleolus. If the real leg lengths were equal, then a difference in apparent leg lengths would indicate a pelvic obliquity as might be seen with scoliosis. Although it is controversial, leg length discrepancies of as little as 5 mm have been suggested to cause mechanically related dysfunctions

around the pelvis, spine, and hips (Woerman, 1984).

Ortolani Test

The Ortolani "click" sign is a test for a dislocated hip in an infant. The infant is positioned supine with the hips adducted and the hips and knees flexed to 90 degrees (Fig. 22-5A). The examiner's hands are placed around the femoral condyles so that the thumb is on the medial side of the thigh and the index and middle fingers are on the lateral side extending to the level of the greater trochanter. The two hips are then gently abducted and externally rotated towards the table (Fig. 22-5B). A normal hip can be abducted and externally rotated to about 90 degrees, but a dislocated hip has a block to the motion at about 30 to 40 degrees (Gruebel Lee, 1983). If continued pressure is applied to the dislocated hip, a "click" (ie, "click of entrance") will be palpable to the examiner's fingers over the greater trochanter as the femoral head is reduced into the acetabulum. The "click" is thought to be due to the femoral head sliding ("clicking") across the defective posterosuperior acetabular labrum as it is reduced by the maneuver.

Barlow's Test

Whereas Ortolani's sign is performed to test for a dislocated hip, Barlow's sign is used to test for a *dislocatable* hip. The child is positioned in the same manner as in the Ortolani test, and each hip is individually tested. One of the examiner's hands stabilizes the contralateral thigh and pelvis while the other hand grasps the hip to be tested between the thumb and the middle finger. The middle finger is placed laterally over the greater trochanter, and the thumb is placed medially on the inner aspect of the thigh pressing on the femoral head. The hip is abducted as in the Ortolani test and the examiner palpates for a click of entrance. To do the Barlow test, the hip is then adducted somewhat (Fig. 22-6). A dislocatable hip can then be pushed out of the socket, giving a "click of exit," by lateral pressure from the thumb and reduced by medial pressure over the greater trochanter by the middle finger (Gruebel Lee, 1983). This procedure should not be repeated

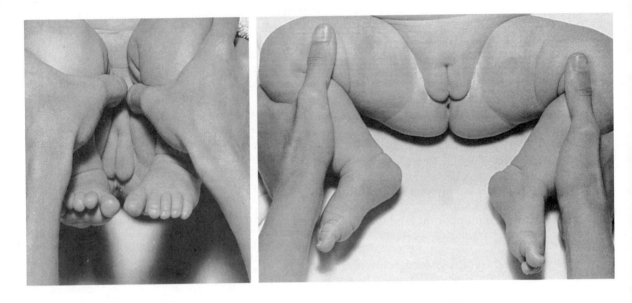

Figure 22-5. *(A)* Starting position for Ortolani's test. *(B)* A normal hip can be abducted to approximately 90 degrees (as shown here), but a dislocated hip will give a "click of entrance" at about 40 degrees of abduction.

Figure 22-6. Barlow's test. A continuation of Ortolani's test, the hip is in about 10 to 15 degrees of abduction. Lateral pressure by the thumb can dislocate the hip, giving a "click of exit."

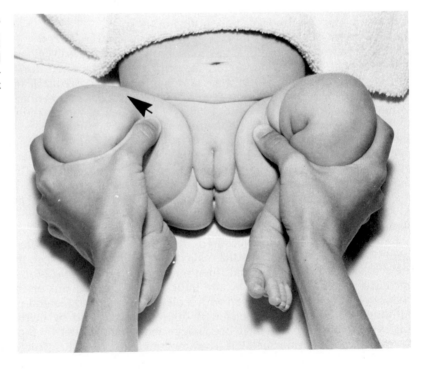

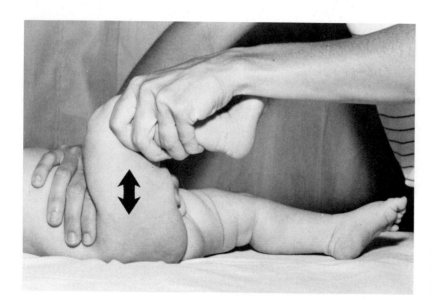

Figure 22-7. Piston test. With a dislocated hip, the thigh will show a "pistoning" effect upon compression and distraction of the joint.

more than twice because it can cause damage to the hip joint structures of the infant.

Piston Test

A pistoning or telescoping movement can be obtained in a child with a dislocated hip. The child lies supine with the hip and knee flexed to 90 degrees. The examiner grasps the knee and thigh of the child with one hand and stabilizes the child's pelvis with the other hand (Fig. 22-7). The thigh is alternately pushed downward toward the table and pulled upward away from the table. A normal hip will show relatively little motion during this test, but a dislocated hip will demonstrate a "pistoning" effect because the femur moves excessively during compression and distraction of the hip joint (Gruebel Lee, 1983).

CONCLUSION

Evaluation of most hip joint problems would not be complete without a careful roentgenographic examination. Certainly, many hip joint problems could not be properly diagnosed without this part of the evaluation. Other tests that the physical therapist may find useful are isokinetic strength testing or various functional tests. The evaluation sequence presented in this chapter, however, outlines an appropriate evaluative procedure to be followed by a physical therapist assessing hip joint dysfunction.

ANNOTATED BIBLIOGRAPHY

Cyriax J, Cyriax P: Illustrated Manual of Orthopedic Medicine, pp 73–86. Boston, Butterworths, 1983 (Provides an excellent discussion of hip joint evaluation.)

Daniels L, Worthingham C: Muscle Testing, 5th ed, pp 38–63. Philadelphia, WB Saunders, 1986 (Provides basic techniques related to manual muscle testing and goniometry.)

Gruebel Lee DM: Disorders of the Hip. Philadelphia, JB Lippincott, 1983 (Discusses evaluation and treatment of many hip joint dysfunctions, and provides an excellent discussion of congenital defects of the hip.)

Kapandji IA: The Physiology of the Joints, 2nd ed, pp 32–36: New York, Churchill Livingston, 1976 (Provides an excellent discussion of the anatomy and biomechanics of the hip joint.)

Magee DJ: Orthopedic Physical Assessment, pp 248–249. Philadelphia, WB Saunders, 1987 (Discusses many special tests related to hip joint evaluation.)

Saudek CE: The hip. In Gould JA, Davies GJ (eds): Orthopedic and Sports Physical Therapy, pp 388. St Louis, CV Mosby, 1985 (This chapter provides an excellent discussion of hip joint evaluation and treatment.)

Singleton MC, LeVeau BF: The hip joint: Structure, stability, and stress. Phys Ther 55:957, 1975 (Reviews hip joint anatomy and biomechanics.)

Tepperman PS: The Hip Joint. Toronto, H Charles Enterprises, 1981 (Provides an excellent discussion of pathological gait problems related to the hip joint.)

Turek SL: Orthopedics Principles and Their Application, 4th ed, pp 1109–1268. Philadelphia, JB Lippincott, 1984 (Discusses evaluation, pathology, and surgical treatment of hip joint problems.)

Woerman AL, Binder-Macloed SA: Leg length discrepency assessment: Accuracy and precision in five clinical methods of evaluation. J Orthop Sports Phys Ther 5:230, 1984 (This article reviews various methods of measuring leg length.)

23 Musculoskeletal Analysis: The Knee

MATTHEW C. MORRISSEY

The knee joint is the most often injured peripheral joint in the human body. Its propensity for injury is mainly due to the large forces applied to this joint in all planes of motion. These large forces result from the long bony levers, the tibia and femur, that converge to form this joint. Of the primary peripheral joints, the knee is farthest from its proximal (hip) or distal (ankle) joints. Added to this are the large forces encountered by this joint in weight bearing. In light of its injury frequency and importance in ambulation, proper care of the injured knee is critical. Proper care consists of two major components: evaluation and treatment. Proper treatment requires not only the use of a satisfactory treatment regimen but also application of the chosen therapeutic measures to the correct structure or structures of the knee. This is solely dependent on proper evaluation.

SUBJECTIVE EXAMINATION

The most effective and easily used method for evaluating the injured knee joint requires classification of the injured knee into one of the four major disabling factors for any joint: inflammation, immobility, instability, and muscle weakness. A perfunctory analysis of each of these factors is initially performed in the subjective portion of the knee examination. The subjective examination assesses the patient's perception of the presence and severity of any of the four major maladies. In addition, it offers insight into the cause of the affliction, and often the most effective method of treatment.

The subjective examination of the knee-injured patient commences with the first visit to the physical therapist and continues throughout the period of treatment. The time devoted to the subjective examination decreases from the first visit, but this portion of the examination is critical up to the last day of treatment. The specific questions related to knee problems that are necessary in the subjective examination should focus on the following factors:

1. Recreation. Investigate the recreational activities that affect the injured knee. Typically, these include walking and sports. If sports activity results in changes of knee symptoms, then specific questions should focus on the type of sport or sports; frequency, intensity, and duration of participation; and level of competition. The sports that are most injurious to the knee are basketball, football, alpine skiing, ice hockey, and volleyball. Patellofemoral pathology is common in all of these sports, especially those that require repetitive jumping. Usually, these patients have pain and weakness as the major problems. The other common injury in these sports is injury to the ligamentous structures of the knee, which results in instability. Injuries of this sort are especially prevalent in sports that require cutting motions in response to other players or objects, whose avoidance can be attained only by rapid

and forceful changes in the direction of movement.

2. Changes in knee symptoms during the day. Any prevalent patterns of knee disability changes in a typical day must be assessed. Specifically, the patient should be asked whether the knee seems better or worse during a particular part of the day: early morning, late morning, afternoon, evening, or night. An increase in symptoms in the early morning indicates that the knee is susceptible to either prolonged static positioning or is being put in irritating positions during the night. An increase in symptoms at any other time of day usually indicates that the knee is susceptible to increased activity. The knee that feels better and is less troubling in the morning indicates that it is in need of proper rest, whereas a knee that feels better late in the day indicates that proper exercise is needed.

3. Medications being taken for the knee problem. Usually these medications are either for pain relief or to decrease inflammation, though a combination of medications for both purposes is not unusual. The use of medications indicates the physician's impression of the severity of the knee problem and also may be a good indicator of the patient's pain level and tolerance.

4. Activities, knee positions, and treatment that increase or decrease the symptoms at the knee. The patient should be asked about different factors that result in heightened symptoms at the knee versus those factors that seem to make the knee feel better. Usually the symptoms that are affected by activity level are pain, swelling, and giving way of the knee. Specific attention should be paid to activities such as ascending and descending stairs, sudden change of direction in walking or from a static standing position, cutting in running, running, bicycling, jumping, and prolonged sitting and standing. Patellofemoral problems and other overuse problems at the knee are exacerbated by ascending and descending stairs, running, bicycling, jump-

ing, and prolonged sitting and standing. Ligamentous injuries usually result in problems with turning in walking and cutting and stopping in running. Meniscal pathology results in difficulty with the same problems as for ligamentous injury. In addition, there may be difficulty with jumping and prolonged standing, that is, activities that either apply large forces of short duration to the meniscal structures or those that apply smaller loads over prolonged periods.

OBJECTIVE EXAMINATION

The objective portion of the examination can be classified into four components with each portion having an evaluative purpose. These four components focus on joint inflammation, immobility, instability, and thigh musculature weakness. A fifth component of the examination may be used to assess any structural abnormalities that may predispose the joint to injury.

INFLAMMATION

Inflammation of the joint can be assessed by evaluation of joint swelling and by palpation of structures for unusual tenderness and temperature changes. To assess joint swelling, circumferential measures of both legs should be performed at the knee joint line and at a point 5 cm proximal to the joint line. These should be performed with the knee at or near full extension. Bilateral assessment allows comparisons in the circumference of the injured and uninjured knees and gives you an indirect estimate of the volume of the joint. Subsequent measurements are useful in appraising changes in the amount of swelling in the joint.

The two other components of joint inflammation that may be easily assessed in the clinic are changes in temperature or tenderness, or both, of specific joint structures. These changes can be assessed through palpation of the injured and uninjured knees. Attainment of this skill requires determination and perseverance by the novice clinician. An excellent resource is Hoppenfeld's book, *Physical Examination of the Spine and Extremities* (1976).

In palpating the many structures of the knee, note tenderness that may be present in the injured knee but absent in the uninjured knee. This tenderness is rated on a scale that ranges from no tenderness (or within normal limits) to mild, moderate, and severe tenderness. More precise and accurate analysis of the level of tenderness is usually of little value unless the assessment is being used in clinical research. Temperature differences between the two knees are measured using the same scale as for palpation, though assessment is made of more general areas (eg, medial knee).

For palpation of specific structures the surface anatomy of the knee may be divided into anterior, posterior, medial, and lateral quadrants. Palpation of the anterior knee focuses on the extensor mechanism, which includes the following structures:

1. Tibial tubercle
2. Infrapatellar tendon
3. Inferior pole of the patella
4. Prepatellar bursa
5. Superior border of the patella
6. Quadriceps tendon
7. Medial border of the patella
8. Medial retinaculum
9. Medial patellar facets
10. Lateral patellar border
11. Lateral retinaculum
12. Lateral patellar facets

A systematic method of palpating these structures includes palpating the first six structures from inferior to superior and then palpating the medial and lateral structures. This requires that palpation be initiated at the tibial tubercle and proceed in a cephalic direction by way of the infrapatellar tendon, inferior pole of the patella, prepatellar bursa (superficial surface of the patella), superior border of the patella, and quadriceps tendon. These structures should be palpated with the knee at or near full extension. To assist in palpation of the inferior pole of the patella, the knee should be placed in slight flexion and an inferiorly directed force

should be applied to the superior border of the patella. Using the fingers of the other hand, the pole may then be easily palpated. In injury of the extensor mechanism unusual tenderness may occur at one or more of the anterior structures. The most typical areas of undue tenderness occur at the tibial tubercle, infrapatellar tendon, inferior pole of the patella, and the medial patellar structures.

The most difficult structures to palpate in the anterior quadrant are the medial and lateral patellar facets. The most effective method for palpating these two areas is with the knee in an extended position. To palpate the medial patellar facet, the patella should be forced medially and the face of the patella should be rotated laterally. This may be accomplished with a manually applied force on the lateral portion of the anterior patella in a posteromedial direction. The fingers of the other hand should be used to palpate the medial facet with a posteromedial approach to the posterior surface of the patella. The direction of the force on the patella and the approach to the posterior patella is opposite to that described when palpation is focused on the lateral patellar facet (Fig. 23-1).

Another important consideration in palpation of the anterior structures is assessment of the presence of an inflamed plica. A plica is a synovial fold and is a normal variant in the knee. The three most common plicae are the suprapatellar, medial shelf, and infrapatellar plicae. The most commonly inflamed is the medial plica. To investigate this plica, one finger should be placed on the patella with a second finger placed on the medial femoral condyle. Palpation should occur between these two landmarks and any unusual inconsistency of the underlying tissue in combination with unusual tenderness is indicative of this inflamed synovial fold.

The posterior structures of the knee palpated in a typical knee examination include (1) origin of the gastrocnemius muscle, (2) popliteal fossa, and (3) popliteus muscle. Palpation of these structures is best performed with the patient in the prone position. Both heads (medial and lateral) of the gastrocnemius may be pal-

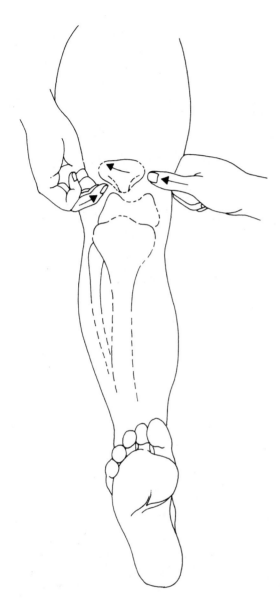

Figure 23-1. Palpation of the lateral patellar facet. (After Hoppenfeld S: Physical Examination of the Spine and Extremities, p 178. New York, Appleton-Century-Crofts, 1976)

pated by following this muscle superiorly from its muscle belly. Isometric plantarflexion and knee flexion with the knee in 90 degrees flexion may be useful in delineating these structures.

The popliteal fossa is the large area located between the tendons of the semitendinosus (medial border) and biceps femoris muscles (lateral border) superior to the gastrocnemius heads. Unusual swelling in this area may be caused by the presence of a popliteal cyst or, as it is more commonly known, Baker's cyst. This cyst usually represents a distention of the gastrocnemius-semimembranosus bursa.

A structure that is too often forgotten in palpation of the knee is the popliteus muscle. Locating the origin of this muscle is possible by first placing one finger on Gerdy's tubercle and another on the lateral epicondyle. The popliteus origin lies between these two landmarks.

The medial structures that require attention in palpation of the knee are as follows:

1. Pes anserinus insertion
2. Conjoined tendon of the pes anserinus
3. Individual tendons of the pes anserinus
4. Medial joint line
5. Medial meniscus
6. Medial femoral condyle articulating surface
7. Adductor magnus
8. Adductor tubercle (adductor magnus insertion)
9. Medial collateral ligament

The medial and anterior structures of the knee are the most commonly tender structures in knee joint pathology. Systematically, the medial structures should be palpated inferiorly to superiorly as listed above. Under this system, the pes anserinus will be palpated first. Tenderness of the pes insertion and conjoined tendon indicates overuse of this structure, which occurs because it functions both as a passive stabilizer of the medial knee and as an active stabilizer of the knee against external forces that cause tibial external rotation or anterior tibial translation, or both. Palpation of the separate tendons of the pes anserinus can be performed posterior to anterior from the semitendinosus to the gracilis and, finally, the sartorius.

The medial joint line and adjacent articulating surfaces may be palpated next. Of importance here is palpation of the medial meniscus and its attachment to the medial tibial plateau and palpation of the articulating surface of the medial femoral condyle. Palpation of these structures should be performed with the knee in different positions of flexion. The best position for palpation is in 90 degrees flexion with the patient sitting on the edge of a treatment table. With the tibia in external rotation, an inferiorly directed force offered to the medial meniscus should be applied along the anteromedial line. A superiorly directed force on the distal femur from this position is useful in palpating the articulating surface of the medial femoral condyle. These medial joint line areas are commonly involved in knee pathology. Of special note is the area of the coronary ligaments where they attach the anterodistal medial meniscus to the tibial plateau. Increased tenderness of these structures is common in anterior instability of the knee. Perhaps the excessive forward translation of the medial tibial plateau is causing the overlying femoral condyle to pull the medial meniscus posteriorly, thus resulting in stretching of the anterior attachment of the meniscus at the tibial plateau.

The adductor magnus muscle inserts on the superior surface of the medial femoral epicondyle at the adductor tubercle. This bony prominence and conjoined tendon are easily palpated.

One of the most important structures of the medial knee is the medial collateral ligament (MCL). It is a large ligament that runs from the superior to the inferior medial knee area. This ligament should be palpated from its proximal attachment at the medial epicondyle to its distal attachment at the medial tibial flare (Fig. 23-2).

Palpation of the lateral knee focuses on the following structures:

1. Fibular head
2. Biceps femoris muscle distal tendon
3. Gerdy's tubercle
4. Iliotibial band

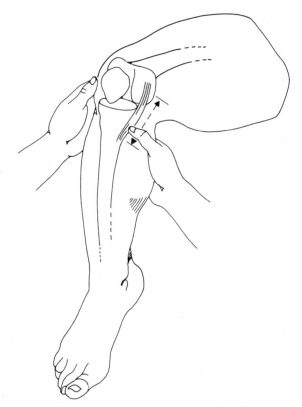

Figure 23-2. Palpation of the medial collateral ligament. (After Hoppenfeld S: Physical Examination of the Spine and Extremities, p 181. New York, Appleton-Century-Crofts, 1976)

5. Lateral joint line
6. Lateral meniscus
7. Lateral femoral condyle articulating surface
8. Lateral collateral ligament

Tenderness of these structures is less common than tenderness in the anterior or medial structures. These structures may be palpated inferior to superior in the order listed with the original point of reference at the easily located fibular head. Proximal to the fibular head the distal tendon of the biceps femoris muscle may be palpated. Locating this structure can be facilitated by having the patient perform an isometric contraction of the hamstrings with the knee in 90 degrees of flexion.

At the level of the lateral epicondyle, by slowly moving the fingers anteriorly off the biceps tendon to the next tendinous structure, the iliotibial (IT) band may be located. Following this tendon distally to its insertion, a bony prominence on the anterolateral tibia surface may be located. This is Gerdy's tubercle. This tubercle and the distal IT band are the common location for the iliotibial band friction syndrome that is most prevalent in running athletes.

The lateral joint line may be palpated in a similar manner as the medial joint line with the knee positioned in 90 degrees of flexion. This joint line may be located most easily in this position by starting at the inferior pole of the patella and moving the fingers laterally. To palpate the lateral meniscus from this position the tibia should be externally rotated and the force of the fingers should be directed inferiorly parallel to the axis of the tibial shaft. In contrast, a superiorly directed pressure on the proximally located lateral femoral condyle is used to palpate the articulating surface of this condyle.

The small, round, and cordlike lateral collateral ligament is most easily palpated with the patient in the crossed-leg position. This consists of placing the lateral malleolus of the leg being palpated on the superior area of the opposite leg while in the bent-knee sitting position. In this position of knee flexion, and femoral abduction and external rotation, the ligament may be located by following its path from the fibular head to the lateral femoral condyle.

A complete palpation examination of the knee is helpful in evaluating the predominant problems of the injured knee. In general, significant tenderness of knee structures is indicative of a primary problem of inflammation. More specific analysis of the most tender structures, useful in delineating the pathology causing the knee disability, will be discussed later.

IMMOBILITY

Decreased mobility of the knee joint is common in most pathologies of the knee. It is probably least common in the overuse pathologies where pain with activity predominates and most common in the traumatic injuries such as ligament sprains where pain and swelling predominate. Open joint surgery of the knee joint often results in a hypomobile knee, especially if immobilization of the knee is required postsurgically.

Of the two planes of motion at the knee (sagittal and transverse), detection of poor mobility in the knee is easiest in measuring sagittal plane motion (ie, flexion and extension). Evaluation of this motion may be done both passively and actively, though passive measurement is preferred. Although the patient may be put in a number of positions to measure passive knee range of motion, reliable and accurate measuring depends upon consistency in the method of measurement more than the actual position used. One of the more useful methods for measuring passive extension is to place the patient in the long sitting position with an object such as rolled-up towel placed under the Achilles tendon of both legs to prevent friction of the heel on the table from hindering the motion. The patient is then instructed to relax both knees to his comfort and measurement of knee extension in both extremities is performed. Measurement should be executed from a lateral position with the use of a goniometer. For ease of measurement normal knee extension is set equal to 0 degree, while hyperextension receives a positive value (eg, +5 degrees) and limited knee extension measures receive negative values (eg, −10 degrees).

To measure passive knee flexion range of motion the patient is placed in a supine position. The hip is flexed to 90 degrees followed by passive knee flexion from an extended position as the lower leg is supported. Again, measurement should be done bilaterally from a lateral view. Values in this measurement range from 0 degree (no flexion) to 150 degrees (full flexion). If the setting is appropriate, this measure may be best performed with the patient in the supine position with both feet propped on a wall. Gradual flexion of the knee being tested may be performed with the wall and contralateral leg offering support against gravity to prevent sudden motion.

Measurement of knee motion in the transverse plane (internal and external tibial rotation) is much more difficult and less useful in management of knee injury. Instead of precise goniometric measurement of mobility in this range, it may be useful to compare both knees for positions of the tibia relative to the femur as the knee is actively extended. Tibial rotation should also be noted with the knee placed in a passive position of knee extension. Abnormalities in tibial rotation in either of these tests may be indicative of some type of internal knee derangement, such as a meniscal tear.

The mobility of the musculature that crosses the knee is another important component of the knee evaluation. Specifically, mobility tests of the gastrocnemius, hamstrings, and rectus femoris are useful. Gastrocnemius length can be measured by passive dorsiflexion of the ankle in two knee positions: extension and 90 degrees flexion. An increase in ankle dorsiflexion with the knee flexed versus the knee extended position is indicative of gastrocnemius tightness.

The hamstrings muscle length may be measured by applying knee extension and hip flexion stretches to this group, which is responsible for knee flexion and hip extension. To do this the patient should be lying supine. With the contralateral extremity stabilized, the unilateral hip should be flexed while the knee is maintained in extension. The end of hamstrings range is usually noted by a springy end-feel and complaints by the patient of a stretch pain behind the knee. Goniometric measurement lateral to the hip for hip flexion range is noted. A useful variation of this test consists of stabilization of the contralateral leg against the table as the patient lies supine while the hip is flexed to 90 degrees with the knee flexed. While manually holding this position of hip flexion, the knee is extended until the hamstrings become taut, which usually results in the same complaint of a stretch pain behind the knee. The amount of knee extension in this position is measured and recorded. Immobility of the gastrocnemius and hamstrings has been

noted in patients suffering from overuse injuries of the knee extensor mechanism. The possibility exists that tightness in these knee flexor structures may require greater force production by the quadriceps in achieving knee extension. This would result in greater tension on the extensor apparatus and greater compressive forces at the patellofemoral joint.

Rectus femoris muscle length can be measured by applying hip extension and knee flexion forces to the extremity while the pelvis is stabilized. This is performed by placing the patient in a supine position with the legs hanging off the edge of the table. The patient is instructed to pull one knee up against his chest and to maintain this position. The opposite extremity is first positioned in hip extension against the table, and then the knee is passively flexed until the patient complains of a stretch pain in the anterior thigh, indicative of stretch of the rectus femoris. The knee angle is measured, recorded, and then compared to a similar measurement of the opposite extremity.

INSTABILITY

The most difficult portion of the knee examination is stability testing. This portion is difficult because of the large number of tests available and because of the difficulty in gaining clinical ability in measuring joint play. Regardless, stability assessment represents a vital component of the knee evaluation. Systematic assessment of passive stability of the knee should be performed for each quarter of the knee: anterior, posterior, medial, and lateral. Then, stability of combinations of these quarters should be performed to assess rotatory stability, eg, anterolateral stability.

Anterior and posterior stability can be assessed with the patient either supine or sitting with both hips and knees placed in a flexed position. The drawer test is performed with the knee in 90 degrees flexion and the tibia in neutral rotation. The therapist then applies an anteriorly directed force on the posterior surface of the proximal tibia to assess anterior stability (Fig. 23-3). A force in an opposite direction on

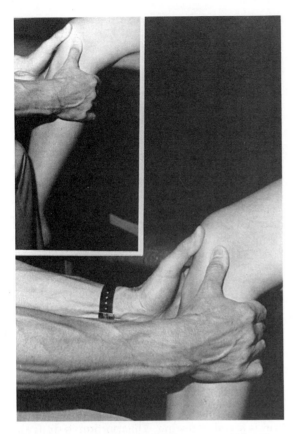

Figure 23-3. Straight anterior drawer test. (After Henning CE, Lynch MA, Glick KB: Physical examination of the knee. In Nicholas JA, Hershman EB: The Lower Extremity and Spine in Sports Medicine, Vol I, p 781. St Louis, 1986, The C.V. Mosby Co.)

the anterior surface of the proximal tibia is applied to assess posterior stability (Fig. 23-4). Anterior instability is more common than posterior instability and is more easy to detect using the drawer test. The clinician must note any posterior sag of the tibia when the knee is positioned for the performance of the drawer tests. If this is left undetected the drawer test will be incorrectly positive for anterior instability and the posterior instability will remain undetected.

Modifications of the anterior drawer test may be useful for further analysis of knee stability. By placing the tibia in external rotation and applying an anteriorly directed force to the

knee, anteromedial stability may be assessed. Applying a similar force to the knee with the tibia internally rotated is useful in measuring anterolateral stability. And finally, an anterior drawer test with the knee in a more extended position (20 to 30 degrees flexion) is useful for further analysis of anterior stability (Fig. 23-5). This last test is known as the Lachman's test for anterior knee stability.

The tests for medial and lateral stability are performed with the patient in a supine position. These tests require application of valgus

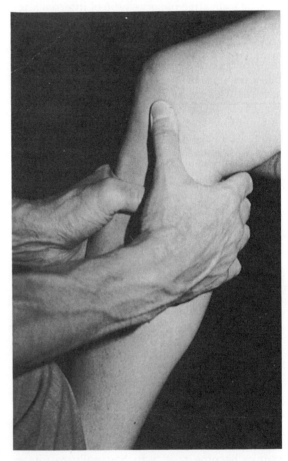

Figure 23-4. Straight posterior drawer test. (After Henning CE, Lynch MA, Glick KB: Physical examination of the knee. In Nicholas JA, Hershman EB: The Lower Extremity and Spine in Sports Medicine, Vol I, p 786. St Louis, 1986, The C.V. Mosby Co.)

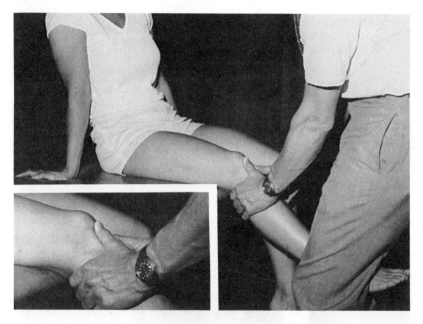

Figure 23-5. Lachman's test for anterior stability. (After Henning CE, Lynch MA, Glick KB: Physical examination of the knee. In Nicholas JA, Hershman EB: The Lower Extremity and Spine in Sports Medicine, Vol I, p 782. St Louis, 1986, The C.V. Mosby Co.)

and varus stresses to the joint with the knee in different positions in the sagittal plane. The easiest method of applying these tests consists of first positioning both knees in 30 degrees flexion by placing the therapist's hand under the distal end of the femur. Valgus and varus forces are then applied bilaterally and any differences noted (Figs. 23-6 and 23-7). The knees are then placed in full extension and the test is repeated. Instability of the medial knee from valgus forces with the knee in 30 degrees flexion is indicative of injury to the medial collateral ligament and medial capsule. Medial instability with the knee in full extension is indicative of injury to the medial collateral ligament, medial capsule, posteromedial capsule, and the anterior and posterior cruciate ligaments. Lateral instability to varus stress with the knee flexed 30 degrees indicates injury of the lateral collateral ligament and the lateral capsule. Lateral instability with the knee in extension indicates injury of the lateral collateral ligament, posterior and anterior cruciate ligaments, and the arcuate complex.

A number of additional tests are available to measure rotatory stability. Of these, I have found the pivot shift test to be most useful.

This test measures anterolateral stability, that is, the integrity of the anterior cruciate ligament, arcuate complex, and lateral capsule. This test requires placement of valgus and internal rotation forces on the tibia as the knee moves from a position of extension to flexion and tibial internal to external rotation (Fig. 23-8). A pop at the lateral joint during this test is indicative of movement of the lateral tibial plateau from a position of excess internal rotation, ie, anterolateral instability, to its normal position.

MUSCLE WEAKNESS

Assessment of muscular weakness is useful because injury to a joint frequently results in muscular weakness. Rehabilitation usually consists of resistance training of the appropriate musculature. Strength assessment is usually focused on the quadriceps and hamstrings because these muscles are important in knee function and their torque-producing capacity can most easily be assessed. Often forgotten but also of great importance is the torque-producing capacity of the tibial internal and external rotators. Their function in knee sta-

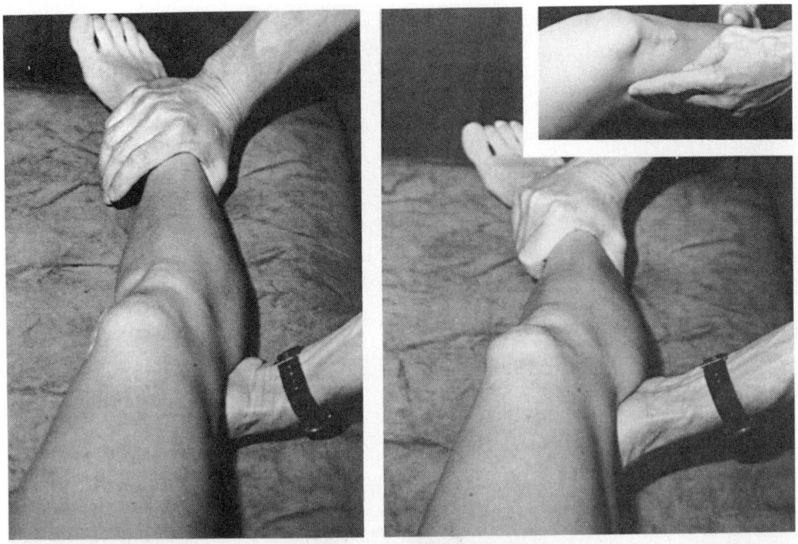

Figure 23-6. Varus test for lateral knee stability. (After Henning CE, Lynch MA, Glick KB: Physical examination of the knee. In Nicholas JA, Hershman EB: The Lower Extremity and Spine in Sports Medicine, Vol I, p 784. St Louis, 1986, The C.V. Mosby Co.)

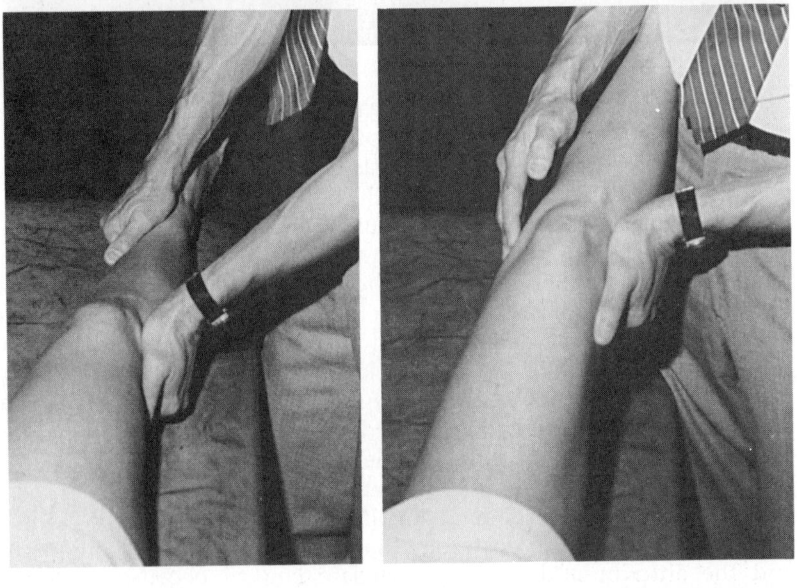

Figure 23-7. Valgus test for medial knee stability. (After Henning CE, Lynch MA, Glick KB: Physical examination of the knee. In Nicholas JA, Hershman EB: The Lower Extremity and Spine in Sports Medicine, Vol I, p 783. St Louis, 1986, The C.V. Mosby Co.)

bility and immobility is poorly understood, as is the effect of knee injury on their torque-producing capacity.

A useful and easy method for assessing the integrity of the thigh musculature is circumferential measures of this portion of the lower extremity. Circumferential measurements at 5 and 20 cm proximal to the superior border of the patella should be assessed. The distance from the patella of the most proximal measure may need to be decreased in short patients. These measurements are useful because a significant positive correlation exists between thigh circumferential measures and isokinetic performance of the quadriceps and hamstrings. This is not to imply that circumferential measures can replace more sophisticated tests of thigh muscle strength. Rather, in the ab-

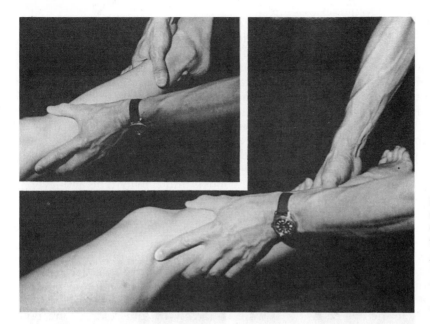

Figure 23-8. Pivot shift test. (After Henning CE, Lynch MA, Glick KB: Physical examination of the knee. In Nicholas JA, Hershman EB: The Lower Extremity and Spine in Sports Medicine, Vol I, p 791. St Louis, 1986, The C.V. Mosby Co.)

sence of other testing devices or when resistance testing is contraindicated, circumferential measures are easily applied and useful.

Interpretation of circumferential measures is best performed by making bilateral comparisons. A smaller thigh circumference is usually indicative of quadriceps weakness more than hamstrings weakness, because the quadriceps is usually affected most in thigh atrophy. Care must be taken in interpreting the measurement closest to the knee joint because this measure may be affected by knee joint swelling.

Quadriceps reflex inhibition is either difficulty or an inability to actively contract the quadriceps muscle. It is most prevalent in the acute stage of injury when pain and swelling persist and after prolonged immobility of the knee joint. A simple method to assess this problem is to palpate the quadriceps muscle during an isometric contraction in the terminal knee extension range of motion (0 to 30 degrees). The relative strength of the contraction should be compared to the uninjured quadriceps and rated comparatively as normal, good, fair, poor, and no contraction. Reflex inhibition appears to be most prevalent in the vastus medialis oblique head of the quadriceps.

Isokinetic testing of thigh musculature torque-producing capacity may be useful, but is not necessary for proper knee evaluation. The major problem in using resistance testing occurs with patients who have pain with resisted knee motion, especially knee extension. When pain is present during contraction the pain may inhibit the patient's ability to offer a full effort of the contraction. As a result, the test becomes an evaluation of pain level and pain tolerance instead of muscle torque-producing capacity. Worse than this is the possibility that the testing may exacerbate pain and swelling of the knee joint.

If isokinetic testing or any other form of resistance testing is used, the therapist must consider the following in testing the concentric strength of the quadriceps and hamstrings.

1. Speed of testing. Slow-speed testing (<120 degrees/sec) should be avoided because the great forces applied to the joint, especially the patellofemoral joint, may exacerbate knee inflammation and offer excess force to articular surfaces such as the posterior patella. These articular structures are especially susceptible after injury because

of the negative effects of joint swelling and immobility common in injury. Another consideration is specificity of training relative to limb speed. The normal speed of knee extension in walking is approximately 230 degrees/sec, and greater speeds are expected in faster activities such as running. Speed specificity would indicate that slow-speed testing offers little information on the functional ability of the knee and is thus unnecessary.

2. Measurement of pain. Patients should be instructed to offer maximum effort within their pain tolerance. It may be useful to measure pain level in each contraction by use of a visual analogue scale. This scale is a straight line with "no pain" marked at one end and "the worst pain ever experienced" marked at the other end. The patient marks the scale at a point that best describes his pain relative to the two ends of the spectrum. It is important to measure pain because it has a major effect on the individual's ability to maximally contract the muscles.

3. Pain/swelling as testing guides. At no time should testing be continued if the patient's pain or knee swelling is increasing significantly during testing.

4. Contralateral testing and warm-up. The uninjured extremity should be tested first and proper warm-up offered to both extremities. Warm-up may consist of multiple submaximal contractions of the quadriceps and hamstrings on the isokinetic unit or perhaps stationary bicycling.

5. Comparisons in assessing thigh muscle strength. The strength of the quadriceps relative to the hamstrings is dependent on test speed, because the hamstrings become stronger relative to the quadriceps as test speed is increased. At slow speeds, such as 60 degrees/sec, the hamstring/quadriceps ratio in Cybex testing should be approximately 60% and should increase to approximately 100% at top speeds of 300 degrees/sec. These values vary because of a number of factors, and are presented for testing without consideration of the effects of gravity. It is more useful to compare the performance of the injured side musculature to the uninjured side, because the uninjured side may be considered "normal." In cases where the uninjured side may not be normal, that is, in cases of prior injury to the uninjured side or in circumstances where decreased activity has affected both lower extremities, the peak torque to body weight ratio should be calculated and compared to norms for individuals of the same age, gender, and activity type and level.

6. Parameters used in analysis. A number of parameters may be measured in isokinetic testing. These range from the most commonly used measure, peak torque, to less common measures such as torque acceleration energy and power. Peak torque may be defined as the maximum torque output, or highest point on the torque curve, as the joint is forced by muscular contraction through the range of motion. For the most accurate comparison of one muscle group to another or for comparisons of the strength of a particular muscle group from one test session (eg, presurgical) to another (eg, postsurgical), the torque value at a specific angle should be used for analysis. Using this measure assures control over two testing variables that greatly affect torque production: joint angle and muscle length.

STRUCTURE

Inspection of the structure of the lower half of the body, including the knee, is necessary in a proper knee evaluation. This inspection is used to assess any structural abnormality that may affect the function of the knee. Analysis should begin at the foot, where the posture of the ankle-foot complex should be evaluated bilaterally in standing. Excess pronation of the foot, indicated by an externally rotated foot and fallen arch, has a major impact on knee function. Foot pronation can cause problems of the knee extensor mechanism as well as medial knee pain. In a number of cases, correction of the pronation problem results in immediate relief of medial knee pain in standing, walking, or running.

Structural analysis of the knee is performed with the patient walking, standing, and supine. Special attention should be focused on knee valgus/varus form in walking, standing, and lying. Excess valgus or varus has important implications for injury to the extensor mechanism and knee collateral ligaments. Valgus is common in medial knee and extensor mechanism injuries and varus is indicative of lateral knee pathology. The amount of tibial rotation should be assessed in standing and supine. Usually tibial rotation is measured by assessing the position of the tibial tubercle relative to the inferior pole of the patella with the knee in full extension. In normal knees the tibial tubercle should lie in a vertical line that is just lateral to a vertical line that bisects the inferior pole. Unusual amounts of tibial rotation may be correlated with poor knee function, especially as it pertains to the mechanics of the extensor mechanism.

With the patient in a supine position, the length of the infrapatellar tendon and Q angle may be measured. These measurements also have important implications for the function of the extensor mechanism. The length of the infrapatellar tendon is measured and compared to the length of the patella. A length ratio of 1:1 is considered normal. Patella baja is descriptive of an infrapatellar tendon that is shorter than the patellar length, while patella alta describes an infrapatellar tendon that is longer relative to the patellar length.

The Q angle may be described as the angle formed by the resultant line of pull of the quadriceps muscle group and the infrapatellar tendon. Measurement consists of drawing two lines on the patient that estimate the line of pull of these two structures. The infrapatellar tendon pull is estimated by drawing a straight line running from the tibial tubercle up the middle of the infrapatellar tendon to the mid-patella and from there up the anterior thigh. The pull of the quadriceps is estimated by drawing a line from the anterior superior iliac spine to the midpoint of the patella. The angle formed by these two lines superior to the mid-point of the

patella, an angle that opens superiorly, is described as the Q angle. The normal Q angle equals 15 degrees, while values greater than 20 degrees are indicative of an excess lateral pull on the patella. This excess pull is detrimental to extensor mechanism function and may result in injury to this vital portion of the knee.

The final component of the structural examination to be discussed is a simple analysis of general joint mobility. Specifically, hypermobility is assessed and includes examination of the knee, elbow, shoulder, and thumb. At the knee and elbow, hypermobility is indicated by hyperextension of previously uninjured joints. Shoulder hypermobility is indicated by excess external rotation at a position of 90 degrees abduction. Many patients with either ligamentous injury or extensor mechanism disorders have general joint hypermobility.

ANALYSIS OF THE RESULTS OF THE EXAMINATION

One of the more difficult parts of the examination is the last portion, which consists of synthesis and analysis of the results of the examination. One method to clarify this often confusing element of the examination is to quickly review the notes taken during the examination and mark with an asterisk (*) those findings that you have found to be most significant. Using these most important findings of both the subjective and objective examination, the major problem of the patient should be determined. These major problems can be classified into one of the following:

1. Inflammation (pain and swelling)
2. Immobility
3. Instability
4. Muscular weakness

Based on the classification chosen, the treatment program for the patient can be planned. For example, the hypomobile patient can be treated with manual stretching and exercise to increase mobility. Typically, the patient progresses through several classifications, except for immobility and instability, which are often mutually exclusive. The key to effective progression of the patient in physical therapy is frequent reevaluation of the patient to assess the most accurate description of the problem, followed by application of procedures deemed most appropriate for the condition.

COMMON KNEE INJURIES

Patients with the most common injuries of the knee have characteristic subjective complaints and objective findings. To describe these characteristics, knee injuries will be divided into two major categories: traumatic and nontraumatic injuries. Traumatic injuries are those that result from one or several major insults to the knee joint. One example is a tear of the knee ligaments in an alpine skiing mishap. Nontraumatic injuries, also known as overuse or microtraumatic injuries, result from numerous, repetitive minor insults such as would occur at the knee in running. A satisfactory subjective examination usually results in the detection of the injury as either traumatic or nontraumatic, and this is verified with the objective examination.

Traumatic Knee Injuries

Within the traumatic injury category, the most typical knee injuries include ligament sprain, meniscal damage, or both. Clinical characteristics of the major types of ligament damage, anterior cruciate (ACL) and medial collateral ligament (MCL) sprain, as well as meniscal injury will be described.

Anterior Cruciate Ligament Sprain
The subjective examination of the patient with an ACL injury usually consists of a report that the original injury occurred in sports activity, typically a pivot injury that may have been combined with body contact with another player or during a fall in skiing. Prolonged positioning in knee extension usually exacerbates knee pain. The patient complains of difficulty or inability to cut in running or pivot in walking, or both. For an anteromedial instability, pivoting or cutting in a direction opposite of the injured knee is troublesome. For anterolateral instability, movement in the direction towards the injured leg is difficult. During the subjective examination, the patient complains of difficulty in stopping during running.

Findings of the objective examination may consist of knee swelling, especially in the acute phase. Palpable tenderness follows a pattern that is dependent upon the specific instability disabling the knee. For example, anteromedial instability usually results in palpable tenderness of the medial structures, whereas anterolateral instability consists of lateral tenderness. Also of note during the palpation examination is frequent tenderness of the posterior, posterolateral, and posteromedial tendon structures. Perhaps these tendons become inflamed from overuse in resisting anterior translation of the tibia.

The ACL-injured knee may become hypomobile and, typically, extension is limited, especially in the acute stage of injury. The examination of knee stability should be positive for at least one of the three types of anterior instability: straight, anterolateral, or anteromedial. As is true in most knee injuries, muscular weakness is prevalent in the quadriceps. Finally, no preexisting structural abnormalities are consistently present in injury of this type. This is true in all of the traumatic injuries.

Medial Collateral Ligament Sprain
Findings in the subjective examination of the patient with a MCL injury consist of injury onset with a valgus load applied to the knee in falling, especially in sports such as skiing. A component of tibial external rotation during the fall is common. This injury may also result from a lateral blow to the knee with the foot planted during participation in a contact sport. Although most of these injuries result from traumatic incidents, unusual weakness of the quadriceps because of inactivity or another injury may result in stretching of the MCL. Positioning the knee in valgus may be irritating, and the patient will report pain relief with varus positioning. Pivoting away from the injured leg in walking and running is usually disabling for the patient.

The objective examination consists of swelling, especially medially, in the acute phase, and palpable tenderness of the MCL and associated medial knee structures. Knee mobility is limited in the end of range of knee flexion and extension, especially when the tibia is externally rotated. The stability examination is positive for medial knee instability, and this represents the most important finding of the examination. Quadriceps weakness is prevalent, and resisted exercise of the quadriceps is usually painful in terminal extension as the tibia is "screwed home" into external rotation. This "screw home" mechanism irritates the MCL, which is stretched with knee extension and external tibial rotation.

Meniscal Damage

Injury to the meniscus is much more difficult to assess in the knee evaluation when compared to ligamentous injury. This is because the external measurements used to determine injury, such as stability testing, are less definitive in this injury. Evaluation is further clouded by the fact that meniscal damage often occurs concurrently with ligament injury. The usual mechanism for injury consists of a pivoting or jumping injury that may occur in an activity of daily living or sport. Symptoms are exacerbated with prolonged standing or further jumping and the pain is described as a deep ache in the "middle of the knee," a complaint that is common in ACL injury as well.

Swelling is prevalent in the early stage of recovery, and tenderness is at and about either the medial or lateral joint line for medial and lateral meniscus injury. End of range flexion and, more typically, extension are limited and painful because these positions represent the closed-packed positions of the joint that result in greater compression of the menisci and articular cartilage. The menisci are important in knee stability, but passive stability tests are not sophisticated enough to detect meniscal damage. Muscle performance of the quadriceps is usually affected most. Typically, there are no structural abnormalities of the lower body that predispose the patient to this type of injury.

Nontraumatic Knee Injuries

The most common nontraumatic injury of the knee is overuse of the extensor mechanism.

Problems in overuse usually begin insidiously and are not related to a particular incidence of falling or trauma. These problems normally result from repetitive stresses on a particular structure that forms the weak link in the kinetic chain. These overstresses often result from a structural abnormality in the lower extremity.

Extensor mechanism disorder is a global term that embraces a number of diagnoses, such as chondromalacia patella and jumper's knee. Typically, these problems occur in either athletes (recreational and competitive) who are involved in a large amount of running, jumping, or bicycling, or they occur during rehabilitation of the knee after injury of a different nature. Other findings in the subjective examination include exacerbation of knee pain with prolonged weight bearing during standing, walking, running, rising from sitting, stair ascension and descension, and prolonged sitting with the knee in flexion. Each of these represents an activity that places major forces on the extensor mechanism. Relief is gained by positioning the knee in slight flexion and with rest. Typical of overuse injuries, continued activity exacerbates the pain. This pain is usually present late in the day, while pain is at its minimum in the morning when the patient complains of minor stiffness in the knee.

Because overuse problems are primarily pain problems, an important component of the objective examination is assessment of pain with palpation. The extensor mechanism structures, especially the tibial tubercle, infrapatellar tendon, and inferior pole, are sensitive to palpation. In addition, the medial knee structures may also become involved. Knee immobility is usually not present, though hamstrings and gastrocnemius tightness may be a cause and should be evaluated. Instability testing is negative, and muscle weakness persists in the quadriceps. Evaluation of actual quadriceps weakness is very difficult because of the persistence of pain with resistance to knee extension.

The structural examination is crucial in gaining a complete understanding of the extensor mechanism disorder. It is not unusual to find excessive foot pronation, tibial rotation (usually external), and an exaggerated Q angle. Furthermore, patella baja or alta may present, as well as general joint hypermobility.

CONCLUSION

Successful treatment of any joint is dependent upon a thorough musculoskeletal evaluation. I have described four of the most common problems of the knee. More useful than describing additional specific knee problems is to categorize signs and symptoms presented by the patient into a "chief complaint" or major problem description, such as knee immobility. Subsequently, treatment is planned in accordance to the predominant difficulty in the knee. It is critical to remember that physical therapists treat the physical manifestations of joint injury, not the diagnosis that is used to describe the injury. A diagnosis is not as reliable and offers less information than the specific physical disabilities impairing the patient's musculoskeletal function.

ANNOTATED BIBLIOGRAPHY

Henning CE, Lynch MA, Glick KR: Physical examination of the knee. In Nicholas JA, Hershman EB (eds): The Lower Extremity and Spine in Sports Medicine, p 765. St Louis, CV Mosby, 1986

(This excellent chapter is useful for both the new and the experienced therapist. Though it is focused on athletic injuries of the knee, it is valuable for proper evaluation of any knee injury. A number of illustrations are used to describe knee evaluation, and these are especially useful for knee stability testing.)

Hoppenfeld S: Physical examination of the knee. In Hoppenfeld S: Physical Examination of the Spine and Extremities, p 171. New York, Appleton-Century-Crofts, 1976

(The bible of physical examination. The excellent illustrations of palpation of the knee are especially useful.)

24 Musculoskeletal Analysis: The Foot and Ankle

HELEN PRICE

The ankle and foot complex is one of the most biomechanically intricate and most frequently ignored segments of the musculoskeletal system. The challenge for the physical therapist is to understand the elaborate interaction of the structural and functional elements of the ankle and foot complex in dynamic versus static activity. Only by integrating basic anatomy and normal biomechanics can one ascertain the effects tissue dysfunctions create, and more precisely which foot pathologies cause which patient complaints. Astute observation skills and subtle manual skills are needed by the physical therapist for successful evaluation and management of the foot and ankle complex.

The ankle and foot complex provides a stable base for weight bearing, serves as shock absorber and force converter for the lower extremity in gait, becomes a rigid lever upon which the body pivots during propulsion, and provides kinesthetic feedback for balance and coordination. The interaction of the 26 foot bones, with the supporting muscles, ligaments, and connective tissues allow for such a spectrum of activity to exist.

The ankle and foot complex is functionally divided into the hindfoot, midfoot, and forefoot. These units will be discussed briefly to assist you in an understanding of structure and movement that is preparatory to a musculoskeletal evaluation of the foot and ankle. The reader is referred to *Gray's Anatomy* (1980) and Kapandji (1970) for an extensive review of anatomy and joint arthrology.

ANATOMY AND BIOMECHANICS

HINDFOOT

Inferior Tibiofibular Joint

The inferior tibiofibular joint is a syndesmosis joint and allows for tibiofibular spread with slight lateral rotation and superior glide of the fibula during ankle dorsiflexion. The existence of this joint play is critical for normal talocrural movement and subsequent gait activity. The joint is stabilized by the anterior and posterior tibiofibular ligaments and the interosseous ligament.

Talocrural Joint

Joint Type: Uniaxial, modified hinge joint

Axis of Motion: Oblique transverse axis; lateral malleolus is slightly posterior and inferior to the medial malleolus.

Range of Motion: 20 degrees dorsiflexion to 50 degrees plantarflexion

Capsular Pattern: Limited in plantarflexion more than dorsiflexion, coupled with hard end-feel

Close-Packed Position: Full dorsiflexion

Resting Position: 10 degrees plantarflexion, midway between inversion and eversion

The talocrural joint allows for ankle dorsiflexion and plantarflexion. The talus may also rotate and tilt slightly within the mortise during these movements. The amount of dorsiflexion is obviously affected by the position of the knee. Normal gait requires that there be 10 degrees of dorsiflexion and 20 degrees of plantarflexion when the knee is extended. Many persons lack the necessary 10 degrees of dorsiflexion, and compensate through early heel-lift in the gait cycle or excessive genu recurvatum.

The structure of the ankle mortise with elaborate ligamentous reinforcement indicates that the talocrural joint is constructed for stability. The joint is supported medially by the strong deltoid ligament and laterally by the anterior talofibular ligament, the posterior talofibular ligament, and the calcaneofibular ligament. By understanding the function of each ligament, the examiner can identify the involved structure if ligamentous support is lost. Table 24-1 lists the ligaments about the ankle and foot with the movements each ligament limits in normal function. The anterior talofibular ligament is the most frequently injured ligament, occurring with an inversion-plantarflexion sprain. As a whole, the lateral ligaments are more vulnerable.

The most frequent dysfunctions at the talocrural joint include (1) limited dorsiflexion because of shortening of the gastrocnemius muscle, or shortening of inert structures, thus preventing tibiofibular spread, and (2) hyper-mobility within the joint from loss of ligamentous support.

Subtalar Joint

Joint Type: Modified multiaxial joint

Axis of Motion: Oblique axis from postero-lateral plantar aspect to an anteromedial dorsal aspect

Range of Motion: Supination should be twice the amount of pronation.

Capsular Pattern: Limited calcaneal inversion or varus

Close-Packed Position: Supination

Resting Position: Neutral

The axis of the subtalar joint and the joint structure of three articulating facets allow for movement to occur in all three cardinal planes simultaneously. Calcaneal inversion, adduction, and plantarflexion will always be in combination and result in subtalar supination. Calcaneal eversion, abduction, and dorsiflexion will always be in combination and create subtalar pronation (Fig. 24-1). For evaluation purposes, a distinction must be appreciated between the triplanar motions and more pure motions of calcaneal inversion and eversion. Calcaneal inversion and eversion (Fig. 24-2) will be the recorded measures, which, in combination with forefoot movement, will reflect

Table 24-1. Purposes of Each Ankle or Foot Ligament

LIGAMENT	MOTIONS CHECKED
Deltoid	Takes displacement in all directions, particularly inversion and lateral rotation
Calcaneofibular	Posterior displacement of foot, dorsiflexion
Posterior talofibular	Posterior displacement of foot
Anterior talofibular	Anterior displacement of foot, medial tilting of talus, plantarflexion
Lateral and cervical talocalcaneal	Subtalar inversion
Medial and interosseous talocalcaneal	Subtalar eversion
Plantar calcaneonavicular	Supports medial aspect of longitudinal arch
Long plantar	Supports lateral aspect of longitudinal arch
Dorsal, plantar, and interosseous	Support interconnecting tarsal bones

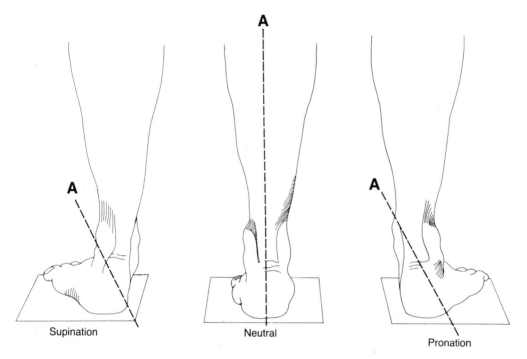

Figure 24-1. Open kinetic chain, triplanar movement of pronation and supination (A, oblique axis of motion of the subtalar joint—anterior, superior, and medial to posterior, inferior, and lateral). (After Donatelli R: Normal biomechanics of the foot and ankle. J Orthop Sports Phys Ther 7:92, © by American Orthopaedic Foot Society, 1985)

the triplanar motions of supination and pronation.

The primary functions of the subtalar joint are to accommodate the body to uneven terrain and to help absorb and convert rotational and shear forces created by the tibia during gait.

MIDFOOT

Talocalcaneonavicular Joint

Joint Type: Multiaxial, ball-and-socket joint

Calcaneocuboid Joint

Joint Type: Biaxial, sellar joint

Cuneonavicular Joint and Intercuneiform Joints

Joint Type: Plane synovial joints

Cuboideonavicular Joint and Cuniocuboid Joint

Joint Type: Fibrous joints

Capsular Pattern for the Midfoot: Limited plantarflexion, dorsiflexion, medial rotation, and adduction, without limit of lateral rotation or abduction

Close-Packed Position for the Midfoot: Supination

Resting Position for the Midfoot: Neutral or slight pronation

The talocalcaneonavicular joint and the calcaneocuboid joint are functionally described as the transverse tarsal or midtarsal joint. Some authors discuss separately the talocalcaneonavicular joint as it relates to subtalar motion. The reader is referred to Norkin and Levangie

Posterior View

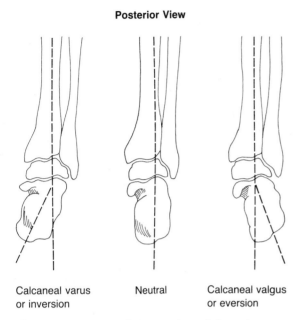

| Calcaneal varus | Neutral | Calcaneal valgus |
| or inversion | | or eversion |

Figure 24-2. Monoplanar motion of the calcaneus measured in an evaluation.

(1983). The axis of motion for the transverse tarsal joint is similar in orientation to the subtalar joint axis except with less vertical inclination. Movement at this joint is triplanar and results in either supination or pronation.

A clear understanding of transverse tarsal motion in the non-weight-bearing and weight-bearing position is necessary for adequate management of the midfoot. In the non-weight bearing position, an open kinetic chain, motion at the transverse tarsal joint coincides with subtalar motion. When the subtalar joint supinates or pronates, the transverse tarsal joint will also supinate or pronate. More importantly, in the weight-bearing position, a closed kinetic chain, the transverse tarsal joint counteracts subtalar pronation, thereby promoting total foot contact. That is, subtalar pronation is neutralized by transverse tarsal supination. This creates an unlocked, flexible foot. With subtalar supination, the transverse tarsal joint becomes locked, cannot counterrotate, and may move into additional supination (MacConaill and Basmajain, 1969). Some compensation for mid-

foot supination can occur at the tarsometatarsal joints.

The motions of the remaining midfoot joints are minimal, or for the intercuneiform joints, nonexistent. Gliding occurs and promotes foot adaptation to surface contours. The joint play movements will be assessed solely through manual articulations and not with active or passive range of motion measures.

Substantial ligamentous support exists for the midfoot joints. Abnormal lengthening of the spring ligament significantly affects the integrity of the longitudinal arch.

FOREFOOT

Tarsometatarsal Joints and Intermetatarsal Joints

> Joint Type: Plane synovial joints
>
> Axes of Motion: Each ray (tarsal bone and adjacent metatarsal) has its own oblique axis; the first and fifth rays are most oblique; the third ray approximates the frontal plane.
>
> Range of Motion: Minimal gliding
>
> Close-Packed Position: Supination
>
> Resting Position: Neutral

Motion of the tarsometatarsal and intermetatarsal joints is slight gliding of the bones upon one another to accommodate to the ground and to transmit forces directed through them. Only the first metatarsal has an additional joint motion of conjunct rotation that accompanies plantar glide. This allows for better first ray adaptability to the ground. Movement at these forefoot joints is reflected by a concomitant increase or decrease in the transverse arch of the foot.

Tarsometatarsal motion is directed by the hindfoot and midfoot activity. The tarsometatarsal joints adapt in proportion to the amount and direction of forces moving distally to allow total forefoot contact across the metatarsal heads. For example, supination of the hindfoot will be offset by first ray plantarflexion and fifth ray dorsiflexion. With extreme lower extremity abduction in the weight-bearing position, the tarsometatarsal joints counterrotate relative to the hindfoot, again, to provide ground contact of the forefoot.

Metatarsophalangeal Joints

Joint Type: Condyloid joints

Axes of Motion: Transverse and longitudinal axes

Range of Motion: first MTP—45 degrees flexion, 70 to 90 degrees extension, 10 degrees abduction; second to fifth MTP—45 degrees flexion, 40 degrees extension, 10 degrees abduction

Capsular Pattern: first MTP—marked loss of extension, slight loss of flexion; second to fifth MTP—variable

Close-Packed Position: Full flexion

Resting Position: 10 degrees extension

The important function of the metatarsophalangeal joints in the participation in gait. As weight is transmitted to the forefoot, the metatarsophalangeal joints assume an extended position. This creates tension across the plantar aponeurosis, thereby increasing the longitudinal arch, and adding to a rigid structure of the foot. This action, described as the windlass effect, allows for absorption of 60% of weight-bearing stresses.

Interphalangeal Joints

Joint Type: Hinge joints

Axis of Motion: Transverse axis

Range of Motion: Proximal IP—90 degrees flexion, 0 to 10 degrees extension; Distal IP—5 to 10 degrees flexion, 40 degrees extension

Capsular Pattern: Limited extension more than flexion

Close-Packed Position: Full extension

Resting Position: Slight flexion

Motion at the interphalangeal joints occurs to assist in maintaining foot stability and balance. Activity is prevalent in static postures more than during gait.

PLANTAR ARCHES

The plantar arches should now be mentioned because they involve elements of the hindfoot, midfoot, and the forefoot. A transverse and longitudinal arch is created when you twist a rectangular plate such that the posterior edge of the plate is vertical and the anterior edge is horizontal (Fig. 24-3). Thus, in standing, the horizontal metatarsal heads have twisted 90 degrees relative to a vertical calcaneus. The medial aspect of the longitudinal arch is controlled by the verticality of the calcaneus, is statically maintained by the plantar ligaments, and is dynamically supported by the anterior and posterior tibialis muscles.

The lateral aspect of the longitudinal arch and the transverse arch, at the plane of the tarsometatarsal joints, reflect true architectural arches. The cuboid and third cuniform serve as the structural keystones.

Functionally, pronation of the subtalar joint results in a flattening of the medial aspect of the longitudinal arch and of the transverse arch. This position can lead to excessive foot mobility and abnormal gait biomechanics.

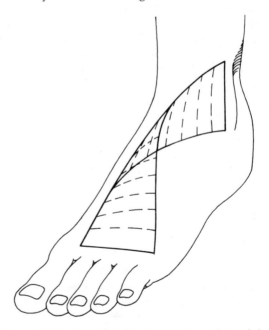

Figure 24-3. Twisted osteoligamentous plate of the foot, resulting in a longitudinal and transverse arch. (After Norkin C, Levangie P: Joint Structure and Function: A Comprehensive Analysis, p 354. Philadelphia, FA Davis, 1983)

GAIT

During gait, the ankle-foot complex serves as a base of support, a shock absorber, an adapter to uneven terrain, and a rigid lever for propulsion. Understanding which actions occur during each phase of gait is important for thorough gait analysis. The normal gait cycle consists of a stance phase, occurring 60% of the time, and a swing phase, occurring 40% of the time. This implies that the ankle-foot complex is weight bearing, reflecting a closed kinetic chain, and then non-weight bearing, reflecting an open kinetic chain within each gait cycle.

Stance Phase

At heel strike, the subtalar joint pronates, creating a non-rigid, pliant midfoot that can absorb excessive vertical compression forces and accommodate the dynamic internal rotation of the lower extremity. With the completion of heel contact, pronation ceases and midstance is initiated. The lower extremity externally rotates and the subtalar joint regresses from pronation to neutral. At midpoint of midstance, the ankle-foot complex is at its most neutral position with the metatarsal heads in horizontal alignment and fully contacting the surface. Moving from midstance to heel-lift, the subtalar joint begins supinating and the midfoot becomes increasingly more rigid. The intrinsic and extrinsic muscles of the foot also assist in stabilizing the midfoot. With continued forward motion, the talocrural joint plantar flexes, the subtalar joint completes supination, the midfoot is locked, and the metatarsophalangeal joints are extending. The foot has become a rigid lever for propulsion, and the limb is ready for toe-off.

Swing Phase

Following toe-off, the ankle-foot complex is relieved of all weight-bearing stresses. Dorsiflexors clear the toes at midswing, and in preparation for heel strike the subtalar joint is in the beginning stage of pronation.

EXAMINATION

When evaluating the ankle and foot complex, three basic premises should be kept in mind.

1. Ankle and foot pain usually arise from local pathology and rarely refer pain proximal to the knee.
2. The ankle and foot complex must be assessed both statically and dynamically, in weight-bearing and non-weight-bearing positions.
3. Ankle and foot dysfunction frequently lead to, or occur simultaneously with, knee, hip, sacroiliac, and/or lumbar dysfunction.

SUBJECTIVE EVALUATION

As with any patient complaint, extracting critical information about the complaint and the patient's medical history leads to a more successful assessment of the joint pathology. After determining the age, sex, and occupation of the patient, the following information should be ascertained.

1. What is the patient's complaint? Most complaints will be of pain, but others may be swelling, sensory changes, pressure, tightness, or feelings that the ankle wants to give way. Complaints of "giving way" suggest proprioceptive compromise and will frequently be seen following severe ankle sprains.
2. Where is the complaint felt? Because ankle or foot pathology is fairly reliable, an exact description of the complaint site is critical. You should be able to narrow the choices of pathology by identifying probable structures beneath or around the complaint site. Sensory changes should be differentiated by dermatomal distributions, peripheral nerve distributions, or vascular supplied areas.
3. Was the onset traumatic or insidious in nature? The ankle is frequently subject to traumatic injury and the foot is commonly subject to biomechanical stresses or overuse problems. With traumatic injuries, have the patient describe the mechanism of injury. Visually duplicating an image of the injury can suggest involved tissues. Ankle inversion injuries typically lead to capsular and ligamentous compromise. Eversion injuries create more severe pathologies and

frequently lead to fractures. If the injury was traumatic, did swelling occur? If so, have the patient describe the location. You may be able to differentiate between an intracapsular and extracapsular lesion. Swelling that is localized reflects an intracapsular lesion, with the injured tissues lying beneath the swelling.

4. What brings on the complaint? Is the complaint activity related or time related? If activity provokes the complaint, have the patient be as specific as possible in describing the situation. You can then relate the activity to the biomechanical demands placed upon the ankle and foot, for example, during the phases of the gait cycle. If the patient reports a time delay between activity and onset of complaint, you need to consider muscle weakness, overuse problems, vascular compromise, or neural compression. A new sport activity may create different demands on the foot or ankle of which the patient is unaware. Problems secondary to an increase in the duration of an activity, such as an increase in running distance, suggest overuse problems.

5. What type of shoes does the patient wear? Women who frequently wear high-heeled shoes can develop shortening of the gastrocnemius and forefoot deformities. Shoes without an appropriate heel counter or arch support can allow increased pronation and subsequent arch flattening, creating excessive demands upon the plantar aponeurosis and plantar ligaments. Patients should be reminded to bring their shoes with them for inspection and possible modification.

6. How does uneven terrain affect the complaint? Hard terrains like asphalt may be more problematic than soft terrains. Inclines and declines place different demands upon the talocrural and subtalar joints.

7. How has the initial complaint changed? Is the pain getting worse? Has swelling increased or decreased? Are abnormalities in sensation changing in intensity or surface area?

8. Is there any pertinent medical history or previous injury? Systemic conditions such as rheumatoid arthritis, gout, diabetes, and collagen diseases can show concomitant foot pathologies. Congenital defect or deformities can create long-standing biomechanical dysfunction.

9. Have x-ray films been taken? X-ray films are essential in identifying skeletal compromise or structural malalignment. The examiner is directed to Kleiger, Greenspan, and Norman (1982) for relevant analysis.

Some specific nontraumatic complaints can suggest common foot pathologies. Pain on heel strike can suggest a bone spur. Swelling or pain or both at the back of the heel can be Achilles' tendinitis or calcaneal bursitis. Pain on the sole of the foot at the metatarsal head region suggests plantar fasciitis, Morton's neuroma, or metatarsalgia. Pain at the first metatarsophalangeal joint can indicate the presence of a bunion, hallux rigidus, or gout (Hoppenfeld, 1982). Pain at sites of shoe contact can be from corns or calluses from hammer toe, mallet toe, or claw toe deformities (Fig. 24-4).

OBJECTIVE EVALUATION

The examiner should always compare one side of the body to the other side for symmetry and asymmetry using the nonpathological side as the norm.

Observation

As mentioned previously, you must observe the ankle and foot in the weight-bearing and non-weight-bearing positions. Observation should be made from the anterior, posterior, and lateral sides. In the weight-bearing position, you should note the following:

1. Distribution of weight right to left and heel to toe (50% to 60% of the body weight should be borne in the heel);
2. Amount of out-toeing (5 to 18 degrees is normal);
3. Calcaneal verticality (position should be neutral, no varus or valgus);
4. Integrity of plantar arches (midfoot should not splay; the medial aspect of the longitu-

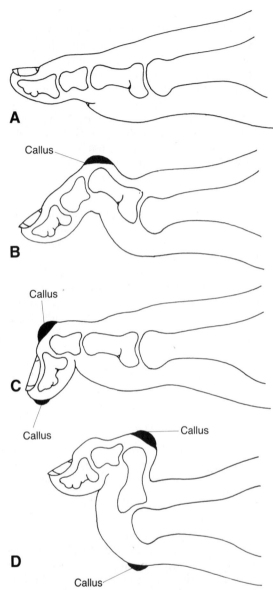

dinal arch should be maintained such that the navicular tubercle falls on a line that passes through the medial malleolus and first metatarsal head);

5. Forefoot alignment and ground contact (note forefoot abduction, hammer toes, mallet toes, claws toes as shown in Fig. 24-4, or excessive abduction of the first phalanx); and

6. Standing posture, checking bony landmarks and total body alignment (abnormal hip medial rotation can create in-toeing or foot pronation; excessive hip lateral rotation can result in an elevated longitudinal arch; knee valgus can create calcaneal malalignment).

In the non-weight-bearing position, or sitting, the same observations are made, with the expectation that the foot will rest in slight supination. Failure of a pronated foot to assume any supination suggests a rigid foot structure and lack of mobility.

Inspection

With the patient sitting or supine, the ankles and feet are analyzed for skin and soft tissue problems. You should note the following:

1. Skin color and moisture (discrepancies can suggest abnormal vascularization, abnormal sympathetic activity, or systemic pathologies);

2. Swelling (presence of ecchymosis identifies tissue bleeding; the coloration can be related to the stage of healing);

3. Size and location of corns and calluses or open lesions (these reflect areas of abnormal biomechanical stress and/or vascular compromise);

4. Integrity of toenails (nails should be relatively smooth, flat, and should blanch momentarily with pressure; abnormalities suggest vascular compromise or systemic disease); and

5. Wear patterns of the patient's shoes, areas of breakdown inside and outside the shoes, and the integrity of the toe box.

Figure 24-4. *(A)* Normal toe. *(B)* Hammer toe. Note flexion deformity of the proximal interphalangeal joints. The distal interphalangeal joint is in neutral position or slight flexion. *(C)* Mallet toe. There is flexion contracture of the distal interphalangeal joint. The proximal interphalangeal and metatarsophalangeal joints are in neutral position. *(D)* Claw toe. The proximal and distal interphalangeal joints are hyperflexed and the metatarsophalangeal joint is dorsally subluxed. (After Jahss MH: Disorders of the Foot, p 212. Philadelphia, WB Saunders, 1982)

Active Movements

By having the patient perform functional active movements you can assess the tolerance of the ankle and foot to motion, and the range of motion in the weight-bearing position. The patient should assume each of the positions identified below and then take several steps with the ankles and feet held in that position. Use your judgment to decide whether the patient should perform these activities in the parallel bars. Patients have a tendency either to use the bars for upper extremity support, which alters overall body balance, or feel somewhat boxed in by the bars. Walking near a plinth is recommended.

1. Foot Flat. Have the patient walk at a normal cadence, and look for any abnormal biomechanics as discussed with talocrural movements and mechanics in each phase of the gait cycle. If a patient reports pain or dysfunction while running, you must observe the gait mechanics with the patient running. Use of a treadmill would be helpful for such observations.
2. Tip-toes. With plantarflexion the calcaneous should invert and the longitudinal arch should increase. Inability to toe walk requires further assessment of the gastrocsoleus group and lumbar screening to rule out neural compromise. Recall that neural compromise can be irritation or compression at the nerve root proximally, or compression distally as in peripheral nerve entrapments.
3. On Heels. If the patient cannot keep the toes up, you should consider dorsiflexor weakness or neural compromise. Lack of dorsiflexion suggests distal tibiofibular joint dysfunction or a shortened gastrocsoleus muscle group.
4. Supination. The patient should step on lateral borders of the feet. If the patient loses balance, proprioceptive feedback from the ligaments and muscles may be deficient. This is common following ankle sprains.
5. Pronation. The patient should step on the medial borders of the feet. This is an awkward movement to perform. A tendency for the foot to lose pronation during midstance is acceptable.

Active movement should also be checked in the non-weight-bearing position, preferably sitting, to assess muscle recruitment, coordination, and range of motion. Check movements as follows: (1) ankle dorsiflexion and plantarflexion; (2) foot supination and pronation; and (3) toe flexion, extension, and abduction.

Passive Movements

Passive motion is tested in sitting, except for subtalar inversion and eversion, which is assessed with the patient prone. In addition to measuring the range of motion, each movement should be tested for an end-feel. The normal end-feel for all ankle and foot movements is firm ligamentous or capsular in nature. You are referred to Norkin and White (1985) for a review of goniometric measurements and end-feel assessment of the ankle and foot. Additional critical instructions are provided below.

1. Ankle Dorsiflexion and Plantarflexion. Test dorsiflexion with the knee flexed to assess the talocrural end-feel. If the knee is extended, you will more likely be testing the extensibility of the gastrocnemius muscle. Be sure that your distal hand applies dorsiflexion force through the talocrurual joint only, by placing your hand at the midfoot and not the forefoot.
2. Subtalar Inversion and Eversion. For easy reference, draw a line bisecting the calcaneous and Achilles' tendon when measuring subtalar inversion and eversion (Fig. 24-5).
3. Foot supination and pronation
4. Toe flexion, extension, and abduction

Resisted Movements

The examiner looks for either pain or weakness with the requested maximal isometric contraction. The ankle and foot should be in the neutral position to avoid pinching or stretching any inert structures. In addition to checking contractile integrity, myotome testing is done simultaneously for the nerve roots listed. Re-

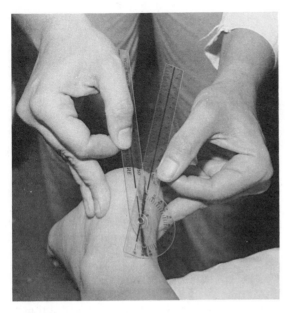

Figure 24-5. Measuring calcaneal inversion and eversion.

sisted movements are tested in sitting with the left and right extremities tested simultaneously for easy comparison. If you find an asymmetry in strength, recheck by testing each ankle or foot individually.

1. Tibialis anterior (L4) and tibialis posterior muscles
2. Peroneus tertius, brevis, and longus muscles (S1)
3. Extensor hallucis longus (L5) and extensor digitorum muscles
4. Toe flexor muscles
5. Gastrocnemius and soleus muscles (previously tested with tip-toe walking, S2)

Active, passive, and resisted movements are analyzed according to the principles of Cyriax's Selective Tension Testing. Differentiation between contractile and inert tissues are then made.

Joint Play Movements

Assessment of joint play movements becomes a critical component of the examination because the ankle and foot complex is mostly an osseous structure controlled by connective tissue, ligaments, and long tendons from muscle bellies proximal to the ankle. Three general principles apply for assessing joint play movements at the ankle and foot.

1. The range and quality of each articular glide must be compared to the uninvolved side to determine hypermobility or hypomobility.
2. Keep each joint in neutral or loose-packed position when performing a glide to prevent premature tissue tightening.
3. Impart very slight distraction prior to any glide to prevent jamming of the articular surfaces.

A description of each joint play movement to be assessed follows with diagrams for clarification. The patient is positioned in the supine position for every assessment.

Inferior Tibiofibular Joint
Anterior-Posterior Glide. The patient should be supine with the hip and knee each flexed 45 degrees, and the foot resting on the table. You stand facing the patient, cradle the lateral malleolus between thumb and medial border of your index finger, and stabilize the tibia with your other hand. Glide the fibula anteriorly and posteriorly (Fig. 24-6). Excessive motion suggests stretching or rupture of the ligaments attached to the fibula.

Talocrural Joint
Talar Distraction; Anterior-Posterior Glide. The patient's leg should be relaxed and will stabilize itself as you begin distraction. Interlace your fingers and cradle the talus so that your fifth digits are across the talar neck, your web spaces surround the medial and lateral sides of the foot, and your thumbs cross the sole of the foot. Pull the talus toward your chest to get distraction (Fig. 24-7). The amount of play reflects the overall freedom of the talocrural joint.

To test anterior and posterior glide, move to the side of the table, stabilize the tibia and fibula with your hand that is proximal to the patient, and grasp the talus and calcaneus with the other hand. Hold the calcaneus in slight eversion to lock it against the talus. Be sure not

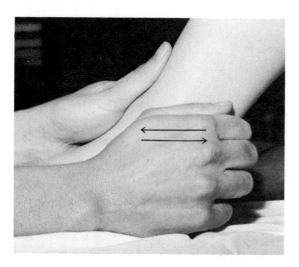

Figure 24-6. Anterior-posterior glide at the inferior tibiofibular joint.

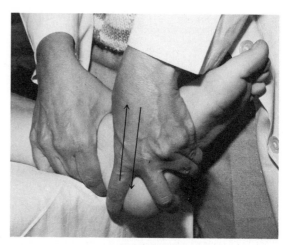

Figure 24-8. Anterior-posterior glide at the talocrural joint.

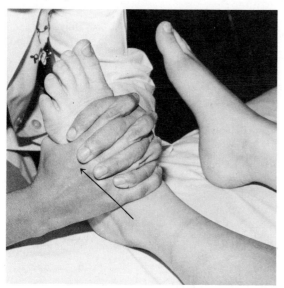

Figure 24-7. Distraction at the talocrural joint.

to squeeze the tibia and fibula together, or the talus will not be able to spread them apart. Glide the talus in an anterior and posterior direction (Fig. 24-8). Excessive anterior glide incriminates the anterior talofibular ligament. Limitation of anterior glide results in decreased plantarflexion, whereas limitation of posterior glide results in decreased dorsiflexion.

Subtalar Joint

Inversion-Eversion Tilt; Dorsal-Plantar Rock. Sit with your back to the patient and bring the patient's leg around your hip so that the knee is flexed to 90 degrees and the foot is in your lap. Stabilize the talus by crossing the talar neck with your thumb, with thumb web across lateral malleolus, and wrapping your fingers around the lower leg. Hold with your other hand so that the thumb is on the medial calcaneus and the fingers are on the lateral calcaneus. Tilt the calcaneus into valgus or inversion and varus or eversion (Fig. 24-9). Excessive valgus suggests compromise of the deltoid ligament, particularly the tibiocalcaneal ligament. Excessive varus incriminates the calcaneofibular ligament.

Maintain the stabilizing hand in the same position, and now cradle the calcaneus in the palm of the other hand. Rock the calcaneus in a dorsal and distal direction and then in a plantar and proximal direction (Fig. 24-10). Some joint play must exist in all four directions for the subtalar joint to adapt to uneven terrain appropriately.

Talonavicular Joint

Dorsal-Plantar Glide; Rotation. Stabilize the talus and calcaneus by placing your hand that is proximally located with the thumb across the

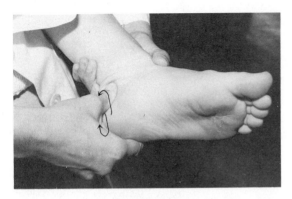

Figure 24-9. Inversion-eversion tilt at the subtalar joint.

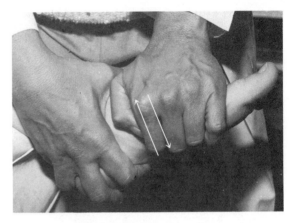

Figure 24-11. Dorsal-plantar glide at the talonavicular joint.

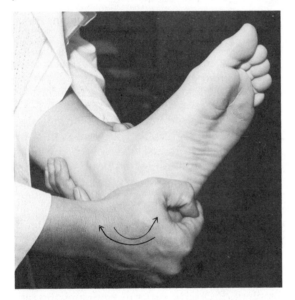

Figure 24-10. Dorsal-plantar rock at the subtalar joint.

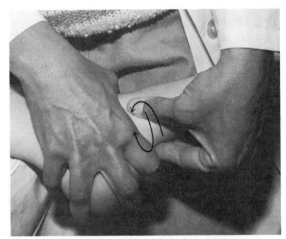

Figure 24-12. Rotation at the talonavicular joint.

neck of the talus and fingers hugging the calcaneus. Locate the navicular and place the hyperthenar eminence on the dorsal surface, wrap your index finger around the medial border, and place the pad of your index finger on the plantar surface of the navicular. Your stabilizing and articulating hands are butted against each other. You may need to displace the stabilizing hand slightly forward to prevent the right and left first metatarsophalangeal joints from hitting one another. (This will be a principle for appropriate hand placement through-

out the foot.) Glide the navicular in a plantar and dorsal direction with your arm locked in extension (Fig. 24-11).

For rotation, hold the navicular with the finger pads and slightly spin the navicular in a clockwise and counterclockwise position (Fig. 24-12).

Naviculocuneiform Joint
Dorsal-Plantar Glide. Repeat the general procedure outlined for navicular glide, with the hand most proximal on the patient now stabi-

lizing the navicular and the hand most distal mobilizing the cuneiforms as a unit in dorsal and plantar glide (Fig. 24-13).

Calcaneocuboid Joint

Dorsal-Plantar Glide. Place your hand that is located proximally on the patient so that the thumb crosses the talar neck, the thumb web encases the lateral calcaneus, and the fingers surround the calcaneus. Hold the cuboid with your other hand so that the hyperthenar eminence is on the dorsal surface and the index finger wraps around to the plantar surface of the cuboid. Glide the cuboid in a dorsal and plantar direction (Fig. 24-14).

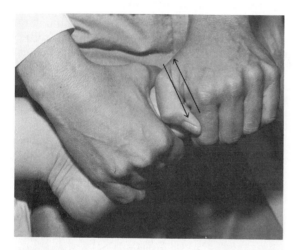

Figure 24-13. Dorsal-plantar glide at the naviculocuneiform joint.

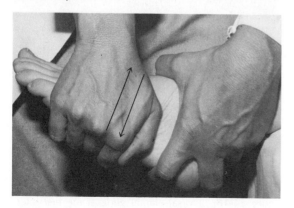

Figure 24-14. Dorsal-plantar glide at the calcaneocuboid joint.

Tarsometatarsal Joints

Dorsal-Plantar Glide; Rotation. On the medial aspect of the foot, stabilize the cuneiforms by placing the hyperthenar eminence on the dorsal surface and wrapping your index finger around to the plantar surface. Your other hand will hold the first and second metatarsals, and subsequently glide the metatarsals in a dorsal and plantar direction (Fig. 24-15). On the lateral aspect of the foot, stabilize the cuboid by placing the hyperthenar eminence on the dorsal surface and wrapping your index finger around to the plantar surface. Your other hand will hold the fourth and fifth metatarsals and glide them in a dorsal and plantar direction (Fig. 24-16).

For rotation, bridge your stabilizing hand across the dorsum of the cuneiforms and the cuboid. Place your other hand so that your fingers stretch across the dorsal surface of the metatarsals and your thumb is on the plantar surface of the foot. Rotate the entire forefoot clockwise and counterclockwise to simulate conjunct supination and pronation movement (Fig. 24-17).

Intermetatarsal Joints

Dorsal-Plantar Glide. Stand below the patient's foot. Stabilize the second metatarsal with your thumb along the plantar surface and your finger pads along the dorsal surface of the bone shaft. Holding the first metatarsal in a

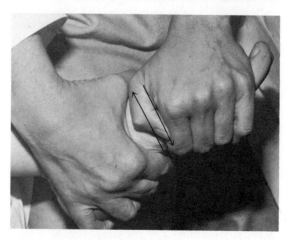

Figure 24-15. Dorsal-plantar glide at the cuneiform-metatarsal joint.

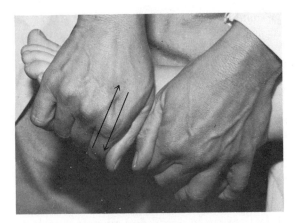

Figure 24-16. Dorsal-plantar glide at the cuboid-metatarsal joint.

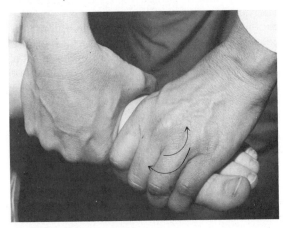

Figure 24-17. Forefoot rotation.

similar fashion with the other hand, glide the first metatarsal in a dorsal and plantar direction (Fig. 24-18). Stabilize the second metatarsal again by switching hands, and now mobilize the third metatarsal on the second. Repeat the general procedure and mobilize the fourth metatarsal on a stabilized third metatarsal, followed by mobilizing the fifth metatarsal on a stabilized fourth metatarsal.

Metatarsophalangeal and Interphalangeal Joints
Dorsal-Plantar Glides; Distraction; Rotation. For each joint, stabilize the proximal segment and glide the distal segment. There is slightly more

glide in the plantar direction than in the dorsal direction. Distraction is performed by pulling the distal segment longitudinally away from the stabilized proximal segment (Fig. 24-19).

The critical determination for joint play movement in the ankle and foot is identifying hypermobility or hypomobility when compared to the uninvolved side. Because the patient is supine throughout this portion of the evaluation, you will find making comparisons easier if you test each joint on the uninvolved side and then the involved side, back and forth, rather than testing one entire foot at a time.

Neuromuscular Evaluation

Having tested the myotomes, reflexes and sensation are assessed. The Achilles' tendon reflex tests the integrity of the S1 nerve root. This is

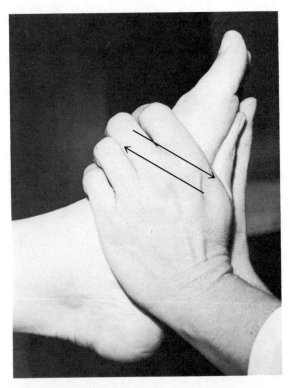

Figure 24-18. Dorsal-plantar glide at the first intermetatarsal joint.

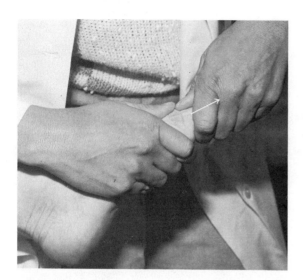

Figure 24-19. Distraction of the first metatarsophalangeal joint.

tested by striking the Achilles' tendon briskly, with the knee in the flexed position.

A sensory check is made by passing your hands over each aspect of the patient's leg and foot. The patient keeps her eyes closed and is asked, "Does this feel the same or different?" Any discrepancies are reassessed and further delineated with a pinwheel, or any instrument used for sharp-dull testing. You can determine if the sensory disturbance results from peripheral nerve or nerve root compromise based on the pattern of sensory change. Dermatomal patterns suggest nerve root irritation or compression, whereas cutaneous sensory pattern deficits suggest peripheral nerve problems. Sensory abnormalities at the ankle and foot frequently arise from lumbar spine dysfunction or entrapment of the common peroneal nerve.

Palpation

The examiner must develop competent palpation skills as a necessary tool in ankle and foot assessment. Palpation can clarify conflicting data gathered in the objective exam. By palpating bony landmarks, protuberances, tendons, ligaments, muscles, and blood vessels, the examiner can visualize the structure of the patient's ankle and foot. The reader is referred to

Hoppenfeld (1976) for a description and visual depiction of important structures.

SPECIAL TESTS

Volumetric Measures

Distal extremity swelling resulting from ankle sprains or vascular problems should be monitored throughout the management period. Circumferential measurements are tedious, time consuming, and are not reliable. The amount of edema can be objectively assessed through volumetric measurements. The distal extremity is submerged in a water-filled container. The displaced water is collected and measured in a graduated cylinder (Fig. 24-20).

Footprint Recording

If the examiner needs a clear picture of the weight-bearing loads directed through the foot, a pressure-sensitive footprint may be beneficial. The Harris pad provides such a footprint. Pressure is reflected by the ink-stained areas. The darker the area, the greater the amount of compression by the foot at that site. This is an important tool when fabricating orthotic devices for biomechanical adjustment or when managing an insensitive foot. The footprint can be taken in standing or during gait.

Thermography

Temperature measures may be used to clarify circulatory compromise. A thermogram gives a visual representation of temperature patterns of the foot. The thermography unit has plates of liquid crystals that heat according to contact surface temperatures and create a color array based on that temperature. Comparisons for normal foot temperature patterns can be made, as well as analyzing the thermal patterns for symmetry (Fig. 24-21).

Proprioception Evaluation

A multiaxial balance evaluator (MABEL) can be constructed by the therapist. This device counts the number of times a patient moves out of static balance as well as the length of time out of balance (Decarlo and Talbot, 1986). The data can be analyzed for asymmetry, which

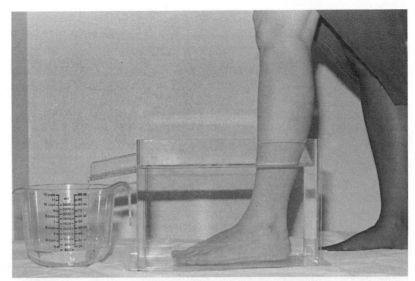

Figure 24-20. Circumferential assessments using volumetric measurements.

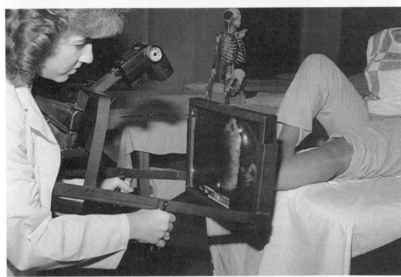

Figure 24-21. Thermography unit used to qualify foot temperatures, with the resulting visual image.

would reflect kinesthetic feedback to the central nervous system. Initially this assessment would indicate a need for proprioceptive reeducation, and over time could indicate the success of a rehabilitation program (Fig. 24-22).

CONCLUSION

The ankle and foot complex deserves critical attention with any lower extremity pathology.

This complex may be the primary site of the patient's complaint or may be a major contributory factor to all other lower quarter problems. Successful management depends on a comprehensive evaluation assessing static and dynamic activities, combined with sound deductive reasoning to identify the pathological tissues. Although the ankle and foot complex is a challenge to understand, alleviating foot pain or resolving a biomechanical problem wins much gratitude from any patient.

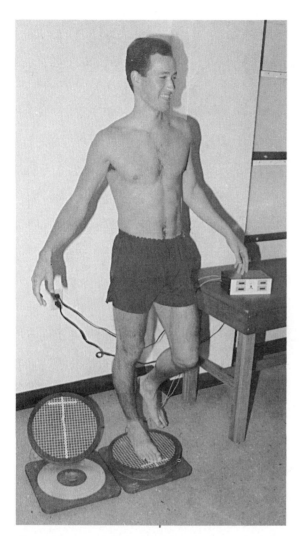

Figure 24-22. Multiaxial balance evaluator for bilateral ankle proprioceptive analysis.

ANNOTATED BIBLIOGRAPHY

DeCarlo MS, Talbot RW: Evaluation of ankle joint proprioception following injection of the anterior talofibular ligament. J Orthop Sports Phys Ther 8:70, 1986 (Describes the multiaxial balance evaluator used to assess an individual's balance, which should be a reflection of ankle proprioception. Specifications are available through the authors.)

Hicks JH: The mechanics of the foot: The joints. J Anat 87:345, 1953 (Early concepts of foot mechanics which remain true, although some of the information is outdated.)

Hoppenfeld S: Physical Examination of the Spine and Extremities. New York, Appleton-Century-Crofts, 1976 (This text illustrates various joint evaluations. Pictures and descriptions of palpatory landmarks are the best feature. Refer especially to Chap. 8.)

Hoppenfeld S: Physical Examination of the Foot by Complaint. In Jahss MH (ed): Disorders of the Foot. Philadelphia, WB Saunders, 1982 (A readable review of general patient complaints of foot pain with illustrations for clarification. Refer to Chap. 5.)

J Sports Phys Ther 7(3):91–114, 1985; 9(1):3–39, 1987 (These two issues of this journal provide significant reading for various ankle and foot topics. Articles by Donatelli are excellent, and review normal and abnormal biomechanics of the foot and ankle. Other topics include gait biomechanics and pathomechanics, peroneal influences on pathology, stability through ankle tapping and orthoses, and painful heel etiologies.)

Kapandji IA: The Physiology of the Joints: The Lower Limb, Vol 2. New York, Churchill Livingstone, 1970 (The ankle and foot complex is analyzed from an engineering and biomechanical focus. Drawings enhance the presentation, although the text can be somewhat confusing. This reference is a must for joint physiology.)

Kleiger B, Greenspan A, Norman A: Roentgenographic Examination of the Normal Foot and Ankle. In Jahss MH (ed): Disorders of the Foot. Philadelphia, WB Saunders 1982 (A cursory review of common ankle and foot pathologies evidenced on x-ray films. Very readable with good illustrations. See Chap. 6 especially.)

MacConaill MA, Basmajian JV: Muscles and Movements: A Basis for Human Kinesiology. Baltimore, Williams & Wilkins, 1969 (An excellent reference for human kinesiology, in particular, the discussion of gait.)

Norkin C, Levangie P: Joint Structure and Function: A Comprehensive Analysis. Philadelphia, FA Davis, 1983 (Chap. 10 contains a conceptual difference in presentation of the talocalcaneonavicular joint that may be consistent with other ankle and foot research.)

Norkin C, White D: Measurement of Motion: A Guide to Goniometry, pp 90–112. Philadelphia, FA Davis, 1985 (A concise and well-illustrated presentation of goniometric assessment.)

Phys Ther 59:7–33, 1979 (This special issue reviews the insensitive limb. Various articles identify good evaluative procedures along with treatment suggestions.)

Root MC, Orien WP, Weed JH: Clinical Biomechanics: Normal and Abnormal Function of the Foot, Vol 2. Los Angeles, Clinical Biomechanics Corp, 1977 (A good reference for general overview of the mechanics of the foot, including typical abnormalities in foot function.)

Williams PL, Warwick R (eds): Gray's Anatomy, 36th ed. Philadelphia, WB Saunders, 1980 (Chaps. 3 to 5 provide a detailed description of the osseous structures, the relevant musculature, and the arthrology for the ankle and foot complex. An excellent anatomical reference.)

25 Musculoskeletal Analysis: The Temporomandibular Joint and Cervical Spine

BARBARA BOURBON

In this chapter I will present an orderly and logical scheme to assess temporomandibular joint dysfunction and the influence of the cervical spine upon this dysfunction. Temporomandibular joint disorders result in signs and symptoms that may involve not only the jaw, but the ears, face, and neck, thereby disrupting the functions of chewing, hearing, speaking, and swallowing. Conversely, cervical spine disorders result in signs and symptoms that may involve not only the neck but the entire arm and shoulder girdle as well as the head and face, thereby altering pain-free movement of the appendicular skeleton and head. Thus, this chapter will outline the approach to the assessment of the cervical spine and temporomandibular joint.

To understand the normal function and consequent dysfunction of the cervical spine and temporomandibular joint, it is helpful to consider the evolutionary and developmental adaptions that have occurred within the stomatognathic system. This complex system includes the temporomandibular joints, the bony framework of the face, the muscles of mastication as well as the tongue and facial musculature, and the limiting ligaments and supporting dentoalveolar tissue that house and stabilize the teeth. The phylogenetic development of the craniofacial system is important in order to understand the functional relationship between the masticatory system and the cervical spine. The evolutionary changes emphasize the importance of posture on the head and neck.

Phylogenetic specialization of the facial framework and subsequent morphologic adaptations of the masticatory musculature have resulted in a powerful posterior bite, with a concomitant horizontal overbite. This overbite or overjet is recognized as the distance in the horizontal plane between the lingual, or tongue, surfaces of the upper teeth and the labial, or lip, surfaces of the lower teeth. Early hominid occlusion was that of an incisal edge-to-edge contact. Among Eskimo populations, dental occlusions have changed from incisal edge-to-edge contact to an overjet position within a single generation following the introduction of soft-cooked diets.

Another trend in the phylogenetic development of the hominids is the reduction of the facial skeleton under the cranium; this tendency is referred to as klinorhynchy. This trend is related to the development and expansion of the cerebral frontal lobes and the increasing use of teeth for grinding and slicing. The trend toward klinorhynchy, coupled with the acquisition of bipedal posture, finds the contents of the pharynx caught between the cranial base and the encroaching posterior surfaces of the maxillae and the pterygoid plates. To prevent this encroachment from becoming acute, the maxillary portion of the face has tended to be smaller. Additional biomechanical adaptations have resulted in a complex temporomandibular joint with a ginglymoarthrodial, or gliding hinge joint, replacing the quadripedal pure hinge mechanism of the temporomandibular joint.

Due to the acquisition of bipedal posture and the ability to speak, humans have had to sacrifice stability and simplicity of the temporomandibular joint for mobility and complexity. The upright posture necessitates extreme condylar translation to prevent jaw opening from interfering with the structures in the anterior part of the neck. In addition, speech requires functional versatility among the muscles of mastication, deglutition, and vocalization.

The resultant narrowing of the space between the pharynx and the mandible as humans acquired the bipedal posture has reduced the space available for mandibular movement during jaw opening. The temporomandibular joint apparently adapted by incorporating a forward glide during opening, thus moving the mandible farther forward, thereby providing room for the widest possible gape during mandibular depression.

The proximity of the temporomandibular joint to the pharynx and cervical region results in a uniquely interdependent relationship between these two regions. Trauma or dysfunction of one group of muscles, namely the prime movers of the mandible or accessory muscles such as the suprahyoid or infrahyoid muscles, may adversely affect all cervical supporting musculature. Conversely, trauma to the cervical region as in a whiplash injury may manifest as signs or symptoms of temporomandibular joint dysfunction. This structural, as well as functional, interdependence makes it imperative to consider both regions when evaluating either region.

ANATOMY AND BIOMECHANICS

CERVICAL SPINE

The body's most complicated and mobile articular system is designed for mobility at the expense of stability. Seven cervical spinal vertebrae are all held together by 14 zygapophyseal joints, 5 intervertebral discs, 12 joints of Luschka, and a musculoligamentous system that provides enormous maneuverability and range of motion and supports the entire head.

The cervical spine has three functions: (1) its articulating vertebral facets allow for the head's range of motion; (2) it furnishes support and stability for the head; and (3) it provides housing and transport for the spinal cord and vertebral artery.

The cervical spine has two functional units unique and dissimilar from the others: the upper two segments, the occipito-atlanto (skull and first cervical vertebra) and the atlanto-axial (C1-C2) units. The units below the axis (C2) consist of an anterior weight-bearing, shock-absorbing portion and posterior gliding section. The remaining cervical segments (C3-C7) have their respective vertebral bodies separated by a shock-absorbing fibrocartilaginous intervertebral disk. This disk is a self-contained fluid elastic system that absorbs shock, permits intermittent compression, and allows fluid displacement within its elastic container.

The posterior portion of the functional unit is composed of a neural vertebral arch, two transverse processes, a central posterior spinous process, and paired articulations. These paired posterior facet joints (Fig. 25-1), otherwise known as apophyseal or zygapophyseal, are lubricated by synovial fluid within the joint capsule. The joints of Luschka are located anterior to the functional unit and are also known as the uncovertebral joints (Fig. 25-2).

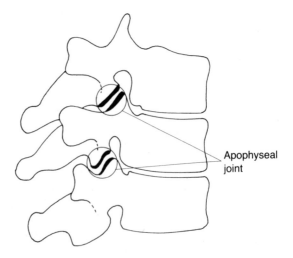

Apophyseal joint

Figure 25-1. Typical facet joint.

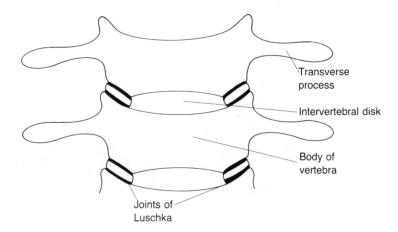

Transverse process

Intervertebral disk

Body of vertebra

Joints of Luschka

Figure 25-2. Joints of Luschka.

All segments of the neck move synchronously, but the direction and degree of movement varies at different segmental levels. The major degree of flexion, extension, and rotation occurs between the skull and the atlas and between the atlas and the axis. Below the axis the extent of movement is dependent upon ligamentous laxity and the distortion and compressibility of the intervertebral discs.

Movement in the anterior-posterior plane of flexion and extension occurs between the occiput and the atlas, producing the "yes" nod. Flexion occurs in the range of 10 degrees and extension, 25 degrees. Therefore, the head can move through a 35 degree range without neck participation. In lateral flexion and rotation of the head and neck, the occiput and atlas (C1) move as one.

The greatest rotational movement of the cervical spine occurs between the atlas (C1) and the axis (C2). The normal cervical spine provides approximately 140 degrees of rotation from right to left. More than 50% of this motion is provided by the articulation between C1 and C2. Between C2 and C7, movements of flexion, extension, lateral side-bending, and rotation are possible. Flexion and extension occur as a "gliding" movement of the upper upon the lower vertebrae. Anterior, or flexion, and posterior, or extension, movements occur as a relatively pure motion. Lateral side-bending causes ipsilateral rotation, and rotation initiates ipsilateral side-bending, or lateral flexion.

Although the greatest amount of movement in the cervical spine takes place between C1 and C2 (as much as 90 degrees), the most active and most mobile region lies between C4 and C6. This is also the region of maximum static curvature, and thus maximum stress.

The cervical region serves as a relatively narrow elastic support for the 12-pound human head. The ligaments remain the sole support of the head when the muscles are overpowered or fatigued. The ligaments connecting the occiput to the atlas are dense and broad, protecting the entrance of the spinal cord through the foramen magnum into the skull. The remaining segments of the cervical spine from C2 to C7, and the disk's annulus, are reinforced by the anterior and posterior longitudinal ligaments. You may wish to refer to an anatomy text for a complete description and review of these structures.

CERVICAL MUSCULATURE

The neck muscles may be divided into two major functional groups: those that flex and extend the head, and those that flex and extend the cervical spine. The capital (head) flexors flex the head upon the neck and are recognized as the longus capitis, the rectus capitis anterior and lateral, and the suprahyoid muscles. The head extensors attach to the skull and move the head upon the neck; they are recognized as the longissimus capitis, semispinalis capitis, and the splenius capitis muscles.

The cervical flexors attach exclusively upon the cervical vertebrae and have no functional attachment to the skull; they are the anterior and middle scalenes and the head and neck muscle, the sternocleidomastoid. The cervical extensors originate and attach upon the cervical spine and alter the curvature of the cervical spine; they are the longissimus cervicis, semispinalis cervicis, and the splenius cervicis muscles.

TEMPOROMANDIBULAR JOINT

The temporomandibular joint, located just anterior to the external auditory meatus and the cartilaginous tragus of the ear, is the articulation between the condylar process of the mandible, and the mandibular fossa and the articular eminence of the temporal bone. Because the condyle translates from the concave mandibular fossa to the convex eminence of the temporal bone, the shape and the relationship of the articulating surfaces, and the space between them, change with functional movements. These changing surfaces are accommodated by a flexible interarticular disk. The joint is surrounded by a capsule lined with synovium and subdivided into separate and distinct compartments. A larger, superior synovial compartment includes the articulation of the undersurface of the temporal bone with the superior surface of the fibrocartilaginous disk. A smaller, inferior synovial compartment is composed of the inferior surface of the fibrocartilaginous disk and the articular surface of the mandibular condyle.

Laterally, the capsule is thickened by the temporomandibular ligament. Medially, the capsule is thin and loose. Posteriorly, the capsule is loose and attached to the disk by highly elastic tissue that is innervated and vascularized. The anterior portion of the capsule is attached to the superior head of the lateral pterygoid muscle. Tendinous fibers from this superior belly of the lateral pterygoid muscle pass through the capsule to insert onto the disk.

Mandibular Movements

Basically, two types of mandibular movement can be identified: rotation and translation.

Mandibular movements guided by the temporomandibular joints and muscle activity occur as a series of interrelated three-dimensional rotational and translational movements.

Rotation

The mandible has three axes of rotation: a medial-lateral axis, an anterior-posterior axis, and a longitudinal axis (Fig. 25-3). Rotation about a mediolateral axis causes opening and closing and occurs between the condyle-articular disk portion of the lower joint compartment. This mediolateral axis of rotation provides a hinge movement in the sagittal plane for rotation, which occurs during the first few degrees of opening.

Mandibular movement about an anterior-posterior axis occurs when one condyle moves

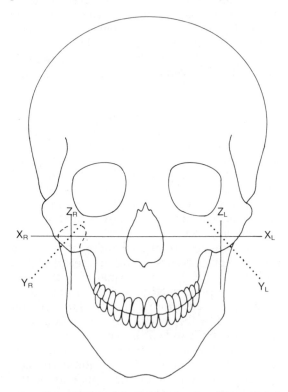

Figure 25-3. Axes of rotation for the right and left temporomandibular joints: X_R–X_L, axes of motion in the sagittal plane; Y_R–Y_L, axes of motion on the frontal plane; and Z_R–Z_L, axes of motion in the transverse plane.

inferiorly while the opposite condyle remains relatively stationary. This motion occurs in the frontal plane and produces a lateral side-to-side shift, or lateral deviation.

Motion about the longitudinal or vertical axis of rotation occurs when one condyle moves anteriorly about an axis through the opposite condyle. This motion occurs in the horizontal plane.

Translation

Gliding movements occur in the superior compartment between the inferior surface of the temporal bone and the superior surface of the disk. Translation occurs during the downward and forward movement of the disc-condyle complex, in a forward or protrusive movement. A return of this complex to the upward and backward position is referred to as the retrusive movement.

Functional Movements

The biomechanics of the temporomandibular joint are determined by the morphology and structural arrangement of its parts as they relate to the demands of function. These bilateral ginglymoarthrodial joints, suspended by strong temporomandibular ligaments, are capable of linear, sliding movements down and around the articular eminence.

As the condyles continue to rotate, the mandible glides forward on the disk. This disk remains between the anterior slope of the condyle and the articular eminence. As the translatory phase begins, the upper surface of the articular disk slides down against the articular eminence, rounds the crest, and moves forward along its anterior plane. During the closing phase, the upper surface of the disk retraces the sliding movement back to the resting position. During this return phase the disk rotates anteriorly until the cycle has been completed.

Protrusion-Retrusion

Protrusion occurs when the mandible is moved forward with the teeth separated. This forward movement of the mandible takes place in the superior joint compartment, consisting of disk and condyle moving downward and forward.

Retrusion is the return phase of the translatory cycle with the retracing of the disk and condyle back to the rest position. Retrusion beyond the rest position rarely amounts to more than 3 mm and is not in a functional position.

Lateral Deviation

During lateral excursion the disk and condyle of the nonworking joint move medially as they approach the articular eminence. During a simple lateral movement, there is motion occurring about the sagittal, horizontal, and vertical axes.

MASTICATORY MUSCULATURE

The intrinsic mandibular prime movers include four pairs of varying-shaped muscles that directly influence mandibular movements. Three of these, the masseter, medial pterygoid, and temporalis muscles, exert their power in a vertical direction, acting as powerful mandibular elevators. The lateral pterygoid muscle, oriented in a horizontal plane, pulls the mandible forward in a protrusive movement.

Of the extrinsic muscles of mastication, only the digastric and geniohyoid muscles exert a direct pull on the mandible, pulling it in a posterior and inferior direction, thereby retruding and depressing the mandible. The remaining suprahyoid muscles, the mylohyoid and stylohyoid along with the infrahyoid group, and the cervical musculature are recognized as extrinsic muscles of mastication. These extrinsic muscles are responsible for maintenance of postural alignment of the skull with respect to cervical alignment (Fig. 25-4).

SUBJECTIVE EXAMINATION

As in all evaluations, a clear chronological history is essential to the therapist's understanding of the patient's problem, its etiology, and its impact on the patient's life. A complete history must include a review of the patient's medical and dental care. Relevant trauma must also be identified. In addition, the patient's psychological make-up can greatly influence temporomandibular joint pathology. Finally,

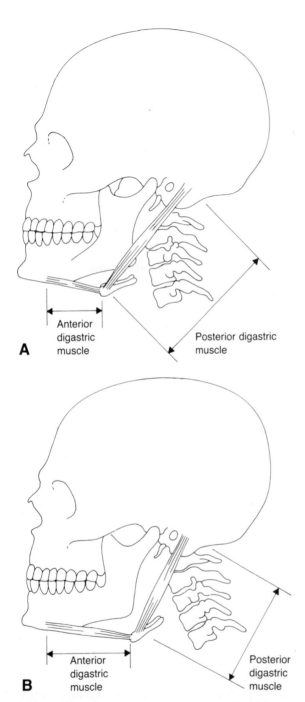

Figure 25-4. The extrinsic muscles of mastication are responsible for maintaining postural alignment of the skull with respect to cervical alignment. *(A)* Normal alignment. *(B)* Forward posture.

the patient's occupation and daily habits may be relevant to the problem. Pertinent points in each area of the history are presented below.

MEDICAL HISTORY

A medical history should include any arthritic condition. If ear, nose, or throat symptoms such as tinnitus (ringing in the ears), sinusitis, cysts, or polyps are reported, consultation with an otorhinolaryngologist should be considered. Additional medical information, past and present, should be sought such as surgery, fractures or sprains. The therapist should also check for endocrine disorders, particularly hypothyroidism because temporomandibular joint symptoms appear to show a correlation with hypothyroidism in women. Any complaints that suggest a medical problem should be identified and appropriate consultations requested. Allergies to medication and the type of drugs currently being taken should be listed.

DENTAL HISTORY

A dental history should indicate previous temporomandibular joint treatment and results as well as any familial tendency toward temporomandibular joint dysfunction. Pain symptoms should be recorded including date and location of onset, type or quality of pain, and triggering devices of pain.

Oral symptoms other than pain would include clenching and grinding habits, muscle fatigue, gingival bleeding, and facial swelling. Vertigo and syncope should be noted with respect to frequency and duration.

Ear symptoms related to temporomandibular joint dysfunction would include tinnitus, popping and whooshing noises on opening and closing, stuffiness in the ear, and changes in hearing patterns.

TRAUMA

Recent or past episodes of trauma may shed light upon the etiology of the dysfunction. Should trauma occur between the thoracic inlet and the cranial base, it can disturb sympathetic and cranial nerves, veins, arteries, and lymphatics. As a consequence cerebral congestion, faulty cerebrospinal fluid (CSF) metabolism, weakened tissues, headaches, and neuralgias may occur.

Acute trauma may result in sprains of the cervical region caused by whiplash injury. Trauma of the masticatory musculature may be due to prolonged opening of the mouth as a result of extended dental treatment, extractions, tonsillectomies, or intubations.

Chronic trauma is often the result of untreated acute conditions such as malocclusion, missing teeth, or faulty restorative and orthodontic treatment.

STRESS

Stress increases physiological tension within skeletal muscle. The chronically tense muscle, in a state of perpetual overuse, will react by becoming an intensely painful, sore muscle. In time, manifestations of this pain-dysfunction syndrome may become evident by occlusal wear, tooth mobility, unilateral mastication, abnormal swallowing patterns, muscle tenderness, and aberrant sounds within the temporomandibular joint.

OTHER CONSIDERATIONS

Habits such as bruxing (grinding of teeth), pipe smoking, tongue thrusting, and pencil chewing can offset the normal pattern of masticatory behavior and lead to asymmetrical muscle activity and mandibular malalignment.

Occupational postures such as the static, exaggerated kyphotic seated position of the computer operator, typist, or student places undue stress upon the temporomandibular joints due to the stretch upon the suprahyoid muscles as a result of the forward head posture.

OBJECTIVE EXAMINATION

Objective assessment must include the following elements: (1) evaluation of posture; (2) palpation of muscles and joints; (3) assessment of range of motion; (4) assessment of joint play within the temporomandibular joint; (5) assess-

ment of muscle function, and (6) a neurological assessment. Each element is described below.

POSTURE

The patient should be properly draped, and placed in a good light. Observe the patient's posture while she is sitting, standing, and walking. Check it from the front, back, and side. Note such anatomic details as scapular height, spinal curves, head tilt, and head posikion. Specifically observe the extent of cervical lordosis, thoracic kyphosis, and lumbar lordosis.

Observe the patient for any abnormal appearance, such as extreme height or shortness, an unusually long or short neck, retracted mandible, crooked teeth, or a high palate. These as well as facial asymmetry, abnormal facial development, and asymmetric bone and muscle development suggest congenital anomalies of the cervical spine.

Typically, the patient with temporomandibular joint dysfunction, and with emotional overtones, will exhibit a posture of elevated shoulders, forward head, stiff neck and back, and have shallow restricted breathing.

PALPATION

Cervical Region

Palpate the anterior and posterior cervical triangles for the brachial plexus and examine the site of the subclavian artery. Deep palpation allows examination of the transverse process of the atlas.

In the anterior triangle, identify the following landmarks. The hyoid bone is adjacent to C3, the thyroid cartilage is at the level of C4.

Observe the levator scapulae, trapezii, rhomboids, and scalene muscles and the superior angle of the scapula, checking for atrophy, weakness, and neurological signs. Observe the deltoid, supraspinatus, and infraspinatus for atrophy. Examine the skin for color, scars, temperature, and ecchymosis. Palpate the carotid arteries and determine the pulse rate. Examine the sternocleidomastoid muscles and their angles relative to head and neck alignment (each should be approximately 45 degrees). Mark sites of tenderness with a felt-tip pen and try to correlate with local structures.

Facial Region

Palpate the skin for warmth, tenderness, moisture, and mobility. Palpate the muscles of mastication for tenderness, pain, consistency, mobility, and signs of spasm. Palpation of the muscles of mastication should routinely include the origin and insertion of the masseter, temporalis, medial pterygoid, and origin of the lateral pterygoid muscles. In addition, a cursory examination of the muscles in the maxillofacial region should be palpated, including the facial muscles, sublingual and suprahyoids, and the infrahyoid muscles.

Temporomandibular Joint

First, palpate the joint extra-auricularly by palpating the condylar heads immediately anterior to the tragus of the ear. Do this with the mouth closed, then again with the mandible in a relaxed state with a free-way space discernible between the maxillary and mandibular incisors (front teeth). You should feel a forward drift of the condylar heads during opening. The posterior aspect of the joint can best be palpated intra-auricularly through the external auditory meatus. Pain and tenderness in this region suggest a capsulitis. Abnormal capsular thickening, warmth, and swelling should be noted.

Palpation should be performed bilaterally so that a comparison of both joints can be made and any symmetrical movements recorded. Palpable clicking, popping, or snapping should also be noted. Note the type of sound associated with the movements and the particular phase of movement in which it occurs. Palpation should be performed during all movements: opening, closing, lateral deviation, protrusion, and retrusion.

RANGE OF MOTION

Cervical

With the patient sitting, observe the movement of the entire cervical spine in flexion, extension, lateral flexion, and rotation. Determine the passive ranges of motion and then see if you can actively provide overpressure to increase them. Next, test all four motions against resistance to observe the patient's strength and to determine whether muscle contraction against resistance produces pain. Your goal is to produce signs and symptoms that will identify the pain-sensitive structure for a precise diagnosis. Determine whether the shoulder or any structure within it is contributing to dysfunction or pain.

Temporomandibular Joint

Observe the general patterns of active range of motion, elevation, depression, lateral deviation, protrusion, and retrusion for freedom of range and symmetry. Ascertain where in the range pain occurs. Masticatory pain is typically not well localized. It may be felt in and around the joint or ear and often it is felt diffusely through the face, teeth, jaws, and mouth.

Note the type of end-feel as well as the presence of pain and spasms. Determine the strength by applying resistance to mandibular opening, protrusion, and lateral deviation. Pain arising in the lateral pterygoid muscles may be provoked by resisted deviation to the nonpainful side.

CAPSULAR PATTERNS

Temporomandibular Joint

Record the restrictions of movement and asynchronous patterns of movement; measure the maximal maxillary to mandibular incisal opening. Lateral movements should be recorded because these movements are often limited earlier and to a relatively greater degree than vertical motions. Abnormal or premature translatory movements will be evident by a reduction of incisal overjet and excessive prominence of the condylar heads.

Note whether pain is provoked when the jaws are in occlusion and when the patient is asked to bite against a tongue blade on one side. Such tests help distinguish muscle spasms from diskitis and retrodiskitis. Abnormal capsular thickening, warmth, and swelling should be noted.

One of the most common intracapsular dysfunctions of the temporomandibular joint is the internal derangement of the articular disk. This is most commonly characterized by anterior displacement of the disk and a posterior superior displacement of the condyle. The most common signs of internal derangements are: (1) reciprocal clicking, (2) the locking condition, and (3) osteoarthritic conditions.

Two specific pathologic conditions of the temporomandibular joint must be recognized. One is in relation to a hypermobile joint with excessive translatory glide that induces sounds in the joints like reciprocal clicking, subluxation, or dislocations. The second is locking in the joint that is characterized by hypomobility; that is, a joint that exhibits limitation of opening mainly restricted to rotation in the joint with an average opening of 25 mm. The locking of the joint, or close-lock, can be of two major types. One is the shortening of the periarticular connective tissue as a defensive mechanism. With passive stretch, one sees a considerable increase in range of motion with a gummy endfeel. The second is a close-lock caused by an anterior displacement of the disk. This is characterized by a posterior-superior displacement of the condyle with a limitation of opening and a hard end-feel (Fig. 25-5). Passive stretch will produce little or no increase in range of motion. Approaches to treatment in these two situations of hypomobile and hypermobile joints are quite different.

ASSESSMENT OF MUSCLE FUNCTION

Deviation of the mandibular incisal path during opening is a shift from midline in opening with a return to midline position upon completion of mandibular elevation. This differs from deflection, which implies a discursive movement from a straight path but terminates in the deviated path. These aberrant postures often reflect masticatory muscular dysfunction.

Mandibular Elevators

Marked restriction of mandibular vertical opening may be due to pain or myospasm within the masseter muscle; unilateral masseter in-

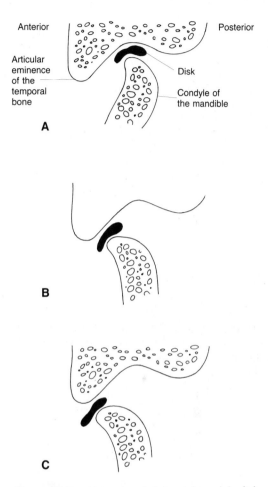

Figure 25-5. Normal and abnormal condyle disk relationships: *(A)* normal closed position, *(B)* normal open position, and *(C)* anterior disk displacement.

volvement tends to deviate the mandible toward the affected side. Myofascial trigger points in the muscle refer pain to the lower jaw, molar teeth, and maxilla. When acute, the trigger zones restrict opening to one and one-half knuckle measurement. Normally, a patient opens sufficiently to place three of his knuckles into the incisel opening.

Headaches appear to be a common symptom of temporalis muscle involvement, with pain felt throughout the temple, along the eyebrow, behind the eye, and in the maxillary teeth. With pain or tenderness noted in the posterior fibers of the temporalis muscle, the mandible may exhibit a zig-zag deviation during opening and closing.

Referred pain from the medial pterygoid muscle is found in the tongue, pharynx, hard palate, and ear. Fullness in the ear may be associated with medial pterygoid movement as it relates to the tensor veli palatini muscle and the subsequent opening of the eustachian tube. Chewing or clenching the teeth often produces increased pain within the medial pterygoid muscle. Mandibular opening is usually restricted, and unilateral involvement produces deviations of the mandible toward the opposite side.

Mandibular Depressors

Pain within the temporomandibular joint may be a reflection of referred pain from the lateral pterygoid muscle. Malocclusion with premature occlusal contact may reflect hyperactivity of this muscle, and bruxism may be either the cause or result of this overuse. Marked deviation from midline during opening is away from the side of the affected lateral pterygoid muscle. With temporomandibular joint pain-dysfunction syndromes, the lateral pterygoid has been reported to be more tender to palpation than any other masticatory muscle.

Pain arising from the posterior belly of the digastric muscles radiates into the upper part of the sternocleidomastoid muscle to the pharynx and larynx. Pain referred from the anterior belly of the digastric radiates to the four lower incisor teeth. Coughing, swallowing, and retrusion of the mandible strongly recruit the digastric muscles. Therefore, these motions may be performed to check for digastric muscle integrity. Involvement of the posterior belly of the digastric tends to pull the mandible to the same side. The anterior digastric may be tested by pulling down the corners of the mouth aggressively enough to tense the anterior neck muscles. If positive, this motion will activate incisal toothache. Trigger zones in the posterior belly of the digastric are common when trismus, caused by masseter tension, has become chronic.

Tongue

Normal excursion of the tongue includes placement of the tongue outside the oral vestibule with protrusion and lateral deviation being uninhibited by a restrictive frenulum. Protrusion should be midline and lateral deviations balanced side to side; these motions test the integrity of the extrinsic musculature.

Intrinsic tongue movements alter the shape of the tongue and should provide for a variety of configurations. Elevation of the tongue during swallowing should be followed by tongue depression. The tongue rest position should be noted behind the central incisors.

Accessory Muscles

The remaining suprahyoid muscles, the stylohyoid, geniohyoid, and mylohyoid muscles assist in mandibular depression. Their action can best be noted by palpating the excursion of the hyoid bone with the mandible fixed, and conversely their movement upon the mandible with the hyoid bone fixed.

The infrahyoid muscle group, which acts upon the hyoid bone by depression or fixation of the hyoid bone, often manifests such symptoms as sore throat, pain upon talking, and shoulder pain caused by omohyoid splinting.

Cervical Muscles

In the first, most superficial layer of posterior cervical muscles the upper, middle, and lower fibers of the trapezius muscles are located. The upper fibers of the trapezius refer pain unilaterally upward along the posterolateral aspect of the neck to the mastoid process and are the major source of "tension neckache." Additional referred pain extends to the angle of the mandible.

The fibers of the middle trapezius often refer a burning pain between the medial borders of the scapulae and the spinous processes of C6-T2. The lower trapezius refers pain along the paraspinal muscles from the mid-thoracic to the high cervical region. The adjacent mastoid process, acromion process, and subscapular region may be the sites of an annoying deep ache with hyperactivity of the lower trapezius.

The common complaint of "stiff neck" is more often the result of myospasms in the levator scapulae muscles. Pain radiates from the base of the neck to the vertebral border of the scapula and shoulder posteriorly. The patient tends to hold the neck rigid, with the head tilted toward the involved side; neck rotation is restricted with the face turned toward the side of pain; neck flexion is blocked at the end of movement and extension is usually unaffected.

The deeper splenius capitis and the splenius cervicis muscles usually refer pain from the vertex or occiput, respectively. Hyperactivity of the splenius cervicis and levator scapulae may completely block rotation to the ipsilateral side. Often pain in the orbit and blurring of vision are associated with splenius cervicis myospasms. Postural stresses such as chronic forward head activate these muscles. Trauma such as rear-end collisions invariably involves trigger zones in these muscles.

The third and fourth layers of the posterior musculature include the semispinalis capitis, semispinalis cervicis, and longissimus capitis in the third layer, and the multifidus and rotatores in the fourth layer. The trigger points in these areas refer pain and tenderness to the suboccipital region and to the superior border of the scapula. Palpable tenderness is often noted over the back of the head and neck. Pressure of the head upon a pillow is often intolerable. Should the greater occipital nerve become involved, numbness, tingling, and burning pain in the scalp may be reported.

With posterior cervical involvement, patients often hold the head and neck rigid with the shoulder dramatically elevated. Head and neck flexion and rotation are restricted. Should the involvement be on one side, the head and neck are flexed to that side.

The deepest layer of posterior cervical muscles are the four suboccipital muscles. Pain referred from these muscles extends from the occiput to the eye and forehead and is of a deeper quality in the upper neck region. Generally head and neck mobility are not markedly affected. Deep tenderness is elicited upon palpation.

The anterior cervical muscles include the scalene group, longus coli, and the sternocleidomastoid muscles. Myospasms of any of the anterior, middle, or posterior scalene muscles may refer pain anteriorly to the chest, laterally to the upper extremity, and posteriorly to the medial borders of the scapula and mid-scapulae region. The referred pain on the left may be mistaken for angina pectoris. When taut, the anterior and middle scalene muscles often entrap part of the brachial plexus at the thoracic outlet with subsequent neurological symptoms of numbness and tingling in the hand.

A common complaint from scalene involvement is deep aching soreness in the neck and arm muscles. The patient may be observed kneading the extremity in an attempt to wring out the soreness. Lateral side-bending to the contralateral side is restricted and painful. Neck rotation is painful at the extreme range on the ipsilateral side.

The sternocleidomastoid muscle has two components that evoke two distinct sensory disturbances. The sternal division refers pain to the vertex, occiput, face, eye, throat, and sternum. The clavicular division usually involves symptoms such as frontal headaches and earaches, including proprioceptive dizziness related to posture and disturbed equilibrium. Neck pain and stiffness are not common features of sternocleidomastioid involvement.

NEUROLOGICAL ASSESSMENT

If the patient's pain is constant, severe, unrelieved, and disabling, and results in sleeplessness, a neurological screening should be included in the objective examination.

Testing for Nerve Root Compression

Use the quadrant position to alter the size of the intervertebral foramina and determine if the nerve roots can be compressed. Start with head extension so that the inferior facet of the vertebra above glides posteriorly on the facet of the vertebra below, narrowing the foramen. If this produces shoulder pain or paresthesias, or numbness, *go no further!* The nerve root has already been compressed in the foramen.

If these symptoms do not appear, add lateral flexion, which closes the foramina toward the side of flexion and opens it on the opposite side. If no symptoms appear, add full rotation, which maximally closes the foramen on one side and opens it on the opposite side.

Individual Roots

First and Second Cervical Roots. The first intervertebral disk lies between the second and third cervical vertebrae. Therefore, pain in the head cannot be due to a disk lesion at the upper two joints because they do not contain a disk. This pain may be an example of extrasegmental referred pain from the dura mater. Joint pain from C1 may spread to the vertex of the skull or from C2 to the temple, forehead, and behind the eye.

Third Cervical Root. The third cervical root is seldom affected. However, when involved, it produces unilateral pain in the neck, and numbness around the ear and posterior part of the cheek.

Fourth Cervical Root. The pain spreads outward from the mid-neck and is concentrated at the shoulder. A horizontal band of cutaneous analgesia, 2 to 4 cm wide, may be found along the spine of the scapula, the mid-deltoid area, and the clavicle like a half-loop. No muscle weakness is discernible.

Fifth Cervical Root. The pain extends from the scapula area to the front of the arm and forearm as far as the radial side of the hand, but it does not extend to the thumb. Pins and needles are not commonly present. Weakened muscle groups are the deltoid and biceps. The biceps jerk may be sluggish or absent.

Sixth Cervical Root. The pain spreads down the front of the arm and forearm to the radial side of the hand, and pins and needles are reported in the thumb and the index finger. Weakened muscles include the biceps brachialis, supinator, and extensor carpi radialis. The biceps jerk is sluggish or absent.

Seventh Cervical Root. The seventh cervical root is the most common root affected. Pain extends from the scapular area down the back of the arm to the fingertips. Pins and needles are usually felt in the index, long, and ring fingers. The outstanding weak muscle is the triceps. In addition, both the radial flexors and extensors may be weakened. Cutaneous analgesia is often found on the dorsum of the long and index finger.

Eighth Cervical Root. Painful areas include the low scapular region, the back and inner surface of the arm, and the inner forearm. Pins and needles are usually felt at the long, ring, and little fingers. The weak muscles are the ulnar deviators of the wrist, the extensor and adductor muscles of the thumb, the extensor muscles of the fingers, and the adductor of the digits. Cutaneous analgesia may be noted at the fifth finger.

First Thoracic Root. Most patients with symptoms attributable to the first thoracic root are usually suffering from some other disorder, such as cervical rib, secondary vertebral neoplasm, or pressure on the median or ulnar nerve. If the lesion is at this level, pain is felt diffusely in the lower scapular area and spreads down the inner aspect of the arm to the ulnar border of the hand, where pins and needles and slight numbness may be noted.

Trigeminal Nerve

The functions of the trigeminal nerve are determined by testing the corneal reflex, sensation over the face, and the motor strength in the masseter, temporalis, and pterygoid muscles. The afferent portion of the corneal reflex may be elicited by gentle stroking of the cornea with a wisp of cotton. Under normal circumstances, an immediate blink response occurs bilaterally.

Sensation over the face is tested with bilateral simultaneous stimulation using touch and pin prick to differentiate acuity between the two sides. Motor function is assessed by having the patient clench the jaws tightly while temporalis and masseter muscles are palpated. The pterygoids are tested by lateral resistive movement. Both the afferent and efferent portions of the jaw jerk reflex are located in the trigeminal nerve.

Facial Nerve

The facial nerve, which is the seventh cranial nerve, supplies efferent fibers to the muscles of facial expression and the posterior belly of the digastric. Secretomotor fibers pass to the lacrimal gland and the mucous membrane of the nose, nasopharynx, palate, and pharynx. Other fibers pass to the chorda tympani, which mediates taste from the anterior two thirds of the tongue.

With facial weakness, the patient may present with loss of nasolabial fold, sagging of the lower eyelid, and inability to close the eye. Facial weakness may be detected during smiling when the corners of the mouth are drawn to the unaffected side.

Glossopharyngeal Nerve

The ninth cranial nerve supplies (1) motor fibers to the stylopharyngeus muscle, (2) secretomotor fibers to the parotid gland, (3) sensory fibers from the back of the tongue and pharynx and carotid sinus, and (4) taste and general sensation from the posterior one third of the tongue.

Sensation over the posterior third of the tongue and pharyngeal wall may be tested by touching these areas with a cotton applicator. The gag reflex consists of elevation of the palate and retraction of the tongue with contraction of the pharyngeal muscles when the posterior pharyngeal wall is stimulated. Absence of the gag reflex may occur in hysteria as well as lesions to the ninth cranial nerve.

Hypoglossal Nerve

The hypoglossal nerve, which is the twelfth cranial nerve, supplies motor fibers to the muscles of the tongue. Upon examination, the patient is asked to protrude the tongue, which should be in the midline. With lower motor neuron lesions, the tongue is deviated toward the side of the lesion when the patient is asked to protrude the tongue. The strength of the tongue muscles may be checked by asking the patient to push on the cheek against resistance of the examiner's hand. The protruded tongue should be examined for atrophy, which produces increased wrinkling and some loss of bulk on the side of the lesion. Tremor of the tongue muscles should be differentiated from fasciculations. Tremor is rhythmic, whereas fasciculations are random contractions of individual motor units within the tongue.

When normal movements of the tongue are impaired, resulting dysrhythmias and incoordination are easily recognized as explosive, thick speech.

INTERPRETATION OF FINDINGS

The findings from the assessments described above should lead to (1) the identification of the source of pain; (2) an understanding of the underlying mechanisms causing the pain; (3) a plan of care to reduce or eliminate the pain; and (4) a plan to nullify or reduce the effects of the pathological mechanisms. In the case of temporomandibular joint pathology, use of the syndromes described by McKenzie for low back pain can be helpful in identifying the source and mechanism of pain production. The three syndromes presented by McKenzie are particularly pertinent in the temporomandibular joint. They are described below as they apply to temporomandibular joint pathology.

The *postural syndrome* presents a pattern of pain resulting from prolonged, undue stress on otherwise normal tissue. The prolonged forward head posture causes the suprahyoid muscles to pull the mandible posteriorly, or retrusively, causing decreased vertical dimension in the temporomandibular joint and increasing the stresses on the joint and causing pain. In the postural syndrome, restoration of normal posture normalizes the joint stresses and eliminates the pain, and no further intervention is indicated. However, it should be noted that an isolated "postural syndrome" is rare, because prolonged poor posture will ultimately lead to adaptive changes in the tissue. These changes often lead to a *dysfunction syndrome.*

A dysfunction syndrome presents with pain at the end of ranges of motion *and* abnormal ranges as the result of changes in surrounding soft tissue. For example, the reduced vertical dimension secondary to poor posture is often followed by capsular restriction and muscle tightness, leading to limited range of motion of the temporomandibular joint.

Because of its unique structure and in particular its disk, the temporomandibular joint is prone to *derangement syndromes* in which the normal articular alignment is disrupted. Joint sounds such as popping and clicking associated with abnormal movement of the disk are telltale signs of derangement. Clicking suggests violation of the rules of synovial joints, which are friction-free joints. An audible click on opening indicates condylar movement as it snaps under the posterior band of the disk and falls into its normal relationship on the concave surface of the disk. An audible click on closing indicates a posterior slide of the condyle to the posterior band of the disk with resultant anterior displacement of the disk.

Reciprocal clicking is classified as early, intermediate, or late depending upon the degree of opening at which the click occurs. A joint that produces a clicking sound is a mobile joint, because a locked joint does not click. If the click occurs in the end range of opening, this indicates anterior disk displacement to a greater degree than if the click occurred at the beginning of opening. Locking occurs when the disk becomes lodged anterior to the condyle.

When a grinding sound is recognized in the joint, this crepitus is suggestive of surface wear of either cartilage or condyle, and indicates possible degenerative arthritis.

By classifying the patient's complaints according to these three syndromes—*postural, dysfunction,* and *derangement*—the examiner has identified the source of pain (articular or soft tissue) and has essentially defined the underlying mechanisms. Thus, outlining a plan of treatment is straightforward. The goals for treatment are generally to reduce pain and to improve function.

ANNOTATED BIBLIOGRAPHY

Bell, WE: Temporomandibular Disorders: Classification, Diagnosis, Management, 2nd ed. Chicago, Year Book Publishers, 1985 (As the name implies, a good reference for classification, diagnosis, and mangement of temporomandibular joint dysfunction.)

Cyriax JH: Manual of Orthopedic Medicine. Boston, Butterworths, 1983 (A comprehensive hands-on approach to the evaluation of the cervical spine. Also ties together cervical spine evaluation with temporomandibular joint symptomatology.)

Friedman MH, Weisberg J: Temporomandibular Joint Disorders. Baltimore, MD, Quintessence Publishing, 1985 (A comprehensive interaction and appropriate use of the team approach between a dentist and a physical therapist.)

Gelb H: Clinical Mangement of Head, Neck, and TMJ Pain Dysfunction. Philadelphia, WB Saunders, 1977 (A general introduction to the management of TMJ dysfunction with contributions reflecting a multidisciplinary approach. The last chapter is devoted to physical therapy. Given the year of publication, 1977, and the lack of team approach as it applied to physical therapy, it serves as a milestone for dental and physical therapy teamwork.)

Hoppenfeld S: Physical Examinations of the Spine and Extremities. New York, Appleton-Century-Crofts, 1976 (A concise, descriptive, hands-on approach to evaluation and treatment techniques of the cervical spine.)

Kapandji IA: The Physiology of the Joints, Vol 3. New York, Churchill Livingstone, 1974 (Descriptive analysis of the cervical spine and its biomechanical relationship to the temporomandibular joint. Excellent text for comprehension of postural alignment and dysfunction.)

McKenzie, Robin: The Lumbar Spine. Walkanae, New Zealand, Spinal Publications Ltd, 1981

Neff PA: Occlusion and Function: A Teaching Aid, 4th ed. Washington, D.C., Georgetown University, 1980 (Excellent visual analyses of anatomy, biomechanics, and dysfunction of the stomatognathic system. May also be purchased in slide form for visual teaching presentation.)

Shore NA: Temporomandibular Joint Dysfunction and Occlusal Equilibrium. Philadelphia, JB Lippincott, 1976

Sicker H: Oral Anatomy. St Louis, CV Mosby, 1949 (Fundmental text for dental terminology and relationships within the stomatognathic system.)

26 Musculoskeletal Analysis: The Thoracic Spine

GAIL M. JENSEN

Symptoms referred to the thoracic spine can mimic a wide variety of disorders, many of which are visceral in origin. Thus, the evaluation process is critical in determining whether the signs and symptoms are mechanical and dependent on activity and rest, or whether the problem lies beyond the realm of physical therapy. The upper thoracic spine is further complicated by the discrepancy between dermatomes and myotomes. The scapula and muscle overlying the scapula area are derived from middle and lower cervical segments. The skin overlying these structures and the ribs is derived from thoracic segments. Therefore, pain felt in the upper, posterior thorax could have a cervical or thoracic origin. The cervical spine must be ruled out as a source of symptoms before determining that the problem is thoracic (Cyriax). You can now understand why treatment of the thoracic spine would depend on both a thorough evaluation and an understanding of applied anatomy.

APPLIED ANATOMY

JOINTS AND MUSCLES

Mechanically, the thoracic spine is less mobile than other regions of the spine. The direction of the facet or apophyseal joints for T1 through T10 is close to frontal plane and should allow for free lateral movement. However, motion is limited by the sternum and rib cage. Movement between adjacent vertebrae is also limited by relatively thin intervertebral disks (Moore).

Several joints must be considered when examining the thoracic spine. The intervertebral joint is a fibrocartilaginous joint. The facet or zygapophyseal joints are classified as plane, synovial joints. The costovertebral joints between the ribs and vertebral bodies and the costotransverse joints between the ribs and transverse processes are both synovial joints. The costovertebral joints allow for plane-type movement. The costotransverse joints where the neck and tubercles of the ribs articulate with the transverse processes (except for ribs 11 and 12) allow for both rotation and gliding movements (Moore). The joints on the anterior thorax include (1) the sternocostal joints between the costal cartilage and the sternum and (2) the costochondral joints between the costal cartilages and the depressions at the ends of the ribs.

The muscles of the thorax, which both initiate and control movement, are mostly arranged in layers. An easy way to remember the posterior trunk muscles is that they are categorized by layer, area, function, and direction. The layers from deep to superficial are the rotators, multifidus, semispinalis, and sacrospinalis. These layers are incompletely separated. In the anterior thorax there are also layers of muscles, which are external and internal as well as intercostal. Refer to a standard anatomy text for a complete description and review of these structures.

The spinous processes of the thoracic spine are easily palpable, but you must remember that they slant downward. The spinous process of T1 is very prominent; it is more prominent than C7 when the neck is flexed. The middle seven or eight thoracic segments have the tip of the spinous process at the same level as the lamina of the vertebra below. This is not true for the upper two or three thoracic segments or the lower two or three segments, where the lower margin of the spinous process lies about on the same level as the lower edge of the same vertebral body. The seventh thoracic segment is usually the source of greatest angulation in the thoracic spine, and for that reason is referred to as the transitional vertebra (Grieve, 1981.)

MECHANICS

Figure 26-1 illustrates the average amount of movement for each level of the thoracic spine. As you can see, flexion and extension are greater in the lower thoracic spine and rotation is greatest in the upper thoracic spine. The close-packed position of apophyseal joints is extension and the open-packed position is semiflexion (MacConaill and Basmajian).

Lateral flexion and rotation of the spine are almost inseparable, that is, lateral flexion and rotation occur together. *Coupling* is a term that refers to this consistent rotation about one axis when another motion is occurring about a sec-

ond axis. In the upper thoracic spine, the coupling pattern is rotation occurring with lateral flexion. Rotation occurs so that the spinous processes move toward the convexity of the curve or away from the side of lateral flexion. In the middle thoracic spine, the coupling movements are somewhat inconsistent. An interesting phenomenon is seen in scoliotic spines, where the direction of rotation of the spinous process is always toward the concavity. White and Panjabi's book *Clinical Biomechanics of the Spine* is an excellent source for further reading on the coupling pattern in scoliosis.

SUBJECTIVE EXAMINATION

Remember that pain in the thoracic area can mimic conditions not treatable by physical therapy. Therefore, a thorough subjective examination before proceeding with the objective exam is essential. The following are some questions that should be considered. These are in addition to the other major components of the subjective examination.

1. The patient's age and occupation is important. Certain conditions affect specific age groups. For example, adolescent osteo-

Figure 26-1. Representative values for average range of motion for flexion-extension, lateral flexion, and rotation for the thoracic spine. (After White AA, Panjabi MM: The basic kinematics of the human spine: A review of past and current knowledge. Spine 3:12, 1978)

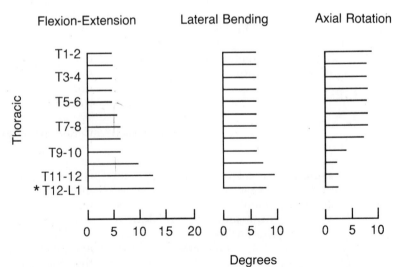

chondrosis, or Scheuermann's disease, is likely to occur in teenagers and ankylosing spondylitis is often detected in the young adult. You also need to know what kind of activities a patient does throughout the day, and the various postures he assumes when engaged in these activities.

2. Ask about the onset of present symptoms. Was the onset sudden or gradual? Is there a tendency for recurrence? Does a postural problem appear to be developing as a result of certain positions or activities? A patient with ankylosing spondylitis may have a characteristic history of morning stiffness and improvement with exercise.

3. Have the patient describe the site of the symptoms. Remember, there are several joints that could be the sources of symptoms (eg, costovertebral, intervertebral, costotransverse, and costochondral). Remember that lower cervical problems can refer pain to the mid-thoracic area, and T1 and T2 can refer pain into the upper extremity.

4. Make certain you find out what, if any, changes of symptoms occur with a deep breath or cough. Symptoms that are intercostal, muscular, costal, or pleural could cause pain with inspiration and expiration, whereas cardiac problems are not likely to provoke pain with deep breathing. Cyriax believes that a deep breath is more likely to cause pain than a cough in thoracic joint problems.

5. You should ask about the presence of paresthesia or anesthesia. There are few occurrences of nerve root compression in the thoracic spine, but be on guard for other causes of symptoms, such as a thoracic neuroma or neuritis.

6. Although it is unlikely, inquire about the presence of any spinal cord signs, such as bilateral tingling in the feet or a gait disturbance.

7. You should ask about general health, other medical conditions, and medication. For example, patients who are known to be osteoporotic or who have been receiving long-term steroid therapy would require

caution in handling during the objective examination.

OBJECTIVE EXAMINATION

OBSERVATION

With the patient standing in good light, observe the patient's general posture and shape of the thoracic spine. Look for any deviations in the spine (eg, kyphosis or scoliosis). Is there a localized kyphosis or dowager's hump? Is there an angular kyphosis (kyphosis at one level), which is characteristic of a collapsed vertebra? A flat lumbar spine with a lower thoracic kyphosis may indicate a past adolescent osteochondrosis. An absence of a lumbar lordosis with marked thoracic kyphosis is often present in ankylosing spondylitis. A number of curve patterns could be present in scoliosis. Look for any asymmetry at the level of the shoulders, scapula, and pelvis. Check the patient's arm hang or the distance between trunk and upper extremity. Observe the patient from lateral and anterior aspects as well. What is the relationship of the head to the neck? Are there any chest deformities, such as barrel chest (the diameter of the chest appears increased) or funnel chest or pectus excavatum (a depression of the sternum and ribs).

CLEARING OTHER JOINTS

As in all evaluations, you must think about surrounding areas that may refer symptoms to the area you are examining. In the case of the thoracic spine, the examination should begin with the neck. To eliminate the neck as a source of symptoms, have the patient perform these active cervical movements: rotation right and left, lateral flexion right and left, and flexion and extension. First, each movement is done actively by the patient, and then you apply gentle overpressure. The overpressure allows you to assess the joint end-feel and make sure no symptoms are referred to the thoracic spine by these movements.

DURAL SIGNS

Neck flexion stretches the dura mater, and therefore is considered a test for irritation of the dura in thoracic problems. Pain felt in the thoracic region with neck flexion is likely to be the result of a thoracic joint problem. Cyriax calls this a "dural sign." Another dural sign Cyriax describes is scapular approximation. He theorizes that this movement pulls T1 and T2 nerve roots upward, which may bring on pain. A specific test for T1 mobility is done by having the patient place her arm in 90 degrees of abduction, then flex the elbow to 90 degrees. This should not bring on any symptoms. Then have the patient flex her elbow fully and place her hand behind the neck. This movement pulls on the T1 nerve root. If there is involvement at this thoracic level, pain would be referred to the scapular area or arm.

ASSESSMENT OF JOINT MOVEMENT

In the clinic, it is best to organize your examination in a sequence that allows for the least amount of positional change for patients, that is, moving from standing to sitting to supine. I have grouped the tests according to categories that were discussed in the introductory section.

Active Physiological Movements

Active physiological movements are assessed with the patient standing. These movements include lateral flexion right and left, and extension and flexion. It is important to use your observational skills. Ask yourself where the motion occurs? Is it in the thoracic spine or somewhere else? Is the movement symmetrical? (For example, in forward flexion a nonstructural or functional scoliosis will disappear as the patient flexes. This is in contrast to a structural scoliosis, where you will see a rib hump or flaring of the rib cage because of abnormal vertebral rotation and other structural changes.) Also, try to have the patient localize thoracic spine movement. For example, when you test forward flexion, instruct the patient to start bending from the head, slowly. You can then watch for movement or lack of movement at each segment.

In extension and lateral flexion, do you see a smooth curve or does it appear that some segments are moving more than others? Bilateral limitation of lateral flexion in the elderly is normal, but in young patients it is rare and may suggest serious disease (Cyriax). With all of these active movements, once the patient performs a pain-free movement, you must then apply overpressure. If the movement is not pain free, note when in the movement and where the pain occurred. You will also want to have some measure of these active movements for reassessment purposes. Various methods of measuring spinal mobility, such as tape measures and goniometric methods using inclinometers or spondylometers, are being developed and improved.

Trunk rotation is best tested with the patient sitting. This eliminates movement at the hip. First, have the patient cross his arms. Then stand in front of the patient so you can stabilize the patient's knees between your own knees as he rotates. Cyriax states that normal range of motion for rotation is roughly 70 degrees actively and 90 degrees passively. Methods used to measure thoracolumbar rotation have included tape measures or inclinometers. It has been difficult with these methods, however, to produce reliable and valid results. With rotation, therapists often report an estimate of total movement, cited as a percentage or fraction. Rotation is one of the most frequent movements to reproduce pain with thoracic joint problems. If you are dealing with a joint problem, it would be unusual not to be able to reproduce pain with rotation.

Passive Physiological Movements

In the thoracic spine, passive physiological movements can also be assessed. This is testing of the intervertebral movement or the movement between each vertebrae. Here, you collect information about how the joints move. For example, do they move too little or too much? What is the quality of the movement? Are any symptoms present? Testing of flexion and extension can be done easily with the patient sitting. Flexion and extension in the upper thoracic spine is tested by having the therapist use one hand to move the patient's head passively while the other hand palpates for the movement. The middle finger should be placed between the spinous processes while the index finger palpates the upper margin of the lower spinous process (Fig. 26-2). Ask yourself what you are feeling. What is the quality of the movement? Is it too much movement (hypermobile) or too little (hypomobile)? Lower thoracic movement (T4-T12) is tested in the same manner, except the patient now holds his hands behind the neck, or may have his arms crossed with his hands resting on his shoulders. The therapist then supports under the patient's elbows and passively moves and palpates for movement as before. Lateral flexion is tested in much the same way, except the therapist must now grasp the trunk and continue to move down the thorax as the movement does (Fig. 26-3). The palpating hand is at the level being examined and the tip of the middle

finger is at the far side of the interspinous space of the joint being tested (Maitland).

Rotation can be tested either with the patient sitting or sidelying. It is easier to stabilize the patient in the sidelying position. The patient's hips and knees are flexed. You place your forearm in line with the spine to help stabilize the pelvis, and again the middle finger is palpating upward against the undersurface of the interspinous space. The other arm rotates the trunk from above the level tested (Fig. 26-4) (Maitland).

Passive Accessory Movements

Passive accessory movements commonly used in the examination and treatment of the thoracic spine are central and unilateral posterioanterior movements. Simple posterioanterior movements can also be done on joints of the

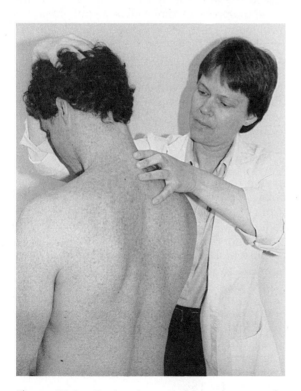

Figure 26-2. Testing intervertebral movement for flexion and extension in the upper thoracic spine (T1-T3).

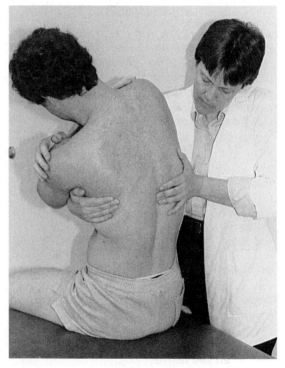

Figure 26-3. Testing intervertebral movement for lateral flexion.

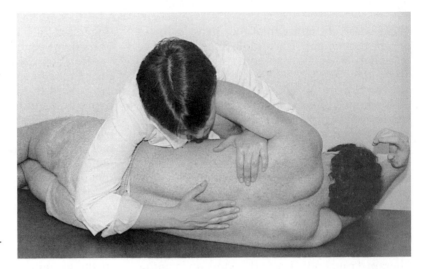

Figure 26-4. Testing intervertebral movement for rotation.

anterior trunk (eg, costochondral or sternocostal joints).

SOFT TISSUE ASSESSMENT

Assessment of contractile structures or muscle is done through resisted isometric tests or static tests. Resisted side flexion is best done with the patient standing. The therapist stands at the patient's side with one foot between the patient's feet. You then place one arm around the patient's shoulders, and your other hand pulls down on the patient's arm that is closest to you. The patient then attempts to side flex away from you (Fig. 26-5). Resisted flexion and rotation are best tested with the patient sitting, and resisted extension with the patient prone. More specific testing for these muscle groups can be done using standard muscle testing procedures.

Cyriax provides these guidelines for pain on resisted tests with the thorax:

1. Pain in the front of the chest with resisted adduction: pectoral muscles
2. Pain on breathing: intercostal muscles
3. Pain at the back of the chest with resisted adduction: latissimus dorsi
4. Pain with resisted rotation: inferior posterior serratus (rare) or oblique abdominals
5. Pain with resisted flexion: rectus abdominus

It is important to remember that muscle lesions do not refer pain from the posterior thorax to the anterior or vice versa. If this is the case, the problem may well be a joint or visceral problem.

In the thoracic area, there are several areas to palpate. You are looking, as always, for spasm, tenderness, temperature changes, bony alignment, and a feeling of crepitus or thickening. Palpation of both anterior and posterior structures should be done as part of the examination.

NEUROLOGICAL EXAMINATION

Nerve root involvement is rare in the thoracic area. Of course, symptoms can be referred from other areas, which must always be a consideration. Dermatomes in this area overlap and tend to follow the ribs. The plantar response must be checked for any signs of pressure on the spinal cord or the presence of an upper motor neuron lesion. Keep in mind that T1 root pain and weakness, as the result of a joint problem, is rare. If these signs are present, it is more likely to be the result of serious pathology, such as a neoplasm (Pancoast's tumor) or pressure from a cervical rib.

SPECIAL TESTS

If you suspect other problems or pathologies, here are some examples of other special tests.

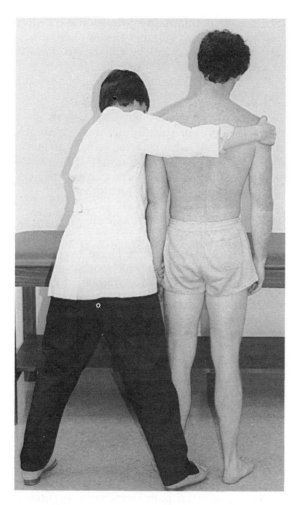

Figure 26-5. Testing resisted side flexion.

Thoracic Outlet

The Adson or scalene maneuver is used to test the state of the subclavian artery. To perform this test, you take the patient's radial pulse, then have the patient take a deep breath and hold it. Next, have the patient extend her neck and turn her head toward the side being examined. In a positive test, you would feel a change in the radial pulse. In some patients the effect is greater when the head is turned toward the opposite side, so try both positions. Another test for this area is the costoclavicular test. Here, the costoclavicular space is narrowed by approximating the clavicle to the first rib. The

patient assumes the exaggerated military position by drawing her shoulders down and backward. Again, if the radial pulse is changed with reproduction of the symptoms, it is a positive test.

Chest Expansion

When you have some indication that there may be restriction of the chest, you should take an objective measure. For example, in a patient with ankylosing spondylitis, you would want to document the mobility of the chest cavity. A common level for measurement is the fourth intercostal space. Have the patient exhale, and then inhale. A normal difference between inspiration and expiration is anywhere from 3 to 7.5 cm (Magee).

FUNCTIONAL ASSESSMENT

Functional movements that reproduce the patient's symptoms should also be part of your objective examination. This information provides good reassessment measures that are relevant to both you and your patient. The functional activities that are likely to aggravate thoracic problems are rotational movements, a combination of flexion and rotation, or sustained unsupported sitting.

INTERPRETATION OF FINDINGS

It is important to remember that few people have "normal thoracic spines." There is often reduced accessory joint movement and local tenderness present in the thoracic spine. The following is by no means an exhaustive list of possible problems of the thoracic spine, but only an introduction. Refer to other sources such as Cyriax or Grieve for more comprehensive information.

POSTERIOR JOINT PROBLEMS

Areas of posterior joint problems include the intervertebral joint, facet, and costotransverse or costovertebral joint. Significant clinical findings may be the following:

1. Onset of the symptoms may be sudden or gradual.

2. Pain is usually dependent upon activity and posture.
3. Pain may radiate anteriorly along the costal margin.
4. A deep breath is likely to hurt more than coughing, whereas a cough may hurt more in a pleural or intercostal muscle problem.
5. Trunk rotation is likely to reproduce symptoms.

RIBS AND INTERCOSTAL MUSCLES

Following fracture of a rib, localized pain usually lasts six weeks at most. Pain that persists may be due to an intercostal muscle problem.

Intercostal muscles often are injured from a direct bruise or specific sport. There may be pain with resisted flexion and rotation and active trunk extension (which stretches the muscle).

THORACIC NEUROMA

Thoracic neuroma should be suspected when the patient has nerve root pain with or without central pain. The patient will also have pain with a deep breath, cough, laugh, neck flexion, and scapula approximation. Active movements may demonstrate that side flexion away from the painful side is limited and painful, and rotation in either direction is painless. The patient may also have a patch of numbness or spinal cord signs.

ANKYLOSING SPONDYLITIS

Signs of ankylosing spondylitis are often present in the history. The typical patient is a young adult under the age of 40 years, with an insidious onset of pain in the thoracolumbar area. The duration of pain is often greater than three months. Pain is associated with morning stiffness and improves with exercise. Ankylosing spondylitis has a 7:1 predominance in males.

ADOLESCENT OSTEOCHONDROSIS

In the patient with adolescent osteochondrosis, a round hyphosis usually appears in the second decade of life. Active extension can be limited and painless, whereas flexion, lateral flexion, and rotation may be full range. Passive extension is limited.

NEURITIS

Neuritis of the spinal accessory nerve, long thoracic nerve, or subscapular nerve may give rise to constant scapular ache, which can last as long as three weeks. In contrast, if this trunk pain was the result of herpes zoster, vesicles would appear in three to four days.

TIETZE'S SYNDROME OR ACUTE COSTOCHONDROSIS

Acute costochrondrosis, or Tietze's syndrome, is an irritation of the costochondral junction. Common symptoms are as follows:

1. Pain can follow persistent cough or bronchitis.
2. There may be pain with a deep breath.
3. Pressure on the sternum may reproduce pain at the affected joints.
4. There may be swelling or localized swelling of the costal cartilages.

CONCLUSION

It is important to be very careful when evaluating the thoracic spine. Remember, it can be the source of referred pain from many organs. A careful evaluation will pinpoint whether the problem is of musculoskeletal origin.

ANNOTATED BIBLIOGRAPHY

Cyriax J: Textbook of Orthopaedic Medicine: Diagnosis of Soft Tissue Lesions, Vol I, 7th ed, pp 295–327. London, Bailliere Tindall, 1983 (Cyriax's Volume I contains an excellent section on the thoracic spine. It includes a thorough discussion of differential diagnosis and provides a brief overview of Cyriax's evaluation for the thoracic spine.)

Grieve G: Common Vertebral Joint Problems, pp 31–35, 232–249, 326. New York, Churchill

Livingstone, 1981 (An excellent source for reading more about spinal pathologies. The book also contains Grieve's approach to evaluation and treatment of patients with spinal musculoskeletal problems.)

Grieve G (ed): Modern Manual Therapy of the Vertebral Column. New York, Churchill Livingstone, 1986 (Presents detailed information on the structure and function of the spine as well as information on evaluation, treatment, and clinical considerations. It would be an excellent resource for expanding your knowledge of the spinal area. Several chapters also deal specifically with the thoracic spine.)

MacConaill MA, Basmajian JV: Muscles and Movement, pp 13–44. Huntington, NY, Robert E Krieger Publishing, 1977 (Some excellent basic material on the mechanics of the thoracic spine.)

Maitland GD: Vertebral Manipulation, 5th ed, pp 233–258. Boston, Butterworths, 1986 (The chapter on the thoracic spine provides a thorough description of Maitland's approach to evaluation and treatment of patients with thoracic musculoskeletal problems.)

Magee DJ: Orthopedic Physical Assessment, pp 142–169. Philadelphia, WB Saunders, 1987 (A valuable source for anyone doing musculoskeletal evaluation. The chapter on the thoracic spine is well done, concise, and easy to understand. The approach to evaluation is a synthesis of several different philosophies.)

Moore K: Clinically Oriented Anatomy, pp 1–36. Baltimore, Williams & Wilkins, 1980 (An excellent anatomy resource. Moore has taken Grant's *Atlas* material and combined it with many relevant clinical examples. The section on the trunk and thoracic spine is well done.)

White AA Panjabi MM: Clinical Biomechanics of the Spine, pp 44–49, 74–77, 91–93. Philadelphia, JB Lippincott, 1978 (A classic in the field. Both the text and illustrations are presented in a style understandable to any clinician with some basic knowledge of biomechanics. The authors continue to do research and publish in this area.)

27 Musculoskeletal Analysis: The Lumbar Spine and Lumbopelvic Region

SUSAN S. SMITH

The human spine is a magnificent structure that simultaneously provides stability, flexibility, strength, coordination, and protection. In both form and function, the human spine is one of the most interesting and complex structures in the neuromusculoskeletal system. Because it is a unique and central unit, pain and loss of function in this area is integral to the individual's ability to function. As with any complex system, there is greater potential for dysfunction here than in other areas of the musculoskeletal system. Consequently, back injuries are one of the most frequent causes of work absenteeism. Billions of dollars are spent annually for medical care, disability claims, lawsuits, absenteeism, and back care products that range from mattresses to exercise equipment.

Management of low back disorders consists of a broad range of diagnostic testing and treatment. Treatment includes, but is not limited to, bed rest, medication, manipulation, surgery, exercise, bracing, education, acupressure, reflexology, heat, cold, electrical modalities, biofeedback, injections, psychological counseling, or combinations of these methods. The variety and controversy surrounding treatment strategies, and the huge sums of money spent on low back pain, serve as unfortunate reminders that low back pain remains an unsolved puzzle.

Treatment strategies frequently have been based on the clinician's philosophy and training rather than on the patient's *signs* (objective, reproducible observations and measurements obtained by the clinician) and *symptoms* (subjective information related by the patient). Low back pain has different causes, and effective treatment must be based on the results of the evaluation of the patient. The purposes of this chapter are to briefly review anatomical structures, identify basic examination procedures, provide an examination format, describe rationale for the examination procedures for evaluating the lumbar spine and pelvic girdle, and to explain how the results of the examination are used to evaluate or assess the patient's problem. Various specific treatments are discussed elsewhere in this and other texts.

ANATOMY

Knowledge of lumbar and lumbopelvic regional anatomy is essential. Therefore, a very brief anatomy review is presented here.

OSSEOUS (BONY) TISSUE

The 33 bones of the spinal column are divided into five areas. The lumbar spine consists of the lowest five mobile vertebrae, and the sacrum consists of five fused vertebrae. The lumbar spine is concave posteriorly, or lordotic, and the sacral spine is convex posteriorly, or kyphotic. These curves provide balance and strength. An increase in the normal curves increases flexibility, whereas decreased curves tend to have less flexibility.

Lumbar Spine

The bodies of the lumbar vertebrae are columnar and kidney shaped. Their function is to support weight. The ends of the bodies are also articular. The vertebral arch consists of two short, broad pedicles emanating from the posterior body and united posteriorly by two laminae. The arch encloses the vertebral foramen, forming a canal, and functions to house and protect the spinal cord. This canal is triangularly shaped in the lumbar spine. The lumbar transverse processes are relatively slender, pointed, and horizontal, and the spinous processes are large, quadrangular, and horizontal. These processes, or projections, serve as levers and as muscle attachments. The four articular processes (two superior and two inferior) face lateromedially, and therefore are aligned in a sagittal plane, except at L5 where the articular processes are aligned slightly more frontally. Each articular process is surfaced with an articular facet. Therefore, the term *facet* is not synonymous with the name of the joint. Unique to the superior articular processes in this region are the mammillary processes for the origin of the multifidus and the accessory processes on the transverse processes for the insertion of the longissimus, psoas, and quadratus lumborum muscles.

Intervertebral Foramen

Above the pedicle is the superior articulating notch, and below the pedicle is the inferior articulating notch. When two adjacent vertebrae are in articulation, the two adjacent vertebral notches form the intervertebral foramen for the exiting spinal nerve and intervertebral vessels. These vertebral vessels provide nutrients to and remove waste from the dura, ligaments, and vertebral bodies. Spur formation within the foramen can decrease the size of the foramen and compress spinal nerves.

Lumbopelvic Region

The bones of the lumbopelvic region consist of the fifth lumbar vertebra, the right and left ilia, and the sacrum. The ilium is composed of three segments: the ilium, ischium, and pubis. Important landmarks of the ilia include the iliac crests, anterior superior iliac spines (ASIS), posterior superior iliac spines (PSIS), and pubic tubercles. The sacrum is formed by the fusion of five vertebrae and is wider superiorly than inferiorly and broader anteriorly than posteriorly. The sacrum is perforated by four pairs of foramina. Sacral bony landmarks important for palpation include the sacral hiatus, sacral cornu, and spinous processes of the sacral vertebrae, or median crest. The pelvises of men and women differ significantly because of the childbearing capabilities of women. The male pelvis is more upright and the ilia are more vertical with a narrower base. The female pelvis is broader, and the ilia are shorter, more oblique, and tend to angle inward.

JOINTS

Joints are formed by the articulation of two or more bones. Joints and their accompanying soft tissue structures are the functional units of the skeleton.

Lumbar Spine

The joints of the lumbar spine are composed of the two adjacent inferior and superior articular processes of the L1-L5 vertebrae. These are called zygapophyseal joints (or apophyseal joints). Also, the bodies of adjacent vertebrae articulate with each other by means of the intervening disk. The disk partially determines the amount of movement in adjacent vertebrae, but the direction of the movement is determined by the apophyseal joints. As reviewed previously, the L1-L4 articular processes are aligned lateromedially, permitting movement primarily in the sagittal plane (ie, flexion and extension) and severely restricting lumbar rotation. The alignment of these joints also allows the intervertebral disks to bear weight in the lumbar spine in the erect posture, and the apophyseal joints to bear more weight in the laterally flexed position and during rising from the flexed position. The lower articular processes of L5, which face more frontally, bear weight even in the upright position.

Lumbopelvic Region

Joints of the lumbopelvic region are the right and left L5-S1 apophyseal joints, the L5 body articulating with the S1 body, the right and left sacroiliac joints, and the pubic symphysis. As noted above, the L5-S1 apophyseal joints are directed more frontally and are weight bearing, as is the articulation of the L5 and S1 bodies, which facilitates transmission of weight from the trunk to the pelvis. The two sacroiliac joints are formed by the sacrum articulating with each ilium. The pubic symphysis is an amphiarthrodial joint formed where the pubic bones of each pelvis articulate anteriorly. The hip joints are also considered with the pelvis because ground forces reach the pelvis through the hips. Decreased hip joint range of motion can alter lumbopelvic mechanics.

NONCONTRACTILE TISSUES

Articular Cartilage, Capsules, and Synovial Lining

The apophyseal joints are covered with smooth, shiny hyaline cartilage. This cartilage is somewhat compressible in young persons, but the compressibility and thickness decrease with age. The articular capsules encompass all apophyseal joints and consist of both white fibrous and yellow elastic tissue. The capsules support and protect the synovial membrane, and function with the ligaments to direct and limit joint movements. The elasticity of the capsule prevents the capsule from being pinched between two articular surfaces during movement, and also stabilizes the spine by helping articulating facets to maintain approximation with each other (the close-packed position). The joint capsules are lined with synovium. The synovial lining contains villi or interarticular protrusions, frequently called *meniscoid inclusions*. During an abnormal movement, these meniscoid inclusions can become trapped between the articular cartilages and painfully block movement.

Ligaments

Ligaments are fibrous, noncontractile structures that are partially responsible for maintaining static stability of joints by limiting or modifying movement.

General and Lumbar Ligaments

The anterior longitudinal ligament, posterior longitudinal ligament, ligamenta flava, interspinous ligament, and supraspinous ligaments are common to most areas of the spine, including the lumbar spine. The anterior longitudinal ligament (ALL) extends along the anterior surface of the vertebral column from the occiput to the sacrum. The ALL adheres to the anterior vertebral bodies and to the disks. Functionally, the ALL becomes taut with extension, slack with flexion, and reinforces the anterior disks during lifting. The posterior longitudinal ligament (PLL) is located in the spinal canal and descends along the posterior surface of the vertebral bodies and disks from C2 or C3 to the sacrum. The PLL adheres to the disks at each level, but it is not attached to the vertebral bodies. The lateral expansions over the disks are thinner than the central portions, which may explain why posterior disk protrusions move more laterally than centrally. Notably, the PLL narrows as it descends, and becomes so narrow in the lumbar spine that it protects the disks only minimally during lifting. The PLL becomes taut with spinal flexion and slack with extension.

The ligamenta flava are paired ligaments extending between adjacent laminae, and their lateral borders blend with the apophyseal joint capsules. Because they are elastic, the ligamenta flava assist in returning the spinal column to the erect position and in preventing the synovial capsule, lining, and meniscoid bodies from being nipped between the joint surfaces of the apophyseal joints during flexion. Hypertrophy of the ligamentum flavum can compromise the spinal cord and emerging nerve roots. The interspinous ligament is a loose ligament located between adjacent spinous processes. Functionally, it limits spinal flexion. The supraspinous ligament is located between and on the tips of adjacent spinous processes. This ligament may end at L4. Functionally, the supraspinous ligament limits flexion and some rotation. Tension of this ligament is palpated during some spinal passive mobility testing.

Two additional structures unique to the lumbar spine are the iliolumbar ligaments and the thoracolumbar fascia. The iliolumbar ligaments are located at L5 and sometimes L4. These ligaments traverse from the transverse processes to the iliac crests just above the PSIS. They are divided into superior and inferior bands. The superior band stabilizes L5 (and L4, if present) during flexion. The inferior band checks extension of the involved vertebral bodies. They also restrict lateral flexion and rotation. The thoracolumbar fascia is not technically a ligament, but it is a very strong and important noncontractile structure in this region. The fascia spans from the iliac crest and sacrum to the thoracic region. During flexion, the thoracolumbar fascia resists excessive flexion, and it assists with initiating and enhancing extension.

Lumbopelvic Ligaments

Primary stabilizers of the pelvic region include the anterior and posterior sacroiliac ligaments, sacrospinous ligaments, and sacrotuberous ligaments. The anterior sacroiliac ligaments support the anterior aspect of the joints, while the posterior aspect is surrounded by the posterior sacroiliac ligaments. The sacrospinous ligaments cross from the ischial spine of the anterior inferior sacrum, and the sacrotuberous ligaments attach at the ischial tuberosity and traverse to the inferior sacrum. These ligaments check flexion of the sacrum. Two ligaments—the superior and inferior ligaments—surround the pubic symphysis. The iliofemoral, ischial femoral, and pubofemoral ligaments of the hip are also important to consider in this region.

Disks

The intervertebral disks consist of an annulus fibrosus and a nucleus pulposus. Disks provide for distribution of forces and some intervertebral movement. The annulus fibrosus consists of 12 to 20 layers of fibers that crisscross with alternate layers of fibers aligned in the opposite direction, similar to a radial tire. The nucleus pulposus is a mucopolysaccharide gel with water-binding capability, making it nearly incompressible. When the nucleus pulposus degenerates because of age or damage, the water-binding capabilities decrease. Movement of the nucleus within the annulus is controversial; however, in a normal disk, the nucleus may displace minimally in a direction opposite a compressive force on the annulus. For example, spinal flexion causes an anterior compressive force, which may displace the nuclear material posteriorly. Migration is more apparent with damage to the annulus. This proposed nuclear movement is an important concept in McKenzie's (1981) treatment approach for derangement (diskogenic) syndromes.

Nerves

The spinal nerves originate from the spinal cord within the vertebral canal and exit through the intervertebral foramen. At descending levels the nerves exit at increasing downward angles; therefore, the lumbar nerves have more potential for compression than nerves at higher levels. These nerves and their roots may be irritated or compressed, resulting in distal signs and symptoms.

CONTRACTILE TISSUES

Contractile tissues consist of the muscle, the musculotendinous junction, the tendon, and the bony insertion of the tendon. Space does not permit a review of the anatomy of the numerous contractile tissues associated with the lumbar and sacral areas. However, the more significant muscle groups are listed below with a notation of their possible importance in spinal conditions.

General and Lumbar

Contractile tissues common to most areas of the spine and lumbar area include the following muscles, or muscle groups.

The trapezius and latissimus dorsi together span the entire spine from the occiput to the sacrum. Combined, they position the shoulder and retract it during lifting. The latissimus also attaches to the thoracolumbar fascia and helps tense this important tissue. The erector spinae consist of the iliocostalis, longissimus, and spinalis. If the iliocostalis and longissimus are tight or in spasm, these muscles can restrict breathing. Also, these important spinal extensors (and rotators) are required for lifting, especially if performed with a lumbar lordosis. Patients with chronic low back pain frequently demonstrate weakness of the erector spinae. The interspinalis, intertransversarii, and multifidus provide sensory monitoring, intrinsic stability, and assist with extension, lateral flexion, and rotation, respectively. Spasm or tightness of the intertransversarii can compress the exiting peripheral nerves. The quadratus lumborum helps maintain the pelvis in a neutral position during gait and assists with lateral trunk flexion. Tightness of the quadratus lumborum can restrict rib cage expansion and lateral flexion in the direction opposite the tight muscle. The abdominal muscles consist of the rectus abdominis, internal and external obliquus abdominis, and the transversus abdominis. The abdominal muscles compress the abdominal contents, increase intraabdominal pressure, stabilize the pelvis, and attenuate force, particularly during the first phase of lifting. The rectus is an important trunk flexor, the obliques are important rotators, and the transverse abdominals are important lateral flexors. The latter also assist in creating tension on the thoracolumbar fascia. Although known mostly for their role as hip flexors, the *psoas* muscles also act on the lumbar spine, causing a lordosis when contracted.

Lumbopelvic and Hip

Twenty-eight muscles attach on the pelvis, with the majority located on the ilium. No muscle groups specifically move the sacrum; however, muscles that insert and originate on the ilium and sacrum can, when positioned in certain ways, create force on the pelvic bones sufficient to alter their position. In addition to some of the muscles noted above, such as the abdominals, the length and strength of the muscles listed below must be checked when evaluating the lumbopelvic region.

Tightness of the tensor fasciae latae, rectus femoris, and adductors magnus, brevis, and longus can each cause an anterior torsion, or rotation of the ilium. The adductors also can affect the pubic symphysis. The iliopsoas (iliacus and psoas) is stretched when the hip is extended, causing an inferior and posterior stress on the superior lateral pubic ramus. This can cause an anterior torsion of either ilium. The gluteus minimus, medius, and maximus are mainly hip abductors and extensors, but also act to keep the pelvis level while the opposite leg is in the swing phase of gait. Tight hamstrings can create an increased posterior torsion of the ilium. The piriformis has a strong sacral attachment and can alter proper sacral function if tight or weak. The gracilis, quadratus femoris, sartorius, obturators externus and internus, and the superior and inferior gemelli are also muscles that can alter the biomechanics of pelvic motion.

BIOMECHANICS

Equally important to knowledge of the anatomy of the lumbar and lumbopelvic regions is an understanding of the biomechanics.

LUMBAR REGION

When the spinal mechanics are balanced, the spine is straight when viewed from the front or back, the pelvis and shoulders are nearly level, and the thoracic and sacral kyphotic curves, and the cervical and lumbar lordotic curves reciprocate. These curves increase the ability of the vertebral column to withstand axial compressive loads. If the pelvis is not level, the vertebral column is forced to bend sideways, causing compensatory curves and adaptive shortening of the soft tissue supporters to maintain the eyes in a horizontal plane.

Spinal movements occur in the spine generally around an axis located posterior to the center of the intervertebal disk. As noted previously, the intervertebal disks dissipate forces and to some extent determine the amount of spinal motion, whereas the plane of the articulating facets determines both the direction and the amount of movement. A spinal segment has six degrees of freedom, that is, the vertebral body can move six ways: compression and distraction along the longitudinal axis; anterior and posterior gliding in the sagittal plane; flexion and extension tilting around a frontal axis; lateral tilting around a sagittal axis; sidegliding in a frontal plane; and rotation in the horizontal plane about a vertical axis. Most spinal movements are a combination of these motions. However, spinal movements occur according to certain laws, which were described by Fryette (Saunders, 1985). In general, in the lumbar and thoracic spine, rotation and lateral flexion occur opposite to each other except in full flexion or extension, in which case rotation and lateral flexion occur to the same side. Also, if motion is introduced into a segment in any plane, motion in all other planes is reduced. However, persons can voluntarily perform movements that override these laws.

Most lumbar flexion and extension occurs at the lower lumbar (L4-L5-S1) segments. Saunders (1985) lists the total L1-L5 motions as 5 degrees of rotation, 20 degrees of lateral flexion, 40 to 43 degrees of flexion, and 30 to 40 degrees of extension. These ranges differ somewhat from those cited by Mayer (1984) and by Paris (1979).

LUMBOPELVIC REGION

The normal lumbosacral angle is 140 degrees with a sacral inclination angle of 30 degrees. This arrangement reduces the shear forces of the superincumbent body weight. Increasing the lumbosacral angle increases lordosis and increases shear forces in the spine. A more vertical sacrum decreases the lordosis and creates a more rigid spine.

Each sacroiliac joint is sometimes considered as being two joints: the iliosacral (IS), which is the ilia moving on the sacrum, and the sacroiliac (SI), which is the sacrum moving within the ilia. Movement of the SI joints is somewhat controversial. However, in general, the position of the sacrum is determined by forces from the spine above (trunk forces), and the ilium is controlled by movement of the femur and the ground forces.

Normal physiological movement of the sacrum consists of flexion (nutation) and extension (counternutation) of the sacrum on the ilium. As the lumbar spine begins to flex the pelvis is rotated anteriorly over the hips, the sacrum begins to extend within the ilia. Simultaneously, there is a backward movement of the pelvis on the hips in the horizontal plane, which maintains the center of gravity over the feet. As the person returns to standing, the lumbar spine becomes concave, and the pelvis derotates and shifts forward.

The sacrum can also rotate on oblique axes of motion. These axes pass obliquely through the sacrum from the upper right corner to the lower left corner (right oblique axis) and from the upper left corner to the lower right corner (left oblique axis). The sacrum can either rotate left on the left oblique axis or rotate right on the right oblique axis, depending on the lumbar vertebrae. For example, if the lumbar spine is laterally flexed left, trunk forces reach the sacrum in the right anterolateral corner, causing the sacrum to assume an adapted position of left rotation on the left oblique axis (Fig. 27-1).

The ilium, as mentioned, is controlled by movement of the femur. The most extreme movement of the sacroiliac (iliosacral) joints occurs during standing from sitting.

At heel strike during the beginning of the

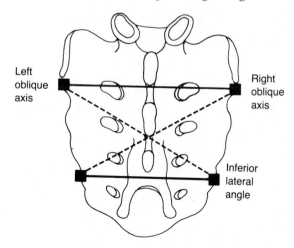

Figure 27-1. Multiple axes of the sacroiliac joint.

stance phase of gait, the ilium posteriorly rotates on the sacrum, progressing to an anterior rotation as weight bearing occurs. This movement is accentuated during running. In addition, an upslipping of the ilium can occur as a result of ground forces. If the ground forces are equal, movement of the ilium on the sacrum is symmetrical. However, if the ground forces are unequal, as in cases of leg length discrepancies or abnormal lower extremity mechanics, adaptive changes occur.

When one leg is shorter, every time that person steps on the short leg, the pelvis drops a distance equal to the amount of the leg length discrepancy. The amount of force transmitted up through the foot increases because of the increased distance to the ground. The asymmetrical forces cause sacral and lumbar adaptive changes that render the lumbopelvic area susceptible to soft tissue injury.

A weak abdominal wall can also cause asymmetrical forces from the ground up and from the trunk down. Weak abdominals cause the ilia to migrate anteriorly, and increased lumbar lordosis results. The posterior apophyseal joints become weight bearing and vulnerable to increased wear. Therefore, proper balance of the strength and length of muscles in the lumbopelvic region is essential in treating problems in this area.

ETIOLOGY AND PATHOLOGY OF SPINAL DYSFUNCTION

The etiology and pathology of spinal dysfunction is a complex and controversial subject with sufficient information to fill a textbook. However, without some knowledge of etiology and the clinical features of various pathologies, an examination cannot serve its purposes. Etiological factors include the following: trauma (eg, strains, zygapophyseal joint subluxations, surgery, disk herniation, fractures); faulty mechanics (eg, habitual postural strain, hypomobility); congenital disorders (transitional vertebra, hemivertebra, hereditary predisposition); inflammatory disorders (eg, ankylosing spondylitis); metabolic disorders (eg, osteopor-

osis); circulatory disorders (eg, abdominal aortic aneurysms); infections; toxicity; benign and malignant tumors; and psychoneurotic problems (eg, pain memory, malingering) (Paris, 1979).

Pathologies can be considered according to the structure involved. For example, joint disorders include sprains, subluxations, hypomobilities, hypermobilities (instabilities), inflammations, and degenerative changes. Muscle disorders include secondary guarding and spasm, strains, contusions, inflammation, and adaptive changes in strength and length. Disk disorders include herniation, protrusion, and degeneration. Disorders involving neural structures include disk herniations with nerve root compression, inflammation, impingement, and nerve root adhesions.

Each pathology is represented by a set of signs and symptoms. However, more than one tissue may be involved. The process of aging leads to hypomobility and frequently to accompanying cumulative postural changes, osteoporosis, and obesity. Also, one tissue may be traumatized initially and lead to secondary changes in other areas. A healed disk herniation may have caused decreased mobility, decreased muscle flexibility, and a loss of trunk and leg strength. Paris (1979), Saunders (1985), and Cyriax (1969) present key clinical information about various pathologies.

GENERAL EXAMINATION CONCEPTS

''Examination'' in this section refers to the acts of inspecting, measuring, screening, and checking. ''Evaluation'' or ''assessment'' refers to the process of interpreting the results of the subjective and objective examinations. Therefore, we do evaluate patients, but we also perform subjective and objective examinations.

EXAMINATION GUIDELINES

The following guidelines may be helpful to remember while performing the evaluation.
1. Most patients have real problems, which should be treated as such unless proven otherwise. Although some people may

take unfair advantage of worker's compensation and other benefits, persons with legitimate problems are often made to feel that they must prove they have a problem. Also, fear (often, inadvertently facilitated by medical management) and general lack of understanding of pain and dysfunction may cause some people to attribute a number of unrelated causes and symptoms to their current problem. One task of the evaluation is to sort through the patient's presentation of the problem. Additionally, some clinicians have a preset clinical picture of how a patient with back pain should behave. If instead of moaning and moving slowly, the patient leaps off the examination table, the clinician may assume the patient does not have a problem. Such a patient's symptoms are perhaps less irritable, but not necessarily less present or limiting.

2. The examination should be as inexpensive and simple as possible. More extensive tests and specialists should be reserved for those patients who need a more in-depth examination. Results of the subjective examination assist in determining the contents of the objective examination. A patient who does not complain of radiating leg symptoms probably does not require sensory or reflex testing.

3. The examiner needs to keep an open mind during the examination and avoid jumping to conclusions about the patient's problems before finishing the examination. Patients may have more than one problem, that is, more than one site or tissue may have sustained injury. Also, secondary problems may result from acute or chronic dysfunction. Often, a combination of poor posture and overuse contributes to the injury or prevents recovery.

4. The abnormal objective findings should be *measured* when possible. Most of the purposes for examination (eg, basis for significant change, determining ability, and investigating efficacy of treatment) can be served only with quantification. However, at this time, some aspects of the examination defy measurement.

Finally, remember that evaluation is an ongoing process. Patients should be evaluated not only initially, but also before, during, and after each treatment. They should also be reevaluated retrospectively after a series of treatments, before discharge, and on follow-up visits, if those are indicated.

EXAMINATION SEQUENCE

The examination needs to be thorough, logical, and efficient. The sequence is determined by the content, time and equipment available, and the *irritability* of the patient's condition, that is, the ease with which the patient's symptoms are aggravated and the length of time required for the symptoms to subside to their customary level (Maitland, 1986). One of the most difficult aspects for the novice is learning to arrange the sequence of the examination according to patient position rather than by the type of information being obtained. Some therapists will acquire all information needed (ie, strength, flexibility, and passive accessory movements) supine, then reposition the patient sidelying and then prone, and repeat the process. This prevents excessive patient movement and is more efficient. However, this approach is not only difficult for the novice, but is often difficult for the patient, who is asked to respond alternately to different requests and procedures (ie, sometimes the patient is asked to describe pain patterns, then asked to "hold" in muscle testing, then asked to relax as the examiner performs passive mobility testing). Similarly, the examiner must be thinking about all the different types of tests to be performed in each position. The detailed sequence suggested in Table 27-1 is a compromise between patient movement and examination content. Expectations for patients are fairly similar, and they return to the supine, sitting, and standing positions anyway to get up from the examination table.

EXAMINATION

The examination itself consists of gathering subjective data (symptoms) and objective data

Table 27-1. Sequence and Specific Examination Content for Low Back and Sacroiliac Examinations*

Sitting

1. General observations

2. Subjective examination
   Description of symptoms
   Location of symptoms
   Current history
   Site-specific questions
   Previous history
   General medical history
   Personal information

Standing

1. General observations
2. Postural examination
   a. Posterior view: body build, scars, stance, waist angle, lateral shifts, scoliosis, levels of shoulders, scapulae, iliac
      crests, PSIS, gluteal folds, trochanters, and fibular heads, calcaneal angles, longitudinal arches
   b. Lateral view: head carriage, spinal curves, pelvic angle, trunk inclination angle, observations of hips, knees, and
      ankles
   c. Anterior view: chest configuration, levels of ASIS, observations of hips, knees, and ankles
3. Anthropometric features
   Weight-bearing leg lengths from umbilicus and from ASIS to medial malleolus
4. Active movements (ROM, quality of movements, effect on symptoms, overpressure)
   Flexion
   Extension
   Lateral flexion
   (Rotation, if performed standing)[†]
   Sidegliding
   Prolonged flexion
   Repeated flexion, extension, sidegliding
   Combined movements
   Lateral shift correction
   Forward flexion test
5. Squat to stand clearing test

Sitting

1. Active movement: rotation (if not performed in standing)[†]

Supine

1. Active movements: effect on symptoms
   Supine lying
   Flexion
   Prolonged flexion
   Repeated flexion

Prone

1. Active movements: effect on symptoms
   Prone lying
   Extension
   Repeated extension
   Lateral shift correction

*Evaluation content is determined by the subjective examination, irritability of the condition, and so forth; therefore, the clinician is advised to omit
inappropriate examination components.
[†]Rotation may be performed in sitting or in standing positions.

2. Palpation
   a. Bony landmarks: lumbar spine, ilia, and sacrum
   b. Soft tissue: skin, subcutaneous tissue, muscles, ligaments
      Temperature
      Tissue tension
      Spasm
      Tenderness
   c. Passive movements
      Lateral flexion
      Rotation
      Iliac torsion
   d. Accessory movements
      Sacral springing
      PA gliding and rotation
   e. Nerve sensitivity test
      Posterior knee bend
   f. Muscle testing
      Gluteus maximus, hamstrings, middle and lower trapezius

Sidelying

1. Passive movements
   Flexion-extension
2. Flexibility (muscle length)
   Tensor fascia latae
3. Muscle testing
   Transversus abdominis, gluteus medius, tensor fascia latae, adductors

Supine

1. Palpation
   Bony landmarks: ASIS, pubic tubercles
   Soft tissue
2. Anthropometric features
   Non-weight-bearing leg lengths from umbilicus and ASIS to medial malleolus
   Leg circumferences, if atrophy noted
3. Clear hips, knees, and check ROM
4. Passive movements
   ASIS rocking
   (Torsion tests, if not performed in other positions)
5. Accessory movements
   SI provocation tests (also to clear SI joint)
6. Flexibility (muscle length)
   Latissimus dorsi; pectoralis major and minor, iliopsoas, hip adductors, gracilis, hamstrings (with simultaneous SLR test), tensor fascia latae, rectus femoris, gastrocnemius, soleus
7. Upper motor neuron check
   Babinski test
8. Check subtalar mobility, clear ankle
9. Functional sit-up test
10. Muscle testing
    Abdominals: rectus and obliques, iliopsoas, quadratus lumborum

continued

Table 27-1. (continued)

Sidelying (Opposite Side)

1. Flexibility (muscle length)
   Tensor fascia latae
2. Muscle testing
   Transversus abdominis, gluteus medius, tensor fascia latae, adductors

Sitting

1. Neurological examination
   Sensation
   Reflexes
   Selected resisted muscle testing (if not done during rest of exam)
2. Muscle testing
   (Iliopsoas), quadriceps femoris, hip internal and external rotators, anterior tibialis, peroneals, extensor hallucis longus
3. Special tests
   Distraction-compression

Standing

1. Muscle testing
   Heel-toe walking (or gastrocnemius, soleus, and anterior tibialis tests)
2. Balance
   Stork standing
3. Gait (or running) examination

Other (Tests with Equipment)

1. Muscle testing
   Trunk, torso
2. Endurance
3. Function
   Lifting capacity
   Simulated activities
4. Fitness
   Submaximal stress testing
5. Other

---

*Evaluation content is determined by the subjective examination, irritability of the condition, and so forth; therefore, the clinician is advised to omit inappropriate examination components.
†Rotation may be performed in sitting or in standing positions.

(signs). This information is then integrated into an assessment, from which a plan is formulated.

SUBJECTIVE EXAMINATION

A key point to remember when performing the subjective examination is to *listen* carefully. Often, the patient with a spinal disorder will *tell you how to treat* it successfully, especially if the results of your objective examination concur with the patient's subjective statements about the location, onset, and behavior of the pain.

Questions should be simple (eg, no technical terms), short, specific, one at a time, and unbiased (ie, questions that will not elicit a particular response). Be sure the patient answers each question you ask. If not, rephrase the question. The therapist must impose a controlled structure to prevent the patient from providing irrelevant detail, but at the same time allow for and listen to spontaneous comments that can be quite important.

In addition to obtaining information, the subjective examination should convey to the patient that you *care*. This is accomplished by being gentle, rephrasing questions to assist the patient to answer, making eye contact, smiling, touching appropriately, and communicating nonverbally, such as by sitting down. Also, observe the patient's nonverbal communication, and simultaneously compare it to her verbal communication. In addition to eliciting precise information, observing and communicating are also part of the objective examination.

The content of the examination consists of the description and location of the symptoms, current history, behavior of the symptoms, previous history, if any, of this problem, site-specific questions, and general medical history. The selective rationale for obtaining information about these areas is discussed below. The order of the subjective examination can vary, and sometimes order is cued by the patient's starting point. Usually the patient wants to tell you about the pain first; therefore, an opening question might be, "What is the problem causing you to seek care?" The patient will probably respond by explaining the nature of the symptoms.

The symptoms and their location are often recorded on a body chart. In some clinics, the patient fills out a body chart indicating the location, description, and intensity of the symptoms. Sometimes it is helpful to have the patient's own diagram. However, the patient's diagram does not replace the therapist's drawing, which should be more anatomically precise.

Description of Symptoms

Patients usually complain of one or more of the following general problems: pain, stiffness, weakness, "giving way," loss of function, spasms, numbness or tingling, fear of progressive deformity (eg, scoliosis), instability, or hypersensitivity. The patient may have been referred after surgery, injection, or other treatment. The specific words selected to describe symptoms may have some diagnostic significance; however, these are only one piece of a puzzle and conclusions cannot be based on descriptions alone.

Diskogenic pain tends to be deep, diffuse, poorly localized, and segmental. A dull, aching pain that is well localized may describe ligamentous pain. Tight, tired, diffuse, cramping, and burning may describe muscular pain. A zygapophyseal joint sprain may be described as sharp, well defined, superficial, and unilaterally referred. Dural pain tends to be described as knife-like, and has extrasegmental reference. *Tingling* (pins and needles) and *numbness* should be differentiated. If the patient describes numbness, ask if there is an area of skin that can be touched or pricked without being felt. Repeatable joint noise, such as popping or slipping, may suggest instability, soft tissue scarring, or joint surface abnormalities. Painless weakness following a specific myotome distribution may indicate a neurological deficit, whereas generalized weakness may be the result of disuse.

Intensity can be described, at least from the individual patient's perspective, by using a zero to ten scale. *Zero* means no symptoms. The patient is asked, "On a scale from zero to ten, with ten being the worst imaginable pain, what is the level of your pain now?" Some patients need to be pressed for a specific number. Next, ask the patient to give the range of the pain for a specified duration. Using a numerical scale such as this assists in determining the patient's perception of the severity and serves as a method of reporting the extent of change.

Location of Symptoms

Concurrent with ascertaining the nature of the symptoms, the patient is asked the exact location of the symptoms. A precise spot can overlay the cause of the pain, or if deeper could indicate a sclerotome. Larger, more generalized pain areas suggest disorders of other structures. Pain is more frequently referred distally than proximally. However, location of pain is not a reliable indicator of the site of the problem. For example, spinal joint disorders are usually unilateral, but can refer pain great distances. Diskogenic symptoms can be bilateral across the spine and can refer symptoms bilaterally or unilaterally. Inflammation and muscle spasm tend to spread from the original site. Sacroiliac symptoms frequently include point-specific pain, tenderness at the sacral sulcus, and occasionally radiating leg pain.

The patient may cite his primary symptoms and not mention leg pain, for example. If the patient does not volunteer the information, you must ask about other associated symptoms—in this case, particularly in the buttocks or legs.

Current History

The next line of questioning relates to how long the patient has had the symptoms (to determine the stage of the disorder) and whether the symptoms began suddenly or gradually. The specific time frame must be defined. If the symptoms began suddenly, was there a specific injury such as an accident, fall, or twist? How severe was the trauma, and does it correlate to the severity of the complaints? If the symptoms began gradually, then predisposing factors or an incident may have been the cause. Predisposing factors might include overuse, fatigue, unaccustomed activity, prolonged posture, heredity, a virus, smoking, or the cumulative effects of poor biomechanics, stress, exposure to vehicular or other vibration, poor posture, or general deconditioning. Patients usually try to blame a specific incident. However, an incident may be the precipitating event, and the cause may actually relate to the predisposing factors. Also, have the symptoms changed, and are they getting worse, better, or staying the same? The effect of other treatments should be noted for possible inclusion in, or exclusion from, the treatment program.

Behavior of Symptoms

A most important aspect of the subjective examination is determining the behavior of the symptoms. Behavior refers to the relationship of the symptoms to rest, activities, and positions; ease of irritability; constancy; changes in site and intensity; frequency; duration; and periods of relief. Ask if the symptoms are constant or intermittent. If constant, do they vary in intensity with certain activities or positions? Record specifically how long an incident lasts and when it comes on. If the patient states that

the symptoms begin after standing for 10 minutes, then the specific time can be used as a comparison for change with treatment. The effects of rest, bending, sitting, rising from sitting, standing, walking, and lifting need to be noted. The ease with which the symptoms began, the length of time they last, and how long they take to return to their previous level help determine the irritability. The therapist is looking for common denominators. A patient may state that his pain is aggravated by sitting, bending, lifting, brushing his teeth, shaving, and driving to work. The positions and movements common to these activities involve lumbar flexion. Diskogenic pain is typically aggravated by sitting and forward flexion, whereas standing and walking, which involve lumbar extension, tend to relieve the pain. However, walking may aggravate zygapophyseal joint pain. Sacroiliac symptoms may be aggravated by weight bearing on the side of the lesion, sitting on the ischial tuberosity on the involved side, and rising from sitting to standing.

Musculoskeletal symptoms are generally aggravated by specific positions and movements, and are relieved by rest. Symptoms unchanged with rest and unrelated to specific movements or postures may indicate more serious pathology.

Site-Specific Questions

Special questions should be asked based on the anatomical and physiological aspects of a particular area. For example, gynecological problems can cause back symptoms. Therefore, women need to be asked if back symptoms are related to the menstrual cycle. Because space-occupying lesions of the spine are usually aggravated by coughing or sneezing, the therapist must inquire about these sudden exertions.

Previous History

The previous history of this problem should be obtained, including the cause, duration, treatment, and result. The course and frequency of any successive bouts should also be determined.

General Medical History

Questions about the general medical history are to help determine any precautions or contraindications for treatment, or whether the problem is truly musculoskeletal in origin. These include questions about general health; unexplained weight loss; previous surgeries; cardiac problems; tingling or numbness of the feet, hands, or genital region; bladder disturbances; osteoporosis; and current medications.

Personal Information

Personal information including age, gender, and occupation may already have been obtained from admitting records. Some disorders are age- or gender-related. True disk herniations are rare after age 50 because the disks have generally degenerated. Most forms of ankylosing spondylitis are more prevalent in men. In addition to the more obvious personal information, the actual positions and activities required for a particular job may vary within the same job title and cannot be assumed. Additionally, it is important to note the patient's avocational activities, general activity profile (sedentary, light, moderate, or heavy), job satisfaction, and goals.

PLANNING THE OBJECTIVE EXAMINATION

Before beginning the objective examination, the therapist should consider the subjective findings. Were the patient's statements about the onset, nature, location, intensity, and behavior of the symptoms consistent? Which statements need to be checked in the objective examination? Are special tests indicated? How irritable does the condition seem? What precautions need to be considered? It may be helpful to list the possible causes of the problem, that is the underlying joints and muscles, and the referring structures. Also, what mechanical problems could have caused the problem or could predispose the patient to recurrences? These need to be examined. The preventive concept means treating more than just the symptoms of the problem. An inexperienced therapist will need more time for planning. In fact, it may be a good idea to leave the patient for a few minutes in order to plan, check reference texts, or consult colleagues. Checking does not reflect poorly on the therapist, but *not* checking does.

OBJECTIVE EXAMINATION

The therapist's purpose is to reproduce the *comparable signs,* or those combinations of movements or positions that most accurately reproduce the patient's symptoms (Maitland, 1986). The patient must be sufficiently undressed to examine the entire spine and legs.

General Observations

Initial observations are made immediately upon meeting the patient and while conducting the subjective examination. How did she rise from sitting? Does she limp? Does she sit still or shift constantly? How is her sitting posture? Does she use a cane or wear a brace? Because disk pressure is high when sitting, a patient with disk pain may prefer to stand during the examination. Ligamentous pain tends to become more pronounced with prolonged postures; therefore, this person may shift constantly.

Posture and Anthropometric Features

The postural examination consists of observation and palpation posteriorly, laterally, and anteriorly. The patient is usually asked to stand facing away from the examiner. The patient's unstructured stance is noted. In this habitual stance the patient may be compensating for a number of postural asymmetries. Therefore, it will be easier to detect these problems if the stance is structured, that is the patient should stand with the feet hip-width apart and perpendicular to a line on the floor, and with the shoulders relaxed. Figures 27-2 *A* and *B* show a dramatic example of the difference between structured and unstructured stance.

Observations made posteriorly include body build, scars, stance, waist angle, lateral shifts, and scoliosis. The levels of the shoulders, scapulae, iliac crests, posterior superior iliac spines (PSIS, which are also palpated for

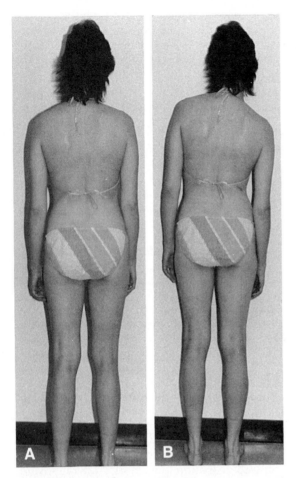

Figure 27-2. *(A)* The patient's habitual, unstructured stance. *(B)* The patient's posture when her stance is structured to eliminate compensatory mechanisms.

asymmetries in depth), gluteal folds, trochanters, fibular heads, calcaneal angles, and longitudinal arches are either observed or palpated. Forward head carriage and the amounts of kyphosis, lordosis, pelvic angle, and trunk inclination angle are best viewed from the side. Areas of possible decreased or increased mobility can be noted now, and confirmed later in the examination. The chest configuration is viewed anteriorly, and the levels of the anterior superior iliac spines (ASIS) are palpated. The hips, knees, and ankles are also observed.

Because asymmetry is the "norm" rather than the exception, assessing the significance of asymmetry is difficult, especially at this point in the examination. One common asymmetry is that the shoulder on the side of the dominant hand is usually slightly lower than the shoulder on the nondominant side; therefore, a possible abnormal finding is a lower shoulder on the nondominant side. The therapist can begin thinking about the possible effects of structure on mechanics and in relationship to the patient's symptoms. For example, some asymmetries in the leg seem to be the body's attempt either to correct or respond to asymmetry. Supination of the foot functionally increases leg length; pronation decreases leg length; and knee hyperextension increases leg length. Various knee angles (genu varus or genu valgus) affect symmetry, particularly if one leg demonstrates a greater deviation than the other. A functional or structural leg length discrepancy may cause lateral flexion of the lumbar spine away from the short leg and necessary rotation toward the short leg side. This causes approximation of the zygapophyseal joints on one side with unilateral disk compression and asymmetrical stress.

If ipsilateral discrepancies in the levels of the iliac crest, ASIS, PSIS, and the trochanter are noted, lengths of either the limb segments or the total leg length are measured. Typically, leg lengths are measured in two ways and in two different positions to distinguish functional and structural differences. Leg lengths are measured in the weight-bearing (standing) position and in the non-weight-bearing (supine) position from the ASIS to the medial malleolus and from the umbilicus to the medial malleolus on each leg. Leg lengths are difficult to measure reliably, but leg length discrepancies may be a significant finding particularly with sacroiliac problems where pelvic mechanics may be significantly altered. For example, a posterior iliac torsion may accompany an actual long leg on the same side. Circumferential measurements are taken if atrophy or hypertrophy are noted in the legs during the postural examination.

Active Movements

The patient is asked to perform a series of active spinal movements, first in standing and sitting, then in supine and prone (see Table 27-1). The purposes of the active movement examination are to determine the total spinal range of motion, note the range at various spinal segments, observe the quality of the movements, and ascertain the effect of movement on the patient's symptoms.

The usual protocol is to instruct the patient to "bend forward slowly as far as possible *starting with your head*." The clinician observes the movement and the recovery to the upright position. This procedure is repeated in each direction of movement including flexion, hyperextension, right and left lateral flexion, and right and left rotation. The therapist may need to view flexion and hyperextension posteriorly and laterally; therefore, these movements may be performed more than once.

Range of Motion

The overall range or quantity of movement as well as the location of the movement is determined. Are various segments hypomobile (ie, lack the normal curve)? Are there adjacent hypermobile segments (ie, sharply angled curves)? Are these segments symptomatic? True lumbar flexion and hyperextension

ranges of motion (versus the composite lumbar and hip movement) are measured.

One technique to measure total range of motion and true lumbar range of motion in flexion and extension is with the use of two pendulum goniometers (inclinometers). In this technique one pendulum goniometer is zeroed at T12 and the other is zeroed on the sacrum (S1). The patient is asked to flex or extend the back. The T12 goniometric reading represents the total range of motion in either flexion or hyperextension. The difference between the T12 measure and the S1 measure represents the range of motion of the lumbar segment. The lumbar lordosis should merely flatten with flexion, not become kyphotic (hypermobile). However, if it does not flatten, hypomobility is noted (Fig. 27-3).

Reports of normal range of motion of the lumbar segment vary; however, Mayer and coworkers (1984) reported approximately 55 degrees of flexion and 27 degrees of hyperextension in normal subjects using inclinometers. New, computerized devices for measuring spinal range of motion, such as the Electronic Digital Inclinometer (EDI 320) (Cybex, Division of Lumex, Inc., Ronkonkoma, NY) are becoming available.

Some therapists prefer to have the patient sit to observe spinal rotation because the pelvis

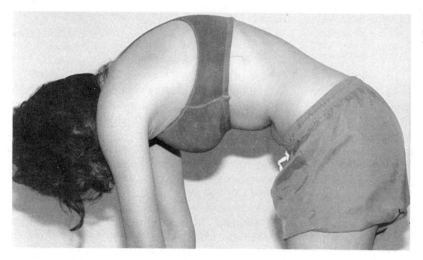

Figure 27-3. Hypomobility of the lumbar spine in flexion. The lordosis should flatten.

is better stabilized. Alternatively, the pelvis can be manually stabilized posteriorly in standing. As rotation occurs in one direction, lateral flexion occurs in the opposite direction in the lumbar spine. The spinous processes also move opposite the rotation. Both the spinous processes and the lateral flexion movements are observed during rotation. Attempts to measure lumbar spine rotation and lateral flexion reliably have not been very successful. However, the technique using two pendulum goniometers described above can be adapted, or the EDI 320 can be used for lateral flexion measurements. Range of these movements is frequently described as within normal limits, or minimally, moderately, or severely restricted according to bilateral comparisons. An alternative method of reporting is to envision the full arc of motion in quadrants or percents and describe movement restriction in those terms. For example, most people can laterally flex sufficiently to touch their fingertips to the lateral side of the knee (full arc of motion for lateral flexion).

To determine active sacroiliac (iliosacral) movement, the examiner palpates the migration of the PSIS bilaterally with the thumbs while the patient slowly flexes approximately 30 degrees forward. If there is *less* movement on one side, the PSIS on that side will move upward and forward sooner and farther than the opposite PSIS. This procedure is called a *forward flexion test*, and it may be performed with the patient sitting.

Quality

Quality refers to the smoothness and uniformity of the patient's movement throughout the spine. Movement quality can be observed simultaneously with measuring the range of motion, or while determining the effect of movement on the symptoms. Is the movement smooth? Are there deviations during or at the end of the movement? Deviations might suggest unilateral hypomobility, a posterolateral disk protusion, or unilateral hamstring tightness. Figure 27-4 demonstrates a movement deviation.

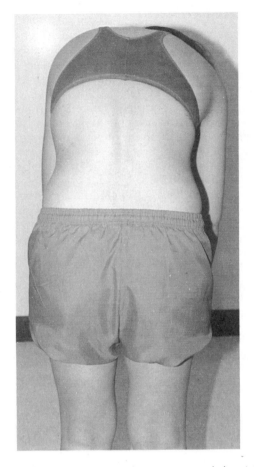

Figure 27-4. Movement deviation toward the right with trunk flexion.

Effect on Symptoms

The patient is asked to explain the effect of each movement on the position, location, and intensity of the symptoms, including changes in radiating pain. Particularly important are those movements that *centralize* the pain (cause the pain to move toward the midline), and those movements that cause the pain to increase or move distally away from the spine and into the buttocks and legs (McKenzie, 1981).

Instead of rotation and lateral flexion, McKenzie (1981) describes a combination of these movements called *side-gliding*, which is performed toward the right and toward the left. This movement is performed in standing by stabilizing the patient's shoulders and instructing the patient to glide the hips laterally while keeping the shoulders parallel to the floor. The effects of prolonged posture (holding a position 30 seconds or longer) and repeated movement (10 repetitions or more) are noted particularly in flexion, extension, and side-gliding. In other words, do the symptoms get better, get worse, or remain unchanged during single, repeated, or prolonged movements or positions? Do the effects on movement correlate with the patient's description of symptoms? The effects of single and repeated movements and prolonged positions are also obtained with the unloaded spine in supine (supine lying, double knees to chest) and prone (prone lying, prone on elbows, press-ups).

If the patient demonstrates an acute postural problem such as a lateral shift or hypolordosis, attempts are made to correct the posture, and the effects of the correction are determined. Sometimes gradually correcting a lateral shift will centralize diskogenic pain. Figures 27-5 *A* and *B* show a lateral shift and a lateral shift correction.

Repeated flexion will typically cause increased peripheral symptoms in disk protrusions, but may actually relieve joint hypomobilities. A "slipping" sensation may indicate hypermobility. Sometimes combinations of movement are required to elicit a comparable sign and to achieve relief. This is especially true if the patient describes a particular movement combination that is painful or is similar to that which occurred at the time of injury. Hyperextension with rotation is frequently painful over an involved sacroiliac joint.

Passive Movements

Passive movements further help to determine the tissue involved. During passive movements the noncontractile tissues are stressed while the contractile tissues remain at rest.

Physiological Passive Movements

The same movements (flexion, extension, lateral flexion, and rotation) tested actively in the lumbar spine are tested passively to check intersegmental mobility and the effect of movement on the symptoms. Because of body weight considerations, the sidelying and prone positions are frequently used to check physiological passive movements in the lumbar spine and sacroiliac joints. Passive mobility of the sacroiliac joints consists of ASIS rocking, and anterior and posterior torsions of the ilia. ASIS rocking consists of placing your palms on the patient's ASIS area and gently rocking the ASIS backward to feel the movement symmetry. Passive movements are graded using a six-point scale described in Chapter 19, Musculoskeletal Analysis: Introduction. Grading passive mobility requires palpation skill, practice, and experience; however, even then, reliability from one rater to another is low.

Additionally, the passive motions of the bilateral lower extremities, especially the hips and subtalar joint, are checked. Restrictions in hip and subtalar ranges of motion frequently accompany sacroiliac problems.

End-Feel

The end-feel (type of restriction felt at the end of the patient's available range) is determined by feeling the end of the motion. Cyriax (1982) describes various types of end-feels.

Accessory Passive Movements

Accessory movements are involuntary motions necessary for full, painless voluntary range. Spinal accessory movements include posteroanterior (PA) glides, segmental rotation, and traction/compression. PA glides and rotation movements are tested using *spring tests*. PA glides in the lumbar spine are performed with the patient prone, using either the thumb or the pisiform area of the hand to apply a springing movement to each spinous process and the sacrum. Rotation is tested similarly, but a unilateral force is applied to each transverse process. Distraction is a force applied to separate joint surfaces slightly, and compression approximates joint surfaces. Compression and

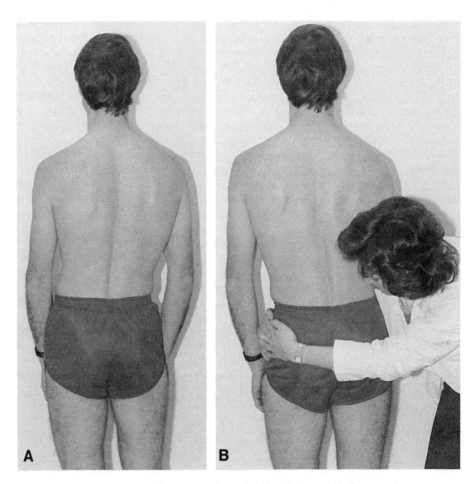

Figure 27-5. *(A)* Patient with an acute lateral shift. *(B)* Lateral shift correction.

distraction in the lumbar spine and sacroiliac joints are used more frequently to provoke symptoms than to detect mobility. In fact, they are called *provocation tests* and are described later in the special tests section.

Bony and Soft Tissue Examination

The bony and soft tissue examination consists of palpation and tests of flexibility, strength, and muscular endurance.

Palpation
Palpation is used to determine the position and condition of skin, subcutaneous tissue, muscle, musculotendinous junctions, ligaments, joint lines, and bony prominences. Palpation is performed bilaterally with the patient prone (not lying on any pillows) and supine. The examiner begins distal from the immediately symptomatic area to gain a feeling for the patient's normal tissue. Palpation is performed lightly and progresses more deeply, with the examiner noting temperature, tissue tension, muscle spasm, tenderness, swelling, nodules, and painful areas. Structures that may be palpated with the patient prone include skin, subcutaneous tissue (using a *skin-rolling* test), the erector spinae, gluteus maximus, piriformis, supraspinous and infraspinous ligaments, iliolumbar ligaments, posterior sacroiliac ligaments, L1-L5

spinous and transverse processes, obturator foramen, sacral hiatus, sacral cornu, sacral spines, inferior lateral angles, sacral sulcus, and PSIS. Structures palpated in the supine position include the ASIS position and the pubic tubercles.

Palpation is particularly necessary for determining pelvic girdle dysfunction. For example, the position of the sacrum is palpated to determine if rotation has occurred about either of the two oblique axes. If the sacrum is rotated left about a left oblique axis, the cornu on the left will feel more prominent, whereas the right cornu will feel deep. In the case of a posteriorly rotated right ilium, the right PSIS will feel more prominent and the right pubic tubercle will appear higher. Sponginess and increased tissue tension over the sacrum is frequently associated with dysfunction. All structural asymmetries need to be correlated to the patient's symptoms. Again, asymmetry alone does not necessarily correlate with the patient's problem.

Flexibility (Muscle Length)

Shortening of various muscle groups, especially hip and two-joint muscles, can contribute to or occurs in response to a variety of postural and joint dysfunctions. Tightness may not cause specific disorders, but tightness may result from other forces and may aggravate certain conditions. For example, tight hamstrings may restrict hip mobility and increase the strain on lumbar and lumbopelvic structures. Unilateral hamstring tightness is frequently associated with a posteriorly rotated ilia. Rectus femoris tightness is associated with hyperlordosis. Associated muscles usually checked for length include latissimus dorsi, iliopsoas, hip adductors, gluteus medius, tensor fascia latae, piriformis, rectus femoris, hamstrings, soleus, and gastrocnemius.

Strength

The muscles involved with posture, spinal movements, the pelvis, and lower extremities may need to be checked for possible weakness or imbalance. These tests are in addition to the selected resisted tests in the neurological screening section. Strength testing of these additional muscle groups may need to be deferred if the spinal condition is irritable. These tests are not diagnostic, but rather are performed for the purpose of setting treatment goals such as increasing stability, correcting posture, reducing strain, and preparing to return to work. Some specific muscles to be checked are included in Table 27-1.

Strength testing is difficult because strength is poorly defined and varies with different types of contractions, muscle lengths, body positions, and so forth. Also, the validity of strength testing is largely unknown. Therapists typically use manual isometric testing techniques; however, a trend exists toward the use of force transducers, isokinetic, and other mechanical devices. Trunk strength in particular is difficult to determine with manual techniques.

Numerous companies manufacture isolated trunk testing devices. Most of these are relatively new, and reliability and validity have yet to be established. Devices range from isometric to isokinetic. Most research thus far has been done with Cybex isokinetic devices (Cybex, Division of Lumex, Inc., Ronkonkoma, NY).

Mayer and co-workers (1985), using Cybex instrumentation, demonstrated generalized trunk flexor and extensor weakness and an imbalance between the muscle groups in patients with chronic low back pain. They further demonstrated that increased isokinetic trunk strength (among other variables) correlated with return to work. Generally, these devices and measurements obtained need further investigation.

Endurance

Endurance refers to the ability of a muscle or muscle groups to perform repetitively. Muscular endurance testing is not indicated with an acute problem, but may be important with postoperative and chronic problems before discharge and return to work. Of particular interest in these cases is the endurance of the trunk musculature and all the muscle groups involved in lifting. Endurance tests range from simple (observation and counting during a repetitive lifting task) to sophisticated measures of endurance using various forms of strength testing equipment.

Other Factors
Other measures of motor performance including power, work, coordination, and speed may also be important. However, little is known about the contribution of these factors to function.

Neurological Screening
A quick screening of sensation, muscle strength, and reflexes is performed if the patient complains of pain or numbness in the buttocks or legs.

Sensation
Light touch and pinprick are tested by dermatomes, usually at a distal point in the dermatome, and compared to the uninvolved extremity. Many of the references listed at the end of this chapter include dermatome reference charts. If a sensory loss is found, sensation is examined in more detail.

Reflexes
Deep tendon, or myotactic, reflexes are checked if numbness is present. The lower extremity reflexes checked include the infrapatellar tendon (knee-jerk) reflex, representing the L3-L4 neurological level, and the Achilles' tendon (ankle-jerk) reflex, representing the S1 level. Reflexes are checked bilaterally and graded from zero (absent) to four-plus (hyperactive). A grade of three-plus is considered normal.

Selected Resisted Muscle Tests
Selected resisted muscle testing is performed manually primarily to check the integrity of the innervation to the muscle groups. Selected muscles representative of spinal nerves are checked. These usually include L1-L2, psoas and iliacus; L3-L4, rectus femoris; L4, anterior tibialis; L5, extensor hallucis longus; S1 (L5), peroneals; S1, gluteus maximus; and S1-S2 gastrocnemius-soleus. Hand-held force transducers or other mechanical devices may offer greater reliability and discrimination, as well as the ability to use the numbers statistically for research or statisical analysis on individual patients.

Nerve Sensitivity Tests
Several tests can be used to stretch the spinal cord, cauda equina, sciatic, or femoral nerves. Three are the *straight leg raising test* (SLR), the *Kernig test* (head to chest), and the *prone kneebend test* (PKB).

The SLR is used to reproduce back and leg pain. With the patient supine or sitting, the examiner passively flexes the hip with the knee straight. Normal straight leg raising is about 80 degrees. Positive SLR for sciatic nerve problems usually occurs between 30 and 60 degrees, but must be differentiated from hamstring stretch pain. Movement in the range above 50 to 60 degrees stresses the supporting structures of the pelvis and can also cause symptoms. Dorsiflexing the foot during straight leg raising will further stretch the sciatic nerve and may produce the comparable sign. Occasionally, symptoms are aggravated when the opposite leg is raised.

The Kernig test is also designed to stretch the spinal cord. With the patient supine, the patient forcibly flexes the head toward the chest. Pain suggests nerve root involvement or dural irritation.

A PKB test is passive knee flexion with the patient prone to hyperextend the hip. This test is similar to the SLR test, but stretches the femoral nerve. Therefore, it is used if pain or other symptoms are present in the upper lumbar spine or in the L1-L3 dermatomal region. Pain from this test must be differentiated from rectus femoris stretch pain.

Balance
Proprioceptive problems, associated with injuries and after surgery in peripheral joints, may also be a problem in the spine. Body stability and postural sway can be tested using a simple stork standing test; however, measurements of displacement using a force platform, digital balance board, or an Equitest (Neurocom International, Inc., Clackamus, OR) can provide more objectivity and sensitivity.

Upper Motor Neuron Tests

Patient complaints of numbness or ataxia warrant a check to rule out upper motor neuron lesions. The Babinski test elicits a pathological reflex and can be used as a quick screen.

Special Tests

Special tests are those specific to a particular region of the body. Some of these tests are discussed as either lumbar or sacroiliac tests, but yield information about both body sites.

Lumbar Tests

A *distraction test* for the spine is a neurological test as well as a mobility test. Traction is applied to the spine with the patient sitting. The therapist stands behind the patient, reaches under the patient's axillae to grasp the patient's crossed arms at the wrists, and leans the patient backward (Fig. 27-6). This test may produce relief from spinal nerve impingement, disk pain, or zygapophyseal joint pain. Because distraction is not specific, this technique may be more helpful in determining if traction might be a beneficial treatment than it is to differentiate problems.

Compression of the spine consists of applying a downward force on the patient's shoulders to determine if pain is reproduced. Additional special tests are described in the bibliography at the end of this chapter.

Sacroiliac Tests

Distraction and *compression* tests are also performed at the sacroiliac joint and symphysis pubis. To compress the symphysis pubis and simultaneously gap or distract the sacroiliac joints, the patient is supine lying. The examiner places her hands on the ASIS with arms low and parallel and then compresses the pelvis by pushing inward (Fig. 27-7). Little, if any, movement can be perceived, but this distraction test may provoke sacroiliac symptoms. A similar test is frequently performed with the patient sidelying.

Compression of the sacroiliacs with simultaneous gapping of the symphysis pubis is also performed with the patient supine. The examiner places her hands on both ASIS medially

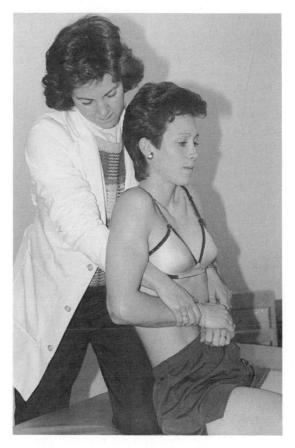

Figure 27-6. Distraction test for the lumbar spine.

with arms crossed and exerts an outward and downward pressure (Fig. 27-8). Again, this is a provocation test.

The functional sit-up test is similar to the standing forward flexion test, except that the lower extremity is stabilized on the treatment table, and the position is non-weight-bearing. To properly align the pelvis for the functional sit-up test, the patient flexes his hips and knees, placing his feet flat on the table, then lifts (bridges) his hips, lowers, and subsequently straightens his legs. The examiner stands at the foot of the table and places her thumbs immediately distal to the medial malleoli bilaterally, noting their position. If a right posterior torsion of the ilium is manifested, the

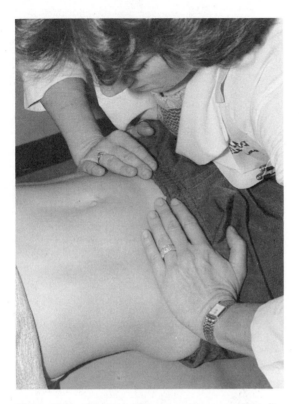

Figure 27-7. Therapist demonstrating a sacroiliac distraction provocation test.

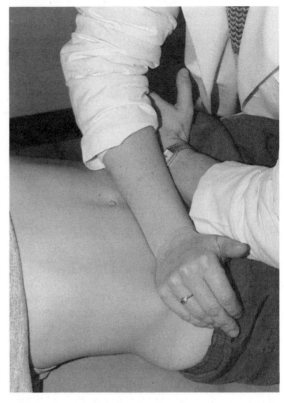

Figure 27-8. Therapist demonstrating a sacroiliac compression provocation test.

acetabulum will be retracted and the right medial malleolus will appear shorter than the left (ie, assuming there is no actual leg length difference). The patient then moves to a long-sitting position. As the patient bends forward during supine to sitting, the spine ligamentously locks each successive segment. As flexion arrives at the sacrum, if the right sacroiliac joint is immobile normal accommodation cannot occur, and the sacrum and ilium will move together. Thus, the acetabulum is moved forward and the right leg will appear to lengthen, causing a distal migration of the medial malleolus. The opposite events occur if the ilium is hypomobile in anterior torsion (Porterfield, 1985). The hip clearing tests described next are also important in stressing the sacroiliac joints.

Joint Clearing

Clearing a joint is examining it to determine whether or not it is involved in the patient's problem. To determine if a joint is normal may entail repeated quick movements, sustained overpressure at end of range, compression, and combined movement testing. There are active and passive clearing tests. A quick active test is squatting on the heels from standing and returning to standing. This quick test requires the extremity joints to go through full active range of motion with minimal back involvement.

Passive clearing may include tests for the lumbar spine, sacroiliac joints, hips, knees, and ankles. Some tests involve more than one joint or area, which may permit either clearing two areas simultaneously or, in some cases, the inability to distinguish the specific areas involved. Changes in symptoms or pain should be noted. If a comparable sign is produced, more in-depth examination is needed.

Lumbar clearing tests include active and passive movement tests with overpressure, compression, and distraction tests described earlier. Sacroiliac clearing includes the compression, distraction, torsion tests, sacral springing, and some of the hip clearing tests described below.

Hip clearing tests are the hip flexion-adduction-internal rotation test and the flexion-abduction-external rotation test (Fabere's test). The hip is placed in one of these positions, and overpressure and perhaps compression forces are applied. Hip tightness frequently accompanies sacroiliac dysfunction on the same side.

The knee is cleared by a check of the medial and lateral collateral ligaments using a varus and then a valgus stress on an extended knee, by gliding the tibia anteriorly and posteriorly with the knee flexed (drawer), and by overpressure in end-range movements.

To clear the ankle, the talus is glided anteriorly and posteriorly between the tibia and fibula, and overpressure is applied at end-range inversion and eversion.

Function

Various functional activities may need to be assessed for the purposes of treatment in both acute and chronic problems. In a patient in the acute stage, an activity may be aggravating the condition. One of the first treatment principles is to reduce or eliminate aggravating activities.

Gait

A gross gait analysis is particularly useful with sacroiliac problems in determining asymmetries in transferring and accepting force on the weight-bearing skeleton (Porterfield, 1985). The patient is instructed to walk 20 feet back and forth about four times, and the gait is viewed from each plane. Running may also need to be evaluated. A treadmill is useful for examining walking and running.

Activities of Daily Living, Work, and Play

Evaluating functional activities may be as simple as observing the patient's sitting posture and movements while sitting at a simulated desk arrangement. The therapist may observe activities or positions consistent with those that aggravate the condition. More complex assessment involves task analysis and measurement with work simulators and lifting devices. The purpose of functional analysis includes eliminating activities, modifying activities, or preparing the patient to perform activities.

Fitness

General cardiovascular fitness has been shown to correlate with low back problems. Therefore, fitness assessment may be appropriate in chronic conditions, particularly if the patient indicates a desire to improve in this area. A description of stress testing is outside the purview of this chapter.

ASSESSMENT (INTERPRETATION)

The most important and the most difficult step in the evaluation process is the assessment or interpretation of the findings. Novice clinicians may panic because the assessment seems so overwhelming and so critical. A misassessment can mean mistreatment, which wastes time and money, and perhaps even causes harm. Both the novice and the experienced clinician may feel hopelessly lost in a jigsaw puzzle of seemingly unrelated pieces of information, in this case called signs and symptoms. As in completing a jigsaw puzzle, the clinician must look for similarities among the pieces and "fit" them together to form a big picture, that is, the pathology or syndrome. For this reason, knowledge of anatomy, function, and clinical features is essential. The difference between knowledge and lack of knowledge in these areas is like putting together a puzzle while you look at the picture on the box, versus putting together a puzzle without the benefit of a picture. Of course, the exact clinical picture in low back pain is often not known, which is the challenge. As in solving a puzzle, part of the satisfaction is gained in the process of figuring it out, and not just in accomplishing the task. Given adequate background knowledge and a thorough examination, the assessment process can be described in the six overlapping steps discussed below.

CORRELATION OF SUBJECTIVE AND OBJECTIVE FINDINGS

The patient's subjective statements about the history and symptoms should match each other and the clinician's objective findings. For example, severe symptoms are rarely directly attributable to minor trauma. Predisposing factors must have been present and need to be detected. If the patient complains that pain is aggravated by flexion-type activities, then the active movement examination should support this statement.

CLASSIFICATION OF THE TISSUE INVOLVED

The clinician compares a fairly consistent set of signs and symptoms with the clinical features of various pathologies, and again looks for a match. Remember that more than one diagnosis can be manifested simultaneously, and that structures interact, causing secondary problems. Sometimes, because of a patient's response to a specific treatment, the original tissue type implicated cannot be the one involved, and a reassessment is required.

DETERMINATION OF STAGE

The stage of the disorder refers essentially to the duration and type of symptoms manifested, although some symptoms remain in an acute stage longer than expected. Paris (1979) describes five stages: (1) *immediate*—the first few minutes following trauma and before the onset of guarding; (2) *acute*—from minutes up to one to two days following the onset, characterized by worsening of the condition; (3) *subacute*—the symptoms begin to decrease, and function increases; (4) *settled*—the condition is stable, and corrective therapies are more effective; and (5) *chronic*—months or years in duration, and represents a poor response to treatment or lack of appropriate treatment. The type, aggressiveness, and sequence of treatment is determined largely by the stage of the disorder.

FORMULATING CLINICAL IMPRESSIONS

Forming a clinical impression involves deciding which factors are primarily responsible for the dysfunction, and which factors occur secondarily. Treatment partially depends on these determinations. This step also includes estimating the prognosis and the treatment time required, and recommending if physical therapy services are appropriate.

PROBLEM IDENTIFICATION

Once impressions, prognosis, and appropriateness of physical therapy care are determined, the precise problems requiring treatment are defined. Frequently, the tissue, stage, impression, and problems are stated in one or two sentences, for example:

> This patient has chronic, grade 5 (hypermobile) posterior rotation of the left iliosacral joint apparently secondary to a leg length discrepancy on that side, and perpetual overuse from running 45 miles per week during the last five years. The patient is well motivated, accustomed to exercise, and should respond well to treatment.

ESTABLISHING GOALS

A few global, functional long-term goals are determined, supported by specific, measurable short-term treatment goals. Short-term goals include the estimated time required to achieve the goals, and the method of determining whether a goal has been reached. An example of a short-term goal is "Increase passive PA gliding mobility of L4-L5 from grade 2 to grade 3 in three treatment sessions."

The next steps, of course, are developing and implementing an individualized treatment plan based on the problems identified during the examination. Once treatment has started, evaluation begins again.

ANNOTATED BIBLIOGRAPHY

Cyriax J: Textbook of Orthopaedic Medicine: Diagnosis of Soft Tissue Lesions, Vol 1, 8th ed. London, Bailliere Tindall, 1982 (A classic text describing clinical examination techniques for differential diagnosis of soft tissue lesions by systematic stressing of potentially involved tissues. Included are the signs and symptoms of various soft tissue lesions.)

Kendall HO, Kendall FP, Boynton DA: Posture and Pain. Baltimore, Williams & Wilkins, 1952 (This book is divided into four parts: evaluation of postural alignment, analysis of mobility, treatment of painful postural conditions, and a discussion of developmental and environmental factors affecting posture. The authors emphasize the role of faulty posture and body mechanics in painful conditions.)

Maitland GD: Vertebrae Manipulation, 5th ed. London, Butterworths, 1986 (Discusses systematic assessment of different spinal levels, including the use of combined movements. The sections on history-taking and communication are particularly organized and detailed. The text also includes a glossary of terms, principles and applications of manipulative technique based on signs and symptoms, and case history examples.)

Mayer TG, Gatchel RJ, Kishino N et al: Objective assessment of spine function following industrial injury: A prospective study with comparison group and one-year follow-up. Spine 10:482, 1985 (This study won the 1985 Volvo Award in Clinical Sciences. Quantitative functional capacity measures and degree of effort were used to guide the treatment of 66 chronic low back pain patients. These patients were compared with a group of 38 chronic pain patients who did not receive the treatment program. Results demonstrated that functional capacity measures collected for the treatment group improved in approximately 80% of the patients, and at one-year follow-up, this group had approximately twice the number of patients who returned to work compared to the control group.)

Mayer TG, Tencer AF, Kristoferson S et al: Use of non-invasive techniques for quantification of spinal range-of-motion in normal subjects and chronic low-back dysfunction patients. Spine 9:588, 1984 (Presents a simple method to separate and measure the components of the compound sagittal motions of the hips and spine using inclinometers. Normal subjects and chronic low back pain patients were tested and differentiated. Comparisons of this technique and measures of radiographic flexion-extension films demonstrated no statistical difference between the radiographic and the inclinometer techniques.)

McKenzie RA: The Lumbar Spine: Mechanical Diagnosis and Therapy. Waikanae, New Zealand, Spinal Publications Ltd, 1981 (Presents a three-category classification and differentiation system for mechanical low back pain: postural syndrome, dysfunction syndrome, and derangement syndrome. The author advocates postural correction for the first disorder, and usually self-treatment of dysfunctions and derangements using the patient's own movements. The discussions of predisposing and precipitating factors, the centralization phenomenon, and the effects of various spinal movements are essential reading. Treatment procedures are described for each of the three mechanical low back syndromes. Except in rare cases, derangements are initially treated using principles of spinal extension, for which McKenzie is best known, and progress through spinal flexion.)

Paris SV: Course Notes: The Spine: Etiology and Treatment of Dysfunction Including Joint Manipulation, 1979. (These are the course notes and handouts that accompany the spinal manipulation courses (S1-S3) given by Paris and colleagues and sponsored by the Institute of Graduate Health Sciences. The notes consist of outlines, article reprints, explanatory materials, and illustrated manual therapy techniques. Specifically, they include the history of manipulation, a review of anatomy and spinal mechanics, descriptions of spinal dysfunctions organized by structure, evaluation, treatment concepts [especially manipulative techniques taught in the courses], appendix, and references.)

Porterfield JA: The sacroiliac joint. In Gould JA, Davies GJ (eds): Orthopaedic and Sports Physical Therapy, pp 550–580. St Louis, CV Mosby, 1985 (Reviews the relevant anatomy and biomechanics of the lumbosacral region and describes the procedures for evaluating this area, organized by body position. Treatment is discussed, including the use of the sacral support belt developed by the author.)

Saunders HD: Evaluation, Treatment and Prevention of Musculoskeletal Disorders. Minneapolis, Anderberg-Lund Printing Co, 1985 (The author takes a comprehensive approach, emphasizing the role of examination and assessment. Includes sections on the principles of orthopaedic physical therapy; evaluation of musculoskeletal disorders; basic spinal biomechanics; pathology and treatment concepts for the spine, extremities, and temporomandibular joint; spinal mobilization; traction; orthotics; and educational programs for back care. Suitable for entry-level therapists.)

28 Neuromuscular Analysis

GEORGE E. CARVELL
JESSIE M. VAN SWEARINGEN

Physical therapists use neurological assessments to ascertain whether functional deficits are related to nervous system dysfunction. Clinical testing of neurological function can help to localize the problems and guide the therapist in choosing and implementing effective therapeutic interventions. In this chapter we will introduce some basic clinical measures of nervous system function performed by the physical therapist and the rationale for interpretation of the test results.

It is assumed that the reader has prior knowledge of the anatomy, physiology, and pathology pertinent to the normal and abnormal nervous system. You will recall that the nervous system can be divided into a peripheral nervous system (PNS) and a central nervous system (CNS) (Brodal, 1981; Daube and co-workers, 1986).

The PNS includes cells in the peripheral ganglia, including autonomic, dorsal root, and cranial nerve ganglia and their axons. It also includes motoneurons, which project their axons into cranial or peripheral nerves, and supportive cells such as Schwann cells that produce peripheral nerve myelin and have important reparative functions in injured peripheral axons. The CNS includes all the neurons and their projections that remain within the brain and spinal cord. It also includes supportive cells, primarily glial cells, found in the brain and spinal cord. Glial cells perform metabolic, nutritive, and other support functions including myelination of CNS axons. Glial cells react to CNS injury, but, unlike Schwann cells, may actually impede regeneration of neural pathways.

The CNS contains gray matter where neuron cell bodies are located. Diseases that produce damage to gray matter structures will result in death of neuron cell bodies. Neurons are amitotic, that is, neurons that die will not be replaced. Death of neurons means a loss of the integrative signal processing that characterizes normal neuronal function. It should not be surprising that large nervous system lesions produce permanent damage and lasting signs and symptoms of neurological dysfunction.

The CNS is also composed of white matter, which contains axons that carry information over short or long distances from one part of the nervous system to another. Diseases that affect central nervous system axons produce a disconnection of neural signal distribution. If axons are severely damaged they will degenerate. *Functional* regeneration over long neural pathways is virtually nonexistent in the CNS, but may occur in the PNS. Central white matter lesions producing axon degeneration will result in permanent loss of prior connections, typically resulting in lasting signs and symptoms of neurological dysfunction.

However, there is increasing evidence for plasticity, even in the adult nervous system (Bishop, 1982; Kaas and co-workers, 1983). Plasticity refers to structural or functional adaptation of the nervous system to changes within the internal or external environment.

Plasticity is part of normal development through the life cycle. Some adaptive processes may occur during a very narrow window in the life cycle. Exposure to changing conditions in the environment outside of this window will have little or no effect in triggering adaptive processes. For example, a patient with congenital cataracts may have normal vision restored if the cataracts are removed *early* in life. But, if the cataracts are not removed until the patient is an adult, although the eye is restored to normal function the patient will not have restoration of normal vision. Unfortunately, the time table for maturation and potential for adaptation of the motor system is more elusive. Often we are not sure if the window is open or closed for adaptive changes in motor circuitry in patients of different age groups. Although behavior may change in a patient, the neural correlate of this adaptive response is often difficult to specify. Much time and effort have been and will continue to be expended in research devoted to identification of triggers, windows, and neural events associated with plasticity.

The nervous system also responds to injury. Because the nervous system distributes its processing among related, but separate, neural centers, most injuries produce both local and projected changes in neuronal connections and integrative functions. These changes may either assist or hinder recovery of function. Therefore, a lesion restricted to one motor area (eg, motor cortex) will not obliterate motor function because motor function is distributed among many regions of the CNS. However, the lesion will produce qualitative and quantitative changes in motor function resulting from local damage in the motor cortex and disconnections with remote motor centers located in the brain and spinal cord. What we see clinically are the functions that initially survive the lesion and, later on, those functions that recover following adaptive changes over time.

Physical therapists should actively explore therapeutic interventions that will enhance neurological recovery. As a general rule, one would expect lesions restricted to small regions of the white matter to have the best opportunity for functional recovery. Larger lesions, especially those affecting vital gray matter structures, have more drastic and permanent neurologic sequelae.

Data contributing to a patient's neurological assessment are provided by many members of the health care team. These data help to establish the site and, if possible, the pathogenesis of the nervous system dysfunction. Subsequent treatment should be implemented by the appropriate health care professionals with goals that are mutually set by the health care team and, whenever possible, by the patient. Periodic evaluation of progression or regression should be based on appropriate documentation of the results of therapeutic interventions.

The physical therapist typically has frequent, direct contact with patients who have suspected or diagnosed neurological disease. These contacts include assessment and intervention to improve function. Therefore, the physical therapist may have a pivotal role in recognizing subtle or drastic changes in function of the patient over time. Judgment and documentation of recovery of function must be based on objective measures. Some of these current clinical measurements are well established, valid, and reliable, whereas others carry only the weight of empirical "dogma" based on historical insights or deductions from clinical observations. This state of the art and science percolates down through all the health professions. Health care providers must use judgments based on empirical data if cause-and-effect scientific rationale is not fully established. These limitations should not be a barrier to clinical practice, but a spark for cooperative endeavors to improve the tools by which we evaluate and treat persons who have suffered neurological impairment.

Neurological assessment should be based on the best information available. Information is available to the physical therapist from medical records, written and verbal information from other health professionals, information from family or other caretakers, and, most importantly, information from the patient. Information from the patient should include chief complaint(s), history of current and past illness(es), observation of physical and mental function, and objective testing of neurological function. In the following sections of this chapter we will present methods used to evaluate specific neurological dysfunctions, briefly discuss the importance of the testing procedures, and note how information from evaluation may guide your subsequent treatment of the patient.

MOTOR TESTING

Normal human movement is a result of the coordinated activity of multiple divisions of the nervous system. Often, specific tests are used to evaluate the function of one of the divisions of the motor system. However, information flow in the nervous system typically occurs over interconnected serial and parallel pathways. Thus, a single movement may represent the concurrent action of multiple neural centers.

OBSERVATIONS AT REST

Motor system testing begins with observations of the patient at rest. The therapist initially notes any asymmetry of the size of muscles or muscle groups. Asymmetry of muscle size may reflect the manner in which the patient has used or not used the muscles. Such patterns of use may result in a loss of muscle volume or muscle atrophy. The presence of muscle atrophy requires further evaluation of specific muscles and muscle groups through manual muscle testing and functional testing.

The position of the limbs or the trunk at rest may indicate the balance of activity between agonist and antagonist muscle groups about a joint. For example, a lesion within higher brain centers may release the inhibition of the tonic descending inhibitory input from brain stem centers to the spinal cord motor centers, and result in a predominance of extensor muscle activity. This imbalance of activity between extensor and flexor muscle groups tends to alter joint positions and yield a more extended posture. Observing joint positions

maintained at rest may also provide the therapist with information concerning weak or painful movements. To avoid or prevent movements in the direction of pain or weakness, patients may "splint" joints or use abnormal muscle activity to hold a specific joint position.

In addition to observing too much or too little muscle activity, the therapist should be alert to abnormal muscle function at rest. Fasciculations or spontaneous twitches of a muscle at rest are characteristic of certain lower motor neuron disorders or muscle injuries.

The therapist's suspicions derived from observing the patient at rest are confirmed by observing the individual in action. The ability of the person to move or be moved, to manage a load, and to perform activities involving sequencing motor acts for functional goals must be assessed.

ACTIVE MOVEMENT

Beginning the motor testing with active movement testing involves the patient early in the evaluation process and allows time for the patient to adjust to the evaluator and the novel situation prior to hands-on testing. Because active movement testing requires performance, the patient's willingness to move, communication skills, attentiveness, and body awareness are often apparent. For the person with difficulties in comprehending verbal requests, demonstrating the action desired may help avoid biasing the assessment of the motor system because of a communication disorder.

Active movement testing allows the therapist to observe a minimal functional level of muscle force production and range of movement. In addition, observing active movement permits the therapist to assess the ability of the nervous system to initiate, maintain, guide, and terminate movement.

In general, the therapist performs the active movement testing by asking the patient to move a particular body part from a specified starting position to an identified end point. For example, you might say to the patient, "Arms straight at your sides, palm of the hand facing forward, thumbs leading, lift your arms out to the side and over your head." As traditionally performed, active movement testing challenges a person's ability to produce task-oriented, isolated movements.

Fractionation, or the production of individual muscle contractions, demonstrates a unique aspect of human motor control. The inability to fractionate typifies the disordered movement characteristic of a corticospinal tract lesion. The person may exhibit gross, full, or partial limb movements in place of the specified isolated movement, such as a "raking" grasp movement of the hand and arm instead of a pincer grasp mechanism for retrieving an object.

Assessing Quality of Movement: Cerebellar Disorders

Normal, unloaded active movements of a body part from a starting position to a designated end point occur smoothly from start to finish. Both quantity and quality of active movement are essential features to observe. Moving a limb accurately to a target requires the return of information from the ongoing peripheral movement to the motor centers of the brain to guide the evolving motion (feedback-assisted movement). Under the direction of a normal nervous system, fast movements of large amplitude compromise accuracy. In contrast, the therapist should expect greater accuracy of the patient performing slow movements of small amplitude.

Accuracy of movement is an important factor in evaluating involvement of the cerebellum. Accuracy is a qualitative aspect of movement; problems with accuracy should alert you to the possiblity of a cerebellar disorder. Other qualitative aspects of movement associated with cerebellar lesions include delays in initiating (difficulty starting) and terminating a movement. Difficulties in moving, such as starting and stopping, and errors in the direction and velocity of movements represent ataxia or the decomposition of movement associated with cerebellar lesions. Errors in performing the range of movement requested, such as past pointing (dysmetria), and the in-

ability to continue repetitive alternating movements that require switching between agonist and antagonist muscles (dysdiadochokinesia) are qualitative changes in motor control also observed following cerebellar deficits. Another movement disorder attributed to cerebellar dysfunction, dyssynergia, involves difficulty performing compound movements, such as moving an entire limb in a specified pattern. Of course, not all of these qualitative movement changes are present in every patient with cerebellar disease.

Motor responses more consistently noted following cerebellar lesions include transient weakness in certain voluntary movements. The weakness resolves as the person, given enough time, often produces an appropriate muscle force for the given movement. For example, the patient asked to lift his arm overhead may lift the arm partially through the range, appear to "stall," and then, if not interrupted and encouraged to continue to attempt the movement, eventually produces sufficient muscular contraction to complete the range of motion.

The patient with cerebellar disease frequently demonstrates difficulty in holding a limb at one point in the range of motion. This holding motion requires the patient to produce and maintain muscle force output over time. Inability of the individual to hold the limb steady may be due to weakness, fatigue, or a proprioceptive problem. A manual muscle test of the functional muscle group may rule out weakness as the responsible factor. If muscle fatigue were the primary factor for the patient's inability to hold the limb steady, the limb would fall in the direction of the pull of gravity. Most likely, the patient also would report the sense of failing effort for the task. True "drift" of the limb refers to movement of the limb from the static position in directions other than the direction of gravitational pull (ie, up or out). The inability of the patient to prevent drift from the limb hold position with the eyes closed suggests a primary proprioceptive problem (deficit in position sense; see discussion later in this chapter). However, test performance may improve for the patient with the eyes open, because visual feedback may enable the patient to compensate with conscious, voluntary muscle contraction to maintain the steady limb position. If weakness and fatigue are primary causes of limb drift from the hold position, most likely the failure to sustain the limb position would occur with the eyes open as well as closed.

Assessing Quality of Movement: Basal Nuclei Disorders

Similar to the signs and symptoms noted after cerebellar disease, the qualitative aspects of movement change noticeably after basal nuclei disease. The role of the basal nuclei in movement concerns the strategic control of movements, that is, helping to select what motor acts should occur, in which order, and when appropriate. In contrast, the cerebellar function might be summarized as the moment-to-moment adjustment and timing of motor acts.

A loss of strategic movement control in persons with basal nuclei lesions results in what appears to be poorly planned and involuntary movements. For instance, the patient may be unable to string together the movements needed to rise from sitting to standing in a smooth, continuous movement despite having adequate joint range, muscle force, energy, and motivation. The involuntary movements range from rapid, large, flowing motions to the marked, short, oscillating movements characteristic of certain tremors. Thus, lesions of the basal nuclei disrupt the control and organization of movement, sometimes yielding lots of movement and at other times fixing the patient in a particular posture, as if frozen.

The patient with Parkinson's disease suffering from a depletion of dopaminergic neurons in the substantia nigra illustrates many changes in motor function related to loss of normal basal nuclei control. At rest, the patient with Parkinson's disease displays a characteristic tremor, often described as "pill rolling" of the fingers. The tremor may not be restricted to the distal limb (forearm and hand), but may include proximal limb (upper arm), head, and even trunk movements. The tremor typically decreases or disappears with volitional movement such as picking up a glass of water to drink. Tremor may also decrease with performance of a cognitive task, such as adding or subtracting numbers, and during sleep.

Passively moving the limb of a patient with basal nuclei disease elicits a motor response characterized by fluctuations in joint stiffness (cogwheel rigidity). An alternative motor response would be a generalized increased resistance to passive limb movement (plastic rigidity). The different forms of resistance to passive movement are described more fully in a later section on passive movement testing. During active movement, the signs of rigidity increase with increasing patient effort because co-contraction of flexor and extensor muscles also increases.

The most disabling motor symptom of Parkinson's disease is bradykinesia, or slowed movements. Bradykinesia may be severe enough to result in poverty of movement, a common descriptor of the lack of movement observed in the patient with Parkinson's symptoms. The slowed movement disorder prolongs reaction time for initiating, switching, or halting movements stimulated by external environmental stimuli or internal, willed movements. The patient's motor programs (sequence of motor acts) for movement tend to lose energy (de-energize) with repetition of the sequential motor task. Thus, the typical patient with basal nuclei involvement exhibits difficulty maintaining a repeated pattern of movement, such as the reciprocal movements performed during walking. The deficit in producing appropriate joint torque combined with too much co-contraction tends to immobilize the person in a certain posture (poverty of movement), and severely reduces associated movements of a given activity, such as arm swing during gait.

The typical festinating gait of the patient with Parkinson's disease illustrates the overall waning of motor output with repetition. In the festinating gait, the patient's center of gravity appears to be leading the forward movement. As a result, the person attempts to increase the walking speed and use momentum to catch up to the body's center of gravity. The patient is unable to stop the increasingly rapid shuffling gait, and loses control of the gait pattern. Changing directions or slowing on approach to a chair presents a major problem for the Parkinson's patient, whose ability to plan ahead for motor output and adapt motor programs appears severely compromised. Similar difficulties in managing motor output and adapting changes in speed and torque are readily observed in the patient's speech and feeding motor activities. The speech pattern may be one of slowed sound production and mumbling as a result of reduced lip movement. Chewing food may be characterized by slowed jaw action and the decline of jaw and tongue movements with repeated chewing motions.

In contrast to the poverty of movement or bradykinesia of the patient with Parkinson's disease, the involuntary movements (dyskinesias) characteristic of other basal nuclei diseases usually involve too much movement (hyperkinesia) or an alternation between too much and too little movement. Choreiform movements may completely disrupt the resting posture of a patient afflicted with Huntington's disease. The involuntary jerky movements characteristic of choreiform movement may occur in the head, face, trunk, or limbs. Another form of dyskinesia, athetoid movement involves slower, sinusoidal, writhing involuntary movements. Athetoid movement interferes with the patient's attempts to make voluntary movements. Attempts to move by the athetoid, cerebral palsy patient, for example, yield too much movement of the agonist and antagonist, sometimes resulting in co-contraction. Thus, joint position becomes stabilized when movement is desired. Alternatively, the production of too much movement of the agonist and antagonist may at other times be demonstrated as greater range of motion than necessary for the movement task. In some persons with athetoid cerebral palsy, periods of little or no motor responsiveness are followed by excessive movement, a condition known as fluctuating dystonia. Wild, flailing movements of the limbs constitute the hemiballistic movement of persons with subthalamic lesions. Though inappropriate for the

specific functional activity motivating the movement, the movements appear normal with respect to the muscle groups activated and the movement patterns. Practically speaking, the muscle activity produces nice movement, but in the wrong place, at the wrong speed, and at the wrong time! If severe, hemiballism may prevent the person from sitting still or sleeping.

PASSIVE MOVEMENT

Active movement testing provides information concerning an individual's willingness to move and a general idea of the quantitative and qualitative aspects of motor control. Passive motion testing serves to clarify the impression of the client's capacity for movement by indicating structural or functional limitations of the movement range. To obtain accurate data from passive motion tests, the client must be relaxed. Relaxation is difficult, particularly for the aware person who is unfamiliar with the therapist and the conditions that have brought the two together. For example, patients are like all of us when we are exposed to unfamiliar settings or are experiencing pain. The typical response to such experiences is an increase in muscle tension throughout the body, and a decrease in expression of movement and thoughts. With the patient in this state, determining full passive range of motion, palpating the muscle accurately, and even reliable patient reports of daily functional abilities becomes a problem. Thus, passive motion may need to be reevaluated in subsequent sessions when the client is more comfortable, to substantiate the initial passive movement evaluation findings.

Aside from comfort, key factors in performing passive movement testing and obtaining accurate findings include the positioning and stabilization of the patient's body and moving parts and the verbal and nonverbal directions for movement given. Position the patient so that mechanical factors, such as a two-joint muscle stretched simultaneously over both joints, do not restrict passive movement. Clothing, equipment, or even the therapist may also pose artificial restrictions to the passive movement. Positioning and stabilization of areas proximal or distal to the passive testing should be standardized, or at least noted. Repeat evaluations of passive movement should occur under similar conditions of position and stabilization.

Structural limitations to the passive range of motion usually have a distinctive end-feel at the end of the available range of motion: bone to bone (approximation of two hard surfaces), soft tissue approximation (compression of soft tissues), capsular (leathery nature with little give), muscular (like capsular, but with slightly more give), and springy (feeling of rebound). Functional limitations to the range usually result in an empty end-feel (no restriction to movement felt; patient's subjective report halts the passive movement). An empty end-feel, often associated with severe pain, prevents the patient from allowing the therapist to move the part to the point of resistance.

Noting and comparing the reaction of the limb muscle to passive movement provides information about the state of the muscle. The muscle reaction may be sensitive to the velocity of the limb displacement. For example, the muscle that exhibits an increased resistance to a rapid passive movement but little or no reaction to a slower passive movement demonstrates spasticity (a velocity-sensitive stretch reflex). In contrast, rigidity (an increase in joint stiffness with passive movement) does not change with changes in the velocity of the movement. As mentioned previously in relation to Parkinson's disease, a muscle resisting a passive movement of the limb through the range of motion demonstrates plastic rigidity. Another type of rigidity, referred to as cogwheel rigidity, presents as an unusual resist-give-resist-give pattern of reaction to the passive movement. This interrupted stiffness pattern of cogwheel rigidity may represent a tremor (oscillatory movement) imposed on rigidity (an increase in joint stiffness with passive movement).

RESISTED MOVEMENT

In a sense, active and passive movement testing convey the readiness and potential of the neuromuscular system to perform. The addition of a load or resistance asks the neuromuscular system to "perform under pressure." A muscle or muscle group is activated to produce force to move a load through a distance, ease the movement of a load through a distance, or prevent movement (maintain a position against resistance). Key elements of normal, purposeful resisted movement are the capacity to produce an adequate force, and the ability to isolate force production to the appropriate muscles, to build and adjust force output to variations in the resistance, and to protract force output over time (endurance).

Keep in mind that neuromuscular activity requires the support of the cardiovascular, respiratory, and digestive systems for fuel and waste product removal, particularly when stressed. As a functional measure, force output of a group of muscles varies with a person's age, history of activity, physical dimensions, and subjective factors such as pain, comprehension, and attention. Thus, the determination of normality based on resisted testing relies on the evaluator's synthesis of a number of potential variables.

Physiologically, the isolation of a force to a specific muscle results from discrete activation of pyramidal tract neurons (PTN) in the motor cortex for the flexor or extensor muscle resisted. Therefore, positioning and stabilization of the patient and therapist for resisted testing is important in isolating the test to a specific muscle or muscle group function. The site of the functional origin of the muscle of interest must be stabilized. The therapist should apply resistance in the opposite direction of the torque produced by the activation of the muscles of interest. Subtle changes in hand position for resisted testing may lead to errors in interpretation of dysfunction. For instance, if the therapist's hand placement for resistance to wrist extension is applied to the back of the client's hand, slightly to the radial aspect, the resulting resistance torque is in a flexion and adduction direction. Such a resistance isolates the radial wrist extensor muscle function, innervated primarily by axons of the C7 nerve root. Should the therapist be unaware of the radial shift of hand position, the interpretation of resisted wrist extensor testing could be normal, overlooking a C8 nerve root involvement indicated by ulnar wrist extensor weakness.

Pyramidal tract neurons appear to respond to the torque (tendency of a force to produce rotation about an axis) created by the load. The quantity of torque produced in response to a given resistance is graded normal if equal to a level of force expected for the person's size, age, and physical condition; mild weakness when the force produced seems under expectations for the individual, but within functional limits; severe weakness when the individual initiates muscle contraction and the force produced counteracts the resistance of gravity, but fails to reach functional levels; or complete paralysis when no detectable movement of the muscle occurs. (See manual muscle testing texts for specifics of resisted test performance and grading.)

Subsets of PTNs in the motor cortex respond for different aspects of torque production elicited by the resistance: (1) the rate of force production, (2) the maintenance of a steady-state level of force output, and (3) intermediate properties related to adjusting the speed and force of resisted movement. If the PTNs are functioning normally, the therapist would expect to observe some of the following responses to resisted testing. When resistance to a flexion movement is unexpectedly increased in midstream, co-contraction of flexors and extensors results in the initial stretch reflex flexor response. This co-contraction may represent an attempt to "reset" the level of muscle stiffness needed to manage the load. If the added load is sustained, the person should maintain the flexor torque output at the reprogrammed level. Inability of the client to demonstrate any of the above aspects of torque management suggests involvement of the PTN output.

In addition to quantitative information regarding force output of a muscle group, resisted testing enables the therapist to evaluate certain qualitative characteristics of human neuromuscular performance. During resisted testing the therapist asks the patient to match the resistance offered to his movement by holding the resisted limb at a certain position against a constant force (steady-state force production). The patient should also demonstrate the ability to adjust the level of force readily to an increased resistance (reset the level of muscle stiffness). Subsets of PTNs in the motor cortex are known to alter their activity to control the rate of force development, and thus the speed of movement, while other subsets of PTN control the steady-state level of force. Thus, lesions of the corticospinal region may result in the patient experiencing difficulty adjusting the rate of maintenance of a steady-state output of force of a muscle or group of muscles.

Not all movements occur under cortical control. The central nervous system seems to be able to switch control to subcortical centers depending on injury, disease, or the attentive and emotional state of the person. In the case of insult to the motor cortex, efficient and accurate resisted movement may be lacking. However, more general patterns of movement or rhythmic contractions may occur with adequate force development and speed. Qualities such as being able to adjust muscle stiffness to respond to unexpected changes in resistance may be impaired. Thus, the person with cortical involvement may display activation of multiple limb muscles in response to an isolated resistance. For example, when the therapist asks the patient to flex his wrist against resistance, the patient may respond with a total upper limb flexion pattern. Often these patients may accomplish the task as requested, while reporting a major increase in the effort required.

In addition to quantitative and qualitative characteristics of resisted movement, the pattern of weakness among structurally and functionally related muscles or muscle groups provides the therapist with insight into localizing the involved structure of the nervous system. Often, over time, the patient practices and the nervous system compensates for a weak muscle or weak link in a sequence of muscle contractions for a certain task-oriented movement by substituting with synergist activation or the combined activation of more than one muscle. For example, the patient who has a spinal cord injury at the C6 level may produce elbow extension for support of her body weight on her hands with the combined action of the shoulder external rotators and the shoulder flexors (C5-innervated muscles). Alternatively, the patient may alter normal posture or altogether avoid the use of weak muscles in movement. The patient with a cerebral vascular accident (CVA) resulting in hemiparesis may externally rotate his entire leg from the hip to avoid the use of a weak quadriceps muscle in stabilizing the knee during the stance phase of gait. The therapist becomes a detective in observing and recognizing motor substitutions or compensatory patterns.

Discovering an abnormally weak muscle should direct the therapist to examine more closely muscle groups innervated by the same branch of a peripheral nerve, the same peripheral nerve, a division of the same cord of a nerve plexus, the same trunk of a plexus, or the same nerve root level of origin of innervation. Sensory changes, particularly in related dermatomes, and deep tendon reflexes of relevant muscles are important correlative information in determining a specific level of nervous tissue damage.

Thorough evaluation of neuromuscular function includes evaluating muscle force production by asking the patient to perform repetitive contractions. A certain muscle group may demonstrate normal force production initially. However, upon the patient repeating the movement several times, the therapist notices a progressive deterioration of the force produced. For example, patients with myasthenia gravis typically respond in this manner to repeated contractions.

In contrast, single forceful muscle contractions are normally followed by relaxation of the muscle. Abnormally slowed relaxation following such muscle contraction is characteristic of myotonia.

FUNCTIONAL MOVEMENT

Beyond the individual tests of motor system performance and control, which aid the clinician in focusing on the involved area of the nervous system, the ultimate test of the motor system is performance of an activity involving movement of the entire body. Functional movements require accurate integration within and cooperation among multiple CNS "motor" centers. This distributed parallel and serial processing of motor acts requires planning, programming, and correct execution of simultaneous and sequential motor acts. Although the neural code(s) for the motor system is still largely unknown, research suggests that interconnected neuronal pools form cooperative networks that rely upon feedforward and feedback information. For example, while about two thirds of PTNs code aspects of ongoing motor execution of willed motor acts, the remaining one third of PTNs are coding the motor set for *subsequent* action. Therefore, it should not be surprising that functional activities can be distorted by lesions in widely separated "motor" and "sensory" brain areas.

Asking a patient to walk or perform activities of daily living during evaluation offers the opportunity to observe function. Observing functional activities provides valuable information for assessing the client's problems and planning the treatment program. In evaluating functional activity performance the intent is to determine what activities remain functional, what aspects of functional activities can be accomplished with substituted movements or external assistive devices, and what is the client's motivation for achieving movement competence.

Performances of gait and standing balance involve all areas of the motor system and typically illustrate a variety of altered patterns of movement caused by diverse neurological disorders. Many of the gait patterns resulting from diseases of the nervous system are distinctive and associated with a particular disorder.

While observing gait, quality and quantity of movement plus posture, balance, and effort exhibited should be noted and recorded. For example, the patient with hemiplegia often demonstrates generally reduced movement of the involved limbs. The involved lower extremity may be dragged or circumducted in the swing phase as a consequence of the functionally lengthened and less mobile extremity (eg, the stiffly held knee, or the foot plantarflexed because of foot drop). In addition, movement in the lower limb is often triggered by proximal trunk movements. The hemiplegic patient's involved arm may be held close to his abdomen in a semiflexed position.

The patient with spastic paraparesis may demonstrate an even greater reduction of movement characterized by a scissors gait. In a scissors gait, forward progression is slowed and awkward, and the patient drags both feet along the ground, knees scraping together as the adducted legs cross one in front of the other. As described previously, in relation to Parkinson's disease, a festinating gait presents an even more striking reduction of the quantity of limb movement.

By contrast, patients with cerebellar disorders frequently demonstrate gait patterns displaying excessive limb or body movement with postural instability. The person with a cerebellar gait (ataxia) walks with a widened base of support, and rather loose limb movement with irregular limb advancement and foot placement. If the ataxic patient is asked to stop suddenly or turn around, he often demonstrates reeling and marked unsteadiness.

Persons with muscular dystrophy or spinal muscle atrophy often demonstrate a waddling gait, resulting from pelvic girdle muscle weakness. This waddling gait is characterized by increased lumbar lordosis, a bulging abdomen, and increased trunk sway (side to side) to compensate for the pelvic girdle muscle weakness.

A person with weakness of the ankle dorsiflexors demonstrates a distinctive slapping of the foot after heel contact, unilaterally or bilaterally. Similarly, a steppage gait, which is characteristic of a person with severe bilateral foot drop, results in a high-stepping action with the foot flopping and the toes often dragging. Bilateral foot drop and the steppage gait may result from diverse conditions, for example, peroneal nerve damage, alcoholic neuritis, or progressive muscular atrophy. Alterations in the rhythm of a gait are most often associated with pain (limping or painful gait). The patient gently places the painful limb on the ground and rapidly advances the uninvolved leg in order to reduce the time of weight bearing in pain. Persons with hysterical gaits present a bizarre mixture of the previously described patterns, including alternation between wild, lurching, large movements and slowed, small, exaggerated actions with little limb movement.

Some involuntary movements are noted during other phases of the neurological exam, but are best assessed during performance of functional activities. The amplitude, frequency, rhythm, nature, and condition of occurrence of involuntary movements should be recorded. Tremors are involuntary movements resulting from a disruption of the normal agonist-antagonist activation pattern for a movement, and cannot be prevented by the conscious effort of the patient. Difficulty terminating contraction of antagonistic muscle groups delays initiation of the agonist, alters the terminal joint position, and leads to oscillations of a joint or several joints. Tremors may occur at rest (static tremors), throughout the range of movement (action tremors), or most marked toward the end of a movement (intention tremors). Static tremors of the head and hands are rapid in rate, small in amplitude, and generally disappear with purposeful movement. Examples include the senile tremor observed in a number of older people or the "pill-rolling" movement of the fingers and hands (and sometimes affecting the limbs, lips, and tongue) of the patient with Parkinson's disease.

Action tremors are associated with a variety of diseases, including metabolic or toxic disorders. The tremor may vary from a fine movement of the hand during writing or when grasping an object, to a much larger movement of the hands. Interestingly, essential or benign familial tremor, though sometimes gross, does not disrupt fine movements such as threading a needle. The gross, bizarre tremor of the hysteric patient tends to be inconsistent and may disappear when the patient's attention is diverted.

The primary cause of intention tremor is a

lesion of the cerebellum or the brain stem connections of the cerebellum. Depending on the severity of the lesion, the patient may have some degree of static tremor as well. However, the tremor worsens towards the end of a movement. This patient experiences major difficulty with writing and feeding because movements are inaccurate and uncontrolled.

SUMMARY OF MOTOR TESTING

Interpreting the collection of signs and symptoms noted during motor testing to arrive at some conclusions about the area and extent of motor system dysfunction is often difficult. Motor pathways significantly overlap with regard to anatomical targets and functional roles. In addition, the variability of each person's nervous system and life experiences, which may imprint or mold nervous system function, means similar lesions in different persons produce varying pictures of dysfunction. However, some degree of predictability allows the association of certain signs and symptoms with a particular level, area, or pathway of the motor system. An overview of the influence of a lesion to either of the two major descending pathways (ventromedial and dorsolateral) appears in Figure 28-1.

Clinical descriptions of motor testing results commonly classify motor system lesions as upper motor neuron or lower motor neuron. Both types of lesions cause muscular weakness.

Disruptions of the lower motoneuron (LMN) in the ventral horn of the spinal cord and its motor axon frequently present with disorders of movement involving single muscles. The clinician may observe fasciculations (twitches of groups of muscle fibers) of the involved muscle and the appearance of muscle atrophy. Deep tendon reflexes are hypoactive or absent, and the affected muscles lack the normal resting tension of healthy muscle, which is prepared to contract when called into action. Thus, the affected muscles in LMN disorders are more compliant to passive stretch. In addition, nerve conduction changes and EMG evidence of denervation accompany LMN disease. The ability to isolate muscle contractions is preserved in muscles with a manual muscle test grade of poor or better.

The upper motoneuron (UMN) syndrome results from lesions that disrupt neurons in the motor cortex, or neurons that give rise to the descending brain stem pathways, or the axons of these neurons that convey descending commands to spinal cord segmental centers. In contrast to LMN lesions, general features of the UMN syndrome include groups of muscles rather than single muscles, affected lack of fasciculations, and lack of muscle atrophy. Deep tendon reflexes heighten and the resting muscle tension appears increased. The combination of increased deep tendon reflexes and muscle stiffness is associated with the condition known as spasticity.

Spasticity describes the condition of increased sensitivity of the affected muscles to passive stretch. In spasticity, the passively moved limb resists the movement; the resistance of the moved limb is proportional to the velocity of passive movement. As previously reviewed, spasticity arises in part from the stretch reflex and frequently occurs with the clasp-knife phenomenon (the tendency for muscle tension to decline abruptly after an initial vigorous resistance to passive movement). Disruption of direct and indirect descending motor pathways to spinal cord lower motoneurons leads to a hyperreflexic state in UMN disease. A positive Babinski sign in the lower extremity and the Hoffman sign (described in the following section on reflexes) in the upper extremity are considered reliable signs of disruption of the descending motor pathways.

The loss of modulating descending information (which normally travels in the corticospinal and brain stem pathways to segmental motor centers) results in decreases in the force and speed of muscle contraction, alterations in muscle stiffness, and a loss of fine, skilled movement control. Lesions of the motoneurons of the cerebellum and basal ganglia affect the quality of movement. Such lesions disrupt smooth, coordinated movement, sequencing of motor acts, and motor programming. As a result, purposeful movements are often poorly timed and the force of movements may wane, leaving the performance of tasks incomplete. In

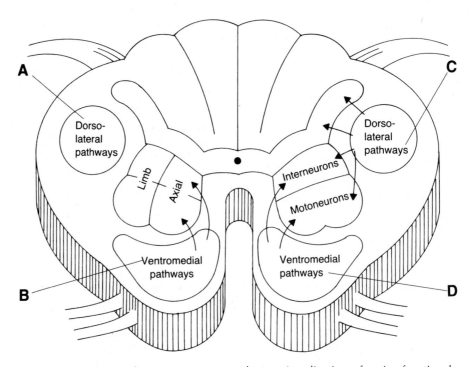

Figure 28-1. Descending motor system pathways. Localization of major functional groups of the motor system at the spinal level. Typical functional deficits associated with lesions to specific groups are as follows. (*A*) Loss of distal limb movements greater than proximal. The patient is unable to fractionate movements of the distal limb muscles, and manual dexterity is compromised. Lesions of this area at the spinal level may or may not produce upper motoneuron signs and symptoms. (*B*) Loss of axial and proximal limb muscle control. The patient has difficulty maintaining balance and posture, and stabilizing and producing sets of movements of the trunk and limbs, such as in the alternating pattern of muscle activity of human locomotion. Lesions of this area are accompanied by upper motoneuron signs. (*C*) Lesions of axons affect flexor and extensor muscles. Alterations in segmental and projected reflexes may result. Effects of damage to axons are primarily observed in unilateral movement responses. (*D*) Lesions of axons in this area tend to disrupt grouped muscle function or sets of muscles, as in a synergy. Most of the descending information in the region has strong bilateral influences on movement responses.

addition, involuntary movements frequently are present when the lesion involves the cerebellum and basal ganglia. Clinical signs of upper and lower motoneuron lesions are summarized in Table 28-1.

REFLEXES

A typical method for evaluating sensory-motor integration is the testing of reflexes. A reflex in the classical sense is a stereotyped response to a given adequate stimulus. Some of these reflexes have a simple segmental reflex arc, such as the monosynaptic phasic stretch reflex or deep tendon reflex. The entire reflex arc of the deep tendon reflex is well established from receptor to effector. Other reflexes, such as the short-latency flexion reflex (withdrawal reflex), may utilize a number of different types of receptors. The withdrawal reflex has complex

Table 28-1. Signs and Symptoms of Lower and Upper Motoneuron Lesions

Lower Motoneuron

Flaccid paresis (plegia)

Fasciculations observed in involved superficial muscles

Atrophy of affected muscles

Increased compliance of muscles to passive stretch

Decreased or absent deep tendon reflex

EMG evidence of denervation

Retention of the ability to isolate muscle contractions

Upper Motoneuron

Spastic paresis (plegia)

Increased deep tendon reflex

Positive Babinski and Hoffman signs

Velocity-sensitive increase in resistance to passive stretch

Loss of the ability to isolate muscle contractions (loss of fractionation)

Increased tendency for inappropriate stereotypic movement patterns with volitional effort

---

interconnections over multiple spinal levels and typically produces a response in multiple muscles. Even more complex reflexes, such as the tonic neck and long loop stretch reflexes, require more extensive interconnections between the spinal cord and the brain.

SOMATIC REFLEXES

Deep Tendon Reflex: Testing Segmental Motoneuron Excitability

One of the most commonly tested reflexes is the monosynaptic phasic stretch reflex or the deep tendon reflex (DTR). DTRs are usually symmetrical for homologous muscles on either side of the body at any one testing. If the patient is not relaxed, if the limb is not supported adequately, or if the muscle is not on slight stretch, test results will vary.

The most reliable and commonly tested DTRs include the biceps brachii jerk (BJ), the triceps brachii jerk (TJ), the brachioradialis jerk (BrJ), the quadriceps femoris or knee jerk (KJ), and the triceps surae ankle jerk (AJ). The muscles of mastication innervated by the trigeminal nerve (jaw jerk, JJ) are often included in testing; however, results may vary in normal subjects because relaxation of these muscles is often dif-

ficult to achieve, especially when the evaluator is approaching the face with a reflex hammer.

It is important to strike the tendon briskly and firmly. Don't peck at the tendon like a bird pecks at birdseed. When the Achilles' tendon of a relaxed, alert person is tapped with a reflex hammer with adequate intensity and velocity, a brief twitch response will typically be evoked from the triceps surae muscles (the AJ response).

Some persons who have no clinical signs of a neurologic disorder have persistent and profound hypoactive DTRs. One technique that has been used to enhance the DTR response is the Jendrassik maneuver. The Jendrassik maneuver is performed by having the subject strongly contract muscles remote to the tested muscle in an attempt to facilitate the DTR. For example, if a person has hypoactive lower extremity DTRs, have him clasp his hands together and perform an isometric contraction of his upper extremities while you tap the lower extremity tendon. A similar procedure can be performed when testing upper extremity DTRs. In this case have the person cross his legs and push one leg against the other, producing an isometric contraction in the lower extremities. Then tap the tendon of the upper extremity muscle you wish to test. The timing is important, so that the subject should begin contracting the distant muscles just prior to the tendon tap. The Jendrassik maneuver is thought to have its effect through a generalized facilitation of spinal motoneurons (irradiation or overflow).

The most sensitive receptor for the DTR is the primary ending of muscle spindles located in the stimulated muscle.

The primary ending of the muscle spindle is innervated by the group Ia afferent axon. The Ia axon is the largest, most heavily myelinated axon in the peripheral nerve. Therefore, it has a very low threshold for excitation by electrical stimulation, and rapidly conducts impulses back to the alpha motoneurons in the spinal cord.

If you stimulate the tibial nerve in the popliteal fossa with a low-threshold electrical pulse, the Ia axons will be excited and conduct a synchronous volley of impulses back to the spinal cord. The Ia afferent impulses monosynaptically excite the alpha motoneurons in the S1 and S2 spinal cord segments. You can then record a monosynaptic reflex response from the triceps surae muscles. This electrically induced monosynaptic reflex is called the H-reflex. By maintaining constant stimulation parameters, you can now observe changes in the level of motoneuron excitability by recording the relative amplitude of the H-reflex when other inputs to the motoneurons vary. Figure 28-2 shows an electromyogram recording of the H-reflex in the triceps surae of a person with an intact nervous system.

The magnitude of the monosynaptic H-

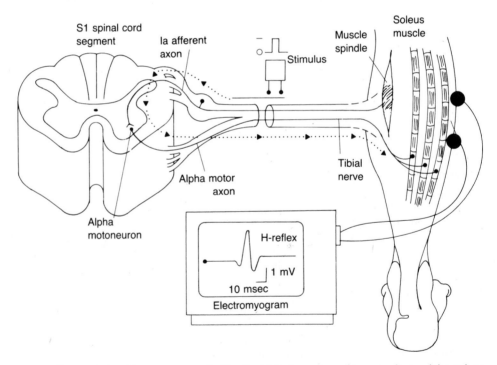

Figure 28-2. The monosynaptic H-reflex. Electromyographic recordings of the soleus monosynaptic H-reflex elicited by electrical stimulation of Ia afferent axons in the tibial nerve. This reflex excites alpha motoneurons located in the S1-S2 spinal cord segments. Submaximal stimulation is utilized to evoke a response from low-threshold Ia afferent axons.

reflex and the DTR may vary across the normal population and may also change from time to time within the individual subject because of normal fluctuation in CNS excitability. For example, a *slight* volitional contraction of the plantarflexors may facilitate the motoneurons (see Fig. 28-3A). Influences on spinal motoneurons may be disturbed in patients who have UMN pathology. Figure 28-3B shows a loss of facilitation of the H-reflex when a patient with multiple sclerosis attempts to contract the planterflexors volitionally. On the other hand, volitional contraction of the antagonist dorsiflexors reciprocally inhibits the motoneurons innervating the plantarflexor muscles in a normal subject. Figure 28-4A shows almost complete inhibition of the triceps surae H-reflex when a normal subject contracts the dorsiflexors. By contrast, a patient with multiple sclerosis has incomplete reciprocal inhibition (Fig. 28-4B).

Abnormal Deep Tendon Reflexes: Signs of Sensory Motor Dysfunction

The normally fine-tuned sensory-motor integration may be altered by nervous system disease, resulting in abnormal stretch reflex responses. Peripheral nervous system disease that alters the conduction of impulses over large myelinated axons will reduce or eliminate the DTR. Both the Ia sensory axon innervating the primary ending of the muscle spindle and the A alpha motor axon innervating the muscle's motor units are large myelinated axons. Thus, reduced or absent DTRs may be an early indicator of pressure on a nerve or a demyelinating neuropathy. Loss of a large population of motoneurons or loss of a large percentage of muscle fibers will result in a loss or deficit in the efferent (motor) portion of the reflex arc. Persons with lower motoneuron disease or late-stage muscle disease will have reduced or

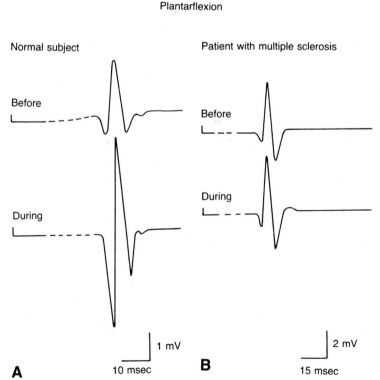

Plantarflexion

Normal subject

Patient with multiple sclerosis

Before

Before

During

During

1 mV

2 mV

A 10 msec **B** 15 msec

Figure 28-3. Facilitation of the monosynaptic H-reflex. Electromyographic recordings of the soleus H-reflex before and during slight volitional contraction of the plantarflexors. (A) A strong facilitation of alpha motorneurons in an individual with an intact nervous system. (B) A poor facilitory response consistent with upper motoneuron weakness. Note difference in scale between A and B.

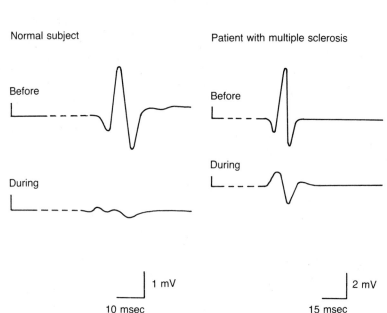

Figure 28-4. Inhibition of the monosynaptic H-reflex. Electromyographic recordings of the soleus H-reflex before and during slight volitional contraction of the dorsiflexors. (*A*) Normal reciprocal inhibitory effects. (*B*) Incomplete reciprocal inhibition associated with an upper motoneuron lesion. Note difference in scale between *A* and *B*.

absent DTRs even though the sensory system is intact.

DTRs are altered following CNS lesions to descending motor pathways or to motor areas in the cerebral cortex. These lesions produce upper mononeuron signs and symptoms. Lesions to descending motor pathways may occur in the white matter at all levels: supratentorial, brain stem, or spinal cord. One of the most common sites of involvement is the internal capsule of the cerebral hemisphere. Loss of axons in descending motor pathways here will produce upper motoneuron signs and symptoms typical of a stroke.

For a period immediately following injury to the spinal cord (spinal shock) or to the motor cortex or its corticofugal (descending) pathway (eg, stroke), reflexes including the DTRs are transiently absent or hypoactive. Following this period of reflex suppression, DTRs can become hyperactive in patients with upper motoneuron lesions. Tapping the tendon of the muscles affected by such a lesion results in a spastic reflex response. Hyperactive DTRs may

be manifested by a single brisk, abnormally large twitch response or by repeated twitches (clonus) (see below). The repeated twitches indicate an oscillation in the stretch reflex circuitry. Moreover, in some patients with severe spasticity the response may not be limited to the tested muscle, but may overflow to include a number of synergistic or sometimes even antagonistic muscles in that limb. An irradiated DTR response is a significant finding because it suggests profoundly abnormal integration within and among segmental motor centers. If a patient has hyperactive DTRs, the physical therapist should further check the sensitivity of the stretch reflex.

To determine the sensitivity of the stretch reflex, the physical therapist should tap the muscle belly instead of its tendon with the reflex hammer. A normal person will have no response or a barely visible twitch. A patient who has spasticity will show a brisk twitch response to this procedure. The physical therapist should also check other less commonly tested muscles in patients who have spasticity.

For example, striking the adductor tendons on the medial distal thigh will produce an exaggerated DTR. Similarly, tapping the long finger flexor tendons at the wrist or palm in patients with spasticity typically produces exaggerated DTRs.

Responses to Sustained Passive Stretch

The physical therapist should perform passive range of motion to the limbs to establish whether ROM is normal and pain-free. Once the normal ROM is assessed, you should increase the velocity of passive motion within the pain-free range. A normal person may have a slight stretch response to higher velocity stretches of a muscle. A patient with a spastic muscle will have an exaggerated stretch response that typically increases in magnitude with increasing velocity of stretch. This exaggerated stretch response may be felt as a sudden rise in tension, which "melts away" with increasing length of the muscle. This sudden increased tension followed by decreased tension is known as the "clasp-knife" phenomenon.

A second type of abnormal response to a high-velocity sustained muscle stretch is a clonic muscle response. Clonus may occur when the spinal circuitry involved in the stretch reflex is unstable. A sustained stretch impedes shortening of the muscle and muscle spindle following the exaggerated twitch, and thus "reloads" the spindle reflex, resulting in a rhythmic 5 to 8-Hz oscillation (clonus). Normal (unfatigued) persons do not typically have an oscillatory response to a sustained stretch. However, patients with an upper motoneuron disease no longer have adequate CNS mechanisms to dampen a response to an imposed stretch stimulus.

If the patient has brisk DTRs, it is imperative that the physical therapist check for clonus. Clonus may occur in any spastic muscle. However, three muscle groups most commonly show clonus in a patient with spasticity: the triceps surae, the quadriceps femoris, and the long wrist and finger flexors. When checking for clonus in the triceps surae, you should perform the test with the knee extended as well as flexed to help distinguish between clonus in the soleus versus the gastrocnemius muscles. To check for clonus of the quadriceps, the physical therapist should push the patella distally (and sustain the stretch) with the knee slightly flexed. If there is clonus, the physical therapist should place his fingers in the palm of the patient's hand, stabilize the forearm, and then rapidly extend the wrist (with a sustained stretch). The wrist will oscillate if there is clonus.

Hyperactive DTRs and abnormal responses to imposed passive stretch in patients with spasticity provide evidence of an upper motoneuron lesion. However, these responses do not allow you to predict the ability of the patient to use the spastic muscles functionally. For example, a patient may have exaggerated stretch reflexes during passive stretch of the muscle, but may still be capable of actively contracting that muscle during a functional activity.

Interestingly, although the patient with an upper motoneuron lesion has an exaggerated segmental phasic stretch reflex, she may not have an intact longer latency long-loop stretch response (Fig. 28-5*B*). It is this longer latency "functional" stretch response (FSR) that appears to be important in postural control and facilitation of volitional movements. If a normal person has a reasonably brisk DTR response, the physical therapist may actually feel two responses to a high-velocity sustained stretch if the person volitionally contracts the muscle being stretched slightly (especially the triceps surae). The first response is the short latency monosynaptic phasic stretch reflex (DTR) and the second response is a long-loop FSR response (latency of about 90 to 110 msec for the triceps surae). Interestingly, the FSR and subsequent "volitional" response are susceptible to instruction-dependent motor set, so that telling the patient to resist the imposed stretch will alter the FSR and later "volitional" EMG (see Fig. 28-5*A*). By contrast, instructing the patient to "yield" to the stretch often reduces or abolishes these long latency responses (see Fig. 28-5*C*). A patient with an upper motoneuron lesion often has an exaggerated phasic stretch

Figure 28-5. Short and long latency responses to sustained muscle stretch. Electromyograms show short latency (phasic stretch reflex) and long latency functional stretch reflex (FSR) responses of the soleus muscle in a normal person (*A, B*) and in a patient with spastic paresis (*C*) following a sustained stretch of the plantarflexor muscles. In *A* and *C* the individual was asked to resist the sustained stretch. Note the strong FSR and volitional response of the healthy subject (*A*) and the exaggerated phasic reflex but weak FSR and volitional response in the patient with spasticity. When the normal individual was asked to yield to the sustained stretch ("Don't resist"), the FSR is reduced and the volitional component is absent. The electromyogram of the patient with spasticity would look very similar to that shown in *C* when asked to yield to the sustained stretch (not shown).

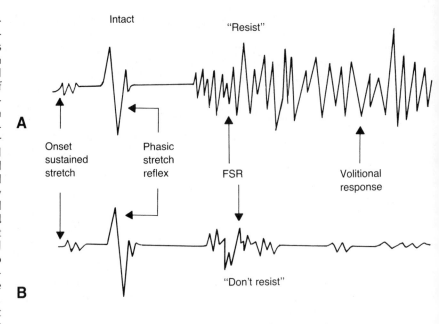

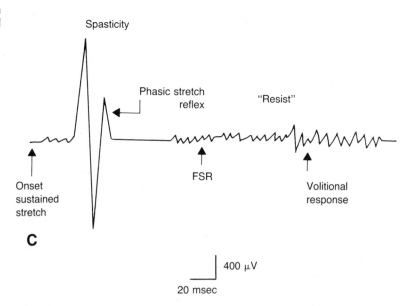

reflex response, but a weak or absent long latency FSR, and a weak or absent volitional response during resisted lengthening contractions (see Fig 28-5B). Functional weakness in spastic muscles may at least partially be due to inappropriate "resist" and "yield" instructions to the spinal cord from higher motor control centers.

Vibration of a spastic muscle will often produce an inappropriate reflex response and typically interferes with the ability of the patient to control the spastic muscle. Vibration of a muscle will often result in a slowly building tonic vibration reflex (TVR) in the vibrated muscle. This TVR is a long-loop reflex requiring interconnections among neurons at different levels within the CNS. In addition to the TVR response, vibration produces a burst of afferent impulses into the spinal cord, which presynaptically inhibits the Ia axon inputs to the alpha motoneurons. In a normal subject a reduction in the monosynaptic H-reflex occurs *during* the period of vibration (with a rebound facilitation of the H-reflex as soon as the vibration stops) (Fig. 28-6*A*). However, a patient with multiple sclerosis shows little or no effect of vibration on the monosynaptic reflex (see Fig. 28-6*B*). This suggests that there is improper CNS control of incoming peripheral afferent input onto spinal motoneurons in patients with upper motoneuron disorders.

Extensor Plantar Responses: Sign of Babinski

Certain types of cutaneous input may produce abnormal reflex responses in patients who have interruption of descending motor pathways. Extension of the big toe with or without fanning of the other toes in response to stroking of the sole of the foot is known as the sign of Babinski, and is considered a reliable clinical sign of upper motoneuron pathology. The stimulus to elicit the Babinski sign should be a firm stroking from the heel along the lateral plantar surface continuing medially to the ball of the foot (Fig. 28-7). The stimulus should not be so light a touch as to produce a tickling sensation, nor should it be painful. Use caution with patients who have sensitive feet or easily damaged skin. Some clinicians use the thumbnail, some use a key, and others use a wooden applicator to stimulate the extensor plantar response. Some clinicians also insist that the foot should be warm to get reliable test results. The physical therapist should always repeat the test to confirm results.

The same extensor plantar response may be elicited by other types of cutaneous stimuli. For example, stroking the lateral border of the foot produces a response (Chaddock sign)

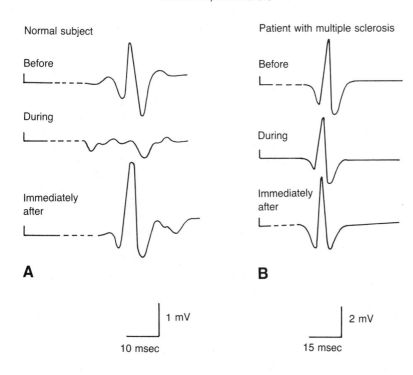

Vibration of plantarflexors

Normal subject

Before

During

Immediately after

A

Patient with multiple sclerosis

Before

During

Immediately after

B

1 mV

10 msec

2 mV

15 msec

Figure 28-6. Effects of muscle vibration on the H-reflex. Electromyograms of the soleus muscle H-reflex before, during, and immediately after vibration of the plantarflexor muscles. Vibration normally inhibits the monosynaptic reflex during the period of vibration. A rebound facilitation occurs immediately after cessation of vibration. This inhibition does not occur in a spastic muscle during vibration and there is little postvibration facilitation of the H-reflex. These results suggest inadequate central nervous system control of peripheral input in spasticity.

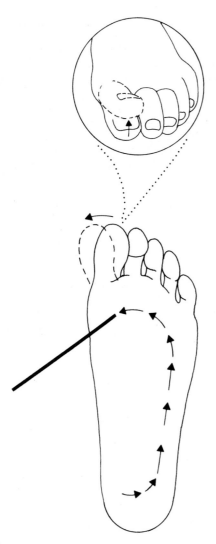

Figure 28-7. Pathological reflex: sign of Babinski. Stroking the sole of the foot in a line from the heel to the lateral plantar surface to the ball of the foot normally produces no response or a flexion of the toes. An extension of the big toe (*inset*) with or without flaring of the other toes is a pathological response that occurs in patients with upper motoneuron disorders.

similar to the Babinski. These cutaneous stimuli may also evoke a general flexor reflex: ankle dorsiflexion and hip and knee flexion. The normal response to these stimuli is flexion of the toes or no motor response.

Hoffman Sign of the Upper Extremity

A pathological reflex similar to the sign of Babinski can be elicited in the upper extremity of a patient with an upper motoneuron lesion. Snapping the fingernail of the middle finger will cause a flexion response of the index finger and flexion/adduction of the thumb (Fig. 28-8). This positive Hoffman sign is considered to be an upper extremity equivalent of the extensor plantar response in the lower extremity. The Hoffman sign is negative in normal persons (no response). The Babinski and Hoffman reflexes in patients with lesions of descending motor pathways suggest an alteration of the normal integration of central and peripheral sensory influences on segmental motor centers.

Abdominal Reflex

Other superficial cutaneous reflexes, such as the abdominal reflex, may be altered by upper motoneuron disease. Stroking the skin over the abdominal muscles normally elicits a contraction of the underlying abdominal musculature. This reflex may be lost following upper motoneuron lesions. However, the results may be quite variable for persons with normal or altered CNS; therefore, it is not considered a very reliable test.

Grasp Reflex

Normally, cutaneous input to the palm and volar surface of the fingers provides tactile cues that are vital to active touch. These sensory inputs may facilitate or inhibit muscles used in manual dexterity. For example, cutaneous receptors in the fingers detect shear forces and proprioceptors provide cues to alter finger position and muscle force. These sensory inputs help to regulate finger torque required to hold a styrofoam cup. A dynamic interplay between sensory and motor signals allows one to hold the cup firmly enough to prevent it from slipping out of the grasp, but lightly enough to avoid crushing it. Active touch interplay is dependent upon intact cortical control.

A proximal to distal firm stroking of the palm and fingers of a patient with a contralateral frontal lobe lesion may elicit a mass finger

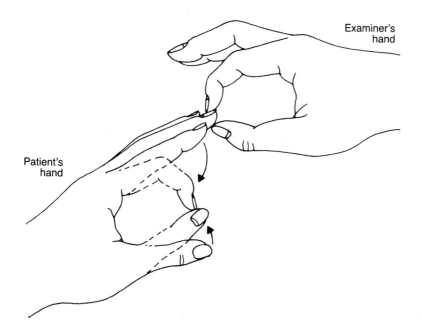

Examiner's hand

Patient's hand

Figure 28-8. Pathological reflex: Hoffman's sign. Flicking the nail of the middle finger normally produces no reflex response. A positive Hoffman's sign of finger and thumb flexion occurs in patients with upper motoneuron disorders. This pathological reflex in the upper extremity often accompanies a positive Babinski response (see Fig. 28-7) in the lower extremity of patients who have spastic hemiplegia or spastic quadriplegia.

flexion response called the grasp reflex. The exact mechanism that produces this pathologic grasp is not known, but is thought to occur if the pre-motor frontal cortex has been destroyed. A mass grasp with inability to release the grasp volitionally will obviously interfere with hand function.

Extensor Thrust

Other types of cutaneous input may produce other patterns of abnormal motor responses. Pressure on the ball of the foot (from weight bearing on a plantarflexed foot or manual pressure) may elicit a strong extensor motor pattern (extensor thrust) in persons with interruption of descending pathways. This response may be variable depending upon the position of the lower extremities or body posture when the stimulus is applied. For example, if a patient with spasticity attempts to rise from a sitting position, the spastic limb(s) may suddenly go into a full extensor pattern. This extensor pattern will typically include ankle plantarflexion and inversion, hip and knee extension, and often trunk extension and hip adduction. Altering the combination of joint, cutaneous, and

muscle receptor input will effect this response. For example, the physical therapist may help to minimize this extensor thrust by preparing the patient to rise from sitting. This includes placing the foot in a dorsiflexed position, and flexing the knee, hip, and trunk before attempting to rise from sitting. The physical therapist may also alter the patient's footwear so as to minimize pressure on the ball of the foot and mechanically assist in maintaining a dorsiflexed ankle position. The extensor thrust may be very strong in some patients. Pressure on the ball of the foot from the foot pedals on a wheelchair may actually cause the person to fall out of the wheelchair. Wheelchair modifications and positioning will be an important aspect of treatment for these patients.

Withdrawal Reflex

We are all aware of the withdrawal reflex, which occurs when we are subjected to a painful (noxious) stimulus. This reflex is a normal protective response. For example, if we step on a sharp object, we will flex the limb out of harm's way. This flexion reflex includes ankle dorsiflexion and knee and hip flexion in the stimulated limb, and typically extension in the opposite weight-bearing limb. These withdrawal reflexes are adaptive in normal persons. Descending pathways from the brain stem and the cerebral cortex help to control the spinal flexion reflex. A patient who has a normal nervous system may still be able to walk despite a painful callus on the bottom of his foot.

It is now known that non-noxious cutaneous input may facilitate different muscle groups. Depending upon the current status of the activity in the CNS, either flexor or extensor muscle groups may be facilitated by cutaneous input. For example, non-noxious cutaneous input to the foot during weight bearing actually facilitates the extensor muscles and inhibits the flexor muscles of that limb. However, the same cutaneous input will facilitate the flexor muscles and inhibit the extensor muscles during the non-weight-bearing swing phase of gait. The effect of cutaneous input during transition phases of gait may either prolong or facilitate the transition from swing to stance, or vice versa. This suggests that peripheral sensory input complements but does not dominate CNS control of functional movements. Patients who have lesions involving descending pathways have lost this normal balance between peripheral and central influences on interneurons and motoneurons. These patients may have uncontrolled reflexes that may interfere with normal functional activities. For example, a patient with spinal cord injury may have an uncontrolled flexion reflex when touched even lightly on the foot. Similarly, a callus on the bottom of the foot of the hemiparetic side of a patient who has had a stroke may set off reflexes that make walking impossible. Therefore, it is extremely important to prevent skin breakdown and minimize or eliminate other sources of noxious stimuli in these patients. If the therapist is considering use of electrical stimulation to facilitate motor responses during functional activities, he should remember that this stimulation will trigger a shower of sensory impulses into the nervous system. Thus, electrical stimulation may either help or hinder the desired motor response.

Tonic Brain Stem Reflexes

Tonic brain stem reflexes, such as the tonic neck reflex (TNR) and tonic labyrinthine reflex (TLaR), are normally well integrated within the adult nervous system. Overt expression of these reflexes is usually not seen except perhaps under conditions of physical stress (eg, athletic competition or heavy work of muscles to fatigue) or unusual environmental conditions (eg, inverted body position). However, overt tonic reflexes resulting from changes in the position of the head relative to the body or the neck may emerge in patients with supraspinal lesions of descending motor pathways. The inability to suppress limb reactions to changes in body or head postures may seriously impede normal movements; thus, these tonic reflexes should be assessed and considered when formulating treatment plans for these patients.

The physical therapist should check the patient who has upper motoneuron disease for emergent TNR responses. One method of testing is to turn the patient's head passively to the right or left. If there is a strong TNR response, turning the patient's head to the right will result in elbow extension on the right and elbow flexion of the left. Responses may be seen at other joints of the upper and lower extremities, but the most reliable indicator is the change in posture at the elbow joint. If the patient cannot volitionally suppress these responses, they are termed "obligatory" TNR responses and indicate a significant loss of cortical control mechanisms. For many patients with upper motoneuron disorders, the TNR responses only emerge periodically when the CNS is engaged in motor activity. For example, a stroke patient with a right hemiparesis may suddenly have an increased flexion of his elbow while walking if he looks at his therapist, who is assisting on the patient's left side. In this case, only the right elbow may show an overt reaction so that no change in tension is felt by the therapist holding the left arm. Some patients may demonstrate TNR responses only when the motor system is working under stress. For example, a stroke patient with a right hemiparesis is performing a PNF diagonal pattern with the left upper extremity. As the patient visually tracks the moving hand, there may be no overt TNR response until the patient becomes fatigued or the therapist applies sufficient resistance to slow or halt the movement pattern. Under all these conditions, it is impossible to rule out contributions by the labyrinthine apparatus.

Testing for the TLaR may be done by placing the patient in an inverted (head-down) position. Under this condition, extensor activity of limbs and trunk is increased, but a rigid whole body extensor response should not normally occur. *Caution* must be taken because this head-down position also affects baroreceptors and autonomic regulation. Sudden swings in blood pressure and heart rate are *not* tolerated by patients with compromised cardiovascular function. It should be obvious that attempts to produce a restricted labyrinthine stimulus are impractical by routine clinical testing, and patient reactions to static or dynamic (rotary) head and body stimulation must be interpreted cautiously.

Changes in the position of the head and neck will stimulate the labyrinthine receptors in the inner ear (innervated by the vestibular division of the eighth cranial nerve), and proprioceptors located in the cervical apophyseal joints and in the deep neck muscles. If the patient's eyes are open, visual motion cues are also relevant stimuli. Although visual input may be easily eliminated, it is difficult to separate the contribution of neck or labyrinthine receptors in any motion of the head, neck, or body unless one or the other type of receptors are completely eliminated. There is good evidence that neck proprioceptive and labyrinthine input are normally integrated and tend to cancel each other's effect in most functional movements of the head and neck.

VISCERAL REFLEXES

The visceral nervous system consists of a neural and a humoral component including the sympathetic and parasympathetic autonomic outflow as well as the hypothalamic-pituitary neuroendocrine neuraxis. Examination of the autonomic nervous system should include testing of the parasympathetic components of cranial nerves III, IX, and X (see discussion of cranial nerve testing) and thoracolumbar sympathetic and sacral parasympathetic outflow at the spinal level. Peripheral nerves contain postganglionic sympathetic C fibers, so autonomic function should be assessed related to peripheral nerve innervation patterns (see Fig. 28-1).

Tests for Autonomic Function

1. Check heart rate and take blood pressure. Watch for signs of postural hypotension, which may lead to falls.
2. Ask the patient about bowel and bladder function and, if appropriate, sexual function, and check for signs of parasympathetic dysfunction.
3. Observe the patient for the following signs of sympathetic hyperactivity: excessive sweating; elevated blood pressure (may reach dangerous levels!); tachycardia, arrhythmias, or "palpitations"; flushing, or pale or mottled skin appearance; piloerection ("goose bumps"); nasal stuffiness; and pounding headache.
4. Observe the patient for signs of sympathetic dystrophy (loss of sympathetic nerve function), such as edema; trophic changes (changes in skin and nail texture, changes in skin color, loss of hair); poor peripheral temperature regulation (skin may feel cold); lack of sweating (skin is dry and does not respond to warming).
5. Observe the patient for Horner's syndrome, which includes miosis (pupillary dilation), ptosis (partial drooping of the eyelid), anhydrosis (lack of sweating), and flushing of face. This syndrome results from a lesion in the descending sympathetic pathway in the lateral medulla or lateral spinal cord or from a lesion of the T1 cord, T1 root, or cervical sympathetic plexus.
6. Observe the patient for difficulties with swallowing; listen for hoarseness of the voice.
7. Ask the patient or consult the medical

record for signs of GI disturbances: nausea, vomiting, changes in GI motility (ie, diarrhea, constipation).

Autonomic and somatic inputs converge on interneurons in the intermediate spinal gray areas. Output from these interneurons affects both visceral and somatic motoneurons. Therefore, changes in the pattern of afferent input from the viscera may affect somatic function. An example is the effect of constipation or a full bladder on the level of hyperreflexia in the patient with a spinal cord injury. A physical therapist may notice a sudden increase in muscle spasms in a spinal cord patient who has a distended bladder. Similarly, a decubitus ulcer in such a patient may increase limb reflexes, as well as produce uncontrolled reflex emptying of the bowel and bladder. It is critical to check for bladder obstruction or other possible causes of sympathetic hyperreflexia in persons who have a high thoracic or cervical cord injury, because the autonomic overactivity may be life threatening.

Autonomic dysfunction may be related to pharmacologic treatments. Many neurological patients have cardiovascular or respiratory disease, and many of the drugs used in treating these diseases will also affect neurological function. For example, side-effects of sympathomimetic cardiovascular drugs may include not only peripheral autonomic signs and symptoms (eg, sympathetic hyperactivity), but may also affect CNS function because receptors for these drugs may not be limited to smooth or cardiac muscle. These sympathomimetic drugs may make the patient anxious, disturb his sleep, or even alter his moods and emotions. The patient's behavior may become more impulsive and movements may actually be more jerky and uncoordinated. Similarly, certain drugs used to treat neurologic/psychiatric illness have side-effects that affect the visceral system. For example, L-dopa is a common pharmacologic treatment for Parkinson's disease. However, L-dopa may be used not only by dopaminergic axon terminals in the striatum, but also by postganglionic sympathetic neurons, which convert L-dopa into norepi-

nephrine. Sympathetic dysfunction is a common side-effect of L-dopa treatment in patients treated for Parkinson's disease. Side-effects may also include difficulty sleeping, hallucinations, and other psychiatric disorders. Because certain dopaminergic pathways and noradrenergic pathways have been implicated in some mental disorders, it may not be surprising that L-dopa (which may be converted to dopamine or to norepinephrine) has psychologic side-effects.

BALANCE, EQUILIBRIUM, AND RIGHTING

Humans have a unique ability to maintain an upright bipedal posture and move from that posture in a well-controlled manner. We are often unaware of the harmonious interactions among sensors, neural, and musculoskeletal elements contributing to postural reactions. Postural stability may become obvious (sometimes in the pit of the stomach) under conditions that may result in bodily harm (eg, a fall). We may also pay attention to body position when attempting to maintain an unusually difficult posture or move within a demanding, changing environment. Gymnasts and ballet dancers are well aware of the effort expended in postural control. Astronauts must learn to fight nausea and motion sickness. Virtually every level of the nervous system is involved in balancing the body mass and, not unexpectedly, many types of nervous system dysfunction will alter normal postural control. It is interesting that a cat with high brain stem transection can walk or even run on a moving treadmill, but only if its body is physically supported. Thus, we know that the brain stem alone is not sufficient for dynamic postural control.

The goal of upright posture is to maintain the center of gravity over the base of support. Obviously, the level of difficulty increases as the base of support decreases (eg, standing on one foot) and as the center of gravity shifts farther away from the center of the base support. An obvious solution to inadequate postural control is to lower the center of gravity and broaden the base of support, for example, by crawling on all fours rather than using bipedal locomotion.

Postural control is taxed more heavily as conditions become more complex. If we are standing on a solid, nonslippery surface that is not moving, we can generate adequate torque through foot contact to maintain balance even if we are *gently* pushed. If we are pushed off balance by a larger perturbing force, we must then either move the hips and trunk to maintain balance or take a step to regain balance. When we take a step, we are shifting the center of gravity over a new base of support. This is normally a graceful, well-controlled postural transition in human locomotion. Changing the support surface on which we stand will also increase the challenge of maintaining postural support. If standing on a narrow beam, we can no longer produce adequate torque through the feet to maintain balance, and we must then shift weight more proximally by moving the trunk and hips. Similarly, a compliant support surface (eg, a deep pile carpet with foam rubber padding, or deep snow, or sitting on a large ball) may require a different strategy for postural adjustments.

Changes in visual context may further tax the system. A patient with marginal control of balance may be more likely to lose his balance if visual context is removed (eg, if lighting is dim or peripheral vision is reduced). This may also be true if visual context becomes too complex (eg, rapidly changing scenery).

Motion of the support surface will trigger responses to maintain balance (Nashner, 1982). Small perturbations trigger less drastic responses where the feet maintain contact with the support surface. Postural reactions reduce body sway by adjusting the center of gravity over the base of support. Larger perturbations may require stepping to regain balance. In this circumstance, we must adjust the center of gravity to a new base of support position. The most difficult circumstance would be those postural control mechanisms called upon when both the body and the support surface are moving (eg, attempting to walk to a seat in a bus that is accelerating or decelerating).

Assessing the cause of balance deficits is a difficult task because postural control is so widely distributed in the nervous system. There are three major requirements for normal postural control. First, we require sensors to establish our position relative to the environment.

Second are the CNS centers that access inputs, coordinate and program adequate responses, and then distribute the motor commands to the appropriate spinal segmental motor centers.

The third major requirement for normal postural control is an adequate neuromuscular output and the articulated skeleton upon which the muscles act.

The most important sensors are surface contact cues from cutaneous receptors; proprioceptive input from the neck, trunk, and limbs; and cues about head position from vestibular and visual inputs. Loss of one or more of these sources of information may not obliterate postural control, but will certainly increase the dependence upon the remaining senses and increasingly challenge the neural control system. A simple test, the Romberg, is used to evaluate the ability of the patient to maintain balance when visual cues are removed. The Romberg test requires first that the person be able to stand erect with feet together and eyes open and not lose her balance. If the subject cannot maintain this position with eyes open, then the Romberg test cannot be performed. The Romberg test is positive when the subject loses her balance with eyes closed *but not* with eyes open.

The physical therapist should instruct the patient to stand with feet together and arms folded over the chest. The physical therapist guards the patient with eyes open and observes the patient's balance for about 15 seconds. If the patient maintains his balance, then the physical therapist instructs the patient to close his eyes and maintain his balance. Again, the physical therapist must guard the patient closely. The patient should be able to maintain this posture for about 15 seconds (or longer). It is not unusual for a normal person to sway more with eyes closed than with eyes open. The test is positive only if the patient cannot maintain balance with eyes closed. Thus, the Romberg is used to test the ability of nonvisual cues (proprioceptive, cutaneous contact cues, and vestibular cues) to compensate when vision is occluded.

The Romberg is stated to be a test for sensory ataxia. If the patient performs satisfactorily, one can further tax the system by having the patient stand on a compliant surface such as a wheelchair cushion (high-density foam, air cushion, or liquid/gel cushion). These cushions are designed to distribute forces, and therefore will provide less reliable somatosensory input. A normal subject can maintain balance on these surfaces with eyes open and closed (although sway may increase). Persons with marginal maintenance of balance under standard Romberg testing (large sway, but no loss of balance) may be unable to retain balance under these more challenging conditions (Shumway-Cook and Horak, 1986). Obviously, if a patient has a positive result on the Romberg test, one should correlate this finding with signs of proprioceptive and cutaneous sensory loss from the lower extremities and signs of vestibular involvement. (Note: Many patients with vestibular disorders may be unable to assume the feet-together station with eyes open.)

We are normally capable of regaining balance (getting the center of gravity centered over the base of support) if our posture is perturbed. If the center of gravity does not extend beyond the limits of the base of support, we adjust by synergistic muscle contractions with the feet stationary. However, if the center of gravity is displaced outside of the base of support, we must then alter the base of support by stepping, or by reaching out to stabilize ourselves so that we will not lose our balance. These reactions typically occur within 85 to 180 msec, suggesting that these responses are not segmental reflexes (Nashner, 1982). Segmental reflexes have a shorter latency. Furthermore, these reactions to perturbation of balance are adaptive, synergistic responses, which suggests access to an internal reference system. Muscles are not recruited individually. Groups of muscles are coupled in synergistic motor patterns set by CNS control mechanisms.

These synergies are thought to be centrally programmed and "called up" according to the context of the postural situation (Nashner, 1982).

Sensory inputs and motor commands are thought to be integrated in a number of different areas within the CNS. Lesions of most (if not all) supraspinal motor centers cause disturbances in balance. Brain stem lesions, cerebellar lesions, basal ganglia lesions, and cerebral cortical lesions all affect postural control. For these patients, the sensory inputs may still be intact and access the internal postural reference system, but the coordination, programming, or distribution of motor commands are disturbed. Unlike normal persons, these patients may respond with inappropriate timing, sequence, or selection of muscular responses. For example, if the surface on which one stands is suddenly shifted posteriorly (slightly), the normal response consists of a synergy between distal and proximal muscles of the lower extremities to reverse the body sway and bring the center of gravity back over the base of support. The initial response occurs distally and proceeds proximally in normal persons. Stroke patients may reverse the order so that proximal muscles respond before distal muscles. This results in a destabilizing postural reaction. Patients with cerebellar disease may no longer have appropriate reciprocity between agonist-antagonist activation, and may fall. Cerebellar patients often react similarly with eyes open or closed, suggesting a difficulty in organization of the correct output rather than a deficit in access to sensory input.

It should be no surprise to physical therapists that adequate muscular strength is required for postural control. Muscles weakened by peripheral nerve damage, primary muscle disease, or disuse will tax the neural control system and the musculoskeletal system. Orthopedic dysfunction may then disrupt the output stage or the input stage if proprioceptors no longer function properly. A patient with an ankle sprain may be at greater risk for subsequent ankle injuries or even for falls unless treatment includes postural rehabilitation. Exercises should be incorporated to challenge the ankle's stability in dynamic weight-bearing postures.

Tests of postural control are usually incorporated into assessment of sitting balance, standing balance, transfers, gait, and so forth, but the reasons for deficits seen during these functional tasks may not always be apparent. Tests of "righting and equilibrium reactions" have been utilized by physical therapists to assess balance and postural control. These tests incorporate different positioning of the patient (lying, sitting, standing). The physical therapist then perturbs the patient's posture and observes the patient's reaction. This test may be performed with the patient positioned on a nonmoving, stable surface (eg, standing in parallel bars, or sitting on a raised mat table) or on a surface that moves (eg, a large therapeutic ball or an equilibrium board). Equilibrium boards have a flat surface on which the patient lies, sits, or sometimes stands, and a cylindrical bottom. The physical therapist tilts the board, guards the patient, and observes the reaction to the tilt. The typical response to these perturbations is the adjustment of one's posture to maintain a head-up position and to maintain a visual perspective that is parallel to the horizon. Thus, the patient attempts to maintain a head position normal to gravity. The perturbation of the patient or of the moving surface should not be so excessive that it produces protective stepping or reaching responses.

For example, if a normal person is seated on an equilibrium board and gently tilted laterally, he will laterally bend the trunk towards the "uphill" side so as to maintain a head-erect position. If he must reach out or step to "catch his balance," the perturbation was too severe and produced a protective reaction. A patient who has had a stroke may not react appropriately. He may not bend his trunk, and his head may tilt towards the downhill side. If the perturbation is large enough, he may fall. For some patients, even a very mild tilt may elicit a protective reaction. Inappropriate reactions may also be found with patients who have cerebellar, vestibular, brain stem or basal ganglia disorders.

The reactions are difficult to assess. The physical therapist can see an abnormal reaction, but without other specific measures will have difficulty in sorting out the precise reason for the abnormality. Was the abnormal response caused by functional weakness, delays in response, inappropriate groups of muscles responding, inaccurate sensory information, loss of appropriate body image mapping in the brain, inappropriate sensory motor integration, or other causes?

Future methods of clinical assessment of posture and balance may incorporate measures of force, EMG, and motion analysis to critically assess and better target therapy to improve function. More specific clinical measures of balance deficits will allow us to zero in on the exact center of the problem rather than blasting the surround with a shotgun approach (Nashner, 1982; Shumway-Cook and Horak, 1986; Horak, 1987).

SENSORY TESTING

As every parent knows, children can ask the most provocative questions. How do we see? How do we hear? How do we feel things? The simplest answer is that we see with our eyes, we hear with our ears, and we feel things with our hands. The intuitive child soon learns, however, that there is more to our senses. She can "see" in her dreams. She can "see and hear" heroes in action in her favorite book. She can still "feel" her legs moving after removing her skates, and she can "feel" pins and needles in her fingers after bumping her "funnybone." There is more to our senses than receptors.

The brain forms perceptions and interprets events. Loss or distortions of sensations may result from damage to receptors, peripheral nerves, sensory pathways in the CNS, or neural centers in the CNS that process sensory information. The physical therapist also should realize that descending pathways from the cerebral cortex and from the brain stem can modify incoming sensory inputs. For example, a large number of corticospinal tract axons synapse on cells in the dorsal horn of the spinal cord. The dorsal horn contains cells that process and relay sensory information. The "highest" level of the brain may regulate the flow of sensory signals as they enter the CNS. Similarly, neural centers in the brain stem send descending signals to the dorsal horn to modulate the transmission of pain. Both limbic and nonlimbic cortical areas may also modulate the processing of information in sensory cortical areas.

Selective attention, motivation, habituation, sensitization, and gating of sensations during specific movement patterns will shape what we feel, and will provide state-dependent behavioral outcomes associated with sensory experiences. Obviously, the normal CNS has the capability to "hear" what it wants to "hear" and disregard the rest. We have the exquisite capability to explore our surroundings actively and discriminate subtle differences in stimulus features rapidly. Sensations may guide or trigger a behavior, and behavior may alter sensations that enrich our knowledge of and provide for our interaction with the world.

Clinical examination of conscious sensations requires a conscious, alert, and cooperative subject. Standard clinical tests demand attention to and recognition of the sensory input, judgment of critical features of the sensory experience (ie, perception), and an appropriate behavioral response. The correct response may be as simple as identifying the presence or absence of a stimulus. Other responses require a forced-choice testing paradigm (eg, "Hot or cold?" "Sharp or dull?"). Still other testing procedures require a more complex sensory-motor integration response, such as the active matching test for proprioception. Thus, the requirements for testing conscious sensations include not only the sensory system but also "higher" integrative centers and the motor system.

Most clinical tests of sensation are screening tests that provide a relatively crude assessment of the exquisite capabilities of our sensory system: the windows to our world. More sophisticated equipment is available for sensory testing. Although this equipment provides accurate quantitative data, it is expensive and impractical for routine clinical testing.

The following section of this chapter will focus on evaluation of general somatic sensations originating from receptors located superficially or deep within the body wall and the limbs. Figures in textbooks often depict somatosensory representations in the brain as static maps where the body surface is represented as a two-dimensional homunculus. The homunculus emphasizes two important concepts. First, the anatomical relationships of body parts to one other are maintained from the periphery to their central representation. Secondly, the map is distorted so that more neural space is allotted to those body parts that have the highest peripheral innervation density (eg, digits of the hand and the lips). This topographic, though distorted, neural representation of the sensory periphery forms the basis for our ability to localize the source of tactile stimulation of the body. The particular neural networks that are most active and the patterns of activity within them depends on (1) the location of excited receptors and (2) the ensemble of sensory receptor types activated. Spatiotemporal features of receptor populations provide a dynamic "signature" within the appropriate portions of the somatotopic maps. Recent evidence suggests that this signature is modifiable. For example, changes in the pattern of input over time may alter the signature. Loss of peripheral input may reorganize not only the signature, but also the slate upon which the sensory inputs are signed (Kaas and co-workers, 1983; Whitsel and co-workers, 1988).

CLINICAL SENSORY TESTING

Classical testing for sensation includes sharp-dull, hot-cold, vibration sense, two-point discrimination, position sense, graphesthesia, stereognosis, and light touch. Most neurology texts describe the first two tests (sharp-dull, hot-cold) as specific for the spinothalamic (anterolateral) pathway and the next five tests (vibration sense, two-point discrimination, position sense, graphesthesia, and stereognosis) as specific for the dorsal column-medial lemniscal (spinal lemniscal) pathway. The final test (light touch) has been ascribed to either or both anterolateral and spinal lemniscal pathways.

A summary of clinical sensory testing is presented in Figure 28-9. The information from the test correlates known neuroanatomical and neurophysiological representation of the somatic sensation with clinical dysfunction associated with different pathologies.

LIGHT TOUCH

The classical test for light touch is to dab a "wisp" of cotton onto the skin and ask the subject to report when and sometimes where she has been touched. This test activates multiple receptor types, and thus involves multiple afferent fiber sizes and multiple ascending sensory pathways. More than one somatosensory cortical area receives responses from light touch. Thus, there is redundant neural circuitry for place coding of general tactile sensations. Be sure to test more than one site in the appropriate dermatomes and peripheral nerve territories. Because innervation density will vary across the skin surface, the patient's report of sensation will also vary. Receptor type varies according to glabrous (nonhairy) versus hairy skin. Response to light touch stimulation will also vary if there is scar tissue or callus. In addition, skin temperature may also affect responsiveness. A cold skin area may show a depreciation in light touch.

If repeated tests show no response to light touch within a given area, look for a specific anatomical pattern. For example, if a patient cannot feel light touch sensation on the palmar surface of the index and middle fingers of one hand, the problem might be a median nerve lesion. This loss of sensation could also occur with a C6-C7 cervical root problem, so one must check the ulnar nerve territory (ring and index fingers) and the radial nerve territory (dorsum of the hand) as well as the more proximal C6-C7 cutaneous areas on the lateral border of the forearm. The physical therapist should confirm findings from light touch testing with other tests (ie, other sensory tests), muscle tests, and an orthopedic screening exam for cervical spine disease. Results from these tests should be compared to the contralateral side. More specific tests of the PNS (nerve conduction and EMG needle exam) may also be indicated if abnormalities follow a peripheral nerve or root pattern. It is unlikely that an anatomical distribution of sensory loss for only the palmar index and middle finger skin would be caused by a CNS lesion.

If light touch sensation is abnormal in multiple nerve and root territories in the arm and leg on one side of the body, this would suggest a supratentorial lesion of the contralateral hemisphere of the brain or possibly a lesion of the contralateral side of the brain stem in the posterior fossa. Obviously, one would look for other abnormalities characteristic of a cerebral or brain stem lesion in these cases.

If light touch sensation is abnormal in all four extremities distally but not proximally, this would suggest a peripheral polyneuropathy. Loss of light touch and all other sensations plus a loss of motor control below a certain segmental level suggests a spinal cord lesion.

A pattern of sensory loss involving the palm of the hand and the proximal phalanges (but not the distal phalanges) that follows no anatomical or functional neural representation suggests a psychogenic dysfunction rather than an organic somatic pathogenesis.

If your patient reports presence or absence of light touch sensation at all sites tested, you cannot conclude that sensation is normal. The quality of the patient's sensory experience will also provide information about lesions in the sensory system. For example, a subject may report an odd or abnormal sensation or demonstrate a considerable delay in reporting the sensation. These evaluative reports could indicate disordered somatosensation. Abnormalities reported in light touch sensation could help to localize a peripheral nerve disease or an extensive CNS lesion (eg, complete spinal cord transection or an extensive parietal lobe lesion). However, reported abnormalities in light touch sensation are unlikely to help the therapist localize a single root lesion or an incomplete lesion of somatosensory pathways.

TWO-POINT DISCRIMINATION

The two-point discrimination test is the classic test for determining thresholds of spatial locali-

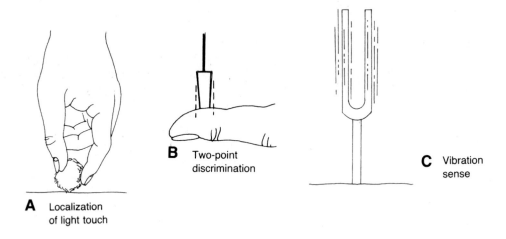

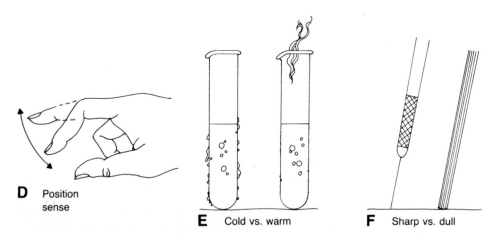

Figure 28-9. Clinical testing of somatosensation. The therapist asks the patient the following questions. (A) "Without looking, tell me when and where I touch you." Can the subject localize superficial touch sensation? (B) "Without looking, tell if you feel one or two points touching you." Repeat, decreasing distance between points. Note the spatial resolution of tactile detail (forced choice). (C) "Without looking, tell if you feel touch or vibration." If sensed, "Tell when vibration ceases." What is the lower limit for detecting low-threshold, high-rate stimuli (forced choice)? (D) "Without looking, tell me if your finger is moving up or down." Decrease size of displacement in middle of range. Note the direction of passive limb displacement (forced choice). (E) "Without looking, tell if the object touching you feels cold or warm." Note the direction of the thermal gradient applied to the skin (forced choice). (F) "Without looking, tell if the object touching you feels sharp or dull. Does it feel like a pin prick (forced choice)?"

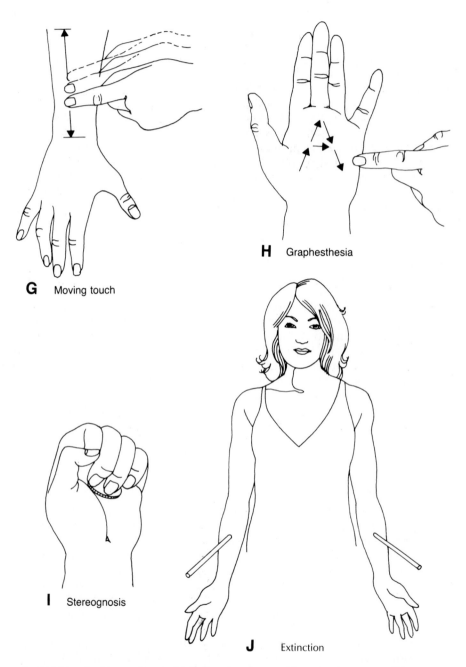

G Moving touch

H Graphesthesia

I Stereognosis

J Extinction

(*G*) "Without looking, tell me which direction the touching stimulus moves." Note the direction. (*H*) "Without looking, tell me what letter I am drawing on your skin." Note whether subject can identify it. (*I*) "Without looking, tell what object I have placed in your hand." Note whether subject can manipulate and identify the object. (*J*) "Without looking, tell me where I touch you—right, left, or both arms." Note whether subject recognizes unilateral versus simultaneous bilateral touch (forced choice).

zation. The test employs a divider or compass with blunted tips. The examiner simultaneously applies two tips at decreasing distances until one tip is reported rather than two. Because the purpose of this test is to determine precise stimulus localization, it has been interpreted as a dorsal column-medial lemniscal discriminative sensory test. However, the location of testing on the body and manner in which the stimuli are delivered can affect the minimal distance threshold. For example, the digits have a very small threshold (2 to 3 mm) of discrimination between two points, whereas more proximal body sites may have large distances as a threshold. Lesions restricted to the dorsal columns (eg, in multiple sclerosis) do not obliterate two-point discrimination. However, threshold distance may be at least transiently increased. It is likely that multiple receptor types are activated and both large and small primary afferent fibers carry relevant information into the CNS. Two-point discrimination sensation most likely includes both the ipsilateral spinal lemniscal and the contralateral anterolateral pathways, and is perceived by interaction among multiple somatotopic sensory areas in the cerebral cortex.

Although this test was once thought to be a definitive test for stimulus localization involving the dorsal column-medial lemniscal pathway, it is now believed to be a relatively crude measure of discriminative sensation. This test is probably best reserved for serial testing in persons with peripheral nerve lesions involving the hand. The physical therapist can then compare changes in two-point discrimination over time to document recovery of sensory function. Serially testing the uninvolved hand can serve as a control for errors related to the limitations of the testing technique.

VIBRATION SENSE

Classical testing of vibration sense involves applying a tuning fork to bony prominences, fingernails, and toenails. The tuning fork is tapped to set it vibrating and the handle (not the vibrating portion) is placed against the patient's skin. The subject is asked to report the sensation felt. The best tuning fork frequency to use is 256 Hz, although 128 Hz is adequate and usually produces a larger magnitude vibration. Because the vibration (or striking the tuning fork to start vibration) will produce audible cues, the examiner should randomly apply the tuning fork to a bony prominence both with and without vibration present. The subject should be able to discriminate between touch or pressure and actual vibration, which may be reported as vibrating, buzzing, humming, and the like. If possible, show the subject what the vibration feels like in an area where sensation is thought to be intact. The therapist should also estimate the magnitude of vibration required for perception by asking the patient to identify when the vibration stops. The examiner should then match the sensation reported by the patient to a comparable body site on himself. The patient's reported minimal amplitude of vibration detection should closely match that of the examiner. Use caution in interpreting results in elderly subjects, because vibration sense is often diminished in the distal lower extremities even when there are no obvious signs of nervous system disease.

The most sensitive receptor for vibration at 256 Hz is the pacinian corpuscle. Meissner's corpuscles located in dermal papillae are most sensitive to lower frequency (30 to 40 Hz) "flutter," but may have a high-threshold response to higher frequencies. Pacinian corpuscles are located at the junction of the dermis and the underlying subcutaneous tissue, in the periosteum of bone, and in the mesentery of the gut. However, some joint and muscle (spindle and Golgi tendon organ [GTO]) proprioceptors are also sensitive to high-frequency, low-amplitude vibrations. All of these receptors are innervated by large myelinated primary afferents. The central projections of some of these primary afferents ascend in the dorsal columns, and therefore represent a rapid conduction system to the conscious level through the dorsal column-medial lemniscal pathway. However, transection of the dorsal columns does not eliminate vibration sense, as other ascending pathways also carry this information rostrally. Vibration, when applied to bony prominences or the nails, is conducted mechanically over a wide area. Individual pacinian corpuscles are exquisitely sensitive to vibration and have large receptive fields. Therefore, vibration sense is *not* a good localizing test of sensory deficits. Vibration testing is a good test for large primary afferents and rapid conducting ascending pathways. Vibration sense may be diminished in peripheral nerve disease affecting large fibers (eg, demyelinating peripheral neuropathies), or in central demyelinating disease (eg, multiple sclerosis). Following a peripheral nerve injury, functional reinnervation of pacinian corpuscles is one of the last sensations to return. Serial testing of vibration sense may help the physical therapist to follow functional recovery of sensation mediated by remyelinated nerve fibers.

POSITION SENSE

The classic test for proprioception is passive joint displacement. Although any joint can be tested, the distal extremity joints (eg, fingers, toes, wrist, ankle) are used most routinely in neurological exams. Because the physical therapist is interested in the function of all joints, position sense testing should not be limited to the distal extremities. For example, even a slight loss of proprioception at the hip may affect posture and gait.

Position sense testing should be performed with minimal skin contact to minimize extraneous tactile cues. For example, the examiner should hold the patient's finger on the radial and ulnar surface rather than on the dorsal and volar surface. The patient is asked to identify in which direction the joint is displaced, (eg, ''Up or down?''). For most extremity joints, normal persons can sense a slight displacement of several degrees or less in a specific direction in the middle of the joint range at a moderate speed of movement.

The muscles that move the joint should be relaxed to ensure the examiner is eliciting a sensitive measure of passive motion. Slight contraction of a muscle will engage other receptors, such as the GTO, which are very sensitive to changes in tension. Both muscle and joint receptors contribute to proprioception. Recent evidence suggests that joint receptors contribute most of their input at the extremes of joint motion. Therefore, small passive displacements at the middle of joint range will provide the most discriminative test of position sense. A deficit in position sense is indicated if the therapist must increase the range of joint displacement before the patient recognizes the change in position. A patient with greater proprioceptive loss either will detect motion only at the extremes of motion or will detect the direction of motion only when contracting muscles surrounding the joint. A complete loss of proprioception would be indicated by a 50:50 (chance) ratio of correct responses even with large displacements into the end of the range.

A depreciation of proprioception could indicate dysfunction of joint or muscle receptors. Both types of receptors may be affected by aging or by musculoskeletal disorders. Loss of position sense could also indicate disease in large myelinated primary afferents, disruption of spinal lemniscal ascending pathways, or dysfunction of sensory processing centers at a higher level. Although proprioception has been classically linked to the dorsal column-medial lemniscal pathway, interruption of the dorsal columns alone does not obliterate conscious proprioception.

WARM-COOL

Classical testing of thermal sensitivity involves a forced-choice discrimination between warm versus cool thermal gradients. It is important that the amount of surface area the testing tool touches on the skin is the same so that nonthermal cues (touch/pressure) do not interfere with testing results. The use of ''hot'' and ''cold'' tap water provides a temperature difference that is adequate for the test. Variances in the patient's skin temperature at the time of the test could affect the outcome. Thermal stimuli evoke a response in small primary afferent fibers. Information about thermal gradients is conveyed to the brain primarily, if not exclusively, by the anterolateral pathway. This information may be localized by nerve impulses carried in the contralateral spinothalamic tract.

SHARP-DULL

Another classical forced-choice test is used to determine if a noxious stimulus (sharp) can be distinguished from touch/pressure (dull). The pinprick utilized in this test should be applied with sufficient pressure to deform the skin surface without drawing blood. A random presentation of a blunt or sharp stimulus should be applied to skin areas that include dermatomes and peripheral nerve territories you wish to test. Theoretically, the contact surface area for sharp versus blunt stimuli should be reasonably similar. However, typically the blunt stimulus area is much larger than the sharp stimulus area (eg, pin end versus clasp end of a safety pin).

The critical feature of the sharp versus dull test is to distinguish a cutaneous zone where pinprick is not sensed as a discrete sharp sensation. As previously discussed, differences in skin composition may affect results. A prior painful stimulus applied to a tested area also may alter the threshold for pinprick sensation. Because a ''dull'' touch sensation utilizes multiple aspects of the sensory neuraxis, the dull test by itself is not discriminative. The ''sharp'' sensation more specifically utilizes nociceptors, small fiber afferents, and the anterolateral pathway. However, loss of ''sharp'' sensation in an area does not exclude the possibility of feeling pain in that area. The pain experience incorporates a more extensive neuraxis than merely conscious awareness of a pricking sensation. A selective dulling of pinprick sensation could indicate involvement of small fiber afferents, the anterolateral system, or prior activation of pain suppression mechanisms in the CNS (self- or externally induced).

If the crossed spinothalamic tract is cut (eg, by a surgical anterolateral cordotomy to relieve chronic pain), only crude thermal and pain sensibilities may remain on the contralateral side of the body. Thus, a patient with a left anterolateral cordotomy in the thoracic cord may experience dull, aching, or burning pain in the right lower extremity and may be able to distinguish temperature changes only for very hot or very cold thermal stimuli. Additionally, the patient may complain of the diffuse, unpleasant nature of these stimuli. These crude thermal and pain sensibilities are thought to be carried by a polysynaptic pathway that survives the cordotomy. This pathway includes information that projects from the spinal cord to the brain stem reticular formation. This crude sensation is relayed from the brain stem to cells in the thalamus, which in turn have a diffuse projection to many forebrain structures including the hypothalamus and other limbic areas.

MOVING TOUCH

Clinical testing of moving touch is not always included in a routine sensory exam. Brushing along the patient's skin surface produces a specific spatiotemporal pattern of neural activity within or across peripheral receptive fields. The subject is asked to determine the direction of the moving touch (forced choice). A camel's hair brush or even light stroking by the examiner's finger is an adequate suprathreshold stimulus. A medium-velocity stroking (about 5 to 35 cm/sec, as when petting an animal) should suffice, but the optimal velocity and distance have yet to be determined for clinical testing of all body sites. Considering the variation in the innervation density and the cortical representation of the digits (especially fingers) compared to the proximal limb or the trunk, a 1- or 2-cm starting distance should be adequate for the fingers, twice that for the palm, and perhaps five to ten times that for the proximal limb. Discrimination of moving touch requires an intact dorsal column-medial lemniscal pathway and intact somatosensory cortical areas, which process spatiotemporal tactile information (parietal cortex).

GRAPHESTHESIA

A higher level test of spatiotemporal tactile discrimination is the identification of letters or numbers drawn on the skin surface. This test assumes that the patient can cognitively recognize the printed symbols. For example, a person who has been blind since birth may not be familiar with written numbers and letters; however, he may be quite familiar with Braille and, in fact, depends upon tactile spatiotemporal cues to read.

To examine graphesthesia, clearly trace a letter or number across the surface of the patient's skin with your finger. You should trace the symbol as if the person were reading it on a page, that is, don't trace upside down or inverted symbols. The spatial limits for this test are not well defined, but tracing within a 1- to 2-in square should suffice for the palm of the hand. The tracing may have to be larger on more proximal body parts. In any event, the lines drawn on the skin should be separated sufficiently to provide a "black on white" mental image of the symbol. You should use a moderate speed in forming the symbols. This test requires the undivided attention of your patient. Normal persons who do not fully concentrate on the testing situation may reduce their recognition "score" to as low as 70% accuracy.

Graphesthesia is dependent upon information flow in the dorsal column-medial lemniscal pathway, cortical perceptual processing of information, and sensory memory (a neural "afterimage"). Patients who have damage to the dorsal columns, medial lemniscus, ventral posterior thalamus, or the parietal lobe will have dysgraphesthesia or agraphesthesia in the affected receptive fields.

ACTIVE TOUCH: STEREOGNOSIS

Active touch is a phenomenon whereby the sensory periphery of our body has contact with and interacts in a meaningful way with the environment. For example, movement and sensation are intertwined in the exploration and manipulation of objects. Finger movements alter tactile and proprioceptive inputs and sensory feedback guides the sequence of motor events. The ability to manipulate tools has expanded the range of work the hand can perform. As one develops skill, one develops a "feel" for the tool such that it becomes part of

the hand, an extension of the body image. For example, when turning a screw in wood one can feel the contact of the tip of the screwdriver in the slot of the screw head and one can sense the torque generated from tip to handle, that is, the sensory-motor system is extended to the tip of the screwdriver. Refinement of active touch is provided by *experience*. A mechanic can judge torque applied to a bolt in much finer detail than a person who doesn't know the difference between a crescent wrench and a ratcheting socket wrench. That's why therapists improve manual skills by repeated clinical practice.

Stereognosis is tested clinically by asking the patient to identify common objects placed in the hand. The patient must manipulate the object to define its texture, size, and three-dimensional form. Commonly used objects are keys, coins, rings, paper clips, and closed safety pins. If the patient has the motor capability (including coordination) to move the digits dexterously, then an inability to identify the objects correctly would suggest a dysfunction in sensory processing.

Astereognosis may occur with severe deafferentation, a lesion of multiple ascending pathways, or a parietal lobe lesion. The patient who can localize touch, has good position sense, can recognize the direction of moving touch, and has good motor strength, but has astereognosis, probably has a lesion in the posterior parietal lobe, or, less likely, a lesion of frontal cortical areas involved in the planning of a motor sequence (eg, the supplemental motor area).

BODY IMAGE AND SPATIAL PERCEPTIONS

As we mature, we develop a bilateral and reasonably symmetrical body image, although we often develop preferences related to laterality (eg, handedness). Body image is a complex phenomenon with both "physical" and "mental" parameters. These parameters are dynamic rather than static. Our physical body changes and our mental image of our being undergoes alterations with age, experience, changes in health, and often self-imposed or societal "best-fit" models of body image.

We relate body image to the external world in at least four dimensions (three-dimensional space, and each dimension as it relates to time). These relationships help us to define up, down, vertical, horizontal, midline, right, and left within a changing environment. These spatial relationships are plastic. For example, normal adults wearing prism glasses can adjust to right-left or up-down reversals *over time,* and then can adapt back when prism glasses are removed.

Patients with lesions of the posterior parietal or adjacent temporal and occipital cortex may have significant distortions of body image. These patients may ignore, dissociate, or even reject portions of their body image and the relationship of body image to the external world. Their perceptual body map may no longer represent their physical body map. Their "mental" abstractions regarding the external world and interactions of the body within it may no longer coincide with physical parameters of the self in space. Some of these patients may have mild alterations of body image. For example, they may be able to receive input from a restricted portion of the body and determine body relationships to a restricted portion of the environment, but may become easily confused in the presence of competing stimuli. These patients may pay attention to only one modality (eg, visual input only). They also may be unable to recognize competing inputs within *one* modality from different portions of the body or external environment; for example, failure to recognize simultaneous tactile input to both sides of the body. Thus, body image deficits may become most evident when crossing the midline, using multiple sensory cues in learning, increasing the complexity of the environment or behavioral task, or with a novel environment.

Some relatively simple body image and spatial perception tests should be done when cerebral dysfunction is evident. The normal school-aged child or adult should be able to recognize tactile input to body parts, and subsequently name them. The normal person should be capable of recognizing the presence of two simultaneous and *competing* sensory inputs (test for somatosensory extinction).

Another test of the extinction phenomenon can be used for visual space. First, determine the extent of the patient's right and left visual fields (see later discussion of visual field testing). The examiner then wiggles fingers in one visual field or both visual fields and asks the patient to identify where he sees the wiggling fingers. The patient's inability to perceive competing stimuli on the involved side of the body or competing stimuli between uninvolved and involved sides of the body suggests a lack of access to or integration of distributed neural processes that govern the formation of the dynamic internal reference system of the body scheme and its relation to extracorporeal space. The patient has a perceptual deficit.

An active matching test is a crude method of testing proprioceptive extinction. The examiner moves one of the patient's limbs passively into a position (if weakness is present, move the paretic limb), and then asks the subject to close his eyes and precisely match that limb position with the same limb on the opposite side. The test is made more complex by using multiple joint positions. A person with perceptual distortions may be capable of reproducing simple, single-joint, single-plane position changes, but may be unable to actively match compound multiplane limb positions. Knowing of this loss of complex proprioception would obviously be important if the therapist were trying to teach a complex motor pattern (eg, a PNF diagonal).

Normal persons are aware of the relationship of the body to the vertical plane. Whether the head or body is upright or tilted normally, one can determine when a pencil is oriented 90 degrees to the horizon. If this simple test cannot be completed, this suggests a distorted perception of the patient's internal reference to verticality. You should also tilt the person to right-left and forward-backward, and ask him to identify when he feels upright (vertical). An inability to define this simplest of references to "which end is up" may seriously compromise efforts to recover bilateral, symmetrical function.

There are a number of paper and pencil tests for perceptual defects. In one test, the patient is asked to draw a man, house, or clock to assess proper spatial relationships. A person with a distorted body image may draw a man with missing limbs or displaced limbs. A loss of normal perceptual symmetry may result in drawing a clock that is incomplete, or that has all the numbers compressed to one side of the clock face.

Perceptual deficits may directly affect the ability to make proper judgment in moving through space and may be a major obstacle to achieving independent function. A number of rehabilitation centers now incorporate "cognitive rehabilitation" by psychologists, therapists, and others. These efforts are directed at improving higher brain functions to increase capabilities for independent living. However, little is known about the neural basis for these "cognitive" higher functions and even less is known about how these functions are altered in cerebral disease.

Therapists who have worked with patients with organic brain diseases are often aware of changes in the capacity of certain persons to make proper judgments in planning, programming, and then executing complex behaviors. Some of these patients have normal findings on perceptual testing and good sensory and motor recovery of function, but still are incapable of choosing appropriate behaviors according to circumstances or when planning daily activities. These judgmental defects are frustrating because they are among the most difficult to document objectively and are equally difficult to treat.

CRANIAL NERVE TESTING

Localizing the level of the lesion or dysfunction within the CNS assists the therapist in determining potential disabilities. Because the majority of cranial nerve nuclei and related integrative centers reside in the brain stem, cranial nerve testing provides a useful means of delineating the brain stem level of involvement. The clinical exam for cranial nerves can rule out involvement of a particular nerve by examining some unique aspect of that nerve's function (eg, jaw jerk reflex, cranial nerve V) or examining composite functions that several cranial nerves share (eg, extraocular eye movements, cranial nerves III, IV, VI). Sophisticated tests for vision, hearing, and vestibular senses now exist. Physical therapists perform only simple screening tests to localize the dysfunction and to draw attention to cranial nerves deserving a more in-depth evaluation by the appropriate specialist. In this section, brief screening tests for cranial nerve functions are presented or described. The therapist should interpret the findings of the clinical examination of cranial nerves in relation to the anatomical brain stem location of the cranial nerve or cranial nerve nuclei (Kandel and Schwartz, 1985).

SMELL: CRANIAL NERVE I

Simply asking the client to recognize familiar odors, such as wintergreen or fresh coffee grounds, adequately examines the sense of smell. It is important to use nonirritating odors for the test. Lack of smell, or anosmia, is difficult to interpret with regard to the involved structure because of the close association of the olfactory system with the limbic lobe of the brain. Thus emotions, memory, and motivation may influence the perception of odors.

VISION: CRANIAL NERVE II

Thorough evaluation of vision is the role of a specialist in ophthalmology. However, clinically useful information for the physical therapist and some information about visual capacity can be obtained from a test of peripheral vision. The examiner's finger or an object held in the fingers is moved from behind the client's head toward the field of vision as the client looks straight ahead. The point in the visual field at which the person first sees the object should be roughly full and comparable on both sides. A visual field deficit, such as when the patient has a larger field of vision on one side than the other, or homonymous hemianopsia, may be recognized by the test (Chusid, 1985).

EYE MOVEMENTS: OCULOMOTOR SYSTEM AND CRANIAL NERVES III, IV, AND VI

First, observe the patient's eyes at rest, noting pupillary size, shape, and signs of ptosis (drooping of the eyelid), drifts of both eyes (conjugate), or a drift of one eye suggesting an extraocular muscle imbalance. An "H" test of eye movements requires the patient to perform eye movements in the six cardinal planes of gaze. Beginning at the midpoint of the horizontal bar of the H, the patient looks to one side, then the other (medial and lateral rectus muscles). At the end of eye movement range to one side, the patient looks up and down (testing the superior and inferior rectus muscles of the laterally deviated eye, and the inferior and superior oblique muscles of the medially turned eye). Repeating the up and down gaze on the opposite side completes the exam. During the H test, note observed weakness or complaints of diplopia (double vision), which are often associated with extraocular muscle weakness. The test for nystagmus follows, with the client following the examiner's finger to the extremes of range in the sagittal and transverse planes. Rapid to and fro eye movements (nystagmus) indicate an abnormality, but it is not uncommon to observe a few small jerks at the extremes of lateral gaze. Evaluating the pupillary light reflex involves shining a light in one eye and watching for the direct response (eye blink) of that eye, and the consensual response or eye blink of the opposite eye. The optic nerve provides the afferent limb of the reflex; a lesion of the optic nerve eliminates both the direct and consensual responses of the reflex.

The patient's ability to adjust gaze from a distant point to the therapist's finger positioned a few inches in front of his nose tests for convergence, or the accommodation reflex. Pupillary constriction normally occurs with accommodation.

TRIGEMINAL REFLEXES: CRANIAL NERVE V

Assessing the sensory function of the trigeminal nerve includes testing the patient's ability to detect pinprick and light touch of the skin of the face, and demonstrating an intact corneal reflex. Testing the corneal reflex (afferent limb via cranial nerve V, efferent limb via cranial nerve VII to the levator palpebra muscle) involves the patient gazing to one side while the cornea is gently touched by a wisp of cotton brought to the eye from the side opposite of gaze (not a particularly comfortable stimulus for the patient). The normal response constitutes a prompt eye blink of the stimulated eye.

The jaw jerk reflex, performed by tapping the patient's chin with a downward motion and watching for the normal response (closing when the jaw is open or opening when the jaw is closed), relies on intact motor function of cranial nerve V. Observing deviation of the mandible from the midline during opening or closing may indicate a unilateral weakness of the pterygoid muscles (innervated by the trigeminal), but the deviation may also result from temporomandibular joint dysfunction.

FACIAL: CRANIAL NERVE VII

Facial asymmetry noted while a person talks, smiles, frowns, whistles, looks pensive, or shuts tightly and opens the eyes, indicates a lesion of cranial nerve VII. Bell's palsy is a complete unilateral facial paralysis as a result of a viral attack on the seventh cranial nerve. Patients with Bell's palsy often report noticing a drooping of one side of the face when looking in the mirror early in the morning after rising.

AUDITORY AND VESTIBULAR SYSTEMS: CRANIAL NERVE VIII

Audiometry provides the best evaluation of hearing. However, a cursory test involves the person's ability to hear the sound of a watch ticking, or the sound produced by rubbing the thumb and forefinger together near the ear. Normally, hearing acuity is comparable from one side to the other.

Clinical evaluation of vestibular function is performed only when cranial nerve VIII or brain stem disease is suspected, or the patient demonstrates a sensory ataxia. Difficulty balancing and increases in postural sway during one- or two-foot balance with the eyes shut or in semidarkness are characteristic of a vestibular disorder. Nystagmus toward the involved side and vertigo may accompany loss of balance.

PHARYNGEAL AND LARYNGEAL REFLEXES: CRANIAL NERVES IX AND X

Alterations in speech sounds and swallowing difficulty illustrate lesions of cranial nerves IX and X. A soft, breathy voice implies a weakness of the oropharyngeal muscles (cranial nerve IX), whereas a hoarseness of the voice suggests laryngeal muscle weakness (cranial nerve X). Palatal weakness, an additional symptom of a lesion of cranial nerve X, is noted by observing a deviation of the uvula toward the uninvolved side of the larynx. If the ninth cranial nerve is intact, the gag reflex results in contraction of the pharyngeal muscles in response to stroking the back of the patient's throat gently with a tongue depressor blade.

In addition to the isolated functions of cranial nerves IX and X, the function of these nerves may be evaluated through motor activities involving the integration of the motor output of several cranial nerves. Phonation and articulation involve the coordinated function of multiple nerves in pronouncing even one word. The following example illustrates the complexity of motor output in pronouncing "capacity."

   CA—posterior pharynx; cranial nerves IX and X

   PA—lips; cranial nerve VII

   CI—tongue; cranial nerve XII

   TY—masticatory muscles and tongue; cranial nerves V and XII

Multiple cranial nerve function also occurs in the act of chewing and swallowing food. These functions require the muscles of mastication (cranial nerve V), the tongue muscles (cranial nerve XII), and the pharyngeal muscles (cranial nerves IX and X) to work together. Alterations in the taste of food may imply involvement of cranial nerves VII and IX, because of the role of these nerves in the innervation of the taste buds of the tongue.

SPINAL ACCESSORY: CRANIAL NERVE XI

Weakness of the sternocleidomastoid muscle provides the best check of cranial nerve XI function. Strong and pain-free resisted cervical rotation is the normal response. Axons of cranial nerve XI may be compressed by space-occupying lesions in the region of the foramen magnum.

LINGUAL FUNCTION: CRANIAL NERVE XII

Signs of dysfunction of the hypoglossal nerve include unilateral weakness of the tongue, resulting in deviation of the protruded tongue toward the side of the lesion. Atrophy and fasciculations of the tongue may accompany the weakness when the lesion involves the lower motoneuron, as in amyotrophic lateral sclerosis.

SPECIAL CONSIDERATIONS DURING TESTING

Evaluating the nervous system becomes more difficult when the patient is unable or unwilling to cooperate with directions from the therapist. Such patients require the evaluator to observe keenly for assumed postures, demonstrated movements, movement involved in functional activities, and the presence or absence of elicited reflexive movements.

The patient with an altered consciousness may be severely limited in his capacity to respond. Disorders of alertness may exhibit varying degrees of limitations to responses. The causative lesion usually involves the consciousness system localized in the reticular formation of the medulla, pons, and midbrain regions and the hypothalamus of the diencephalon. Altered consciousness affects motor performance through changes in response to sensory stimuli, depression of reflexive behaviors, and variations in vital signs, particularly patterned respiratory function. For instance, lesions involving the medullary centers usually result in sustained inspiratory or expiratory phases of respiration. Lesions of the descending motor system higher in the neuraxis may result in a breathing pattern of rapid shallow breaths followed by periods of apnea (no breathing). This breathing pattern is known as Cheyne-Stokes respiration.

Varying levels of consciousness following brain insult may be observed by the therapist. The patient may be in a deep coma in which there is no response to even noxious stimuli; absence of reflexive behavior; slowed, irregular pulse; and periodic respirations varying in rate and depth. In successively improving levels of consciousness, the patient may demonstrate increasing reflexive behavior and motor responses to less intense stimuli, gradual regularization of pulse and breathing patterns, and gradual recovery of awareness.

The patient who is alert but uncooperative requires the evaluator to be direct and simple with requests for movements and persistent and repetitive with testing. Evaluation sessions should be limited to short periods with frequent breaks in order to keep the client's attention focused during testing. Observing the uncooperative client or child when he is unaware of the observation may provide information about the client's real functional capacity. Children often demonstrate their motor capabilities in functional or task-oriented activities. Demonstrating the movements you wish the client to perform along with giving verbal descriptions of the movement may provide an image for the uncooperative client, who may knowingly or unknowingly repeat the movement at a later time. A demonstration may also erase the "fear of the unknown" that may be blocking the patient's cooperation.

Gathering accurate data is essential to any patient evaluation if the data are to be used to plan the treatment program. Reliability of the neurological evaluation of the uncooperative patient can be attained by repeating evaluation procedures in subsequent meetings and gathering data by using more than one testing approach. Factors that may confound neurological evaluation of uncooperative patients relate to the "state" of the client. Motor output is shaped from a repertoire of neuronal activity. The state of the client at any one time may alter the balance of activity in neuronal centers and result in an altered motor output or behavior. An overexcited person may perform more accurately if his excitement (emotion) is lowered by the quieting tone of the therapist's voice and

touch, diminished background noise, and a calm environment. In contrast, the sedate client may need an arousing environment to demonstrate true motor potential. Evaluating any difficult patient requires the therapist to control the patient-therapist interaction, exhibit patience, be direct and repetitive with requests, and be an accurate observer of all patient activity.

CLINICAL ELECTROPHYSIOLOGICAL TESTING

Clinical electrophysiological testing typically incorporates assessment of peripheral nerve conduction of motor and sensory axons and the assessment of neuromuscular integrity by electromyography. EMG testing involves use of a needle electrode, as opposed to surface electrodes commonly used in kinesiologic EMG, EMG biofeedback, and nerve conduction testing.

NERVE CONDUCTION TESTS

Peripheral nerve conduction testing typically includes recording of both motor and sensory waveforms evoked by supramaximal stimulation of the appropriate peripheral nerve. The most commonly tested nerves include the median, ulnar, peroneal, tibial, sural, and radial nerves. However, most peripheral nerves can be tested, including some of the cranial nerves.

A typical setup for a motor nerve conduction test of the median nerve is illustrated in Figure 28-10. Surface electrodes record the compound muscle action potential, or M-wave, from the abductor pollicis brevis. The M-wave is the summed muscle response of all innervated motor units in the muscle. It is evoked by supramaximal stimulation of the median nerve at two different sites: the wrist and the elbow. The M-wave is amplified and displayed on a cathode ray oscilloscope screen (Fig. 28-11). The waveform then can be examined and measurements taken. Many clinical NCV/EMG machines now have sophisticated

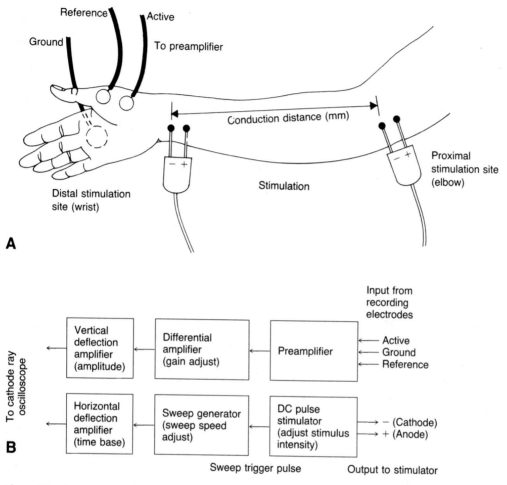

Figure 28-10. Motor nerve conduction testing. (*A*) The sites for stimulation and recording for testing nerve conduction in alpha motor axons of the median nerve. (*B*) The basic instrumentation needed for nerve stimulation, biological signal amplification, and display of the evoked response.

methods to process the signal, store the signal, and calculate measurements.

A motor nerve conduction velocity (NCV) can be calculated for the wrist to elbow segment of the median nerve by measuring the distance between the stimulation sites and then dividing that distance (in millimeters) by the difference in conduction time (in milliseconds) between the distal latency (wrist) and the proximal latency (elbow) of the M-waves. Other waveform parameters are measured

such as the amplitude, duration, and sometimes the area under the curve of the M-wave (see Fig. 28-11). There are a number of good references that describe in detail both techniques and interpretation of electrophysiological testing (Hammer, 1982; Kimura, 1983).

Two major types of nerve conduction waveforms (motor and sensory) are recorded from surface electrodes. Motor nerve conduction is recorded from a distal muscle, and the evoked M-wave response is a compound mus-

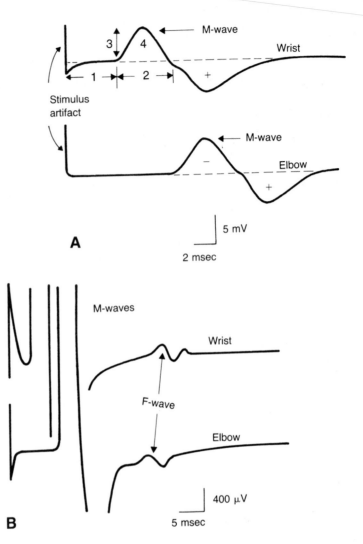

Figure 28-11. Evoked motor nerve conduction waveforms. (*A*) An oscilloscope trace of the motor response (M-wave) of the abductor pollicis brevis muscle with supramaximal stimulation of the median nerve at two stimulus sites (wrist and elbow). Note the identical waveform shape for wrist and elbow stimulation. (*B*) The longer-latency, smaller-amplitude F-wave, which can be seen only with a higher amplification and slower sweep speed settings. (*1*, latency for conduction of the fastest axons; *2*, duration of the initial negative phase of the waveform; *3*, amplitude of the initial negative peak of the waveform; *4*, area under the curve of the initial negative phase of the waveform. These same parameters are measured for the M-wave evoked by stimulation at the elbow.)

cle action potential (MAP). Sensory nerve conduction is recorded from the peripheral nerve, and thus represents a compound nerve action potential (NAP). In both cases, the MAP and the NAP represent the summed response to stimulation of only A-sized nerve fibers (large myelinated axons), and therefore do not represent the response of the dorsal root C or sympathetic C fibers to the peripheral nerve. The compound MAP is the evoked response of all the extrafusal muscle fibers in the muscle, that is, all intact A motor axons are stimulated and all innervated motor units contract synchro-

nously. Therefore, the motor response is large and relatively easy to record; the motor units act as built-in physiological amplifiers because each motor axon discharges multiple muscle fibers. The sensory waveform, however, is very small and somewhat difficult to record because it represents the summation of small electrical signals produced by a relatively small population of individual A fibers in the peripheral nerve. Therefore, in early peripheral neuropathies that affect the large fibers, one may find an abnormal or absent sensory response even though the motor response is within normal limits. A peripheral nerve disorder that selectively affects the smaller unmyelinated C fibers will not be detected by routine motor and sensory nerve conduction testing. Peripheral nervous system disease that affects *only* small fibers is not as common as the disorders that affect large or large and small peripheral axons.

Abnormalities in nerve conduction may result from impaired nerve impulse transmission or failure of nerve impulse transmission. Impaired nerve impulse transmission results in a prolonged conduction time (increased latency, slowed nerve conduction velocity, prolonged duration of waveform) through the involved segment(s) of the nerve. Impaired nerve conduction may result from demyelination, which slows but does not block impulse transmission or impulse conduction over immature regenerating axons. A block of nerve conduction may result from a transient physiological block (eg, transient ischemia), or from anatomical changes such as severe demyelination or axonal degeneration. Waveform changes associated with a partial block in nerve conduction include a decrease in amplitude and possibly duration, a decrease in waveform area, and possibly a breaking up of the waveform shape into separate smaller peaks.

Most peripheral neuropathies produce a combination of impaired impulse transmission or failure of impulse transmission in multiple axons in multiple peripheral nerves. A local entrapment or peripheral nerve injury will produce a more restricted pattern of pathophysiology. Motoneuron disease (lower motoneuron pathology) will produce a failure of nerve conduction in motor but not sensory axons. CNS disorders typically do not directly produce a deficit in peripheral nerve conduction. Nerve conduction changes may not be evident immediately after an injury in which a nerve is severed if stimulation and recording are distal to the lesion. Both motor and sensory waveforms may be elicited for three to five days following the injury. At that time, the neuromuscular junction fails and the motor waveform will fail (complete injury). A sensory waveform may persist for another 24 to 48 hours. Obviously, stimulation proximal to a complete lesion and recording distally will produce no sensory or motor response. EMG evidence of denervation also does not occur immediately (see below).

EMG EXAMINATION

The EMG needle exam is a means for evaluating the status of skeletal muscle fibers and their marriage to motor axons (motor units). The trained eyes and ears of the experienced electromyographer look and listen for signs of marital bliss or discord. The typical exam has three stages. The first stage includes the sights and sounds of the muscle fibers as the needle is advanced into the muscle. This insertion activity causes mechanical stimulation of muscle action potentials and injury potentials to the small number of damaged muscle fibers. It normally sounds like static on a radio and lasts only as long as the needle is actually moving. The absence of insertional activity suggests either a technical error or absence of viable muscle fibers in the area of the muscle that is sampled. An increased insertional activity (which outlasts the time of needle insertion) suggests an abnormal instability of muscle fibers resulting from a denervation hypersensitivity or sarcolemmal hyperirritability caused by certain types of muscle disease (eg, myotonia, myositis, or periodic paralysis).

After the cessation of needle insertion, the sampled muscle is electrically silent in a normal (and relaxed) person. The absence of any sights or sounds of electrical activity in a muscle at rest is an important sign of a happy neuromuscular family. Spontaneous discharges of fibrillation potentials, positive sharp waves, or complex repetitive discharges in a muscle *at rest* are signs of pathology and suggest that all is not well between the motor axon terminals and the motor end plates of the muscle fibers, or that the sarcolemma is hyperirritable. Fasciculation potentials in a resting muscle may or may not indicate a pathologic condition. It is important to note that these signs of neuromuscular discord (spontaneous potentials) do not typically begin until 15 to 21 days after the onset of the lesion. The abnormal potentials appear only after adequate time for biochemical alterations in the sarcolemma, the end plate zone of the denervated muscle fibers, and acetylcholine receptor proteins. The one major exception to this rule is the electrical activity seen at rest when the needle is next to an intramuscular nerve. In this case, potentials will be seen after the needle stops moving. However, the potentials are characteristically different from those mentioned above, and typically, the patient will complain of intramuscular pain. Both the electrical activity and the pain will cease as the needle is moved away from this site in a normal muscle.

In the last stage of the EMG exam, the sights and sounds of the muscle during volitional effort are assessed. The electromyographer will assess the waveform parameters of individual motor units and also the pattern of motor unit recruitment. When the patient is asked to contract the muscle with minimal effort, one or several motor units can be seen and heard. The normal motor unit potential has normal parameters of amplitude, duration, and shape and typically has fewer than four phases. There should be a sharp take-off from baseline (rapid rate of rise) and a distinct "popping" sound. If there are no viable motor units within the immediate surrounding territory, distant motor units may be heard as a muffled sound of low-amplitude potentials that have a slow rate of rise. As the contraction continues, each motor unit retains its identity and can be seen again and again (as long as the needle does not move).

Abnormal motor units will have abnormal parameters. The electromyographer will specifically look for repetition of individual motor units to make sure that the parameters of the motor unit do not change. For example, a motor unit with more than three to four phases (polyphasic motor unit) could indicate peripheral neuromuscular disease. Therefore, it is important to distinguish whether the waveform seen on consecutive sweeps has a consistent polyphasic shape or whether the abnormal shape actually represented the incidental overlap of two motor units that happened to be recruited at the same time. An abnormally large motor unit suggests an enlarged motor unit territory caused by axon collaterals of surviving motor units "rescuing" nearby denervated muscle fibers. Intramuscular collateral sprouting of axons from surviving motoneurons to innervate adjacent denervated muscle fibers suggests that some message of "separation anxiety" is shared between involved and intact motor units. The source of this message and how the information is communicated are still unknown, although a retrograde transported "trophic" factor has been suggested by some researchers. The expanded motor unit territory may result from an incomplete peripheral nerve injury or motoneuron (lower motoneuron) disease. These potentials may have normal or abnormal shapes, and normal or, more often, a prolonged duration. Abnormally small motor units with an increased number of phases and short durations suggest that the motor unit territory is decreased, that is, that there are fewer viable muscle fibers remaining in each motor unit, as might occur in muscle diseases. Normal amplitude but highly polyphasic potentials with increased durations suggests an asynchronous activation of muscle fibers within the motor unit. This asynchrony may be caused by immature regenerating axonal branches that conduct impulses at different speeds, resulting in asynchronous activation of different muscle fibers within the motor unit.

A normal person, when asked to increase muscular tension, will recruit already activated motor units at a higher rate *and* will begin to recruit other motor units. If a person has lost motor units because of peripheral nerve disease or a lower motoneuron lesion, the small population of remaining viable motor units must now compensate by drastically increasing their firing rates to match the effort required. Therefore, the electromyographer will see fewer different motor units but will see the same motor units repeated again and again at a high rate of response. If a person has fewer muscle fibers per motor unit (as in muscle disease), then a demand for increased effort will require a larger than normal number of motor units to be activated to produce a small rise in tension. If many different motor units are discharging at the same time, the motor unit potentials begin to overlap and individual motor units can no longer be distinguished (interference pattern). Normally, this interference pattern builds gradually and a high level of overlapping of motor unit potentials does not occur until high levels of tension approaching maximal effort are achieved. An early interference pattern is characteristic of patients in early stages of muscle disease. During the later stages of muscle disease, there are so few viable muscle fibers that interference is incomplete and is clinically associated with extreme weakness.

If there are only a few or no motor units recruited with demands for increasing volitional effort, then one of two conclusions can be reached. The subject is not applying adequate volitional effort (because of fear, pain, upper motoneuron disease, conversion reaction, and so forth), or he has no motor innervation to use (severe peripheral nerve injury or lower motoneuron disease). The electromyographer may then try to recruit the muscle not as a prime mover, but as a synergist in another type of movement to see if any motor units are present in that muscle. The electromyographer must also adequately sample other territories within that muscle and other related muscles. Subsequently, the electromyographer must correlate other clinical and electrical findings with the results of the EMG exam. The ability of the clinician to perform a comprehensive electrophysiological evaluation requires not only didactic knowledge in applied anatomy, physiology, kinesiology, neuroscience, electrophysiology, and pathology, but also substantial clinical experience and expertise.

The clinical electrophysiological exam may also incorporate testing of long latency waveforms, which allows the examiner to assess more proximal segments of nerve fibers, including impulse conduction through nerve roots. One of the testing procedures is the Hoffman or H-reflex. This H-reflex should not be confused with the Hoffman sign of the upper motoneuron lesion. The H-reflex is thought to be a monosynaptic reflex. The H-reflex incorporates impulse conduction to the spinal cord from the Ia axons innervating muscle spindles and impulses conducted to a muscle in alpha motor axons originating from alpha motoneurons in the spinal cord. Both the afferent Ia axons and the efferent alpha motor axons are large diameter, heavily myelinated, and rapid conducting. The Ia axons have the lowest threshold for electrical excitation. The H-reflexes are therefore elicited with submaximal stimulus intensities. At supramaximal stimulus intensities, the H-reflex disappears. The action potentials conducted towards the spinal cord from the site of stimulation collide with the reflex-generated action potentials, and this collision nullifies conduction of impulses in the alpha motor axon (see Fig. 28-2). H-reflexes can be reliably tested in the lower extremity, but are rarely observed in upper extremities in adults. Interestingly, the H-reflex appears to be prominent in upper and lower extremities in infants. Because this test is based on a central synaptic excitatory process, it is subject to influence by a number of peripheral and central influences on alpha motoneuron excitability. Loss of the H-reflex in the triceps surae muscles correlates with S1 nerve root lesions, and has proved beneficial in evaluating suspected S1 impingement syndromes and peripheral nerve injuries that affect the nerve roots, such as Guillain-Barré syndrome.

Another mechanism to assess the most proximal portion of the motor nerve is supramaximal stimulation of a peripheral nerve and recording from a distal muscle (as in motor NCV testing), a longer latency response called the F-wave (see Fig. 28-11).

The F-wave is a small-amplitude response that occurs at a similar latency to the submaximally stimulated H-reflex. However, unlike the H-reflex, the F-wave has greater variability in latency and amplitude with successive stimulations. Note in Figure 28-11 that the latency of the F-wave decreases as the stimulation site is moved proximally. This is exactly what would be expected, because there is a shorter conduction distance to the alpha motoneurons at the more proximal stimulus site. Protocols have been developed to estimate the conduction velocity of the most proximal portion of motor axons, that is, in the plexus and ventral roots (Kimura, 1983). The F-wave survives dorsal rhizotomy and is thought to be the result of an antidromal invasion of the motoneuron, which triggers an action potential at the axon hillock *if* the electrical membrane properties are ideal. Therefore, the F-wave is not thought to be a reflex response, but a "backfiring" of motoneurons in the spinal cord. Thus, the F-wave includes nerve conduction in the most proximal portions of motor axons. A condition that tends to facilitate the F-wave is a slight voluntary contraction, which presumably produces a subthreshold depolarization of a number of motor units. The antidromic action potential may then further depolarize the cell to fire an orthodromic action potential. These depolarizing inputs must compete with significant hyperpolarizing inputs, especially recurrent inhibition from Renshaw cells. This explains the variability and small size of the F-wave. Unlike the H-reflex, the F-wave can be elicited in virtually all motor nerves tested clinically and provides a window to conduction in the most proximal portions of the motor axons, including the ventral roots. An abnormal F-wave may be found in peripheral nerve or ventral root lesions or in motor neuron (lower motoneuron) disease.

A more recent method of assessing central sensory pathways is to utilize averaged evoked potential recordings following visual, auditory, or somatosensory stimuli. Electrodes are placed on the scalp or neck to record the volume conducted potentials from the appropriate sensory pathways. Scalp-recorded potentials evoked from contralateral peripheral nerve stimulation are called somatosensory-evoked potentials (SEPs). Scalp recordings from repeating visual pattern displays are called visual evoked potentials (VEPs), and scalp or neck recordings of auditory click stimuli are called auditory-evoked potentials (AEPs). Investigators have attempted to correlate the origin of the different phases of this complex of evoked potential waveforms, but as yet there is still disagreement regarding the origins of different phases in the potential. However, delays seen in the early components of the evoked responses have been positively correlated with the presence of central demyelinating disease (eg, multiple sclerosis) and with other selected CNS disorders. Although this technique offers hope for a closer look at central neuronal pathways, evoked potential recordings still have limited clinical applications and provide only a relatively crude measurement of CNS function.

CONCLUSION

It is imperative that physical therapists who evaluate and treat neurologically involved patients have a working knowledge of applied neuroscience. The problems brought to the physical therapist by these patients rarely have simple solutions. Indeed, one of the most pressing issues in the practice of physical therapy is how we *objectively* define the problem. If we cannot justify therapeutic interventions based on both scientific rationale and empirical data, our practice will be limited to technical procedures imposed by others.

The most fundamental question to be answered by the neurological evaluation is whether the signs, symptoms, and dysfunctions of the patient are caused by nervous system disease. In some cases, there are obvious clues of direct nervous system involvement. The site and extent of the lesion(s) are easily distinguished by modern methods of diagnostic testing that supplement the clinical evaluation (eg, in the case of a localized parietal lobe tumor). Other cases may defy systematic investigation as to the exact source of the problem (eg, unsteady balance and gait of unknown origin).

Beyond the determination that a patient's loss of function is correlated to nervous system disease, the physical therapist must employ clinical testing to look for systematic patterns of neurological involvement. These patterns may reveal what systems are involved (eg, motor, sensory systems) and what anatomical areas are involved (eg, cerebellar dysfunction or peripheral nerve pathology).

LOCALIZATION OF NERVOUS SYSTEM DYSFUNCTION

The nervous system can be clinically subdivided into four levels: peripheral, spinal, posterior fossa (brain stem and cerebellum), and supratentorial (superficial and deep structures of the cerebral hemispheres). Certain anatomical landmarks are used to separate these levels: for example, the tentorium cerebelli separates the supratentorial and posterior fossa brain, and the foramen magnum separates the posterior fossa brain from the spinal cord. The PNS includes all neurons and their processes located external to the brain stem or the spinal cord. That is, all cranial and spinal nerves are part of the peripheral nervous system. Some neuroscientists include the lower motoneurons located in the motor nuclei in the brain stem and spinal cord as part of the peripheral nervous system.

The presence or absence of certain neuro-logical signs and symptoms will help the physical therapist to localize the level or levels of nervous system dysfunction. Table 28-2 summarizes some of the signs and symptoms associated with each of the four levels of the clinically subdivided nervous system. The deficits listed for each level are based on the localized functions of the structures at that level.

Note that both sensory and motor dysfunctions may result from lesions at any level of the nervous system: supratentorial, posterior fossa, peripheral, or spinal. The sensory and motor systems are contiguous across all levels of the nervous system. Other dysfunctions are typical of only one level of the nervous system. For example, higher level dysfunction such as communication disorders (eg, aphasia, agraphia, alexia) or disorders in spatial perceptions (eg, unilateral sensory neglect, distortions of body image) occur only with supratentorial lesions. Similarly, cranial nerve deficits

Table 28-2. Clinical Localization of Neurological Dysfunction

SUPRATENTORIAL	POSTERIOR FOSSA		SPINAL	PERIPHERAL
	Brain	*Cranial Nerves*		

Major Structures

1. Right and left cerebral hemispheres: limbic and nonlimbic cerebral cortex, internal capsule, optic radiations	1. Brain stem: deep reticular nuclei locomotor regions, eye movement control centers, autonomic nuclei, descending and ascending projection pathways to and from spinal cord	1. Cranial nerve nuclei/pathways and cranial nerves III through XII	1. Spinal gray: local interneurons, projection neurons, motoneurons (somatic and autonomic)*	1. Ganglia: dorsal root and autonomic ganglia
2. Deep structures: basal ganglia, limbic nuclei and pathways, thalamic nuclei	2. Cerebellum and associated nuclei/pathways		2. Spinal white: intersegmental connection pathways, long ascending and descending projection pathways	2. Superficial and deep sensory receptors
				3. Effector organs, somatic skeletal muscle, autonomic cardial and smooth muscle, glands
				4. Peripheral axons: roots, rami, plexi, nerves

Localizing Signs and Symptoms

1. Higher function deficits: aphasia, alexia, agraphia, acalculia, memory deficits, dementia	1. Reduction of consciousness with decerebrate posturing (upper motoneuron signs)	1. Diplopia	1. Combined upper motoneuron and lower motoneuron signs with or without sensory deficits	1. *No* upper motoneuron signs
		2. Unilateral opthalmoplegia plus loss of direct light reflex		2. Lower motoneuron signs with or without sensory deficits

continued

Table 28-2. (continued)

SUPRATENTORIAL	POSTERIOR FOSSA		SPINAL	PERIPHERAL
	Brain	*Cranial Nerves*		

Localizing Signs and Symptoms

2. Spatial perceptual defects 3. Spastic hemiparesis (plegia) of face,[†] arm, trunk, leg (upper motor neuron signs) with hemisensory deficits of same side of face and body plus homonymous hemianopsia 4. Abnormal involuntary movements: chorea, athetosis, ballism. Plastic or cogwheel rigidity combined with hypokinesia and resting tremor.	plus dilated and fixed pupils (nonreactive to light) 2. Ipsilateral facial paresis (plegia) plus contralateral hemiparesis (plegia) of arm, trunk, and leg 3. Ipsilateral hemisensory deficits for face plus contralateral hemisensory deficits for arm, trunk, and leg 4. Internuclear opthalmoplegia 5. Dysmetria, ataxia, dysdiadochokinesia, and intention tremor 6. Speech deficits: slurring of words, explosive irregular speech pattern with no loss of linguistic content, no prior history of speech defects 7. Akinesia (head and body) plus neurologic breathing pattern, and no response to sensory input, eyes open	3. Hemisensory deficits in face 4. Unilateral paresis (plegia) of facial muscles 5. Vertigo 6. Tinnitus 7. Nystagmus 8. Atrophy and fasciculation of tongue 9. Misarticulation of consonants with no defect in syntax or linguistic content	2. Spastic quadriplegia with anesthesia in same segmental levels plus bowel and bladder dysfunction 3. Restricted zone of bilateral pain and temperature deficits with lower motoneuron signs in upper extremities plus upper motoneuron signs (central cord syndrome) in lower extremities sparing bowel and bladder function 4. Spastic paraplegia with anesthesia of lower extremities and bowel and bladder dysfunction 5. Flaccid paraparesis with loss of pain and temperature sensation in lower extremities, but at least partial preservation of touch, pressure, vibration sense, and proprioception in lower extremities, plus bowel and bladder dysfunction (anterior cord syndrome) 6. Unilateral upper motoneuron signs, and spastic paresis of lower extremity with discriminative sensory loss in that extremity plus loss of pain and temperature in opposite extremity (hemisection of cord)	3. Motor (lower motoneuron), autonomic, and sensory deficits all within specific peripheral anatomical pattern (root-plexus-nerve) 4. Radicular pain, paresthesia within specific peripheral anatomical pattern in extremity 5. Horner's syndrome: ipsilateral miosis, partial ptosis, anhydrosis, flushing of face with no upper motoneuron sign or facial sensory deficit 6. "Glove and stocking" distal sensory deficits, atrophy, and weakness of distal muscles and trophic skin/nail changes distally in all four extremities 7. Flaccid paraplegia with sensory deficits in lower extremities with or without bowel and bladder dysfunction

*Some neurologists consider alpha motoneurons as part of the peripheral nervous system.

†Sparing of frontalis muscle.

and cerebellar deficits suggest lesions involving the cranial nerves or cranial nerve nuclei located in the brain stem and the cerebellum within the posterior fossa of the skull. Loss of sensory and motor function below a well-defined segmental spinal level suggests a spinal cord injury. Patients with this loss will show no evidence of brain dysfunction. Lesions restricted to the PNS are unique in that input and output of neural signals are interrupted, but central integrating functions are preserved. Patients with restricted peripheral nerve lesions have no signs and symptoms of CNS dysfunction typical of spinal, brain stem, cerebellar, or higher level supratentorial brain involvement.

Your evaluation should reveal not only "classical textbook" signs and symptoms, but also should identify each patient's specific problems that accompany the variability of pathologic insults seen in human disease.

Individualized treatment plans should be based on the actual presenting problems of each patient, not the expected constellation of neurological sequelae "defined" for a diagnostic group. The physical therapist must use professional talents to accomplish patient care goals within the confines of a health care delivery system that is increasingly based on diagnostic grouping of "typical" patients.

ANNOTATED BIBLIOGRAPHY

Adams RD, Victor M: Principles of Neurology. New York, McGraw-Hill, 1985 (This is a comprehensive, detailed examination of neurology as a clinical specialty. It is a foundation text of clinical neurology. Comprehensive examination of all types of neurological disorders includes diagnosis, prognosis, pathological features, clinical features, and current treatment regimes. Neurological examination is related to the identification and localization of neurological dysfunction.)

Barr ML, Kiernan JA: The Human Nervous System: An Anatomical Viewpoint, 5th ed. Philadelphia, JB Lippincott, 1988 (This book provides a fundamental overview of nervous system structures, pathways, and their supportive structures. Cytology, neuroembryology, and reaction of neurons to injury are introduced. Clinical correlates of nervous system disease are included in some chapters.)

Bishop B: Neural plasticity I–IV. Phys Ther 62(8):1122; 1132, 62(9):1274, 62(10):1442, 1982

Brodal A: Neurological Anatomy in Relation to Clinical Medicine. New York, Oxford University Press, 1981 (This is a classic text replete with detailed anatomy and descriptions of connectivity within the nervous system. Clinical neurological deficits are explored in depth. This text is based on years of scientific investigations in the laboratory and the clinic. Virtually every point is exhaustively referenced. This is not a reference for therapists who have only a casual interest in neuroscience.)

Brooks VB: The Neural Basis of Motor Control. New York, Oxford University Press, 1986 (An integrated review of how the nervous system controls movement, this book requires the reader to have background knowledge of neuroanatomy and neurophysiology and have experienced movement.)

Carpenter MB, Sutin J: Human Neuroanatomy. Baltimore, Williams & Wilkins, 1983 (No annotated bibliography that includes reference to human neuroanatomy would be complete without this book. There is no substitute for the overview and detail in neuroanatomy given in this text. Illustrations are excellent and the text is well documented by classical and modern references to neuroanatomical studies. If the therapist wants a condensed version of this book, *Core Text of Neuroanatomy* by Malcolm B. Carpenter, Baltimore, Williams & Wilkins, 1985 would be an excellent reference text for the library.)

Chusid JG: Correlative Neuroanatomy and Functional Anatomy, 19th ed. Los Altos, CA, Lange Medical Publishers, 1985 (A source for concise but thorough structural and functional aspects of human nervous system function as related to a clinical understanding of the neurologically involved patient.)

Daube JR, Reagan TJ, Sandok BA et al: Medical Neurosciences: An Approach to Anatomy, Pathology and Physiology by Systems and Levels. Boston, Little, Brown & Co, 1986 (The authors have subdivided the nervous system into clinically relevant subsystems and levels. The focus of this text is on clinical manifestations of nervous system structure and function. Clinical correlations focus on localization of function implied by nervous system pathology involving different subsystems or levels.)

Hammer K: Nerve Conduction Studies. Springfield, IL, Charles C Thomas, 1982 (This book provides step-by-step techniques for performing nerve conduction testing and shows examples of abnormal waveforms that result from specific types of peripheral nerve pathology.)

Horak FB: Clinical measurement of postural control in adults. Phys Ther 67:1881, 1987

Kaas JH, Merzenich MM, Killackey HP: The reorganization of somatosensory cortex following peripheral nerve damage in adult and developing mammals. Annu Rev Neurosci 6:325, 1983

Kandel ER, Schwartz JH: Principles of Neural Science, 2nd ed. New York, Elsevier, 1985 (A foundation text of human neuroanatomy and neurophysiology, written with the premise that behavior results from neural activity.)

Kimura J: Electrodiagnosis in Diseases of Nerve and Muscle: Principles and Practice. Philadelphia, FA Davis, 1983 (This is a comprehensive text for clinicians who utilize electrophysiological techniques to evaluate neurological patients. Both principles and application of those principles are discussed in detail including instrumentation and techniques for routine and special nerve and muscle testing procedures. Neuromuscular disorders are discussed in relation to electrophysiological testing.)

Mancall EL: Alper and Mancall's Essentials of the Neurologic Examination. Philadelphia, FA Davis, 1981 (This book describes the clinical examination of neurological function. Both subjective and objective testing are included. This text also includes interpretation of clinical findings, applicability and interpretation of laboratory tests, and correlating findings to functional anatomy.)

Nashner LM: Adaptation of human movement to altered environments. Trends in Neuroscience 5:358, 1982

Pryse-Phillips W, Murray TJ: Essential Neurology. New York, Medical Examination Publishing, 1978 (This is a "no-frills" introduction to neurology. There is an excellent chapter on the neurological examination and a wealth of clinical experience evolves in those chapters that characterize and categorize nervous system disease.)

Shumway-Cook A, Horak FB: Assessing the influence of sensory interaction on balance: suggestions from the field. Phys Ther 66:1548, 1986

Whitsel BL, Favorov O, Tommerdahl M et al: Dynamic processes govern the somatosensory cortical response to natural stimulation. In Lund JS (ed): Sensory Processing in the Mammalian Brain: Neural Substrates and Experimental Strategies. New York, Oxford University Press, 1988 (in press)

29 Cardiovascular Analysis

ELLEN HILLEGASS

The physical therapist analyzes the patient's cardiovascular system to assess dysfunction or physical disability that would create limitations in movement. In this chapter, I will describe the evaluative procedures used to provide information on specific cardiovascular pathology. The physical therapist is specifically assessing the heart valves, coronary arteries, pressure in the vascular system, electrical activity, and effectiveness of the muscle pump of the heart.

Objective information on the patient's cardiovascular system is derived from significant data obtained from the following procedures: thorough review of the patient's medical record, interview of the patient, performance of an initial physical examination and follow-up monitored ambulation, blood pressure measurement, interpretation of the electrocardiogram, and results of exercise testing and other evaluative testing.

MEDICAL RECORD REVIEW

The purpose of the medical chart review is to extract pertinent information to develop a data base on the patient. Based on this information, the physical therapist performs the appropriate evaluation and develops the optimal treatment plan. The therapist should focus the review of the medical record by identifying the following significant information:

1. Diagnosis and date of the event
2. Symptoms upon admission and since the patient's admission
3. Other significant medical problems
4. Medications
5. Risk factors of heart disease
6. Chest roentgenograms
7. Laboratory data
8. Electrocardiogram and serial monitoring
9. Hospital course since the event; defined as complicated versus uncomplicated, according to the criteria of McNeer and colleagues (1975)
10. Occupation
11. Family situation/home environment

DIAGNOSIS AND DATE OF EVENT

The physical therapist needs to know the primary diagnosis as well as any additional diagnoses made since the hospital admission to determine the patient's appropriateness for treatment and the need for monitoring the patient's responses. Specific cardiovascular diagnoses that indicate some form of cardiac dysfunction include coronary artery disease, congestive heart failure, arrhythmias, valvular dysfunction, coronary artery bypass surgery, angioplasty, syncope, hypertension, angina, peripheral vascular disease, or atherosclerosis. For example, patients with a history of coronary artery disease would be appropriate for treatment, but should be monitored for abnormal responses to exercise. However, when presented with a patient admitted with a diagnosis of "Rule out myocardial infarction," the physical therapist should review the chart for documentation of a definitive diagnosis and level of activity before proceeding with any treatment and monitoring of responses.

The date of the event identifies the acuteness of the situation for the physical therapist. The date of the primary event or diagnosis is often documented in the history and physical examination written by the physician; however, the date of the secondary diagnosis or subsequent events may be discovered by reading the physician's progress notes or physician's orders, or both. Patients with acute cardiac dysfunction will need to have activity restricted, and probably need close monitoring when activity is initiated.

SYMPTOMS

Cardiac symptoms may be described as occurring anywhere above the waist. These symptoms are described differently by each patient. Classically, any discomfort, such as chest pain, tightness, shortness of breath, palpitations, indigestion, and burning may be considered cardiac symptoms. Reviewing the patient's symptoms upon admission and during hospitalization provides the therapist with awareness of those symptoms that are to be assessed as cardiac versus noncardiac. Orders for ambulation or cardiac rehabilitation may be given to attempt to reproduce the symptoms and assess the patient's responses when the symptoms occur. Therefore, admitting symptoms are important data gained from the chart review.

OTHER MEDICAL PROBLEMS

The therapist needs to assess other medical problems that may interfere with evaluation or treatment of the patient. Other diagnoses including pulmonary, orthopaedic, or psychological dysfunction may affect the treatment program. For example, a patient with a history of chronic tobacco use may be limited by his pulmonary capacity rather than his cardiac condition. A patient may have been diagnosed with a hiatal hernia prior to this admission, and thus may not believe he has a cardiac problem.

MEDICATIONS

The medications the patient is currently taking as well as those that have been prescribed during the hospitalization are usually listed in the chart. The medications provide information about the patient's present or recent past cardiovascular abnormalities, including angina, hypertension, arrhythmias, and heart failure.

Because medications will affect the patient's responses to exercise, the physical therapist must become familiar with the broad categories of cardiac medications, understand the indications for their use, and know their side-effects (Table 29-1). Nitrates or anti-anginal medications are used for their vasodilating effects on the cardiovascular system. Patients are often given nitroglycerin tablets to use sublingually (or nitroglycerin spray to use on the tongue) during an acute angina attack. Because the vasodilation is nonspecific, both the venous and arterial systems are affected, with some vasodilation occurring in the coronary arteries. With systemic vasodilation, preload and afterload on the heart are also decreased. Therefore, the common side-effects of nitrates are hypotension and dizziness.

Diuretics are usually the "step-1" drugs for treatment of high blood pressure. Diuretics decrease serum sodium and volume (water) from the blood. Common side-effects of diuretic use include low sodium levels, hypotension, metabolic alkalosis, and hypokalemia (which can lead to life-threatening arrhythmias).

Beta adrenergic receptor blocking drugs are the commonly used "step-2" medications used for decreasing blood pressure and decreasing the work on the heart (by also decreasing the heart rate). Therefore, beta-blocking medications will blunt the heart rate and blood pressure responses to exercise. However, beta blockers also decrease the force of contraction of the heart muscle. Patients receiving beta blockers may therefore develop failure of the muscle pump with exertion. Other side-effects

Table 29-1. Medications

Common Antiarrhythmia Drugs	***Calcium Antagonists***
Lidocaine (intravenous use only)	Nifedipine (Procardia)
Quinidine	Verapamil (Isoptin, Calan)
Procainamide (Pronestyl, Procan SR)	Diltiazem (Cardizem)
Disopyramide (Norpace)	
Flecainide (Tambocor)	***Diuretics***
Mexiletine (Mexitil)	Furosemide (Lasix)
Tocainide HCl (Tonocard)	Triamterene (Dyazide)
Bretylium (Bretylol)	Hydrochlorthiazide (Moduretic)
Amiodarone (Cordarone)	Methyclothiazide (Enduron)
Enkaid	Bumetanide (Bumex)
	Hydrochlorothiazide (Maxzide)
Antianginal Drugs	
Nitroglycerin (Nitrolingual spray, NTG, Nitro-Bid, Nitrodur, Transderm-Nitro)	***Inotropic Agents***
	Digitalis
Deponit	Digoxin (Lanoxin)
Isosorbide dinitrate (Sorbitrate, Isordil)	Amrinone (Inocor)
Beta-adrenergic Receptor Blocking Drugs	***Other Antihypertension Drugs***
Timolol (Blocadren)	Prazosin (Minipress)
Propranolol (Inderal, Inderide)	Enalapril (Vasotec)
Nadolol (Corgard)	Methyldopa (Aldomet)
Metoprolol (Lopressor)	Reserpine
Atenolol (Tenormin)	Captopril (Capoten)
Pindolol (Visken)	Hydralazine (Apresoline)
Acebutolol (Sectral)	Minoxidil
Labetalol (Trandate)	Labetalol (Normodyne)

include bronchospasm in patients with chronic obstructive pulmonary disease, blocked hypoglycemic response in diabetics, insomnia, fatigue, and impotence. Beta-blocking medications are widely used in the post-myocardial infarction (MI) patient because research has shown that these medications decreased the morbidity and mortality after MI (Frishman, 1981).

Should the first two steps of antihypertensive treatment prove ineffective in controlling blood pressure, "step-3" drugs, vasodilators, are added to the medications. These antihypertension medications have potent side-effects, including hypotension, insomnia, extreme fatigue, and impotence.

Antiarrhythmia medications are used to control life-threatening arrhythmias by decreasing the incidence of premature ventricular contractions (PVCs), couplets, and the like. Some antiarrhythmia medications specifically act to decrease the incidence of sustained ventricular tachycardia. Side-effects of these medications include nausea, diarrhea, symptoms suggestive of systemic lupus erythematosus, and proarrhythmia (increasing frequency of arrhythmia). Calcium antagonists are used in patients with hypertension, coronary artery spasm, and supraventricular arrhythmias. Calcium antagonists perform three functions: (1) decrease smooth muscle contraction of the artery walls (decrease muscle spasm), (2) vasodilation, and (3) decrease supraventricular arrhythmias. Common side-effects include hypotension, dizziness, and conduction delays including atrioventricular block.

Digoxin is the most commonly used inotropic (meaning that it affects contractility) medication used to improve the force of contraction of the heart muscle. Patients with congestive heart failure or rapid ventricular response to supraventricular arrhythmias (atrial fibrillation or atrial flutter) are usually started on positive inotropic agents. Positive inotropic medications can cause changes on the resting electrocardiogram. Toxic levels, if they develop, can cause gastrointestinal side-effects, arrhythmias, hypotension, and renal failure.

RISK FACTORS

The history and physical report usually describes the patient's risk factor profile for heart disease. Awareness of the patient's risk factors enables the therapist to develop goals for the patient's long-term treatment as well as identify other rehabilitation team members to whom the patient should be referred. Table 29-2 lists the risk factors of heart disease. Detailed information on risk factors can be obtained from the Framingham study (Kannel and co-workers, 1971).

CHEST ROENTGENOGRAM

The main indication for review of the chest roentgenogram is the presence or absence of signs of congestive heart failure or cardiac enlargement. Patients with abnormal chest roentgenograms have more complicated cardiac dysfunction. The chest x-ray film provides general information regarding overall heart size and individual cardiac chamber enlargement, size and configuration of the major vessels, presence of any calcification on the major cardiac structures, and changes in the lungs and thorax secondary to cardiac or pulmonary disease.

The x-ray report is usually a written description of any increased vascularity, interstitial edema, or pulmonary edema, which provides information on the presence of heart fail-

Table 29-2. Risk Factors of Heart Disease

Hypertension
Smoking
Elevated serum cholesterol
Family history of heart disease
Stress/Type A personality
Sedentary
Obesity
Male sex
Age
Diabetes

(Kannel WB, Castelli WP, Gordon T et al: Serum cholesterol, lipoproteins, and the risk of coronary heart disease: The Framingham Study. Ann Intern Med 24:1, 1971)

ure. Cardiomegaly (cardiac hypertrophy) is enlargement of the heart.

Chest x-ray films may also indicate some degree of pulmonary dysfunction.

LABORATORY DATA

Laboratory data provide important objective information regarding the clinical status of the patient with cardiac dysfunction. The laboratory data specific to the patient with cardiac dysfunction include cardiac enzymes, blood lipids (cholesterol and triglycerides), hemoglobin, and prothrombin time.

Cardiac Enzyme Levels

Evaluation of specific serum enzyme levels contributes to the definitive diagnosis of myocardial necrosis. When damage has occurred to the myocardium, intracellular cardiac enzymes are released into the circulation. Their presence can be measured by serum blood tests. The enzymes of diagnostic importance are creatine phosphokinase (CPK), lactic dehydrogenase (LDH), and serum glutamic-oxaloacetic transaminase (SGOT). In addition, isoenzymes, which are different forms of the same enzyme, have been found to be more conclusive of specific muscle cell necrosis. The most specific isoenzyme for cardiac muscle necrosis is CPK-MB fraction, but LDH-1 is also conclusive for cardiac necrosis.

The enzymes and isoenzymes increase

Table 29-3. Cardiac Enzymes

	NORMAL SERUM LEVEL VALUES (IU)*	ONSET OF RISE (HR)	TIME OF PEAK RISE (HR)	RETURN TO NORMAL (DAYS)
CPK	55–71†	3–4	33	3
LDH	127‡	12–24	72	5–14
SGOT	24	12	24	4

*1 IU is the amount of enzyme that will catalyze the formation of 1 μmol of substrate per minute under the conditions of the test.
†CPK MB, 0%–3%
‡LDH-1, 14%–26%
(Smith AM, Theirer JA, Huang SH: Serum enzymes in myocardial infarction. Am J Nursing 73(2):277, 1973)

within the first 36 hours after myocardial injury. The enzymes elevate and peak at different rates, and are further described in Table 29-3.

Blood Lipid Levels

Hyperlipidemia (elevated lipid levels) is considered a risk factor contributing to coronary artery disease. Thus, the concentration of cholesterol and triglycerides in serum plasma needs to be assessed. The American Heart Association defines elevated cholesterol levels as those above 200 mg/100 mL. Elevated triglyceride levels are defined as those above 150 mg/100 mL. Elevated cholesterol levels are associated with ingestion of cholesterol and saturated fats as well as hereditary influences. Elevated triglyceride levels are associated with increased carbohydrate ingestion and often accompany diabetes mellitus.

Some clinical laboratories provide more detailed information on cholesterol levels by dividing the total cholesterol level into the component parts of high-density lipoproteins (HDL) and low-density lipoproteins (LDL). An increased ratio of total cholesterol to HDL identifies a person at an increased risk of heart disease (Table 29-4). High levels of LDL also increase a person's risk of heart disease.

Other Laboratory Tests

Hemoglobin values are important for the therapist to know because hemoglobin is an important component of the oxygen transport system. Hemoglobin values are measured in concentration on the blood (in grams per 100 mL of blood). Normal range of hemoglobin for females is 12 to 16 g/100 mL, and for males 14 to 18 g/100 mL. Low levels of hemoglobin indicate the myocardium must work harder to transport more oxygen to the tissues even when the body is at rest. It is important to determine the hemoglobin value in every patient because it defines the oxygen-carrying capacity of the blood.

Prothrombin times have recently become an important component of the patient's data base because of the procedure of streptokinase infusion that is currently being performed in some hospitals. Prothrombin time (PT) and partial thromboplastin time (PTT) measure

Table 29-4. Total Cholesterol to HDL Cholesterol Values

TOTAL CHOLESTEROL/HDL	RISK OF HEART DISEASE
Men	
3.43	½ Avg
4.97	Average
9.55	2× Avg
23.39	3× Avg
Women	
3.27	½ Avg
4.44	Average
7.05	2× Avg
11.04	3× Avg

(Gordon T, Castelli WP, Hjortland MC et al: Diabetes, blood lipids, and the role of obesity in coronary heart disease risk for women. Ann Intern Med 87:393, 1977)

blood coagulation. Streptokinase infusion is a means of dissolving clots that may critically block a coronary artery and induce a myocardial infarction. It may be done intravenously or directly into the coronary arteries. Streptokinase infusion is used as an anticoagulator in an acute event. After the initial streptokinase infusion is performed, intravenous heparin is started. As a result, PT and PTT must be monitored closely to determine the therapeutic ranges of anticoagulation.

In general, all electrolyte levels should be monitored during hospitalization because disturbances in these would affect the patient's performance. Sodium (N), potassium (K), and carbon dioxide (CO_2) are the most important electrolytes to monitor. Hydration, medications, and disease can affect these values. For example, patients receiving diuretics need to have potassium monitored closely, because many diuretics deplete potassium by their action on the kidney. Dangerously low levels of potassium (<3.5 mEq/L) can cause serious, life-threatening arrhythmias. Low levels of CO_2 can create an alkalotic state and cause dizziness and muscle weakness.

ELECTROCARDIOGRAM AND SERIAL MONITORING

The electrocardiogram (ECG) provides valuable information regarding the viability of the heart muscle and the rhythm of the heart. The ECG will show previous myocardial injury, hypertrophy of the heart muscle, and any delays in the generation of the cardiac impulse. Serial monitoring during hospitalization provides a historic record of the patient's cardiac rhythm. Details of the electrocardiogram will be discussed later in this chapter.

HOSPITAL COURSE

A thorough review of the medical record should reveal pertinent information regarding the patient's clinical course after a myocardial infarction. Patients with serious complications within the first four days of the myocardial infarction have a higher incidence of mortality or late serious complications. Table 29-5 lists the serious complications defined by McNeer

Table 29-5. Criteria for a Complicated Post-Myocardial Infarction Hospital Course

Any of the following within the first four days after event
Ventricular tachycardia or fibrillation
Atrial flutter or fibrillation
Second- or third-degree atrioventricular block
Persistent sinus tachycardia (>100 beats per minute)
Persistent systolic hypotension (<90 mm Hg)
Pulmonary edema
Cardiogenic shock
Persistent angina/extension of infarction

(McNeer JF, Wallace AG, Wagner GS et al: Circulation 51:410, 1975)

and co-workers (1975). Patients who are characterized as uncomplicated have a low incidence of morbidity and mortality after the cardiac event.

OCCUPATION

Identifying the type of work the patient currently performs provides for setting realistic goals and planning for return to work, if this is possible. For example, a patient who has experienced a massive complicated myocardial infarction may not be an appropriate candidate for return to a job requiring heavy lifting, and may need referral for vocational rehabilitation.

FAMILY SITUATION AND HOME ENVIRONMENT

A supportive family is important to the success of the rehabilitation of the patient with cardiovascular injury. A support system can improve a patient's ability to respond to disease, but a negative home environment can deter the patient's rehabilitation. Early assessment of the family situation and involvement of the family in the patient's care provides for optimal rehabilitation.

PATIENT INTERVIEW

After the medical chart review, the patient interview is the first step in the physical therapist's initial evaluation. The purpose of the interview is to gather important information about the patient's present complaint, history of medical problems and symptoms, the patient's report of risk factors, the patient's understanding and adjustment to the chief problem, psychological status, the patient's perception of the condition, goals for rehabilitation (both occupation and leisure), prior level of activity, and family situation (support system).

An important component of the interview is the ability to establish effective communication and rapport with the patient. Simple, open-ended questions using language easily understood by the patient and family should elicit the answers the therapist seeks. For example, the physical therapist might ask, "What did your discomfort feel like and where was it located when you were admitted to the hospital?" Listening is essential for learning about the patient's understanding of the problem as well as his adjustment to the problem.

DESCRIPTION OF SYMPTOMS

The patient's description of his symptoms provides the therapist with terminology to use with the patient for optimal understanding in the future (eg, chest tightness, burning, indigestion). Using questions to elicit a full description of the symptom will assist the therapist in establishing a baseline of information on the type and severity of the symptom. This is valuable in assessing future symptoms the patient may perceive. Sample descriptors and questions for assessing symptoms are listed below.

Location: Where did the symptom originate? Did it radiate?

Quality: How did it feel? Was it "like" something else?

Quantity: How intense was it?

Chronology: When did it start? How long did it last?

Setting: What were you doing when it started?

Aggravating or alleviating factors: Did any-

thing make the symptoms worse? Better?

Associated symptoms: After the original symptom, did any other symptoms appear? (Proceed through descriptors again.)

Questions regarding the patient's history of cardiac symptoms, including factors that aggravated or alleviated the symptoms, provide information on the suddenness of the problem and the amount of denial the patient may have experienced prior to the incident. A person who had numerous symptoms before hospitalization will more likely accept the problem, compared with the person who, without warning, experienced a sudden acute event.

RISK FACTOR PROFILE

Often a thorough risk factor review is not present in the medical chart review. During the interview the therapist can review the patient's risk factors (see Table 29-2) and gain significant information about the patient's social and family profile. This interview will help identify individual problem areas that can be focused on in the educational program.

PATIENT'S UNDERSTANDING OF THE DISEASE

A basic level of understanding of coronary disease and its manifestations by the patient is imperative for the patient's rehabilitation. The patient may have misguided or biased beliefs about the disease and his prognosis based on previous experiences with friends or family. An assessment of the patient's understanding provides a baseline for beginning an educational program for both the patient and the family.

The patient's level of knowledge will also affect his motivation to modify his life-style as needed to prevent further cardiovascular problems. For example, a patient may believe that smoking was not what caused his cardiac event because his parents smoked and they lived until they were 90 years old. This patient would not be motivated to stop or decrease smoking if his level of understanding is not improved before hospital discharge.

PSYCHOLOGICAL STATUS

Denial and depression are two of the most common psychological reactions associated with a major health problem such as heart disease. The physical therapist and the nurse are the two health care professionals who have the most contact with the patient during hospitalization. Thus, they are usually the ones who have a keen awareness and understanding of the patient's psychological adjustment. An early assessment of the patient's psychological status will allow early intervention by the appropriate team member, for early resolution and optimal rehabilitation.

REHABILITATION AND LEISURE GOALS

Assessment of the patient's prior level of activity, including leisure and occupational activities, allows the therapist to develop realistic and practical goals. Early discussion of goals often removes misguided fears of how patients with cardiac conditions are able to perform. When the patient's goals are not considered by the physical therapist, the patient is less likely to comply with his overall rehabilitation program.

FAMILY SITUATION

A supportive environment is optimal for total rehabilitation, but often family stress is present in the patient's risk factor profile. Frequently financial obligations are involved in the family stress. Assessment of the family situation provides the therapist with an awareness of possible factors that may limit the patient's rehabilitation. If this information is not already available from a medical chart review, it may be obtained from the patient or from family members who are present during the patient interview. Another source for this information is the nurse on duty, who is often aware of the family interrelationships. Consultation with other health team members may be an impor-

tant component of the rehabilitation of the patient with family problems.

PHYSICAL EXAMINATION

The physical examination is the second step in the initial evaluation of the patient. The physical examination requires the physical therapist to use skills in inspection, palpation, percussion, and auscultation where appropriate.

Inspection includes visual examination of all parts of the body, including musculoskeletal integrity, skin color, respiration, jugular venous integrity, and facial expression. Musculoskeletal abnormalities should be documented because they may affect the treatment program. Skin color shows oxygenation of the tissues, and particular attention should be focused on the distal extremities. Skin color reflects either cardiac output, vascular supply, or oxygen-carrying capacity of the blood. Respirations per minute can be assessed as abnormal if they are less than 12 per minute or greater than 15 per minute. Rapid respirations indicate physiological or emotional distress. Facial expressions, including a look of serious concern, pain, and widened eyes often project an appearance of distress.

CHEST WALL EXAMINATION

Palpation is performed to evaluate chest wall discomfort and circulatory status of the patient. Palpation is performed on all areas of the upper chest including anterior, posterior, and lateral regions of the thorax. Often, patients may develop musculoskeletal pains from bed rest or after a cardiac event; such pains can be isolated from true cardiac pains by palpation. Pulses in the extremities are also important to palpate during the initial evaluation because of the diffuseness of coronary artery disease. Patients with diabetes and peripheral vascular disease often have diminished pulses in the feet and legs.

Palpation of the heart, including point of maximal impulse and heart sounds, is usually performed by the more advanced clinician or the cardiologist and is not within the scope of this chapter.

Percussion is performed on patients to determine the amount of air or solid material in the underlying lung. This procedure is reserved for patients with congestive heart failure and for those cardiac patients with any underlying pulmonary problem.

Auscultation, which is the technique of listening, is performed in a quiet setting, using a stethoscope to provide information about the heart and lungs. The therapist should be able to differentiate between normal and abnormal heart and lung sounds. Normal heart sounds are audible with the ear to the chest wall or with a stethoscope, and they sound like "lub-dub." The first heart sound (S1) is associated with the closure of the mitral and tricuspid valves, whereas the second heart sound (S2) is associated with the closure of the aortic and pulmonic valves.

Abnormal heart sounds include murmurs, S3, and S4 heart sounds and rubs. Murmurs are classically described as a "swishing" sound heard most often between S1 and S2, although murmurs have been occasionally detected following S2. Murmurs often indicate heart valve dysfunction. The third heart sound (S3), if present, is audible immediately following the second heart sound. S3 indicates decompensated heart functioning or heart failure if heard in an older person or someone with heart disease. S3 is also called a ventricular gallop. S3 is considered a physiologically normal sound if heard in healthy children, young adults, or in the athlete. The fourth heart sound (S4) is heard immediately preceding the first heart sound and is associated with increased resistance to ventricular filling. S4, also known as an atrial gallop, is frequently heard in persons with hypertensive heart disease, coronary artery disease, and myocardiopathy. (Refer to Hearst (1978) for further information on heart sounds.)

Abnormal lung sounds include crackles, wheezes, rubs, and bronchovesicular and bronchial breath sounds.

During the cardiac evaluation, the therapist is performing auscultation for sounds of heart failure. Auscultation of heart and lung sounds is a clinical skill that can be learned with frequent practice.

SELF-CARE EVALUATION

Following the chest wall examination, the therapist is ready to perform an initial evaluation of the patient's responses to exercise. The self-care evaluation is an assessment of responses to the following situations: at rest (supine), sitting, standing, activities of daily living (dressing, hair combing, teeth cleaning), ambulation, and Valsalva's maneuver.

This initial assessment is made as early as three days after the myocardial infarction. If the patient has not had a myocardial infarction, the assessment may be made when the patient is considered stable. During the above activities the patient's heart rhythm and heart rate are monitored by the physical therapist, who watches the telemetry. Blood pressure and cardiac symptoms are also monitored during all the activities. Heart and lung sounds are evaluated before and after each activity. These responses are recorded and then interpreted both for the therapist's use and for the patient's chart (Fig. 29-1).

The self-care evaluation is terminated anytime during assessment of the activities if abnormal responses are identified that would make continuing the evaluation inappropriate or unsafe. Upon conclusion of the self-care evaluation, an individualized program of monitored ambulation is initiated if the responses were assessed as safe or appropriate. Studies have shown that the heart rate, blood pressure, and ECG responses with ambulation during the self-care evaluation strongly correlate with the responses that occur with the patient's monitored ambulation program (Butler, 1983).

MONITORED ACTIVITY AND AMBULATION

Following the self-care evaluation, the therapist develops a program for the patient's rehabilitation that includes both exercise and edu-

Name _____ John Doe _____

Hospital number _____

Risk factors: High BP _____ Family History _____X_____ Overweight _____

Smoking _____X_____ Diabetes _____ Age _____45_____

Lack of exercise _____ Stress _____X_____

Diet (elevated serum cholesterol) _____X_____

	Comments	HR	BP	Arrhythmias
Rest (supine)		100	110/70	None
Sitting		108	108/70	None
Standing		110	100/68	Rare PVC
ADL activity		120	100/60	2 PVCs
Ambulation		126	90/60	8 PVCs
Valsalva		Held		
After activity		108	108/70	None

ECG recordings _____

Interpretation

  Patient demonstrated sinus tachycardia throughout rest and all activities. Patient demonstrated orthostatic hypotension to sitting and standing, but demonstrated an abnormal blood pressure response to ambulation (hypotension). Patient also demonstrated increased frequency in arrhythmias with activity. Activity is being held on this patient because of abnormal responses (arrhythmias, blood pressure) to activity.

Therapist _____ Date _____

Figure 29-1. Self-care evaluation.

cation. Day-to-day evaluations of the patient's responses to activities are made by the physical therapist to revise the exercise program for each patient. Daily assessment of the heart rate response, symptoms, heart and lung sounds, blood pressure response, and ECG monitoring are important evaluations used to guide the patient's daily activity.

  The normal heart rate response is a gradual increase in heart rate with increased activity or work load. A linear relation exists between heart rate response and work load and oxygen consumption. Patients taking cardiac medications, particularly beta blocking agents, will demonstrate a blunted heart rate response. In addition, maximal heart rate declines with age, which can be predicted from the simple equa-

tion used to determine maximal heart rate: 220 minus age.

  Symptoms to be observed during the monitored ambulation include any chest, cervical, or jaw discomfort that develops during exertion, shortness of breath, leg fatigue or discomfort, or dizziness. Symptoms are evaluated in relation to the other responses to activity.

  The physical therapist should be able to detect any differences in heart and lung sounds if auscultation of the heart and lung sounds is performed before and after activity. Although the therapist is not expected to be able to interpret all heart sounds, he should be able to hear gross abnormalities, such as murmurs and loud S3 gallops, and should be able to detect noticeable changes with activity.

Blood pressure measurement should be performed at rest, during the activity, and after the activity. The resting blood pressure should be measured in the position the patient will be performing the activity. For example, if the patient will be walking, a resting standing blood pressure should be obtained. If the patient will be bicycling, a resting sitting blood pressure should be obtained. Optimally, the activity blood pressure should be obtained while the patient is exercising. If the patient stops exercising, the blood pressure should be obtained within 10 seconds of stopping the activity, because the blood pressure can drop in 10 seconds. With patients who are ambulating, blood pressures can be taken while they mark time in place to get an accurate activity level reading.

Single-lead ECG monitoring is performed to obtain information about the patient's heart rhythm with activity and after activity. The patient's pulse may be palpated to identify any irregularities in rhythm. However, definition of the irregularities and their clinical significance cannot be made by palpation alone. Increased frequency or severity of ventricular arrhythmias requires immediate medical attention because these patients may be at risk for cardiac arrest or an ischemic episode.

SPECIFIC TESTS

BLOOD PRESSURE MEASUREMENT

Arterial blood pressure is an overall reflection of the function of the heart as a pump. The arterial blood pressure is defined as the systolic pressure (pressure exerted against the arteries during the ejection cycle) and diastolic pressure (pressure exerted against the arteries dur-

ing rest). Factors affecting the blood pressure include the cardiac output, peripheral resistance, distensibility of the arteries, volume of blood in the system, viscosity of the blood, and neural input.

Normal blood pressure in the aorta and arteries is defined as less than 140 mm Hg systolic and less than 90 mm Hg diastolic (Table 29-6). Blood pressure can be measured directly using a catheter inserted into the brachial artery or indirectly using a sphygmomanometer.

Blood pressures are usually taken on the upper arm with the distal margin of the cuff approximately 3 cm above the antecubital fossa. Palpation is performed to locate the brachial artery pulse. This is the location for auscultation (or palpation) of the blood pressure. Following inflation of the cuff, auscultation of the first audible sound designates the systolic pressure, whereas the diastolic pressure is the value when the sounds become muffled.

Blood pressure may differ between like extremities, with change of body position, or with activity. Changes between like extremities may reflect uneven peripheral resistance, either vasomotor tone or occlusion. Changes with body position may reflect vasomotor tone, venous return, and the effects of gravity. Measurement of blood pressure with activities reflects the functioning of the heart as a pump with the activities. Therefore, it is imperative that the physical therapist knows normal blood pressure responses to exertion and can identify abnormal responses.

Problems exist in accurate measurement of blood pressure with activity because of the rapid drop in pressure that occurs when a patient stops performing the activity (change occurs within 10 to 15 seconds). The technique of measurement of blood pressure during an

Table 29-6. Definition of Resting Blood Pressure

	NORMAL	BORDERLINE	HYPERTENSIVE
Systolic (mm Hg)	<140	140–150	>150
Diastolic (mm Hg)	<90	90–100	>100

(American Heart Association Guidelines)

activity or immediately following an activity requires practice to assure accuracy.

Normal Responses

The normal systolic response to increasing levels of exertion is to increase, whereas the normal diastolic response is a maximal change of 10 mm Hg increase or decrease from resting value (Fig. 29-2). Adult females generally demonstrate a slower rate of rise in the systolic blood pressure as compared with adult males.

However, systolic blood pressure rises in response to increased work load on the body as a result of an increase in cardiac output to meet the demands of the activity. Peripheral resistance to blood flow is reduced during exercise as a result of the hypothalamus detecting the increased temperature in the body occurring from exercise. The thermal effector response to internal heat is vasodilation. The diastolic pressure changes very little because of the peripheral vasodilatation that occurs with exercise. Younger persons and trained athletes may demonstrate a progressive decrease in the dia-

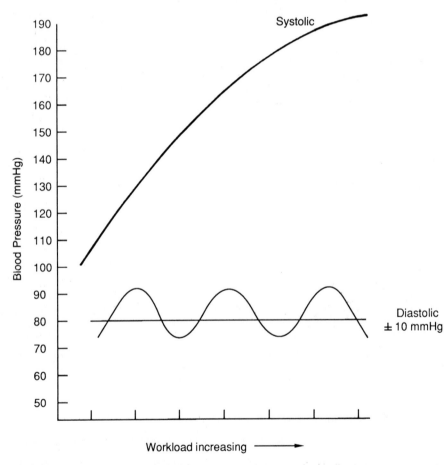

Figure 29-2. The systolic blood pressure gradually rises with a gradual increase in work load. The diastolic blood pressure should change very little with an increase in work load (+/− 10 mm Hg).

stolic pressure with exercise as a result of increased peripheral vasodilatation. This fall in diastolic pressure is considered a normal response in the young and the athlete, but not in older persons.

Additionally, the normal systolic and diastolic blood pressure response to endurance activity (maintenance of the same or similar work load) is to remain constant or decrease slightly. This indicates the body has achieved a steady-state condition and the circulation has accommodated to the work load.

Abnormal Responses

If the therapist knows and understands the normal blood pressure responses to exertion, identifying the abnormal responses will be easy. Abnormalities can exist with both the systolic and diastolic responses to exertion. The abnormal responses are first defined, and then the mechanism of action and clinical implications are described.

Systolic Responses

Hypotensive systolic blood pressure and blunted blood pressure are the two abnormal responses to increased activity. Hypotensive systolic blood pressure response can be described as a rise in blood pressure at submaximal levels, followed by a sudden progressive decrease in systolic blood pressure despite increasing levels of work (Fig. 29-3). Exertional systolic hypotension has been correlated

highly with cardiac pathology. Related pathology includes perfusion defects on exercise thallium tests and severe coronary disease or poor ventricular function, or both, as documented by coronary angiography (Hakki and colleagues, 1986).

A blunted blood pressure response can be described as a slight increase in systolic blood pressure at low levels of exertion followed by a failure to rise with increasing levels of work. This definition does not apply to persons who are undergoing any medication therapy (Fig. 29-4). Bruce and co-workers (1977) have reported that a failure to reach a systolic blood pressure of 130 mm Hg at peak effort when no medications are in use indicates high risk of future sudden death.

Patients must be identified who regularly take cardiac medications, especially beta blocking agents. These patients will demonstrate what appears to be abnormal responses (particularly blunted responses) when it is the medication that is affecting the blood pressure response.

Another abnormal response cited in the literature is found in subjects with normal resting blood pressures who develop abnormally high systolic pressure with exercise. These persons have an increased risk of developing clinically significant hypertension (Dlin and co-workers, 1983).

Abnormal responses to endurance activity involve either a continous rise or continous fall

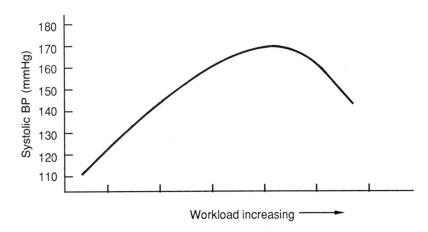

Figure 29-3. An abnormal blood pressure response to an increase in work load. Greater than 2.5 mph work load caused the systolic blood pressure to decrease continually, demonstrating a failure of the heart muscle to meet the demands.

Workload increasing ⟶

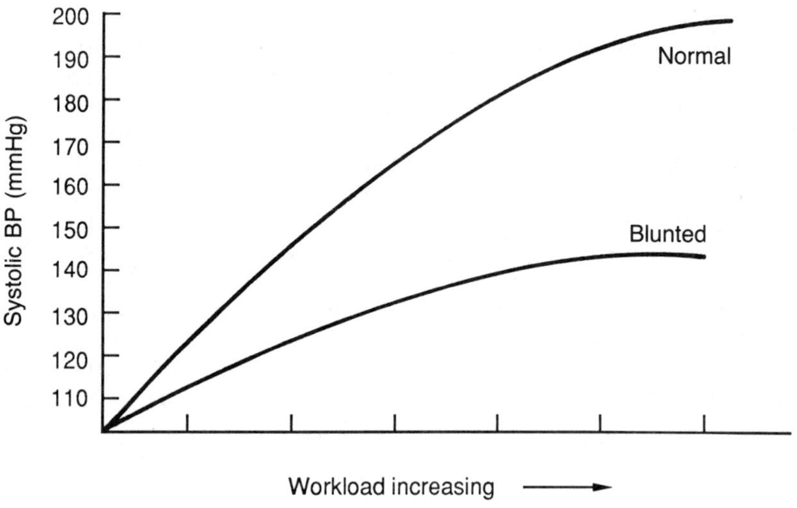

Figure 29-4. The blunted blood pressure response, or very gradual rate of rise in systolic blood pressure, is seen typically when patients are taking beta blocker medications. If the patient is not taking these medications, and the blood pressure response is blunted, this demonstrates an abnormal blood pressure response.

in systolic blood pressure. Persons with abnormal responses to endurance activity have a higher incidence of dysfunction of the ventricular wall or a problem with the tissues' ability to extract oxygen from the circulation.

Mechanism
When the blood pressure suddenly starts to decrease with increasing levels of exertion or resists rising, the underlying cause can be understood by reviewing normal cardiac physiology. Blood pressure is indicative of cardiac output and peripheral resistance. Therefore, a drop or flat systolic response indicates either the cardiac output is failing to meet the demands of the system or the peripheral resistance is decreasing rapidly. According to the literature, hypotensive or flat systolic blood pressure responses are caused by a failing cardiac output. Because cardiac output depends upon heart rate and stroke volume, if the stroke volume becomes unable to increase beyond a certain level of work, then the demand to maintain or increase the cardiac output is placed on the heart rate. Unfortunately, the heart rate is unable to maintain an increased cardiac output, and the blood pressure drops as a result.

Clinical Implications
Identification of abnormal systolic responses to activity (increasing work load or endurance) is

essential information for the physical therapist to know about the patient. Although restriction of activity might not be necessary, patients with abnormal systolic blood pressure responses will need to be monitored closely during actvity. The treatment plan may need alterations in the duration and intensity of work to be performed. Decisions regarding the amount of supervision the patient needs when performing activity can be made safely following interpretation of blood pressure responses. Finally, the patient may need to be educated about symptoms and limitations to be aware of while performing the exercise program.

Diastolic Responses
A progressive rise in diastolic blood pressure beyond 15 mm Hg is an abnormal response to increased work load (Fig. 29-5). Although not documented in the literature, this finding is based on clinical experience. In addition, a sustained elevation of the diastolic blood pressure during the recovery phase of activity is an abnormal response.

One theory regarding the mechanism of a progressive rise in diastolic blood pressure is that there is a need for increased driving pressure into the coronary arteries, which creates a demand for increased diastolic blood pressure. The need for an increased driving pressure exists when blood flow through the coronary

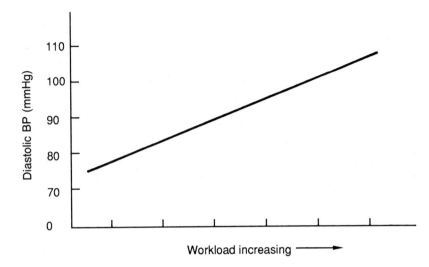

Figure 29-5. The normal diastolic blood pressure response to an increased work load is a change of +/− 10 mm Hg. A progressive rise in the diastolic pressure with an increase in work load is an abnormal response.

arteries is below the level needed to meet the demands of the myocardium (usually because of blockages in the arteries). Despite the lack of documentation of this abnormality, the physical therapist should be aware of the normal response and be sensitive to a progressive rise in diastolic pressure as an abnormal response.

ELECTROCARDIOGRAM

Basic electrocardiography is a subject that requires in-depth study beyond the scope of this chapter. In this chapter I will explain the electrocardiogram, including its limitations and indications for use, and provide some basic principles. Other sources recommended for detailed discussion of dysrhythmias and conduction defects are Mariott (1972) and Schamroth (1982).

The electrocardiogram is a graphic tracing of the electrical forces produced by the heart (Fig. 29-6). The electrical activity of the heart is recorded from the skin by sensitive monitoring equipment. Normal electrical activity causes depolarization of specialized muscle cells, which in turn causes progressive contraction of the myocardial cells (because of rapid migration of sodium ions into the cell, and migration of potassium out). Following complete depolarization, the myocardial cells repolarize (re-

covery phase, where the movement of potassium ions is into the myocardial cells). It is the depolarization and repolarization of the myocardial cells that are recorded on the electrocardiogram.

The sinoatrial (SA) node is located in the posterior wall of the right atrium and initiates

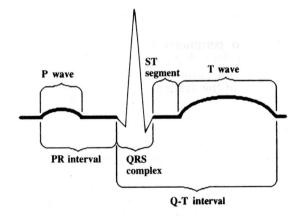

Figure 29-6. The P wave represents atrial depolarization and contraction. The QRS wave represents ventricular depolarization and contraction. The T wave represents ventricular repolarization. The PR interval starts at the beginning of the P wave and ends at the beginning of the QRS wave. The ST segment begins at the end of the S wave and goes to the beginning of the T wave.

the electrical impulse for cardiac stimulation. Once initiated, the wave of depolarization proceeds through both atria and is represented on the electrocardiogram as the P wave. Depolarization continues to the atrioventricular (AV) node, where a one-tenth second pause occurs before the AV node is stimulated. This one-tenth second pause is for the blood to pass from the atria into the ventricles. The pause in conduction time is represented as the PR interval on the electrocardiogram.

The depolarization continues from the AV node down the AV bundle of His to the bundle branches, which consist of a left bundle (with an anterior and posterior division) and a right bundle. The electrical impulse terminates in the Purkinje fibers. Depolarization of the AV bundle, bundle branches, and Purkinje fibers is represented on the electrocardiogram as the QRS complex. The QRS complex thus represents the stimulation of the ventricles.

Following the QRS complex is a pause, which is represented on the electrocardiogram as the ST segment. This normally appears as the flat piece of baseline between the depolarization of the ventricle (QRS complex) and the repolarization of the ventricles (T wave). Repolarization provides for the regaining of the negative charge within the cell (movement of potassium ions out of the myocardial cells to allow for another wave of depolarization.

Understanding deflections of the QRS complex is important for identifying abnormalities in the tracings. Positive deflections are recorded above the baseline, and negative deflections are recorded below the baseline (Fig. 29-7).

The electrocardiogram is recorded on graph paper with the smallest divisions (or squares) 1 mm long and 1mm high. Time is represented on the graph paper by 0.04 seconds between each small square and 0.2 seconds between the large squares (Fig. 29-8). It is important to know the amount of time on the electrocardiogram to determine the duration of the waves or the intervals (eg, the PR interval) as well as to identify a six-second strip of paper for defining heart rates and arrhythmia detection.

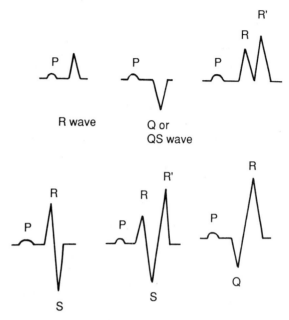

Figure 29-7. Possible QRS complexes. Each ECG tracing is different; for example, a QRS tracing may not have any downward deflection. Therefore, one would call the wave an R wave only. The first downward deflection of the QRS is always called a Q wave. The first upward deflection is always called an R wave, and the first downward deflection after the R wave is an S wave.

The standard electrocardiogram consists of tracings from six limb leads and six chest leads. The six limb leads are I, II, III, aV_R, aV_L, and aV_F. They are connected to six different electrodes on the body. The six chest leads of the electrocardiogram are monitored simultaneously from six different positions on the chest, and are numbered from V_1 to V_6 from the patient's right chest wall to the left side. The waves on the tracings look different in the various leads because the electrical activity is monitored from different positions. Monitoring activity from different angles gives a much better perspective of the electrical activity of all views of the heart.

Electrocardiograms are reviewed for the following general reasons: (1) heart rate, (2) rhythm, (3) hypertrophy (atrial or ventricular), and (4) ischemia, injury, or infarction.

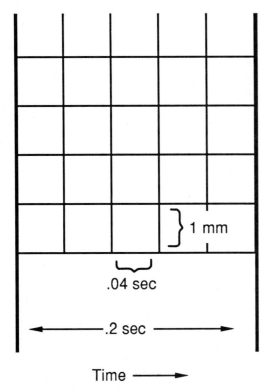

{ 1 mm

.04 sec

.2 sec

Time ⟶

Figure 29-8. Each small square on the ECG paper represents 0.04 seconds horizontally or 1 mm vertically. Each large square (five small squares) represents 0.2 seconds horizontally.

The heart rate can be determined rapidly by one of two methods. A six-second portion of an electrocardiograph recording provides a method of counting the number of QRS complexes present in six seconds. The number of QRS complexes in six seconds is then multiplied by 10 to determine heart beats per minute. The alternative method is to find a specific R wave that falls on a heavy black line. Count off "300, 150, 100, 75, 60, 50" for each heavy black line that follows. Where the next R wave falls in this counting method gives the actual heart rate. For example, if the next R wave is found on the third black line that follows, the therapist would count 300, 150, 100 and find the heart rate to be 100 beats/minute. These specific numbers must be memorized to

determine rapid heart rates from graph paper.

Rhythm is determined by examining the electrocardiogram for abnormalities in any of the waves. Dysrhythmias are then identified by any aberrance from normal. Examination of the electrocardiogram should include the following: evaluation of the P wave, PR interval, QRS complex, R to R wave interval, ST segment, and T waves. More detailed descriptions of examining the electrocardiogram can be found in Mariott's text (1972).

Hypertrophy refers to an increase in thickness of the cardiac muscle. Signs of atrial hypertrophy can be noted by examing the P wave on the electrocardiogram (diphasic P wave found on the tracing from electrocardiogram chest lead V_1). Signs of right ventricular hypertrophy are noted by changes found on lead V_1 (large R wave, S wave smaller than R wave, and R wave tracing found on lead V_1 gets progressively smaller in the tracings from leads V_2, V_3, and so on). Signs of left ventricular hypertrophy are shown in the tracing from lead V_1 (deep S wave) and in the tracing from lead V_5 (tall R wave). If the sum of the depth of the S wave in lead V_1 plus the height of the R wave in lead V_5 is greater than 35 mm, left ventricular hypertrophy is present.

An acute myocardial infarction is usually preceded by ischemia and injury to the myocardium, and can be determined through examination of ECG wave forms. However, ischemia, injury, and infarction may occur independent of each other. Ischemia (decreased blood supply) is represented on the electrocardiogram as inverted T waves in the absence of other abnormalities. Injury to the myocardium indicates the acute event of infarction and is represented by an elevated ST segment (located above the baseline). Following the acute event, the ST segment will return to the level of the baseline, and if the injured myocardium has not received blood supply, infarction occurs. Infarction is defined by the presence of a significant Q wave (1 mm or one third the height of the QRS complex). All leads should be checked for the presence of significant Q waves. The presence of a significant Q wave indicates that a myocardial infarction has occurred sometime in the past. Defining when the infarction occurred when a Q wave is present is beyond the capabilities of an ECG alone. Clinical follow up is necessary to determine the age of the infarct. Diagnosis of infarction is also difficult when certain conduction defects are present, such as bundle branch blocks (when conduction throughout the bundle branches, a part of the heart's conduction system, is partially obstructed).

The presence of a Q wave in certain leads indicates the area of heart muscle that was infarcted. The presence of a Q wave in V_1, V_2, and V_3 indicates an infarction in the anterior portion of the left ventricle. The presence of Q waves in leads I, aV_L, V_5, or V_6 indicates an infarction in the lateral portion of the left ventricle. An inferior infarction is represented by Q waves in leads II, III, or aV_F, or all three. A posterior infarction is suspected when a large R wave is present in V_1 or V_2 (Table 29-7).

EXERCISE TESTING

Exercise testing is a noninvasive method of measuring cardiovascular responses to increased activity. Originally, exercise testing was used to measure functional capacity, or as a means to evaluate abnormalities of coronary circulation. Currently, exercise testing is used for a variety of other patient management problems. Indications for exercise testing include the following:

- Evaluation of chest pain suggestive of coronary disease

- Determination of prognosis and severity of disease
- Evaluation of the effects of medical and surgical therapy
- Screening of latent heart disease
- Evaluation of dysrhythmias
- Motivating a patient to change life-style to reduce risk of coronary disease
- Assessment of functional capacity
- Screening to provide an exercise prescription
- Evaluation of hypertension with activity

Exercise testing involves systematically and progressively increasing the oxygen demand on the myocardium and evaluating the responses to the increased demand. The technique varies with different modes of exercise chosen and different protocols used by the examiner. Formal testing includes the following modes of exercise: walking up and down steps, exercising on a stationary bicycle, and walking on a treadmill with variable speeds and inclines. Informal testing is done to screen for exercise programs on a group basis, and includes tests such as the Cooper's 12-minute run for distance, the pulse recovery test, or the 1.5-mile run for time.

The clinical monitoring tools used during exercise testing include continuous electrocardiographic monitoring, blood pressure, heart rate (often extracted from the ECG recording), patient-reported or demonstrated symptoms, and heart and lung sounds. Multiple-lead electrocardiographic monitoring previously de-

Table 29-7. 12-Lead ECG Changes and Area of Infarction

ECG CHANGES	AREA OF INFARCTION
Q or QS in V_1–V_3	Anteroseptal
Q or QS in V_1–V_6	Anterior
Q or QS in I, aV_L, V_5, V_6	Anterolateral
Q or QS in I, aV_L	Lateral
Q or QS in II, III, aV_F	Inferior
Increased R waves in V_1, V_2	Posterior
ST segment depression, No Q waves, T wave inversion	Subendocardial

scribed in this chapter is used to depict electrical activity from different anatomical locations of the heart. Detection of both dysrhythmias and ischemia can be recorded from the ECG. Ischemia is defined as deviations from the baseline of the ST segment during exercise testing. Highly sophisticated laboratories may also directly measure oxygen uptake using computerized oxygen analyzers.

The most important safety factor in exercise testing is a knowledgeable and experienced examiner in charge of performing the test. Safety precautions include discussing and having the patient sign a consent form, knowing when to exclude a patient from performing the test, when to terminate a test, what to do in the event of an abnormal response or situation, and having available the necessary equipment and supplies to manage an emergency (eg, defibrillator, drugs, and crash cart).

Most institutions adopt a standard protocol to use to compare the response of patients to their previous tests and to the tests of other subjects. Testing procedures require a 12-lead electrocardiogram to be performed before any exercise test. The patient is then connected to the electrocardiograph for continuous monitoring during the test. Normal procedure is to monitor a minimum of six leads during the test. Pretest procedures include taking a risk factor history; assessing the patient's symptom history; and performing a resting evaluation of blood pressure, heart rate, heart and lung sounds, and ECG. The exercise is initiated and the work load is increased according to the chosen protocol. Subsequently, the patient is continuously monitored using the clinical monitoring tools listed above. Upon request by the patient or when an abnormality is identified in one or more of the parameters being measured, the test is terminated. The patient is continuously monitored in the recovery period until pretest values are achieved. A written report documenting and interpreting the results is prepared following the test.

Maximal and Submaximal Stress Testing

Protocols used are either described as maximal or submaximal. The difference between the type of protocol exists in the termination point of the test. Submaximal tests are terminated upon achievement of a predefined end point (unless symptoms otherwise limit completion of the test). The predefined end point may be either a certain percentage of patient's predicted maximal heart rate, or when a certain work load is achieved (eg, 2.5 mph and a 12% grade). A special subset of submaximal testing is low-level testing, performed on patients during the recuperative phase after myocardial injury or coronary bypass surgery.

Symptom-limited maximal stress testing is most often used to measure functional capacity as well as to diagnose coronary disease. The protocol for testing involves a progressive work load until the patient perceives an inability to continue because of some limiting symptom such as shortness of breath, chest pain, or leg fatigue.

Protocols are also described as continuous versus intermittent. Intermittent testing provides progressive work loads with short rest periods interspersed to give the subject time to recover and decrease the amount of peripheral fatigue. Continuous tests provide progressive work loads until the test is terminated.

Contraindications to Testing

Although a knowledgeable examiner in charge of the test is essential, knowing who should *not* be tested is essential for safe testing. Thoroughly evaluating the patient before testing will screen for any contraindications to testing. Absolute contraindications to maximal stress testing include the following:

- Recent myocardial infarction
- Acute pericarditis or myocarditis
- Resting or unstable angina
- Serious ventricular or rapid atrial arrhythmias (ventricular tachycardia, couplets, atrial fibrillation, atrial flutter)
- Second or third degree heart block
- Overt congestive heart failure (pulmonary rales, third heart sound)
- Any acute illness

In addition to the absolute contraindications, the general clinical status of the patient must be considered before determining whether or not the stress test is contraindicated. The following relative contraindications should be considered on an individual basis:

- Aortic stenosis
- Patients with known left main coronary artery disease (or left main equivalent coronary disease)
- Severe hypertension (defined as greater than 220 mm Hg systolic at rest or greater than 150 mm Hg diastolic at rest or both)
- Idiopathic hypertrophic subaortic stenosis (IHSS)
- Severe depression of the ST segment on the resting ECG
- Compensated heart failure

Testing Protocols

The most commonly used protocols in maximal stress testing involve the stationary bicycle or treadmill. Blood pressures are easier to auscultate on the stationary bicycle than the treadmill. The bicycle also takes up less room, and requires very little patient coordination to operate. The greatest disadvantage of the stationary bicycle, however, is that bicycling is not a daily functional activity for most persons. Therefore, patients will develop muscular fatigue faster because they are using different muscle groups that are not as "trained" as the muscles used for walking. These persons will therefore not achieve the best results, because the maximal heart rate may be well below what is considered diagnostic (85% of predicted maximal heart rate).

The treadmill is large, requires a patient to have balance and coordination, and is very noisy, making blood pressures difficult to auscultate. However, because walking is a functional activity, the muscles will not fatigue as fast as with biking, and therefore the treadmill is considered to have greater diagnostic capabilities.

The two most common treadmill protocols are the Bruce protocol and the Balke protocol. The Bruce protocol (Table 29-8) is probably the most widely used and provides normative data in the form of a nomogram to calculate functional aerobic impairment. Because of the rapid increases in speed and grade, and the fact the subject starts on a 10% grade, the average time a subject actually exercises during the test is between 6 and 10 minutes. The Balke protocol requires a longer time to perform and is used more widely with athletes, especially runners. The advantage to using the Balke protocol is the very gradual addition of an incline (no incline is present when the test is started), which is more representative of normal running. The test starts at 3.3 mph on level surface, and a 2% incline is added every two minutes.

The most widely used bicycle testing protocol is displayed in Figure 29-9. This protocol may be used intermittently rather than continuously because of the peripheral fatigue that develops.

Table 29-8. Bruce Treadmill Protocol

STAGE	TIME (MIN)	SPEED (MPH)	GRADE	MET*
I	3	1.7	10%	4–5
II	3	2.5	12%	6–7
III	3	3.4	14%	8–10
IV	3	4.2	16%	11–13
V	3	5.0	18%	14–16
VI	3	6.0	20%	17–19

*1 MET = resting metabolic rate = 3.5 ml of oxygen per kilogram of body weight per minute.

(Ellestad MH, Myrvin H: Stress Testing Principles and Practice. Philadelphia, FA Davis, 1986)

Bicycle Testing Protocol

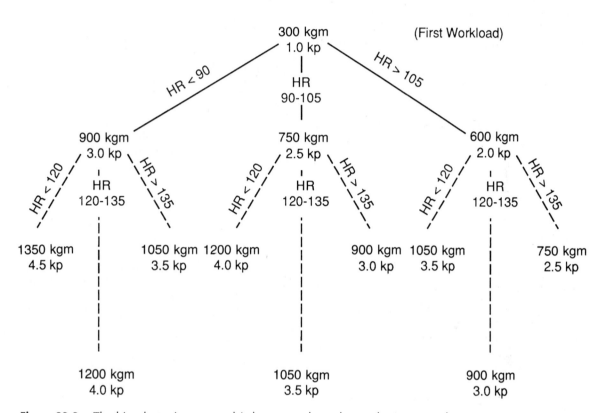

Figure 29-9. The bicycle testing protocol is heart rate dependent; subsequent work loads are adjusted depending upon the heart rate at the previous work load (HR, heart rate). (Golding LA, Myers CR, Slinning WE (eds): The Y's Way to Physical Fitness, rev ed. Chicago, The YMCA of the USA, 1982)

Safety

Stress testing should be done in a setting where emergencies can be expertly treated and managed efficiently. Continuous monitoring of ECG, blood pressure, and symptoms should be performed. An emergency medication kit along with a crash cart with appropriate equipment should be present and updated when necessary. A DC defibrillator should be present and functioning properly. Examiners performing the testing should be trained in emergency techniques and the use of the defibrillator. Written protocols should be available describing emergency procedures to be followed.

Reasons for Terminating the Testing Protocol

The examiner administering the stress test must be continually observing the patient and the monitor during the test to decide when the test should be terminated. Guidelines for termination of the test include the following:

Increasing frequency or pairing of premature ventricular contractions or development of ventricular tachycardia

Rapid atrial arrhythmias, including atrial fibrillation or atrial flutter

Development of second- or third-degree heart block

Increased angina pain (level two on a scale of one to four)

Hypotensive blood pressure response (20 mm Hg or greater decrease)

Extreme shortness of breath

Dizziness, mental confusion, or lack of coordination

Severe ST segment depression. The American College of Sports Medicine recommends termination with 2 mm or more, but some will proceed with changes of greater magnitude if the patient looks and feels good.

Observation of the patient reveals pale and clammy skin.

Extremely elevated systolic or diastolic (or both) blood pressure associated with symptoms

Upon achievement of predicted maximal pulse rate. It is usually safe to proceed with the test beyond the predicted maximal pulse if the patient is able and willing to continue, and in the absence of other indications to terminate the test.

Leg fatigue or leg cramps

Patient requests termination of test.

Interpretation

Once the test is concluded, the results are written on a worksheet (Fig. 29-10) to provide data for the interpretation. The following parameters are necessary to obtain for a thorough interpretation:

1. Time on test
2. Limiting factors (reason for termination)
3. Presence or absence of chest pain at peak exercise: usually defined as positive, negative, or atypical for angina or extreme shortness of breath
4. Maximal heart rate achieved
5. Blood pressure response
6. Arrhythmias: description of when they occurred, and what type
7. ST segment changes: usually described as

positive, negative, equivocal, or indeterminate for ischemia
- Positive: 1.0 mm or greater horizontal or downsloping ST segment depression
- Equivocal: >0.5 mm but <1.0 mm horizontal or downsloping ST segment depression
- Negative: <0.5 mm horizontal or downsloping ST segment depression
- Indeterminate: unable to measure accurately because of the presence of any of the following: bundle branch block; medication (digoxin); resulting ST changes on the ECG; or myocardial hypertrophy

8. Heart sounds: notation of pretest and posttest sounds
9. Functional aerobic impairment: can be determined from a nomogram if the Bruce treadmill protocol is used. This is used as a comparison to normal values to determine impairment in functional capacity.
10. R wave changes: amplitude changes are considered to be additional diagnostic information in interpreting exercise test results. The normal response to exercise is a decrease in R wave amplitude. If no change or an increase in R wave amplitude occurs with exercise, the patient with coronary artery disease is considered to be at an increased risk for developing a cardiac problem in the future.
11. Maximal oxygen consumption ($\dot{V}O_2$) can be calculated using formulas if not directly measured during the test.

The final assessment of the stress test should define whether the outcome of the test was normal or abnormal and provide reasons why the outcome of the test is abnormal. Although the physical therapist may not actually perform the stress test, obtaining the interpretation of the results will provide valuable data for developing an exercise prescription. The interpretation will also provide valuable information regarding safety during exercise for the patient.

Prognostic Value

Stress testing is used as a noninvasive screening device for detecting coronary disease. Its

Name _____John Doe_____ Date _____

Age __46__   Sex __M__   Height __5'10"__   Weight __190 lb.__

Diagnosis _____ Reason for test __chest pains__

Protocol __Bruce__

Time of test __8 AM__   Time last cigarette _____   Time last meal __12__

Medications __None__   Time last dose _____

Physician _____

RESULTS

12-Lead ECG interpretation __Normal__

Minutes completed __7.05__   Limiting factor(s) __Leg fatigue__

Rest HR __84__   Rest BP __140/96__   Heart sounds __Normal__

Maximum HR __170__   Maximum BP __190/102__

BP Response __Diastolic hypertension throughout__

Chest pain __None__

Summary of ST segment changes __Negative for ischemia__

Summary of arrhythmias __Rare PAC throughout__

Physical work capacity __Poor, 30% below predicted functional aerobic impairment__

Remarks/recommendations __Patient needs an exercise program to decrease blood pressure and improve functional aerobic impairment.__

Interpreted by _____ Date _____

Figure 29-10. Worksheet for results of stress test.

accuracy in diagnosing coronary disease is limited by the fact that it is a noninvasive test, and therefore only reflects metabolic and electrical changes in the heart. Therefore, studies evaluating the specificity and sensitivity of stress testing have provided valuable information describing populations where testing is most accurate in identifying disease and the severity of disease (Ellestad, 1986). Sensitivity is the measure of reliability in identifying the presence of disease. Specificity is the measure of reliability of stress testing in identifying the population without disease. In general, testing demonstrates greater sensitivity and specificity in males over age 40 years than in females. Fe-

males generally demonstrate a greater percentage of false-negative tests. It is beyond the scope of this chapter to describe the predictive values for populations. However, the reader is referred to the article by Diamond (1984) on the use of Bayes' theorem to aid clinical judgment in predicting the risk of developing coronary artery disease.

Stress testing is also limited by the variability between examiners conducting the test. Problems with testing include strict adherence to protocols and encouraging the patient to perform to maximal effort, interpretation of ST segments, and interpretation of symptoms.

Several studies have attempted to identify

single parameters and combinations of variables that could define the subset of persons with more severe disease (Ellestad, 1986). Ischemia reflected by ST segment depression early in exercise has been correlated with more severe disease than when it occurs at peak exercise. Goldschlager and co-workers (1976) demonstrated an increased incidence of subsequent myocardial infarctions when ST segment depression occurred at light work loads. Severity of coronary disease has also been correlated with length of recovery time after exercise for the ST segment to return to normal. Ellestad (1986) identified a population with more serious prognosis of disease when the magnitude of ST segment depression was considered.

A subset of persons at high risk for progression of angina, myocardial infarction, or death was identified by Ellestad. Persons with normal ST segments at peak effort, but who achieved maximal heart rates considerably below their predicted pulses (bradycardic heart rate response or chronotropic incompetence) demonstrated high risk of progression of angina, myocardial infarction, or death. The tendency was to describe the test results as normal because the patients in Ellestad's study did not demonstrate ischemic changes.

The presence of angina pain gives added significance when the patient demonstrates ST segment depression during exercise. Ellestad described a double risk of subsequent coronary events in patients with angina and ST segment depression compared to patients without angina but with ST segment depression.

The incidence of sudden death is increased in two subsets of patients: those unable to exceed a maximal systolic blood pressure of 130 mm Hg, and those with increased frequency and severity of arrhythmias during testing.

Calculating a probability score from the combination and weighting of clinical variables from the exercise test will identify the subsets of individuals at greater risk for coronary events. Many institutions are in the process of developing multiple variable analyses that will increase the predictive value of exercise testing (Weiner and co-workers, 1984).

Thallium Stress Testing

The use of radioactive nuclear dye for detection of perfusion defects has provided clinicians with an even greater body of information that can be obtained from the exercise stress test. Current practice involves injecting radioactive thallium during peak performance in a stress test. Following the injection of the nuclear dye, a minute of exercise is required for circulation of the dye. After the dye has circulated, the patient is returned to a supine position and passed under a nuclear scanner for the purpose of evaluating perfusion of the heart immediately after exercise. The subject returns three to four hours after the exercise test to again lie under a nuclear scanner to evaluate perfusion of the heart during the delayed post-exercise period of time.

Indications for uses of thallium injection with stress testing include detection of myocardial infarction and transient myocardial ischemia. Myocardial areas supplied by narrowed coronary arteries may demonstrate normal thallium uptake at rest, but when injected during exercise may show decreased concentration compared to normally perfused areas. This indicates perfusion defects that may not have been demonstrated on the electrocardiogram during the exercise test. If a region is absent of thallium uptake at rest and does not change after injection during exercise, myocardial infarction or scarring, or both, is assumed to be present in that particular region. Thallium stress testing appears to be more sensitive than exercise electrocardiography in identifying patients with coronary disease.

Low-Level Exercise Testing

Low-level exercise tests are usually performed on patients who have recently had a myocardial infarction or undergone coronary bypass surgery. The test has been performed as early as five days after myocardial infarction or surgery (Blessey, 1976), but more likely is performed prior to discharge from the hospital. Some physicians prefer to wait until anywhere from two to three weeks after the cardiac incident before administering low-level exercise testing.

Low-level exercise testing is useful in predicting the subsequent course of a myocardial infarction and bypass surgery and for identifying the high-risk patient. The high-risk patient is the patient with increased risk of morbidity or mortality as a result of myocardial ischemia or poor ventricular function. When the high-risk patient is identified, the decision on optimal medical management or surgical intervention is more clearly defined.

Exercise-induced ST depression of 0.2 mm or greater on low-level exercise tests was identifed as the single most valuable indicator of prognosis after myocardial infarction, according to the regression analysis by DeBusk. In addition, early onset of ST segment depression is related to increased incidence of coronary events. Starling and co-workers (1981) demonstrated a significantly increased risk of death after myocardial infarction when both ST depression and angina were produced during early exercise testing. Exercise-induced angina alone was associated with subsequent coronary artery bypass surgery.

Exercise-induced arrhythmias may be an indication for therapeutic management prior to hospital discharge. Sudden death was reported to be 2.5 times higher in patients who manifested ventricular arrhythmias during low-level exercise testing (Theroux and colleagues, 1979).

Other variables of minor prognostic significance after myocardial infarction include inappropriate blood pressure response, maximum heart rate, and maximum systolic blood pressure achieved.

Low-level exercise testing can also provide information useful for optimal medical management after myocardial injury or surgery including treatment for angina, arrhythmias, or hypertension, and is used in screening for cardiac rehabilitation programs (Ibsen and colleagues, 1975). Activity level can be prescribed on the basis of the results of the low-level exercise test for rehabilitation both at home and in the hospital.

Not all patients are appropriate candidates for low-level exercise testing. Safety of exercise testing early after myocardial infarction has been a topic of debate because of the traditional medical belief that a recently damaged myocardium is prone to further injury, including rupture, aneurysm, extension of infarction, and susceptibility to serious arrhythmias. However, safety of exercise testing was documented as early as 1973. Knowledge and adherence to contraindications to testing optimize the safety of this test (Table 29-9).

Institutions may vary in the choice of low-level exercise protocol. However, a progressively increasing work load from 2 MET (a multiple of the resting metabolic rate) to approximately 6 MET is used. The most common protocols are the modified Naughton and modified Bruce (Tables 29-10 to 29-12).

Safety in exercise testing patients early after a myocardial injury also requires knowledge of reasons for test termination. Institutions vary in their specific criteria for termination, but the general criteria for terminating a low-level exercise test are listed below.

- 17.5 mL O_2/kg (5 MET)
- 70% to 75% of age-predicted maximal heart rate
- Fatigue or dyspnea
- Level 1 angina (first perception)
- Maximal heart rate of 120 to 130

Table 29-9. Contraindications to Low-Level Testing

Unstable angina or angina pectoris at rest

Severe heart failure (overt left ventricular failure on exam with pulmonary rales and S3 heart sound)

Serious arrhythmias at rest

Second- or third-degree heart block

Disabling musculoskeletal abnormalities

Valvular heart disease

Blood pressure >180/105

Patient refuses to sign consent form

(Starling MR, Crawford MH et al: Predictive value of early postmyocardial infarction modified treadmill exercise testing in multivessel coronary artery disease detection. Am Heart J 102(2):169, 1981)

Table 29-10. Modified Naughton Treadmill Protocol

	TIME							
	0 min	3 min	6 min	9 min	12 min	15 min	18 min	21 min
Speed (mph)	2	2	2	2	2	3	3	3
Percent grade	3.5	7	10.5	14	17.5	12.5	15	17.5
MET	3	4	5	6	7	8	9	10

Table 29-11. Ellestad Submaximal Protocol*

STAGE	SPEED (MPH)	GRADE (%)	TIME (MIN)	MET	TOTAL TIME (MIN)	$\dot{V}O_2$ (ML/MM/KG)
1	1.5	0	3 min	2.8	3	6
2	1.5	4	3	3.2	6	9
3	1.5	8	3	3.7	9	12
4	1.7	10	3	4.0	12	15
5	2.0	12	3	5.0	15	20

*Pre-discharge low-level test after myocardial infarction.

Table 29-12. Modified Bruce Submaximal Protocol

STAGE	SPEED (MPH)	GRADE (%)	TIME (MIN)
1	1.7	0	3
2	1.7	5	3
3	1.7	10	3
4	2.5	12	3

- Frequent (nine per minute) unifocal or multifocal PVCs, paired PVCs, ventricular tachycardia
- ST segment depression of 1 to 2 mm
- Claudication
- Dizziness
- Decrease in systolic BP of 10 mm Hg below peak value
- Hypertensive BP: systolic > 200, diastolic < 110

There is a psychological benefit to both the patient and the discharging physician from a pre-discharge exercise test. Improvement in exercise performance following a myocardial infarction has been related to improvement in patient's self-confidence as a result of a successful, uneventful pre-discharge exercise test. The test can potentially differentiate between chest wall and angina pain for both the physician and patient.

In summary, low-level exercise testing soon after myocardial infarction is a safe, non-invasive method for evaluating the functional capacity for physical activity; for detecting arrhythmias, angina, and hypertensive responses; for optimal medical management; and for predicting the risk of subsequent cardiac events.

ADDITIONAL INVASIVE AND NONINVASIVE TESTS

Various other tests may be performed that can provide more definitive information on the patient's cardiac condition. Tests are ordered for the following reasons:

1. to obtain a correct diagnosis on the patient and identify complications;
2. to provide information concerning prognosis in the patient with known disease;
3. to identify subclinical disease; and

4. to provide information to assist in monitoring complicated treatment

This section will define and describe other diagnostic tests of the cardiovascular system.

Holter Monitoring

Continuous 24-hour electrocardiograph monitoring of a patient's heart rhythm is essential to the diagnosis and management of episodes of cardiac arrhythmias and corresponding symptoms. Twenty-four hour electrocardiograph documentation must be reliable to capture, recognize, and reproduce any abnormality in heart rhythm, particularly those that threaten life or cardiac hemodynamics.

A patient's rhythm can be monitored by means of a transcutaneous tape recorder applied to the patient's chest wall. The patient wears the Holter monitor for 24 hours while performing normal activities (except bathing). The patient records the activities that are performed, as well as any symptoms that may be felt during the 24 hours. Once the recorder is removed from the patient, the tape is processed by reproducing the recording on paper for visual inspection. Continuous monitoring systems must provide reproductions of cardiac rhythms with very little artifact.

Based on a review of the recording and the related symptoms or activities, the physician interprets the results of the Holter monitor. The physical therapist must review the interpretation of the results to determine if modifications are needed in the patient's activities. For example, patients with life-threatening arrhythmias recorded by the Holter monitor should be withheld from physical therapy activity until treatment for the arrhythmia is initiated or modified.

The indications for use of the Holter monitor include identifying symptoms possibly caused by arrhythmias, describing the arrhythmias (including their frequency and severity), and evaluating anti-arrhythmia therapy and pacemaker functioning. A common practice is to perform Holter monitoring routinely before discharging any patient who has had a myocardial infarction.

Echocardiogram

Echocardiography is a noninvasive procedure that uses pulses of reflected ultrasound to evaluate the functioning heart. A transducer that houses a special crystal emits high-frequency sound waves and receives echoes when placed on the chest of the patient. The returning echoes, reflected from a variety of intracardiac surfaces, are displayed on the ultrasonographic equipment. The echoes are displayed in the order in which they strike the transducer. Therefore, the echoes from a surface close to the transducer are displayed more superficially than echoes from a more distant cardiac surface.

Placement of the transducer is in the third to fifth intercostal space near the left sternal border. The technician tilts the transducer at various angles so that the echo beams can scan the segments of the left ventricle.

Two types of echocardiographic instruments are now used in cardiology: the M-mode and two-dimensional instruments. The M-mode instrument uses a transducer containing one crystal that emits a single beam of sound. Narrow images of cardiac structures are produced but no lateral view is available. The two-dimensional instrument uses a transducer with one or more crystals that are either mechanically rotated or electronically fired. Two-dimensional instruments produce a wide-angle view of several areas of the heart, allowing for easier visualizations of certain cardiac structures. Two-dimensional echocardiography has become the primary imaging instrument because of its ease of use and rapid report of results.

Important information can be obtained from the echocardiogram, including ventricular cavity size, thickness of the interventricular septum, estimation of diastolic, systolic, and stroke volumes, functioning of the valves, and motions of individual segments of the ventricular wall.

Assessment of the performance of the heart muscle itself, especially regional functioning of the left ventricle, is a valuable application of echocardiography as is evaluation of a variety of signs and symptoms. Echocardiography can quantify volumes of the left ventricle, estimate an ejection fraction, and analyze motion of the valves and heart muscle.

Diagnosis of a variety of signs and symptoms as well as ventricular function is easier as a result of echocardiography. Echocardiography can provide reliable data for the following diagnoses: (1) pericardial effusion; (2) cardiac tamponade; (3) idiopathic congestive cardiomyopathy; (4) hypertrophic cardiomyopathy; (5) mitral regurgitation; (6) mitral valve prolapse; (7) aortic regurgitation; (8) aortic stenosis or bicuspid aortic valve; (9) vegetations on valves; (10) intracardiac masses; (11) ischemic heart disease; (12) left ventricular aneurysms; (13) ventricular thrombi; (14) proximal coronary disease; and (15) congenital heart disease (valvular heart disease and great vessel abnormalities).

Vectorcardiogram

The vectorcardiogram records the electrical activity of the heart. The vectorcardiogram differs from the electrocardiogram in that the vectorcardiogram records a three-dimensional display and the electrocardiogram records on a single plane. Three planes are used in vectorcardiography: frontal, sagittal, and horizontal.

The patient is connected to eight surface electrodes, which are connected to the vectorcardiograph machine. The tracing is recorded during relaxed breathing. The electrical vector forces generated by the heart are displayed for photographic or written recording. Vectorcardiograms are then interpreted by the physician.

Vectorcardiography is not frequently used because the equipment is expensive and there is little need for the data obtained from the procedure; however, its advantages involve the need for a more definitive diagnosis or picture of the electrical activity of the heart. Indications for use of vectorcardiography include myocardial infarction, injury or ischemia, conduction defects, atrial and ventricular hypertrophy, and whenever axis deviation is described on the electrocardiogram.

Vectorcardiography is indicated in myocardial infarction or injury to determine the actual location and size of the injured or infarcted area. Occasionally, conduction defects or ventricular hypertrophy can mask the location and the size of the injury. With the loss of ventricular tissue, there is a loss in vectorial forces generated by these areas. The infarcted area is inert. The overall vectorial forces are dependent on the location and size of the infarcted area. Therefore, the sequence of the electrical activity will be altered. In the case of ischemia, the ST vectors reflect the abnormality and are directed away from the injury. A vectorcardiogram performed on a patient with anterior injury will demonstrate vectors displayed posteriorly. Vectorcardiograms are particularly useful in the patient with diffuse subendocardial injury to identify a more specific location of injury.

Vectorcardiograms are more sensitive to identifying right ventricular hypertrophy than electrocardiograms are. Right ventricular hypertrophy can be masked in the electrocardiogram, especially if any axis deviation exists. Vectorcardiograms are also beneficial in differentiating conduction defects, including bundle branch blocks and hemiblocks.

Cardiac Catheterization and Angiography

Cardiac catheterization provides extremely valuable information for the diagnosis and management of patients with cardiac disease. The general goal of cardiac catheterization is to obtain objective information that can (1) establish or confirm a diagnosis of heart disease, (2) demonstrate the severity of the disease and assess prognosis, and (3) determine guidelines for optimal management of the patient, including medical and surgical management and a program of physical exercise.

Cardiac catheterization indicates the insertion of a catheter into the cardiovascular system to measure pressures or perform angiography (anatomic evaluation). The specific procedure includes catheterizing the right and left sides of the heart, contrast angiography, and sometimes intervention with drugs or pacing.

The procedure is done in a cardiac catheterization lab or in a special room in the x-ray department. The patient undergoes cardiac catheterization while awake but under sedation. The procedure involves inserting the catheter into the brachial artery or the femoral artery, depending upon the cardiologist's expertise with an individual technique. The catheters are then passed into the great vessels and cardiac chambers under fluoroscopic control. Pressures are taken and cardiac output is measured to assess valve competency and myocardial function. Finally, radiopaque contrast medium is injected into the chambers and then into the coronary arteries (and sometimes the aorta). The passage of the contrast is followed and filmed for closer evaluation when the procedure is completed.

Upon completion of the cardiac catheterization, the cardiologist reviews the films to assess ventricular function and the severity of coronary artery stenosis. The degree of stenosis in each arterial segment is graded during the review of the film, with total occlusion being 100%. Problems with interpreting the cardiac catheterization film include the fact that angiography is only two dimensional, and the film interpretation is subjective. Therefore, error may be present in evaluation of the film. However, cardiac catheterization has greater sensitivity than other noninvasive procedures mentioned previously.

The data obtained from cardiac catheterization are listed below.

- Cardiac output
- Shunt detection
- Angiography
    Coronary angiography
    Ventriculography
- Left and right heart pressures
    Right atrial, 0 to 4 mm Hg
    Right ventricle, 30/2
    Pulmonary artery, 30/10
    Pulmonary artery wedge, 8 to 12
    Left ventricular end-diastolic, 8 to 12
- Ventricular ejection fraction (estimated)

Specific diagnoses that can be made as a result of cardiac catheterization include (1) severity of coronary artery disease (degree of stenosis); (2) left ventricular dysfunction or aneurysm or both; (3) valvular heart disease and the severity of the dysfunction, including aortic valve stenosis or regurgitation, mitral valve stenosis or regurgitation, and pulmonic valve dysfunction; (4) pericardial disease; (5) myocardial disease, including cardiomyopathy; and (6) congenital heart disease.

Controversy exists as to the indication for performing cardiac catheterization. Some critics in the medical field believe the catheterization technique is overused, and believe less invasive procedures should be used before catheterization. However, others quote the fact that coronary angiography is the only test that provides information about the actual site, extent, and severity of obstruction in coronary artery disease. Cardiac catheterization has greater predictive accuracy in assessment of coronary artery disease than exercise testing. It also may be used to confirm diagnoses from other noninvasive tests. Cardiac catheterization must be performed before any surgical intervention. Common practice demonstrates that coronary angiography and ventriculography are being performed on the majority of patients following acute myocardial infarctions to assess severity of disease and amount of ventricular dysfunction resulting from the infarction.

ERGONOVINE STIMULATION

Coronary artery spasm has been demonstrated to play a role in the manifestation of ischemic heart disease. To document coronary artery spasm, one must demonstrate significant or total narrowing of a segment in an artery that may or may not have partial arteriosclerotic narrowing. If increased narrowing of the artery occurs, and the narrowing is relieved with the administration of a vasodilator, then coronary artery spasm has been documented. Spasm is rarely documented with coronary angiography (3%). Therefore, because the angiography does not frequently induce the spasm, ergonovine stimulation has become an important diagnostic test for coronary spasm.

Ergonovine stimulation is done in the cardiac catheterization laboratory, or in the coronary care unit if previous angiography studies have demonstrated normal coronary arteries. Either intravenous injections in incremental doses of ergonovine, or a single bolus of ergometrine, is given while a patient is continuously monitored for electrocardiographic or hemodynamic changes. The patient is monitored throughout the injections until a maximal dosage is given or until the patient experiences symptoms.

When ergonovine stimulation is performed in the cardiac catheterization laboratory, repeat angiography is performed when symptoms or changes develop, and treatment with vasodilators is initiated after spasm is documented. In the coronary care unit, the patient is treated with vasodilators when the electrocardiogram changes or the patient complains of symptoms. When a positive response occurs to ergonovine stimulation, a patient will then be managed medically with medications that reduce or prevent the occurrence of spasm.

Ergonovine stimulation is used when coronary spasm is suspected, particulary in a patient with documented electrocardiographic changes during symptoms or with documented ischemic episodes and a normal coronary angiographic study. The test has a high degree of sensitivity and specificity for coronary spasm.

CONCLUSION

Effective evaluation of the patient with cardiovascular dysfunction requires thorough medical record review, patient interview, physical examination, and review of invasive and noninvasive tests. After collecting all the clinical information, the physical therapist will be able to develop a safe program to improve exercise tolerance. Thorough evaluation is essential for the initial prescription. In addition, ongoing evaluation is essential for the safety of the patient as well as the effectiveness of the therapeutic treatment.

ANNOTATED BIBLIOGRAPHY

Abouantoun S, Ahnve S: Can areas of myocardial ischemia be localized by the exercise electrocardiogram? A correlative study with thallium-201 scintigraphy. Am Heart J 108:933, 1984 (An excellent discussion of the improvement in diagnosis of myocardial ischemia with the use of thallium injection during exercise testing. Gives credibility to exercise testing as an excellent noninvasive tool for identifying those at risk of myocardial infarction.)

Bigger JT, Weld F, Rolnitzky L: Prevalence, characteristics and significance of ventricular tachycardia detected with ambulatory electrocardiographic recording of late hospital phase of acute myocardial infarction. Am J Card 48(5):815, 1981 (Discusses serious arrhythmias, including the incidence and importance of early detection. Also discusses classical signs and symptoms associated with ventricular tachycardia.)

Blessey RL: Aerobic capacity and cardiac catheterization results in 13 patients with exercise bradycardia. Abstract Med Sci Sports Exerc 8:50, 1976 (Describes an important clinical phenomenon not documented in the literature that describes a group at high risk for coronary artery disease but without blatant exercise test results for coronary disease.)

Bruce RA, DeRouen T, Peterson DR et al: Noninvasive predictors of sudden death in men with coronary heart disease. Am J Card 39:833, 1977 (An excellent discussion of signs and symptoms that demonstrate an individual's risk for sudden death.)

Butler SM: Phase one cardiac rehabilitation: The role of functional evaluation in patient progression. Master's Thesis. Atlanta, Emory University, 1983 (An excellent reference documenting the importance of monitored ambulation as a guide for progression in a phase I cardiac rehabilitation program rather than the "step formula.")

Cooper KH: A means of assessing maximal oxygen intake: Correlation between field and treadmill testing. JAMA 203:201, 1968 (A classic reference correlating results of exercise performance with exercise testing performance to identify an individual's level of fitness or aerobic impairment.)

DeBusk RF, Davidson DM, Houston DM et al: Serial ambulatory electrocardiography and treadmill exercise testing after uncomplicated myocardial infarction. Am J Card 45:547, 1980 (Documents the safety of early exercise testing after a myocardial infarction. Parameters and endpoints are outlined.)

DeBusk R, Haskell W: Symptom limited versus heart rate limited exercise testing soon after myocardial infarction. Circulation 61(4):738, 1980 (A classic reference documenting the safety of exercise testing soon after a myocardial infarction, as well as parameters to be measured during the test and endpoints to use for stopping the test.)

Diamond GA: Bayes' theorem: A practical aid to clinical judgment for diagnosis of coronary artery disease. Prac Card 10(6):47, 1984 (A classic article describing the combinations of risk factors that improve the diagnostic probability of exercise testing.)

Dlin RA, Hanne N, Silverberg DS et al: Follow-up of normotensive men with exaggerated blood pressure response to exercise. Am Heart J 106(2):316, 1983 (Describes the subtle predictors of individuals who develop long-term hypertension. A good description of normal and abnormal blood pressure responses to exercise.)

Ellestad MH: Stress Testing Principles and Practice. Philadelphia, FA Davis, 1986 (A very important and classic reference that provides information on all normal and abnormal responses to exercise, and then puts all the information into interpretation of an exercise test. Good discussion of ST segment responses, blood pressure responses, stress testing protocols, and significance of abnormal responses.)

Ericsson M, Granath A, Ohlsen P et al: Arrhythmias and symptoms during treadmill testing three weeks after myocardial infarction in 100 patients. Br Heart J 35:787, 1973 (Discusses predictors of morbidity and mortality after myocardial infarction discovered with early exercise testing after myocardial infarction. A classic reference documenting the need for early exercise testing.)

Fein S, Klein N, Frishman W: Prognostic value and safety of exercise testing soon after uncomplicated myocardial infarction. Cardiovasc Clin 13(3):279, 1983 (Classic article on the safety of early exercise testing after myocardial infarction, and the important information derived from the results that demonstrate increased risk for morbidity and mortality.)

Frishman WH: Beta-adrenoceptor antagonists: New drugs and new indications. N Engl J Med 305:500, 1981 (Excellent reference on these cardiac medications, their indications for use, side-effects, and effects on exercise responses.)

Fuller CM, Raizner AE, Verani MS et al: Early post myocardial infarction treadmill stress testing. Ann Intern Med 94:734, 1981 (Classic article about the importance of early exercise testing after myocardial infarction, including its safety and prognostic value.)

Goldschlager H, Selzer Z, Cohn K: Treadmill stress tests as indicators of presence and severity of coronary artery disease. Ann Intern Med 85:277, 1976 (Commonly used reference describing the prognostic value of stress testing to identify coronary artery disease. A good discussion of interpretation of testing.)

Hakki A, Munley BM, Hadjimiltiades J: Determinants of abnormal blood pressure response to exercise in coronary artery disease. Am J Card 57:71, 1986 (Identifies blood pressure responses to exercise, normal versus abnormal, and the prognostic value of these responses.)

Hearst J: The Heart. New York, McGraw-Hill, 1978 (A classic reference on every aspect of the cardiovascular system. Excellent sections on anatomy, physiology, cardiac diagnostic tests, and transplants.)

Holloszy JO, Oscai LB, Mole PA et al: Biochemical adaptations to endurance exercise in skeletal muscles. Adv Exp Med Biol 11:51, 1971 (Describes the peripheral effects of aerobic exercise. Discusses the mitochondria, capillaries, and metabolism.)

Ibsen H, Kjoller E, Styperck J et al: Routine exercise ECG three weeks after acute myocardial infarction. Acta Med Scand 198:463, 1975 (A classic reference on the safety of exercise testing early after a myocardial infarction.)

Irving JB, Bruce RA, DeRouen TA et al: Variations in and significance of systolic blood pressure during maximal exercise testing. Am J Card 39:841, 1977 (Discusses blood pressure response to exercise, as well as the prognostic value of blood pressure response during exercise testing.)

Irwin S, Techlin JS: Cardiopulmonary Physical Therapy. St Louis, CV Mosby, 1985 (A good reference on pathophysiology of cardiac and pulmonary disease, evaluation techniques for therapists, diagnostic results, and treatment plans for cardiac and pulmonary patients. Excellent descriptions of phase I, II, and III cardiac rehabilitation programs.)

Jelinek VM, Ziffer RW, McDonald IG et al: Early exercise testing and mobilization after myocardial infarction. Med J Aust 2:589, 1977 (Classic reference on safety and prognostic value of early exercise testing after myocardial infarction.)

Kannel WB, Castelli WP, Gordon T et al: Serum cholesterol, lipoproteins, and the risk of coronary heart disease: The Framingham study. Ann Intern Med 74:1, 1971 (A classic and important reference describing risk factors of heart disease and the role of cholesterol. Excellent reference list.)

McNeer JF, Wallace AG, Wagner GS et al: The course of acute myocardial infarction. Circulation 51:410, 1975 (A classic and important reference describing the difference between complicated and uncomplicated myocardial infarctions. A good discussion of the hospital course of myocardial infarctions.)

Mariott HJ: Practical Electrocardiography, 6th ed. Baltimore, Williams & Wilkins, 1972 (An excellent reference on arrhythmias. Good pictures of examples and their prognostic value. Also a good discussion of other abnormalities identified on 12-lead ECGs.)

Markiewicz W, Houston N, DeBusk R: Exercise testing soon after myocardial infarction. Circulation 56(1):26, 1980 (A classic reference on early exercise testing, discussing the safety of and prognostic value.)

Miller D, and Borer J: Exercise testing early after myocardial infarction: Risks and benefits. Am Med 72:427, 1982 (Discusses early post-myocardial infarction exercise testing, including risks and benefits; prognostic value for morbidity and mortality.)

Pitt B, Thrall, J: Thallium-201 versus Technetium-99m pyrophosphate myocardial imaging in detection and evaluation of patients with acute myocardial infarction. Am J Card 46:1215, 1980 (Discussion and description of cardiac diagnostic testing for myocardial infarction and ischemia.)

Poyatos ME, Lerman J, Estrada A et al: Predictive value of changes in R-wave amplitude after exercise in coronary heart disease. Am J Card 54(10):1212, 1984 (Demonstrates the value of other parameters that should be observed during exercise testing to increase the sensitivity of testing.)

Rerych SK, Scholz PM, Newman GE et al: Cardiac functioning at rest and during exercise in normals and patients with coronary artery disease. Ann Surg 187:449, 1978 (Discusses the physiology of the heart, as well as how a disease process will impair normal functioning.)

Robb GP, Marks HH: The value of the standard 2-step exercise test in detecting coronary disease in a follow-up study of 1000 military personnel. Research Report AMSGS-21-54, Army Medical Service Graduate School, Walter Reed Army Medical Center, 1957 (A classic reference demonstrating the value of an alternate mode of exercise testing to detect coronary disease.)

Schamroth L: An Introduction to Electrocardiography, 6th ed. Oxford, England, Blackwell Scientific Publishers, 1982 (An excellent source to learn arrhythmias, 12-lead ECGs, and abnormalities on the ECG. Very good pictures of arrhythmias and descriptions of their significance.)

Starling MR, Crawford MH, Kennedy GT et al: Predictive value of early post-myocardial infarction modified exercise testing in multivessel coronary artery disease detection. Am Heart J 102(2):169, 1981 (Documents the safety and value of early exercise testing after myocardial infarction.)

Stein RA, Walsh Frank F et al: Clinical value of early exercise testing after myocardial infarction. Arch Intern Med 140:1179, 1980 (Documents the safety and value of early exercise testing after myocardial infarction.)

Sutton DC, Davis MD: Effects of exercise on experimental cardiac infarction. Arch Intern Med 48:1118, 1931 (An excellent reference demonstrating the safety of exercise early after myocardial infarction. A good discussion of cardiac physiology and pathophysiology.)

Theroux P, Waters D, Halphen C et al: Prognostic value of exercise testing soon after myocardial infarction. N Engl J Med 301(7):341, 1979 (Another classic reference documenting the safety and prognostic value of exercise testing early after a myocardial infarction.)

Weiner DA, Ryan TJ, McCabe GH et al: Prognostic importance of a clinical profile and exercise test in medically treated patients with coronary artery disease. J Am Coll Cardiol 3(3):772 1984 (Medical management of the patient with coronary artery disease, emphasizing the signs and symptoms that indicate need for further diagnostic testing. A good discussion of the need to follow the patient closely and alter medical management immediately.)

Wessler S, Zoll PM, Schlesinger MJ: The pathogenesis of spontaneous rupture. Circulation 6:334, 1952 (An excellent discussion of cardiac anatomy and pathophysiology following a myocardial infarction.)

30 Respiratory Analysis

LINDA CRANE

The ability of physical therapists to assess or analyze movement dysfunction and physical disability resulting from disorders of the pulmonary system is *vital* for safe and effective clinical practice. The role of physical therapists in the assessment, prevention, and treatment of pulmonary dysfunction is unique because of the combination of knowledge and skills they bring to a variety of clinical settings. The blend of biological, kinesiological, pathological, psychosocial, and clinical sciences strongly enhance the unique role of physical therapists in managing patients with pulmonary dysfunction, regardless of the nature of the problem.

In this chapter, I will describe assessment and evaluation procedures physical therapists use to analyze movement dysfunction and physical disability that result from acute or chronic disorders of the respiratory system. Procedures for testing dysfunction of other body systems, such as the cardiovascular, musculoskeletal, and neuromuscular systems, will also be included, but only as they relate *specifically* to patients with pulmonary disorders. I believe it is necessary to preface this chapter, which deals exclusively with a physical therapist's assessment of patients with pulmonary dysfunction, with a brief discussion of the interrelationship of the heart and lungs.

The anatomic and physiologic relationship of the cardiovascular and respiratory systems precludes any serious attempts to discuss them as separate entities. It is helpful to think of the right and left atrioventricular halves of the heart separately, each followed by a vascular network and capillary bed. Functionally, the pulmonary vascular and systemic vascular systems lie between the right and left sides of the heart.

The intimate interrelationship and interdependency of the heart and lungs under normal conditions is carried through and intensified in conditions of increased stress (as with exercise) and pathology. Wasserman and Whipp described the interaction of physiologic mechanisms during exercise. The interlinking and interdependence of the systems necessary to deliver oxygen to the working muscles and rid the body of the waste products of metabolism is presented in Figure 30-1. A breakdown or problem anywhere in the "system" will interfere with gas delivery and removal, and ultimately affect function.

Any chronic or acute problem (with significant disruption in function) in either the cardiovascular or respiratory systems will result in pathological changes in the other system. An example would be the patient with chronic lung disease who commonly develops right-sided heart failure (cor pulmonale). Another example is the patient with an acute myocardial infarction who suddenly develops pulmonary edema.

The author wishes to thank photographer Stephen Weymouth of the Media Services Department at the University of New England for his outstanding contribution to this chaper.

548

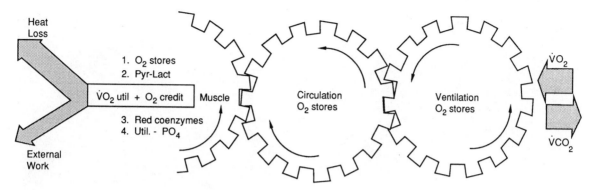

Figure 30-1. The interaction of physiologic mechanisms during exercise. The gears represent the functional interdependence of the links in the system.

Physical therapy assessment of a client with pulmonary dysfunction should routinely include some components of a cardiovascular assessment. Many clinical signs and symptoms of pathology of either system are similar and must be differentiated. A therapist analyzing movement dysfunction and physical disability of a patient with a pulmonary disorder always needs to be mindful of the interrelationship of the two systems. Appropriate and individualized clinical judgment improves with practice and experience, and emphasizes the premise that physical therapy is both a science and an art.

LABORATORY, RADIOGRAPHIC, AND SURGICAL TESTS

In this section, I will discuss tests and measures physical therapists do not commonly perform, but use as a basis for assessment and planning.

CHEST ROENTGENOGRAM

Chest x-ray films provide the clinician with a static assessment of anatomic abnormalities. Roentgenograms are used initially to screen patients for abnormalities and provide a baseline assessment for repeated exams, and to monitor progress and effects of treatment. Chest roentgenograms enhance the clinical ex-

amination by pinpointing the exact location of abnormalities such as atelectasis and infiltrates.

The ideal chest roentgenogram is a posterior-anterior (PA) chest film taken at a distance of six feet with the patient in the upright position after performing a full inspiration. The six-foot distance enhances sharpness and reduces magnification of images on the film. The full inspiration and upright position allows the diaphragm to descend to its lowest position, revealing more lung. Gravitation of fluid in the pleural space to the more dependent areas of the thorax is more readily identified in an upright than a supine film. The PA direction of x-rays from the source of the film (PA is shot posterior to anterior) results in less magnification of the heart, because the heart is located more anteriorly in the thorax. Figure 30-2 presents a normal PA chest roentgenogram.

Portable equipment is used for patients who are too sick or unstable to be transported to the x-ray department. Portable equipment allows for AP chest roentgenograms (the film is behind the patient and the x-ray source in front). The quality of a portable AP film is generally poorer because positioning and cooperation of the patient are difficult to obtain and the distance is usually shorter. The direction of the x-rays through the thorax also tends to magnify the cardiac-mediastinal shadow.

Lateral chest views are extremely impor-

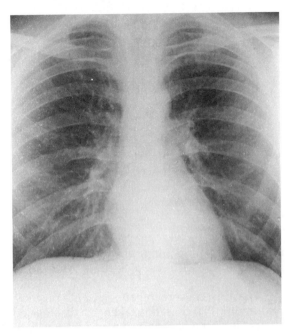

Figure 30-2. Normal posterior-anterior chest roentgenogram.

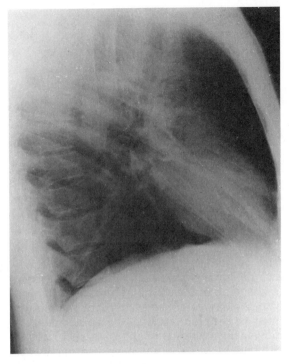

Figure 30-3. Lateral chest roentgenogram.

tant to identify disease processes behind the heart and posterior in the thorax. Anatomically the upper, middle, and lower lobes overlap each other in the frontal plane. The lateral view therefore provides a third dimension, which can assist in accurately locating a lesion. A lateral chest roentgenogram is presented in Figure 30-3.

The silhouette sign occurs when two separate structures next to each other have similar densities, obliterating the border between the two. Normally the diaphragms, heart borders, and mediastinum have densities that contrast significantly with aerated lung. Lung pathology in lobes and segments adjacent to these structures increases density, and the contrasts are lost. Those silhouette signs are extremely helpful in localizing lung pathology in patients from whom only a single AP film, taken by a portable x-ray unit, is available.

Interpretation of chest x-ray films requires a thorough knowledge of thoracic anatomy and

familiarity with normal chest films. Abnormalities on chest x-ray films associated with pulmonary dysfunction generally include changes in density, size, and configuration of the lungs, heart, and mediastinum or diaphragms. Examples of chest roentgenogram signs and their common corresponding pathologies can be seen in Table 30-1.

Chest roentgenograms can be taken from various other views than those already described. Views such as oblique (from right front to posterior left of patient or vice versa), decubitus (patient lying down and x-ray beam parallel to the floor), and lordotic (from posterior to anterior with the x-ray beam aimed at an upward angle) are used for specific purposes to assist in verification or elucidation of findings.

Chest roentgenograms are important adjuncts to the physical examination to assist physicians in diagnosis of a variety of thoracic conditions. For the physical therapist, data

Table 30-1. Chest Roentgenogram Signs and Associated Pathologies

ROENTGENOGRAM SIGNS	PATHOLOGY
Increased radiolucency Loss of vascular markings to chest wall Deviation of trachea from the midline	Pneumothorax
Density: patchy and irregular	Pneumonitis, fibrosis, or neoplasm
Density: segmental or lobar Air bronchogram Silhouette sign	Pneumonia
Shift of hilum towards side where lung appears smaller; linear densities	Atelectasis
Butterfly densities	Pulmonary edema
Straight line (air-fluid level) Blunted costophrenic angle	Pleural effusion

provided by chest roentgenograms initially assist in treatment planning by identifying specific locations of lesions, and subsequently indicate effectiveness of therapeutic interventions.

ARTERIAL BLOOD GASES

Arterial blood gas (ABG) values are invaluable to any clinician managing patients with pulmonary disease. Blood gas measurements are sensitive indicators of a patient's changing physiologic state. The two major reasons for monitoring ABGs are to determine (1) if a patient is adequately oxygenated and (2) the acid-base status of a patient (both ventilatory and metabolic).

Blood samples for ABG determination must be obtained using extremely precise and careful methods to ensure accurate and reliable results and to minimize potential problems of the invasive procedure. Specimens are usually drawn through an indwelling arterial catheter (usually in the radial artery) or by arterial puncture (usually the radial, brachial, or femoral artery). A sample of approximately 2 to 4 mL of arterial blood is drawn into a heparinized syringe. The sample is placed in ice and quickly analyzed in a calibrated blood gas analyzer.

To interpret a set of ABG values, a therapist must have normal values for comparison of the patient to the normal population. In Table 30-2, commonly accepted normal ranges of ABG values as described by Shapiro and colleagues are presented.

Evaluation of the ventilatory and metabolic acid-base status is the first step in ABG interpretation. The ABG values of pH, partial pressure of carbon dioxide ($PaCO_2$), and plasma bicarbonate (HCO_3) indicate if a patient's acid-base status is primarily ventilatory or metabolic and what level of compensation has occurred. The seven primary acid-base classifications are presented in Table 30-3. Base excess (BE) reported in milliequivalents per liter (mEq/L) is considered to be a true nonrespiratory reflection of acid-base status. The adequacy of alveolar ventilation is directly reflected by $PaCO_2$. The "cornerstone" of acid-base status is the pH value. It is this value that the body systems valiantly attempt to maintain within normal range. Physiologic mechanisms to maintain pH homeostasis are generally ventilatory or metabolic in nature. The clinical significance of acid-base regulation is that cellular metabolism functions appropriately only within a narrow range of pH.

Once blood pH is altered, the body attempts to normalize it. The lungs regulate CO_2 (acid) and the kidneys regulate HCO_3 (base). The respiratory and renal systems will attempt to *compensate* for an abnormal pH. An extremely important "rule" for this compensa-

Table 30-2. Normal Ranges of Arterial Blood Gas Values

BLOOD GAS VALUE	LABORATORY NORMAL RANGE
pH	7.35–7.45
$PaCO_2$	35–45 mmHg
HCO_3	22–28mEq/L
O_2 saturation	>90%
PaO_2	>80 mmHg*

*Adult and child; normal values for neonates and elderly persons are lower.

Table 30-3. Seven Primary Blood Gas Classifications

CLASSIFICATION	PaCO₂	pH	[HCO₃]p	BASE EXCESS
Primary Ventilatory				
1. Acute ventilatory failure	↑	↓	N	N
2. Chronic ventilatory failure	↑	N	↑	↑
3. Acute alveolar hyperventilation	↓	↑	N	N
4. Chronic alveolar hyperventilation	↓	N	↓	↓
Primary Acid-Base				
1. Uncompensated acidosis	N	↓	↓	↓
Uncompensated alkalosis	N	↑	↑	↑
2. Partly compensated acidosis	↓	↓	↓	↓
Partly compensated alkalosis	↑	↑	↑	↑
3. Compensated alkalosis or acidosis	↑ or ↓	N	↑ or ↓	↑ or ↓

°Arrows indicate depressed or elevated values; N is normal.
(Reproduced with permission from Shapiro BA, Harrison RA, Walton JR: Clinical Application of Blood Gases, 3rd ed, p. 135. Copyright © 1982 by Year Book Medical Publishers, Inc., Chicago)

tion is that *neither system will overcompensate.* For example:

> A patient with mild chronic lung disease and an acute lower respiratory infection is admitted to the hospital with a pH of 7.32, PCO₂ of 55, and HCO₃ of 24 (acute respiratory acidosis). The renal system will attempt to compensate for the respiratory acidosis by adding bicarbonate to the blood. Several hours later the ABGs might be pH of 7.35, PCO₂ of 55, and HCO₃ of 30. If you were analyzing this second set of values, and if you knew nothing about the patient, you would have to decide between chronic respiratory acidosis and compensated metabolic alkalosis. The key to correct decision making in this example is that the pH is towards the acid side of the normal range (7.35–7.45). The "rule" that body systems do not overcompensate means that the correct interpretation is *not* compensated metabolic alkalosis because the pH, in that case, would have to be *greater than* 7.40.

Fortunately, we do not interpret blood gases in isolation. The patient's medical history and clinical course provide invaluable information to assist in ABG interpretation.

Evaluation of oxygenation includes an assessment of hypoxemia (PaO₂ only) and blood oxygen transport (PaO₂, blood oxygen content, and hemoglobin-oxygen affinity). Assessment of hypoxemic state can be directly determined by the arterial oxygen tension (PaO₂). Adequacy of blood oxygen transport is much more complicated and includes assessment of the patient's clinical status as well as arterial blood gases.

Hypoxemia can accurately be assessed only when the patient is breathing room air. According to Shapiro and co-workers, relative degrees of hypoxemia in patients under 60 years of age are mild (60–80 mm Hg) and moderate (40–60 mm Hg). For every year above 60, one mm Hg should be subtracted from these values. Severe hypoxemia exists at *any* age if a PaO₂ is less than 40 mm Hg.

Assessing the adequacy of blood oxygen transport, which impacts on the oxygen state of the tissues, involves arterial oxygen tension, oxyhemoglobin affinity, and blood oxygen content. The partial pressure of oxygen in arterial blood determines the pressure gradient between the capillaries and tissues. The bond of hemoglobin and oxygen is affected by many factors including pH, body temperature, and phosphorylase enzyme systems. The stronger the affinity or bond of oxygen and hemoglobin, the less effective a pressure gradient of blood and tissue oxygen is in transferring oxygen to the tissues (see example below). Blood oxygen content, which includes both the oxygen carried by hemoglobin and oxygen dissolved in plasma, is affected by all the factors described above that affect arterial oxygen tension and oxyhemoglobin affinity. The presence of anemia would also affect blood oxygen content.

To assess blood oxygen transport, the therapist analyzes the *patient* and *all* of the ABG values with special emphasis on PaO_2 and oxygen saturation. It is important to realize that although a patient could demonstrate oxygen values that do not appear to be alarming, his clinical condition could be serious indeed! For example:

> A patient has a PaO_2 of 65 mm Hg and O_2 saturation of 89% with a $PaCO_2$ of 45 mm Hg, HCO_3 of 48 mEq/L, and *p*H of 7.6. This patient is dangerously hypoxic because a severe uncompensated metabolic alkalosis has shifted the oxyhemoglobin dissociation curve to the left, and the affinity of hemoglobin for oxygen is so strong that sufficient oxygen is not delivered to the tissues.

Clinical signs of hypoxia include increased heart rate, increased respiratory rate, cyanosis, and restlessness. Patients with significant respiratory or metabolic problems should be closely observed for these signs along with ABG determination.

Arterial blood gas values can provide a physical therapist with invaluable information for planning appropriate and safe treatments. It is important that a physical therapist is *aware* of a patient's ventilatory, acid-base, and oxygen status no matter what the goals of therapy are. Blood gas determination in the acute care setting can also be an important indicator of the effectiveness of a treatment designed to improve airway clearance and ventilation.

PULMONARY FUNCTION TESTS

Pulmonary function testing is an essential component of the clinical assessment of a patient with known or suspected respiratory disease. Tests of pulmonary function vary from simple bedside spirometry to complex plethysmography and dilution techniques in a sophisticated laboratory. Abnormal pulmonary function tests (PFTs) indicate the *effects* of pathology and are often more sensitive indicators than chest roentgenograms and physical examinations. Specific pathologic processes and etiologies cannot be determined by PFTs, only alteration in function.

The two major types of PFTs include (1) those that detect mechanical abnormalities of the lungs and chest wall, and (2) those that detect problems with gas exchange. For the purposes of this chapter, only tests related to the ventilatory function of the lungs and chest wall will be discussed in any detail.

Static properties of the lungs and chest wall, such as volumes and capacities, reflect the condition of the elastic properties of the system. The total lung capacity (TLC), which is the total volume the lungs can hold, is subdivided into capacities and volumes. A capacity is composed of more than one volume. An example would be the functional residual capacity (FRC), which is made up of the residual volume (RV, volume remaining in the lungs after a complete expiration) and expiratory reserve volume (ERV, volume that can be further expired after a normal tidal expiration). The subdivisions of lung volumes in normal adults are illustrated in Figure 30-4. Normal values of static volumes and capacities vary with age, body size, and gender. Textbooks on respiratory physiology and pulmonary function testing include tables of normal values, which are used to compare values obtained from patients.

Vital capacity (VC), which is the volume of air expired maximally after a maximal inspiration, is the most common static measure of pulmonary function. Any condition that decreases lung or chest wall compliance (distensibility) will reduce vital capacity.

1. A patient with an enlarged liver and fluid in the abdomen (ascites) will demonstrate a reduced VC because the diaphragm will be restricted and the patient will not be able to inspire to his full capacity.
2. A patient with emphysema has lost elasticity of the lung tissue, and this air is trapped

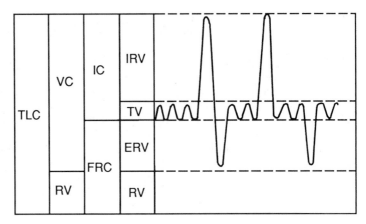

Figure 30-4. Illustration of normal lung volumes and capacities.

during expiration. This trapped air increases the residual volume, which decreases the VC.

Dynamic properties of the lungs and chest wall, or flow rates of air moving in and out of the lungs, reflect the condition of the nonelastic properties of the system. Dynamic volumes are a measurement of volume over time. The most common test of maximal expiratory flow is the forced expiratory volume in one second (FEV_1) or the volume expired in the first second of the vital capacity. The volume expired in one second is usually related to the vital capacity and expressed as a ratio or percent. Normal values of FEV_1/FVC are greater than 70%. A ratio less than 70% is indicative of obstructive lung disease.

Other commonly measured flow rates include the maximal midexpiratory flow rate (MMEFR), peak expiratory flow rate (PEFR), and inspiratory flow rate. The MMEFR is the average flow during the middle half (25% to 75%) of the FVC. The MMEFR is particularly helpful when the patient's effort does not appear to be maximal. Approximately the first 200 mL of a maximal expiration primarily depends on the patient's effort. Therefore, if flow is measured after the first 25% of expiration (at least 200 mL), it will more accurately reflect how flow is affected by pathology. Inspiration flow is even more effort dependent than expiratory flow, and is therefore more unreliable.

Maximum voluntary ventilation (MVV), or maximum breathing capacity (MBC), is an indicator of the *overall* mechanical disorders of the lungs and chest wall. In this test patients breathe as hard as they can, in and out, for approximately 12 seconds (Fig. 30-5). Decreased MVV can be indicative of either obstructive or restrictive lung disease, depending on the pattern.

Measurement of static and dynamic mechanical function is done by spirometry. The patient breathes through a mouthpiece attached to a spirometer, which has a recording device. The patient should be instructed carefully and wear nose clips to increase accuracy. Performing a forced expiration can induce

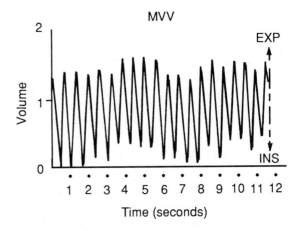

Figure 30-5. Example of normal maximum voluntary ventilation (MVV) pattern.

coughing and bronchospasm. If this happens, the test is delayed until the patient is breathing normally once again.

The American Thoracic Society has established standards for pulmonary function testing, which should be followed if the test is to be accurate and reproducible. Two important aspects of the procedure include (1) testing standing if at all possible and (2) repeating the test one or two times so that there are at least two tests within 5% of each other. Because PFTs are effort dependent, the values are *not* averaged. The best of the two or three trials is the value that is recorded. The three measurements that are standard in a spirometry assessment are FVC, FEV_1, and MVV. All other measures can be calculated from these.

Therapists can easily test pulmonary function at the bedside. A small hand-held spirometer (Fig. 30-6) that measures VC is the easiest and least expensive method. A portable, computerized spirometer (Fig. 30-7) is more expensive and slightly more complicated, but can measure dozens of PFT parameters. Volume incentive spirometers (Fig. 30-8) can be used to estimate inspiratory capacities. Cherniack and colleagues describe other simple bedside techniques to assess pulmonary function. One example is timing the forced expiration time during auscultation with a stethoscope. Normally, expiratory time is less than four seconds. A longer forced expiratory time is indicative of moderate to severe obstructive lung disease.

Pulmonary function test values are primarily used by the physical therapist to follow the progression of altered respiratory mechanics in chronic lung and musculoskeletal disease and as an objective way to document effectiveness, or response to therapeutic maneuvers in more acute respiratory disorders.

OTHER TESTS USED TO ASSESS PULMONARY DYSFUNCTION

Special laboratory tests, radiologic examinations, and surgical diagnostic techniques are used to assess the specific diagnosis and extent of a pulmonary disease or condition that affects the respiratory system. Some of these tests are

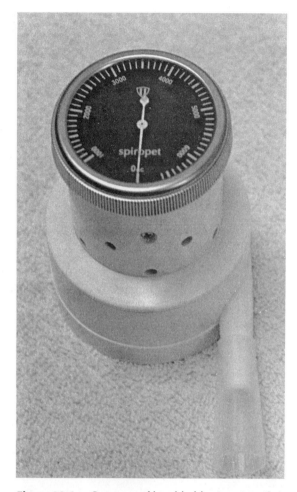

Figure 30-6. One type of hand-held spirometer (Spiropet), which measures vital capacity.

commonly used to screen patients who exhibit certain clinical symptoms and signs of pulmonary dysfunction. These so-called screening tests tend to be readily available and relatively inexpensive. Other tests are less readily available, are more expensive, and may carry a greater risk for the patient. These tests are used only when *specifically* indicated and when other, more routine, procedures will not yield a definitive diagnosis.

In this chapter I will present and discuss only the tests that physical therapists are most likely to encounter. The common screening

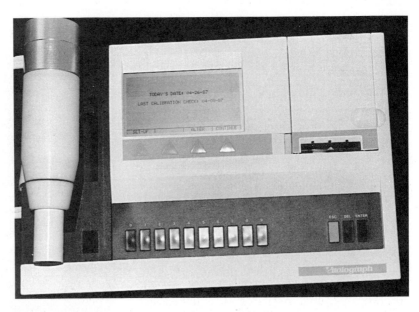

Figure 30-7. Compact computerized spirometer (Vitalograph).

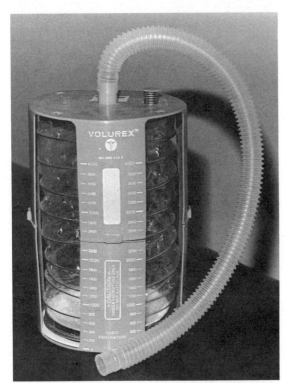

Figure 30-8. Example of a volume incentive spirometer (Volurex).

tests to be discussed include blood counts and cultures, body temperatures, sputum cultures, and sweat tests. The procedures to be discussed that are less routine include sonography, tomography, lung scintigraphy, gallium scanning, pleural fluid analysis, and surgical tests such as direct laryngoscopy, bronchoscopy, and biopsy.

A physical therapist managing patients with pulmonary dysfunction must understand the nature and implications of these diagnostic tests. The information provided by these procedures often affects the treatment plan, because they clarify indications, contraindications, and precautions for certain physical therapeutic interventions.

Blood analyses are the most common laboratory tests performed for diagnosis of pulmonary disease. The complete blood count (CBC) qualifies the cellular components (red and white cell counts) and determines hemoglobin concentrations and hematocrits. An elevated white blood cell (WBC) count indicates systemic infection. The type (or types) of WBC that is increased is determined by the type of infection. Red blood cell (RBC) count, hemoglobin concentration, and hematocrit analysis indicate the oxygen-carrying capability of the blood. Examples of normal values are presented in Tables 30-4 and 30-5.

Blood cultures may be ordered if a patient is suspected of having septicemia or bacteria in the bloodstream. It is imperative that the sample does not become contaminated by skin bacteria. Therefore, the technique must be as sterile as possible. Results of blood cultures take 24 to 72 hours before specific pathogens can be identified.

Elevated body temperature, measured orally or rectally, usually indicates the presence of infection. An elevated temperature is often the first indicator of an acute pulmonary problem, such as pneumonia and atelectasis. A patient who is at risk for developing a pulmonary complication or problem and who spikes a temperature is often immediately assumed to have a pulmonary problem. Unfortunately, this assumption is often made without supporting evidence. A therapist who works with "at risk" patients (ie, postoperative thoracic and abdominal surgery) should be aware that infection or inflammation of other body systems may be the cause of the temperature. Some examples of differential reasons for an elevated temperature include urinary tract infection, thrombophlebitis, and normal reaction of the body to major surgery. Although a fever may not have a pulmonary etiology, it usually does. Changes

in fever can be useful clinical indicators of effectiveness of physical therapy treatment of these conditions.

The sweat test is presently the definitive diagnostic laboratory test to confirm a diagnosis of cystic fibrosis. In cystic fibrosis (CF) both sodium and chloride concentrations are elevated in the sweat. Sweat testing involves a procedure called pilocarpine iontophoresis. Pilocarpine chemically induces sweat, which is collected in gauze pads and carefully analyzed for chloride and sodium concentration. It is essential that the sweat test be done according to recommended standards for as accurate an assessment as possible. Generally, two positive tests (levels greater than 80 mEq/L) are required to confirm a diagnosis of CF. Early diagnosis is important in CF, but it is more difficult to do a sweat test on an infant. Insufficient amounts of sweat often affect the accuracy of the test in very small babies.

Cytological and bacteriological evaluations of sputum samples provide assistance for differential diagnosis and enable identification of the specific bacterial pathogen. A sputum culture also provides a mechanism to test for which antibiotics the infecting organism is sensitive to and which it may be resistant to. The physical therapist may participate in collection of sputum for analysis, and therefore should be

Table 30-4. Normal White Blood Cell Values*

CELL TYPE	NORMAL PERCENT OF TOTAL WBCs
Neutrophils	50–70
Eosinophils	<1
Lymphocytes	25–33
Monocytes	4–6

*Total white cell count: <10,000/mm^3

Table 30-5. Normal Red Blood Cell Values

	MALES	FEMALES
Red cell count (venous blood)	4.5–6.2 million/mL	4.2–5.4 million/mL
Hematocrit	42%–54%	38%–46%
Hemoglobin	14–18 g/dL	12–16 g/dL

aware of the recommended collection procedures of the laboratory or institution where she practices. The four types of tests performed on a sputum sample are presented in Table 30-6.

Sonographic testing is noninvasive and without radiation hazard. Ultrasonography is used to detect pulmonary abnormalities such as pleural effusions, tumors, and other masses. Sonography can assess density so masses can be determined to be solid or fluid. One drawback of sonography is that the sound waves cannot penetrate deeply in the lungs.

Tomography, a series of cross-sectional x-rays, can more accurately detect pulmonary lesions deep in the lungs or mediastinum. Thoracic computed tomography (CT) uses a computer to convert the x-ray data to high-resolution images. A radiopaque contrast agent can be administered to differentiate blood vessels. Thoracic CT is a very sensitive and accurate evaluation tool.

Lung scintigraphy comprises two separate tests: a ventilation scan and a lung perfusion scan. Ventilation scanning involves inhalation of a radioactive gas and a series of recordings of the wash-in, equilibrium, and wash-out phases. Lung perfusion scans involve intravenous (IV) injection of a radiopaque contrast agent. Ventilation and perfusion lung scans can assist in identifying and differentiating airway obstruction, unequal gas distribution, and blood vessel obstruction such as a pulmonary embolus. Lung scans are not anatomically specific (as the CT scan is), but give a qualitative indication of ventilation and perfusion patterns in the lungs.

Gallium scans involve IV injection of radioactive gallium citrate and waiting 24 to 48 hours before scanning. Both benign and malignant neoplasms take up gallium (as do some normal organs and inflammatory lesions). Gallium scanning can help to identify the *location* of primary tumors, inflammatory lesions, and metastatic neoplasms. A more specific diagnosis of any of these conditions requires testing in addition to the gallium scan.

Pleural fluid analysis requires aspiration of fluid from the pleural cavity, or thoracentesis. This invasive procedure carries a risk of infection and pneumothorax. Aspiration of accumulated pleural fluid may be therapeutic in itself because it decreases lung compression by eliminating the trapped fluid. Pleural fluid is analyzed for abnormal cells or other factors and is cultured for pathogens. A chest roentgenogram is usually taken immediately after the thoracentesis to rule out pneumothorax.

Definitive diagnoses of some respiratory disorders require more invasive surgical procedures such as direct laryngoscopy, bronchoscopy, and lung biopsy. These procedures carry increased risk to the patient for infection, hemorrhage, pneumothorax, and other postoperative complications.

Direct laryngoscopy is performed with a fiberoptic endoscope or laryngoscope inserted through the mouth or nose and pharynx. The vocal cords and larynx can be examined for tumor, edema, scar tissue, foreign bodies, and congenital malformations (such as a tracheal web). Benign tumors and foreign bodies can be removed and tissue biopsies obtained (during the laryngoscopy).

Bronchoscopy can also be both a therapeutic and a diagnostic procedure. As an evaluative technique, bronchoscopy involves insertion of a metal or fiberoptic bronchoscope into the trachea and bronchi to visualize possible tumors, foreign bodies, and sites of bleeding. Sputum and tissue specimens can be obtained

Table 30-6. Sputum Analysis Tests

TEST	ASSOCIATED PATHOLOGY
Gram's stain	Lower respiratory infection
Acid-fast stain	Tuberculosis
Culture and sensitivity	Lower respiratory infection
Cytologic testing	Tumor, granuloma, inflammation

through a bronchoscope for laboratory examination.

Lung biopsies are performed to confirm diagnoses of benign or malignant tumors and other diseases of lung tissue. Biopsies can be done by means of a needle, transbronchially during bronchoscopy, and through a surgical incision (open biopsy). Needle and transbronchial biopsies are less invasive than open biopsy, but are limited by the small amount of tissue that can be obtained. If the lesion is not close to the tracheobronchial tree, a needle biopsy is not feasible. General anesthesia and a thoracic incision are required for an open biopsy. These conditions can increase a patient's risk for complications. Biopsy specimens are examined histologically to identify the cell type and the condition of the tissue.

THE CHEST EVALUATION

In this section I will describe the five major components of the chest evaluation and some specific and applicable components of assessing other systems as they relate to a patient with pulmonary dysfunction. Discussion of the chest evaluation also includes special considerations for assessing infants and children. Special considerations for evaluating a patient preoperatively are also discussed.

The five components of a chest evaluation are (1) inspection and observation, (2) auscultation of the lungs, (3) palpation, (4) mediate percussion of the chest wall, and (5) cough assessment.

INSPECTION AND OBSERVATION

The inspection and observation component of the chest evaluation is common to *any* evaluation a physical therapist does for any patient. However, when assessing a patient with pulmonary dysfunction, specific areas are emphasized. As a clinician with many years experience, I *cannot overemphasize* the importance of the visual inspection. Therapists must pay attention to the subtle changes in clinical appearance that are often indicative of clinical state. In my experience it is not unusual for a patient's clinical appearance to change, indicating an acute event, even *before* the monitors can record the changes in physiologic state.

Assessment begins before a word is exchanged between a therapist and patient. As a patient enters the department or clinic or while the therapist enters a patient's room, cubicle, or home, the therapist generally observes posture or position, the face, and the extremities.

Posture abnormalities and positioning may be indicative of habit, acute distress, chronic respiratory disease, or musculoskeletal problems. Initial observation of a patient's posture and position can provide valuable clues to clinical state. A patient who is reclined and obviously resting comfortably is quite different from the patient who is anxious, dyspneic (short of breath), and leaning forward.

In a hospital bed, patients will most often be positioned in the semi-Fowler's position (Fig. 30-9). Most patients with respiratory dysfunction prefer a head-up or inclined position of the head and trunk, which allows diaphragmatic excursion without significant resistance of the abdominal contents, which shift slightly downward with gravity.

Normal abdominal muscle contraction is essential for the diaphragm to return to its elevated resting position. Patients with spinal cord injury involving the abdominal muscles (T10-T12 and above) have greater diaphragmatic excursion in the supine position than the erect position. This is because when supine, the abdominal contents push the diaphragm to a higher resting level. Thus, supine is a more mechanically advantageous position and results in more efficient breathing in these patients. In sitting and standing, patients whose abdominal muscle cannot contract against gravity require external abdominal support to ensure adequate inspiratory capacities.

Patients with chronic lung disease who have altered chest wall biomechanics secondary to air trapping and loss of elasticity are often more dependent on accessory muscles to increase chest wall excursion. Most accessory muscles of ventilation attach to the shoulder

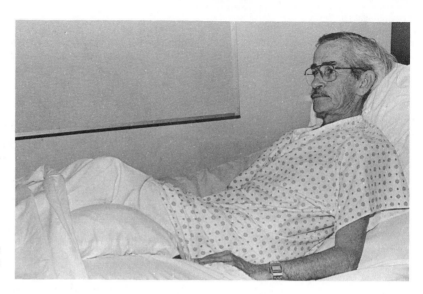

Figure 30-9. Patient in the semi-Fowler's position in a hospital bed.

girdle and neck as well as to the thoracic cage. This is why, when acutely distressed, these patients lean forward and support their upper extremities to stabilize their shoulder girdles so the accessory muscles can pull the thoracic cage upward or outward and increase thoracic capacity (Fig. 30-10). These actions are all compensatory for the loss of adequate diaphragmatic function. Although the use of accessory muscles is less efficient with respect to oxygen consumption, it may be necessary and unavoidable.

Observation of a patient's position can also contribute to more appropriate interpretation of other components of the chest evaluation. An example would be the patient who is positioned supine and upon auscultation has rales or decreased breath sounds over the posterior-inferior lung fields. Positioning could be contributing to these abnormal and adventitious (extra) breath sounds.

Therapists should also note whether a patient is frequently found in one particular position every time the patient is visited. This may indicate a need to work with the nursing staff and the patient to ensure changes in positioning, which can be essential to optimal management.

Abnormal posture may indicate musculo-skeletal anomalies, which can either contribute to pulmonary dysfunction or result from the pulmonary problem. Several musculoskeletal anomalies of the spine and rib cage can inter-

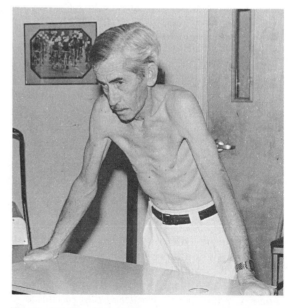

Figure 30-10. Forward-bending or professorial posture assumed by some patients with chronic lung disease.

fere with normal excursion and result in restrictive patterns. The most common of these conditions are scoliosis, kyphosis, and ankylosing spondylitis. Pulmonary function is often not compromised unless the deformities are moderate to severe.

A kyphotic posture can also be the result of chronic obstructive lung disease, particularly if the patient uses anterior accessory muscles to assist ventilation (eg, pectoral muscles). The therapist should also note body type and proportions such as obese or cachectic. State of consciousness may also be important to document if the patient is not alert and oriented.

Face, Head, and Neck

Observation of the patient's face, head, and neck can yield many clues about clinical state. Expression or demeanor can be very revealing, leading the examiner to sense the patient's emotions and nonphysical problems and ask appropriate questions. The face is the most important area to look for skin color changes. Central cyanosis, which results in a bluish discoloration of the skin and mucous membranes, can be detected by observing the perioral skin and mucous membranes of the mouth (in patients with dark brown or black skin, cyanosis can be detected by observing the mucous membranes). Cyanosis is indicative of greater than 5 g% of unsaturated hemoglobin (generally associated with an oxygen saturation of less than 80% and arterial oxygen tension of less than 50 mm Hg). Cyanosis is an important but unreliable sign of hypoxia. Patients with anemia (fewer red blood cells) could be hypoxic but not appear cyanotic, and patients with polycythemia (too many red blood cells) could appear cyanotic and not actually be hypoxic. A sudden change in skin color, especially pallor, is indicative of acute distress and may signal underlying pathologic changes. Redness in the face can sometimes indicate hypertension.

Another clinical sign of respiratory distress noted in the face is flaring of the nasal alae. Many clinicians think this is seen only in infants, but it is not. Nasal flaring can occur at any age.

Spontaneous pursed-lip breathing (PLB) is a clinical sign of chronic obstructive pulmonary disease (COPD), which indicates an attempt to alleviate air trapping. A patient may breath out against pursed lips (Fig. 30-11), thereby theoretically increasing intra-airway pressure, delaying collapse of small airways, and decreasing air trapping. The exact physiologic effects of PLB are controversial. I am certain, however, that the patients who use this technique spontaneously must derive physiologic benefit. I believe patients use PLB to relieve the sensation of dyspnea by attempting to decrease functional residual capacity (FRC).

When observing the neck, the therapist looks for jugular vein distension (JVD) and prominence of the sternocleidomastoid (SCM) muscles. Distended neck veins in a patient whose head and trunk are inclined at least 45 degrees, with the head up, are abnormal. In a patient with chronic lung disease this can be indicative of cor pulmonale (right-sided heart failure). If the patient has associated cardiovas-

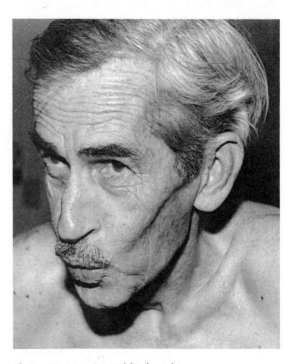

Figure 30-11. Pursed-lip breathing.

cular disease, JVD can also indicate congestive heart failure (CHF). The SCM muscles are commonly used as accessory muscles of ventilation, and therefore may become hypertrophied.

Extremities

The fingers and toes of patients with chronic lung disease should be inspected for signs of clubbing. Digital clubbing involves the obliteration of the normal base angle of the nail (angle formed by the root of the nail and nail is usually about 160 degrees) and bulbous enlargement of the terminal phalanges. Clubbing is most commonly associated with chronic tissue hypoxia, bronchogenic carcinoma, bronchiectasis, and cystic fibrosis. The final stage of digital clubbing is hypertrophic pulmonary osteoarthropathy. The wrist and ankle joints are most commonly involved, with painful swelling and inflammation.

Local cyanosis of the nail beds and digits is *not* indicative of cardiac or pulmonary dysfunction. The fingers and toes can be blue because of cold or vasospasm.

Chest Wall

The chest wall is the next area to be inspected for signs of pulmonary dysfunction. Examination of shape and configuration of the rib cage and sternum may reveal some deviations or deformities. Congenital deformities have little direct effect on pulmonary function, although they may be associated with other congenital or acquired signs and conditions. Pectus carinatum (pigeon chest), pectus excavatum (funnel chest), and bifid sternum are the three congenital deformities that might be observed.

The barrel-shaped chest is characterized by an anterior-posterior diameter equal to or greater than the transverse diameter. A barrel chest is usually acquired and is associated with COPD and air trapping. As RV and FRC increase, the rib cage, sternum, and diaphragm all are eventually prevented from returning to their normal resting positions. These changes result in several biomechanical and functional problems, which will be discussed in detail later in this chapter.

Occasionally, asymmetry of right and left chest wall motions can be detected through observation of the chest. More often symmetry must be checked through palpation of lateral rib cage motion.

Some patients with COPD exhibit abnormal or paradoxical rib cage motions during breathing. The paradoxical indrawing of the lateral rib margins during inspiration is called Hoover's sign. Hoover's sign is attributed to the more horizontal pull of the fibers of the flattened diaphragm on the lower ribs. Another observed paradoxical motion of the chest in patients with COPD is an indrawing of the lower sternum in early inspiration. Based on a study by Gilmartin and Gibson, this motion is thought to be caused by relaxation of the abdominal muscles that contract (abnormally) during expiration in patients with COPD and hyperinflation.

Observation of breathing patterns, rates, and ratios are an important part of assessing a patient with pulmonary dysfunction. Various patterns of breathing that can be observed are presented in Table 30-7. The rhythm and depth of the respirations are the important characteristics of breathing pattern.

Determining the rate of respirations is accomplished by counting respirations for a full minute. Because respiratory rate can be altered consciously, it is essential that the patient be unaware that you are counting. The easiest way to accomplish this is to count respirations directly after counting heart rate while continuing to palpate the radial pulse. One note of caution: Patients who are monitored in intensive care units often have digital readings of respirations and heart rate. These rates are generally unreliable because of a high incidence of artifact, which is interpreted as a breath or beat. It is always advisable to measure heart rate and respirations *directly* in these patients.

Inspiratory:expiratory time ratio is normally 1:2. Pulmonary disease can either shorten inspiratory time or lengthen expiratory time. While assessing respiratory rate, the therapist should also time the inspiratory:expiratory ratio.

Table 30-7. Breathing Patterns

TYPE	PATTERN	ASSOCIATED CONDITIONS (EXAMPLES)
Eupnea	Normal rate and rhythm	Normal
Apnea	Absence of breathing	Prematurity; CNS dysfunction; upper airway obstruction
Tachypnea	Faster rate; regular rhythm	Fever, anxiety, exercise
Bradypnea	Slower rate; regular rhythm	Sleep; respiratory decompensation; narcotic effect
Cheyne-Stokes	Gradually faster and deeper with alternating periods of apnea	CNS dysfunction
Biot's	Faster and deepr breaths with abrupt pauses	Spinal meningitis
Kussmaul's	Faster and deeper breaths without pauses	Metabolic acidosis

Special Considerations for Infants

Observation and inspection of infants primarily involves identification of specific signs of respiratory distress, skin color (as previously discussed), and breathing pattern. Neonates and infants have less compliant lungs, more compliant rib cages, and narrower airways. These factors combine with others to result in marked increases in work of breathing when pulmonary dysfunction is present. Babies also tend to respond to respiratory compromise by increasing rate rather than depth of ventilations.

Signs of infant respiratory distress include rib cage retractions (suprasternal, subcostal, substernal, or intercostal), nasal flaring, expiratory grunting, stridor (loud inspiratory noises indicating upper airway obstruction), and head bobbing. Cyanosis is also a sign, but pallor is more common. Prolonged periods of sternal retractions can result in acquired pectus excavatum in some infants.

In terms of the breathing pattern, tachypnea (rapid respiratory rate) may also accompany other signs of respiratory distress. Conversely, in premature infants, apnea (cessation of breathing) may be the most apparent clinical sign. Newborns normally have irregular patterns of breathing, so pauses up to 5 to 10 seconds are not unusual or pathological.

It is also important to note if the infant coughs or sneezes spontaneously. Sneezing is generally a more common reflexive response in infants than coughing. Both reflexes, as well as the gag reflex, are protective of the airways because there are serious potential consequences if these reflexes are depressed or absent.

AUSCULTATION

The second major component of the chest evaluation is auscultation (listening to chest sounds) with the aid of a stethoscope. Auscultation is an extremely important skill for physical therapists. Skills in differentiating lung sounds and identifying signs of pathology require practice listening to many chests, both healthy and pathological. Lung sounds are divided into breath sounds, adventitious sounds, and voice sounds. Auscultation is an extremely sensitive assessment and is convenient and noninvasive. Auscultation of the chest is also more subjective than many more sophisticated assessment techniques. Reliability of auscultation depends on many factors, including the stethoscope used, position of the patient, the skill of the evaluator, and effective and accurate communication and documentation.

Stethoscopes vary significantly in construction and cost. The less expensive stethoscopes are not adequate, and the most expensive models are not necessary. Basically the stethoscope should be short (12 to 14 inches), thick walled, and have *both* a bell and diaphragm that are sturdily constructed (Fig. 30-12). The diaphragm needs to be at least 1.5 inches in diameter (for an adult stethoscope). The earpieces are molded plastic or rubber and need to fit properly and comfortably for the evaluator to auscultate adequately. Most manufacturers will exchange earpieces for a size that fits properly.

Technique

When auscultating the chest, the diaphragm portion of the stethoscope is usually used because it is designed to pick up the higher-pitched lung sounds. The bell is generally used to auscultate lower-pitched heart sounds, occasionally smaller areas of the chest wall, or infant chests (when a smaller stethoscope is not available).

The position of the patient can influence airflow, and therefore should be optimized for the best possible assessment. Whenever possible, the patient should be sitting with the feet supported. Occasionally, patients cannot be elevated or sitting, so lung fields are auscultated with the patient sidelying. In this situation it is extremely important that the therapist listen to both lung fields with each area auscultated uppermost. If both lung fields are auscultated

with the patient lying on the same side, it is likely the lower lung fields will be interpreted as having decreased breath sounds when compared to the upper lung fields.

Lung sounds vary to some extent from one person to another. It is therefore best to compare sounds between right and left lung fields in the same patient. Patients with diffuse, bilateral pathology will not have a baseline to compare against. The more experience and practice the evaluator has, the more reliable the assessment will tend to be. I recommend that before auscultating chests of patients with pathology, therapists should auscultate many normal chests as a basis for interpretation.

Auscultation generally progresses superior to inferior and side to side. The general surface area projection for each bronchopulmonary segment (except medial basal, which has no surface projection) should be auscultated. To do this, the evaluator must be familiar with surface anatomy of the chest and the location of the borders and fissures of the lungs.

The patient should be instructed to breathe deeper than normal and with the mouth open (Fig. 30-13). If there is excessive chest hair, friction of the diaphragm of the stethoscope against the hair when the chest is moving will cause sounds that mimic rules (crackles). If the hair is wet, the distortion will usually be eliminated. Never try to auscultate over clothes,

Figure 30-12. Adult-size stethoscope with diaphragm and bell.

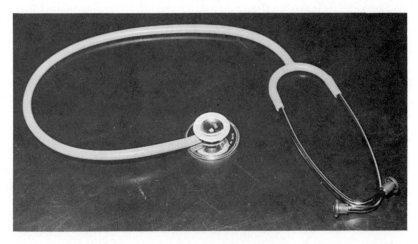

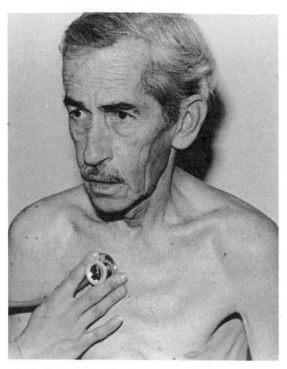

Figure 30-13. Patient breathing through the mouth during auscultation.

and be sure to hold the stethoscope firmly against the chest wall, preferably over an intercostal space.

Terminology

The key to effective communication among health care providers with respect to chest aus-cultation is semantics. There has long been confusion when communicating auscultation findings between health care professionals because several different terms are used for adventitious lung sounds.

Three categories of lung sounds will be discussed in this chapter: breath sounds, adventitious sounds, and voice sounds. Normal breath sounds are the sounds created by air flowing through the tracheobronchial tree. Adventitious sounds are created when air flows through secretions and narrowed airways. Voice sounds are created when the patient's vocalizations are auscultated.

Breath Sounds

Of the four types of normal breath sounds, only three are generally auscultated routinely. Table 30-8 presents the normal breath sounds and where they are commonly heard. Tracheal breath sounds are not often auscultated unless the patient is suspected of having an upper airway problem. The normal sounds produced as air flows through the branching and progressively narrowing airways constitute *normal* breath sounds *when they are heard over their appropriate associated areas of the chest wall.*

Bronchial breath sounds are normally heard over the manubrium and on either side of the manubrium. Bronchial breath sounds are loud, high pitched and tubular, or hollow and harsh. There also is a gap or hesitation between inspiration and expiration with expiration heard predominantly. Bronchial breath sounds

Table 30-8. Normal Breath Sounds

BREATH SOUNDS	QUALITY OF SOUNDS	LOCATION
Bronchial	Loud, high pitched, and hollow or harsh; hear full inspiration and expiration	Manubrium Either side of manubrium
Bronchovesicular	Softer and lower pitched than bronchial; hear full inspiration and expiration	Sternum and either side of sternum Between the scapula Apex of the right lung
Vesicular	Soft and breezy; low pitched; hear full inspiration and one third of expiration	Peripheral lung areas (except apex of right lung)

are created by air flowing through the larger airways.

Bronchovesicular breath sounds are normally heard just distal to the central airways over the upper sternum, on either side of the sternum, posteriorly between the scapulae, and over the apex of the right lung. Bronchovesicular sounds are a slight variation to bronchial breath sounds, but are softer and lower pitched. They also have no gap or hesitation between the inspiratory and expiratory components, with each component heard equally. Bronchovesicular breath sounds are created as air moves through some larger airways *and* some alveoli. These sounds are harder to differentiate from bronchial and vesicular sounds and are therefore not used very often clinically.

Vesicular breath sounds are heard over the rest of the peripheral lung fields. Vesicular sounds are low pitched, soft, and breezy. They have a predominant inspiratory component, and the expiratory sound is fainter and disappears approximately one third of the way through expiration. Vesicular breath sounds are created by air moving through very small airways and alveoli.

Abnormal breath sounds are noted when bronchial and bronchovesicular sounds are heard over the periphery where normally vesicular sounds should be heard. In lung pathology, alveoli may be occluded, filled with exudate, or collapsed. When these changes occur, the sound transmitted to the stethoscope is airflow proximal to the pathology, which is transmitted to the chest wall. If the distance for transmission of sound is great or the pathology blocks the sound, absent or very decreased

abnormal sounds will be noted. The normal vesicular sounds can also be diminished due to pathology or hypoventilation.

The first thing a therapist should determine when performing chest auscultation is if the breath sounds are normal (vesicular except in the specific locations previously noted), abnormal (bronchial or bronchovesicular over peripheral lung fields), diminished, or absent. The therapist then considers assessing adventitious sounds.

Adventitious Sounds

Adventitious sounds are extra sounds produced by pathological processes in the airways, lungs, and pleura. These processes include secretions, edema, fibrosis inflammation, bronchospasm, atelectasis, tumor, and other pathologic changes that cause obstruction, turbulence, and friction during ventilation. Adventitious sounds, if heard, are always abnormal and are superimposed on breath sounds. The terminology I use to describe adventitious sounds in this chapter is based on recommendations of the Ad Hoc Joint Committee on Pulmonary Nomenclature of the American Thoracic Society and the American College of Chest Physicians in 1975. I also indicate the recommendations of the International Lung Sounds Association (1976). The terms and their classifications are presented in Table 30-9.

Rales are discontinuous sounds that are also referred to as crackles. These sounds are likely created when air bubbles pass through secretions. They are also heard when airways suddenly pop open, such as when atelectatic areas are inflated, and collapsed larger airways are opened early in inspiration. In the above

Table 30-9. Adventitious Lung Sounds

RECOMMENDED TERM*	CLASSIFICATION	QUALITY	ALTERNATIVE TERM
Rales	Discontinuous	Fine Medium Coarse	Crackles
Rhonchi	Continuous	High pitched Low pitched	Wheezes Rhonchi

*Ad Hoc Joint Committee on Pulmonary Nomenclature, American Thoracic Society and American College of Chest Physicians (1975); International Lung Sounds Association (1976)

situations, rales are heard predominantly during inspiration. The rales heard early in inspiration tend to be coarse and loud and usually reflect larger airway seretions or collapse. Late inspiratory rales are fine and higher pitched, and reflect pathology in the terminal bronchioles and alveoli.

Rales can also be heard throughout all of inspiration and expiration with diffuse lung parenchymal fibrosis. This sound is likely created by stretching and relaxation of fibrotic tissue during breathing.

Rhonchi are continuous sounds, also referred to as wheezes. Continuous adventitious sounds are created because of narrowing of the airways. Rapid airflow is necessary for the rhonchal sound to be created. Rhonchi are most commonly heard during expiration. This is probably due to the fact that further narrowing of the airways occurs during expiration (even in normal lungs). Rhonchi can be high pitched or low pitched, usually depending on the location of the narrowing. High-pitched rhonchi usually originate in the smaller airways and low-pitched rhonchi in the larger airways.

Stridor is a continuous type of adventitious sound heard during inspiration and without the aid of a stethoscope. Stridor is associated with upper airway obstruction (eg, croup, laryngeal spasm).

A pleural friction rub is a loud creaking or grating sound heard during both inspiration and expiration. This sound is associated with inflammation of the pleural surfaces, which rub together.

Voice Sounds

Voice sounds or vocal resonance is often checked once some abnormality in breath sounds has been noted. Sound is carried best through a solid and least through air. Vocalizations of the patient with normal lungs are therefore usually distorted and muffled when listening over the lung periphery. The three types of voice sounds most commonly assessed over abnormal lung are bronchophony, egophony, and whispered pectoriloquy.

Bronchophony is elicited by having the patient give a nasal-type vocalization, such as saying "99" or "A, E, I, O, U" and auscultating bilaterally. Bronchophony is a loudening and more clear detection of the spoken voice than normal.

Egophony, another abnormal voice sound, occurs when the patient is saying "Eeeee. . ." and the sound is transmitted as "Ay. . .". Whispered pectoriloquy is when the patient's loud whisper of "one, two, three, four" (which normally would be distorted and faint) sounds through the stethoscope as if the patient is whispering in the evaluator's ear. All of the abnormal vocal resonances are often associated with consolidation, pleural effusion, and atelectasis.

Special Considerations for Infants

Auscultation of infants is a more gross assessment because sounds are transmitted over shorter distances and through less dense tissue. Therefore, it is important not to assume that a pathological condition is located in a particular lobe or segment (or even lung, in premature infants) based only on auscultation. Confirmation by a chest roentgenogram is essential in this population.

Auscultation of infants will be more successful if an appropriate size stethoscope is used. Pediatric and a neonatal stethoscopes are illustrated in Figure 30-14. If an infant is crying, auscultation *cannot* be interpreted. Having a parent or other trusted person hold the infant during auscultation may assist in calming the baby (Figs. 30-15 and 30-16). Neonates and premature infants should be auscultated with their heads in the midline position. If the head is turned, breath sounds may sound diminished in the lung field opposite to the direction the head is turned.

The Mechanically Ventilated Patient

If the patient has an endotracheal or tracheostomy tube and is being mechanically ventilated, special considerations need to be made for auscultation. The breath sounds of a ventilated patient will sound louder and harsher. Often, adventitious sounds are heard, especially rales. These rales could mean secretions

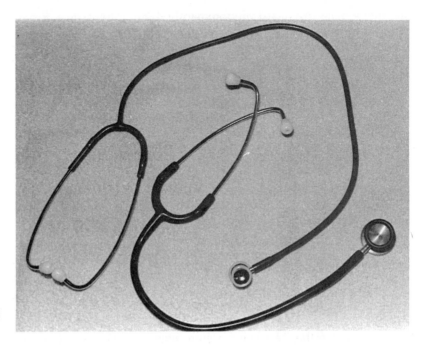

Figure 30-14. Pediatric and neonatal-sized stethoscopes.

in the patient's airways, or fluid in the artificial airway or the ventilator tubing, which collects as the warm, humidified air condenses. Optimize auscultation of these patients by emptying the tubing of condensed fluids and suctioning the airway (if necessary) to clear secretions. If a patient is breathing "in between" ventilated breaths (as in intermittent mandatory ventilation, or IMV), listen to and interpret the nonmechanical breath sounds whenever possible. Many times the nonmechanically ventilated breaths are too weak to give an accurate assessment of the quality of the sounds.

PALPATION

The third major component of the chest evaluation is palpation. Palpations of patients with pulmonary disease are done for several different reasons. They include palpating for mediastinal shift, chest wall motion and symmetry, diaphragmatic motion, tactile fremitus (vibrations), and chest wall pain. Palpation is the natural follow up to inspection to either confirm or rule out a suspected abnormality. Palpation is also a sensitive assessment of superficial struc-

tures and vibrations projected to the surface. Physical therapists traditionally use their hands to assess, treat, and communicate with their clients. Manual assessment techniques are as essential to management of patients with pulmonary dysfunction as they are to patients with neurologic and musculoskeletal problems.

Mediastinal Shift

Mediastinal structures are not rigidly fixed and are subject to pressures within the thorax. The most superficial structure associated with the mediastinum is the trachea. When mediastinal structures shift to the right or left, the bronchi and trachea are pulled and the shift can be palpated in the suprasternal notch. The trachea is normally oriented centrally in the suprasternal notch. The therapist can gently palpate soft tissue "space" on either side of the trachea still within the notch (Fig. 30-17). When the trachea shifts, the examiner will be pushing on the trachea itself on one side or the other just medial to the sternoclavicular joints.

The shift of mediastinal structures deviates

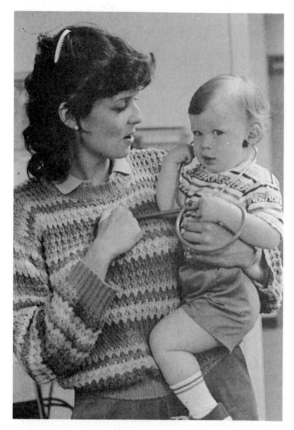

Figure 30-15. The mother of a young child can introduce him to unfamiliar objects, such as the stethoscope.

volves palpation with both hands. The upper and mid-lung fields are palpated anteriorly and the lower segments posteriorly. Cherniack and colleagues describe the most common method for palpating chest cage movement.

Palpation of the upper segments is accomplished with the fingers of both hands over the trapezius at the base of the neck bilaterally (Fig. 30-18). The thumbs meet anteriorly at the midline below the clavicles. As the patient inspires deeply, the thumbs move apart. It is very important during all of these palpations that the palms are firmly pressing the chest wall. The examiner observes both the distance the thumbs separate and whether the distance is equal bilaterally (symmetry).

The middle segments are palpated similarly, with the fingers placed in the posterior axillary folds and the thumbs meeting anteriorly just below the nipple line (Fig. 30-19). This palpation may not be possible to do for female patients with large breasts because the examiner's hands could not be properly positioned and it would be uncomfortable for the patient.

Lower rib cage excursion is palpated poste-

away from space-occupying lesions, pneumothoraces, and hemothoraces. Conversely, the mediastinum will shift toward the side of a large area of atelectasis or unilateral fibrosis.

To properly palpate for a mediastinal shift, the patient should be sitting or lying down with the neck slightly flexed and the chin in the midline. This palpation is not routinely included in a chest evaluation, but is added when a possible cause of a shift is suspected.

Chest Wall and Diaphragmatic Motion

Chest wall and diaphragmatic motion can be easily palpated. Palpation of these motions is qualitative, not quantitative. Manual qualitative assessment of chest wall excursion in-

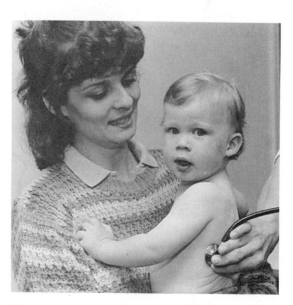

Figure 30-16. Auscultation of an infant or small child is easier when his mother holds him.

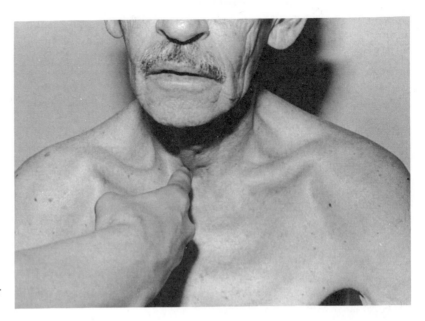

Figure 30-17. Palpation for mediastinal shift.

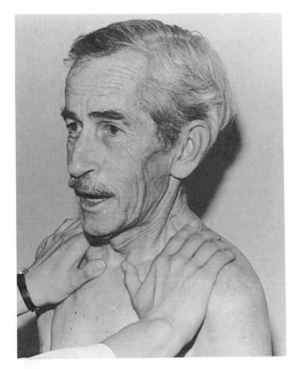

Figure 30-18. Palpation for upper chest wall motion.

riorly with the fingers placed in the anterior axillary folds and the thumbs pulled together and meeting medially over the vertebral spinous processes below the scapulae (Fig. 30-20). It is important that the underlying skin be pulled medially while the thumbs are pulled together.

These qualitative palpations are especially helpful in detecting abnormalities of inspiratory expansion of the chest wall and as a pretreatment and posttreatment screening for increased chest wall mobility.

Some situations require more objective measurements, such as the following:

1. Measure the chest wall diameter with a cloth tape measure at the level of the xyphoid process of the sternum (Fig. 30-21). Take measurements at full inspiration and full expiration. The difference between the two values quantitates chest wall excursion. The normal excursion is approximately 2 to 4 inches in adult males.
2. The sternal angle can be measured with a standard goniometer with the axis at the xyphoid-sternal junction (usually a groove or notch) and the arms aligned with the

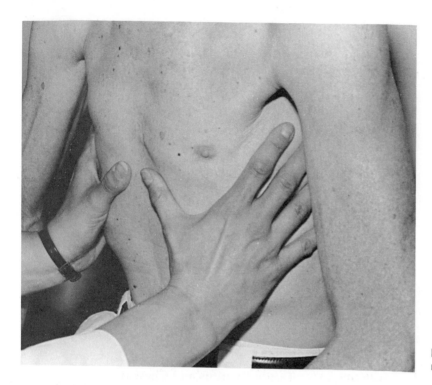

Figure 30-19. Palpation for middle chest wall motion.

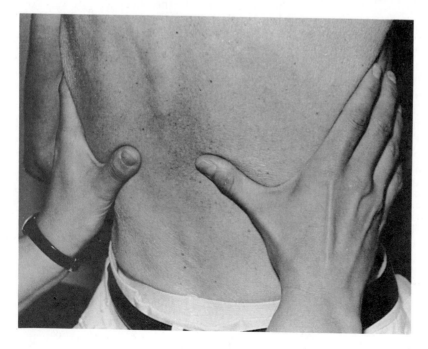

Figure 30-20. Palpation for lower chest wall motion.

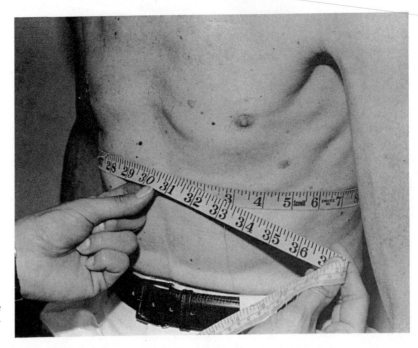

Figure 30-21. Quantitative measurement of chest wall motion using a tape measure.

lower margins of the ribs. Measurements are taken at full inspiration and full expiration. Normal values do not exist for these measurements at this time.

The *diaphragm* contributes to the upward and outward motion of the lower ribs when it is aligned in a normal resting position, which is dome shaped with the peripheral fibers in apposition with the rib cage. This alignment (Fig. 30-22) allows the diaphragm to pull the lower ribs upward. The outward motion occurs because of the "bucket-handle" motion of the lower ribs as they are pulled upward. This action of the diaphragm can be palpated by placing the hands over the lower rib cage anteriorly and laterally with the thumbs resting along the costal margins (pointing up and inward). As the patient inspires fully, the thumbs should move apart (Fig. 30-23). The flattened diaphragm loses the above described action on the lower ribs. In patients where the diaphragm is very flattened, the lower rib margins may be pulled paradoxically inward. In this case, the thumbs would move closer together during inspiration.

Tactile Fremitus and Chest Wall Pain

Tactile fremitus involves palpation of vibrations transmitted to the chest wall during vocalization by the patient. Voice sound created by saying vowels or "99" are normally palpated by placing the palm (Fig. 30-24) or side of the hand (Fig. 30-25) over the chest wall (overlying *lung* tissue). Vocal fremitus will be increased, decreased, or absent over areas of diseased lung tissue.

Palpation of the chest wall is also done to detect or rule out abnormalities such as subcutaneous emphysema and to evaluate chest pain.

Subcutaneous emphysema (SCE) is palpated as a crepitus or crackling sensation under the fingertips. The presence of SCE is secondary to air being introduced into the subcutaneous space. Subcutaneous emphysema is often palpated around a thoracotomy incision, chest tube sites, and subclavian catheters. In infants, SCE may occur with intubation and positive pressure mechanical ventilation.

Pain in the chest is a common symptom, which could indicate serious cardiac or pulmo-

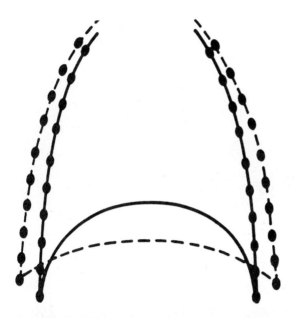

Figure 30-22. Illustration of dome-shaped resting position of the diaphragm. The vertical alignment of the peripheral fibers in apposition to the rib cage results in upward and outward motion of the lower rib cage. (Whitelaw WA: The respiratory pump. In Guenter CA, Welch MH (eds): Pulmonary Medicine, 2nd ed, p 51. Philadelphia, JB Lippincott, 1982)

nary disease, but usually does not. Therefore, it is extremely important to differentiate the many possible sources of chest discomfort. Chest pain of cardiac origin is usually located substernally, with or without radiation to the arms, and is often described as a pressure or weight on the chest. Cardiogenic pain also is often exacerbated by activity or exercise and is relieved by rest or nitroglycerin. The nature of this type of chest pain is usually different from pain referred from other sites. The difficulty is that patients often do not have a frame of reference and usually fear the possibility that they may have angina or be having a heart attack.

The therapist can reassure patients that pain in or about the chest is very common in anyone with pulmonary dysfunction. The therapist can then proceed to assess the location, nature, and reproducibility of the pain.

If the nerve roots are inflamed or irritated, the pain will follow the dermatomal distribution. The nerve root levels that involve the chest, back, and abdomen include C4 (lower neck, shoulders, and clavicular areas) and T2-T12. Possible causes of nerve root pain include herpes zoster, degenerative arthritis, and neoplasms.

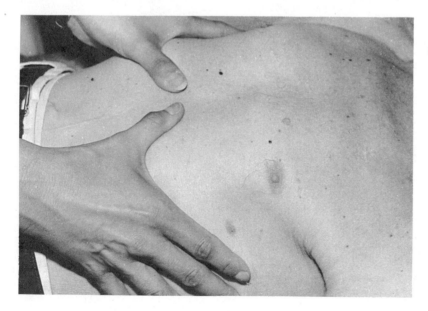

Figure 30-23. Palpation for lower rib cage motion as a result of diaphragm action.

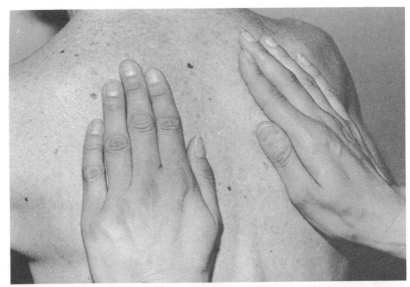

Figure 30-24. Palpation for tactile fremitus with the palms of the hands.

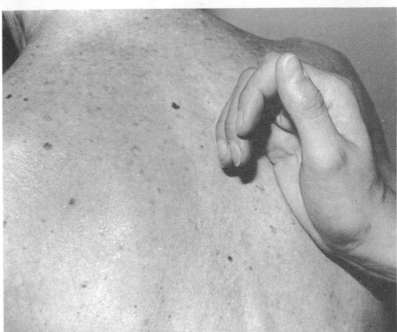

Figure 30-25. Palpation for tactile fremitus with the side of the hand.

Costal cartilage and ribs can be the source of pain. Fractures, subluxation, inflammations, or infections of these tissues are usually exquisitely tender to palpation and very localized. With a rib fracture, grating of the bone ends can often be detected and callus may be palpated if the fracture has healed.

Muscle spasm, strain, and delayed muscle pain after exercise are also sources of chest wall pain. These causes can be differentiated by a history (ie, paroxysmal coughing; recent new exercise or trauma), by deep palpation of the muscle belly, and by offering resistance to the action of the suspected muscle group to try to reproduce the pain.

The parietal pleura can be the source of severe, sharp pain that is worse when the patient takes a deep breath, coughs, or sneezes. Often a pleural rub can be auscultated when the pleura are inflamed.

When assessing chest wall pain, the therapist should first have the patient describe the location, type, and characteristics of the pain and point to the painful area. The area can then be palpated, with firm pressure. The patient should then be asked to cough and take a deep breath to see if those maneuvers reproduce or exacerbate the pain. If appropriate, the assessment should be expanded to rule out other musculoskeletal problems, such as thoracic outlet syndrome, cervical disk problems, or shoulder girdle problems.

MEDIATE PERCUSSION

The fourth major component of the chest evaluation is mediate percussion. Mediate percussion of the thorax is a procedure in which the examiner strikes the middle finger of one hand (which is firmly pressed on the chest wall) with the middle finger of the other hand (Fig. 30-26). This technique is done to produce sound to determine size, position, and especially density of underlying tissues. Mediate percussion is done to reinforce or clarify other evaluative findings and to assess diaphragmatic motion.

Correct technique for mediate percussion requires practice to develop the appropriate quick, staccato motion of the plexor (striking finger) on the pleximeter (the finger that is struck). The distal half of the pleximeter finger is all that should make contact with the chest wall (Fig. 30-27). That finger should be placed in intercostal spaces and not over bone or large muscle masses whenever possible. The wrist of the plexor hand is the fulcrum with no elbow or shoulder motion. Once the pleximeter finger is struck, the plexor should be instantaneously recoiled.

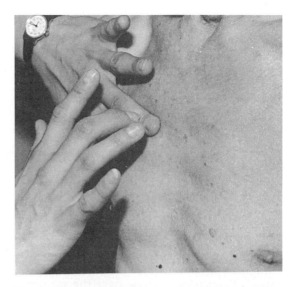

Figure 30-26. Performing mediate percussion over the anterior chest wall.

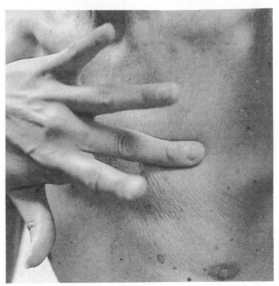

Figure 30-27. The distal half of the pleximeter finger in contact with the chest wall (intercostal space) in preparation for percussion.

The pitch or quality of the sound produced by percussion is what alerts the examiner to the relative density of the underlying tissue (to approximately 5 cm). The more dense the tissue, the duller the sound will be. It is easier to perceive a duller note after a more resonant one. Therefore, it is helpful to sequence mediate percussion so that more resonant areas are percussed first. Thus, if an abnormality is suspected in one area of the lung, the other areas should be percussed first. It is also important to percuss matching areas of the chest wall from side to side to check for unilateral conditions.

Percussion notes over the thorax and abdomen range from flat to tympany. Described in Table 30-10 are the sounds that are normally heard with mediate percussion over the thorax and when they may be abnormal.

Mediate percussion can also be used to detect the extent of the vertical descent of the diaphragm during inspiration. To assess diaphragmatic motion, the patient should be seated. Percussion is done over the posterior chest wall. The pleximeter finger is placed parallel to the plinth or floor. Percussion should progress from resonance to dullness, or superior to inferior. The resting position of the diaphragm is detected first by having the patient breathe out and hold. During the hold, the examiner percusses superior to inferior and

marks the point where the sound becomes dull with a skin-marking pencil. The patient is then asked to take a deep breath in and hold. The percussion procedure is repeated from the first mark downward until the note again becomes dull and that point is also marked. This assessment (Figs. 30-28 to 30-30) should be done bilaterally, especially if there is any reason to suspect paradoxical motion of a hemidiaphragm (one half of the diaphragm that has lost its phrenic innervation).

COUGH ASSESSMENT

The fifth major component of the chest evaluation is assessment of the patient's cough. A cough is both an important and common symptom of pulmonary dysfunction and a technique to improve airway clearance in a patient with secretions. Coughing is therefore both a nuisance and an essential adjunct to the mucociliary transport mechanisms within the airways. Assessing cough as a symptom and its effectiveness helps the therapist determine the most appropriate therapeutic intervention.

A cough can be voluntary or reflex. Cough

Table 30-10. Normal Mediate Percussion Sounds

SOUND	NORMAL LOCATION	PATHOLOGIC LOCATION
Dullness	Liver: On the right side below 6th rib anteriorly and below the 12th thoracic vertebra posteriorly	Over peripheral lung fields with tumor, consolidation, abcess
	Cardiac: Over the sternum and on either side of the sternum anteriorly	
	Visceral: Below the 12th thoracic vertebra on the left side posteriorly	
Resonance	Lung fields: Peripheral lung fields and "strap" areas on the shoulders anteriorly and posteriorly	
Hyperresonance		Over peripheral lung fields when hyperaerated
Tympany	Stomach: Below 6th rib anteriorly on the left	Over peripheral lung fields with pneumothorax

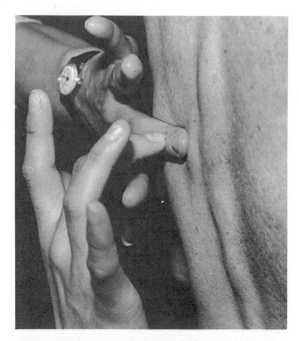

Figure 30-28. Mediate percussion to assess diaphragmatic motion. Initial percussion is for the high (end of expiration) position of the diaphragm.

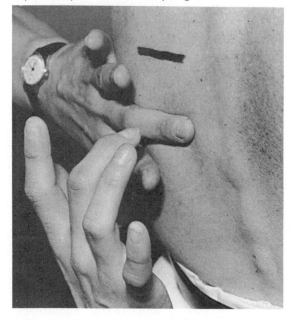

Figure 30-29. Percussion proceeds to find the low (full inspiration) diaphragmatic position.

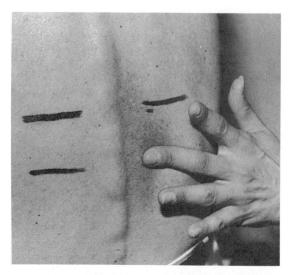

Figure 30-30. Percussion continues on the opposite side to detect differences in hemidiaphragm motions.

reflex receptors are more numerous in the upper airways and around the carina and mainstem bronchi. Studies have shown that coughing is more effective in clearing the first few generations or divisions of the airways.

The cough mechanism has three phases. The overall effect is production of explosive early expiratory flows and reduced large airway diameters. The first phase is the inspiratory phase. A much deeper than normal breath is taken during this phase. The second phase is the "compressive" phase where the glottis closes and the expiratory and abdominal muscles contract, increasing intrathoracic pressures. Phase three, the expiratory phase, is where the glottis opens and air is rapidly and forcefully expulsed with continued contraction of expiratory and abdominal muscles.

Evaluation of cough as a symptom begins with a history and description of the characteristics of the cough. The examiner should look for clues suggestive of etiology by inquiring about the patient's smoking history, allergies, environmental and occupational exposure to irritants, and history of respiratory diagnoses such as asthma, chronic bronchitis, and so on. It is also important to determine if the nature of the cough has recently changed (eg, as in a patient with COPD who develops an acute exacerbation or infection).

The patient should then be asked to describe the characteristics of the cough, including circumstances of onset, type or character of the cough (eg, dry and hacking versus paroxysmal and productive), description of any sputum produced, frequency, and duration. Occasionally patients experience complications or pathological consequences of coughing, especially if the cough is paroxysmal and strong. The following list describes some of the more common complications that therapists need to be aware of.

1. *Pulmonary:* spontaneous pneumothorax; hemoptysis; reversal of mucociliary clearance (in COPD with paroxysmal cough)
2. *Cardiovascular:* hypertension; bradycardia
3. *Central nervous system:* syncope
4. *Musculoskeletal:* rib fracture; costochondritis; intercostal muscle spasm or strain

The assessment of a patient's ineffective cough should concentrate on determining at what phase the cough mechanism is impaired. The inspiratory phase may be insufficient if the patient is unable to take a deep breath. Examples of problems that can interfere with a deep inspiration include chronic lung diseases (obstructive and restrictive), restriction of ventilatory capacity because of neuromuscular or musculoskeletal problems, and splinting after abdominal or thoracic surgery.

Patients who are unable to close their glottises can still cough effectively, but the cough (or huff) requires substantially more muscle contraction and cannot be sustained very long. Central nervous system disorders are the usual cause of incomplete closure of the glottis. The compressive phase may be further impaired by a patient's inability to contract the expiratory or abdominal muscles to sufficiently increase intrathoracic pressure. Weak or paralyzed muscles are the more common reasons for this. The ability to contract the muscles of the pelvic floor is also important for maximum effectiveness of phases two and three of the cough mechanism.

Impairment of phase three, the expiratory phase, may also be caused by pain secondary to recent surgery or trauma. Conditions that decrease expiratory flow rates in general, such as asthma and severe emphysema, can also result in decreased force of the expiratory phase of a cough.

Occasionally miscellaneous factors such as poor motivation, inappropriate posture or position, and very thick mucus also impair cough effectiveness. Once a therapist establishes where in the cough sequence the problem arises, specific compensatory or therapeutic manouvers can be determined.

If the cough is productive of sputum, the volume, consistency, color, odor, and source should be assessed and documented. Assessment of sputum is also important as a reflection of the effectiveness of bronchial drainage treatment.

In neonates, the sneeze reflex is more developed than the cough reflex. Ability to stimulate a cough reflex may be helpful to assess during the initial evaluation of an infant with impaired airway clearance.

PREOPERATIVE ASSESSMENT

Patients who undergo upper abdominal and thoracic surgery are at greater risk for developing postoperative pulmonary complications. A physical therapy evaluation preoperatively should include (but not be limited to) observation and inspection; auscultation; palpation of chest wall motion and symmetry; cough; gross range of motion (especially the shoulders if a thoracotomy incision is anticipated); a preoperative measurement of inspiratory capacity (with an incentive spirometer if it will be used therapeutically postoperatively); a thorough history to help determine increased risk (eg, smoking history); and the patient's activity level.

EVALUATION OF OTHER SYSTEMS

Patients with acute and chronic pulmonary dysfunction often have associated or contributory pathologies or abnormalities of other body systems. Assessments of other systems are discussed in detail in other chapters of this text. This brief discussion of assessments of other systems only serves as a reminder of the more common interrelationships between systems.

CARDIOVASCULAR

Heart rate and blood pressure should be routinely assessed, whether or not the patient has a history of cardiovascular disease. A patient with congestive heart failure may have pedal edema (or presacral edema if on bed rest). Patients with COPD often have tachycardia (to compensate for low PaO_2) and may have frequent premature ventricular contractions (PVCs) on electrocardiogram, especially during exercise.

MUSCULOSKELETAL

Posture should be assessed more formally than by observation in patients who appear to have abnormalities. Range of motion and strength should not be overlooked, especially if the therapist has reason to believe the patient may have limitations secondary to musculoskeletal compromise. Gait can also be assessed if appropriate. Some musculoskeletal abnormalities may affect positioning of the patient for treatment and how well and how soon a patient can be moved out of bed.

NEUROMUSCULAR

Assessment of the patient's general neurologic status is imperative. All central nervous system disorders and most peripheral problems would significantly influence the treatment plan. Paralysis, paresis, spasticity, and flaccidity all may affect the patient's respiratory status. Intracranial pressure may need to be closely monitored in patients with head trauma and other cranial vascular conditions.

DIGESTIVE

A therapist who is preparing to treat a patient in a Trendelenberg's position (head down) needs to know how long it has been since the patient ate. If the patient has a gastrostomy or nasogastric tube, the feeding schedule is important to determine.

EXERCISE AND ENDURANCE TESTING

The general physical therapy goals of exercise training in patients with chronic lung disease are similar to those for all patients with decreased exercise tolerance and reduced functional levels. In contrast, the *mechanisms* by which the goals are accomplished are very different. Similarly, the exercise tests that precede development of an exercise program for a patient with chronic lung disease (CLD) have distinct differences from tests administered to other types of patients.

The literature is currently teeming with new information about respiratory muscles; respiratory muscle function, fatigue, and contribution to dyspnea; and exercise testing and exercise training of patients with pulmonary disease. The fact is, there is still much we do not know about these topics.

EXERCISE TESTING PATIENTS WITH CLD

The types of exercise tests used for testing patients with CLD range from simple to complex. Examples of commonly used exercise tests are described in this section. The advantages and disadvantages of each test are presented. The tests described include treadmill, bicycle ergometer, 12- and 6-minute walk, and 100-m walk. In addition to the above tests, special studies that help determine exercise-induced bronchoconstriction and step tests are briefly discussed.

Monitoring in Pulmonary Exercise Testing

Patients with CLD are generally older (over 50 years of age) and are more likely to have concomitant cardiovascular disease (secondary to age, smoking history, and long-term effects of CLD on the cardiovascular system). Therefore, I strongly recommend that any patient with moderate or severe CLD or one who is over 40 years of age receive an initial monitored, multistage, graded exercise test to rule out significant cardiovascular compromise or symptoms.

Special monitoring techniques for patients with pulmonary dysfunction are discussed later in this chapter. The parameters that can be measured or derived during exercise testing of patients with chronic pulmonary disease are summarized in the following list.

1. Cardiac
   - Electrocardiogram
   - Heart rate
   - Blood pressure
   - Hemodynamic measures (eg, cardiac output, pulmonary arterial pressure, wedge pressure—infrequently done)
2. Respiratory gas exchange
   - Oxygen uptake ($\dot{V}O_2$ and $\dot{V}O_{2\ max}$)
   - Arterial blood gases (PaO_2; $PaCO_2$)
   - Oxygen saturation ($O_{2\ sat}$)
   - Transcutaneous oxygen (TcO_2)
   - Respiratory exchange ratio (R)
   - Anaerobic threshold
3. Ventilation
   - Respiratory rate (RR)
   - Minute ventilation ($\dot{V}_E$)
   - Tidal volume (TV)

Level Course Tests

Exercise tests that use a level course include the 12-minute, 6-minute, and the 100-m walk tests. Walk tests are used to quantify the effects of disease on exercise tolerance (or measure functional impairment) and have been used very successfully in patients with CLD. The advantages of level course tests include low cost, little to no equipment necessary, several patients can be tested simultaneously, easy administration, and no training of the patient is required. Disadvantages include inability to monitor cardiovascular or respiratory signs continuously, space needed for walk course, and increased likelihood of motivation and attitude influences on performance on a self-paced test.

The *12-minute walk test* involves accurate measurement of a "course," which can be indoors or outdoors, but must be level. The distance is usually measured in yards or meters. The patient is instructed to walk as far as pos-

sible in 12 minutes. The distance is then measured and serves as a baseline of exercise capacity. Heart rate, blood pressure, respiratory rate, level of dyspnea, and oxygen saturation should be monitored before and immediately after the test. Studies have shown that at least one or two practice attempts should be provided the first time this test is administered to obtain the most accurate "best effort." During the 12-minute walk, patients may need to stop periodically. This is permitted, but no extra time is allowed. The supervision of this test may include verbal encouragement to optimize performance. It is essential that such encouragement be controlled in some way so subsequent testing can be accurately compared.

It is possible for patients to reach and sustain steady-state values of ventilation and oxygen consumption ($\dot{V}O_2$) during a 12-minute walk test. This has not been demonstrated in shorter timed tests such as the six-minute and two-minute walk tests. Based on my personal experiences with both the 12-minute and 6-minute walk tests, the 12-minute walk appears to be a more accurate reflection of the functional capacity of patients with chronic pulmonary disease.

The *100-m walk test* is another level course test that has been shown to be reproducible, and the results are highly correlated with the 12-minute walk. The 100-m walk differs from the other level course tests in that the distance walked is fixed but the time is variable. When administering the 100-m walk, the patient should be timed for three repetitions of the test with at least 10 minutes' rest between. The time recorded for the third trial is considered the most reliable measure in the 100-m walk test. This test may be preferable when the patient is more severely compromised and may have difficulty completing the 12-minute walk test.

Graded Standardized Tests

Graded exercise tests using a treadmill or bicycle ergometer test exercise tolerance at progressive intensities. Unlike the walk tests, pace (or intensity of work) is imposed. Testing on a treadmill or bicycle ergometer generally allows more complex and continuous physiologic monitoring to take place.

Treadmill Testing

A treadmill is easily calibrated and provides a functional and familiar form of exercise (Fig. 30-31). Patients tend to perform at their highest level of $\dot{V}O_2$ on a treadmill. Disadvantages are that the treadmill is large, noisy, and expensive, and requires familiarizing the patient with the apparatus.

A variety of protocols can be used for testing. Patients with CLD who tend to be limited by their reduced ventilatory capacities generally test better with modified exercise test protocols. The duration of each intensity level affects the patient's ability to reach steady state. The modified standardized protocols decrease duration from three to two minutes. The modified Bruce, Balke, or Naughton protocols can all be used for testing pulmonary patients. Other protocols that involve increasing the speed and not the percent grade may also be better tolerated by the patient with CLD.

Bicycle Ergometer Testing

A bicycle ergometer is smaller and quieter than a treadmill (Fig. 30-32). Monitoring is somewhat easier with an ergometer because less artifact is produced (the patient moves around less). Arterial blood samples can be drawn more easily during a bicycle ergometer test. The major disadvantages are that the seat may be very uncomfortable, and for many patients bicycling is not a familiar activity.

Standardized protocols can be used with a bicycle ergometer. The most common protocols increase work loads at 50 to 100 kilopondmeters/min or 17 W every two minutes.

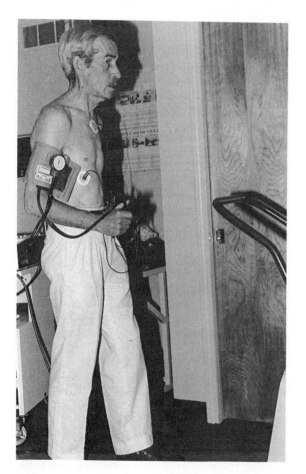

Figure 30-31. Patient on a treadmill for exercise testing.

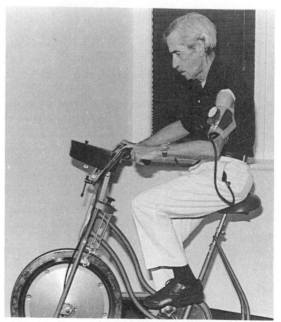

Figure 30-32. Patient on a bicycle ergometer.

Step Tests

Step tests (Fig. 30-33), which are at a single work load or progressive work loads, are frequently discussed in the literature. Advantages include low expense and simplicity. Disadvantages are that monitoring (especially blood pressure) is more difficult or impossible and the work loads tested are often high to begin with. These work loads are usually too high for most patients with CLD. Therefore, it is difficult for a patient with CLD to reach a steady state during these tests. The reliability of these tests is also questionable, because there tends to be a large variation in performance from one trial to another.

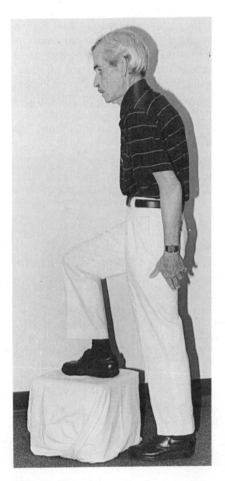

Figure 30-33. Step test.

Tests for Exercise-Induced Bronchoconstriction

Asthma or bronchospasm triggered by exercise is actually probably triggered by airway cooling and drying, which occurs with a high minute ventilation ($\dot{V}_E$). Determination of airway lability in response to exercise is currently done with a combination of pulmonary function tests and an exercise challenge test. Challenge tests for exercise-induced asthma (EIA) are done on both the treadmill and bicycle ergometer using relatively high work loads, which rapidly progress to get the desired effect. These challenge tests are also helpful in testing the effectiveness of certain medications in suppressing EIA.

Use of Oxygen During Exercise Testing

Occasionally patients are exercise tested with low-flow oxygen after they have been previously tested without oxygen. Patients who are hypoxemic at rest (PaO_2 <60 mm Hg) are also tested with oxygen. Oxygen decreases pulmonary vascular resistance and decreases afterload to the right ventricle, enabling an increase in cardiac output. Oxygen use during testing helps determine if the patient benefits from its administration and what concentration the patient should use during exercise training.

SPECIFIC RESPIRATORY MUSCLE TESTS

Patients with COPD have significantly altered respiratory muscle function coupled with increased work of breathing. Table 30-11 presents some major determinants of respiratory muscle energy requirements. Weakness and fatigue of the inspiratory muscles, especially the diaphragm, are therefore common in patients with obstructive disease.

Patients with diseases and abnormalities besides COPD can also exhibit inspiratory muscle weakness and loss of endurance. Some of these conditions include long-term mechanical ventilation; spinal cord injury; extremely deconditioned patients; kyphoscoliosis; and chronic neuromuscular diseases such as Guillain-Barré syndrome, myasthenia gravis, and muscular dystrophy.

Table 30-11. Determinants of Inspiratory Muscle Energy Requirements

Work of Breathing

1. Minute ventilation ($\dot{V}_E$) = tidal volume (TV) × frequency (RR)
2. Lung and chest wall compliance
3. Resistance of the muscles of respiration

Respiratory Muscle Strength and Endurance

1. Length:tension ratio
2. Muscle loss due to atrophy, neuromuscular disease, or malnutrition

Efficiency of the Muscles

1. Deconditioned peripheral muscles
2. Respiratory muscle length, angle of pull, and resistance

(After Braun N: Respiratory muscle dysfunction. Heart Lung 3(4):327, 1984)

Assessment of inspiratory muscle strength (or power) and endurance should be done if abnormality is suspected and quantification is desired. The outcome of specific ventilatory muscle training programs cannot be fully documented without measures that reflect ventilatory muscle strength and endurance. Exercise testing is an indirect method of assessing respiratory muscle function. Direct measurements of strength and endurance are also available.

Testing Respiratory Muscle Strength

Maximum inspiratory (MIP or $P_{I\,max}$) and expiratory pressures ($P_{E\,max}$) are the measures used to indicate strength of the inspiratory and expiratory muscles, respectively. These static pressures provide a quantitative assessment of the potential force available to generate ventilation.

Maximal inspiratory and expiratory pressures are measured with an aneroid vacuum pressure gauge (inspiration) or static pressure manometer (inspiration and expiration).

Maximum inspiratory pressures are measured from either FRC (patient breathes out normal tidal breath before inspiring against the mouthpiece) or RV (patient breathes out as much air as possible before inspiring). Maximum expiratory pressure is measured from TLC (patient takes as deep a breath as possible before expiring). The patient's position can affect the measurement, so it is very important that retesting always occur in the same posi-

tion. The patient should also wear noseclips to prevent inadvertent nose breathing during the testing manouvers.

Measurement of $P_{I\,max}$ and $P_{E\,max}$ is done against an occluded airway, so patients should be warned that they will get resistance and not move any air. Three trials are done for each measurement and the best value is recorded.

Normal values for $P_{I\,max}$ are approximately -80 ± 20 cm H_2O. Maximal expiratory pressures ($P_{E\,max}$) normally have a range of about 140 ± 30 cm H_2O.

Testing Respiratory Muscle Endurance

Endurance of the ventilatory muscles (primarily diaphragm) has to do with how long a patient can breathe at a certain intensity. Intensity in this case can be related to a percent of the maximal voluntary ventilation (MVV) or the resistance to inspiration.

Inspiratory muscle endurance can be tested in a similar manner as graded exercise endurance. Equipment needed includes nose clips and a testing or training device. Inspiratory muscle training devices can be custom made, or commercially available devices can be used (Fig. 30-34). A device like the PFLEX* has six varied diameter resistances for testing.

The patient should be seated comfortably with the nose clips in place. The device is set at the widest diameter or lowest resistance. The

*Health Scan Inc., Upper Montclair, NJ 07043

patient places the mouthpiece in her mouth and breathes in and out at a comfortable rate and depth. After 10 minutes the resistance is increased by dialing the next largest diameter orifice. The test continues in this manner until the patient indicates that she is uncomfortably short of breath or complains of dizziness or a headache. The endurance level is recorded as the number of minutes (out of 10) completed at each setting (or resistance level).

Patients should be warned to anticipate drooling during this test, and tissues should be provided. Water should also be available for the patient once the test is completed.

This test provides a baseline of ventilatory muscle endurance to compare against after training has taken place. This test also helps the therapist determine the appropriate setting (or resistance) to prescribe for the patient's training program. Usually the resistance at which the patient last completed a full 10 minutes during testing is set as the training resistance (eg, if the patient completed four minutes at setting 5, the training setting would be 4).

Resistance to inspiration is best provided by a certain diameter valve through which the patient inhales. The narrower the orifice, the higher the resistance. Some investigators have tried to provide inspiratory resistance with weights over the upper abdomen (with the patient supine). This form of resistance to the diaphragm is only valid for patients with spinal cord injury above the level of T10. If the abdominal muscles are intact, the patient could raise the abdominal weights with assistance from the abdominal muscles, instead of the result of the diaphragm descending against the intra-abdominal resistance created by the external weights.

SPECIAL MONITORING FOR PATIENTS WITH PULMONARY DYSFUNCTION

Impaired ventilatory mechanics and abnormal gas exchange are primary limitations to exercise performance in patients with CLD. There-

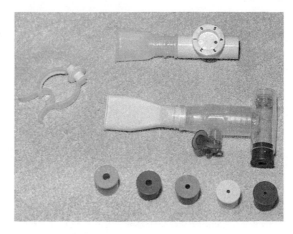

Figure 30-34. Two types of hand-held inspiratory muscle training devices (PFLEX and DHD).

fore, levels of dyspnea and hypoxemia are of great interest to anyone who is evaluating exercise tolerance in these patients. Monitoring of perception of dyspnea, ear oximetry, and transcutaneous oximetry may be done during exercise testing of patients with pulmonary disease.

PERCEPTION OF DYSPNEA

Dyspnea during exercise in a patient with respiratory disease is a complex issue that is currently being widely investigated. Many factors contribute to respiratory effort sensation, including respiratory muscle fatigue and the relationship between inspiratory time and total time of a respiratory cycle.

In patients with lung disease, quantification of level of dyspnea may be a more important indicator of exercise tolerance than heart rate, ECG, and even oxygen uptake. Quantification of the magnitude of dyspnea or breathlessness is generally done using a modified Borg scale (Table 30-12). This scale is a modification of the scale commonly used in exercise testing to quantify overall perception of effort. The scale is an ordinal scale with relative distances between points. At each intensity or at certain time intervals during an exercise test,

Table 30-12. Modified Borg Scale for Perception of Dyspnea

ORDINAL	MAGNITUDE OF DYSPNEA
0	Nothing at all
1	Very slight
2	Slight
3	
4	Moderate
5	Somewhat severe
6	Severe
7	
8	Very severe
9	
10	Maximal

the examiner asks the patient to pick a number from the scale that best reflects the level of breathlessness experienced.

EAR OXIMETRY

An ear oximeter measures oxygen saturation of arterialized capillaries in the pinna of the ear. Ear oximetry is noninvasive and continuous. The earpiece can be held in place during exercise with a special headpiece. Ear oximetry is an important adjunct to ventilatory and hemodynamic monitoring during exercise testing.

One note of caution needs to be made for anyone using an ear oximeter. The relationship between oxygen saturation and PaO_2 depends on pH and $PaCO_2$. Unless an arterial blood gas is drawn to determine blood pH, PaO_2 cannot be directly predicted. The shape of the oxygen-hemoglobin dissociation curve means that PaO_2 can decrease dramatically along the flat portion of the curve with little corresponding change in oxygen saturation. Conversely, oxygen saturation can change dramatically with relatively little decrease in PaO_2 on the steep portion of the curve. An oxygen saturation level of 80% is considered to be a stopping point for exercise because that value usually "sits" on the curve where saturation can drop rapidly.

TRANSCUTANEOUS OXYGEN MONITORING

Transcutaneous monitoring of oxygen and carbon dioxide has been used for several years in pediatric and neonatal intensive care units. Transcutaneous oxygen (TcO_2) monitoring involves placing a heated electrode on the skin where the epidermis is thin (chest, abdomen, or back). The heated electrode arterializes the capillaries and directly measures partial pressure of oxygen. The values of TcO_2 are lower than corresponding PaO_2 values because some gas is absorbed by the skin. The correlation between arterial and transcutaneous oxygen values is very high.

Transcutaneous monitoring is advantageous because it is noninvasive, continuous, and simple. One major disadvantage is the high cost of the monitor (especially when compared to the ear oximeter). Transcutaneous oximetry has more recently been investigated during exercise testing of adults. The correlations between TcO_2 and PaO_2 values before, during, and after exercise in adult subjects were high (0.91–0.96).

Transcutaneous oxygen monitoring is much more sensitive in detecting changes in the upper ranges of PaO_2 (60–100 mm Hg). It is important also that a baseline arterial blood gas be obtained so the ratio between the TcO_2 and PaO_2 values can be determined. This ratio will vary from patient to patient.

CONCLUSION

Physical therapy evaluation and analysis of movement dysfunction and physical disability of patients with pulmonary dysfunction is both unique and interrelated. Some tests and measures are specific for these patients, whereas others are general assessments that are adapted for this patient population.

The execution and interpretation of these assessments require a good understanding of anatomy, physiology, and pathology of the respiratory system. More importantly, the physical therapist must understand how pulmonary dysfunction affects the patient's ability to participate in any therapy program. Physical therapists cannot afford to ignore the respiratory system and still hope to manage their patients adequately. The data obtained from physical therapy evaluation of pulmonary patients are used to develop safe and appropriate treatment programs.

ANNOTATED BIBLIOGRAPHY

American Physical Therapy Association: Physical Therapy Monograph: Respiratory Care. Phys Ther 61(12):1709–1782, 1981; pp 1–78, 1982 (This monograph is from the only special issue on respiratory care published in the physical therapy profession's professional journal.)

American Thoracic Society: Exercise testing in the dyspneic patient. Am Rev Respir Dis [Suppl] 129:SIS100, 1984 (This special issue, the second of two parts, presents important and accurate state-of-the-art information about exercise testing of the patient with pulmonary dysfunction. A wealth of references in one issue.)

Bates B: The thorax and lungs. In A Guide to Physical Examination and History Taking, 4th ed. Philadelphia, JB Lippincott, 1987 (The information and illustrations in this book are excellent and at an appropriate level for physical therapists. The chapter on examination of the thorax and lungs is especially helpful, with an excellent review of surface anatomy.)

Cherniack RM, Cherniack L, Naimark A: Respiration in Health and Disease, 2nd ed. Philadelphia, WB Saunders, 1972 (I consider this book a classic and one of the most important references for all health care professionals who manage patients with pulmonary dysfunction. Presents wealth of information that is complete and for the most part timeless.)

Frownfelter DL (ed): Chest Physical Therapy and Pulmonary Rehabilitation: An Interdisciplinary Approach, 2nd ed. Chicago, Year Book, 1987 (An extremely helpful and clinically oriented reference for physical therapists and other providers of respiratory care. Part two of this text specifically relates to the chest assessment; part three includes impor-tant and unique information on the pulmonary management of patients with neurological deficits; and part four provides helpful information about chest roentgenogram interpretation, pulmonary drug actions, and patients with artificial airways.)

Irwin RS, Rosen MJ, Braman SS: Cough: A comprehensive review. Arch Intern Med 137:1186, 1977 (An excellent review article about cough. Anatomy, mechanics, causes, evaluation, complications, and treatment of cough are included.)

Irwin S, Tecklin JS (eds): Cardiopulmonary Physical Therapy. St Louis, CV Mosby, 1985 (Another excellent clinically oriented reference, written by and for physical therapists.)

Nursing 84 Books—Nurses' Clinical Library: Respiratory Disorders. Springhouse, PA, Springhouse, 1984 (This book is written primarily for nurses, but the level and extent of the content are both very appropriate for physical therapists. Has excellent color photographs and tables and figures that are particularly helpful in understanding the medical and surgical tests and measurements done for patients with respiratory disorders.)

Shapiro BA, Harrison RA, Walter JR: Clinical Application of Blood Gases, 2nd ed. Chicago, Year Book, 1977 (Presents the complicated topic of arterial blood gas interpretation in a complete, clear, and understandable way. The text is clinically oriented and provides many examples.)

Symposium on Exercise: Physiology and Clinical Applications: Proceedings. Clin Chest Med 5(1):1–210, 1984 (The proceeding papers of the symposium contained in this volume provide excellent state-of-the-art references on respiratory muscle function, physiology of exercise, and exercise testing of patients with pulmonary disease.)

Wasserman K, Whipp BJ: State of the Art: Exercise physiology in health and disease. Am Rev Respir Dis 112:219, 1975 (This classic article provides excellent physiologic information regarding the requirements for exercise, the interrelationship of body systems, and the effects of disease on exercise performance.)

31 Integumentary Analysis

SUSAN A. BEMIS
MARTHA L. RAMMEL

In this chapter, we focus on the evaluation of sensorimotor dysfunction caused by defects in the integumentary system resulting from neurovascular ulcers and burn injuries. The physical therapist's role in the management of the patient with integumentary dysfunction emphasizes prevention of secondary sensorimotor dysfunction during both the acute and posthealing phases of such injuries. Although we discuss how to determine the extent, depth, and severity of skin wounds, the physician typically performs these evaluations and includes the results in the medical record. Assessing the *effects* on movement and function of the extent, depth, and severity of skin wounds remains the goal of the physical therapist's evaluation. The information gained through that assessment allows the physical therapist to identify movement dysfunction appropriately and develop a plan of care to prevent secondary dysfunction and to restore lost function.

EFFECTS OF SKIN WOUNDS ON THE STRUCTURE AND FUNCTION OF THE SKIN

Knowing and understanding the structure and function of the skin allows the physical therapist to identify potential secondary sensorimotor dysfunction and potential physiological and psychological problems that affect the physical therapy management of the patient with extensive skin injury. In this section, we relate skin structure and function to movement dysfunction and physical disability.

Skin wounds that involve only the epidermal layer have minimal effect on movement and function. These wounds are caused primarily by overexposure to sunlight (infrared rays), and most often result in decreased movement of the involved parts because of discomfort. Long-term movement dysfunction does not happen because epithelialization of the damaged layer occurs rapidly (within 7 to 10 days).

Wounds that extend into the dermal layer result in moderate to severe dysfunction, depending on the extent and depth of the injury. Such damage affects all of the physiologic functions of the skin: protection from infection, prevention of fluid loss, regulation of body temperature, sensory perception, and determination of self-image. Mild to severe movement dysfunction and physical disability occur because of pain, immobilization, secondary infection, muscle atrophy, and scarring. Healing occurs either by epithelialization from deep epidermal elements (the lining of hair follicles, sweat glands, and sebacous glands) or by skin grafting. These forms of healing require from two to three weeks or several months, depending on the depth and extent of the injury.

Injuries that extend through the dermal layer and into the subcutaneous layer result in moderate to severe dysfunction, depending on the extent of the wound. Such wounds destroy

587

all of the skin elements and disrupt all of the physiologic functions of the skin. Moderate to severe movement dysfunction and physical disability occur. The severity of the dysfunction and disability depend on the extent of the injury and the body part involved. Secondary involvement of the cardiopulmonary, musculoskeletal, and neurosensory systems may also be severe, and can have a great impact on physical therapy management through the acute and posthealing phases.

CLASSIFICATION OF NEUROVASCULAR ULCERS

Skin ulcers are classified according to etiology. Vascular ulcers that result from arterial or venous insufficiency most commonly occur in the distal lower extremities because of small vessel disease. Trophic ulcers (also termed decubitus ulcers or pressure sores) usually occur over bony prominences as a result of impaired sensation. Patients with impaired sensation fail to sense the discomfort associated with excessive pressure and do not shift weight off the involved area, whereas the person with an intact neurosensory system would initiate movement. Further, the vascular structures in denervated skin do not respond as well as normally innervated skin to the ischemia caused by sustained pressure. Thus, trophic ulcers occur. Table 31-1 describes the distinguishing characteristics of arterial, venous, and trophic ulcers.

Evaluation of neurovascular ulcers includes observation and measurement of the lesion, assessment of the vascular integrity of the part, and assessment of the functional ability of the involved extremity. The therapist should carefully document the appearance of the ulcer, noting size, color, location, texture, and drainage. Functional limitations such as range of motion loss, motor weakness, and gait deviations should also be assessed. The therapist should palpate the distal pulses (dorsalis pedis and posterior tibial) to determine the integrity of the arterial system in the lower extremities. Diabetic ulcers commonly occur in the lower leg and foot secondary to the peripheral neu-

ropathy and vasculitis associated with diabetes. Thus, diabetic ulcers may demonstrate characteristics of both vascular and trophic ulcers. These ulcers often become infected because of the increased sugar content in tissue fluids, which provides an excellent medium for bacterial growth. Signs of wound infection may include noxious odor, continuous wound drainage consisting of a viscous or purulent exudate, delayed wound closure, and other signs of inflammation, such as peripheral redness and pain.

Small infected lesions located in the genital or rectal areas may indicate the presence of a fistula. A fistula connects a deeper internal lesion with the skin surface in an attempt to evacuate the infected area. The therapist should estimate the depth of the wound by digital palpation using sterile technique. This information is needed to ensure thorough cleansing and packing of the infected wound.

Other skin ulcerations not necessarily localized over the distal extremities or bony prominences may represent signs of specific dermatological or systemic disorders, such as cancer or rheumatic disease. The location and appearance of these lesions, and the general condition of the skin should be included with the other objective data gathered during the evaluation. If a review of the medical record fails to reveal a notation about the presence or cause of such lesions, the therapist should consult with the patient's primary physician.

CLASSIFICATION OF BURN INJURIES

Each year, over 2 million persons in the United States sustain burn injuries. Of these, at least 100,000 persons require hospitalization (Artz and colleagues). Because of advances in life support measures, development of effective antibacterial topical agents, and improvements in surgical techniques over the past 20 years, more patients survive severe burn injuries. Physical therapists have also become increasingly involved because patients with burns have the potential to develop severe movement dysfunction and physical disability. Effective

Table 31-1. Common Ulcers of the Feet and Ankles

CHRONIC VENOUS INSUFFICIENCY	ARTERIAL INSUFFICIENCY	TROPHIC ULCER

Location Inner, sometimes outer ankle	Toes, feet, or possibly in areas of trauma (eg, the shin)	Pressure points in areas with diminished sensation, as in diabetic polyneuropathy
Skin Surrounding the Ulcer Pigmented, sometimes fibrotic	No callus or excess of pigment; may be atrophic	Calloused
Pain Not severe	Often severe, unless neuropathy masks it	Absent (and therefore the ulcer may go unnoticed)
Associated Gangrene Absent	May be present	In uncomplicated trophic ulcer, absent
Associated Signs Edema, pigmentation, stasis dermatitis, and, possibly, cyanosis of the foot on dependency	Decreased pulses, trophic changes, pallor of the foot on elevation, dusky or cyanotic rubor on dependency	Decreased sensation, ankle jerks absent

(Bates B: A Guide to Physical Examination and History Taking, 4th ed, p 421. Philadelphia, JB Lippincott, 1987)

physical therapy management depends on evaluation of the musculoskeletal, cardiopulmonary, and neurosensory status of these patients.

Regardless of the cause of the injury, the effective management of a patient with burn wounds requires the assessment of the severity of the injury. Five factors influence the severity of a burn injury: (1) extent of the burn wound, (2) depth of the burn wound, (3) age of the patient, (4) past medical history, and (5) part of the body injured. The therapist should consider these factors collectively when evaluating the severity of a burn.

The extent of a burn wound is expressed as a percent of the total body surface area (%TBSA). Emergency care personnel employ one of two methods to determine the extent of a burn wound. Both methods require the use of diagrams that outline the anterior and posterior parts of the body and indicate the percent value of each part. The evaluator draws the location of the burn wound on the diagram, and then calculates the %TBSA based on that drawing.

The rule of nines divides the body into multiples of nine (Fig. 31-1). This method allows rapid calculation of an estimate of the extent of the burn. The head and upper extremities each represent 9% of the body surface. The lower extremities, the anterior trunk, and the posterior trunk each represent 18% of the body surface. These areas account for 99% of the body surface, and the perineum accounts for the remaining 1%. The advantage of the rule of nines lies in its use for a rapid determination of

the extent of a burn injury. However, it does not allow for differences in the proportion of the size of the head and lower extremities in infants and children as compared to adults; thus, it is inaccurate for these age groups.

The Lund-Browder method uses figures and tables that take into account the age-related changes in the proportion of the lower extremities and the head. For example, the head is twice as large in a child compared to an adult, while the proportion of the upper extremities to the trunk remains the same throughout life (Fig. 31-2). Although this method requires more time to determine the %TBSA, it offers a more accurate assessment of the extent of the injury.

Figure 31-1. The rule of nines.

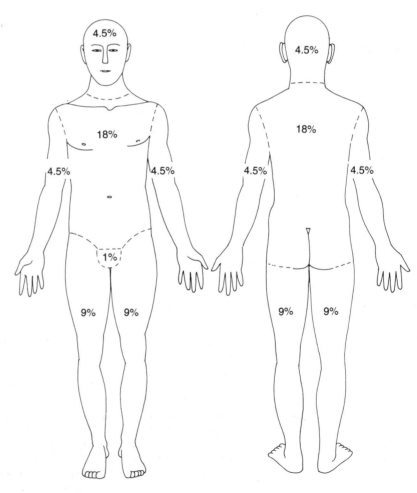

Current terminology classifies burn wounds as either partial-thickness or full-thickness defects. The historical classification of burn wounds into first, second, third, and fourth degree injuries attempted to classify them according to the depth of tissue injury. However, these terms did not accurately describe the depth of injury; rather, they merely described the visual characteristics of the wound. The current classification of partial-thickness wounds includes the categories of first- and second-degree wounds, and full-thickness wounds includes the categories of third- and fourth-degree wounds.

The differential diagnosis of an acute burn wound requires visual and physical assessment of the injured area. The signs and symptoms outlined in Table 31-2 offer the most accurate assessment of the depth of a burn wound during the immediate postburn phase. These signs and symptoms allow an accurate estimate of the depth of a burn wound in most cases. Severe scald burn injuries are an exception, because they may actually cause full-thickness skin loss but appear only as a red, discolored surface. However, the surface of this burn will not blanch and refill with pressure, as a partial-thickness burn would.

Partial-thickness wounds may be classified as superficial or deep. Superficial partial-thickness burns (eg, sunburn) destroy the epidermis, or the epidermis and a thin layer of the

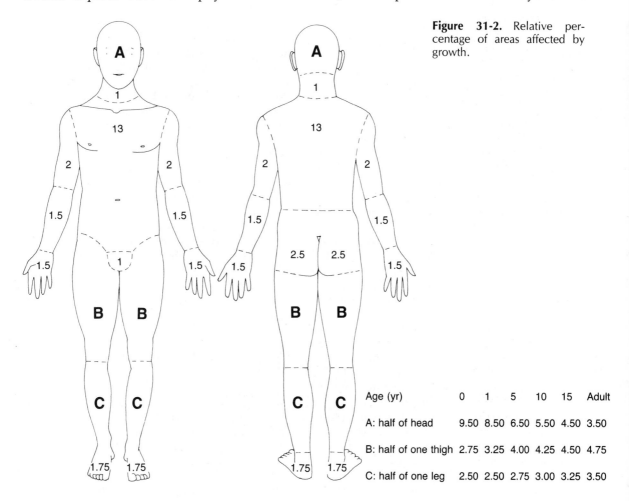

Figure 31-2. Relative percentage of areas affected by growth.

Age (yr)	0	1	5	10	15	Adult
A: half of head	9.50	8.50	6.50	5.50	4.50	3.50
B: half of one thigh	2.75	3.25	4.00	4.25	4.50	4.75
C: half of one leg	2.50	2.50	2.75	3.00	3.25	3.50

Table 31-2. Differential Diagnosis of Depth of Burn Injury

PARTIAL-THICKNESS BURN	FULL-THICKNESS BURN
Sensation	
Normal or increased sensitivity to pain and temperature	Anesthetic to pain and temperature; will not display pain response when hair removed in area of burn
Blisters	
Large, thick-walled; will usually increase in size over first 48 hours	None, or if present thin walled and will not increase in size
Color	
Burn surface red, will blanch with pressure and refill	Burn surface white, brown, black, or red; if red, will not blanch with pressure
Texture	
Skin surface normal or firm; moist	Skin surface firm or leathery; dry

dermis. Although these injuries destroy the superficial dermis, the deeper dermal elements will recover and provide normal skin. A deep partial-thickness burn destroys the epidermis and part of the dermis. Although these burns damage some dermal elements, other dermal elements remain viable and provide tissue for spontaneous healing.

Full-thickness burns destroy all of the epidermis and dermis, and damage the underlying tissue. Spontaneous healing does not occur. This burn wound requires debridement of nonviable tissue and autografting for healing to occur.

The age of the patient sustaining a burn represents the third important factor in determining the severity of a burn wound. Infants and children under two years of age and persons over 60 years of age demonstrate a higher mortality rate than other age groups with injuries of a similar size. Young children and older adults have thinner and more fragile skin than persons in other age groups, which leads to a more severe injury from a like cause. In addition, a poor antibody response to infection in infants results in less resistance and leads to

septicemia. In older adults, exacerbation of latent degenerative processes may lead to severe morbidity and death.

Appropriate assessment of the medical history of the patient with a burn identifies recent or latent disease processes that may become exacerbated by the physiologic stress caused by a burn injury. For example, a full-thickness injury of 20% TBSA results in a more severe injury in the person with diabetes than in a healthy person of the same age. In addition, the presence of a latent or active disease process (eg, cardiac or pulmonary dysfunction) may affect the patient's ability to carry out a physical therapy program during the acute or healing phases.

The location of the burn wound also affects the severity of the injury. Burns of the face, head, neck, and chest lead to an increased incidence of pulmonary problems. Perineal burns tend to become easily infected. Skin thickness varies on the human body: For example, the skin on the sole of the foot, palm of the hand, buttocks, and back is thicker than that of the face, forearm, abdomen, and dorsum of the hand. Burns that involve areas with thinner skin are considered more severe. From the physical therapist's point of view, burns that involve joint surfaces also add to the severity of the injury and increase the potential for long-term dysfunction.

The American Burn Association classifies the severity of burn injuries as minor, moderate, and major (Table 31-3). All persons sustaining major burn injuries and most with moderate burn injuries require hospitalization. Some moderate and most minor burns are easily managed on an outpatient basis.

TYPES OF BURN INJURIES

Excessive heat (thermal) is the most common cause of burn injury. The most common thermal injury occurs when the skin is exposed to flame, often the result of the person's clothing catching on fire. Such wounds have irregular borders, and the depth of the injury varies. Flash burns occur with the sudden explosion or ignition of gases. All exposed surfaces tend to

Table 31-3. American Burn Association Classification of Burn Severity

Minor Burn

15% TBSA* Partial-thickness burn in an adult
10% TBSA Partial-thickness burn in a child
2% TBSA Full-thickness burn in child or adult not involving eyes, ears, face, or genitalia

Moderate Burn

15% to 20% TBSA Partial-thickness burn in an adult
10% to 20% TBSA Partial-thickness burn in a child
2% to 10% TBSA Full-thickness burn in a child or adult not involving eyes, ears, face, or genitalia

Major Burn

25% TBSA Partial-thickness burn in an adult
20% TBSA Partial-thickness burn in a child
All full-thickness burns greater than 10% TBSA
All burns involving hands, face, eyes, ears, feet, or genitalia
All inhalation injuries
Electrical burns
Burn injuries complicated by fractures or other major trauma
All poor-risk individuals: for example, preexisting conditions such as CVA, psychiatric disability, emphysema or lung disease, cardiovascular disease, cancer, diabetes

*TBSA, total body surface area

be burned uniformly, and flash burns usually result in partial-thickness skin damage. Contact burns from hot objects (typically, molten metals) result in deep, sharply circumscribed wounds that destroy all the skin elements and involve underlying structures (ie, muscle, bone, and tendon). Disability in these patients results from the extreme depth of the wound.

Scald burns from contact with hot liquids most often occur in infants and young children. A scald of exposed skin results in a superficial wound that heals with minimal or no scarring in 10 to 14 days. Scalds where the hot liquid remains in contact with the skin for an extended time, such as clothing holding the liquid in contact or immersion of the body part in hot liquid, result in sharply demarcated borders and deep partial- or full-thickness injuries.

Chemical substances, such as acids or strong alkalies, cause tissue damage from the interaction of the chemicals and local tissue components, primarily protein. Damage from exposure to chemicals may continue for long periods unless countermeasures, such as washing with copious amounts of water, occur immediately. Chemical burns may be extensive or circumscribed depending on the area exposed, and may result in partial- or full-thickness damage depending on the emergency care received.

Electrical burns occur when the body is exposed to an electrical current. The burn results from the resistance of the local tissue to the passage of the current. Electrical injuries usually cause well-circumscribed, deep injuries involving the underlying muscle, tendon, and bone. Neurovascular structures are also often involved in the injury, which may result in devascularization of entire muscles despite the skin appearing intact. Severe movement dysfunction and physical disability occur in electrical burns because of the extensive nature of the damage to soft tissues.

PHYSICAL THERAPIST'S ASSESSMENT OF BURN INJURIES

The ability to identify potential movement dysfunction or physical disability depends on the physical therapist's knowledge and understanding of burn wound classification, physiological effects, and wound healing. Appropriate assessment of the wound and its effects occurs during the acute and posthealing phases of a burn injury. In addition, the physical therapist should evaluate the effects of the injury on other body systems.

ACUTE WOUND ASSESSMENT

The purpose of wound assessment by the physical therapist during the acute phase of a burn injury is to identify involved areas that might interfere with normal movement patterns in the musculoskeletal, neurosensory, and cardiopulmonary systems. Acute wound assessment consists of visual and physical assessment techniques, and a review of information in the medical record about the extent and depth of the burn wound, the patient's current status (including vital signs and medications), and the patient's medical history.

Movement dysfunction in patients with acute burn injuries primarily results from the effects of immobilization. The patient may be immobilized because of pain, edema, or scarring. The following examples demonstrate these effects. A full-thickness injury involving the anterior arm and forearm, including the antecubital area, will result in an elbow flexion contracture because of the effects of immobilization caused by pain and scarring that occur with the healing of autografts. Burn wounds of the thorax and posterior trunk, regardless of depth, may interfere with normal chest expansion and lead to decreased ventilatory capacity. Burns that involve the entire surface of an extremity may cause neurovascular problems similar to compartment syndromes because of the presence of edema.

The physical therapist is also responsible, as are other members of the health care team, for monitoring the wound for infection. All burn wounds become infected to some extent because of the bacteria we normally carry on our skin. The presence of bacteria in the burn wound assists in the sloughing of necrotic tissue. However, excessive infection damages viable dermal elements, and may convert a partial-thickness injury to a full-thickness injury if bacterial growth remains uncontrolled. In addi-

tion, excessive wound infection can result in a systemic infection (septicemia), which jeopardizes the patient's life. The therapist should note the amount, consistency, color, and odor of the exudate present in the burn wound during the initial evaluation to form a baseline for comparison in subsequent treatment sessions.

POSTHEALING WOUND ASSESSMENT

Once primary wound healing is complete, either by epithelialization or autografting, the therapist must closely monitor secondary tissue changes when providing appropriate follow-up care. The collagen tissue in a burn scar may require up to two years to mature. During its immature stages, collagen will continue to form abundantly in a disorganized manner, which may produce a hypertrophic scar or *keloid*. Keloid formation most often occurs in dark-skinned persons or in those who sustained deeper tissue damage. This abnormal scar tissue tends to contract as it matures, in a further attempt to "close the wound." Unfortunately, this contraction of the superficial tissues tends to further limit the mobility of underlying musculoskeletal structures.

In addition, the process of wound healing results in a thinner, more fragile skin layer that tends to be drier than normal because it lacks natural oils. This fragility makes the skin more susceptible to recurrent trauma. Permanent loss of pigmentation may also occur with some deep partial-thickness and full-thickness wounds.

The healed burn wound may also demonstrate altered sensation. Most patients experience some degree of itching during the early posthealing stage, which may result from both altered sensation and dryness. Many patients demonstrate a mild hyposensitivity to cutaneous stimuli, whereas others may demonstrate a reactive hypersensitivity. Extreme sensitivity with associated pain and edema may indicate a posttraumatic sympathetic dystrophy (PTSD) or a causalgia, both of which require early intervention to prevent severe functional disability.

Chronic movement dysfunction in the posthealing period may result from many factors, including hypertrophic scarring, prolonged immobilization resulting in joint and muscle contractures, and a fear that excessive movement will retraumatize the healed part. The therapist should not only reassess the *quantity* of the motion present during this stage, but also the *quality* of movement.

ASSESSMENT OF SECONDARY SYSTEMIC PROBLEMS

Movement dysfunction occurring in other systems as a result of burn injuries primarily involves the musculoskeletal, neurosensory, cardiovascular, and pulmonary systems. The magnitude of the problems in these systems depends on the severity of the injury and damage to the skin. Other chapters of this book describe in detail the evaluative techniques for these systems. This section focuses on modifications and precautions necessary in evaluating these systems in a patient with burn wounds. Aseptic technique should be used as a standard precaution during the acute stage of any burn injury, whenever the potential exists for the therapist's hands or evaluation instruments to come in contact with the wound.

Musculoskeletal System

Evaluation of strength of the involved areas in a patient with acute burn injuries yields little data that has an impact on physical therapy management. More importantly, application of resistance to involved extremities increases pain. Manual muscle testing or dynamometer testing remains appropriate for uninvolved areas, but the therapist should pay attention to protecting the burn wounds from undue stress or contact with unsterile surfaces. In evaluating range of motion of the involved areas, the therapist should assure that the goniometer does not come in contact with the burn surface. To prevent wound contamination, the therapist should use a sterilized cloth tape measure when taking girth measurements. Again, the therapist should pay careful attention to aseptic technique.

Evaluation of ambulation ability and endurance in the patient with lower extremity burns requires the application of compression dressings prior to standing. During the acute stage of injury, compression dressings prevent excessive bleeding of the damaged tissue and pooling of blood in the lower extremities. During the posthealing or postgrafting stage, compression dressings prevent damage caused by increased capillary pressure, and, as in the acute stage, pooling of blood in the newly healed skin.

Neurosensory System

During the acute stage, evaluation of neurosensory function of the involved areas should be limited to assessing the depth of the wound as indicated by the absence of a pain response in removing hair follicles from the involved skin. The traditional sensory examination yields little reliable data in the acute phase. In the posthealing phase, the therapist may assess the sensory and motor status of the involved areas by modifying techniques to ensure that the fragile skin will not be damaged. Sharp objects or excessively hot objects should not be used during a sensory examination. Accurate assessment of sharp-dull, hot-cold, and two-point discrimination should be sacrificed to ensure the skin will not suffer damage.

Helm and colleagues report that from 15% to 29% of patients with greater than 20% TBSA burns develop diffuse peripheral neuropathies. Additionally, some persons sustain localized peripheral neuropathies because of improper positioning and overly vigorous stretching programs. Nerve conduction velocity testing may be used to evaluate motor function in the posthealing stage without modifying technique. However, before doing the procedure, the therapist should determine whether or not the electrode gel will irritate the newly healed skin.

Cardiovascular System

Initially, during the acute burn injury stage, cardiovascular function is monitored by means of electrocardiographic monitors and central venous pressure (CVP) lines. However, if the patient requires hydrotherapy for wound cleaning, these monitors are disconnected and the therapist should manually monitor the pulse and blood pressure during the tanking procedure. The blood pressure cuff should be used only on an uninvolved extremity. If the burn involves all four extremities, cardiovascular function can be evaluated by assessing the quality of the pulse. These same precautions apply during the subacute and posthealing stages in evaluating cardiovascular function. Using a blood pressure cuff on an extremity with a newly healed or partially healed wound can damage the skin because of the increased capillary pressure that occurs distally when taking blood pressure.

Pulmonary System

The therapist should carefully monitor the status of the pulmonary system in any patient with burns of the trunk, neck, or face, especially if the burns occurred in a confined or enclosed space. Although the airways rarely sustain direct thermal damage, the pulmonary structures often become involved because the patient inhaled noxious gases and particles of burned matter (soot). The noxious gases and soot cause an inflammatory response, resulting in narrowed airways and increased secretion from the glands lining the airways. Soot around the nose and mouth and singed hairs in the nostrils indicate potential airway involvement. The therapist should be alert to signs of respiratory distress in such patients.

Burns of the trunk, whether circumferential or not, often result in decreased chest expansion. The therapist should assess segmental as well as total chest expansion in these patients. The therapist should use a sterile cloth tape measure and wear gloves when assessing chest expansion. Special consideration of hand placement can keep discomfort at a minimum.

CONCLUSION

In this chapter, we have focused on the physical therapist's role in evaluating movement and function in the patient with skin wounds caused by neurovascular dysfunction and thermal injury. However, we caution the reader against emphasizing evaluation of the thermal injury itself because thermal injuries typically involve other systems beyond the injury site, which can result in greater movement dysfunction.

It is important to remember that the physical therapist's role is the evaluation of movement dysfunction to prevent long-term physical disability. Assessment of the *effects* of the extent, depth, and severity of skin wounds on movement and function remains the goal of the physical therapist's evaluation.

ANNOTATED BIBLIOGRAPHY

Artz CP, Moncrief JA, Pruitt BA (eds): Burns: A Team Approach. Philadelphia, WB Saunders, 1979 (Classic and authoritative text on the team management of the patient with burns. Of particular interest to physical therapists are Sections I, General Considerations; III, Local Care; V, Specific Burns; and VII, General Management and Rehabilitation.)

Bates B: The peripheral vascular system. In Bates B: A Guide to Physical Examination and History Taking, 4th ed, Chap 15, p 406. Philadelphia, JB Lippincott, 1987 (An excellent review of the anatomy and physiology, pathogenesis, and examination of the peripheral vascular system.)

Giuliani CA, Perry GA: Factors to consider in the rehabilitation aspects of burn care. Phys Ther 65:619, 1985 (Review of potential problems encountered in the care of a patient with burns.)

Helm PA, Kevorkian CG, Lushbaugh M, et al: Burn injury: Rehabilitation management in 1982. Arch Phys Med Rehabil 63:6, 1982 (Comprehensive review of the rehabilitative care of a patient with burns. Includes special problems and techniques associated with hand burns.)

Johnson CL, O'Shaughnesy EJ, Ostergren G: Burn Management. New York, Raven Press, 1981 (Emphasizes the physical and occupational therapy management of the burn patient. Excellent, clear discussions of pathology and treatment of burns.)

Salisbury RE, Newman NM, Dingeldein GP (eds): Manual of Burn Therapeutics: An interdisciplinary Approach. Boston, Little, Brown & Co, 1983 (Guidelines for the management of the patient with burns. Excellent chapters on physical therapy, therapeutic recreation, and isolation practices.)

Wright PC: Fundamentals of acute burn care and physical therapy management. Phys Ther 64:1217, 1984 (Excellent review of pathophysiology and general treatment guidelines for the entry-level clinician or the clinician inexperienced in burn care.)

Zane LJ: Evaluation of the acutely ill burn patient. In DiGregorio VR (ed): Clinics in Physical Therapy: Rehabilitation of the Burn Patient. New York, Churchill Livingstone, 1984 (Presents a systematic approach to evaluating the acutely injured patient with burns. Describes medical management and procedures.)

32 Obstetric and Gynecological Analysis

JANET BOWER HULME

The effects of menstruation, pregnancy, and menopause on the responses of body systems are important considerations when evaluating the female patient. This chapter outlines an approach that takes into account these unique aspects of analysis in reproductive, cardiovascular, pulmonary, musculoskeletal, biomechanical, and neurological assessment, and in assessing mental and physical responses to pain and stress. In working with women, particularly pregnant women, the physical therapist must be aware of special considerations. Suggested examinations may be done in whole or in part as appropriate for the individual patient.

EVALUATION OF THE MENSTRUATING PATIENT

UROGENITAL/REPRODUCTIVE EVALUATION

Special Considerations

The therapist should determine from previous medical records or history taking reported problems with urination, that is, changes in frequency, trouble starting or stopping urine flow, pain or burning sensation during urination, color of the urine, or leaking of urine. Pain and burning during urination, increased urinary frequency, or hematuria may indicate urinary tract infection. Leaking urine may be caused by pelvic floor muscle innervation damage, or weak or stretched pelvic floor musculature secondary to pregnancy and vaginal delivery. Stress incontinence and urinary difficulties are common symptoms of cystocele or uterine prolapse.

The therapist should determine the frequency, regularity, length, and flow intensity of menstruation, and the presence of any pain or cramping during menstruation and its effect on the patient's daily routines. Signs of pelvic inflammatory disease and endometriosis (uterine membrane lining located in sites throughout the pelvis or the abdominal wall) include painful or difficult menstruation (dysmenorrhea), pelvic pain, and menstrual disturbances. Sudden cessation of menstruation, abnormal increase in duration or amount of menses (hypermenorrhea), or abnormal frequency of menstruation (polymenorrhea) may indicate the possibility of an ovarian tumor. The therapist should also determine the presence of other symptoms associated with or preceding menstruation, such as swelling of hands and feet, abdominal distention, breast tenderness or fullness, low back ache or pain, pelvic tenderness, depression, fatigue, or emotional lability. These symptoms are often considered indicators of premenstrual syndrome (PMS) pattern.

In menstruating women, the therapist should determine if the patient is presently or has previously been pregnant, and if so, the number of pregnancies and any history of problems during the pregnancies, during the delivery, or postpartum.

In women complaining of pelvic pain, the therapist should determine the onset, duration, and characteristics of the pain. Acute onset may indicate an accident involving pelvic organs (ie, rupture, torsion, internal hemorrhage) or acute inflammation. Gradual onset may indicate endometriosis or a neoplasm. Intermittent or colicky pain often indicates uterine muscle contraction, an ectopic pregnancy, urethral colic, or intestinal obstruction. Dull, throbbing pain may indicate a chronic inflammatory disease or changes related to a pelvic tumor. Cyclic pain is often associated with the menstrual cycle, ovulation, PMS, or dysmenorrhea, whereas a random pain pattern may indicate genital organ pathology. Pelvic pain aggravated or initiated by movements, especially in the lower back, indicates a possible musculoskeletal origin; however, spread of pelvic inflammatory disease or neoplastic disease into the presacral or retroperitoneal area may simulate sciatica.

The therapist should question the patient concerning breast lumps or soreness, any secretions or discharge from the nipples, and any sores or ulcerations of the breasts. Breast examination should be done on a monthly basis by the patient or a medical professional. With the patient sitting or standing, observe the breasts, noting contours, symmetry, and skin consistency. Palpation of the axillae and supraclavicular areas, areola, nipple, and breast tissue is performed, noting masses, nodules, tenderness, and pain. Soreness or gland enlargement caused by PMS will be a temporary phenomenon around the time of the menstrual cycle.

Examination

The following examination most often will be done by the physician or nurse. The physical therapist with special training in obstetrics/gynecology may use the results of the following examination to aid in differential assessment and treatment planning. The lower abdomen, pelvis, and external genitalia are observed for lumps, masses, ulcerations, discolorations, and presence and amount of pubic hair. The labia majora, labia minora, urethral orifice, vaginal orifice, and Bartholin's glands are observed, noting masses, fistulas, abnormal exudate, or redness. The anal opening is observed for any hemorrhoids or protruding pink tissue.

Palpation of the bladder and kidneys is performed. Pain, lumps, or masses are noted. Bimanual palpation of the vagina and uterus and bimanual rectovaginal palpation are performed. Contours, position, and the presence of masses, tenderness, and pain are noted by palpation of the vaginal walls, urethra, cervix, fornices, uterus, ovaries, and rectovaginal septum. Pain with movement of the cervix and ovarian tenderness may indicate pelvic inflammatory disease.

The physical therapist may encounter other diagnostic test results, including the following:

1. Computed tomography is used to identify pelvic masses and pelvic lymph node chains as part of an examination for metastasis of gynecologic cancer.
2. Magnetic resonance imaging can be used for diagnosing carcinoma of the endometrium and for locating adnexal masses.
3. Laparoscopy is utilized in diagnosis of pelvic pain, endometriosis, acute and chronic pelvic inflammatory disease, pelvic masses, and ectopic pregnancy.
4. Ultrasound or sonography is used in gynecology to help confirm physical findings of pathology and assist in specifying pelvic disease.

MUSCULOSKELETAL EVALUATION

Special Considerations

The therapist should determine when during the menstrual cycle the pain or dysfunction occurs, and if it happens on a cyclic or monthly basis. If the patient does not know, the therapist should show her how to use a monthly diary to track the pain, physical activities, and menstrual cycle.

EVALUATION OF THE PREGNANT PATIENT

UROGENITAL/REPRODUCTIVE EVALUATION

Special Considerations

The therapist should determine any presence of or problems with constipation or hemorrhoids. Constipation during pregnancy can be caused by decreased peristaltic action of the intestinal tract resulting from hormonal changes and pressure of the enlarged uterus on the intestines and by decreased expulsive ability of stretched abdominal muscles. Hemorrhoids may be caused by hormonal changes during pregnancy, which relax the vein walls, or by pressure of the uterus on the lower intestine and rectum.

Examination

During pregnancy, both uterine contractions and the height of the top of the uterus (fundus) may be palpated. Uterine contractions are palpated for timing and intensity to provide information on preterm labor or on progression of full-term labor. Recognition of preterm labor is indicated by contractions in a regular pattern less than 10 minutes apart for more than one hour when the patient is at rest. Medical intervention at this point may prevent a preterm delivery. The height of the fundus is an indication of the progression of pregnancy. At the third month, the fundus rises above the symphysis pubis. By the fifth month, it is at the level of the umbilicus. By the ninth month, it is at the level of the rib cage, and during the tenth month, it drops slightly as the fetus settles into the pelvis.

The physical therapist may encounter the following diagnostic test results:

1. Ultrasound or sonography may be used in obstetrics during the second and third trimesters to estimate gestational age, confirm fetal viability, diagnose retarded or accelerated fetal growth, diagnose fetal abnormalities, locate the placenta's implantation site, and guide invasive procedures.
2. Amniocentesis may be used to determine inborn errors of metabolism, chromosomal disorders, disorders of hemoglobin biosynthesis, and neural tube defects of the fetus.
3. Chorionic villus sampling may be used to diagnose fetal genetic and metabolic disorders as early as the first trimester.

CARDIOVASCULAR AND PULMONARY EVALUATION

Special Considerations

When evaluating a pregnant woman, the therapist should determine if the woman has experienced any nausea or vomiting. Her exercise level, daily activity level, and presence of dyspnea during activities should be recorded. The majority of pregnant women experience dyspnea some time during a normal pregnancy, usually during the first or second trimester. Blood pressure readings elevated by 30 or more points systolic or 15 or more points diastolic (or both) are considered high blood pressure during pregnancy. Increases of approximately 5% above the nonpregnant reading are considered normal.

Examination

The therapist observes general appearance including postural deformities, facial expression, and any nose or mouth breathing or nasal flaring. Pregnancy often affects the nasopharynx, causing hyperemia and excessive secretions of the mucosa, leading to possible nasal obstruction, mouth breathing, and nasal flaring.

Consistency of arterial pulses, the presence of edema in the face, hands, ankles, and feet, and the presence of varicose veins are also observed and palpated. Edema during pregnancy can be due to hormonal and circulation changes, or pressure of the uterus on the major vessels transporting blood to the lower extremities. Varicose veins can be caused by the relaxing effect of hormones on vein walls and the pressure of the uterus on abdominal veins, both of which slow the return of blood from the lower extremities. The therapist must also note respiratory rate and patterns, rate and depth of inspiration compared to expiration, use of costal or diaphragmatic breathing, and use of accessory muscles. The rib cage expands during pregnancy and the diaphragm elevates because of the pressure of the growing uterus. Pregnant women naturally breathe more deeply.

Blood pressure should be evaluated in both arms at least once and should be evaluated in three positions: supine, sitting, and standing. A difference between extremities of over 10 to 15 mm Hg suggests arterial compression or obstruction on the side with lower pressure. When changing to a more upright position, a fall in systolic pressure of 20 mm Hg or more when accompanied by other symptoms (ie, dizziness) may indicate orthostatic hypotension.

Aerobic fitness can be evaluated at a submaximal level using the bicycle ergometer or at a maximal level using the treadmill. According to Artal and Wiswell (1986), the bicycle is non-weight-bearing aerobic exercise, so increased weight from pregnancy is not a factor as it is in treadmill testing. The same amount of work in pregnant women may represent greater physiological stress than in nonpregnant women, so submaximal testing is often used. Components to be evaluated every three to five minutes during the activity and also during the recovery period are (1) respiratory rate, (2) heart rate, (3) blood pressure, and (4) perceived exertion. The heart rate during pregnancy normally increases approximately 20% at rest, but decreases approximately 15% during exercise when compared to the nonpregnant state. Other factors to monitor during aerobic activity are lower limb edema, dyspnea, and leg fatigue or cramping. These criteria allow evaluation of a "symptom-limited $\dot{V}O_2$ $_{max}$ test," which approximates actual aerobic capacity. Testing may be conducted at the end of the first trimester, and monthly during the second and third trimesters to determine changes in the pertinent components.

The physical therapist should assess anaerobic fitness during recreational activities and activities of daily living by monitoring heart rate, blood pressure, respiratory rate, dyspnea, and perceived exertion. It is important to evaluate breathing techniques and patterns used during typical activities, checking that the Valsalva maneuver does not occur during exertion, and that exhalation occurs with exertion. As part of any fitness evaluation, fetal heart rate and movement should be assessed before and after exercise.

MUSCULOSKELETAL EVALUATION

Examination

A detailed postural examination should be performed, including observation of standing, long and short sitting, reclining, and squatting. During pregnancy, the center of gravity moves anteriorly, and kyphosis, lordosis, and scoliosis may become accentuated because of this change. Lumbodorsal fasciae become taut, which also may increase lordosis. Enlarged breasts and center of gravity changes increase the likelihood of round shoulders. Hormonal changes increase the capacity of ligaments to be stretched or lengthened, which may result in increased pelvic mobility. Feet become wider and longer, sometimes changing as much as a shoe size. Toeing out increases the base of support during pregnancy and may be caused in part by tight iliopsoas muscles, which can lead to an anterior pelvic tilt, increased lordosis, external rotation of the femurs, and genu recurvatum. Ligamentous laxity caused by hormonal changes may be present for three to four months postpartum or as long as breast-feeding continues.

Assessment of muscle and joint integrity of the trunk should be performed by observing active movement and palpating for condition, position, and mobility. During pregnancy, the L5-S1, sacroiliac, symphysis pubis, and sacral-coccygeal joints are particularly important to assess in relation to pain and dysfunction. It is also important to assess the functional strength of abdominal, back extensor, and pelvic floor muscles during pregnancy because these muscles receive additional stresses from the growing baby, and are also affected by the hormone relaxin. The length and flexibility of neck extensor, pectoral, erector spinae, iliopsoas, hamstring, gastrocnemius, and piriformis muscles should be assessed because postural changes and muscle length are often interrelated. Because the hormone relaxin affects ligamentous length during pregnancy, the rectus abdominis muscle separates or spreads to some degree. This is called diastasis recti abdominis. To test for this separation, the patient is positioned in hooklying, then tucks her chin and lifts her head and shoulders off the surface in a partial curl up. The therapist places two to three fingertips horizontally into the trough created by the division of the two sides of the abdominal muscles above the umbilicus at the widest part of the separation. A two-finger separation between the two sides of the abdominals is considered within normal limits. More than three-fingers' separation (diastasis recti abdominis) is considered an indication for conservative intervention, that is, instructions in protective measures during stressful activities. The separation appears as a gap early in the first trimester of the first pregnancy and as a bulge at the end of pregnancy. The bulge appears earlier in subsequent pregnancies.

BIOMECHANICS EVALUATION

Special Considerations

The therapist should determine activities the patient performs during work and leisure, positions she assumes during these activities, and any associated pain, discomfort, or stiffness.

Examination

The therapist should analyze components of movement patterns and postures during activities, such as (1) lifting and carrying large and small objects, (2) activities of daily living, (3) activities of nightly living, (4) recreational activities, and (5) transition movement patterns from one posture to another (ie, supine to sit, sit to stand, and all fours to stand). Components of the analysis include presence of and changes in the base of support, center of gravity, weight shifts, rotations around the base of support, stabilization points, pelvic position, and assistive devices used. Analysis of gait is essential, because changes in gait are common in pregnancy. A waddling, toe-out gait sometimes is seen during pregnancy and may be caused by hormonal changes that relax the hip and pelvic girdle ligamentous structures.

NEUROLOGICAL EVALUATION

Special Considerations

The therapist should determine the presence and patterns of headaches, problems with muscle strength, balance, coordination, tremors, spasms, numbness, or tingling.

Examination

The therapist should perform a central nervous system screening examination, including isometric strength tests and reflex evaluations to test the integrity of sacral, lumbar, thoracic, and cervical nerve roots. Peripheral nerve tests, including Tinel's test, Phalen's test, and palpation, should be performed when the history indicates a potential problem. Edema during pregnancy, traumatic injuries during labor or delivery, or pressure of the fetal head on nerves during the last months of pregnancy can cause peripheral nerve compression or irritation. The brachial plexus and the median, ulnar, sciatic, femoral, and posterior tibial nerves are commonly affected.

EVALUATION OF MENTAL AND PHYSICAL RESPONSES TO PAIN AND STRESSFUL SITUATIONS

Special Considerations

The therapist should determine what situations are "stressors" for the patient and how the patient has responded to these situations in the past: How did she feel? What did she tell herself? How did she react when she encountered a situation that was totally unexpected or not controllable? In general, the therapist is looking for indications of an internal sense of control and competence instead of an external locus of control, and whether the patient assumes responsibility for the results of her actions in the situation.

Examination

Observation of the patient's responses during exercise, breathing, and relaxation training (which can be viewed as a potentially unfamiliar, stressful situation) provides the therapist with additional information. The therapist assesses risk taking versus safety types of responses and the presence or absence of an internal reward system for approximations of correct behavior during the learning experience.

The therapist observes the patient for areas of tension in the body, methods the patient uses to relax those areas, and breathing patterns at rest, during activities, and when the patient is under stress. These observations are useful in determining treatment approaches that may be particularly effective for the individual patient.

The therapist may also use psychological evaluation reports based on interviews and standardized assessments that provide information about a patient's strengths, weaknesses, adjustment style, and coping resources.

EVALUATION OF THE MENOPAUSAL/POSTMENOPAUSAL PATIENT

UROGENITAL/REPRODUCTIVE EVALUATION

Special Considerations

For the postmenopausal woman, the therapist should determine if there is or has been any bleeding, and if so, when it occurred, its duration and intensity, and its color and odor. The definition of postmenopausal bleeding is bleeding six months beyond the last menses. Postmenopausal bleeding may be caused by estrogen, benign organic lesions, or malignancies, or it may be idiopathic in origin. The therapist should determine from history taking or medical records the frequency and severity of vasomotor instability symptoms (ie, hot flashes, nausea, dizziness, headaches, or night sweats). Sleep deprivation associated with night sweats is another common occurrence that contributes to fatigue, nervousness, irritability, and depression.

Examination

When performing palpation, the therapist should remember that ovaries are not normally palpable in women three to five years past menopause unless the woman is very thin or has an ovarian tumor.

Pelvic relaxation related to atrophy and weakening of connective tissue secondary to estrogen deprivation and aging can result in uterine prolapse.

MUSCULOSKELETAL EVALUATION

Diagnostic test results that the therapist may encounter include single or dual photon absorptiometry, which is used to measure the quantity of bone mineral to evaluate the extent of osteoporosis.

Osteoporosis progresses rapidly at menopause as a result of the decrease in estrogen. The three principal complications of osteoporosis in postmenopausal women are vertebral compression fractures, distal forearm fractures, and hip fractures.

CONCLUSION

Taking into consideration the effects of menstruation, pregnancy, and menopause during the evaluation of all body systems will enable the physical therapist to develop a comprehensive picture of the female patient, and will facilitate development of an optimum management plan. Each patient has unique needs; as therapists, our expertise in selecting the essential examination procedures and interpreting the results on an individual basis will lead to maximizing function and independence for the female patient.

ANNOTATED BIBLIOGRAPHY

Artal R, Wiswell R (eds): Exercise in Pregnancy. Baltimore, Williams & Wilkins, 1986 (A somewhat controversial reference on the effect of exercise on the body systems and the fetus during pregnancy.)

Barten M: Laparoscopic Complications: Prevention and Management. Philadelphia, BC Decker, 1986 (An illustrated reference of laparoscopic procedures, indications, complications, and management.)

Bates B: A Guide to Physical Examination and History Taking, 4th ed. Philadelphia, JB Lippincott, 1987 (Describes sequence and techniques of general external and internal examination of female genitalia and reproductive system, and evaluation of all other systems of the body.)

Danforth D, Scott J, (eds): Obstetrics and Gynecology. Philadelphia, JB Lippincott, 1986 (An in-depth text on pathology, evaluation, medical diagnostic procedures, and medical intervention in obstetrics and gynecology.)

Herron M, Dulock H: Preterm Labor: A Staff Development Program in Perinatal Nursing Care. White Plains, NY, March of Dimes Birth Defects Foundation, 1983 (A resource for preterm labor: its causes, assessment, and intervention.)

Kase NG, Weingold AB: Principles and Practice of Clinical Gynecology. New York, John Wiley & Sons, 1983 (A comprehensive gynecological text that includes descriptions of abnormal menstrual bleeding patterns, pelvic pain, pelvic relaxational prolapse, and premenstrual tension.)

Marchant D: History: Physical examination and breast self-examination. Clin Obstet Gynecol 25: 335, 1982 (An in-depth description of breast examination and self-examination.)

Pitkin R, Scott J (eds): Clinical Obstetrics and Gynecology. Philadelphia, Harper & Row, 1986 (An excellent update on operative obstetrics and the woman during menopause and the years that follow.)

Puhl I, Brown CH (eds): The Menstrual Cycle and Physical Activity. Champaign, IL, Human Kinetics, 1986 (State-of-the-art information on the relationship of menstrual cycle alterations, bone density changes, and physical training.)

Seeds J, Cefalo R: Practical Obstetrical Ultrasound. Rockville, MD, Aspen Systems, 1986 (A current reference on sonography, indications, methods, and management.)

33 Analysis of Renal Dysfunction

GEORGE A. WOLFE

Disease of the kidney is a significant health problem that the physical therapist may encounter as a primary diagnosis or as a sequela of some other disorder. Renal failure, especially in its chronic form, can result in multisystem abnormalities. Pain, edema, structural imbalance, weakness, decreased endurance, and impaired central nervous system control all can arise from decreased renal function, and physical therapy may be indicated in the management of any of these conditions. This chapter has two purposes: first, to outline the information contained in the medical record that the physical therapist should note before conducting an evaluation, and second, to review the assessment tools most likely to be used by the physical therapist treating the patient with renal disease.

REVIEW OF THE MEDICAL RECORD

URINALYSIS

The initial test of any patient with suspected renal disease is urinalysis. Several specific test results assist the physician in making a diagnosis. The presence of abnormally high levels of protein in the urine (proteinuria) is highly suggestive of renal disease. Normally, less than 150 mg of protein should be excreted in the urine over a 24-hour period. However, the therapist should remember that heavy exertion, fever, changes in blood flow, and even emotional stress may also produce transient proteinuria. The presence of blood in the urine (hematuria) may also indicate kidney disease. Normally, less than 1000 red cells per minute are excreted in the urine. Microscopic hematuria will have 3000 to 4000 cells per minute, while greater than 1 million cells per minute is considered gross hematuria. Approximately 15% of patients with gross hematuria suffer from kidney disease; the rest have disorders of the bladder, prostate, or urethra. The presence of casts in the urine indicates inflammation or infection of the kidney. Casts are cylindrical clumps of cells, crystals, or hyaline debris, which derive their form from the renal tubules where they initially are deposited.

GLOMERULAR FILTRATION RATE

The glomerular filtration rate (GFR) is the single most important measurement of kidney function. It measures the amount of blood filtered per minute by the kidneys, and represents the function of approximately 1 million nephrons per kidney. GFR is measured by determining the rate of "clearance" or removal of a substance from the blood or serum by the kidneys. The substance measured must be one that is filtered by the glomerulus but not secreted in the tubules of the nephron. If that is the case, then the clearance equals the GFR. Inulin is a fructose polymer commonly used to determine the GFR, however, it must be administered intravenously. To avoid intravenous administration, endogenous creatinine is often substituted because it is produced by the body at a constant rate, has a stable daily excretion, and has minimal secretion into tubular fluid. Because the serum creatinine level alone should reflect the rate of clearance, it is commonly used as a gross ndicator of renal function. Normal creatinine clearance for a mon is 130 mL/min, and for a woman is 120 mL/min. Normal serum creatinine is 1 mg/dL. Dialysis is generally initiated when the serum creatinine exceeds 10 mg/dL (creatinine clearance, 15-25 mL/min).

BLOOD TESTS

Patients with chronic renal failure who are dependent upon hemodialysis tend to be chronically anemic. A hematocrit level of 20% to 25% is relatively common. The therapist should be aware of the patient's hematocrit and hemoglobin levels, because the degree of reduction of oxygen-carrying capacity will affect the patient's response to the evaluation and ensuing treatment.

Renal disease can have a serious effect on the blood lipid profiles of patients. Elevated levels of triglycerides, total serum cholesterol, and low-density lipoprotein cholesterol coupled with low levels of high-density lipoprotein cholesterol increase the risk for cardiovascular disease in patients with renal disease. The therapist should note the lipid profile if it is available in the medical record, because exercise training programs have been shown to improve abnormal blood lipid levels.

OTHER TESTS

Intravenous pyelography (IVP) can aid in the determination of renal perfusion, function, and anatomy. An iodine-containing contrast medium is administered to the patient. During excretion through the kidney it becomes concentrated as water is reabsorbed in the tubules. Fluoroscopy or multiple roentgenograms then are used to visualize the kidneys and to assess the amount of time involved in the circulation and excretion of the contrast medium. Ultrasonography can be used to determine the location, size, and nature of masses in the kidneys. It can also identify cysts and the presence of

hydonephrosis, and may be used to guide needle biopsy if required. Computed tomography (CT scan) is rapidly supplanting ultrasonography and fluoroscopy as the preferred method for visualizing the kidneys because it produces clearer images and can be controlled more precisely.

Peripheral neuropathy is common in patients with chronic renal failure; therefore, the results of nerve conduction velocity tests and electromyographic (EMG) studies are usually present in the medical record. The physical therapist may be responsible for performing such tests. Any evidence of slowed conduction, denervation, or myopathy should be noted in order to guide the assessment of sensation and muscle strength.

It is also important for the therapist to review the results of radiological studies of the skeletal system. Renal osteodystrophy can result in demineralization and distal resorption of bone. Boney abnormalities must be taken into account while performing the physical therapy evaluation.

Many patients with renal disease develop cardiovascular disorders. These disorders include cardimyopathy, pericarditis, and accelerated atherosclerosis, which can lead to myocardial infarction or stroke. Pulmonary manifestations of cardiovascular problems or of fluid overload may also be present. The therapist must review results of cardiovascular and pulmonary function tests before evaluating the patient.

Several items of interest to the physical therapist are contained in the medical record, and should be considered before assessment of the patient with renal dysfunction. These items are summarized in Table 33-1.

PHYSICAL THERAPY ASSESSMENT

TIMING OF THE ASSESSMENT

Patients with renal disease are often managed by hemodialysis, which requires the patient to be connected to a dialysis machine for approximately four hours, three days a week. The fre-

Table 33-1. Review of the Medical Record of the Patient with Renal Disease

Urinalysis

Proteinuria
Hematuria
Casts

Glomerular Filtration Rate

Inulin clearance
Creatinine clearance
Serum creatinine level

Blood Tests

Hematocrit and hemoglobin levels
Lipid profile

Other Tests

Intravenous pyelography
Ultrasonography
CT scan
Electroneuromyography
Skeletal radiography
Cardiovascular assessments
Pulmonary function

quency and time on dialysis will vary from patient to patient. Changes in fluid volume, electrolyte balance, and acid-base balance occur during these treatments; therefore, the physical therapy assessment should be conducted on a nondialysis day. If this is not possible, it is best to evaluate the patient before rather than after the treatment, because patients often are tired and may experience muscle cramping and nausea after dialysis. Physical therapy assessment during hemodialysis is complicated by the connection of the patient to the machine and by the hypotension, cramping, and nausea experienced by some patients. Similar difficulties may be encountered in the acute renal patient receiving peritoneal dialysis. However, these problems of timing are not as significant in the patient with chronic renal disease managed by continuous ambulatory peritoneal dialysis (CAPD).

MENTAL STATUS

Assessment of the mental status of the patient with renal disease should precede all other assessments. The patient with acute renal failure may have electrolyte imbalances that can result in confusion or dulled sensibility. The patient with chronic failure who is not yet dialyzed can have the same difficulties. In addition, during hemodialysis treatments patients may experience dialysis disequilibrium, which is characterized by headache, nausea, lethargy, and even seizures. Most well-managed patients will not have significant alterations in mental status, but the possibility exists and the physical therapist should determine initially if the patient is able to cooperate in the rest of the evaluation.

DIALYSIS ACCESS

Patients who depend upon hemodialysis require some form of vascular access. This can be an external, Silastic shunt that penetrates the skin and is sutured into an artery and a vein, or it can be an internal fistula created surgically by the anastomosis of an artery and a vein or the implantation of a graft connecting an artery and a vein. The most common location of such devices is the forearm, but other areas may be used because the fistulas may break down or occlude over time. Because a shunt reroutes blood directly from the arterial system to the veins, ischemia may be present distal to its location. The therapist should identify the location of the point of vascular access and determine the relative adequacy of circulation distal to it by observing skin color and comparative skin temperature. It is also important to know the location of shunts because any occlusion or slowing of blood flow through them (eg, when measuring blood pressure) should be avoided because of the possibility of thrombosis. External shunts should always be protected by a bandage and be equipped with clamps to be used in the event of accidental disconnection.

Patients managed by peritoneal dialysis will have a peritoneal catheter. These are Silastic tubes that usually exit the abdominal wall lateral to the umbilicus. A peritoneal catheter should always be adequately dressed and protected by gauze squares taped in place over it. The therapist must note its location and take appropriate precautions to prevent any mechanical trauma to the area.

VITAL SIGNS

It is important to assess vital signs initially and at regular intervals in the patient with renal disease, because autonomic neuropathy may impair the cardiovascular response to changes in posture and to exercise. In addition, most patients with chronic renal disease are hypertensive and medication used to control blood pressure may also affect response to exertion. Tachycardia (rapid heart rate) may also be present because of anemia. Remember that the use of blood pressure cuffs on an extremity that contains an arteriovenous fistula or shunt is contraindicated. Auscultation of the chest should be performed if the medical record indicates the presence of cardiac or pulmonary abnormalities. Friction rubs caused by pericarditis and abnormal breath sounds resulting from pulmonary edema are relatively common in these patients.

SENSATION

Many patients with renal disease experience pain at various times. It is important for the physical therapist to ascertain if the patient has pain at the time of evaluation, or if he has pain at predictable times (eg, during and after dialysis treatments). The type and location of the pain as well as precipitating factors should be noted.

The sensory modalities of superficial pain, light touch, pressure, and proprioception should be assessed in these patients because of the high incidence of peripheral neuropathy. The distal extremities are most commonly affected. Carpal tunnel syndrome is also relatively common, and the sensory evaluation will assist in determining possible etiologies of functional impairment. The physical therapist may also be requested to perform nerve conduction velocity and EMG studies.

RANGE OF MOTION

Passive range of motion should be evaluated to determine if renal osteodystrophy, edema, or prolonged positioning because of weakness has led to any joint restrictions. It is also required as a prelude to manual muscle testing. If boney demineralization is severe, care should be taken during the assessment to decrease the risk of pathologic fractures.

ASSESSMENT OF STRENGTH

Manual muscle testing is an important part of the physical therapy evaluation because peripheral neuropathy and myopathy are common in patients with renal disease. Distribution of weakness can help differentiate between myopathy and neuropathy, because myopathy tends to affect proximal muscles whereas neuropathy causes peripheral weakness. Correlating weakness with the sensory assessment and electroneuromyography will also aid in determining the source of functional loss. Isokinetic evaluation may also be of benefit. There is no contraindication to the application of resistance to the extremity used for vascular access, unless the patient is receiving or has just concluded a hemodialysis treatment at the time of the assessment.

FUNCTION AND ENDURANCE

The functional status of the patient with renal disease will depend upon the degree of problems revealed by the evaluation detailed above. If weakness is severe, walking and other activities may be compromised. A footdrop because of weakness in the dorsiflexors of the ankle is common.

It is possible to assess endurance functionally. However, performance of an exercise stress test is desirable, because many patients function with no difficulty in day-to-day activities, but are unable to perform consistently in the workplace because they become fatigued quickly. A graded exercise test is the best way to determine the aerobic limitations of the patient. Such tests may be done using the treadmill or the bicycle ergometer. However, as is the case for normal persons, the treadmill is a better choice because many patients experience early leg fatigue on the bicycle. Tests can be conducted on a nondialysis day or before hemodialysis. Performance may be impaired in the hours following dialysis treatments because of changes in acid-base balance and blood volume. Patients with lower hematocrit and hemoglobin levels should be expected to demonstrate greater limitation of performance. Average maximal oxygen consumption in patients dependent on hemodialysis has been reported to be 1.30 to 1.35 liters per minute. Symptom-limited maximal graded exercise tests have been shown to be safe for these patients when conducted with normal monitoring procedures.

Because patients with renal dysfunction have multisystem abnormalities, a variety of

Table 33-2. Considerations in the Physical Therapy Assessment of the Patient with Renal Disease

Timing

Influence of dialysis

Mental Status

Electrolyte imbalance
Dialysis dysequilibrium

Dialysis Access

Arteriovenous fistulas
Peritoneal catheters

Vital Signs

Anemia
Hypertension or hypotension
Autonomic neuropathy
Pulmonary edema

Sensation

Pain
Peripheral neuropathy

Range of Motion

Osteodystrophy
Weakness

Strength

Peripheral neuropathy
Myopathy

Function and Endurance

Weakness
Anemia
Cardiovascular impairment
Deconditioning

evaluation techniques must be used. These have been detailed above and are summarized in Table 33-2.

CONCLUSION

Assessment of the patient with renal disease is similar to the assessment of many other types of patients. However, the multisystem involvement experienced by the renal patient makes it imperative to evaluate the entire patient before treatment. The medical record can provide information regarding the extent of renal dysfunction, the degree of anemia, the presence of abnormalities in the blood lipid profile, the degree of skeletal changes, the extent of peripheral neuropathy, and the presence of concomitant cardiovascular or pulmonary abnormalities. Specific areas that the physical therapist should evaluate include mental status, vascular status, vital signs, sensation, range of motion, strength, functional status, and endurance. Once the assessment is completed, an appropriate plan for intervention may be formulated.

ANNOTATED BIBLIOGRAPHY

Asbury AK: Uremic neuropathy. In Dyck PJ, Thomas PK, Lambert EH et al (eds): Peripheral Neuropathy. Philadelphia, WB Saunders, 1984 (Review of neuropathy in the uremic patient, including discussion of evidence for and against its improvement with dialysis.)

Coburn JW Henry DA: Renal osteodystrophy. Adv Intern Med 30:387, 1984 (Thorough review of the boney abnormalities seen in chronic renal disease, and strategies for management.)

Drueke T, LePailleur C, Zingraff J et al: Uremic cardiomyopathy and pericarditis. In Hamburger J, Crosnier J, Grünfield JP et al (eds): Advances in Nephrology from the Necker Hospital, Vol 9, p 33. Chicago, Year Book Medical Publishers, 1980 (Excellent discussion of two cardiac problems and their implications for function.)

Goldberg AP, Hagberg JM, Delmez JA: Exercise training improves abnormal lipid and carbohydrate metabolism in hemodialysis patients. Trans Am Soc Artif Intern Organs 25:431, 1979 (Documents the safety of exercise testing and the effect of training on lipids in hemodialysis patients.)

Goldberg AP, Hagberg JM, Delmez JA et al: The metabolic and psychological effects of exercise training in hemodialysis patients. Am J Clin Nutr 33:1620, 1980 (Documents the safety of exercise testing and impairment of endurance expressed as maximum oxygen uptake.)

Heinemann HO, Maack TM, Sherman RL: Proteinuria. Am J Med 56:71, 1974 (Discusses the variety of causes of proteinuria, including renal disease.)

Noon GP, Short HD: Dialysis access surgery. In Suki WH, Massry SG (eds): Therapy of Renal Disease and Related Disorders. Boston, Martinus Nijhoff, 1984 (Excellent description of various types of fistulas and shunts, and precautions that should be taken in their management.)

Resnick JB, Hamburger RJ: Clinical assessment of renal function. In Flamenbaum WF, Hamburger RJ: Nephrology: An Approach to the Patient with Renal Disease. Philadelphia, JB Lippincott, 1982 (Detailed, but readable discussion of mechanisms of assessment, particularly glomerular filtration rate.)

Russell JM, Resnick MI: Ultrasound in urology. Med Clin North Am 6:445, 1979 (Clearly presented overview of ultrasonography in renal disease.)

34 Assessment of Psychological Factors

ANN HALLUM

The primary goal of a physical therapy evaluation is to identify the patient's specific physical problems and develop a program of treatment. For treatment to be maximally effective, however, the physical therapist must also consider the psychological, social, and environmental factors that may influence the patient's recovery or adaptation to permanent changes in mobility or independence.

Physical therapists seldom need to inquire specifically about the patient's moods, feelings, thoughts, or social-environment situations, because patients usually talk openly about the frustrations and fears related to their injury or illness. With the support of their physical therapists, most patients are able to cope successfully with the recovery process. In some cases, however, psychological, cognitive, social, and environmental factors create major barriers to the patient's rehabilitation. When this situation occurs, a psychological consultation should be requested.

Psychologists can provide the therapist with specific information about the patient's intellectual strengths and deficits. They can also help identify preexisting and present intrapsychic problems, dysfunctional thought processes, and behaviors that might interfere with the patient's motivation. Assessment of the patient's social and environmental circumstances may also be a part of a comprehensive psychological evaluation. When indicated, psychologists can offer direct counseling services to the patients and their families to help them cope with the consequences of illness or disability.

The purpose of this chapter is twofold. First, I will present examples of several comprehensive assessment models that the physical therapist can use when evaluating the psychological, social, and environmental influences that may be affecting the patient. Second, I will introduce some of the assessment measures that psychologists might use when they are asked to work with a patient in a physical therapy setting. I will discuss briefly general measures of personality, measures of specific psychosocial function, measures to assess pain, and measures of intellectual and neuropsychological status.

ASSESSMENT MODELS

An example of an organized plan that can be easily adapted by physical therapists to facilitate assessment of the patient's personal, social, and environmental problems is the patient evaluation grid (PEG) (Fig. 34-1) (Leigh and Reiser, 1985). In this model, three factors—biological, psychological, and social—are assessed against three different time contexts that reflect the patient's present, recent, and background history that might influence attitudes and responses to physical therapy interventions.

The PEG may look overwhelming at first glance, but the items listed in each category are

CONTEXTS			
DIMENSIONS	CURRENT	RECENT	BACKGROUND
Biological	Neurological, muscular, orthopedic symptoms and signs. General health status, stability of vital signs. Medications and pertinent lab values.	Onset of symptoms and signs. Health status prior to onset of symptoms. History of drug and alcohol use. History of present problem.	Family history of illness. Patient's history of disease, injury, surgery.
Personal	Main physical complaint, main psychiatric complaint. Mental status. Physical abilities, limitations. Physical and emotional responses to treatment. Expectations, level of motivation.	Activity level, interests prior to illness or disability. Emotional responses to situation. Coping responses to situation. Social support systems.	Family background, ethnic, cultural background. Family, patient history of psychological problems. Family, patient educational level. Pattern of previous coping.
Environmental	Immediate physical and interpersonal environment. Accessibility of environment (or post-discharge environment—home and work).	Pre-illness, disability environment at home and work. Social environment, family environment.	Early family, cultural environment, peer relationships.

Figure 34-1. PEG: Organization of information. Biological dimensions include physiological components such as neuromuscular, sensory, organ, and central nervous systems, medications, and laboratory values. Personal dimensions include the psychological and behavioral aspects of the person. Environmental dimensions refer to the psychosocial and physical environments of the person. (Adapted from Leigh H, Reiser MF: The patient. Biological, Psychological, and Social Dimensions of Medical Practice, 2nd ed. New York, Plenum, 1985)

only stimulus areas to consider in assessment. For example, if a 25-year-old C6 quadriplegic (secondary to a diving accident) were referred to physical therapy, his therapist might initially decide that a relatively straightforward physical rehabilitation program was in order. However, if the man's PEG (Fig. 34-2) indicated multiple problematic areas related to the patient's preinjury behavior, education level, and family environment, his physical therapist could anticipate the possible psychosocial-environmental problems and arrange for appropriate psychological and social service assistance. This ability to anticipate problems would be particularly important for the therapist who is not working as a member of a comprehensive evaluation and treatment team.

If a patient were referred with a simple back strain, one might have no use for the PEG system. However, if a patient with a simple back strain does not respond well to treatment and there is no radiologic evidence of pathologic findings and no abnormal neurological signs, the physical therapist might stimulate her own thinking about possible psychological, social, and environmental complications by using the PEG approach to problem solving.

Another general outline that can be used by physical therapists as a guide for comprehensive assessment of the factors influencing the patients' response to therapy is the Psychosocial Systems Review. In their system, Schwartz, Tapp, and Brucker (1985) have out-

CONTEXTS			
DIMENSIONS	**CURRENT**	**RECENT**	**BACKGROUND**
Biological	Paralysis—shoulder motion, elbow flexion, pronation, supination, wrist extension intact. Vital signs stable, bladder-bowel incontinence. Bladder infection.	Fracture/dislocation C5-6 on 7-4-88, car-car crash, patient DUI.	Patient no known medical history except ETOH abuse. Father died 2-86 cirrhosis. Mother living.
Personal	Depression, hostility to staff, rejects PT treatment. Refuses to talk with MSW, suicidal statements.	Charged with DUI and manslaughter, driver of other car killed.	HS dropout, worked as delivery man. In ETOH abuse program, but dropped out.
Environmental	Rehabilitation center. Occasional visits by girlfriend.	Lived with girlfriend and her 2 children in one-bedroom second-floor apartment. Temporary employment as delivery man—fired.	Lived in public housing, mother housewife, father occasionally employed as unskilled laborer.

Figure 34-2. An example of a PEG adapted for use in the physical therapy setting. A similar grid system can be used to plan a treatment program that will address all three dimensions.

lined three major systems—the intrapersonal, interpersonal, and social-cultural—that should be considered in a psychosocial evaluation. They have also identified four types of skills needed by a patient in order to function well in each of these systems (Table 34-1).

During this assessment process, if the physical therapist notes that the patient's psychosocial problems may outweigh the therapist's or patient's ability to cope with the situation, a psychologist who is experienced with health-related problems should be consulted.

MEASUREMENT OF PSYCHOSOCIAL FUNCTION

A great deal of research has been done on the psychological assessments measures that I will discuss. Considerable controversy, however, exists among psychologists on the validity of many of the constructs that the measures are purported to assess. My purpose is not to discuss the controversies, but to familiarize you

with some of the typical assessment tools used by psychologists. My underlying purpose is to stimulate you to consider some of these psychological factors that may be influencing the patient's recovery process. Readers interested in the controversies of some of the tests are referred to the bibliography for general texts on psychometics. In this section, I will first discuss some general measures of personality, and second, I will present some measures of more specific psychological functions.

GENERAL MEASURES OF PERSONALITY

A patient's premorbid personality structure is seldom considered in the evaluation of a patient referred to physical therapy. However, the preexisting patterns of behavior may have a major effect on the patient's response to physical therapy interventions.

Two well-known general inventories of personality are commonly used by psychologists: the 16 Personality Factor Inventory (16 PF) and the Minnesota Multiphasic Personality Inventory (MMPI) (Graham and Lilly, 1984).

Table 34-1. Psychosocial Systems Review: General Background

The Psychosocial Systems Review is used to assess three major systems: the intrapersonal (self-system), interpersonal (relations with others), and the social-cultural systems. Each of these general systems can be broken into three important areas:

A. Intrapersonal (self-system)
   Mood-feeling: level and type of everyday emotional reactions
   Thought-speech: patterns of attention, thinking, clarity in speaking
   Values-meaning: personal beliefs, standards, codes of conduct

B. Interpersonal (relations with others)
   Intimacy-belonging: relationships characterized by emotional closeness
   Support-help: availabilty of other people for aid, support
   Boundaries of self—Roles: appropriate definition of social roles (eg, parenthood, professional roles, etc.)

C. Social-Cultural
   Economic: having adequate and predictable sources of income
   Leisure-recreation: having and making adequate use of recreational, relaxing resources
   Community-place: knowing the general resources of one's community; having a sense of belonging to a community

Four general types of skills are needed for a person to function well in the above areas. These are:

A. *Awareness:* being able to perceive one's effect on others, the status of one's relationships, the availability of options for action

B. *Control-management:* ability to manage one's time, energy, and resources to handle daily problems; includes self-control in necessary areas

C. *Problem-solving:* strategies for looking at life problems, searching for alternatives, dealing with obstacles, testing various actions; includes handling emotional stress, social problems, etc.

D. *Negotiation:* skills of asserting one's own rights and wants while recognizing and respecting those of others; using discussion, confrontation, and support to come to mutually beneficial agreements whenever possible

(Schwartz DM, Tapp JT, Brucker B: Behavioral Assessment in Medical Settings. In Schneiderman N, Tapp JT (eds): Behavioral Medicine: The Biopsychosocial Approach. Hillsdale, NJ, Lawrence Erlbaum Associates, 1985)

For both these measures, persons are assumed to have characteristic patterns of behavior or traits that are fairly persistent over time and situations.

The 16 Personality Factor Inventory

The 16 PF is one of the oldest personality tests in use today. This test has been considered appropriate for assessing persons without psychiatric problems and also has been recommended for use with patients who have medical conditions. The test is purported to assess the full range of 16 different personality traits (eg, trusting versus suspicious) that are considered bipolar and are scored on a continuum. An example of a 16 PF profile is shown in Figure 34-3.

Careful analysis of the test profile could help the psychologist and physical therapist identify preexisting personality and behavioral factors that may be influencing the patient's response to the physical therapist or to the treatment program. For example, persons who are usually trusting rather than suspicious may view a physical therapist's suggestions as an attempt to help them, whereas persons who tend to be suspicious may interpret the same suggestions as an attempt to control them. Likewise, a person who is self assured might be able to tolerate the uncertainties and stresses related to a disabling condition better than a person who tends to be generally apprehensive about any new situation.

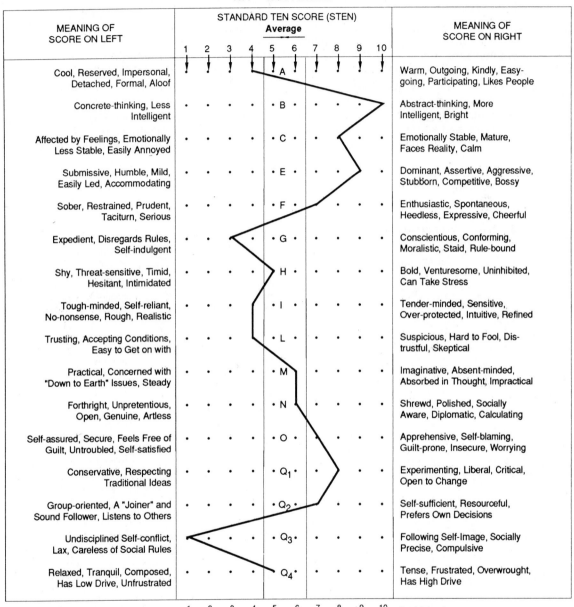

16PF™ TEST PROFILE

MEANING OF SCORE ON LEFT	STANDARD TEN SCORE (STEN) Average										MEANING OF SCORE ON RIGHT
	1	2	3	4	5	6	7	8	9	10	
Cool, Reserved, Impersonal, Detached, Formal, Aloof					A						Warm, Outgoing, Kindly, Easy-going, Participating, Likes People
Concrete-thinking, Less Intelligent					B						Abstract-thinking, More Intelligent, Bright
Affected by Feelings, Emotionally Less Stable, Easily Annoyed					C						Emotionally Stable, Mature, Faces Reality, Calm
Submissive, Humble, Mild, Easily Led, Accommodating					E						Dominant, Assertive, Aggressive, Stubborn, Competitive, Bossy
Sober, Restrained, Prudent, Taciturn, Serious					F						Enthusiastic, Spontaneous, Heedless, Expressive, Cheerful
Expedient, Disregards Rules, Self-indulgent					G						Conscientious, Conforming, Moralistic, Staid, Rule-bound
Shy, Threat-sensitive, Timid, Hesitant, Intimidated					H						Bold, Venturesome, Uninhibited, Can Take Stress
Tough-minded, Self-reliant, No-nonsense, Rough, Realistic					I						Tender-minded, Sensitive, Over-protected, Intuitive, Refined
Trusting, Accepting Conditions, Easy to Get on with					L						Suspicious, Hard to Fool, Dis-trustful, Skeptical
Practical, Concerned with "Down to Earth" Issues, Steady					M						Imaginative, Absent-minded, Absorbed in Thought, Impractical
Forthright, Unpretentious, Open, Genuine, Artless					N						Shrewd, Polished, Socially Aware, Diplomatic, Calculating
Self-assured, Secure, Feels Free of Guilt, Untroubled, Self-satisfied					O						Apprehensive, Self-blaming, Guilt-prone, Insecure, Worrying
Conservative, Respecting Traditional Ideas					Q_1						Experimenting, Liberal, Critical, Open to Change
Group-oriented, A "Joiner" and Sound Follower, Listens to Others					Q_2						Self-sufficient, Resourceful, Prefers Own Decisions
Undisciplined Self-conflict, Lax, Careless of Social Rules					Q_3						Following Self-Image, Socially Precise, Compulsive
Relaxed, Tranquil, Composed, Has Low Drive, Unfrustrated					Q_4						Tense, Frustrated, Overwrought, Has High Drive

A sten of	1	2	3	4	5	6	7	8	9	10	is obtained
by about	2.3%	4.4%	9.2%	15.0%	19.1%	19.1%	15.0%	9.2%	4.4%	2.3%	of adults

Figure 34-3. Sample of 16 PF profile. (Karson S, O'Dell JW: A Guide to the Clinical Use of the 16 PF. Champaign, ILL, Institute for Personality and Ability Testing, copyright © 1976. Reproduced by permission.)

The Minnesota Multiphasic Personality Inventory

The MMPI is the most thoroughly researched and widely administered objective personality assessment instrument. This test has 10 clinical scales that are designed to indicate psychopathology and three validity scales that control for such factors as faking "good" or "bad," carelessness, or malingering. Table 34-2 lists the MMPI scales and some of the characteristics of a person who would score high or low on a particular scale.

Interpretation of the MMPI must be done only by a psychologist sophisticated in its use and scoring because there is no direct, absolute relationship between scores and the patient's psychiatric diagnoses. Inferences about the patient should not be based simply on the name of the scale. Instead, a clinician could infer only that a patient scoring high on a scale would have characteristics similar to other patients who score high on the same scale.

Although used in a variety of health settings, the MMPI appears to serve as a diagnostic aid only if psychological problems such as depression or anxiety are pronounced. It has not been found useful as a tool to assess the psychological mediators of illness such as

Table 34-2. Sample Interpretive Inferences for Standard MMPI Scales

SCALE NAME	SCALE ABBREVIATION	SCALE NO.	INTERPRETATION OF HIGH SCORES	INTERPRETATION OF LOW SCORES
—	L	—	Trying to create favorable impression by not being honest in responding to items; conventional; rigid; moralistic; lacks insight	Responded frankly to items; confident; perceptive; self-reliant; cynical
—	F	—	May indicate invalid profile; severe pathology; moody; restless; dissatisfied	Socially conforming; free of disabling psychopathology; may be "faking good"
—	K	—	May indicate invalid profile; defensive; inhibited; intolerant; lacks insight	May indicate invalid profile; exaggerates problems; self-critical; dissatisfied; conforming; lacks insight; cynical
Hypochondriasis	Hs	1	Excessive bodily concern; somatic symptoms; narcissistic; pessimistic; demanding; critical; long-standing problems	Free of somatic preoccupation; optimistic; sensitive; insightful
Depression	D	2	Depressed; pessimistic; irritable; dissatisfied; lacks self-confidence; introverted; overcontrolled	Free of psychological turmoil; optimistic; energetic; competitive; impulsive; undercontrolled; exhibitionistic
Hysteria	Hy	3	Physical symptoms of functional origin; lacks insight; self-centered; socially involved; demands attention and affection	Constricted; conventional; narrow interests; limited social participation; untrusting; hard to get to know; realistic

continued

Table 34-2. (continued)

SCALE NAME	SCALE ABBREVIATION	SCALE NO.	INTERPRETATION OF HIGH SCORES	INTERPRETATION OF LOW SCORES
Psychopathic deviate	Pd	4	Asocial or antisocial; rebellious; impulsive; poor judgment; immature; creates good first impression; superficial relationships; aggressive; free of psychological turmoil	Conventional: conforming; accepts authority; low drive level; concerned about status and security; persistent; moralistic
Masculinity-femininity	Mf	5	Male: aesthetic interests; insecure in masculine role; creative; good judgment; sensitive; passive; dependent; good self-control	Male: overemphasizes strength and physical prowess; adventurous; narrow interests; inflexible; contented; lacks insight
			Female: rejects traditional female role; masculine interests; assertive; competitive; self-confident; logical; unemotional	Female: accepts traditional female role; passive; yielding to males; complaining; critical; constricted
Paranoia	Pa	6	May exhibit frankly psychotic behavior; suspicious; sensitive; resentful; projects; rationalizes; moralistic; rigid	May have frankly psychotic symptoms; evasive; defensive; guarded; secretive; withdrawn
Psychasthenia	Pt	7	Anxious; worried; difficulties in concentrating; ruminative; obsessive; compulsive; insecure; lacks self-confidence; organized; persistent; problems in decision making	Free of disabling fears and anxieties; self-confident; responsible; adaptable; values success and status
Schizophrenia	Sc	8	May have thinking disturbance; withdrawn; self-doubts; feels alienated and unaccepted; vague goals	Friendly, sensitive, trustful; avoids deep emotional involvement; conventional; unimaginative
Hypomania	Ma	9	Excessive activity; impulsive; lacks direction; unrealistic self-appraisal; low frustration tolerance; friendly; manipulative; episodes of depression	Low energy level; apathetic; responsible; conventional; lacks self-confidence; overcontrolled
Social introversion	Si	0	Socially introverted; shy; sensitive; overcontrolled; conforming; problems in decision making	Socially extroverted; friendly; active; competitive; impulsive; self-indulgent

(Graham JR: The Minnesota Multiphasic Personality Inventory (MMPI). In Wolman BB (ed): Clinical Diagnosis of Mental Disorders: A Handbook. New York, Plenum Press, 1978) chronic anger, which has been cited as a factor leading to chronic heart disease (Karoly, 1985). Information from all the scales may not be helpful to the physical therapist. However, data from the depression and hypochondriasis scales might provide useful insights into the patient's behavior in a physical therapy setting.

The hypochondriasis scale (Hs) is a measure of a tendency to somatize problems or focus obsessively on bodily functions. Persons scoring high on this scale tend to report a large number of multiorgan physical complaints for which they seek professional health care. Subsequently, they often reject the recommended treatment and seek help from a number of other physicians, therapists, chiropractors, or alternative health care providers. They often behave in a dependent and passive manner, yet also express considerable hostility through a cynical, demanding, and complaining attitude. Patients with clearly diagnosed physical problems also tend to score higher on the Hs scale than a person without physical or health related emotional problems, but they score lower than hypochondriacal or somatizing patients.

We have all worked with patients who have behavior patterns similar to persons who have scored high on the Hs scale of the MMPI. These patients are most commonly seen in outpatient clinics where they are treated for various types of chronic pain and musculoskeletal disorders, and less frequently for central nervous system disorders. Although these patients may have a diagnosed physical disorder, their symptoms tend to persist despite repeated therapy sessions with multiple interventions. Unfortunately, if the physical therapist indicates to the patient, in words or behavior, that the patient's problem might be related to psychological issues, the patient's symptoms are likely to increase and the patient will often seek attention from health care providers elsewhere.

Physical therapists can best help these patients if they acknowledge the patient's physical complaints while focusing on developing a warm, trusting relationship. It is often helpful to see this type of patient frequently at first, until the patient feels secure with the physical therapist's attention.

Psychologists treating a patient with hypochondriasis or a somatizing disorder will attempt to determine if the patient's focus on bodily concerns is secondary to stressful life events. Failure to minimize both the underlying stress and the patient's use of somatic rather than verbal communication can lead to prolonged and unsuccessful treatment programs, which actually reinforce somatic responses to stress (Ford, 1983).

In some medical centers or physical therapy group practices, patients with somatizing disorders or chronic pain problems can be treated in a group program led jointly by a psychotherapist and physical or occupational therapist. Because hypochondrical patients often angrily reject any suggestions that their problems have a strong psychological component, this group format allows patients to deal with their physical complaints in an atmosphere where their physical symptoms are not denied, but improvement is strongly reinforced by the group members. In a specialized treatment group, patients often become quite friendly and supportive of one another, and gradually become more willing to share their thoughts and feelings and form positive relationships that are not contingent on illness (Ford, 1983; Moos, 1984).

A strong relationship exists between hypochondriasis and depression. People who score high on the depression (D) scale of the MMPI are characterized as having a persistent, pervasive sense of hopelessness and anxiety about the future, poor morale, dissatisfaction with life in general, and a poor sense of self-confidence.

Patients with a preexisting depressive behavior style or patients with a severe reactive depression who have been unable to regain their preloss or preillness momentum tend to react to their physical problems and the therapy process with persistent exaggerated or inappropriately depressed behaviors (Ford, 1983). These prolonged negative responses in the rehabilitation setting can interfere with the patient's motivation, energy level, sense of competence, and persistence. Cooperation with the staff and compliance with recommendations can be detrimentally affected by depression. Although the MMPI identifies persons with a generalized depressive cognitive-behavioral pattern, depression can also occur as a transitory mental state secondary to a traumatic life event.

Physical therapists often work with patients who are depressed secondary to illness, loss of mobility, or loss of independence. The therapist working with a patient who suffers from loss of function must be able to deal with the patient's grief by talking with him openly about his loss while providing reassurance that his grief is a transitory and common part of the recovery process. While most patients passing through a period of grief over loss will resume a positive state of mind with simple supportive psychotherapy, persons with a prolonged reactive depression or depressive personality style should be referred for more intensive psychotherapy. Working with a psychotherapist can help these patients understand how their depressive patterns of behavior are interfering with recovery.

It is imperative that a physical therapist be aware of the symptoms of depression. No matter how qualified or skilled the physical therapist is, the progress and outcome of treatment is largely dependent on the patient's motivation to improve, cooperation with recommended programs, and sense of self-efficacy (confidence in ability to accomplish a task or behavior). All these factors can be negatively affected by depression. Depressed patients may report problems with sleeping, usually with early morning wakening, loss of interest or pleasure in usual activities, withdrawal from others, physical lethargy, appetite changes, irritability, poor concentration, and feelings of worthlessness, often with recurrent thoughts of death or suicidal intention. If these symptoms are noted by the physical therapist during an intake evaluation or during the treatment sessions, the patient's physician should be informed so that the patient can be referred for appropriate medication and psychotherapy. A simple assessment tool to screen for depression in patients will be described in the next section on measures of specific psychological functions.

The Millon Behavioral Health Inventory

The Millon Behavioral Health Inventory (MBHI) was developed specifically to assess medical-behavioral issues (Millon, cited in Karoly.) The test consists of 20 scales. Eight scales deal with coping styles that indicate interpersonal and personality traits such as level of introversion, sociability, confidence, and forcefulness.

Six scales measure psychogenic attitudes such as chronic tension, premorbid pessimism, and social alienation. The psychogenic attitude scales assess the patient's perceptions about psychological stressors that have been found to exacerbate diseases or conditions, such as heart disease, rheumatoid arthritis, ulcerative colitis, musculoskeletal problems, and chronic pain disorders. For example, a person's tendency toward a negative view of the world is measured by the premorbid pessimism or helplessness-hopelessness scale. Patients who have a tendency to see life negatively are likely to intensify the feelings associated with illness or disability. A pervasive sense of hopelessness and helplessness interferes with successful treatment and has even been indicted as a possible factor in diseases such as multiple sclerosis, ulcerative colitis, and cancer (Karoly, 1985).

In another example, the social alienation scale identifies a patient's real or perceived level of familial and friendship support. Persons scoring high on this scale tend to adjust poorly to hospitalization. Early identification of these problems might allow the physical therapist and medical team to facilitate alternative support systems for the patient.

Three scales identify patients with high levels of somatic anxiety and psychosomatic inclinations, and the last three scales are designed to assist the medical team in identifying patients who might be more susceptible to future treatment problems or difficulties during the course of the illness.

Although the MBHI is a fairly new instrument, it may become a more powerful tool than the MMPI or 16 PF for identification of the interpersonal styles, attitudes, and behaviors that facilitate or endanger recovery from illness or injury (Karoly, 1985). The type of information gleaned from the MBHI might be particularly useful to physical therapists working with patients who are learning to cope with major permanent changes in physical competence and independence. An example of a patient's MBHI profile is shown in Figure 34-4.

MEASURES OF SPECIFIC PSYCHOLOGICAL FUNCTIONS

A great number of instruments have been developed to assess specific psychological factors that are believed to influence behavior. Al-

REPORT FOR: George C. SEX: M AGE: 54

ID NUMBER: DATE:
CODE:

SCALES	SCORE		PROFILE OF BR SCORES (35 60 75 85 100)	DIMENSIONS
	RAW	BR		
BASIC STYLE	1 12	13	XXX	INTROVERSIVE
	2 19	82	XXXXXXXXXXXXXXXXXXXXXXXXXXXXXXXXXX	INHIBITED
	3 19	52	XXXXXXXXXXX	COOPERATIVE
	4 21	22	XXXXX	SOCIABLE
	5 19	32	XXXXXXX	CONFIDENT
	6 17	70	XXXXXXXXXXXXXXXXXXXXX	FORCEFUL
	7 25	43	XXXXXXXXX	RESPECTFUL
	8 21	79	XXXXXXXXXXXXXXXXXXXXXXXXXXXXXXX	SENSITIVE
PSYCHOGENIC ATTITUDES	A 20	70	XXXXXXXXXXXXXXXXXXXXX	CHRONIC TENSION
	B 13	72	XXXXXXXXXXXXXXXXXXXXXX	RECENT STRESS
	C 30	87	XXXXXXXXXXXXXXXXXXXXXXXXXXXXXXXXXXXXXX	PREMORB PESSIMISM
	D 24	76	XXXXXXXXXXXXXXXXXXXXXXXXXX	FUTURE DESPAIR
	E 19	76	XXXXXXXXXXXXXXXXXXXXXXXXXX	SOCIAL ALIENATION
	F 27	90	XXXXXXXXXXXXXXXXXXXXXXXXXXXXXXXXXXXXXXXX	SOMATIC ANXIETY
PSYCHOSOMATIC	MM 16	81	XXXXXXXXXXXXXXXXXXXXXXXXXXXXXXXX	ALLERGIC INCLIN
	NN 10	70	XXXXXXXXXXXXXXXXXXXXX	GASTRO SUSCEPTBL
	OO 22	85	XXXXXXXXXXXXXXXXXXXXXXXXXXXXXXXXXXXXX	CARDIO TENDENCY
PROGNOSTIC	PP 11	59	XXXXXXXXXXXX	PAIN TREAT RESPON
	QQ 12	69	XXXXXXXXXXXXXXXXXXXXX	LIFE-THREAT REACT
	RR 7	80	XXXXXXXXXXXXXXXXXXXXXXXXXXXXXXX	EMOTIONAL VULNER

Figure 34-4. Example of a patient profile on the Millon Behavior Health Inventory (MBH). (Karoly P (ed): Measurement Strategies in Health Psychology. New York, John Wiley, 1985. Reproduced by permission.)

though most of these instruments were originally designed to measure group norms for research purposes rather than to identify an individual's specific behavior, they will be discussed here briefly because of the important concepts they identify.

The State-Trait Anxiety Inventory

The State-Trait Anxiety Inventory (STAI) was developed as a research instrument to measure group differences in the intensity and frequency of anxiety, tension, and apprehensiveness in normal adult populations. The inventory attempts to differentiate between an anxiety trait, which is a general proneness to anxiety, and an anxiety state, which is a more transitory perception of anxiety that a person feels at a particular time and in a specific situation.

The difference between anxiety state and anxiety trait may be an important concept for physical therapists to consider when working with a patient. For example, if a patient exhibits anxiety about his illness or injury and how it will affect his life, the physical therapist can decrease the patient's apprehension by setting aside time to listen to the patient and talk with him about his concerns. During that time, the therapist can give the patient more information about his exercise program, discuss treatment goals, and help the patient identify options for coping with changes in his physical performance and independence level. By making the patient an active force in his physical therapy process, the patient's anxiety will often be decreased while his sense of control and self-efficacy will be increased.

By contrast, the person with an anxiety trait is thought to have a pervasive history of responding to stressful life events with generalized anxiety, worry, and apprehension. Patients with high trait anxiety characteristics might worry about the effect of each new exercise, might be apprehensive about hurting themselves during therapy, might interpret any pain as an ominous sign, and might be pessimistic about their ability to assume independent activity. Patients with chronic or trait anxiety often benefit from counseling or participation in group therapy programs where they can observe other patients with similar problems working effectively within the physical therapy setting.

The Beck Depression Inventory

As noted in the discussion on the MMPI depression scale, depression can have a negative effect on physical therapy outcome. When depression is suspected as a factor interfering with treatment success, use of a screening measure may be appropriate. The Beck Depression Inventory (BDI) is an example of a brief, reasonably nonintrusive assessment measure of a person's current level of depressed mood. The test consists of 21 categories of specific overt behavioral manifestations of depression. In each category, a series of four self-evaluative statements, scored 0 through 3, reflect the level of a person's depressed state (Figure 34-5).

A total score is the sum of scores from each category. Total scores of 0–9 are considered normal, 10–15 mildly depressed, 16–19 moderately depressed, 20–29 moderately to severely depressed, and 30–63 severely depressed. Knowledge of the patient's depression level, as indicated by the total score on the BDI, may help the health team determine if psychotherapeutic and drug interventions would facilitate the rehabilitation process. The BDI can be used as a repeated measure to evaluate changes in the patient's affect over the course of treatment.

Read each group of statements and pick out the statement in each group which best describes the way you have been feeling in the past week, including today. Circle the number beside the statement that you picked.

0 I am not particularly discouraged about the future
1 I feel discouraged about the future
2 I feel I have nothing to look forward to
3 I feel that the future is hopeless and that things cannot improve

---

Figure 34-5. Sample question from the Beck Depression Inventory. (Beck AT, Rush AJ, Shaw BF et al: Cognitive Therapy of Depression. New York, The Guilford Press, 1979)

Multidimensional Health Locus of Control Scales

Another interesting psychological concept for physical therapists to consider is the patient's perceived locus of control for health care. The purpose of measuring locus of control is to determine if the patient perceives that his health is determined predominantly by other people, by chance or by fate (external locus of control), or by factors such as genetic heritage, self-discipline, and sense of self-efficacy in dealing with health issues (internal locus of control). The Multidimensional Health Locus of Control Scale (MHLC) (Wallston and Wallston, cited in Karoly, 1985) is the most widely used assessment tool for measuring locus of control in medical patients.

It is not difficult to imagine how a patient's perceived locus of control could affect her response to physical therapy. A patient who feels that other persons, such as doctors or family members, are responsible for her health may also assume that other persons are responsible for her improvement. Persons with a strong external locus of control for health care tend to be more passive and depressed, responding to an exercise program with minimal energy and poor compliance. Such patients tend to blame any lack of improvement on the physical therapist, on a family member, on lack of time, or even on the weather. However, patients with a high internal locus of control for health would be more likely to feel that their response to therapy is under their own control. They may tend to work with greater vigor, be more compliant with home programs, and be more adaptive to necessary changes in life-style.

Ways of Coping Scale

The way a patient assesses and copes with stress may be a more important factor in the progression of illness or response to treatment than the quantity or quality of stress (Moos, 1984). A patient's coping style can also have a major effect on physical therapy outcome. Coping styles have been conceptualized as being problem focused and emotion focused. These categories, however, are not always clear cut or absolute and should be used primarily as a guide to help us understand a person's coping strategies.

In general, problem-focused coping refers to the plan of action, or behaviors and strategies that a person uses to alter or minimize her sense of stress. For example, prior to discharge from a rehabilitation unit, a woman might arrange for carpenters to build a ramp into her home so that it will be ready for use the day she is discharged.

Emotion-focused coping strategies refer to the processes, such as avoidance, minimization, selective attention, or finding meaning in bad events, that the subject uses to minimize emotional distress. An example might be a patient's belief that his accident was really a blessing in disguise, because now he would be forced to spend more time with his family.

The Ways of Coping Scale—Revised is one instrument designed to identify a person's problem-focused and emotion-focused coping styles specific to a particular event. The scale asks the subjects to respond to 67 statements and indicate whether they used that particular manner of coping in their specific situation (Lazarus and Folkman; 1984). See Figure 34-6 for example questions.

A variation of the Ways of Coping Scale is Tobin's Coping Strategies Inventory, which is being used with medical patients and may have applications to a rehabilitation setting (Karoly, 1985).

Social Support Questionnaire

Patients' responses to chronic pain situations or to changes in physical ability and independence may also be affected by their use of social support systems. Because a person is most susceptible to influence during stressful life events, the way a person deals with the situation may depend somewhat on the support available from significant personal relationships. Types of personal relationships that have been identified are those that provide information, emotional support and guidance, social companionship, and assistance with physical and financial needs.

As with many of the psychological mea-

Please read each item below and indicate, by circling the appropriate category, to what extent you used it *in the situation you have just described* (eg, diagnosis of rheumatoid arthritis).

	Not used	Used some- what	Used quite a bit	Used a great deal
Talked to someone to find out more about the situation.	0	1	2	3
Turned to work or substitute activity to take my mind off things.	0	1	2	3
I reminded myself how much worse things could be.	0	1	2	3

Figure 34-6. Sample questions from the Ways of Coping Scale—Revised. (Lazarus RS, Folkman S: Stress, Appraisal, and Coping. New York, Springer, 1984)

Whom can you really count on to care about you, regardless of what is happening to you? Write in their name or initial.

0) No one
1) E.G. girlfriend   **4)** Fido, dog   **7)**
2) Mother   **5)**   **8)**
3) J.D. work friend   **6)**   **9)**

How satisfied are you with their support? <u>Underline</u> one.

6—very satisfied   5—fairly satisfied   4—a little satisfied   <u>3—a little dissatisfied</u>   2—fairly dissatisfied   1—very dissatisfied

Figure 34-7. Sample questions from Sarason's Social Support Questionnaire. (Sarason IG, Levine HM, Basham RB et al: Assessing social support: The social support questionnaire. J Pers Soc Psychol 44:127, 1983)

surement scales, measures of a patient's social support systems were developed primarily for research purposes and are seldom used for measurement of one person's social support systems. However, these research-oriented measuring tools can make one aware of the types of support that can affect patient function. They also can provide ideas for questioning patients about their social support connections. Sarason's Social Support Questionnaire is an example of a research-based measurement that asks the patient to list up to nine

people to whom he or she can turn for various types of support. An example of several questions from this questionnaire can be seen in Figure 34-7.

By identifying the patient's perceived primary sources of support, the physical therapist may be better able to understand the patient's responses to treatment, develop appropriate treatment goals, and establish realistic discharge plans. For example, if you are treating a generally healthy elderly man with back and hip pain who is not responding to treatment, you may find, when talking with him, that he has no family residing in the area and has no contact with other people except during his walk to the newsstand each morning. For this patient, physical therapy appointments may be the social highlight of his week. A referral to an appropriate senior center for social activities could make a major difference in his response to treatment. In another example, if you found that a teenage girl with a spinal cord injury could not identify supportive peers and listed her parents as her only source of support, you might want to arrange for her to become involved in peer group activities prior to discharge from the rehabilitation unit so that she does not become enmeshed in a family structure that could foster dependence and isolation.

Therapists primarily working with children might review the social support structures of families to help identify whether parental involvement with a handicapped child is markedly limiting their own social interactions. In addition, it is important to determine whether the parents have adequate support systems to help them deal with the complex medical, educational, and social issues related to the child's problems, and whether the child has adequate opportunities to interact with other handicapped and nonhandicapped children.

PAIN ASSESSMENT

Many patients treated by physical therapists experience some degree of pain. With time and treatment, most patients' pain decreases or is completely eradicated. However, some patients continue to experience pain despite extensive treatment by different medical specialists. In some larger medical centers, patients with chronic pain can be referred to pain specialty clinics for evaluation by a neurologist, an anesthesiologist specializing in the treatment of pain, a physical therapist, an occupational therapist, a psychologist, and other specialists, depending on the patient's problem.

When evaluating patients with chronic pain, physical therapists carefully assess the patient's sensory-motor status. They also attempt to determine the character of the patient's pain (eg, burning, stabbing, shooting, constant, intermittent) and to identify conditions that increase the patient's pain, as well as conditions that decrease the patient's pain. The therapist's evaluations, however, seldom focus on the possible psychological factors that are associated with or contribute to the patient's pain.

Personality inventories such as the MMPI or the 16 PF have been used in an attempt to predict how a person will respond to treatment for pain; however, measures such as Melzack's McGill Pain Questionnaire have been developed specifically to assess chronic pain. The purpose of doing a comprehensive psychological assessment of the patient's pain is, in part, to understand the extent of disruption in the patient's life caused by pain, to determine the possible intrapsychic mediators of pain (eg, somatizing or hypochondriacal disorder, depression), to identify the thought processes related to the pain (eg, "I'll never get better," or "I'm too tired to do my exercises"), to review the patient's pain-related behaviors and their interaction with responses of other persons (eg, "I can tell you're in pain when you grimace like that; why don't you just lie down again?"), to assess the effectiveness of the patient's coping methods and support systems, to identify the patient's goals (eg, "I want to get back to work as soon as possible"), and to evaluate the patient's sense of self-efficacy to manage the pain and reach the stated goals ("I want to work, but I don't think I can work an eight-hour day again") (Karoly; Schneiderman and Tapp, 1985).

Although psychologists have developed a number of comprehensive pain assessment questionnaires, the simplest method of assessment that can be used very effectively by physical therapists is the pain diary. With this method, patients are asked to keep a daily record of the intensity, frequency, and type of pain experienced along with a description of the situations or activities that seem to decrease or increase the pain. They also are instructed to monitor the thoughts and emotions that occur prior to the onset of pain, during the pain, or after the pain has subsided. With this self-monitoring system, the assessment team may be able to determine if the patient's pain is related to specific physical activities that biomechanically stress the patient's system or, alternatively, to behaviors, emotions, or cognitions that might suggest a major psychological component. Using the diary technique, the assessment team or a physical therapist can also evaluate the effectiveness of their treatment interventions. An example of one format for a pain diary is shown in Figure 34-8.

TESTS OF INTELLIGENCE AND NEUROPSYCHOLOGICAL FUNCTION

Since cognitive and developmental testing is more strictly the province of psychologists (and some occupational and speech therapists), I will briefly review some of the common tests of intellectual function.

Physical therapists working with children or adults with brain damage know that the patient's ability to cooperate with the treatment program is determined, in part, by the patient's ability to attend to, understand, and respond to verbal, visual, spatial, and tactile instructions. Other factors related to the patients' potential are motivation, emotional stability, and adaptive and judgmental abilities. Although physical therapists working with brain-injured patients often become very clever at finding ways to circumvent the patient's sensory, cognitive, and affective deficits, a thorough understanding of the patient's specific intellectual and neuropsychological problems would facilitate the rehabilitation process.

INTELLIGENCE TESTS

The most common individually administered test of general intelligence in adults is the Wechsler Adult Intelligence Scale—Revised (WAIS—R) (Wechsler, in Graham and Lilly,

Pain Diary					
Week: _____ Circle Day: M T W Th F Sa Su Pain/Stress Scale is 1–100					
Time of Day	Type, Character of Pain	Intensity of Pain (1–100)	Describe Activities Who, What, Where	Feeling, Thoughts, Stresses	Indicate Stress/Pain Reduction Techniques, Exercises, Medications, and Results
6–7 AM					
7–8 AM					
8–9 AM					
9–10 AM					
10–11 AM					
11–12 AM					

Figure 34-8. Truncated example of a pain diary. A complete diary would be divided into one- or two-hour segments from the time the patient arises until the time the patient retires. The last section can be used for reporting nighttime pain.

1984). This test consists of eleven subtests, six centered around verbal skills information, such as vocabulary and arithmetic (Verbal IQ), and five related to performance skills such as picture completion, block design, and digit symbol performance (Performance IQ). The eleven subtests are combined to give a Full Scale Score IQ. Wechsler also developed intelligence tests for children: the Wechsler Intelligence Scale for Children—Revised (WISC—R), appropriate for ages 6 to 16 years; and the Wechsler Preschool and Primary Scale of Intelligence (WPPSI) for children between the ages of 3 years, 2.5 months and 6 years, 7.5 months. Like the WAIS—R, both the WISC—R and WPPSI consist of subtests scored to yield Verbal, Performance, and Full Scale scores of IQ (Newmark, 1985). All the Wechsler scales are designed such that IQs are expressed as deviation scores with a mean of 100 and a standard deviation of 15.

The Stanford-Binet Intelligence Scale (S-B) is another well-known test measuring a subject's current mental functioning. It is most useful for predicting academic achievement or assessing the IQ of children. The Stanford-Binet gives a single IQ score that is a measure of mental (primarily verbal) ability (Graham and Lilly, 1984).

The Bayley Scales of Infant Development was developed for use with infants and young children in the first two and one-half years. The Bayley has 163 items in the mental scale and 81 items in the motor scale. The mental scale assesses factors such as sensory-perceptual activities, object constancy, memory learning, problem-solving ability, and early verbal communication. The motor scale measures degree of control of the body, and gross and fine motor skills. Both the mental and motor scales have been standardized to have a mean of 100 with a standard deviation of 16. The Bayley scales are helpful primarily in identifying infants who are at risk for developing a motor or mental disability; however, the scales are not highly predictive of future behavior on the Bayley or performance on other measures of intelligence.

Because the Wechsler and Bayley require verbal and motor responses and the Stanford-Binet requires verbal responses, they often are not appropriate for measuring the intellectual abilities of persons with speech difficulties, or visual and physical limitations that could impair the ability to manipulate test items. Examples of standardized tests of intelligence that have been used with persons who are limited to finger pointing or "eye pointing" are the Columbia Mental Maturity Scale for children between the ages of 3 years, 6 months and 9 years, 11 months; the Peabody Picture Vocabulary Test—Revised; and the Raven Colored Progressive Matrices. The Stanford-Binet also has been adapted for use with "eye pointing" (Graham and Lilly, 1984).

NEUROPSYCHOLOGICAL TESTS

In some rehabilitation programs for persons with brain damage, psychologists administer comprehensive evaluations of the patient's cognitive, behavioral, and psychological strengths and weaknesses. Therefore, a battery of psychometric tests is used to develop a comprehensive picture of the level and quality of the patient's cerebral function. The Halstead-Reitan Neuropsychological Test Battery (HRB) is the most completely validated test battery to meet these needs. Three versions are available to test patients from age 5 years to adult. The HRB consists of 11 tests, including the age-appropriate Wechsler and the MMPI, which were discussed earlier. The other eight subtests are used to help identify performance on tasks requiring mental skills such as abstract reasoning, concept formation, judgment, mental flexibility, sequencing abilities, perceptual motor tasks such as problems in tactile and kinesthetic feedback, visual scanning, fine motor skills, spatial memory, and right-left dominance. The tests also screen for such deficits as dysgraphia, dyslexia, dysnomia, dyscalculia, dyspraxia, and right-left confusion.

From the subtest scores, a Halstead Impairment Index is computed, reflecting a general level of cerebral dysfunction. Several rating scales have been developed by those who use the battery. The HRB, when used appropriately, can assist members of the rehabilitation team in identifying the patient's cognitive and behavioral assets and deficits, their implications for body functioning, and what types of rehabilitation efforts might be appropriate (Horton and Wedding, 1984).

CONCLUSION

The assessment tools discussed in this chapter are used by clinical and research psychologists to identify a patient's specific preexisting personality style or behavioral patterns or to identify specific psychological factors that might influence the way a person reacts to or copes with stress.

Patients referred for physical therapy must cope with stresses created by their illness or injury. These stresses are caused by such factors as chronic pain, loss of motor function, and changes in the level of independence. Such changes in physical function may affect the person's social interactions, work productivity, and enjoyment of life. It is not uncommon for patients to feel extremely anxious, depressed, or even helpless about dealing with stresses related to their physical problems. If patients also have poor social support systems, preexisting psychopathologic conditions, or a strong external locus of control for health care, they will have difficulty generating the level of physical or psychological energy necessary for rehabilitation. This puts physical therapists in a particularly difficult situation because successful treatment outcome is often dependent on the patient's goal-oriented, active, positive approach toward dealing with the physical consequences of illness or disability.

To be effective, physical therapists must be more than procedurally competent. They must also be experts in motivating their patients to take charge of their own recovery. This can be done by educating patients about their pathologic condition and course of treatment, by developing positive, supportive relationships with their patients, and by helping their patients identify and change psychological factors that may be interfering with their ability to cope successfully with physical problems.

If it becomes evident that psychological, social, or environmental issues are preventing a patient from maximizing his recovery, the therapist should consult with a psychologist, preferably one familiar with behavioral medicine. Often, the psychologist can simply make suggestions that will help the physical therapist deal more effectively with the patient's psychosocial problems. In some cases, however, a full psychological assessment with psychotherapy interventions may be necessary to help the patient recover from or adapt to physical illnesses or disabilities.

ANNOTATED BIBLIOGRAPHY

Ford CV: The Somatizing Disorders: Illness as a Way of Life. New York, Elsevier Biomedical, 1983 (This is a well written, fascinating book covering all aspects of sick role behaviors including hypochondriasis, chronic pain syndromes, malingering, and disability syndromes.)

Goldman J, L'Engle-Stein C, Guerry S: Psychological Methods of Child Assessment. New York, Brunner/Mazel, 1983 (The authors provide a complete text covering most aspects of child assessment such as IQ tests, developmental instruments, projective assessment instruments, behaviorally based measures, and neuropsychological assessment techniques.)

Graham JR, Lilly RS: Psychological Testing. Englewood Cliffs, NJ, Prentice-Hall, 1984 (This introductory text covers the basic principles of tests and measurements. Some of the most commonly used testing techniques are described, illustrated, and evaluated in detail.)

Horton AM Jr, Wedding D: Clinical and Behavioral Neuropsychology: An Introduction. New York, Praeger, 1984 (This book provides a comprehensive view of brain-behavior relationships and the neuropsychological testing techniques used with patients with brain damage. The major tests discussed are the Halstead-Reitan Test Battery and the Luria-Nebraska Test Battery.)

Karoly P (ed): Measurement Strategies in Health Psychology. New York, John Wiley &

Sons, 1985 (An excellent book. The authors discuss the types of assessment tools appropriate for assessing the psychological function of persons in health care settings. Both clinical and research measures are discussed.)

Krueger DW (ed): Rehabilitation Psychology: A Comprehensive Textbook. Rockville, MD, Aspen Systems, 1984 (The editor has compiled papers dealing with topics such as the psychological rehabilitation of physical trauma, psychosocial stressors in coping with disability, sexual rehabilitation, depression and suicide in the disabled, and roles and concerns of rehabilitation professionals.)

Leigh H, Reiser MF: The Patient: Biological, Psychological, and Social Dimensions of Medical Practice, 2nd ed. New York, Plenum Medical Book Company, 1985 (A comprehensive book that details the psychosocial and psychophysiological considerations of being a patient. It also provides a clinical systems approach to assessing the patient and suggestions on managing patient care.)

Moos RH (ed): Coping with Physical Illness. 2: New Perspectives. New York, Plenum Medical Book Company, 1984 (Chapters cover problems related to coping with birth defects, childhood and adult cancer, and other chronic conditions. It also deals with the crises related to hospitalization and treatment procedures, fear of dying, and the stresses encountered by staff.)

Payton OD (ed): Psychosocial Aspects of Clinical Practice, Vol 8. New York, Churchill Livingstone, 1986 (Written by physical therapists, this book contains chapters on professional communication skills, effect of environment and influence of values on patient care, psychological dimensions of illness, and professional socialization. Many examples given are specific to the practice of physical therapy.)

Schwartz DM, Tapp JT, Brucker B: Behavioral Assessment in Medical Settings. In Schneiderman N, Tapp JT (eds): Behavioral Medicine: The Biopsychosocial Approach. Hillsdale, NJ, Lawrence Erlbaum Associates, 1985 (This up-to-date text incorporates sections on psychological and behavioral assessment in medical settings as well as sections on life-styles and health and behavioral aspects of health disorders.)

35 Analysis of Activities of Daily Living

LINDA VAN DILLEN
KATHRYN E. ROACH

As individuals we define ourselves largely by what we do. The ability to perform our day-to-day activities is central to our sense of health and well-being. Health has been defined by Parsons as "A state of optimum capacity of an individual for the effective performance of roles and tasks for which he or she has been socialized." The exact nature of those day-to-day activities may vary greatly from person to person, but certain activities are common to almost everyone. These common activities are often referred to as *activities of daily living* (ADL).

The purpose of this chapter is to provide an understanding of the concepts of function and measurement as they relate to ADL. We will also describe the role of the physical therapist in assessing an individual's ability to perform various ADL and in designing treatment programs to improve that ability. To accomplish this, we will discuss (1) the terminology pertinent to function, measurement, and ADL; (2) the tools and methods used to measure the ability to perform ADL; (3) the factors that influence the ability to perform ADL; and (4) the clinical decision-making process we use to design and implement treatment programs intended to improve the patient's performance of ADL.

DEFINITION OF TERMS

One of the underlying premises of physical therapy is that the goal of the physical thera-pist is to enhance human movement and function. This premise further includes the assessment, prevention, and treatment of movement dysfunction and physical disabilities. To understand this statement, it is important to understand the definition of function.

The term "function" can be used to describe several different phenomena. Function can refer to the action of a body part, such as the function of the upper extremity. Function can also be used to describe the patient's ability to perform ADL. Finally, function can be used to describe a person's performance in all aspects of life.

This third concept of function is subdivided into four separate components. The first is physical function, the area with which physical therapists are most frequently involved. Physical function deals with such sensory-motor tasks as walking, climbing stairs, shopping, housework, and meal preparation. Activities of daily living (ADL) are usually classified as a part of physical function. The second area of function is mental function. This area deals with intellectual or cognitive ability. Memory and reasoning capabilities are examples of mental function. The third area of function is emotional function. Emotional function has been defined by Jette as "a person's affect and effectiveness in psychologically coping with life's stresses." Depression, anxiety, and happiness are factors that reflect emotional function. The fourth area of function is social function. This area is involved with a person's ability to perform various social roles and to establish and maintain human relationships. The ability to be employed outside the home is an example of social function. The term handicap is used to describe the inability to perform accepted social functions.

The term "functional status" can be used to define an individual's performance in any or all of these four categories of function. In physical therapy, the term functional status most commonly refers to performance in physical function. It can also more specifically refer to an individual's ability to perform ADL.

ADL consist of those tasks that are recognized as essential components of everyday life. They are tasks that the person must perform in order to function within the home and within society. ADL can be divided into two categories: basic activities of daily living (BADL), and instrumental activities of daily living (IADL). BADL are tasks that are more fundamental and body oriented. The subcategory of BADL can be further divided into two groups: basic mobility and self-care. Basic mobility tasks include bed mobility, transfers, and ambulation. Self-care tasks consist of such activities as feeding, bathing, and dressing. IADL are more complex and less body-related activities than are BADL. There is less agreement on the range of items included as IADL. IADL can be divided into two categories: activities performed in the home (such as laundry and housekeeping), and activities performed outside the home (such as use of transportation and shopping). Figure 35-1 presents a schema of ADL.

MEASUREMENT OF FUNCTIONAL STATUS

If we define health in terms of a person's ability to perform various roles and tasks, and if the physical therapist's role in health care is to enhance the patient's ability to function in this sense, then functional status must be measured to document both the need for and the effect of physical therapy. From this perspective, functional status is the ultimate outcome measure in physical therapy.

Although the physical signs and symptoms therapists traditionally measure, such as range of motion or pain, may affect a patient's ability to perform ADL, they are not by themselves adequate to describe functional status. Functional status must be assessed as a separate phenomenon. The process of measuring an individual's functional status is complex. Many factors need to be considered when attempting to measure function.

The first decision is whether to use an established, standardized measurement tool or to employ a nonstandardized method. Standardization requires that the items in a measurement tool are uniform and clearly defined. Clear and uniform definition is important in order to provide sufficient information to allow therapists to administer and interpret a measurement tool without requiring any additional outside knowledge. This ensures that two physical therapists with different backgrounds, but equal experience using the measurement tool, will arrive at the same results. Standardized measurement tools usually have rules for assigning numbers to the behaviors being measured.

Standardization in practice is a matter of degree. If a physical therapist always measures something in the same way and describes the results in the same terms, that physical therapist has attained a level of standardization. If a group of physical therapists agree on a method to measure and describe a phenomenon, then they have attained a higher level of standardization. Even formally standardized measurement tools may vary greatly in the degree to which various aspects are defined. Some measurement tools may simply list the number of items to be tested and a method for describing the result. Other measurement tools may strictly define the setting and the manner in which those items will be measured.

The nonstandardized measurement of function is commonplace. This type of measurement has the advantage of being easily tailored to the characteristics of each patient. However, nonstandardized measurement has several disadvantages. A nonstandardized method of measurement can lend itself to incompleteness and subjectivity. It is difficult, if

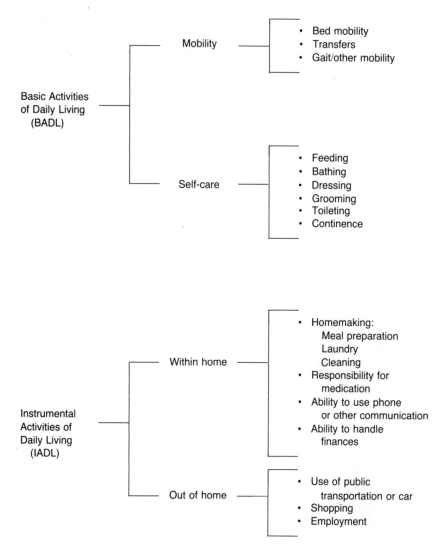

Figure 35-1. Schema of activities of daily living.

not impossible, to use a nonstandardized method of measurement to compare findings between patients, between therapists, or over time.

Ideally, a standardized measurement tool should be both reliable and valid. Reliability addresses whether a measurement tool is consistent in the results it produces. There are two types of reliability. The first is interrater reliability, which deals with the consistency of results obtained by two clinicians measuring the same subject. The second type, intrarater or test-retest reliability, describes the degree to which results are reproducible when the same clinician tests a subject at two different times. If a measurement tool is reliable, then changes that one would obtain from one measurement to another should reflect true differences in the item measured rather than clinician inconsistency or error.

Validity is the ability of a tool to measure what it purports to measure. Establishing the validity of a measurement tool is a complex process, which should begin with testing of its reliability. A measurement tool cannot be valid unless it is also reliable. However, reliability does not guarantee validity.

There are several other characteristics of measurement tools that should be considered when examining functional assessments. The first of these is the measurement dimension. The measurement dimension is an aspect of the measured activity. Measurement dimensions in functional assessment include such things as the degree of difficulty, the amount of pain, and the time required to perform an activity. The rating scale defines the degree or the extent of the measurement dimension. It is critical to match the measurement dimension to the important clinical characteristics of the patient. Measuring the amount of pain experienced may provide a great deal of information when assessing the function of a patient with arthritis. However, the amount of pain experienced is unlikely to provide much useful information when measuring a patient who has suffered a cerebrovascular accident.

Scoring systems are used to assign a numerical value to the patient's performance on a functional assessment. To develop a scoring system, the measurement dimension must be broken down into a rating scale, which consists of levels of performance defined in a way that makes each level as mutually exclusive as possible. A numerical value or score is then assigned to each level. The score for each item may be added for a total score, or items may be grouped into related subsets for which subscores are derived. If the decision is made that one item or subset is more important than another item or subset, then its numerical value can be made relatively greater than the less important one. This process is referred to as weighting.

The second characteristic of measurement tools is mode of administration. Clinicians can obtain information from a functional assessment by direct observation of a patient performing the task, by report from the patient, by report from the family or caretaker, by clinical judgment, or from review of the medical record. Information on some measurement dimensions, such as pain, is difficult to obtain except by patient report. For other measurement dimensions, such as the amount of assistance required, a patient's report may not be as accurate as direct observation. However, direct observation can be time consuming and costly. Direct observation is also limited to the time of the observation and usually best suited to assessment of less complex activities, such as BADL. Direct observation is usually a very reliable method and demonstrates face validity when standardized. Chart audits, clinical judgment, self-administered questionnaires, and standardized interviews are all less time-consuming than direct observation. These are less direct methods of measurement, but allow measurement of more complex activities. All can introduce some degree of subjectivity unless highly standardized.

The third characteristic, focus, is determined by the items to be measured by the tool. Therefore, focus deals with the categories of function addressed, as well as with the nature, and the number of items included within each category. The specific categories of function addressed and the number of items in each category varies greatly from one functional assessment to another.

The fourth characteristic of measurement tools to consider is feasibility. A measurement tool is feasible if it is practical to administer and score in the setting in which it is used. Feasibility is related to the length of time required to administer the measurement tool, and the complexity of administration and scoring.

The fifth and final characteristic is precision. Precision is the degree of refinement with which a measurement tool is defined. In functional assessments, precision is obtained by the choice of items included and by the choice and definition of the measurement dimension. For example, one can choose the measure bed mobility as a single entity, or one can measure its component parts of rolling to either side and transferring from supine to sitting and from sitting to supine. Precision can also be influenced by the definition of the measurement dimension. For example, the measurement dimension degree of assistance required to perform an activity may be divided into three categories: independent, dependent, and unable. To increase precision, degree of assistance may be broken down into five categories: independent, supervision, verbal assistance, physical assistance, and unable.

There is a wide range of functional assessments available. We have already presented some of the advantages of using a standardized assessment. However, before deciding to use any functional assessment, it is important to examine its characteristics carefully to determine if it is suitable for your use.

First, you must determine if the measurement dimension is appropriate for the type of patient you wish to measure. If you are treating an arthritic patient and hope through treatment to decrease the amount of pain that the patient experiences when performing various activities, then the amount of pain experienced is a critical measurement dimension. The use of a different measurement dimension would fail to provide important information.

Second, you must examine the mode of administration in light of the clinical setting and the type of patients to be assessed. Patient or family report of the patient's ability to perform a variety of activities may not be accurate if the patient has recently suffered a major disease or injury and has had no opportunity to attempt those activities.

The third characteristic, focus, is important to consider when you decide exactly what functions you want to assess. A tool that measures only BADL is limited in its use in the home care setting, where IADL becomes an essential part of treatment. The patient may be able to perform all BADL independently but remain dependent in some IADL. A tool that measures only BADL will not reflect this dependency.

The fourth characteristic, feasibility, is critical. A tool's feasibility is dependent on how it is administered and how many activities are measured. If an assessment requires more time than is available to administer it, then its clinical usefulness will be limited.

Finally, it is important to consider a tool's precision. A tool's precision must be adequate to detect degrees of change within the functions measured. This is partially dependent on the degree of change that can be expected in the patient being measured. For example, if a patient's treatment will emphasize training in bed mobility, it is important that the assessment be precise enough to detect change in components of bed mobility. Lack of precision makes it difficult to detect potentially significant degrees of change.

ACTIVITIES OF DAILY LIVING MEASUREMENT TOOLS

The following is a review of four functional status measures most commonly used in rehabilitation. We will discuss characteristics of each tool as well as advantages and disadvantages for their use in various settings. Table 35-1 lists characteristics of these tools.

BARTHEL INDEX AND BARTHEL SELF-CARE RATINGS

The Barthel Index (BI) and Barthel Self-Care Ratings (BSC) are ADL measures (Mahoney). The BI was developed by Dorothea Barthel, P.T., and Florence Mahoney, M.D. The BSC is a modified version of the BI and was developed by Granger and associates. The BI, first published in 1965, is probably one of the best known formalized functional assessments and is widely used in rehabilitation clinics.

The BI is a physical function measure that focuses on self-care and basic mobility. The index includes the following items: feeding, bowel and bladder control, personal toilet, dressing and undressing, wheelchair-to-bed and bed-to-wheelchair transfers, toilet transfers, walking on level surfaces, ascending and descending stairs, and propelling a wheelchair. Both self-care and basic mobility are equally represented.

The measurement dimension employed by the BI is the amount of assistance required to perform each of the defined activities. Ratings

Table 35-1. Characteristics of ADL Measurement Tools

FOCUS	MEASUREMENT DIMENSION	MODE OF ADMINISTRATION	POPULATION APPLIED TO
Barthel Index			
BADL	Level of assistance	Professional judgment, chart audit	Acute care, rehabilitation
Kenny Self-Care Evaluation			
BADL	Level of assistance	Professional judgment, direct observation	Rehabilitation
Katz Index of ADL			
BADL (primarily self-care)	Level of assistance	Professional judgment	Acute care, rehabilitation, institutionalized setting
PULSES Profile			
Physical, emotional, and social function	Level of assistance; impairment	Professional judgment	Acute care, rehabilitation, institutionalized setting

are "independent," "needs help," or "not practical." A person's performance is rated "not practical" if he cannot meet the criteria for "independent" or "needs help." Each item is scored separately. A score is then given to represent how the person performed each item.

The BI uses a weighted scoring system. That is, independent performances of certain items are given more value because they contribute to the person's overall functional status. For example, independence in walking is given 15 points, while independence in feeding is given 10 points. The scores for each item are added together for an overall functional score. The maximum score obtainable is 100. The decision to weight individual items was based on the clinical judgment of those who developed the measure. The developers of the BI maintain that the person who attains a total score of 100 is independent in all the ADL items measured and can perform ADL without attendant care. The mode of administration of the BI is through chart audit and professional judgment.

The original BI has many positive features. It is concise and simply written, which makes it easy to learn. It is also feasible to use in clinical settings because it requires very little time to administer. The scoring system provides information on individual items as well as a total ADL score. The BI has been used in acute care and rehabilitation hospitals. The lack of IADL items on the BI limits its usefulness in home care and extended care facilities. Most of its use has been with chronic disease populations, particularly patients who have had a cerebrovascular accident (CVA) and other patients with some degree of paralysis. Reliability has not been formally reported, but validity has been tested and found acceptable.

The major drawbacks of the BI are lack of precision and questionable reliability. The lack of precision has two sources. First, the small number of items scored and the grouping of several component activities into a single item limits precision. For example, moving from wheelchair to bed and bed to wheelchair includes (1) moving in bed; (2) moving from sit, to supine, to sit; (3) positioning the wheelchair; (4) wheelchair setup for transfer; (5) transferring to and from the wheelchair; (6) approaching the bed to transfer; and (7) performing all of these with safety. For a patient to score 15 for independence in this activity, he must perform independently all of the components just listed. Change in any one of the component activities will not be detected by change in the score. Thus, smaller increments of change in function are not documented.

The second area in which precision is reduced is in the rating scale. The measurement dimension of the BI is level of independence in performance, which is broken down into three levels: "independent," "needs help," and "not practical." The definition of the second level is very broad. It includes all levels of physical and verbal assistance as well as supervision. A person may progress from requiring maximal physical assistance to only verbal cues, and still be rated as "needs help." Thus, change in activity is not reflected by a change in the score.

Reliability can be diminished by lack of adequate definitions of the terminology used in the rating scale and items. Words and phrases frequently used in the practice setting (such as "needs minimal, moderate, or maximal assistance," "requires supervision," "can perform safely," and "performs in a reasonable amount of time") are all used in the BI. Definitions of each term are not supplied. Lack of standard definitions for terminology can introduce subjectivity and result in lack of agreement between therapists and over time.

Modifications in the Barthel Self-Care Ratings made by Granger and his associates have improved both the precision and the reliability of the original BI. Refer to the original resources to evaluate these changes.

KENNY SELF-CARE EVALUATION

The second functional assessment we will review is the Kenny Self-Care Evaluation (Ivenson). The Kenny Evaluation is a physical function measure that focuses primarily on BADL. It is divided into seven major categories: bed activities, transfers, locomotion, dressing, personal hygiene, bowel and bladder, and feeding. Each category is further subdivided into component activities. For example, the major category of bed activities is divided into the following two component activities: moving in bed, and rising and sitting. Each of these activities is then divided into specific tasks, such as shift position, turn to left side, turn to right side.

The measurement dimension for the Kenny Evaluation is the level of assistance required to perform a task. The rating scale ranges from 4, which is defined as completely independent in a task, to 0, which is defined as totally dependent. A total category score (eg, bed activities) is derived by adding each activity score for the category and dividing by the number of activities. A total self-care score is arrived at by adding all of the category scores. According to the developers, patients who attain independence in the defined ADL will be independent in their physical needs at home or in some other protected environment. The mode of administration is direct observation of the patient's performance. Instructions for administration allow the rater to assign scores that seem closest to the patient's average performance, if testing does not appear to be representative of the patient's usual performance. This method is recommended for use with the patient who tends to fluctuate in performance from day to day.

In contrast to the Barthel Index, the strength of the Kenny Evaluation is precision. As illustrated by the description of the scoring system above, precision is achieved by both the detail of the rating scale and the number of component activities and specific tasks into which each category is divided. The Kenny Evaluation provides information on change in each component activity, and this change is reflected in the score.

The organization of the Kenny Evaluation has several advantages. The evaluation facilitates specific treatment planning because each category of ADL is already broken down into component activities similar to those taught in the treatment situation. The evaluation also provides the clinician with information in each category of ADL through the subscores, as well as a total score representing the patient's overall functional status. Because of the nature of the ADL items measured, the Kenny Evaluation is primarily used in clinical rehabilitation settings. Its feasibility in acute care settings is limited by the length of time required to carry out the evaluation. The Kenny Evaluation's use in the home care setting is limited by time, mode of administering the test, and lack of additional functions (ie, IADL).

There are other drawbacks associated with the Kenny Evaluation as a result of its length and detail. It requires a long time to learn how to administer the test accurately. Even though the test is designed for direct observation, the developers do allow the rater to assign scores based on an average performance if testing does not appear to represent usual performance, so interrater reliability may be questioned. Reliability has not been formally reported to date. Some validity studies have been carried out by Shoening and co-workers and reported as acceptable. We refer you to Ivenson and colleagues for further information on the development and use of the Kenny evaluation.

KATZ INDEX OF ADL

The Katz Index of ADL was first reported in 1963 by Katz and his colleagues. The Katz Index is a physical function measure that includes only BADL. Its primary focus is on self-care activities including bathing, dressing, toileting, continence, and feeding. The Katz Index specifically measures only one basic mobility skill, transfers. The measurement dimension is the degree of independence in performance of the BADL items. The mode of administration of the Katz Index is chart audits, patient self report, and professional judgment. Direct observation, in which the therapist watches the patient specifically perform an activity, may be used to supplement the professional's judgment. This may be done when the therapist cannot recall a patient's performance in an activity or feels that he has not observed the patient frequently enough to decide on an average performance.

The original Katz Index has a unique scoring system. For each of the six activities measured, a person scores 1 if he requires no human assistance to complete the item or 0 if help is required. According to the specific activities a person performs independently, a letter ranging from A to G is assigned. For example, if the person is independent in all six self-care activities, he receives a grade of A. If he is independent in feeding, continence, transferring, and dressing and dependent in bathing and going to the toilet, the grade would be C. Given a particular grade, it is possible to determine precisely which activities the person performs independently. The developers have also defined an "other" level for persons who do not fall into this "ordering" of independence in self-care. For further explanation, refer to the original papers by Katz and his colleagues.

Some of the advantages of the original version of the Katz Index are brevity, ease of administration, and ease of learning. This original version of the Katz Index has a worksheet that concisely defines three levels of assistance for each item. These include "independent," "intermediate," and "dependent." The therapist completes the worksheet based on the person's most dependent performance observed in the preceding two weeks. Information recorded on the worksheet is then used to assign a grade of A through G. The worksheet provides the therapist with more detailed information than does the letter grade.

Although not as detailed as the Kenny Evaluation, the Katz Index is better defined than the Barthel Index. Its ratings, (independent, intermediate, and dependent) are easier to learn than the Kenny Evaluation, yet the Katz Index does not lend itself to as much ambiguity as do parts of the Barthel Index. Definitions and levels of performance for each self-care item are written on the worksheet, which facilitates the therapist's rating of the patient. The therapist simply determines the patient's level of performance based on the six ADL items, and then completes the worksheet. The time required to rate the patient depends upon knowledge of the patient's performance over the last two weeks.

Because of its ease of administration, the Katz Index can be used in hospital settings as well as in nursing homes and extended care facilities. The Katz Index could be used in the home care setting as well, but the use of the

Index here is somewhat limited because of the BADL focus.

Because of its unique design, the Katz Index also has some disadvantages. One of the primary drawbacks is decreased precision, which is related to the same features that contribute to its feasibility. As previously mentioned, the Katz Index measures only six ADL items, so an overall picture of the patient is somewhat limited. Because the Katz Index includes basic mobility activities, such as ambulation, as components of a self-care item, the ability to identify changes in just ambulation is lost. It is impossible to determine if a person has achieved independence in ambulation unless the person reaches independence in all the components of dressing or toileting, of which ambulation is a component. The fact that the grading is based on the patient's ability to perform an activity without assistance by another person also limits the precision of the Index. The original version of the Katz Index defines independence as requiring no supervision, direction, or active assistance by another person. A person may have improved in his performance of an item by no longer requiring physical assistance, but may still require supervision for safety. This improvement will not be reflected in the patient's score on the Index.

The original Katz Index has been adapted. The rating scale was redefined and expanded, and numbers were assigned to the rating scale (0, no assistance; 1, uses a device; 2, needs human assistance; 3, completely dependent). Scores for each ADL item can now be identified and an overall ADL score can be derived from adding all the subscores. This allows the tester to identify smaller changes within each ADL and produces an overall ADL score. See Donaldson and co-workers for information on the revised Katz Index.

Reliability and validity testing have been carried out on the original version by Katz and his colleagues. Both have been found to be acceptable. These have not been reported for the adapted version.

PULSES PROFILE

The PULSES Profile, a global functional assessment measure, is included in our discussion of ADL measures because it is commonly used in the medical rehabilitation setting. It is an example of a measure that includes all dimensions of function, that is, physical, mental, emotional, and social. The physical function category measures BADL, both self-care and basic mobility. The Profile was developed by Moskowitz and McCann and was published in 1957. Granger and associates revised the PULSES Profile in 1975.

We will describe the revised version, which has several improvements over the original one. The revised version is clearly defined, measures specific ADL items, and yields a global functional score.

The letters in the title PULSES represent the following categories: P, overall physical condition; U, upper limb function, including self-care; L, lower limb function, including mobility; S, sensory status and communication; E, excretory or bowel and bladder control; and S, situational factors. For each of these subcategories, a four-point rating scale has been defined, with 1 representing no abnormalities in function and 4 representing total dependence in function. Subscores for each category are added for a total score ranging from 16 to 24. We will discuss primarily the two subcategories that deal with ADL measurement, that is, U and L.

The category of upper limb function (U) includes most self-care activities, such as drinking, feeding, dressing upper and lower body, donning and doffing a brace or prosthesis, grooming, washing, and perianal care. Granger and co-workers decided these were functions primarily dependent upon upper limb function. The second ADL category, lower limb functions (L), includes all transfers, ambulation, stair climbing, and wheelchair propulsion.

Of the measures discussed, the PULSES is the least precise in its ability to measure ADL. Precision is lost because multiple component activities are grouped into each of the two categories that deal with ADL. If a person is dependent in any component, he will be rated dependent in the entire category. The score, therefore, does not provide the therapist with information on the specific area of deficit in

ADL. For example, a patient may be independent in feeding, grooming, bathing, and dressing, but may require some supervision in putting on a brace. That patient will receive a score of 3, or "dependent," in self-care activities.

Another drawback of the PULSES Profile is that the rating scale includes both impairment and level of performance within each definition of scoring criteria. For example, a score of 2 in the category of upper limb function is defined as independent in self-care with some impairment of upper limbs. This mixing of concepts (ie, self-care independence and impairment) and lack of clear definitions for some terms can lead to error by the rater. For example, a score of 3 in mobility is defined as "dependent upon assistance or supervision in mobility with or without impairment of lower limbs, or partly independent in a wheelchair, or there are significant architectural or environmental barriers." Impairment and level of assistance are both included within the definition of the rating scale. No definition for the terms "significant" or "impairment" are provided.

The PULSES Profile has correlated positively with other ADL measures, which is proof of one type of validity, but no reliability studies have been reported. The PULSES Profile, particularly the adapted version, gives a more complete picture of overall function of patients than other ADL measures described. It is feasible to use the PULSES in acute care, rehabilitation, and institutionalized settings, but it has limited value in home care because it does not include IADL.

FUNCTIONAL STATUS FACTORS THAT INFLUENCE TREATMENT PLANNING

ADL are classified as a component of physical function. A large number of physical factors influence a person's ability to perform any given ADL. Impairment in one or several physical factors may result in an inability to perform an ADL independently. Most of these physical factors are standardly measured and treated by physical therapists. Strength, joint mobility, balance, coordination, sensation, and endurance are all measured as part of a physical therapy assessment. Before a treatment program is planned it is necessary to examine the contribution of each of these factors to the person's ability to perform ADL. Failure to do so will greatly limit the effectiveness of any treatment program designed to improve ability to perform ADL. For example, a person with Parkinson's disease and a person who has suffered a recent CVA both may be dependent in bed mobility. The physical factors contributing to their inability to perform bed mobility are very different, and the components of their treatment programs should also be very different. The ultimate outcome measure of the entire treatment program remains the ability to accomplish bed mobility.

Although ADL are considered a part of physical function, other areas of function also influence a person's ability to perform ADL as well as the ability to participate in a treatment program. The person's mental function in the form of memory and judgment; emotional function in terms of affect; and social function in terms of his role in society may be critical factors in designing an effective treatment program. For example, two patients who are hemiplegic following a CVA may have very similar levels of physical function. However, they may differ greatly in mental and emotional function. The first person may be highly motivated and cheerful and may demonstrate the ability to learn rapidly all compensatory techniques presented to her. The second person may be severely depressed and unwilling to participate in treatment. He is unable to retain instructions of compensatory techniques. Treatment of the first patient will be directed toward maximizing her strength and teaching her compensatory techniques. Treatment of the second person may involve teaching his caretaker how to manage him. The first person is likely to attain a much higher level of functional status than the second. In another example, two patients who have fractured right hips may come from very different social situations. The first person is a man and lives with his able-bodied wife. His wife willingly assumes all responsibility for bathing and dressing him in addition to doing all the laundry and cooking. The second person is a woman who lives alone. She must learn to accomplish the tasks of bathing, dressing, cooking, and laundry independently because no one is available to perform these tasks for her. Thus, two people with similar levels of physical function, but different social function, attain a very different functional status.

ADL can be viewed as a hierarchy of skills. Certain physical factors such as muscle strength and joint mobility provide the foundation for the basic mobility ADL, such as a sit-to-stand transfer (Fig. 35-2). The ability to perform basic mobility ADL combined with fine motor function as well as certain aspects of mental and emotional function enable a person to perform self-care ADL, such as bathing and toileting. Self-care ADL are more complex than basic mobility ADL. Many of the self-care ADL have a basic mobility component. For example, toileting involves the ability to transfer. It also involves a person's ability to manage his garments. Thus, independent toileting requires that a person be independent in transfers as

well as some aspects of dressing. A person may demonstrate improvement in his ability to toilet independently because he has improved in his ability either to transfer or to dress. It is important to understand the manner in which these ADL are interrelated when designing and evaluating the effectiveness of treatment programs.

Instrumental activities of daily living (IADL) present an even greater level of complexity. The ability to perform the various IADL is influenced by a variety of factors, which fall into the areas of physical, emotional, mental, and social function. The ability to perform some instrumental ADL may also be based on the person's ability to perform other basic and instrumental ADL. For example, for a person to perform the out-of-home instrumental ADL shopping independently, he would need to be independent in basic mobility transfers and ambulation, self-care dressing and toileting, in-home instrumental ADL handling finances, and the out-of-home instrumental ADL use of transportation. Inability to perform any one of these ADL independently would prevent a person from shopping independently. However, if assistance is provided

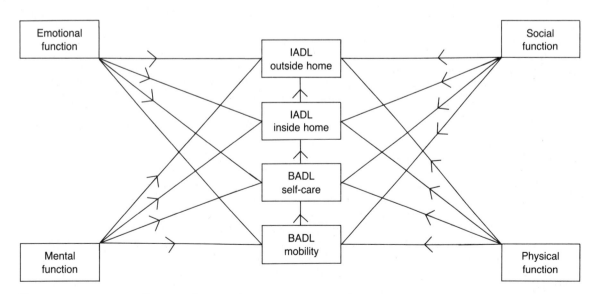

Figure 35-2. Factors influencing functional status.

in one of the component ADL, he may then be able to perform the IADL. For example, a person who is quadriplegic might require assistance with dressing, grooming, and transportation, but if assistance is provided in these areas he could perform the IADL of being employed outside the home.

A physical therapist must ask the following questions in order to design an optimal treatment program to improve a patient's ability to perform ADL.

1. What factors contribute to the patient's inability to perform any given activity of daily living?
2. Which of those factors can be influenced by physical therapy?
3. How likely are those factors to show improvement with treatment and in what period of time?
4. Which factors cannot be influenced by physical therapy?
5. What compensatory techniques are available to counterbalance those factors that are unlikely to improve?
6. Does the patient have sufficient mental function to participate in the treatment program or to learn compensatory techniques?

The following patient case examples are presented to illustrate the problem-solving process used to plan treatment programs designed to improve a person's ability to perform various ADL. These examples will also illustrate the interaction between physical, mental, emotional, and social function, and BADL and IADL.

Example 1

Mrs. S. is a 67-year-old housewife who lives with her 70-year-old retired husband. She was responsible for doing all the cooking, laundry, and housekeeping for the family. She was hospitalized four days ago after having a right CVA, which initially resulted in hemiplegia of the left side. Her left upper extremity (UE) remains totally flaccid, but she has regained some motor function in her left lower extremity (LE). She is, however, unable to move her left

LE against gravity and her movement is somewhat uncoordinated. Her sensation is grossly intact. She requires UE support to balance in sitting and maximal assistance to balance in standing. She is alert, able to follow commands, and has demonstrated the ability to learn. She tires easily, but is cheerful and highly motivated.

Initial assessment of her functional status reveals that she is dependent in bed mobility and transfers and is unable to ambulate. She is also dependent in bathing, dressing, feeding, grooming, and toileting. She is unable to perform any of the IADL.

In order to develop a long-term treatment plan for this woman, we need to review the questions presented earlier in the chapter.

1. *What physical factors contribute to the person's inability to perform any given ADL?* Mrs. S. demonstrates impairment in muscle strength and coordination, balance, and endurance. She is dependent in bed mobility because of decreased strength and impaired coordination. She is dependent in transferring from supine to sit and sit to stand because of impaired strength, coordination, and impaired balance in sitting and standing. She is unable to ambulate because of impaired strength, coordination, and balance. She is dependent in dressing, grooming, bathing, and toileting because of impaired strength and coordination, impaired sitting and standing balance, and dependence in bed mobility and transfers.
2. *Which of these factors can be influenced by physical therapy?* Strength, coordination, balance, and endurance all potentially can be improved by a well-designed therapeutic exercise program. Instruction in basic mobility activities can also improve the patient's performance.
3. *How likely are these factors to show improvement with treatment and in what period of time?* Although it has been a short time since Mrs. S. had her CVA, she has already demonstrated some improvement in motor function. It is reasonable to expect that

this patient will regain additional motor function (ie, strength and coordination), especially in her left LE, in a fairly short period of time. It is also reasonable to expect that Mrs. S. will show improvement in her endurance and her sitting and standing balance over a short period of time.

4. *Which factors cannot be influenced by physical therapy?* Although physical therapy can maximize the use of whatever motor function returns, it cannot produce motor return in the face of overwhelming central nervous system damage. The fact that Mrs. S. has experienced no return in function in her UE indicates that she may have a nonfunctional left UE in spite of everything rehabilitation has to offer.

5. *What compensatory techniques are available to compensate for those factors that are unlikely to improve?* When examining this question, it is important to differentiate between factors that may improve fairly rapidly and those that probably will not improve. For example, this patient's ability to dress is hampered by her impaired sitting and standing balance and by her inability to transfer, all of which are likely to improve in a fairly short period of time. Therefore, it is probably unnecessary to teach her techniques to compensate for these factors. Her ability to dress is also hampered by the lack of motor function in her left UE. Because this patient is unlikely to attain a level of motor function sufficient to allow the left UE to assist with dressing, it is reasonable to teach this patient one-handed techniques to perform dresssing. Mrs. S. was previously responsible for many household tasks that require the use of both UEs. She will need to be instructed in compensatory techniques to allow her to perform these tasks.

6. *How do the person's mental, emotional, and social functions influence her ability to participate in the treatment program or to learn compensatory techniques?* Mrs. S. has demonstrated the ability to learn. This is critical in light of the decision to instruct her in techniques to compensate for the lack of left UE function. She is motivated and cheerful, and is participating actively in treatment. Her social role requires that she perform many household tasks.

Example 2

Mrs. W. is a 74-year-old retired nurse who lives alone. Two months ago she fractured her left hip. She underwent surgical fixation and was not allowed to bear weight for one month. She was discharged from the hospital to a nursing home, but she hopes to return home. She is now allowed to bear weight as tolerated on the left LE. Although she is alert, oriented, and able to learn, she is also depressed, poorly motivated, and very fearful. ROM and strength of her UEs and right LE are within functional limits (WFL). Passive range of motion of the left LE is significantly limited in hip flexion and extension, external rotation, knee flexion and extension, and ankle dorsiflexion. Strength of the left LE is as follows: hip abduction 2/5, hip extension 2/5, hip flexion 2+/5, knee extension 3/5, and knee flexion 3−/5.

Mrs. W. is independent in bed mobility, except that she requires assistance for transferring from sit to supine. She is able to transfer from sit to stand independently. She is able to walk 50 feet with a walker independently, but can walk only 10 feet with a cane with moderate assistance. She requires maximal assistance to climb stairs. She is independent in feeding, but requires assistance for dressing her lower extremities and for tub transfers. She is unable to do her laundry, shop, cook, or use transportation.

We will again review the questions presented earlier in the chapter.

1. *What physical factors contribute to the person's inability to perform any given ADL?* Mrs. W. has difficulty transferring from sit to supine primarily because of weakness in her left hip flexors. She is dependent in ambulation with a cane because of weakness and decreased ROM in her left LE. She is unable to transfer into the tub because of weakness in her left LE. Her inability to

perform LE dressing is related to weakness and decreased ROM in her left LE. Her inability to shop, cook, and do laundry is primarily secondary to her impaired mobility. Because she requires bilateral UE support, she does not have a free hand to carry objects.

2. *Which of these factors can be influenced by physical therapy?* Decreased strength and ROM of her LEs can be potentially improved by an exercise program. Her ability to ambulate with a cane and to climb stairs could be improved by gait training. The ability to ambulate functional distances with the assistance of a cane instead of a walker should enable her to perform the tasks of cooking and laundry independently. The ability to climb stairs and curbs independently with a cane could enable her to use transportation and shop.

3. *How likely are these factors to show improvement with treatment and in what period of time?* There is a reasonable expectation that she should improve with treatment. Given her age, it is also reasonable to expect that progress in some areas may be slow.

4. *Which factors cannot be influenced by physical therapy?* Because of her age and the nature of her injury, she may never regain full strength and ROM.

5. *What compensatory techniques are available to compensate for those factors that are unlikely to improve?* It is important to differentiate between factors that may improve fairly rapidly and those that will improve slowly, if at all. This patient may well regain enough LE strength and ROM to perform transfers sit to supine and LE dressing in a short period of time. However, it may be a long time before she is able to transfer safely into a bathtub, and therefore she may benefit from the use of a bath bench. It may also be a long time before she can walk and carry items in the kitchen; therefore, she may also benefit from a kitchen cart.

6. *How do mental, emotional, and social function influence her ability to participate in the treatment program or to learn compensatory techniques?* Mrs. W. has demonstrated the abil-ity to learn and benefit from instruction; however, she is depressed and not participating fully in treatment. The outcome of her treatment is therefore in doubt. Her treatment is further complicated by her social situation. Because she lives alone, she must attain a very high level of function before she can be discharged home. The alternative would be to arrange for support services to assist with her shopping, laundry, and food preparation.

CONCLUSION

As physical therapists, we need to consider a person's ability to function in performing the activities of daily living when we seek to demonstrate the need for or the effectiveness of physical therapy. In order to accomplish this, we must understand how and why we measure function. If we do not understand measurement, we will not be able to interpret the results we obtain adequately. It is also critical that we understand the way in which all areas of function (ie, physical, emotional, mental, and social) influence a person's ability to perform the activities of daily living. Finally, it is important that we understand how the various activities of daily living are interrelated. When designing treatment programs, physical therapists must consider the role that physical factors and basic mobility ADL play as foundations for the more complex self-care and instrumental ADL.

ANNOTATED BIBLIOGRAPHY

Donaldson S, Wagner C, Gresham G: A unified ADL evaluation form. Arch Phys Med Rehabil 54:175, 1973 (Article on update of the Katz Index.)

Granger CV: A conceptual model for functional assessment. In Granger CV, Gresham GE (eds): Functional Assessment in Rehabilitation Medicine, pp 14–25. Baltimore, Williams & Wilkins, 1984 (Explains the need for and use of functional assessment in rehabilitation.)

Gresham G, Labi ML: Functional assessment instruments currently available for documenting outcomes in rehabilitation medicine. In Granger CV, Gresham GE (eds): Functional Assessment in Rehabilitation Medicine, pp 65–85. Baltimore, Williams & Wilkins, 1984 (Outlines the most frequently used functional assessments and the direction of future research in functional assessment.)

Ivenson IA, Silberberg NE, Stever RC, Shoening HA: Revised Kenny Self-Care Evaluation: A Numerical Measure of Independence in Activities of Daily Living. Minneapolis, MN, Sister Kenny Institute, Abbott Northwestern Hospital, 1977 (A detailed guide to the development and use of the Kenny Self-Care Evaluation.)

Jette AM: State of the art in functional status assessment. In Rothstein JM (ed): Measurement in Physical Therapy, pp 137–168. New York, Churchill Livingstone, 1985, (Reviews measurement principles and physical function measures.)

Kane RA, Kane RL: Assessing the Elderly. Lexington, KY, Lexington Books, 1981 (Thorough reference for all types of functional status measures used in geriatrics.)

Katz S, Ford A, Maskowitz R et al: Studies of illness in the aged. The Index of ADL: A standardized measure of biological and psychosocial function. JAMA 1958:914, 1963 (The original article on Katz ADL Index and theoretical basis for a hierarchy of function.)

Mahoney F, Barthel D: Functional evaluation: The Barthel Index. Maryland State Med J 14:51, 1965 (The original article on development and use of Barthel Index.)

Moskowitz E, McCann C: Classification of disability in the chronically ill and aging. J Chronic Dis 5:342, 1957 (The article on the original PULSES Profile and its use.)

Parsons T: Definitions of health and illness in the light of American values and social structure. In Jaco EG: Patients, Physicians, and Illness. Glencoe, CA, The Free Press, 1958 (An explanation of terminology and concepts relating to health and disease.)

Rothstein JM: Measurement and clinical practice: Theory and application. In Rothstein JM (ed): Measurement in Physical Therapy, pp 1–46. New York, Churchill Livingstone, 1985 (Excellent review of principles of measurement as they relate to physical therapy.)

Schoening HA, Iverson IA: Numerical scoring of self-care status: A study of the Kenny Self-Care Evaluation. Arch Phys Med Rehabil 49:221, 1968 (The original article on validation studies of the Kenny Self-Care Evaluation.)

36 Home Environment Analysis

CANDICE VAN IDERSTINE

The physical design of the environment in which we live is critical to the efficiency and efficacy of our function. When our abilities to operate physically or mentally within an environment are impaired, we have three options:

1. The environment may be adapted;
2. The methods of performing a task may be modified; or
3. We may become dependent on someone else to assist or perform the desired tasks for us.

As physical therapists, we can evaluate the physical capabilities of a patient. We must then coordinate with the patient, his family or caretakers, and the rest of the medical team to decide which of the above options is best for that person. The goal is to assist the person to function at his highest potential. Once we are familiar with the capabilities of the patient, we must then evaluate the environments in which he will be expected to function. Challenges presented in the home environment may facilitate rehabilitation, or may frustrate to the point of forcing unnecessary dependency.

The health care institutions in which therapists work with patients are designed to foster ease in mobility and maximize safety. There is little similarity to the obstacles one must face in the home environment. Although attempts are made at some facilities to simulate a "typical" home, each home is unique. Objective data about the home structure, hallways, doorways, stairs, room sizes, floor plan, site grad-

ing, and access dimensions is critical to determine the level of independence likely to be achieved by the patient.

The period of transition between institution and home is one full of excitement, expectation, and anxiety. This is a critical time for the patient and the family. By identifying and resolving home obstacles, we minimize the fears and frustrations for both the patient and the caretakers and establish an environment where the patient will likely be successful at reaching maximum independent function in the shortest possible time.

It is important to realize that independent functioning in the home does not alter the primary goal of enabling the patient to function successfully in any environment. Facing the home environment is merely the first critical situation for the patient. The success in this environment is a strong basis for predicting success in all other environments.

WHEN TO EVALUATE

The timing of the home evaluation is significant. If at all possible, it is desirable to evaluate the home before the patient returns home. This will enable the necessary modifications to be made prior to the discharge. Early evaluation of the home will facilitate the acquisition of necessary equipment as well as help the discharge planners and social workers determine what services the patient will need at home. In addition, it will give the health care team in the facility treating the patient an opportunity to prepare the patient to deal with the home obstacles that are identified. This can be done in a simulated clinical situation by using tape on the floor to represent walls and doorways. The facility grounds and stairs that are similar to those the patient will face can be used in training. Setting up the patient's room to simulate critical spaces for access in the home will help prepare the patient for mobility in the home.

The patient who does not have the benefit of a predischarge evaluation of the home will still benefit from an evaluation once he is home. Even with the best predischarge evaluation, the therapist will not always anticipate every obstacle. For this reason, a follow-up interview is performed within a few days of discharge. The therapist and patient work to identify and resolve any problems that have become apparent.

CONSIDERATIONS

The three major areas the therapist must consider when evaluating the environment are the patient, the family, and the dwelling. The environment can be adapted in so many ways, with such a high level of technological sophistication, that creativity can far exceed what is practical in a given situation. The therapist's role becomes that of a consultant. Recommendations are made to the patient and family, and they make the final decisions. The therapist determines what assistive devices are available and what structural changes are desirable. It is then up to the patient to determine whether the modification is feasible. Perhaps a homemade version of something unaffordable is possible, or community resources may be available to help finance the necessary modifications.

The following areas should be considered in the evaluation of the home.

THE PATIENT

It is necessary to assess the current medical condition of the disabled person. The therapist must have a clear understanding of the current cognitive and emotional status as well as the strength, available active range of motion, means of mobility, and amount of assistance required for the self-care activities of daily living (ADL) skills and transfers.

Information on the long- and short-term prognosis is necessary. The therapist needs to know the expectation for longevity as well as the likelihood of further return of motor function. It is important to know the current medical restrictions and the length of time they will be imposed. The present and future potential of the person would significantly influence the recommendations for financial expenditures and remodification of the entire family lifestyle that major home modifications may create.

In combination with the prognosis, the premorbid level of function will influence determination of which areas of the home are most critical for access. For example, if the disabled person never prepared meals or did the laundry before becoming disabled, these areas would be of lower priority to access if the disability is anticipated to be short term. On the other hand, if the disability is likely to be permanent, the roles of the members of this same family may be significantly altered. The person who never participated in domestic activities premorbidly may be homebound for extensive periods, while the person previously responsible primarily for the domestic tasks is working at two jobs to sustain an adequate income. The role changes may make kitchen access a priority in order to help the disabled person be a productive member of the household.

It is also helpful to know the premorbid hobbies and leisure activities of the disabled person. When considering rooms in which the person is likely to spend most of his time, this aspect should not be forgotten.

The motivation of the disabled person must also be realistically considered. This often limits a person's functional status more than the disabling condition. It is important to know how the person works with assistive devices. An understanding of how well they accept artificial devices in the home environment is critical before expenditures for such devices are made. The motivation to do things independently, even if it means doing a task in an unconventional way, is something that is best determined by demonstrated behavior. Most people will verbalize the desire to be independent, but when it is time to put forth the necessary effort, they may be unwilling to follow through on tasks that are well within their physical potential. The reasons must be explored, and if it is because of an unwillingness to "associate" with devices for the disabled, the therapist must minimize recommendations for modifications that are not "natural" looking. Fear of failure, laziness, or poor endurance must be considered also.

The financial resources of the disabled person will inevitably be one of the major factors limiting extensive modifications. Although it is necessary to prioritize recommended modifications, it is also necessary to consider fiscally reasonable alternatives. For example, the problem may be that a nonambulatory person has a bedroom only on a level other than the ground floor. Some alternatives may be (1) a stairglide; (2) convert the dining room or family room to a bedroom; or (3) add a room on the lower level. With these alternatives, consideration must be given to the location of the bathroom. Although the bedroom may be moved to the dining room and a curtain or door installed, the person may not be able to bathe and toilet on the same floor. Thus, it may be less expensive to add a stairglide than to add a bathroom.

THE FAMILY MEMBERS

The abilities of family members have a large influence on the extent of some modifications. The family may be very extensive and plan to have someone always with the disabled person. A member of the family who has a home workshop may be willing to make some of the necessary modifications. It is important to have an understanding of the talents and time available to the disabled person from the family, friends, and community.

There must also be an ability and willingness to modify the structure. It is unrealistic to

consider some modifications in a rented home. For example, putting up wall-mounted grab bars by the tub or bilateral stair rails may require written permission of the property owner and can be done only with the owner's permission. The decision to use a temporary ramp or permanent one, or a decision to widen doorways would also depend on the property owner. On the other hand, for some capital improvements, the owner may be willing to absorb some or all of the costs to limit his liability or to keep a good tenant. Tub bars and outside stair rails are examples of improvements the landlord may approve and help finance.

Often a disabled person is forced to move into the home of a family member or friend. The person may own his own home and accept modification suggestions for it, but may feel uneasy about requests for modification in an environment where he already feels intrusive. Thus, it is important to know if the person is going to be in his own home or the home of a caretaker.

The attitude of other members living in the household should be explored. If the patient needs an elevated toilet seat with side rails in the only bathroom, how are the other users going to react to a bedside commode placed over the toilet? Are they going to move it every time they want to use the toilet, so that it will rarely be in place for the patient? Are other members of the household willing to live with rearranged furniture or switching bedrooms? It is an unfortunate fact that a disability places a stress on the family structure. The therapist must be sensitive to the needs of those who will be around the patient and who also must function in the same environment.

THE STRUCTURE

Even some minor modifications require consideration of the structure of the home. Physical therapists are not taught construction techniques or the limitations of the stresses that may be placed on structural materials. The therapist recommends modifications that fit the patient's needs and abilities, and then consults with a licensed home improvement contractor to determine the feasibility of the proposed modifications. There are electrical, plumbing, and structural stability considerations that the contractor also will take into account. There may be simple modifications that family members are willing and able to make. They may be able to put up a handrail or tub rail, but do they know how to avoid cracking the plaster walls or the bathroom tiles? Do they know where to find the studs? Can the walls of a trailer home support the bars? Can the floor of a fiberglass tub support the concentrated pressure of the feet of a tub seat? These are questions that should be directed to the licensed home improvement contractor.

In order to assist the home improvement contractor with the necessary information to get the job done as the therapist intended, some facts about the structure should be requested. Ask about the type of construction, which includes the building type (frame, brick and block, or post and beam). Is it an apartment, a duplex, a townhouse, a trailer home, or a condominium? Note the type of walls (wallboard, plaster, panelled, or tiled).

All the information obtained from the review of the records and interviews with the patient and the family will then be complete. A visit to the home is now scheduled, and an on site evaluation is made. The therapist is armed with sufficient information to know how detailed the home evaluation needs to be. The areas on the home evaluation that can be ignored and the areas of priority access should now be clear. A recording form, a tape measure, and a pen are all that is needed to proceed with the evaluation.

COMPONENTS OF A HOME EVALUATION

EXTERIOR

On arrival at the site, the grading of the land should be noted. A grading of 8% is the maximum safe grade for persons with difficulty ambulating or who are wheelchair users. This means that for every 1 foot the ground rises,

there will be a slope the length of 12 feet to accommodate that elevation.

The walk paths should be noted for their grading and the surface material used. Ideally, there should be no loose gravel or small-unit compact ground material (including bricks). Rough-surface concrete is ideal, but any large cracks or uprisings in the surface should be noted. The distance from car to house door is an important consideration if the patient's endurance is limited. The lighting along these paths is a safety consideration. The location and ease of access to the mailbox will be important to the disabled person. Note how many entrances there are and closely evaluate the one the person is most likely to use to get to and from the car. Note the number and width of steps; location and side of handrails or safe handholds; lighting; presence or absence of an overhang; and number and type of doors, how they open, whether they have spring-loaded hinges, and if they can be operated easily. The threshold height and depth is important to the wheelchair user as well as the ambulatory person. If a ramp is already present, verify the security of the location and construction as well as the grade of the incline.

ENTERING THE HOME

A drawing of the floor plan should be made. This will help organize and orient the therapist and will be a reference later on for orienting the patient to the suggested modifications.

The lighting and the lighting controls are noted for all rooms. Many homes have the same height and type of mechanism for most environmental controls. Measure and note the type now, and note it later for other rooms only if it differs. Some switches may use a rheostat, and it is necessary to note this only if upper extremity impairment will affect the use of the switches, which differ from the standard toggle.

FOYER

The type of flooring in the foyer is important for safety and maneuverability. If throw rugs are present, they will need to be removed or fixed in place. Slate may make a wheelchair difficult to maneuver, and is slippery when wet. A plush carpet is difficult for any type of maneuvering and is difficult to keep clean. Record the number and dimensions of any stairs accessed from the entryway.

LIVING ROOM

Threshold heights and locations are recorded, as are doorway widths in the living room. Flooring type should be noted. The pathway width through the room should be measured, with special note made about any areas less than 36 inches wide. Record what obstructions exist and note how permanent the arrangement is (eg, the television set may have to be by the wall where the antenna wire enters the house, or a cabinet may be fixed such that it requires a carpenter to relocate). Note the type of seating and the height of the seating available if the patient will be using anything other than a wheelchair. Ask if there is a particular seat that the person prefers and examine the chair for security and stability as well as height. Note whether it rocks or reclines, and how the mechanism operates. If there is a television in the room, note what type of dials and controls are used to operate it.

DINING ROOM

The doorway and thresholds of the dining room are examined and measured and the flooring type is recorded. The table height and location of legs are recorded. A wheelchair will fit under a table 2 feet, 6 inches high as long as the legs are greater than 2 feet from the outside edge of the table. The type of legs is important if these minimums are not met, so it can be determined if the table can be safely raised with wood blocks or if they have casters and need to move freely. Look for a captain's chair with arms, and note the length and security of the arms. The access from the kitchen to this room should be checked, especially with respect to the door width and threshold type. Make notes on how easy it will be to get food from the kitchen to the dining room. Can a rol-

ing utility cart be used? Are the pathways wide enough? Keep function in mind as well as considering how much independence the person will need in this area. Count the number and note the location of electrical outlets in the dining room because small appliances may be easier used here (sitting) than in the kitchen.

BEDROOM

The doorway width and threshold of the bedroom are important. The floor plan should also show how the bedroom is accessed from the hall. How much maneuvering space is available to make any necessary turns into the room? What type of flooring material is used, and how is the furniture arranged? The height of the bed and the type of bed frame are important. A bed that is on a metal bed frame with casters is easy to modify, compared to a platform bed or one with a frame that is integral with a headboard or footboard. Note the size of the bed. If necessary, be sure to see if a hospital bed can fit into the room. A standard hospital bed is 36 inches by 80 inches; an extra-long bed is 36 inches by 86 inches. Note which side of the bed is approached to enter. Is there room for the wheelchair? Is there room for toileting with a bedside commode if this is necessary? Be sure to note the location of windows and closets and draw the doors with their "swing" room for planning furniture rearrangement. Measure the closet door width and clothes bar height. The rods should be no higher than 48 inches if wheelchair use is anticipated. Note the type of lighting and how it operates. Does the person have to use the toggle at the entry to operate the bedside light? Do they already have a "touch to turn on" lamp? Is the ceiling lamp the only source of light available? Is a great deal of time anticipated to be spent in this room? If so, is there a suitable chair in the room? If there is a bathroom adjacent to the bedroom, consider that the door may have to be modified to swing into the bedroom. Confined spaces such as closets and bathrooms should not have doors that open in towards the room. If the door opened inwards and the person fell down in the room, he would likely be blocking the only means of access to get help. The type of drawer pulls on the dresser should be noted along with the height of the top and bottom drawers. The therapist can then make recommendations for the best location of the person's clothing.

BATHROOMS

Note the location of all bathrooms that the person will likely need or want access to. Number the bathrooms on the floor plan, and record all the required data on each bathroom. Measure the doorway and note the thresholds and flooring materials, including throw rugs or any nonfixated rugs. Measure sink height and space under the sink if available. Be sure to note any exposed pipes under the sink, which may interfere with leg room under the sink or may cause burns on an insensitive leg. If wheelchair mobility is anticipated, check for these pipes even if a vanity cabinet is currently under the sink. If the vanity is removed for wheelchair access, pipe insulation is necessary for patient safety. Note the mirror location and size. Record the type of faucet and drain controls and the location and type of water controls in the tub or shower. Note the location of the light switch, outlet, towel rack, soap dishes, and any existing grab bars. If there is a tub, note which wall has faucets and measure the width of the edge for a possible clamp-on rail, if needed. Also be sure to note if there are sliding doors, which limit the use of many tub seats. If there is a shower stall, note the threshold height and entry width. Location and access to storage (linen closet) should also be noted. Can the walls in the tub or main area hold grab bars? The toilet height and the space available around the toilet are noted for possible adaptive and assistive equipment. Location of toilet paper should be about 20 inches high. If a wheelchair will be used, measure the maneuvering space in the center of the room.

KITCHEN

The kitchen area is necessary to evaluate even if the person in question has no intention of or ability to prepare full meals. Getting oneself a glass of water or a snack out of the refrigerator may be very important. As mentioned earlier, a person's role in the household may be altered by the disability, and access to the kitchen may be an important part of being a productive member of the family. The therapist must know the doorway widths and the location of the electrical outlets. Check the dimensions and heights of pantry shelves as well as the door opening width. If the cabinets open predominantly in one direction, make a note of this. The stove features are important for operation safety. Measure the height, depth, oven door location and size, broiler location and size, and note whether it is electric or gas. If gas, note the location of the pilot light. The refrigerator door type and the height and number of shelves are important for functional reach. The sink height, basin depth, and faucet style must be considered. Also note if there is any leg space under the sink. If the person must function from a wheelchair, the pipe insulation is also noted. If there is a table in the kitchen, note its height and be sure there is sufficient leg space for the chair the patient will be using. If the kitchen chairs do not have arms, check that one of the dining room captain's chairs will fit under the kitchen table. The location of the garbage container should be recorded. If it requires any special action to open or close the container when it is covered with a lid, the action and amount of force should also be noted. If the person will be doing most of the food preparation from a sitting position, check for a work preparation area that will allow sufficient leg room and height for a wheelchair.

LAUNDRY

The location of the washer and dryer may be in a room already evaluated or it may have a separate area. Be sure to note where it is and who will likely be responsible for doing the laundry. If the patient will need access to the laundry area, an evaluation must be done on this area separately. Note if there are stairs or narrow passages to get to the laundry area. Check the way the machines are loaded (ie, top-load or front-load machines), and note whether or not there is a dryer. Measure the distance of reach necessary to operate the controls and the space available to operate the doors. Note how much reach is needed to get to the bottom of the machines, and how high the clothes need to be lifted to get them into the machines. Check the flooring and access to a light switch and a shelf for storage of the soaps and materials needed for doing the laundry. If the disabled person will be also doing the ironing, check the location of space for ironing and the height range of the ironing board. Measure the height of the outlet, and feel the iron for weight and grip comfort.

ENVIRONMENTAL CONTROLS

The location, number, and type of telephones should be listed. Note whether they are wall mount, or can be pulled to the floor. The type of dialing system of the phone may be important depending on hand function. Note whether the phone is push button or rotary dial, and if it dials from the handset or the base unit.

The thermostat control height and location should be noted. If there is limited maneuvering space around it, this should be measured. If it can only be approached from one side, this too should be noted.

The location and type of cleaning machines should be noted if the disabled person will be performing some of the cleaning functions. Where are the cleaning chemicals stored? What type of floor cleaning method is used? Is a vacuum used, or a mop, or both? Is it a cannister or upright vacuum? How difficult are the controls? Does the person need a dusting mitt or can he grasp a feather duster? These little things can mean a great deal to the disabled person's sense of independence.

CONCLUSION

The occurrence of a disability forces a great deal of change in the life of the person so challenged, as well as in the life-style of family members. It is often very difficult for a family to consider major additional changes, such as modifications of the home. For this reason, it is wise to present the suggested modifications in three catagories:

1. Modifications that are essential to basic safety and strongly advised to be done as soon as possible;
2. Modifications that will greatly enhance the functioning of the person and are highly recommended to be done as soon as reasonable; and
3. Modifications that will enable the person to function better or do tasks with less effort but are not essential in order to live in the evaluated home. These are ideas to make the environment optimal for the challenged person, and are *not* modifications that are essential to safety or basic care and feeding of the person.

Once the therapist has identified the areas needing modification, she must know what solutions to offer. Talents and knowledge of building and carpentry vary from person to person. Whatever the level of knowledge, home evaluations will always present an exciting challenge. Finding just the right solution for the situation is a rewarding experience.

ANNOTATED BIBLIOGRAPHY

Department of Veterans' Benefits: Handbook for Design: Specially Adapted Housing. Washington, DC, Veterans Administration, Publication 26-13, 1978 (Specific design considerations with primarily the wheelchair-bound person in mind.)

Hale G: The Source Book for the Disabled. Philadelphia, WB Saunders, 1979 (Good source of creative ideas for adapting the home with self-help devices for the physically challenged adult or child.)

State of Illinois Capital Development Board: Accessibility Standards Illustrated. Springfield, IL, Capital Development Board, 1978 (Complete guide to standards for access for homes, commercial, and public buildings. Excellent illustrations enhance the understanding and applicability of the standards for various disabilities.)

US Department of Housing and Urban Development: Selected Bibliography on Barrier-Free Design. Washington, DC, US Government Printing Office, 1979 (Annotated bibliography of publications on designing for the disabled. Very comprehensive.)

37 Work Capacity Analysis

GLENDA L. KEY

My goal in this chapter is to show that physical therapists have the skills necessary to work in the industrial therapy setting. Work capacity analysis represents new options for using skills acquired from academic or clinical experiences.

TRADITIONAL VERSUS NONTRADITIONAL PRACTICE AREAS

The traditional physical therapist's environment is usually a medical unit. This could be a physical therapy clinic in a hospital, a long-term care facility, or an outpatient clinic. The dress of the patient ranges from hospital gowns to gym attire. In this setting, physical therapists work with physicians, nurses, and assistants and aides.

The physical therapy intervention is guided by medical standards and focuses on one unit of the body: the back, knee, wrist, or other joint; a muscle group; or an extremity. Treatment is usually one-on-one with a patient. Each treatment lasts approximately one hour. It may occur twice daily in a hospital setting, or once a week in an outpatient clinic. Treatment is usually by physician referral, depending on state regulations and laws.

Traditional measurement guides include goniometric degrees for ranges, grades for muscle strength, and foot-pounds for torque.

Physical therapists work with patients who are categorized by age (pediatric, general, geriatric), body system (orthopedic, neurological, cardiovascular), activity (sports), or body part (back, hand, temporomandibular joint). Often, these categories are further subdivided. For example, a clinic with an orthopedic focus may also have a body part subfocus within that area.

In traditional physical therapy, a typical treatment goal of a patient with a knee disorder may be to decrease or eliminate pain, increase range of motion, and increase strength. In this situation, the therapist provides exercise routines that promote a healing process. Some of the exercises may utilize postures and movements not normally encountered during the patient's activities of daily living.

In contrast, the physical therapist may work in the nontraditional environment of the industrial therapist.

The place of treatment may be where the employee works, in the plant site itself. Or, it may be an outpatient clinic, or a physical therapy clinic that duplicates many facets of the industrial setting. Generally, the environment is a nonmedical unit. The client will be attired in the clothing of the work day. This ranges from the T-shirt, jeans, and sneakers of the assembly line operator to the suit and tie of the executive.

In the industrial setting, physical therapists work more often with nonmedical than medical personnel, including employee, employer, vocational rehabilitation counselor, insurance representative, psychologists, and possibly risk managers and engineering personnel. Industrial therapists may also work with union representatives or other representatives of employee groups.

The treatment is guided by the demands of the work and the setup of the worker environment. The treatment focuses on function and ability of the worker, not a single body unit. The employer needs to know what the employee can do now, not what the knee strength grade is or that the person is lacking the final 10 degrees of extension. Treatment goals must relate to getting the work done in a safe and timely fashion, that is, functional safe ability.

Treatment ranges from one-on-one participation to group education and participation. The goal may be to prevent initial injuries; to treat the worker following an injury; to prevent reinjury; or to sponsor activities that promote health. Group participation can range from group exercise routines to training workshops.

The time required for an intervention is not standard but will vary with the activity being performed. This may range from one hour for a meeting with a worker, to a full-day workshop, to a series of all-day prevention interventions. The initial intervention is usually the first of many. The duration of your relationship with a company can be for greatly extended periods of time as contrasted to traditional treatment having its duration based on rehabilitation recovery of one individual.

Non-physician referral is common within industrial therapy practice. A great deal of work capacity analysis is nonmedical, or ergonometric, treatment. The risk manager, the worker's compensation director, and the insurance representative are only three of the many people who will refer clients to you. They are also very likely to have you come to the industrial site directly.

MEASUREMENT GUIDES

In the industrial setting, the employee is measured by capability in accomplishing given tasks, in addition to the standard physical therapy goals, such as increasing ROM and strength, and improving cardiovascular re-

sponse. For example, when assessing and measuring the client's ability to lift materials between two given heights, the therapist must also consider that the client will be handling materials through a quarter turn arc, totalling a 90-degree angle of movement of those materials. Measurement of ability is also against scales of validity discrimination, repetition of activity, and norms of other profiled injured workers.

Measurement tools will be discussed in detail later, but in brief, clients will first participate in a *functional capacity assessment* of physical abilities. The results of a functional capacity assessment are compared with functional capacity norms of similar employees. The "grade" then becomes the difference between the client's performance on the functional capacity assessment, and what the average or mean response is for that given profile for gender, age, height, weight, and type of job.

The functional assessment data are combined with the *job site analysis* data for both medical and industrial use. The measurement may identify a need for further medical care for the employee, or demonstrate that the job site may need to be modified to meet the needs or limits of the employee's functional abilities.

The primary purpose of *pre-employment screening* is to provide a guide for the acceptance or denial of an individual for employment. The data may be used further to establish programs of capability maintenance, with retesting on specified schedules, usually annually.

Industrial standards provide another measurement tool. Industrial standards can refer to standard heights of counters, tables, and shelves, and standard distances. Meeting industrial standards also means reaching the economic savings goals set by industry. Programs of prevention are graded on their results because decreasing injury rates can decrease employer costs and increase revenues.

The measurement system used in an industrial setting must be complex enough to cover the variables of individual clients yet simple enough to carry out quickly. Measurement tools are more complex in concept than basic goniometric measurements, for example, and with consequences that are much greater. Consider the significance of statistically identifying a client as one who is consciously attempting to manipulate the results of a functional capacity assessment. Or, consider the significance of statistically identifying a client to be a full participator who was previously thought to be a malingerer. The primary measurement is the job itself, and meeting the demands of the job is the goal.

ROLES OF THE INDUSTRIAL THERAPIST

There are many roles the industrial therapist may assume. These roles include (1) assessment role—the injured worker's functional capacity assessment, job site analysis, and pre-employment screening; (2) restorative treatment role—work hardening or work readiness centers, or the industrial-setting clinic; (3) advisory role—case management; and (4) educational role—management workshops, or employee fitness sessions. Assessment and treatment roles may be subdivided into clinical specialty areas, such as an overuse syndrome of the upper extremity, or back care.

These roles are not subject to the same subdividing as some of the traditional physical therapy roles. For example, treatment roles relating to the client's age are not typical in industrial therapy.

The same functional loss in two different patients can have profoundly different effects. If we were to take two men of equal age, height, and weight, each with the loss of the great toe, we might expect the same treatment approach for each. However, the vocational needs of the patient must be carefully identified in order to plan effective treatment. A concert flutist who is missing a great toe has no work-related emphasis on specific toe capabilities. In contrast, the construction worker who walks on high structural beams requires full great toe capability for balance and movement. For these two patients, there should be an entirely different focus in the approach to treatment.

In contrast, injuring a finger may not be as much a part of gainful employment of the construction worker, but is paramount to the needs and life of the flutist. The finger injury of the flutist would be handled considerably different than the finger of the construction worker. Ascertain the patient's needs and wants, and you will be able to design a treatment program for a specific person relative to the exact nature of the job he is to perform. Not only does this give the patient an interest in the treatment, but also affirms that you are spending time where time needs to be spent. In contrast, the construction worker has little interest or need to work with the intrinsic muscles of the hand. Thus, the treatment program for the construction worker may last one half to one third the length of time, as contrasted to the extensive time you may spend with the flutist. Again, the focus is on function, and the philosophy is to treat the patient for his needs and benefit. Your need for both clients may be full restoration of ROM and strength. The construction worker may only want to expend the time and energy to meet the basic needs of gross movement return, but the flutist will probably want a much more extensive program with finer, more precise tools of treatment.

THE PHYSICAL THERAPIST AS THE EXPERT

The physical therapist today possesses the knowledge necessary to be a very valuable participant in the ergonomic world of industrial therapy.

Ergonomics and human factors engineering can be broadly categorized as the practice of designing equipment and environment such that the user can perform the task with minimum stress and maximum efficiency. This includes the operating, servicing, and supporting of the work tasks. My interpretation of design goes beyond that of the equipment and machinery used, to include the design of the activity itself—the biomechanical carrying out of that activity. This must include the most efficient use of the worker, including the neuromusculoskeletal system, the cardiovascular system, and other physiologic and biomechanical considerations.

The physical therapist must be able to analyze movement of the body through anatomical, physiological, and biomechanical principles. The therapist also needs to understand organ systems and body tissue responses to disease and trauma.

The industrial therapist needs to see how the specific disorder is affecting the capability of the individual as a whole unit. The concept can be summarized, "It is the whole body that goes back to work."

JOB SITE ANALYSIS

A job site analysis is a systematic evaluation of a specific job site with the worker performing the job. The site, work area, tools used, machinery operated, and materials handled must be analyzed. The workers' postures and positions while performing job tasks must be studied.

A job site analysis demands measurement of detail: heights, weights, distances, and repetitions. Noise and chemical exposure levels are also required in some locations.

The therapist may be called upon to observe firsthand the relationship between the worker, the job task, the equipment, and the environment. Prior to observing and defining these relationships, let's review the role of each of these and put them into perspective.

1. The role of the worker is based on the capabilities and limitations of the individual person. The role of the worker is not to be defined based on features of the machine.
2. The role of the equipment is to support the worker in accomplishing the job task. The machinery and equipment are to complement the worker's capabilities, thereby relieving stresses and permitting the worker to perform activities beyond the human capabilities.
3. The environment should be such that equipment and worker will each function at the highest capability level. Temperature and sound control may be factors in some industries (Woodson, 1981).

4. The role of the job task is to provide a safe method by which the worker utilizes available resources (supported by the environment and the equipment).

Gathering the details of the requirements of a job puts you in a position to be able to make knowledgeable recommendations in areas of prevention or restoration.

RESTORATION

The treatment plan is built around the individual worker's functional daily activities.

Modalities, exercise routines, and educational sessions are directed at specific functional purposes. The goal may be to provide the strength and stabilization to support a lift of 47 lb from chair to desk level, incorporating a movement of materials from directly in front of the worker to directly at the worker's side.

Tasks that were defined in the job site analysis can be simulated in the clinic. Following a functional assessment to identify starting point recommendations, exercise programs can be built around the patient's job tasks. This is called *work hardening, work conditioning,* or *work readiness.*

PREVENTION

The results of the job site analysis can be compared to the results of the functional capacity assessment of the injured worker. With this comparison you will be able to clearly identify whether the client can meet the varied specific physical demands of the job. If not, you have baseline data that can assist you in bringing the employee from the point of present functional capability to that of preferred, minimum job requirement capability level. The job site analysis becomes a guide for the treatment plan.

According to Worth,* successful and safe placement at the work site is an equation:

Capacity of worker to perform = Job demands

*Unpublished lecture, David Worth, PhD, CPS Rehabilitation Service, 1987.

Functional capacity assessment = Task analysis

Pre-employment Screening

The job site analysis provides the minimum capability standards that the worker will need to meet in the pre-employment assessment. It is a valuable tool used to assist industry in selecting the appropriate employee for the job. Once workers are hired, it is important that they be placed in jobs appropriate for their capability level.

Job Training and Orientation

Training and orientation programs for new or transfer employees can be based on the information from a job site analysis. Basing the training on this analysis will assure that the worker is being introduced to the specific physical requirements of the job. This is important and valuable for all jobs, but becomes critical with high-risk jobs that involve life-threatening factors. For example, a crane operator may be responsible for moving large, heavy, unusually shaped objects high in the air from one point to another, over people who are working below. The cab of the vehicle can be simulated and minimum standard performance requirements can be set based on the job site analysis. The simulated setting can be used as the training ground for the prevention of fatalities and injuries.

The most common form of training for new employees is on-the-job training. This standard process can be improved by simulating work areas and work tasks and requiring that performance competencies be met. Using this process, the employer can be more assured that the new employee has learned the correct and safe procedures to use.

Recommendations

Recommendations for basic modification or redesign of a work station or the job site itself may be based on the job site analysis. Some areas of change can be addressed immediately. For example, work heights are often easy to modify. Also, work-related items within the worksite may require simple placement changes to provide a safer working environment. This can have significant impact on prevention of further injury and thereby support the promotion of safety.

Recommendations to the employee can be made for the purpose of modifying personal movement techniques. Necessary changes in postures and positions of body parts can be identified by comparing the job site analysis with the results of the employee's functional capacity assessment.

The need for specific preventive educational programs may be clearly identified. For example, a higher risk of injury to specific parts of the body may be present. Those risks may be addressed through services and educational programs that you can offer.

In many jobs of high repetition, workers perform the same activities each day. You may consider such work to be boring and undesirable, and you really may not be able to imagine anyone else being happy doing this kind of work. However, this is neither the time nor the place for such a bias. First of all, employees in highly repetitive jobs often operate at a level of skilled intensity to maintain the required quality and quantity standards of their work. Secondly, you are analyzing the job for its physical characteristics, not for its social or psychological rewards. And third, I invite you to enjoy practicing therapy in the industrial setting. It is an environment that allows you to use the complete range of your present knowledge while stretching your skills into new areas.

DESIGNING AND IMPLEMENTING THE JOB SITE ANALYSIS

Familiarity with industry, vocational rehabilitation, and the workers' compensation insurance system is a prerequisite for the industrial therapist. When preparing to analyze the job site, the therapist needs a concise, flexible note-taking format. Figure 37-1 is an example of a basic form. "D.O.T." on the form refers to the *Dictionary of Occupational Titles*. The *Dictionary of Occupational Titles* is a comprehensive, stan-

Ergonomic Analysis

Company Name: _____

Department/Division: _____

Job Title: _____

D.O.T. Title: _____

D.O.T. Number: _____

Contact Person(s): _____

Phone: _____

Analyst: _____

Date of Analysis: _____

I. Job: _____

Task: _____	Motions/Movements Observed	Recommendations
Components:		
a. _____	_____	_____
b. _____	_____	_____
c. _____	_____	_____

Task: _____	Motions/Movements Observed	Recommendations
Components:		
a. _____	_____	_____
b. _____	_____	_____
c. _____	_____	_____

Task: _____	Motions/Movements Observed	Recommendations
Components:		
a. _____	_____	_____
b. _____	_____	_____
c. _____	_____	_____

Figure 37-1. Basic form for job site analysis. "DOT Title" and "DOT Number" refer to the classification in the *Dictionary of Occupational Titles.* (Key Functional Assessment, Inc., Minneapolis, MN 55404)

dardized listing of occupational information including job descriptions and related information for 20,000 occupations, nearly all types of jobs performed in the United States. By incorporating a systematic occupational classification, the dictionary groups occupations according to job tasks and requirements. The dictionary was designed as a tool to facilitate job matching and job placement with worker skills and capabilities.

Other items needed to perform a job site analysis depend upon the depth of the analysis requested. The most frequently used items include the following:

1. Standard 6-ft tape measure
2. Basic athletic-model stop watch
3. Resistance dynamometer for measuring applications of push/pull as well as weighing some job-related equipment and materials.
4. Scale for weighing job-related equipment and materials (bathroom scale is acceptable)
5. Video, Polaroid, or 35-mm camera (optional)

The industrial therapist focuses on partial and full-body movements demanded by the job that may predispose the worker to injury.

The flow chart in Figure 37-2 presents the elements of a basic job site analysis, and demonstrates the process of moving from the largest to the smallest unit of the job.

A task is a unit of activity that is descriptive of more than one action. Each task is broken down into components. A component is the method by which the individual utilizes available equipment. The component is then broken into the respective postures and movements necessary to carry out that specific component.

Figure 37-3 gives an example of analyzing the tasks, components, and individual movements of a job. In this example, pronation and supination of the hand is a motion of the component flipping fish into a bin. The flipping of the fish is, in turn, a component of the task packing. All are elements of the job of wet fish preparation in a fish processing plant.

The next step in organizing a job site analysis adds an additional level of complexity, which may include weight loads, the time of a continuous physical effort or holding time, the time from initiation of a movement to the next

Figure 37-2. Elements of a job site analysis.

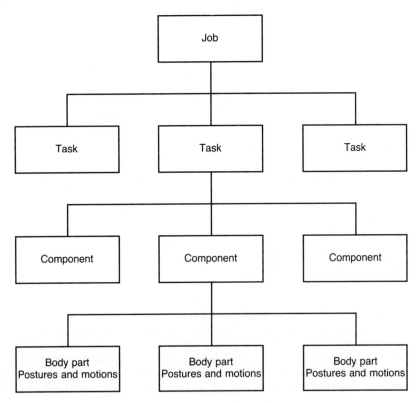

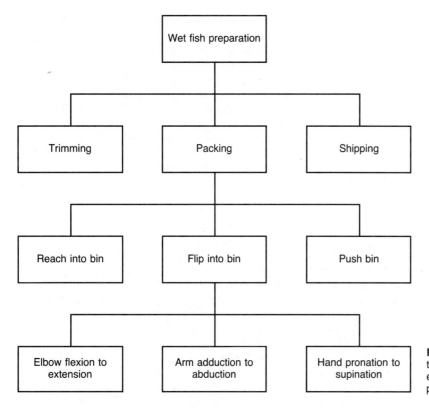

Figure 37-3. Sample analysis of tasks and motions of a job. The example used is the job of wet fish preparation in a processing plant.

initiation of the same movement or cycle time, and the number of repetitions per minute. It may also include graded levels of perceived psychophysical effort. In charting or documenting, one may choose to categorize by body area, body part, muscle group, posture status, or joint involvement.

It is important to remember that a job site analysis focuses on the worker's activities in relationship to the environment. Although machinery or tools may appear to be the "problem," it is the posture and positions that the worker is being placed in that are the focus of your evaluation. For example, your analysis may lead you to recommend that employees perform an activity without bending at the waist. You should not make the issue one of purchasing new equipment when there may also be the option of building platforms to alter the workers' posture.

In the final report, draw attention to the number of times and places the problem occurs, and focus on what has been demonstrated by the worker. Identify the desired postures and positions. The therapist will participate with industry representatives to identify the mode of modification. Modification will be based on the therapist's analysis of the body's abilities and the employer's expertise regarding what is available and feasible to correct the problem, including machinery, tools, space, and budgetary constraints.

WORKER'S FUNCTIONAL CAPACITY ASSESSMENT

The ability to participate in activities at one's highest level of performance is very important for success in both work and personal life. The worker's functional capacity assessment provides objective data regarding the limits within which an individual can safely and productively complete work tasks. This method allows the therapist to construct a "functional" picture to be used in creating an environment most conducive to productivity, based on the client's actual work-related activities and functional capabilities.

"Functional capacity assessment" is a generic term. To better understand the concept, we can define the term by breaking it into its specific words.

Functional implies that the physical therapist is looking at the whole body and how it responds as one unit. The focus is not on individual joints, muscles, or extremities, because it is the whole body that goes back to work. It is important to identify the capability of the whole body, which is affected by the limitations in the area of disorder. These limitations of range or strength or endurance may be the result of any number of system dysfunctions. If the worker's range of motion is 150 degrees instead of 180 degrees, or the muscle grade is 4 instead of 5, the resulting deficiencies may place limits on the capabilities of the entire body. Through the functional assessment process, the capabilities of the individual worker are determined, where previously information and restrictions may have been specific to just a single area of body dysfunction.

Capacity is the measurement of one's full capability. In the functional capacity assessment, the therapist identifies areas of capability with and for the client. The therapist provides capability information in three categories: (1) weighted activities; (2) tolerance activities; and (3) postural activities. Weighted task capabilities include lifting, carrying, pushing, and pulling. Tolerance capabilities include overall workday tolerance as well as shorter durations of tolerance within overall tolerance. For example, sitting tolerance, standing tolerance, and hand or shoulder tolerances are all included within the tolerance to work an eight-hour day. Another important factor to be considered in the category of tolerance is a formula or process for identifying frequency of repetition.

The postural activities category includes specific activities such as bending, stooping, squatting, crawling, stair climbing, reaching, crouching, kneeling, balance, as well as repetitive movements of hands and feet, and neck mobility. These also require capability parameters based on a frequency formula. Not only are specific job-related capabilities identified, the results of a good assessment also include a determination of the worker's capability effort.

Think of the difference of what is available through a functional capacity assessment compared with the traditional focus of a patient's or employee's limitation. A common recommendation may have been "Lifting limitation of 20 lb, no bending or stooping." This provides very little information relating to all the capabilities of the worker, and provides almost no direction relating to the demands of a job.

Historically, the responsibility for identifying a patient's capability level was given to the physician. The patient's medical status was the basis for decisions. As functional assessments have come into practice, identifying safe capabilities is now the responsibility of the therapist. With the functional capacity assessment as a tool, the physician is now able to identify the effect the patient's medical status has on the functional ability level. This joint effort goes beyond the focus on limitations and truly focuses on the capabilities of the individual.

Assessment communicates that amounts are being established and valuations are being made. The word assessment also implies that it is not a test and that acceptance and rejection are not issues. One does not pass or fail a functional capacity assessment.

In assessing safe capability level, the goal is to identify the worker's capability as it currently is. Coaching a client is strictly unacceptable. To direct the client to change postural positions invalidates the accuracy of the capability assessment. At times, it is difficult for the therapist to suspend the role of clinician and act only as an assessor. If the assessment results are biased in any way by the rater, the results will not be accurate and therefore will not be reliable.

The assessment results will provide a great

deal of information that may or may not be addressed at another time. Desired postural adjustments, clinical treatment, and education are appropriately addressed in additional interactions with the client.

Neutrality is extremely important in the concept of the assessment. The assessment protocols must be established such that the client is not being encouraged to do either more or less. Again, bear in mind rater bias. If the rater encourages the client, the rater's results would reflect not the client's effort, but the rater's. However, only the client will be returning to the job, not the client along with the rater. In the interest of scientific clarity, medical safety, and functional application, the rater must remain neutral.

BENEFITS OF THE ASSESSMENT

Physician

Historically, it was the physician's responsibility to provide return-to-work data. Not only were physicians asked when their patients were medically capable of returning to work, but also at what levels of limitations and capabilities. However, most physicians have had no special training in this area. You now have a tool for the physician to use in making determinations of specific limitations. Good judgment and simple measures of strength and mobility are no longer adequate. As our society becomes increasingly litigious, physicians are more reluctant to authorize specific recommendations without benefit of objective, statistically based data. The functional capacity assessment utilizes a standardized process, engineered equipment, thoroughly trained individuals, and data that can be compared on a statistical basis.

Safety of the patient is a concern for the physician. The objectivity and neutrality of a standardized, statistically based functional capacity assessment will allow return to work at given activity recommendations without fear of reinjury of the patient. This relieves the physician of the responsibility and fear of the recommendations being too low, possibly limiting employment opportunities. It also relieves the fear of not making the restrictions severe enough, and exposing the patient to reinjury factors.

As the workers' compensation systems become more complex, physicians are increasingly requested to provide ratings for identifying disability or impairment. These ratings usually have a relationship to insurance coverage. The objective information provided with the functional capacity assessment is useful when establishing these impairment and disability ratings.

Physical Therapist

The therapist will use the data and details identified in the functional capacity assessment to address treatment focus and treatment progression. The data may also be used in advising the client, employer, or other members of the return-to-work team. See Table 37-1 for an overview of the benefits that the functional capacity assessment provides to the therapist.

Treatment Focus

Clinical treatment of the worker may be specifically recommended. For example, instability caused by weakness of the multifidus muscle or a quadriceps muscle may be unmasked as a primary factor limiting the worker's capability. These areas being unmasked will have been identified as limiting factors in the assessment. If addressed through treatment, one would ex-

Table 37-1. Physical Therapist Benefits of the Functional Capacity Assessment

Provides a treatment focus	Body parts, specific strengths and weaknesses
Provides treatment progression guide	Programs of progression; back school, work hardening
Provides for case progression opportunity	Therapist becomes an advisor or consultant to other team members

pect that the worker would exhibit an even higher functional ability level.

Treatment Progression

The client's present functional capabilities coupled with the determination of needed participation level will support intervention to progress the treatment program. This coupling and interfacing of information will provide the basis for recommending work hardening programs, body mechanics education, back schools, job site analyses, psychosocial counseling, and any other appropriate interventions.

On the other hand, this same coupling and interfacing of information may support a recommendation of "no further treatment." This assessment is a very clear statement that the client is working at his highest safe capability of activity, demonstrating the full participation level, and there are no recommendations within your area of expertise for intervention for improvement.

Case Progression

The physical therapist's role on the "team" is significant. The therapist advises the rehabilitation counselor about case progression, the employer about job modification or re-employment of the employee, and the physician about treatment or capabilities.

Employer

The information in a functional capacity assessment can have a high economic impact for the employer.

Previously, information provided to the employer usually included references to limitations in weight, number of repetitions, and tolerance time. Reference to tolerance time may have been applicable to the length of the work day or to sitting or standing, but seldom included specific numerical data.

Tolerance

In the functional capacity assessment, the area of tolerances is addressed first, identifying specifically the number of hours in a work day the individual worker can tolerate. This is then dissected into the component parts of tolerances to include length of time the employee can tol-

erate any of the following: sitting, standing, walking, or hand and shoulder activity. Within these subcategories, time durations are specifically identified. For example, in an eight-hour work day, the client can sit six hours at 40- to 45-minute durations, or stand four hours at 60-minute durations, or walk four hours, frequently, for moderate distances. This type of information provides the employer with a high degree of flexibility when returning an employee to the work site.

Postural Activities

The next area of information provided in the functional capacity assessment concerns postural activities such as bending, stooping, squatting, kneeling, and crawling. In addition to informing the employer that these activities can be done, the assessment should specify a level of frequency. For example, the therapist might state that the client is able to climb stairs 34% to 66% of the eight-hour work day.

In the category of weighted activities, the employer now knows the employee's capabilities of lifting, carrying, pushing, and pulling. If the functional capacity assessment has been designed to match the standards set by industry, the employer knows that the employee has been assessed relative to the needs of the company's own physical plant operation. Information on the worker's capabilities related to industry-specific height, weight, and distance needs will assure that the data will be valuable to the employer.

In the functional capacity assessment, the therapist may compare the employee's results with others of the same demographic profile or health and occupation characteristics. This will show the employer where this employee's profile fits in relationship to other employees of similar profile. If the client's capabilities are comparatively low, further intervention or treatment may be needed. If the profile shows a comparatively high correspondence to the profile of other workers, the employer and insurance company may decide to settle the case, assuming that the client is about as "recovered" as anyone would normally be given his circumstances.

Additional Benefits

The employer experiences additional benefits from performance of a functional capacity assessment and use of the results. The most significant benefit is the decrease in cost and the resultant increase in revenues (Table 37-2).

The employee returns to work earlier because the rehabilitative process is expedited. Treatment decisions can be made with more confidence of success, and thereby proceed more quickly. When an employee returns to productivity, there is immediate financial benefit to the company as well as to the worker. Lost work days are reduced, direct medical costs are decreased, as are the indirect costs of processing the paperwork and workers' compensation premiums. Workers' compensation premiums paid by employers are often based on experience factors. In this system, the amount the company will pay this year is based on a predetermined average that is adjusted according to last year's workers' compensation cost records. The early return of the employee lessens the negative influence of the workers' compensation experience factor on company finances. Medical costs are reduced because further medical tests, physician appointments, and rehabilitation treatments are limited. Unless a situation of too many employees and not enough work existed, the employer spends considerable time and energy to fill a void produced by a missing employee, whether by hiring temporary help, transferring staff on a temporary basis, or requesting overtime of present employees. During this time, the productivity decreases while costs increase.

Indirect costs of a workers' compensation case are four to six times the total direct costs, and these costs are all absorbed by the employer.

Another benefit for the employer is safety. If the employee has been through an objective functional capacity assessment with a statistical base identifying capability and participation levels, the chance of reinjury is diminished significantly. The chance of reinjury for these workers is less than that for those workers who have never been injured.*

The human side of safety is also very important to the employer. In my experience, most employers are genuinely interested in and concerned about employee health and safety. They consider it not only a legal obligation but also a moral obligation to provide a safe environment. This obligation includes hiring and training employees that are physically capable of performing the job.

It is also important that employers be assured of the participation level of an injured employee. A number of unpleasantries evolve with the perception of malingering. When the worker's physical capabilities are confirmed or dispelled, the case moves with expediency.

Vocational Rehabilitation Counselor

The client may have a case manager assisting in the process of returning that client to work. This case manager will usually be a vocational rehabilitation counselor, who coordinates the activities of everyone on the team to assure progression of the case in all aspects.

The benefits of a functional capacity assessment to a rehabilitation counselor also include the client's early return to work, the client's objectively identified capabilities, and the verification of the client's participation level.

Previous to the functional capacity assessment, rehabilitation providers had only the client's perception of his own capabilities and the physician's thoughts based on medical evalua-

*Unpublished data: Client's Work Status Post Key Functional Assessment, Key Functional Assessments, Inc, Minneapolis, MN, 1986.

Table 37-2. Employer Benefits of the Functional Capacity Assessment

Employee returns to work early = ↑ revenues
Known capabilities = safe participation levels = no reinjury = ↑ revenues
Verify level of participation = ↓ cost related to malingering = ↑ revenues

tion and treatment. The data provided through the functional assessments now guide the case progression prior to return to work and after return to work.

Employee

The employee benefits from the functional capacity assessment because the experience of performing the assessment is a reinforcement of his actual capabilities. The results are relevant to home activities, social activities, and work activities. As a result, employees now have clearly defined numerical data to guide decisions as to what activities can be performed and at what level. Should they put the stack of plates up in the cupboard? Should they pick up their grandchild? Should they carry the bag of groceries? Should they carry the tool chest? Should they make themselves sit through the hour of typing or the two hours of a movie? These questions will all be answered for them. The numerical data the client now has can be used as a guide in all aspects of daily life.

The injured individual can now return to work with a clear knowledge of capabilities, knowing specifically how much to do and for how long. Not only does this dissipate some of the fear of reinjury, it facilitates working to full capability level.

Because the client returns to work earlier, he is less likely to become subject to a disability syndrome. A worker's disability syndrome is a neurosis that results in the worker continuing in the role of the patient beyond the point of medical need. This syndrome supports dependency on the workers' compensation system (Hanson-Meyer).

Another benefit of the functional capacity assessment for the client is that when he tests as a "good participator," he is specifically and statistically identified as *not* attempting to manipulate the results. The injured worker is often not trusted. On the job site, supervisors and co-workers may make statements and ask questions inferring that an injured worker may not be as injured as he says he is. The client can now prove to other members of the workers' compensation system, the health care team, and his co-workers that his claim is indeed legitimate.

Insurance Company Representative

Decisions made by insurance representatives have paramount effects on the employee and the employer. Financial authorization for a medical test, a change of physician, the need for a specialist, or an extensive treatment are all in the hands of the insurance representative. Long-term health and employment decisions, sometimes very delicate in nature, are made from the results of the functional capacity assessment.

These decisions have great impact on the welfare and future of the client and the client's family. Historically, these decisions have been based on trust of the involved parties. Objective data to assist in decision making were unavailable. However, the functional capacity assessment provides objective practical data about the functional ability of the whole person.

The benefit to the insurance company case manager or the account manager includes (1) the knowledge of a safe placement of the worker and (2) having closed the file while limiting revenues spent on its closure.

Attorney

The attorney uses the functional capacity assessment to support a position, whether of the plaintiff or the defendant. For the attorney to use information from the functional capacity assessment in representing the client, the assessment must be written in a clear, concise style, and without medical jargon.

CRITICAL COMPONENTS OF THE FUNCTIONAL CAPACITY ASSESSMENT

The components of an injured worker's assessment or a functional capacity assessment may be represented in two different ways.

Physical therapists are most likely to be familiar with a discussion of the technical components. These were presented earlier in this chapter. However, the technical components of an assessment must be presented in a standardized protocol, a series of specific activities following a specific progression.

Equally important, if not more so, than the technical components are the critical components, which are the areas and methods of an assessment that demonstrate a scientific basis. The critical components together provide a system by which statistics can be gathered and data analyzed. The following critical components are necessary in the design of a functional capacity assessment program.

1. *Participation level discrimination.* In the process of a functional assessment, identifying an individual's end results is not sufficient, because these results may not represent the person's full capability. The therapist must be able to identify clearly either that the worker's performance *is* his full capability or demonstrate that he is *not* working at full capability. Participation levels of the client are based on statistical analysis of the results that clearly define the individual's level of psychophysical participation. The assessment analysis cannot be based on a philosophy of treatment, but must be based on scientific data and study utilizing external criteria as well as considering internal consistencies. Double-blind testing techniques are built into validly developed assessments. Double-blind techniques are used so that neither the rater (physical therapist) nor the ratee (client) knows at any point in the protocol what data the client is being measured against. This technique eliminates rater and ratee bias.

2. *Objective protocol.* These include neutrality (no postural coaching); end points established by client's participation, not by therapist influence; double-blind testing techniques; and participation levels that were developed validly.

3. *Standardized protocol.* Frequencies of tolerance, durations, and repetitions are identified. Standards of industry are built into the protocol (specific activities with their qualifiers, including heights and dis-

tances). Safety protocols are established to provide assessment without injury and to prevent re-injury once returned to work. A certification process is used in training therapists to administer assessments. The protocol must be replicable. The coefficient of variance of repeated tests represents the percent error in the test due to measurement procedures. A low percent (5%) represents a high level of repeatability. Finally, inter-rater reliability must be established so that the results will be the same no matter which rater (physical therapist) performs the assessment.

4. *Equipment* is standardized and the same equipment is used by all raters. It is engineered to duplicate functional industrial standards. It is user friendly, and allows clients to participate using their own posture and capability end points. Machine failures and equipment inadequacies must be eliminated from the assessment system to assure safety. Equipment set-ups must be sensitive to space limitations. Finally, equipment must be durable, to be able to stand up to high-repetition and high-impact activities.

5. *Data collection and utilization.* Are functional capacity assessment results being utilized effectively? Are people returning to work at performance levels you identified, and are they tolerating these levels of performance over extended periods of time? Return-to-work studies must be performed. Data must be recorded, and there must be a system for its input and retrieval. Statistical analysis of the data should be available.

6. *Respect for the client.* Explain the purpose of the assessment to the client before testing begins. Emphasize that the functional capacity assessment is not a test. Close the assessment by reviewing with the client the initial data obtained.

The entire process of an assessment needs to be carried out with a feeling of mutual respect between you and the client. The results you obtain often have a significant impact on clients' lives and the lives of their families. The assessment process needs to reflect depth and quality deserving of that level of importance and power.

WORK HARDENING

Work hardening (also known as work readiness or work conditioning) is a restorative treatment process that increases the client's physical, functional capabilities and tolerances specific to select job-related activites. The purpose of a work hardening program is to promote the individual's early and safe return to work.

GOALS

A work hardening program is a restorative plan that includes the goals of improving the following:

- Cardiovascular fitness
- Strength for materials handling
- Endurance for tolerance to hours of a work day
- Endurance for specific materials handling
- General body mechanics techniques
- Body mechanics techniques specific to materials handling or job task
- Utilization of pain control mechanisms

In addition, a work hardening program provides the client with knowledge for prevention of further discomfort or injury.

MAJOR COMPONENTS

Let us look closely at the major components of a work hardening plan that will incorporate the goals identified above. The primary components are chosen for their specificity of application to reach previously identified goals. These components would be selected based on the data identifying the client's areas of need following a functional capacity assessment and after comparing the results of the assessment with the demands of the job. The plan may include any of the following components:

1. *Simulated work tasks:* increasing increments of weights of objects in materials handling, increase repetitions, increase effort time and time of activity, and increase distance of postural end point. Use equipment that is relevant to local industry, and therefore relevant to the work-related needs of the clients. These may include motors, assembly line set-ups, mortar set-ups, carpentry models, supermarket models, and electrical and plumbing models.
2. *Aerobic conditioning:* video tapes, audio tapes, mat exercise programs, stationary bicycle, treadmill, stairs, swimming pool, rowing machine
3. *Postural/body mechanics education:* simulated work tasks, video tapes, audio tapes, slides, one-on-one education format
4. *Flexibility and Stretching Exercises:* simulated work tasks, mat exercise programs, video tapes
5. *Strengthening activities:* simulated work tasks, isokinetic, isometric, or isotonic exercise equipment
6. *Relaxation and pain control training:* biofeedback, audiovisual tapes
7. *Nutrition education:* video tapes

Design a program such that the whole body is focused on function. The postural end points are continually extended, resulting in an increase of functional range of motion. As the weight of the materials handling is increased, the functional strength of the individual increases, as does the tolerance to the weighted activities. Attention is given to areas of weakness as in traditional physical therapy, but the whole treatment program is now based around the functional application of these same concepts.

IMPLEMENTATION

Identify the client's present status through the functional capacity assessment, the goals the client needs to achieve through the job site analysis or job description, and then devise a plan on how to reach those goals progressively through work hardening. The work hardening program focuses on areas of job demand not already met by the worker's present level of capability. The program is specific to activity and work demand; it is not a general conditioning program.

To facilitate the collection of data and the standardization of the program, clear protocols are needed for each phase.

Phase I: Baseline Measurement

The structure of the work hardening program and the progressive development of the client's capabilities is based on two things: (1) the present capabilities of the person as identified by the functional capacity assessment and (2) the requirements of the job. This provides the starting point and the end goal for the work hardening program. Thus, the program begins using information specifically identifying the client's capabilities in the previously detailed areas of weighted activities, postural activities, and tolerances. This information is transferred to activities that address strength and ROM. Postural activities are specific to range of motion, and add significant detail to needed mobility and flexibility capability goals. Information from postural activities is coupled with the frequency determinations to identify the initial baseline in the work hardening protocol.

Tolerance results provide the initial baseline for the individual's tolerance to a standard eight-hour work day. Included in tolerance measurements are present capabilities of sitting or standing tolerances, and hand and shoulder tolerances. As any activity is initiated in the early stages of a work hardening program, it must be designed to begin with the postures and within the tolerance time frames identified on the functional capacity assessment.

Phase II: Treatment Activities

There are three options to formulating the treatment plan. The plan can be based on (1) muscle group conditioning, (2) job-specific simulation, or (3) a combination of the two. Most good work hardening programs combine muscle conditioning and job-specific simulations. The specific protocol for each simulated work task will include weights, repetitions, time elements, distances, and other elements of work demand appropriate to each job. The goal of a simulated work task should be to increase range, strength, tolerances, and endurance while carrying out the work task, so that the activity becomes the exercise. Knowledge of body mechanics and practice of correct postures must become a part of the person's job while they are still in work simulation.

It is primarily through the simulated work tasks that deficiencies are treated. For example, a laborer may need to improve body mechanics, increase strength, and increase mobility and ROM. His job description includes shoveling sand. The simulated shoveling work task may include elements to functionally increase ROM, increase strength, increase mobility, increase cardiovascular fitness, increase tolerance to the work day hours, and body mechanics training.

The patient may demonstrate areas of specific weakness while carrying out the work task. These weaknesses may require specific additional applications of treatment, which may be included as interim goals. For example, if the aim is to increase the endurance or bulk of a specific muscle group, one portion of the work task may be selected for higher repetitions. If the desired response cannot be facilitated through the work task, the appropriate exercise application with traditional exercise equipment would be included in the program until the desired response is reached and the patient is able to incorporate this response into work task activities.

As the participants in work hardening programs increase their functional strength and adapt their posture to their work, they become educated in the relationship between the body and the specific work tasks. They are also emotionally preparing for re-entry into the work world.

Phase III: End Point Measurement

Progress is monitored and final capabilities are identified through a repeat of the functional capacity assessment. It may be necessary to provide only a special purpose assessment at this time. Objective reassessment identifies the changes brought about through the work hardening program. This assessment upon exit provides information about the new capability levels that the individual can tolerate within a job structure. This information is used for two purposes. The more obvious purpose is to give direction for appropriate job placement.

The second purpose for this information is to provide statistical support as to the effectiveness of the work hardening program. You now have "before" and "after" pictures based on data collected through standardized formats and protocols. You may decide to use the before and after data simply to establish the increased capability of this one worker. Or you may gather additional information for predictive purposes. By setting up a follow-up process and gathering information at given intervals, you may track the individuals' work records for a period of time. An information base can be established that includes percentages of those returning to work, staying on the job, and relationships to length of time off work prior to the work hardening program. This information could be compared with data of those individuals *not* going through programs of intervention. You may want to set up ongoing data collection to be used for research that could result in publications. Although you may never "do research," it is extremely important to be able to statistically support the effectiveness of your program. I believe this is important both to your own program and to the development of the profession of physical therapy.

INDUSTRIAL THERAPY CLINIC

What follows is an outline of specific information that can be used as a guideline for setting up an industrial therapy clinic.

1. Equipment needs
   - An assessment station for standardized, statistically based functional assessments
   - Job simulation stations specific to industrial area and client needs; may include motors, sand shoveling area, bricklaying materials, conveyor belt set-ups, assembly jobs, supermarket tasks, parts of automobiles.
   - Restorative treatment and testing equipment (eg, isokinetic machines)
   - Exercycle, rowing machine, stepping machine
   - Time clock
   - Exercise mats
   - Audiovisual materials
2. Space requirements*
   - 1000 ft² working space for initial program; this can accommodate 10 to 12 clients and necessary health care and support personnel.
   - Dedicated space (ie, separate from physical therapy clinic)
   - Open space
   - Nonmedical environment
3. Treatment frequency and duration†
   - Two to six to eight hours per day for each participant
   - Three to five times per week frequency
   - Two to six weeks' duration of program
   - All time factors are contingent on a starting point as identified by the functional capacity assessment, and are modified according to a specific work hardening treatment plan. Goals are based on job descriptions and job site analyses.
4. Treatment teams
   - The return-to-work team may include the physical therapist, patient/employee, employer, rehabilitation counselor, insurance representative, physician, and ergonomist.
   - The work hardening treatment team may include the physical therapist, occupational therapist, physical or occupational therapist assistant, patient (or participant), exercise physiologist, physician, and psychologist.

*Unpublished data, Linda M. Demers, Milliken Physical Therapy Center, Scarborough, ME, 1987.

†Unpublished data, David J. Cegelka, Performance and Assessment Center, Southbury, CT, 1987.

ANNOTATED BIBLIOGRAPHY

Dictionary of Occupational Titles, 4th ed. Washington, DC, US Dept of Labor, Employment and Training Administration, 1977 (Standardized job descriptions and related information for 20,000 occupations grouped according to job tasks and requirements. It was designed to facilitate job matching and placement with worker skills and capabilities. Updated periodically.)

Hanson–Mayer TP: The worker's disability syndrome. Journal of Rehabilitation, p 50, July-August-September 1984

Woodson WE: Industrial systems. In Crawford HB, Fahey G: Human Factors Design Handbook. New York, McGraw-Hill, 1981 (A valuable overview of ergonomics.)

38 Observational Gait Analysis

M. KATIE GILLIS

Walking is a paramount concern for the patient. As physical therapists, we have the obligation and the challenge to assist patients in realizing their highest mobility potential. The purposes of this chapter are (1) to help you to develop observational gait analysis skill through an understanding of normal gait parameters and the pathomechanics of gait and (2) to provide you with a clinically useful system for assessing gait dysfunction. The approach you will learn can be applied to any patient with a movement dysfunction that affects their ability to walk, and is equally applicable to those with an amputation, arthritis, hemiplegia, ankle sprain, multiple sclerosis or any musculoskeletal or neurological condition.

Patients with neuromuscular, musculoskeletal, or cognitive deficits often demonstrate specific manifestations of decreased capacity for physical performance. A common physical performance problem is decreased ambulatory mobility and efficiency with associated deficits in normal gait parameters.

Successful rehabilitation is dependent on competent clinicians who have adequate evaluation skills and the ability to interpret and synthesize evaluative findings. Effective treatment must be founded on a sequential process, which involves accurate identification of a plan to resolve or minimize the problem(s). If this evaluative process is not skillfully and accurately performed, the prescribed and administered treatment may be inappropriate and ineffective.

Therapists in both large and small facilities rarely have available to them elaborate and sophisticated gait analysis systems. These systems require expensive equipment and highly trained personnel, and on a practical basis demand considerable time for acquisition and analysis of data. There is unquestionable need for an effective gait analysis system that not only provides the clinician with the necessary skills to obtain the critical information in a short time, but also enhances the clinician's ability to interpret the findings in terms of functional significance and indications for treatment.

Walking is by its simplest definition a translation of the human body from one point to another by way of bipedal gait. The repetitive pattern of alternating support on one leg and then the other with a heel-toe striding gait may, as Napier (1967) described, be the most significant of the many evolved capacities that separates humans from more primitive hominids.

The cycle of events occurring during gait constitutes a complex sequence of movement patterns, including certain fundamental characteristics of normal walking that are universal. These characteristics provide useful points upon which to base a description of walking.

The walking cycle is represented by the interval between heel strike of one leg and the subsequent heel strike of the same leg. The interval between steps is characterized by two properties, distance and time. Step length and step duration, stride length and stride duration are commonly employed in quantitative studies of normal and pathological gait. Stride length is commonly defined as the distance between two successive footprints of the same foot. Normal adult stride length varies between 140 and 156.5 cm. Stride duration is the amount of time between these same two events. Step length is the distance between two successive footprints, either right to left or left to right, and has a range between 68 and 78 cm. Step duration is the time interval between two successive heel contacts.

Cadence and velocity are additional means of describing the temporal elements of walking. Cadence is usually expressed in steps per minute, and the average normal is 112 to 116 steps per minute. Velocity is the distance walked divided by the time required to cover the distance. The mean normal velocity is 81 m/min as computed from various studies. All of the preceding parameters can be assessed clinically and are valid objective measurements that document and quantify change in a patient's walking ability.

An accurate and systematic approach to gait analysis requires very specific delineation of the phases of swing and stance. The gait cycle should be analyzed in terms of the type and degree of motion occurring in the various segments of the lower limb, pelvis, and trunk.

Historically, gait terminology has been more descriptive of normal gait and has not always been applicable to pathological gait. An example is the use of the term "heel strike." This term is not relevant when describing a person with gait deficits whose initial contact with the floor is toes first. A term that can be applied to any method of floor contact is needed. Additionally, the most commonly used terms to describe the phases of gait—heel strike, midstance, toe off or push off, and swing—are not inclusive of all of the component subphases of the gait cycle. For instance, the period of time following initial contact with the floor is a critical period and needs to be definitively delineated as a separate subphase.

The system of teaching gait that is pre-sented in this chapter is known as observational gait analysis. The terminology used is appropriate to both normal and pathological gait, and the subphases accurately differentiate the gait events during swing and stance. This approach, including the descriptive terminology, was developed at Rancho Los Amigos Medical Center in Downey, California. It is because of my participation in the development and teaching of this method and continued clinical utilization that I strongly advocate its use.

Observational gait analysis is normally taught as a formalized course using slides, normal and pathological gaits shown on film loops, and a number of different patients with various types of gait deficiencies. Gait analysis is a dynamic process and learning is enhanced if your analysis is immediately followed by feedback from an experienced clinician. However, the following sequence and content remains unaltered from material presented in the Rancho Los Amigos course. Throughout this chapter I will make suggestions to the reader, which should help make the information more comprehensible and the process logical. The first step in teaching gait analysis is to identify the various phases of swing and stance and establish the normal joint motions for the trunk, pelvis, hip, knee, ankle-foot, and toes.

COMPONENTS OF NORMAL GAIT

As previously stated, walking requires alternating support on one leg and then the other. This reciprocality requires that weight be accepted in a smooth, fluid manner that does not interrupt continued forward progression. The success of walking depends upon three specific functional tasks, which can be concisely identified as (1) weight acceptance, (2) single limb support, and (3) limb advancement. These tasks are primarily achieved by sagittal joint motions and postures occurring at the hip, knee, and ankle during specific subphases of swing and stance.

Figure 38-1 illustrates the subphases of stance and swing and delineates when each

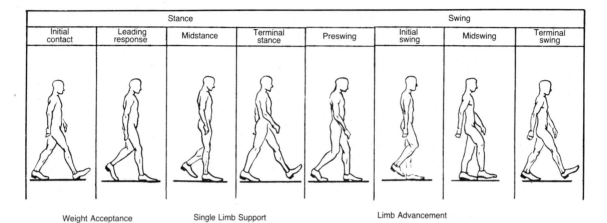

Figure 38-1. Normal gait. (Adapted by permission of Rancho Los Amigos Medical Center, Pathokinesiology Service and Physical Therapy Department)

functional task takes place. I suggest that you review Figure 38-1 to learn the subphases and get a mental picture of the limb's position during each subphase. Note that the right limb is used as the reference limb.

Figures 38-2 through 38-4 define each subphase (weight acceptance, single limb support, swing limb advancement). The line drawings illustrate the collective movements occurring during each subphase. The degree of motion for each segment is stated. Certain motions are *critical* in achieving the intended purpose of each subphase, and are identified. Direct your efforts at this time toward learning the definitions of the subphases, the joint motions that occur, and the motions identified as critical for each subphase. Do not concern yourself with muscle activity for the present. Individual muscle activity will be considered later. These figures are a good learning aid and a quick reference when reviewing segmental motions. In all figures, the reference limb is indicated by solid lines.

Diagrammatic representation of the limb muscle activity, torque, and joint motion is used to present a large body of information concisely and in a readily interpretable manner (Figs. 38-5, 38-6, and 38-7). Each figure presents information on a given segment: ankle, knee, and hip. Each subphase of gait is abbreviated as follows: LR, loading response; MSt, midstance; TSt, terminal stance; PSw, pre-swing; ISw, initial swing; MSw, midswing; TSw, terminal swing. Initial contact is not included because it is only a fractional period of time and the only significant event is how the foot touches the floor. All joint motions during Initial Contact remain the same as in the preceding subphase of Terminal Swing.

The percent of the gait cycle allocated to each subphase is identified. Muscle activity is represented by the darkened areas. Torque measurements reflect the pounds of force created by the muscle activity required to restrain joint movement during specific subphases. The muscle activity and torque measurements Are based primarily on kinesiological studies by Skinner and Perry (1985).

STANCE

Initial Contact

As previously mentioned, initial contact is a very brief period. The anterior tibialis and long toe extensors maintain the ankle in neutral during the initiation of the stance period. This places the foot in a preparatory position for *heel rocker* action, which will occur in loading response.

(Text continues on p. 679.)

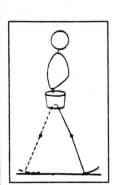

Pelvis   5 degrees forward rotation
Hip   30 degrees
Knee   0
Ankle   0

Critical: Heel first contact

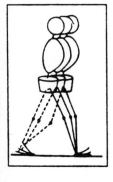

Pelvis   5 degrees forward rotation
Hip   30 degrees
Knee   0 to 15 degrees
Ankle   0 to 15 degrees plantarflexion

Critical: Controlled knee and ankle motion with hip stability

Figure 38-2.   Weight acceptance. Weight is accepted on an outstretched limb while forward momentum and limb stability are maintained. (*A*) Initial contact: The point in time when the foot strikes the ground. (*B*) Loading response: Shock is absorbed as forward momentum is preserved. A foot-flat position is achieved. (Adapted by permission of Rancho Los Amigos Medical Center, Pathokinesiology Service and Physical Therapy Department)

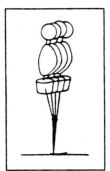

Pelvis   Neutral
Hip   30 degrees to 0
Knee   15 degrees to 0
Ankle   15 degrees plantarflexion to 10 degrees dorsiflexion

Critical: Controlled ankle rocker

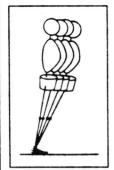

Pelvis   5 degrees backward rotation
Hip   0 to 10 degrees apparent hyperextension
Knee   0
Ankle   10 degrees dorsiflexion to 0
Toes   0 to 30 degrees hyperextension

Critical: Locked ankle heel rise and trailing limb

Figure 38-3.   Single limb support. Body weight progresses over and then ahead of a single, stable limb. (*A*) Midstance: Controlled advancement of the body from behind to ahead of the ankle. Contralateral swing limb provides the momentum. (*B*) Terminal stance: Extreme progression of the body past the MTP heads with a heel rise. (Adapted by permission of Rancho Los Amigos Medical Center, Pathokinesiology Service and Physical Therapy Department)

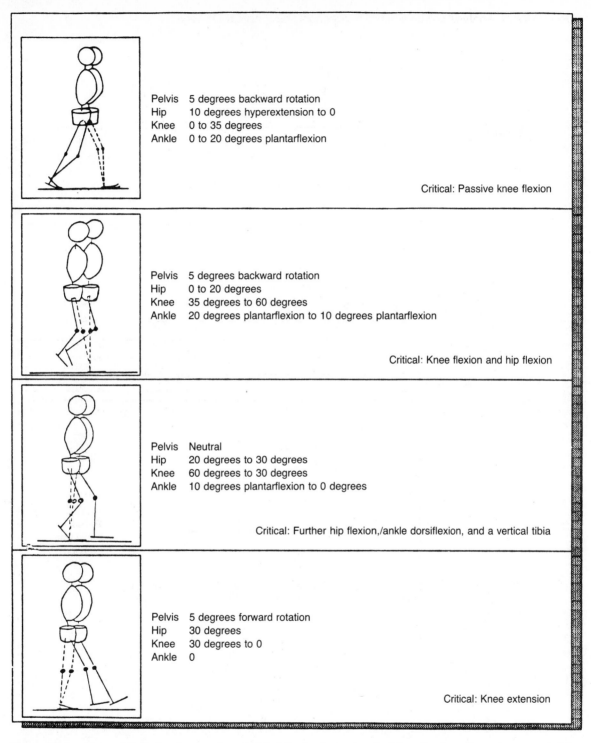

Figure 38-4. The swing limb advances from behind the body to ahead of it as the foot clears the ground. (*A*) Preswing: The foot remains on the floor while weight shifts to the other limb. (*B*) Initial swing: The foot is cleared from the floor as the thigh begins to advance. (*C*) Midswing: The thigh continues to advance as the knee begins to extend. Foot clearance is maintained. (*D*) Terminal swing: The leg reaches out to achieve full step length. (Adapted by permission of Rancho Los Amigos Medical Center, Pathokinesiology and Physical Therapy Department)

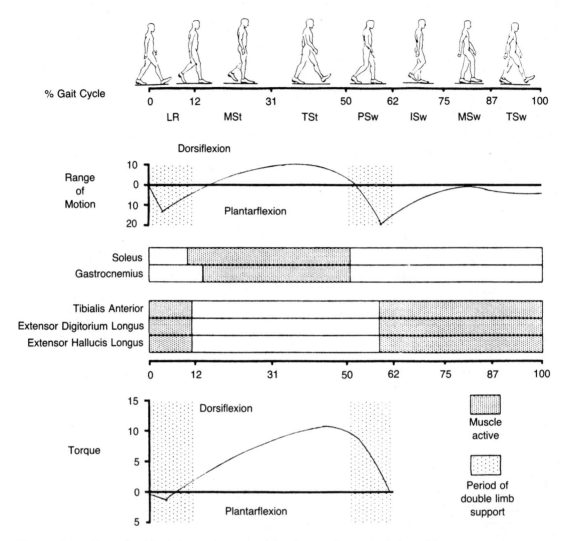

Figure 38-5. Normal ankle: joint motion, muscle action, and torque. (Adapted by permission of Rancho Los Amigos Medical Center, Pathokinesiology and Physical Therapy Department)

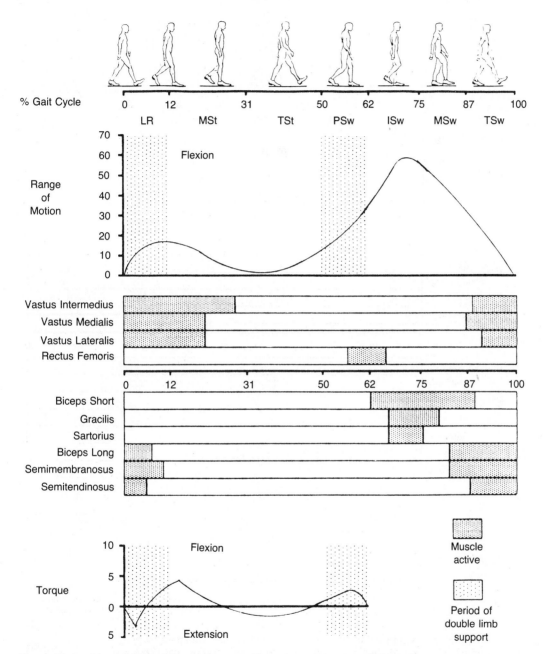

% Gait Cycle

Figure 38-6. Normal knee: joint motion, muscle action, and torque. (Adapted by permission of Rancho Los Amigos Medical Center, Pathokinesiology and Physical Therapy Department)

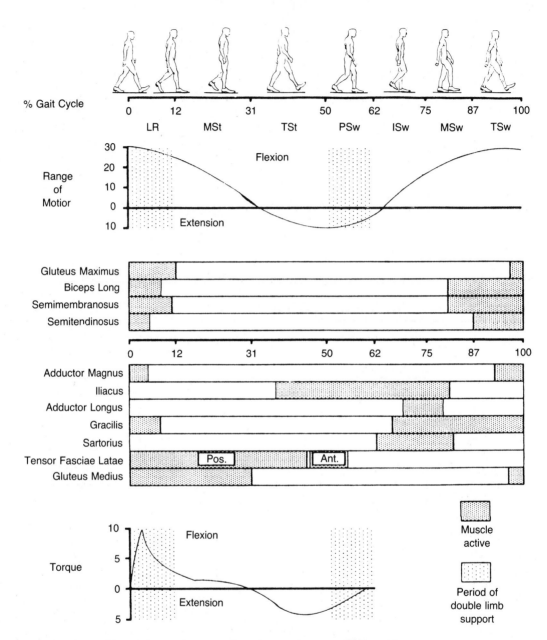

Figure 38-7. Normal hip: joint motion, muscle action, and torque. (Adapted by permission of Rancho Los Amigos Medical Center, Pathokinesiology and Physical Therapy Department)

Loading Response (LR)

At the time of loading response, muscle activity at all segments of the limb counters the flexion threat created by weight acceptance posterior to the ankle joint. Eccentric contraction of the anterior ankle muscles responds to a plantar flexion torque, which is forcing the foot to the floor.

The heel rocker action created by the anterior muscles, pulls the tibia along after the foot, producing forward momentum and flexing the knee. Fifteen degrees of knee flexion is restrained by eccentric contraction of the quadriceps to resist the moderately rapid flexion torque caused by the heel rocker action and the position of the body posterior to the foot. Through controlled plantar flexion and knee flexion, the shock of weight acceptance is absorbed, and limb stability is established while maintaining forward momentum. The hamstring activity present restrains the hip, as described below.

The hip remains in 30 degrees of flexion and the pelvis in 5 degrees of forward rotation. Rapid, high-intensity flexion torque, the second highest torque demand during gait, is counteracted by eccentric gluteus maximus, hamstrings, adductor magnus, and gracilis muscle activity. The pelvis is stabilized in the frontal plane by the gluteus medius, minimus, and tensor fascia lata muscles. Through these actions at the hip, the tendency for trunk flexion to occur is prevented and stability throughout the kinetic chain is preserved.

Midstance (MSt)

During midstance, the ankle slowly flexes to 10 degrees, providing increasing dorsiflexion torque. Soleus and gastrocnemius muscles contract eccentrically to restrain tibial advancement. The body advances over a stable foot and a controlled tibia allowing the knee to extend. This is described as the *ankle rocker.*

Quadriceps muscle activity is only present until the knee extends. An extension torque created by forward momentum of the contralateral swing limb decreases any need for muscle activity to sustain knee extension. An extended knee and controlled tibia contribute to stability during single support.

Hip extension to neutral with pelvic rotation to neutral is created by the momentum of the contralateral swing limb. Consequently, stance stability in the sagittal plane occurs without stance muscle demand from the hip. The pelvis is stabilized in the frontal plane by the abductor muscle group, preventing pelvic drop on the opposite side. Some normal persons, however, appear to be an exception to this by demonstrating an exaggerated and apparently practiced "hip swing." Mild extension torque and adduction torque occurs throughout single limb support.

Terminal Stance (TSt)

In terminal stance, the ankle is locked in neutral to slight dorsiflexion and the metatarsal phalengeal joints extend to 30 degrees. Dorsiflexion torque reaches a peak, producing the greatest demand on any joint during gait. The posterior calf muscles remain active to prevent tibial collapse and allow heel rise as the body weight progresses over the forefoot. The resulting *forefoot rocker* contributes to maximum forward progression for step length. It is extremely important to recognize that three factors are critical in producing this forefoot rocker: a locked ankle, heel rise, and progression over the forefoot, all of which must occur during single limb support. The terminal stance events at the ankle have been universally referred to as "push off." The inaccuracy of this term has been validated by normal force plate studies of below-knee amputees who, because of a rigid ankle, meet the three criteria necessary for a terminal rocker. Obviously, plantar flexor muscles are not creating normal foot floor reactions in these patients.

The knee remains extended as extension torque begins to diminish at the end of this subphase. Stability is maintained without further muscle action.

The hip remains extended to neutral with an apparent posture of approximately 10 degrees of hyperextension. This position is created by backward rotation of five degrees at the pelvis and by extension of the lumbar spine. Note that on the hip analysis form, the motion occurring at this time is actually described as 10 degrees of hyperextension. This is simply because while observing gait, you look for the verticality of the thigh in relationship to the floor. However, it is important to remember that this hyperextension is only apparent. Muscle activity remains the same as during midstance with the exception of the iliacus, which contracts to protect the joint capsule. The fibers of the anterior tensor fascia lata contract late in terminal stance. Mild extension torque exists. The body has advanced past the supporting foot, achieving step length while maintaining stability.

Pre-Swing (PSw)

Although pre-swing is a period of double limb support, it is considered a part of swing because the joint motion that occurs at the knee during this subphase is essential in preparing the limb for advancement and foot clearance during initial swing. During pre-swing, the ankle falls into 20 degrees of plantar flexion, and the metatarsal phalangeal joints extend to 60 degrees. During this period of double limb support, the foot provides balance assistance and no muscle activity is required. A rapid loss of dorsiflexion torque occurs.

Knee flexion to 30 degrees is primarily a passive event, although the gracilis becomes active. Flexion torque is created by loading on the opposite limb and by further advancement of the body past the toes. Knee flexion during the pre-swing subphase is achieved at this time.

The hip remains in neutral extension and the pelvis in backward rotation. Both are primarily passive events. The iliacus and rectus femoris muscles are active. Extension torque is reduced to zero. The limb is prepared for advancement.

Initial Swing (ISw)

The ankle moves to 10 degrees plantar flexion as the anterior ankle muscles prepare the foot for clearance in the next subphase, initial swing.

The knee flexes to 60 degrees and the foot is cleared from the floor. It is during this period that toe drag is most common. In most instances toe drag is the result of inadequate

knee flexion, and not inadequate dorsiflexion as many clinicians believe.

Contribution from the iliacus, adductor longus, gracilis, and sartorius muscles brings the hip to 20 degrees of flexion and the pelvis begins to rotate forward. The pelvis moves in concert with the hip and is rotated forward during hip flexion. Backward rotation of the pelvis accompanies hip extension.

Midswing (MSw)

The ankle achieves a neutral position in midswing secondary to active anterior muscle group activity. This is the key motion that helps to clear the foot.

The tibia reaches a position perpendicular to the floor as the knee extends from 60 degrees of flexion. Momentum is primarily responsible for this passive event although the short head of the biceps femoris remains active for eccentric control.

At the hip, the gracilis continues throughout midswing to help achieve 30 degrees of flexion and creates added momentum to the advancing limb. The sartorius, adductor longus, and iliacus become inactive.

Terminal Swing (TSw)

Anterior ankle muscles remain active to keep the ankle at neutral during the final subphase, terminal swing. This assures an ankle position that will allow heel contact for weight acceptance at the subsequent initial contact subphase.

Concentric quadriceps activity assures knee extension to neutral. The hamstring muscles decelerate the thigh.

The hip posture of 30 degrees achieved during midswing is maintained and 5 degrees of pelvic rotation occurs. Only the gracilis muscle remains active as a hip flexor. The collective motions of hip flexion, pelvic rotation, and knee extension contribute to step length.

After studying the above information, it should be clear that the progressive events of the stance phases accomplish the overall task of providing stance stability during continued forward progression over the supporting foot. The successful completion of the individual phases of swing ensures toe clearance, limb advancement, and forward reaching of the limb for step length.

TRUNK ACTIVITIES

The trunk remains neutral and erect throughout all phases of gait. An erect trunk helps conserve energy by balancing the body weight over the base of support. Contralateral deep trunk extensor muscles contract eccentrically to maintain an erect trunk in the sagittal and frontal planes during weight acceptance. The downward displacement of the trunk at initial contact is met by an upward force exerted on the foot by the floor. This force exceeds body weight and is translated to the pelvis and trunk, and tends to flex the trunk forward because of the relative anterior location of the trunk.

Ipsilateral deep trunk extensor muscles begin contracting in terminal stance to control weight shift. No additional trunk muscle activity is required for limb advancement. There is minimal thoracic rotation (approximately 6.9 degrees) according to Murray (1967), but it is difficult to perceive because of associated movement of the pectoral girdle on the thorax. Therefore, in observational gait analysis, these subtle motions are not scrutinized. Arm swing contributes to forward momentum but is not a prerequisite to walking. The upper extremities do show a distinctive and characteristic relationship to lower limb movements, swinging forward and backward in phase with the direction of the contralateral leg movement (see Fig. 38-1). This rhythmic and reciprocal movement probably contributes to the smoothness of translation.

SUBTALAR JOINT

The axis of motion of the talocrural joint is rotated outward approximately 16 to 20 degrees; as a result, movement between the foot and the leg cannot occur in a sagittal plane. However, motion does occur in a sagittal plane through motion produced at the subtalar joint. No muscles attach to the talus, but the muscles that affect movement at the ankle mortis also cross the subtalar joint, moving it as well. During weight acceptance, approximately 4 to 6 degrees of subtalar valgus occurs, which makes the axis of the mortis joint more perpendicular to the plane of progression, thereby allowing for movement in the sagittal plane.

With the foot fixed on the floor, the tibia rotates internally during dorsiflexion and externally during plantar flexion. Internal rotation with respect to the calcaneus occurs as pronation at the subtalar joint, while external rotation results in supination at the subtalar joint. At initial contact, when the heel first touches the ground, the calcaneus is in valgus. Supination of the forefoot by means of anterior tibialis muscle activity creates a very supple foot to react to irregularities in the terrain. During midstance and terminal stance, when the whole foot is in contact with the floor, the ankle joint is at neutral and supination occurs at the subtalar joint. This causes pronation of the forefoot and provides an intrinsically stable platform for the forefoot rocker occurring during terminal stance.

Motions in the frontal plane are observable, but analysis of foot-ankle motion will not be considered further as part of the basic observational gait analysis system. In those patients with obvious foot-ankle abnormalities, sufficient consideration must be given to the motion and posture of this complex. Kessler and Hertling (1983) review in detail the biomechanics of the subtalar joint during walking.

PATHOLOGICAL GAIT

Human motor behavior represents a superbly integrated and interdependent functional relationship between the nervous, musculoskeletal, and physiological support systems of the body. Motor dysfunction as a result of impairment in any one of these systems can result in a functional penalty manifested as a decrease in movement efficiency, reduced mechanical potential, and inadequate energy to perform motion. When a patient has incoordination of muscle activity, inadequate strength, restricted joint range, poor balance, or inaccurate sensory integration, or if pain is present, deficiencies in gait are inevitable. The extent and type of movement abnormalities are determined by the etiology, the system(s) affected, and ultimately by the degree to which the integrity of motor control is compromised.

Pathological gait can be defined by specific accentuations or suppressions of one or more of the components of normal locomotion. The deviations seen in pathological gait represent a limited aggregate of variable postures and abnormal movements. Through the systematic and comprehensive observational assessment presented in this chapter, these deviations and their resultant penalties can be accurately evaluated and thus treated more effectively.

Five major causes that ultimately determine the conditions of pathological gait are pain, weakness, deformity, sensory disturbances, and disorders of muscle activity related to central nervous system deficits such as increased muscle activity and dyskinesia. Each of these major causes will be briefly discussed and examples given to clarify their potential effect on gait. This will help establish a conceptual foundation for thinking about how these static and dynamic factors can influence the quality of human movement.

PAIN

Pain can exist as a component of both acute and chronic pathological conditions, and when present, may compromise functional movements. Patients with pain avoid activities or motions that exacerbate the pain. The result is a decrease in mobility or fixed joint postures, which lead to more pain and greater dysfunction. The toll of these sequelae on the functional capacity to walk is clearly definable. For instance, unequal stance time is commonly seen as an obvious attempt to minimize stress on a painful joint. Compensatory motion such as laterally leaning the trunk over the limb during stance can decrease the compressive forces at the hip sufficiently to lessen pain during weight bearing. Decreasing the arc of limb movement or the speed of moving the limb during swing is often observed as a means of diminishing pain when walking. If walking is painful for any reason, a decrease in stride length, cadence, and velocity and early unloading of the limb are consistently observable penalties.

WEAKNESS

Paralysis as a result of a musculotendinous lesion or damage to the anterior horn cell axon, myoneural junction, or muscle fiber can have a devastating effect on the ability to walk. However, a patient with extensive muscle weakness can walk if sensation is intact, if sensory integration and central motor control are normal, and if no significant deformities are present. When muscle activity decreases as a result of weakness, the effect may be seen in the eccentric or restraining capacity of the muscle as well as a decrease in concentric activity. An example of loss of restraining muscle activity might be a lack of plantar flexion restraint to control the foot following heel contact, or insufficient quadriceps muscle activity for controlled knee flexion during loading response. Toe drag during midswing is often the result of inadequate concentric activity of the anterior ankle muscles. Lack of limb advancement and lack of forward momentum created by the hip flexor forces during swing may be the direct result of insufficient hip flexor strength. Stance stability is most often compromised by weakness of the lateral hip muscles, and one of two typical gait deviations usually occurs. Either a contralateral pelvic drop or a lateral trunk lean over the supporting limb will be observed. Historically, these deviations have been known as a Trendelenburg and gluteus medius limp, respectively. The most common strength deficit significantly interfering with the stability of the tibia during single limb support is inadequate gastrocnemius-soleus muscle strength. This deficit is usually manifested as a collapsing tibia (excessive dorsiflexion) during midstance and terminal stance. As a result of inadequate tibial stability, forward progression and momentum are compromised, resulting in a decreased step length and slowed velocity.

DEFORMITY

Deformity as a complication of muscle imbalance, increased muscle activity, congenital abnormalities, or amputation is a well-recognized penalty of disability. Restricted joint range can produce definitive gait deviations in the absence of any other contributing factor. Joint restriction in combination with weakness or control deficiencies has an even more dramatic effect on walking. A loss of joint mobility at any segment of the lower extremity is important not only because it interferes with achieving functional activities but it also places secondary stresses at other joints, which must compensate for the mobility loss. More energy is often required to substitute for loss of available motion.

Hypermobility of the lower extremity joints is less frequently observed, although such deviations as an excessive extension range at the knee (hyperextension) or lateral ankle instability (varus) are pertinent examples where function is compromised as a result of a loss of mechanical restraint.

Normal standing posture requires full hip and knee extension and approximately 5 to 10 degrees of dorsiflexion. Body alignment with the center of gravity posterior to the hip axis and anterior to the knee allow hip and knee extension without muscular effort. If this range is not available, additional muscular demands are created. Sustained postures of hip and knee flexion also create additional compressive forces on the joints. A knee flexion posture of greater than 30 degrees is not acceptable to the patient and will eventually cause termination of functional ambulation. Compensatory posture necessitated by deformity is outlined in the following example. If a patient has an ankle plantar flexion contracture of 15 degrees, he must either walk on his toes, which is not a reasonable option, or he must assume an adaptive posture. If the foot remains flat on the floor with the ankle in plantar flexion, the body is aligned behind the foot and loss of balance ensues. To avoid falling backwards, the patient assumes a compensatory forward trunk position, which centers the trunk over the supporting foot. Thus, balance is maintained. This same plantar flexion contracture may cause toe drag during swing. An option the patient may select to clear the foot is to rise onto the contralateral toes (vault), which creates a relative shortening of the swing limb.

SENSORY DISTURBANCES

Impaired sense of joint position is the most significant factor influencing motor control. Without awareness of the limb's position in space or intersegmental relationships, movement control is dependent on visual input or external appliances to dampen or block motion. However, these cannot be adequate substitutions for proprioceptive loss. Common manifestations of position sense deficits are toe drag, medial and lateral ankle instability during stance, or excessive hip flexion during swing.

DISORDERS OF MUSCLE ACTIVITY

Disturbances in motor function caused by disruption of the spinal cord or injury to the brain influence walking in a different fashion. Limb movement is often limited to synergies of flexion and extension, as seen in hemiplegia following cerebral vascular accident, head injury, or hypoxia. As a result, the ability to perform different movement combinations such as hip flexion and knee extension is impaired or lost.

Movement may be distorted as observed in dystonic posturing secondary to birth trauma, genetic errors, or drug overdose. An excessive reaction to stretch, defined as spasticity, is also a concomitant and compromising phenomenon of spinal and central nervous system damage. Brunnstrom (1970) and Bobath (1978) have lucidly described these factors and their effect on gait.

Movement impairment seen in the various syndromes of cerebral palsy is dependent upon the distribution of inappropriate muscle activity. Patients with spastic diplegia manifest a typical standing posture. Increased flexor muscle activity in the lower extremities creates varying degrees of hip and knee flexion. This flexion posture, combined with adductor spasticity, results in the well-known "scissor gait."

If extensor activity is exaggerated, common features are a pillar-like rigidity with weight maintained on the forefoot, varus of the ankle, clawed toes, and difficulty initiating reciprocal flexion and extension of the limb during gait.

Patients with disease of the basal ganglia present a complex of clinical disorders characterized by abnormal involuntary movements or alteration in muscle activity and body postures known as dyskinesias. Dyskinetic motion appears as continuous or sustained displacement of the body's center of gravity through motions of extreme lateral, backward, or forward trunk excursion, extraneous arm and head motions, and alterations in the synchrony and excursion of lower limb movements. The bizarre pattern of involuntary movements seems to defy visual analysis, but the underlying uniformity of postural pattern is striking and can be analyzed by visual assessment.

Individuals with Parkinson's disease, in which rigidity is a major component, usually manifest a flexed posture and a shuffling gait. Stride length and velocity are generally decreased and double limb support may be increased. These patients also have difficulty initiating a step, and once initiated, they may be unable to terminate forward progression, a condition known as festination.

The ability to vary cadence, speed, and step length permits normal persons to adapt, alter, and adjust their walking to meet a variety of conditions. The ultimate penalty of pathological gait is a compromise in efficiency and flexibility with resultant inability to alter the functional parameters of walking.

DESCRIPTIONS OF PATHOLOGICAL GAIT

The terminology used to describe and document gait deviations must be applicable to all types of movement dysfunction seen during walking. It must also be comprehensive enough to encompass the variable deviations that can be observed. The terms presented in this chapter are the result of more than 15 years of clinical trials, formal gait analysis courses, and kinesiological electromyographic studies at Rancho Los Amigos Medical Center.

Tables 38-1 to 38-5 define the terminology of pathological gait for the individual body segments. When reviewing this information, keep in mind your knowledge of the normal events for each of these segments throughout the gait cycle. The definitions are straightforward and will be even more meaningful after you have been introduced to the analysis forms later in the chapter. Each table lists the deviations on the left and defines them on the right. Review the individual segments until the definitions are clear to you. If a definition is not clear, return to the figures representing normal motion for that segment. Recognizing what is normal for the segment at any given time throughout gait makes the definition comprehensible.

OBSERVATIONAL GAIT ANALYSIS FORMS

After you have reviewed the definitions describing gait deviations, the next step in the process of information gathering is to study the gait analysis forms. For the purpose of clarity, these are presented as separate forms, one for each segment. Eventually, all the segments are compiled into one form for clinical use.

Begin your study with the form for the ankle, foot, and toes (Fig. 38-8). Notice that the deviations you reviewed earlier are listed on the left side of the form. Each subphase of swing and stance and the functional tasks are listed across the top of the form. Next, note that there are shaded, open, and dotted spaces opposite each deviation and that these spaces are aligned with a specific subphase. The shaded spaces simplify your observation. You need not consider whether a deviation occurs during this time. You need only consider the open and dotted spaces. A deviation may occur during any subphase that has an opened or dotted space. The presence of a deviation during any subphase means that the normal position or motion expected during that subphase was not achieved. The open spaces reflect the subphase during which the deviation is most significant. The use of dotted and open spaces

Table 38-1. Definitions of Segment Deviations of the Ankle, Foot, and Toes

DEVIATIONS	DEFINITION
Ankle-Foot Segment	
Forefoot contact	Initial contact made with the toes
Foot flat contact	Initial contact made with the entire foot
Foot slap	Uncontrolled plantar flexion at the ankle joint occurring at initial contact
Excessive plantar flexion	Plantar flexion greater than normal for the specific phase
Excessive dorsiflexion	Dorsiflexion greater than normal for the specific phase
Excessive varus	Inversion at the subtalar joint is visible
Excessive valgus	Eversion at the subtalar joint is visible
Heel off	Heel is not in contact with the floor
No heel off	Heel is not off the floor during forefoot contact
Drag	Contact of the toes or forefoot with the floor during swing
Contralateral vaulting	Rising on the forefoot of the stance limb during swing of the reference limb
Toe Segment	
Up	Extension of the toes beyond 5 degrees
Inadequate extension	Less than normal extension for the specific phase
Clawed	Flexion of the toes beyond 5 degrees

Table 38-2. Definitions of Knee Segment Deviations

DEVIATION	DEFINITION
Flexion	
Limited	Less than normal knee flexion for the specific phase
Absent	No flexion of the knee when flexion is normal
Excessive	Flexion beyond normal for the specific phase
Inadequate extension	Less than normal knee extension for the specific phase
Wobbles	Alternating flexion and extension of the knee occurring in a single phase
Hyperextension (knee angle)	Extension of the knee beyond neutral
Extension thrust	Forceful extension of the knee
Valgus	Medial angulation of the knee
Varus	Lateral angulation of the knee
Excessive contralateral flexion	Flexion greater than normal during terminal swing and initial contact of the reference limb

is purely to simplify your learning experience and facilitate use of these forms.

For instance, if the ankle deviation Excess Varus occurs during limb advancement or even during beginning weight acceptance, it is not penalizing. The most crucial time for Excess Varus is during single limb support when an unstable platform could easily result in a fall. As an additional example, look at the line opposite Forefoot Contact and observe that there is only one open space. It is during the subphase Initial Contact that the deviation Forefoot Contact is relevant. If the patient first touches the floor with the forefoot, this space

Table 38-3. Definitions of Hip Segment Deviations

DEVIATION	DEFINITION
Flexion	
Limited	Less than normal flexion for the specific phase
Absent	No flexion of the hip when flexion is normal
Excessive	Greater than normal flexion for the specific phase
Inadequate extension	Less than normal extension for the specific phase
Past retracts	Retraction of the thigh during terminal swing from a previous attained degree of flexion
External rotation	Considered a deviation if other than neutral
Internal rotation	Considered a deviation if other than neutral
Abduction	Considered a deviation if other than neutral
Adduction	Considered a deviation if other than neutral

Table 38-4. Definitions of Pelvic Segment Deviations

DEVIATION	DEFINITION
Hikes	Elevation of one side of the pelvis above level
Posterior tilt	Posterior tilting of the pelvis so that the pubic symphysis is directed upward (flat lumbar spine)
Anterior tilt	Anterior tilting of the pelvis so that the pubic symphysis is directed downward
Lacks forward rotation	Less than normal rotation for a specific phase
Lacks backward rotation	Less than normal backward rotation for a specific phase
Excessive forward rotation	Rotation greater than normal for a specific phase
Excessive backward rotation	Greater than normal backward rotation for a specific phase
Ipsilateral drop	Dropping of the pelvis on the side of the reference limb during swing
Contralateral drop	Dropping of the pelvis on the contralateral side during mid-stance and terminal stance on the reference limb

Table 38-5. Definitions of Trunk Segment Deviations

DEVIATIONS	DEFINITION
Forward lean	The trunk is flexed anterior to vertical axis of the hip
Backward lean	The trunk is hyperextended or posterior to the vertical axis of the hip
Lateral lean (R or L)	Leaning of the trunk to one side
Rotates back	Rotation greater than neutral on the reference side
Rotates forward	Rotation greater than neutral on the reference side

would be checked. The significance of this deviation is that the normal loading response at the ankle cannot be accomplished and the shock absorbing mechanism is diminished.

Consider the deviation of Excess Plantar Flexion. There are many subphases during which this deviation would be inconsistent with normal events at the ankle. If plantar flexion is present during midstance and terminal stance, either definite compensatory movements must occur at other segments to accommodate for alignment of the body's center of

Instructions for Gait Analysis: Ankle, Foot, and Toes
1. Perform gait analysis with least possible bracing and support.
2. Place a check in the appropriate box. With bilateral involvement, use a (R) or (L) instead of a check.

		WEIGHT ACCEPTANCE		SINGLE LIMB STABILITY		SWING LIMB ADVANCEMENT			
		IC	LR	MSt	TSt	PS	IS	MSw	TSw
ANKLE & FOOT:	Forefoot Contact								
	Foot Flat Contact								
	Foot Slap								
	Excess Plantarflexion								
	Excess Dorsiflexion								
	Excess Varus								
	Excess Valgus								
	Heel Off								
	No Heel Off								
	Drag								
	Contralateral Vaulting								
TOES:	Up								
	Inadequate Extension								
	Clawed								

MAJOR PROBLEMS

Weight Acceptance	Single Limb Stability	Swing Limb Advancement
_____	_____	_____

Motions Referred From Other Joints:

External Rotation	☐
Internal Rotation	☐
Abduction	☐
Adduction	☐

Figure 38-8. Gait analysis: ankle, foot, and toes. (Adapted by permission of Rancho Los Amigos Medical Center, Pathokinesiology and Physical Therapy Department)

gravity behind the axis of the ankle, or the patient must walk on his toes. If plantar flexion is present during midswing, toe drag is likely unless movement at another segment is exaggerated.

Refer now to the knee analysis form (Fig. 38-9). Knowing that knee extension is the expected normal during MS and TSt, the deviation Inadequate Extension would be checked in the open spaces if observed during MS or TSt. You might conclude that single limb stability is insufficient and may affect stance ratio, velo-

Instructions for Gait Analysis: Knee
1. Perform gait analysis with least possible bracing and support.
2. Place a check in the appropriate box. With bilateral involvement, use a (R) or (L) instead of a check.

		WEIGHT ACCEPTANCE		SINGLE LIMB STABILITY		SWING LIMB ADVANCEMENT			
		IC	LR	MSt	TSt	PS	IS	MSw	TSw
KNEE:	Flexion: Limited								
	Absent								
	Excessive								
	Inadequate Extension								
	Wobbles								
	Hyperextends								
	Extension Thrust								
	Varus								
	Valgus								
	Excess Contra. Flexion								

MAJOR PROBLEMS

Weight Acceptance	Single Limb Stability	Swing Limb Advancement

Motions Referred From Other Joints:

External Rotation _____
Internal Rotation _____
Abduction _____
Adduction _____

Figure 38-9. Gait analysis: knee. (Adapted by permission of Rancho Los Amigos Medical Center, Pathokinesiology and Physical Therapy Department)

city, step length on the contralateral side, and so on.

All of the segmental gait analysis forms have the same format and are used in the same manner. We will now consider the forms for the hip and the trunk and pelvis (Figs. 38-10 and 38-11). It may be helpful to point out that the deviations described for the trunk and pelvis are mostly compensatory motions. Compensatory motions are the result of inadequate limb function. For instance, if during initial and midswing hip or knee flexion is less than normal, backward lean of the trunk, posterior pelvic tilt, or pelvic hiking might be seen as a means of advancing the limb. Forward lean of the trunk, as previously described, can be compensatory for a plantar flexed ankle, or can be the direct result of inadequate hip extension control or strength, or a hip flexion contracture. Patients with hemiplegia often do not have sufficient proprioceptive acuity or adequate postural responses to assume a less energy-demanding posture and demonstrate a forward trunk during stance as a result of inad-

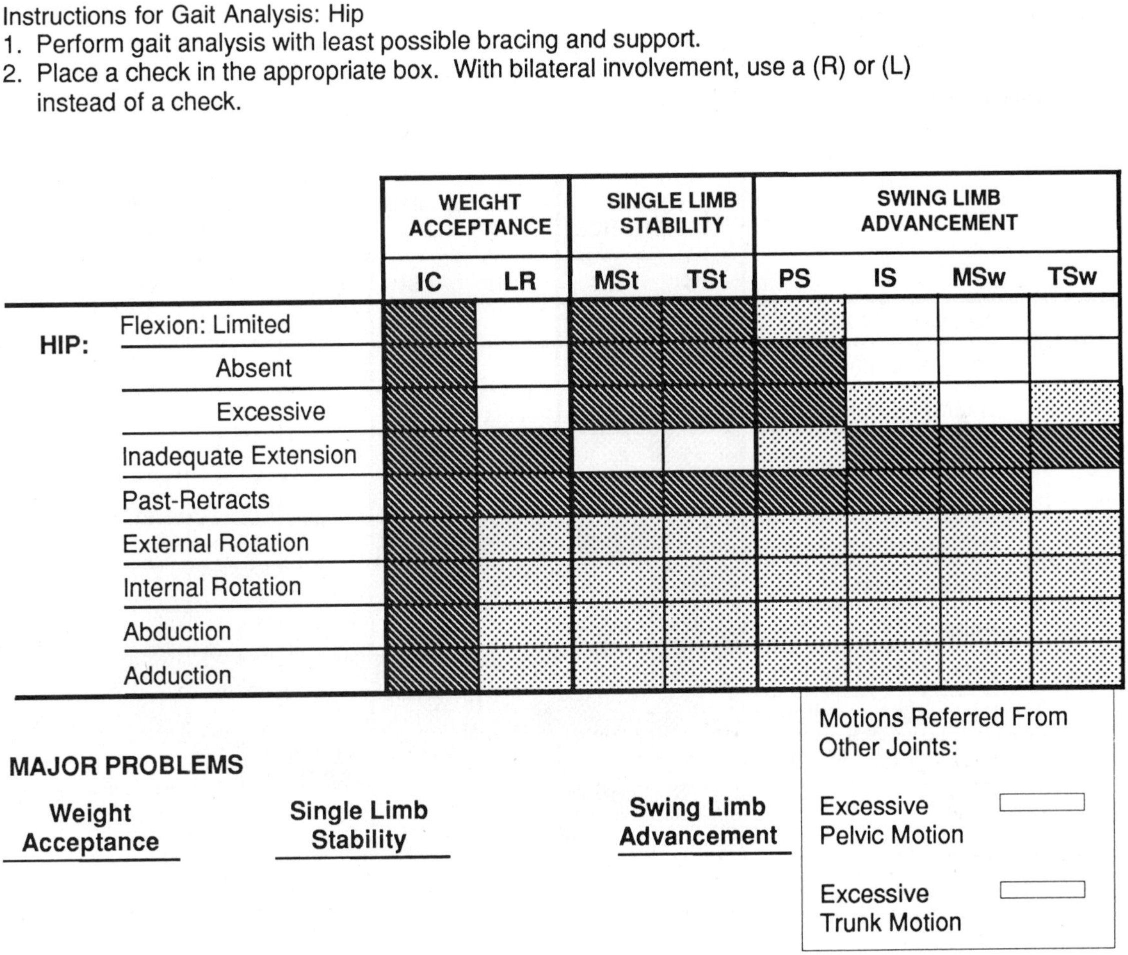

Instructions for Gait Analysis: Hip
1. Perform gait analysis with least possible bracing and support.
2. Place a check in the appropriate box. With bilateral involvement, use a (R) or (L) instead of a check.

		WEIGHT ACCEPTANCE		SINGLE LIMB STABILITY		SWING LIMB ADVANCEMENT			
		IC	LR	MSt	TSt	PS	IS	MSw	TSw
HIP:	Flexion: Limited								
	Absent								
	Excessive								
	Inadequate Extension								
	Past-Retracts								
	External Rotation								
	Internal Rotation								
	Abduction								
	Adduction								

MAJOR PROBLEMS

Weight Acceptance	Single Limb Stability	Swing Limb Advancement

Motions Referred From Other Joints:

Excessive Pelvic Motion ☐

Excessive Trunk Motion ☐

Figure 38-10. Gait analysis: hip. (Adapted by permission of Rancho Los Amigos Medical Center, Pathokinesiology and Physical Therapy Department)

equate hip extension control. In clinical cases where hip extension weakness is the result of a lower motor neuron lesion or muscle disease, such as muscle dystrophy, the patient will have adequate central balance and sensation to substitute with a backward lean of the trunk.

Contralateral drop of the pelvis is a direct result of inadequate lateral hip stabilizers and is not a compensatory motion. However, ipsilateral drop may well be the result of contralateral weakness of the hip abductors during swing of the reference limb. Ipsilateral drop is usually seen as the result of a short ipsilateral

limb as it prepares to touch the floor.

The use of the gait analysis forms helps your evaluation of gait to become more consistent, systematic, and organized. It is very important initially to use these forms when following a segment-by-segment analysis of gait. The most logical way to continue learning about gait analysis at this point would be to observe film loops of each segment in which both normal and pathological walking could be reviewed. Segmental gait analysis requires repetitive observation of patients performing the same walking task over and over. Often pa-

Instructions for Gait Analysis: Trunk and Pelvis
1. Perform gait analysis with least possible bracing and support.
2. Place a check in the appropriate box. With bilateral involvement, use a (R) or (L) instead of a check.

		WEIGHT ACCEPTANCE		SINGLE LIMB STABILITY		SWING LIMB ADVANCEMENT			
		IC	LR	MSt	TSt	PS	IS	MSw	TSw
TRUNK:	Backward Lean								
	Forward Lean								
	Lateral Lean R/L								
	Rotates Back								
	Rotates Forward								
PELVIS:	Hikes								
	Posterior Tilt								
	Anterior Tilt								
	Lacks Forw. Rotation								
	Lacks Backw. Rotation								
	Excess Forw. Rotat.								
	Excess Backw. Rotat.								
	Ipsilateral Drop								
	Contralateral Drop								

MAJOR PROBLEMS

Weight Acceptance	Single Limb Stability	Swing Limb Advancement

Figure 38-11. Gait analysis: trunk and pelvis. (Adapted by permission of Rancho Los Amigos Medical Center, Pathokinesiology and Physical Therapy Department)

tients fatigue or attempt to change their gait patterns, making learning somewhat more difficult for the clinician. Segmental film loops resolve this problem by presenting several steps repeated over and over and without being distracted by observing motion at other joints. This method helps to train your eye and develop a more disciplined approach to analysis. Patient analysis will then be more efficient and accurate. If film loops are not available, you must begin with patients who demonstrate gait dysfunction.

Make several copies of the forms shown here. It is important to select patients who can walk for several minutes before resting, because you will need to observe a much longer time when first learning to analyze gait. Your observation will be easier and more accurate if the patient wears shorts and walks without shoes or supportive equipment when possible. If a cane or walker is needed, you should have someone provide minimal manual assistance during your assessment of the hip and pelvis so that the deviations are not masked by excessive external support.

Analyze one segment throughout all phases of the gait cycle. Begin your observation with the ankle, foot, and toes and proceed proximally as each segment is analyzed.

The full body form is a compilation of the individual segmental forms (Fig. 38-12). Use of this form is suggested after you become familiar with the individual forms. Notice that the three functional tasks are listed to the right on the full body form. Consideration of the major deviations noted during your analysis should always be made with regard to how they interfere or prevent any one task or combination of these tasks.

DETERMINING THE CAUSES OF GAIT DEVIATIONS

After acquiring adequate skill to identify gait deviations consistently and accurately, the causes of the deviations must be determined. The major causes of gait pathology have been alluded to earlier. Through a problem-solving approach, you must now determine which of the five basic factors are responsible for the gait deviations you have observed.

First determine if the three functional tasks (weight acceptance, single limb support, swing limb advancement) have been accomplished. If not, identify what specific deviations are present during the relevant subphase(s). Then you must determine which of these are most significant. In other words, are the deviations observed simply compensatory motions or substitutions, or are the deviations the result of primary limb dysfunction?

You should then use appropriate evaluative procedures (ie, muscle test, range of motion, assessment of sensation and motor patterns) to establish if deformity is present, if strength or sensory deficits exist, or if in-

creased muscle activity or pain may be the primary cause of the deviations identified. Often it is a combination of these factors. The patient's clinical diagnosis will help eliminate some of these considerations.

If you can determine the cause of the major deviations and if corrective measures are possible, such as the use of a cane or ankle-foot orthosis, you should use these to assess their effect on the patient's gait. Remember, during gait analysis the patient should not be wearing shoes and should be wearing as abbreviated clothing as possible. The following is an example of how you would summarize the information derived from a gait analysis.

Case 1

Diagnosis
Hemiplegia secondary to CVA.

Major Gait Deviations
   Ankle: Toe drag ISw
      Excessive plantar flexion MSw
   Knee: Inadequate flexion ISw
      Inadequate knee extension TSw
   Hip: Inadequate flexion MSw, TSw
   Pelvis: Hiking **MSw**, TSw; contralateral drop
   Trunk: Slight forward lean **MSw, TSw**

Reasons for Deviations
   Ankle: Inadequate knee flexion
      Weak flexion synergy
   Knee: Increased quadriceps muscle activity
      Synergy dependent
   Hip: Weak flexion synergy
   Pelvis: Substitution for inadequate limb flexion
      Inadequate hip abductor control
   Trunk: Inadequate hip extension control

Functional Task Deficiency
   Limb advancement
      Single limb support (lateral hip instability)

Penalties Decreased velocity and cadence, unequal stance ratio, and decreased step

(Text continues on p. 694.)

Instructions for Gait Analysis: Total Body
1. Perform gait analysis with least possible bracing and support.
2. Place a check in the appropriate box. With bilateral involvement, use a (R) or (L) instead of a check.

		Weight Accept		Single Limb		Swing Limb Advancement				LIST MAJOR PROBLEMS:
		IC	LR	M St	T St	PS	IS	M Sw	T Sw	
TRUNK	Backward Lean									Weight Acceptance
	Forward Lean									
	Lateral Lean R/L									
	Rotates Back									
	Rotates Forward									
PELVIS	Hikes									
	Posterior Tilt									
	Anterior Tilt									
	Lacks Forw. Rotat.									
	Lacks Bacw. Rotat.									
	Excess Forw. Rotat.									Single Limb Stability
	Excess Bacw. Rotat.									
	Ipsilateral Drop									
	Contralat. Drop									
HIP	Flexion: Limited									
	Absent									
	Excess									
	Inadequate Ext.									
	Past retracts									
	External Rot.									
	Internal Rot.									
	Abduction									Swing Limb Advancement
	Adduction									
KNEE	Flexion: Limited									
	Absent									
	Excess									
	Inadequate Ext.									
	Wobbles									
	Hyperextends									
	Extension Thrust									
	Varus									
	Valgus									
	Excess Cntr. Flex.									Excessive U.E. Weight Bearing
ANKLE	Forefoot Contact									
	Foot Flat Contact									
	Foot Slap									
	Excess Plantar									
	Excess Dorsi									
	Excess Varus									
	Excess Valgus									
	Heel Off									
	No Heel Off									
	Drag									
	Contra. Vaulting									
TOES	Up									
	Inadequate Ext.									
	Clawed									

Figure 38-12. Gait analysis: full body. (Adapted by permission of Rancho Los Amigos Medical Center, Pathokinesiology and Physical Therapy Department)

Table 38-6. Primary Deviations Affecting Weight Acceptance and Single Limb Support

DEVIATIONS	CAUSES	PENALTIES
Hip adduction	Increased adductor muscle activity Inadequate strength of abductors Decreased proprioception	Narrow base of support leading to loss of balance
Contralateral pelvic drop	Weakness or inadequate control of hip abductors	Decreased stance stability Potential loss of balance
Inadequate hip extension	Inadequate hip extension strength or control Hip flexion contracture Increased muscle activity of hip flexors Painful joint Decreased proprioception Secondary to excessive knee flexion posture	Increased energy demand Decreased forward progression; decreased velocity
Inadequate knee extension	Inadequate quadriceps strength or control Knee flexion contracture Increased hamstring muscle activity Increased gastrocnemius muscle activity Secondary to inadequate hip extension or excessive dorsiflexion Painful joint Decreased proprioception	Increased energy demand Decreased stance stability leading to decreased stance time Decreased forward progression and velocity
Knee extension thrust	Inadequate quadriceps control Increased quadriceps muscle activity Secondary to primary ankle instability Increased plantarflexion muscle activity Plantar flexion contracture Decreased proprioception Painful knee (avoids flexion)	Loss of loading response at knee Decreased forward progression and velocity May result in joint problems, pain
Excessive plantar flexion	Increased plantar flexion muscle activity Inadequate plantar flexion strength and control Plantar flexion contracture Decreased proprioception	Decreased forward progression and velocity Need for compensatory postures Increased energy demand Shortened stance time
Excessive dorsiflexion	Accommodation for knee flexion contracture Inadequate plantar flexion strength Decreased proprioception Dorsiflexion contracture (rare)	Stance instability with resultant decreased stance time Compensatory hip and knee flexion resulting in increased energy Decreased forward progression and velocity
No heel off	Inadequate plantar flexion strength and control Painful ankle-foot-metatarsal heads Restricted ankle or midfoot or metatarsal phalangeal motion	Decreased pre-swing knee flexion Decreased forward progression and velocity
Excess varus	Increased invertor muscle activity Decreased proprioception	Unstable base of support with potential for falling and injury Decreased forward progression and velocity
Clawed toes	Increased toe flexor muscle activity Muscle imbalance with weak intrinsics Exaggerated response to compensate for poor balance Toe flexion contracture	Pain resulting from skin pressure and from weight bearing on distal end of toes Decreased forward progession and velocity

Table 38-7. Primary Deviations Affecting Limb Advancement

DEVIATIONS	CAUSES	PENALTIES
Limited or Absent Flexion		
Hip	Increased extensor muscle activity or posturing expecially at knee and ankle Inadequate strength or control of hip flexors Painful joint Decreased proprioception	Decreased forward progression and velocity Decreased step length Compensatory deviations leading to increased energy demands
Knee	Inadequate pre-swing knee flexion Increased knee extensor muscle activity Painful joint Restricted knee flexion range Decreased hamstring muscle strength Decreased proprioception	Toe drag at initial swing
Inadequate knee extension, TSw	Knee flexion contracture Synergy dependent; unable to extend the knee selectively with hip flexion Increased knee flexor muscle activity Dominated by flexor withdrawal response	Decreased step length Decreased forward progression and velocity
Hip adduction	Increased adductor muscle activity Excessive flexor or extensor synergy Decreased proprioception	Swing limb contacts stance limb resulting in potential for fall, decreased forward progression Limb placement in front of the stance limb resulting in a narrow base of support
Excessive plantar flexion, MSw, TSw	Inadequate dorsiflexion strength Ankle plantar flexion contracture Increased plantar flexor muscle activity Excessive extensor synergy Decreased proprioception	Toe drag, MSw Inadequate preparation for initial contact resulting in foot flat or toes first, initial contact; leads to loss of loading response at ankle

length of the reference limb are the resulting penalties.

CAUSES OF MAJOR GAIT DEVIATIONS

Tables 38-6 and 38-7 state specifically which muscles or joints may be involved in a given deviation and delineate the most common causes of the primary deviations that are clinically relevant, essentially those deviations that interfere with or prevent the critical events of each subphase. Primary deviations are the result of pain, deformity, weakness, sensory disturbances, and increased muscle activity. Compensatory deviations are motions or postures that occur as a result of substitution or accommodations for primary deviations, and therefore are not included in the tables.

CONCLUSION

Your use of this material will help you recognize that the most important factors contributing to accurate qualitative assessment of gait are appropriate terminology, a structured format, and a comprehensive delineation of gait deviations. Consistent and disciplined application of the sequential and systematic approach suggested in this chapter will (1) assure you of developing observational skills more quickly, (2) help you develop a more in-depth understanding of intersegmental relationships, and (3) teach you to recognize the functional significance of specific deviations.

The physical therapist, more than any other health care clinician, must be proficient in assessment of movement dysfunction, and most specifically, its effect on gait. Develop this skill; your clinical results will be greatly enhanced and the benefit to your patients will be immeasurable.

ANNOTATED BIBLIOGRAPHY

Bobath B: Introduction; Evaluation of motor patterns and treatment. In Adult Hemiplegia: Evaluation and Treatment, 2nd ed, pp 1–57. London, William Heinemann, 1978 (An excellent resource; clear and thorough description of multiple factors influencing motor pattern, including the effect of abnormalities of muscle tone on standing, walking, and other functional activities.)

Brunnstrum S: Motor behavior of adult patients with hemiplegia, p 7; Gait patterns in hemiplegia, p 101. In Movement Therapy in Hemiplegia. Philadelphia, Harper & Row, 1970 (A description of basic limb synergies and the effect of postural and tonic reflexes and associated reactions on movement.)

Hunt G: Examination of lower extremity dysfunction. In Gould JA, Davies GJ (eds): Orthopedic and Sports Physical Therapy, p 408. St Louis, CV Mosby, 1985 (A discussion of gait analysis with emphasis on the foot, static examination, and pathomechanics. Treatment approaches are also discussed.)

Kessler RM: The ankle and hindfoot. In Kessler RM, Hertling D (eds): Management of Common Musculoskeletal Disorders, p 448. Philadelphia, Harper & Row, 1983 (A good clinical description of ankle and hindfoot biomechanics, with elaboration on function of this complex during gait.)

Murray MP: Gait as a total pattern of movement. Am J Phys Med 46:290, 1967 (Normal values for gait components are presented. A good reference for more detailed information regarding the trunk, pelvis, and upper limbs.)

Napier J: The antiquity of human walking. Scientific American 216:56, 1967 (An anthropological essay discussing bipedal gait from an evolutional viewpoint.)

Saunders MB, Inman VT, Eberhart HD: The major determinants in normal and pathological gait. J Bone Joint Surg 35A(3):543, 1953 (Although of mainly historical interest, this article represents the classic work on normal and pathological gait.)

Skinner SR, Antonelli D, Perry J: Functional Demands on the Stance Limb in Walking. Orthopedics 8:355, 1985 (A description of kinesiological studies supporting the torque values presented in this chapter.)

PART V

Physical Therapy Intervention

39 Improving Flexibility

JAMES E. ZACHAZEWSKI

Movement dysfunction and physical disability are caused by a number of factors. A loss of normal joint range of motion (JROM) or muscle flexibility (MF) are among these factors.

The physical therapist must not only determine which factor or factors are causing the movement dysfunction and resulting physical disability, but more importantly what is the scientific and physiologic basis for the movement dysfunction and physical disability. Once the therapist has determined the scientific and physiologic basis, the appropriate method of clinical intervention may be determined and used.

The purpose of this chapter is to present the physiologic considerations that guide the therapist in determining why a patient has lost range of motion and the ability to move freely and easily. An understanding of the physiologic basis will assist the therapist to determine the appropriate method(s) of clinical intervention to use.

Portions of this chapter have been reprinted with permission from: Zachazewski JE, Reischl SR: Flexibility for the runner: Specific program considerations. Topics Acute Care Trauma Rehab 1:9–27, 1986 and Gossman MR, Sahrmann SA, Rose SJ: Review of length-associated changes in muscle: Experimental evidence and clinical implications. Phys Ther 62:1800–1802, 1982.

DEFINITIONS

The word "flexibility" will be defined as being dependent upon two components: (1) JROM, which is the motion available at any single joint based upon that particular joint's arthrokinematics and the ability of the periarticular connective tissue to deform; and (2) MF, which is the ability of a muscle to lengthen, allowing one joint or more than one joint in series to move through a range of motion.

According to deVries, "Flexibility may be most simply defined as the range of motion available in a joint, such as the hip, or series of joints, such as the spine." Flexibility is specific to a given joint or series of joints and also to a specific person and his activity. JROM is dependent upon the shape and orientation of the joint surfaces, and both JROM and MF are dependent upon the various physiologic characteristics of the muscles, tendons, ligaments, capsule, and fascia about the joint.

JROM and MF play an integral role in human movement. The person must be able to move through a large range of motion with ease and efficiency. Good JROM and MF will allow the tissues to accommodate more easily to the stress imposed upon them, dissipate impact shock, and improve the efficiency and effectiveness of movement. All of these factors assist in preventing or minimizing injury.

Any discussion of flexibility must consider the differences between static and dynamic flexibility. Good static and dynamic flexibility are characteristics of the healthy person who has no movement dysfunction. In the person with movement dysfunction, one or both of these characteristics may be compromised.

Static flexibility is defined by deVries as the measured range of motion available about a joint or series of joints (Fig. 39-1), whereas dynamic flexibility is defined as a measure of the resistance to active motion about a joint or series of joints. As dynamic flexibility decreases, the resistance to the motion (the ease with which that motion may be accomplished) increases.

Human motion is dynamic in nature. The velocity of human motion varies from slow methodical activity, such as walking, to high-velocity, explosive athletic activity (Fig. 39-2). Adequate dynamic flexibility is necessary for the person to maximize performance efficiency and to minimize the chance of microtraumatic

injury. Dynamic flexibility is limited by the ability of the connective tissue to deform easily and by the integration of the neuromuscular system (the contractile elements and their innervation).

The physical therapist must be careful in choosing the terms used to describe the reason for the patient's movement dysfunction. Does the patient suffer from a true *loss of joint range of motion* because of changes in the bony architecture, alignment of the articular surfaces of the joint, true contracture of the periarticular connective tissues, or a joint effusion? Or, does the patient suffer from a *loss of muscle flexibility* about the joint from a decrease in the ability of the muscle and fascia to deform? Static or dynamic losses may be present for either JROM or MF.

The physical therapist should reserve the term "range of motion" to describe what happens concerning the joint's ability to move

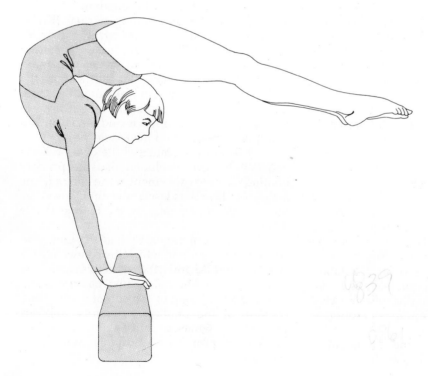

Figure 39-1. Demonstration of static flexibility.

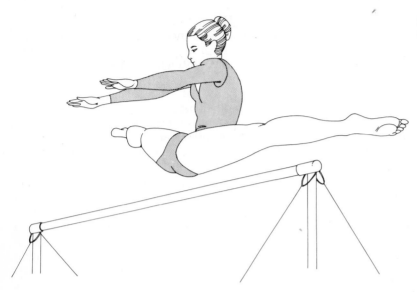

Figure 39-2. Demonstration of dynamic flexibility.

through its anatomic range, while using the term "muscle flexibility" to describe what happens regarding the ability of the muscle and fascia to deform. When evaluating or describing range of motion, the therapist should make certain that any muscle associated with that joint, which crosses two or more joints, is not on stretch because this will tend to limit flexibility, rendering a false impression of the actual JROM.

LIMITING STRUCTURES

JROM available in the normal joint is determined primarily by the bony architecture and the alignment of the articular surfaces. For example, extension of the elbow is ultimately limited by the olecranon fossa, and lateral rotation of the hip is limited when anteversion of the femoral head is present. In a heavily muscled person it is also possible for range of motion to be limited by muscle bulk.

If the bony architecture and alignment of the articular surfaces are normal, the connective tissue structures that surround the joint are the main factors limiting normal JROM. The connective tissues that provide the greatest limitation to JROM may vary depending upon the joint's position in space. Johns and Wright concluded that joint stiffness in the mid-range of joint motion was primarily attributed to the joint capsule. Further resistance was provided by the muscle and fascial sheath and finally by the tendons (Table 39-1).

deVries has recalculated the data of Johns and Wright and concluded that the primary limiting factor to movement at the end of range is the muscle and its fascial sheath, followed by the capsule, and finally by the tendon (Table 39-2).

The physical therapist has the ability to change the manner in which the connective tissues limit JROM and MF. To do this safely and efficiently, the therapist must have a sound working knowledge of the anatomy and composition of the limiting structures, and the methods by which to affect the physical and mechanical properties of the limiting structures.

Table 39-1. Contribution of Tissue Resistance to Joint Deformation (Midposition)*

TISSUE	AT EXTENSION −0.5 RADIAN		AT FLEXION +0.5 RADIAN		PEAK TO PEAK ±0.5 RADIAN	
	g-cm	% Total	g-cm	% Total	g-cm	% Total
Skin	−58	19	−50	−38[+]	8	2
Muscles	−133	43	49	37	182	41
Tendons	−25	8	17	13	42	10
Capsule	−92	30	117	88	209	47
Total‡	−308	100	133	100	441	100

*Frequency of rotation, 0.1 cycle/sec.
+Skin reduced the torque required to flex the joint.
‡Torque in the intact joint.

(Reprinted with permission from Johns RJ, Wright V: Relative importance of various tissues in joint stiffness. J Appl Physiol 17:827, 1962)

Table 39-2. Estimated Contribution of Various Tissues in Resisting Wrist Flexion and Extension in the Cat

TISSUE	TORQUE REQUIRED AT EXTENSION −48°		TORQUE REQUIRED AT FLEXION +48°		TORQUE REQUIRED AT PEAK TO PEAK	
	g-cm	% Total	g-cm	% Total	g-cm	% Total
Skin	−70	11.2	−45*	−8.7	25	2.2
Extensors	−35 ⎫	42.4	0 ⎫	36.9	35 ⎫	40
Flexors	−230 ⎭		190 ⎭		420 ⎭	
Tendon	−70	11.2	170	33.0	240	21
Joint Capsule	−220	35.2	200	38.8	420	36.8
Total	625	100	515	100	1140	100

*Skin aided in flexing the joint.
(Adapted with permission from deVries HA: Flexibility. In deVries HA: Physiology of Exercise for Physical Education and Athletics, 4th ed, p 463. Copyright 1966, 1974, 1980, 1986 Wm C Brown Publishers, Dubuque, IA. All rights reserved. Calculated from the data of RJ Johns and V Wright, Relative Importance of Various Tissues in Joint Stiffness, Journal of Applied Physiology 17:824–828, 1962.)

COMPOSITION OF CONNECTIVE TISSUE

All connective tissues within the body are composed of the same basic structural elements (Table 39-3). Fibrocytes synthesize the proteoglycans and extracellular fibers that make up connective tissue. In hyaline cartilage this function is performed by chondrocytes.

Table 39-3. Structural Components of Connective Tissue

Water
Proteoglycans
Extracellular fibers
  Elastin
  Collagen
  Reticular fibers
Fibrocytes/chondrocytes

COLLAGEN AND ELASTIN

Collagen and elastin are the two extracellular fibers that warrant the consideration of the physical therapist. Collagen and elastin complement each other functionally. Collagen is a fibrous protein and provides the skeletal structure that holds the connective tissue together, enabling the tissue to resist mechanical forces and deformation. Elastin assists in the recovery of a tissue from deformation. Collagen is the primary building block of connective tissue, providing connective tissue with its high tensile strength and the ability to withstand load and deformation. Overall, collagen may be compared to a fibrous suspension bridge. Its load-bearing ability depends upon its structural properties. The structural properties of this fibrous suspension bridge are dependent upon the material properties of the collagen (physical and mechanical properties), the size of the collagen fibril (area and length), and the organization of the fibrils (Fig. 39-3). Therefore, collagen should be the prime target when attempting to improve JROM and MF in the patient with movement dysfunction.

Although collagen is the common building block of the soft tissues, the types of collagen that constitute the tissue vary (Table 39-4). Type I and type III are the most abundant types of collagen found in connective tissue. They are usually found in association with each other, their relative proportions varying with age and pathological conditions.

The biosynthesis of collagen is a compli-

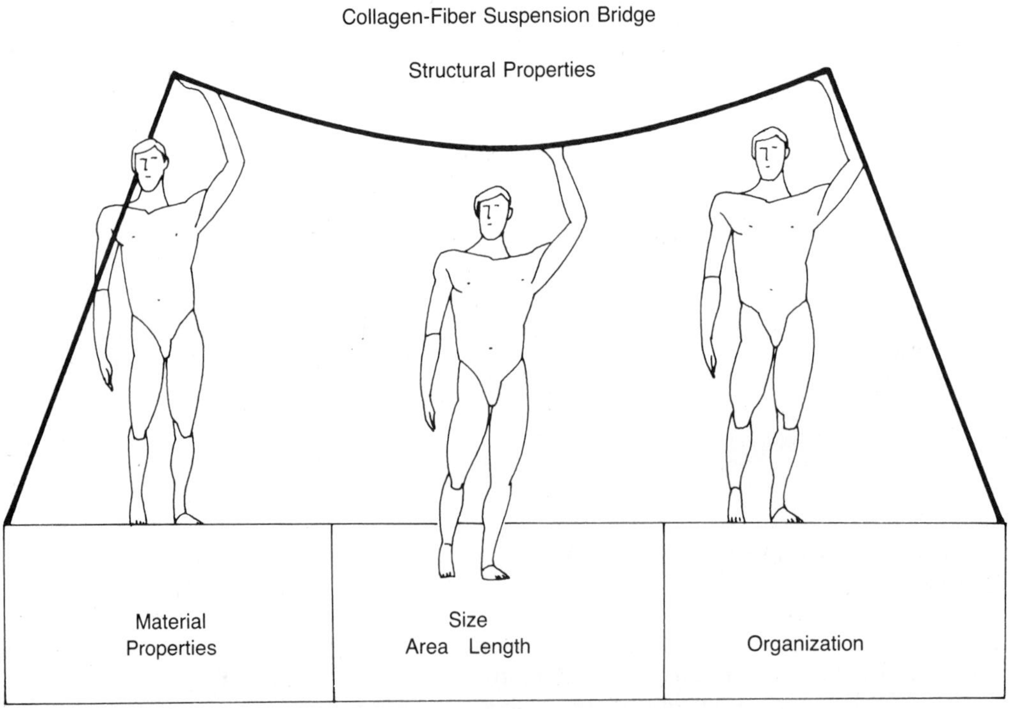

Collagen-Fiber Suspension Bridge

Structural Properties

Material Properties

Size
Area   Length

Organization

Figure 39-3. Collagen acts as a fibrous suspension bridge because of its structural, physical, and mechanical properties. (Reprinted with permission from Woo SLY: Biomechanics of soft connective tissue. Presented at UCLA Department of Kinesiology, Oct 26, 1982.)

Table 39-4. Collagens of Connective Tissue

TISSUE	COLLAGEN TYPE
Skin	I, III
Bone	I
Hyaline cartilage	II
Perichondrium	I, II
Basement membrane	IV
Granulation tissue	I, III
Annulus fibrosis	I, II
Nucleus pulposus	II, I
Muscle	
Epimysium	I, III, IV
Perimysium	I, III, IV
Endomysium	I–III, IV, V
Tendon	
Bundles	I
Endoteninium	III, IV
Joint capsule	I, III
Fascia	I

*Type listed first constitutes the most abundant collagen present.

cated intracellular and extracellular process (Fig. 39-4). Regardless of its genetic type, collagen contains certain amino acids. These amino acids form a single chain of amino acids, termed "protocollagen." During the intracellular process, three chains of protocollagen are synthesized individually and simultaneously. Three protocollagen chains are spontaneously bound together in the form of a right-handed triple helix stabilized by intramolecular hydrogen bonds, forming the molecule procollagen. This triple helix of procollagen is then transported outside the cell membrane. Once outside the cell membrane, extra peptides are removed from the ends of the procollagen, transforming it into tropocollagen. Intermolecular cross-links are then formed between the tropocollagen molecules. Present knowledge suggests that five tropocollagen molecules come together, held by intermolecular cross-links, in a quarter-staggered array. The intramolecular and intermolecular cross-links are quite strong and resistant to external load. These cross-links are responsible for providing collagen with its stability and tensile strength.

Temperatures above approximately 37°C have been shown to have an effect upon the mechanical behavior of the cross-links. Above 37°C, important changes occur that affect their mechanical behavior and allow the cross-links to break more easily and rapidly with less force.

Tropocollagen molecules band together in a characteristic pattern to form a microfibril. Microfibrils come together to form subfibrils and subsequently the collagen fibril, which is the basic load-bearing element of connective tissue. In the relaxed state, collagen has a characteristic crimp structure on the microfibril level (Fig. 39-5). The strength and integrity of the fibril is dependent upon its intramolecular and intermolecular cross-links (Fig. 39-6). This is analogous to the structure of a rope in which strand upon strand comes together to form the rope and give it strength.

The collagen fibrils of any tissue are embedded within the ground substance. The ground substance is composed of glycosaminoglycans (GAG) and water. The GAG are macromolecules with elastic properties that are present in the ground substance (intracellular matrix) of a variety of tissues. In normal tissue this ground substance is a viscous gel-like material that probably provides lubrication and spacing between the collagen fibers at intercept points where they cross. The space between collagen fibers may prevent excessive cross-links between fibers, which could decrease tissue mobility and deformation.

Although ability of a collagen fibril to withstand stress is primarily the result of its cross-links, the fibril's direction of orientation must also be considered (Fig. 39-7). Collagen is able to tolerate a great amount of tensile stress, but it is not capable of supporting significant shear or compressive stress. Therefore, collagen tends to be oriented along its lines of stress.

Tendon, ligament, capsule, fascia, and aponeurosis are all classified as dense regular connective tissue. The collagen fibrils of tendon have the most parallel orientation; therefore, tendon is primarily resistant to tensile stress. A less distinct parallel orientation is evident with ligament and capsule. Fascia and aponeurosis are arranged in multiple sheets or lamellae. Although following a parallel and slightly wavy course within each layer, the direction of orientation of the various layers may differ. Therefore, the fibril orientation of these tissues allows some stress tolerance in a greater number of directions, but still primarily along the collagen's lines of orientation. Loose connective tissue, with its abundant highly hydrated ground substance, is commonly found between muscles and in other sites where mobility is advantageous.

MUSCLE

The joint capsule, ligament, fascia, and aponeurosis are all composed of collagen and act

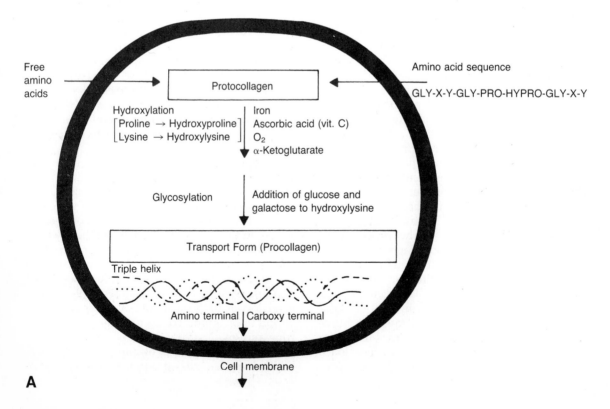

A

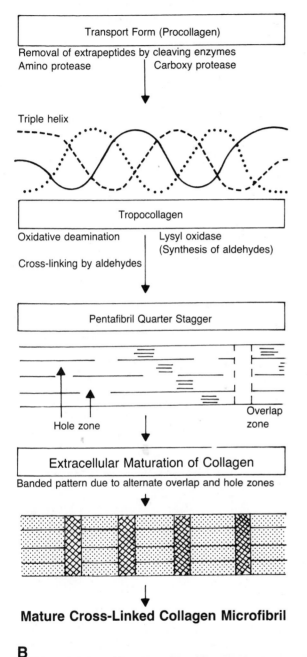

Transport Form (Procollagen)

Removal of extrapeptides by cleaving enzymes
Amino protease | Carboxy protease

Triple helix

Tropocollagen

Oxidative deamination | Lysyl oxidase
(Synthesis of aldehydes)

Cross-linking by aldehydes

Pentafibril Quarter Stagger

Hole zone

Overlap zone

Extracellular Maturation of Collagen

Banded pattern due to alternate overlap and hole zones

Mature Cross-Linked Collagen Microfibril

B

Figure 39-4. Collagen biosynthesis is a complex intracellular *(A)* and extracellular *(B)* process.

as passive restraints to the limitation of JROM. Tendon, considered separately from muscle, also is a passive restraint. Only muscle has active components that may limit JROM and MF. These components are the contractile elements, actin and myosin. When discussing muscle flexibility one must consider both the connective tissue component and the neuromuscular component. Therefore, the question arises: To what extent do each of these structures limit muscle flexibility?

Anatomically, muscle is a complex arrangement of contractile and noncontractile protein filaments. This arrangement makes the task of describing the ability of muscle to deform and recover from deformation difficult.

Muscle has a great amount of connective tissue associated with it (Fig. 39-8). The connective tissue associated with skeletal muscle can be divided into three levels of organization: (1) the endomysium, which represents the association of connective tissue with the individual muscle cell and interconnects to the perimysium; (2) the perimysium, which consists of collagenous septa that surround the fascicles and interconnects to the epimysium; and (3) the epimysium, the layer of connective tissue surrounding the entire muscle fiber.

The endomysium, a delicate connective tissue sheath that invests and separates each muscle fiber, has three components: (1) myocyte-myocyte connectives; (2) myocyte-capillary connectives; and (3) a weave network associated with the basal laminae of the myocytes. The endomysium, found external to the basal lamina and the sarcolemma, is formed primarily of two different-sized filaments, neither of which penetrates into the basal lamina or sarcolemma (Fig. 39-9). The thicker of the filaments (50 μm in diameter) is composed of typical collagen fibers that are arranged predominantly in a longitudinal direction. This orientation may reflect the endomysium's role in providing mechanical support for the fiber's surface and acting as an elastic device for contraction-relaxation cycles. The thinner filaments (20 μm in diameter) intermingle with the thicker filaments and represent immature forms of collagen. Figures 39-9 and 39-10 show the collagenous fibrils that compose the endomysium. These collagenous fibrils do not run only in a parallel direction, but also in various directions over and between muscle fibers. The course and distance between the fibrils varies depending upon the degree of stretch or contraction of the muscle. When the muscle is contracted, the fibrils are close together and at right angles to one another; when the muscle is stretched, they are parallel to the muscle fibers. This arrangement of the connective tissue permits easy displacement of the muscle fibrils and offers increasing resistance to deformation at extreme ranges. The endomysium, arranged as a weave network intimately associated with the basal lamina, may be an important factor in the passive series elastic component of muscle.

Each group of 10 to 20 muscle fibrils, which collectively form a fascicle, is surrounded by a thicker coating of connective tissue called the perimysium. The perimysium is oriented in either a parallel or circumferential direction to the fascicle. The perimysium is composed of varying amounts of collagenous, elastic, and reticular fibers joined with fat cells. The collagen of the perimysium consists of tightly woven bundles of fibers, 600 to 1800 μm in diameter, which interconnect with the fascicles. During passive stretch the amount and arrangement of the connective tissue in the perimysium may be more important than the endomysium. Borg and Caulfield have stated that the perimysium could be a major component of the parallel elastic component of muscle, being important in maintaining proper position of the muscle bundles and distributing the stress associated with passive stretch.

The fascicles of individual muscle are then grouped together and surrounded by the epimysium.

Muscle fibers can exist in three states: relaxed, activated, and rigor. Each state is characterized by tension and stiffness (the change in force produced by a change in length). In a relaxed state, muscle does not generate active force and therefore does not possess a high degree of stiffness. The amount of passive tension that it does show is more or less constant

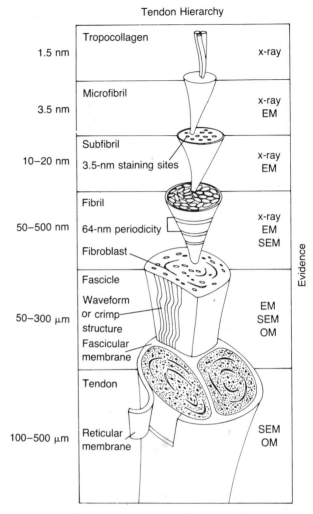

Figure 39-5. Formation of tendon. (Reprinted by permission of Kastelic J, Galeski A, Baer E: The microcomposit structure of tendon. Connect Tissue Res 6:21, 1978. Copyright © Gordon and Breach Science Publishers Inc.)

in a relaxed state. The level of this passive tension will vary proportionally to the muscle's length and will increase as the muscle's length increases. However, the question remains about the source of passive resting tension.

Six anatomic elements are possible contributors to muscle stiffness: (1) adhesions (of one

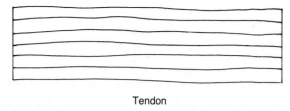

Tendon

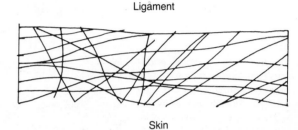

Ligament

Skin

Figure 39-7. Direction of fibril orientation. (Reprinted by permission of Nordin M, Frankel VH: Biomechanics of collagenous tissue. In Frankel VH, Nordin M: Mechanics of the Skeletal System, p 88. Philadelphia, Lea Febiger, 1980)

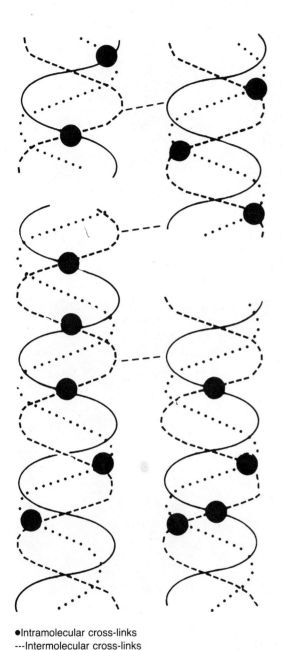

●Intramolecular cross-links
---Intermolecular cross-links

Figure 39-6. Intramolecular and intermolecular cross-links in tropocollagen molecules. (Reprinted by permission of Donatelli R, Owens-Burkhardt H: Effects of immobilization on the extensibility of periarticular connective tissue. J Orthop Sports Phys Ther 3:67–72, © by Williams & Wilkins, 1982.)

fibril to another or between muscle and overlying subcutaneous tissue); (2) the epimysium; (3) the perimysium and endomysium; (4) the sarcolemma; (5) contractile elements within the muscle fiber; and (6) the associated tendons and their insertions.

The exact contribution of each element appears to be unknown; opinion varies widely. A large portion of the passive resting tension of the muscle is due to the connective tissue that lies in parallel with the muscle fibers, although some tension may be attributable to a small proportion of cross bridges between actin and myosin filaments. These cross bridges, according to Hill, are very stable and may have a "long life."

Thus, it appears that both the contractile and noncontractile elements of muscle resist its

Figure 39-8. Connective tissue of muscle. Cross section through human sartorius muscle, showing the connective tissue of the epimysium surrounding the entire muscle, and the perimysium enclosing muscle fiber bundles of varying sizes. (Reprinted by permission of Fawcett DW: Textbook of Histology, p 272. Philadelphia, WB Saunders, 1986)

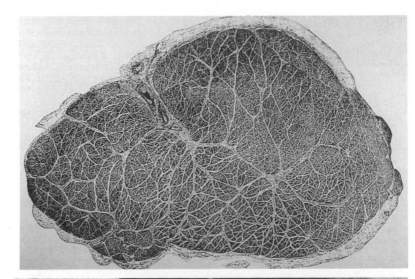

Figure 39-9. Fibrous endomysium, frog sartorius muscle fiber. The fiber surface is covered by a fibrous layer, through which cross striations are visible. (Reprinted by permission of Ishikawa H, Sawada H, Yamada H: Surface and internal morphology of skeletal muscle. In Peachey LD, Adrian RH, Geiger SR (eds): Skeletal Muscle, p 4. Baltimore, American Physiological Society, 1983)

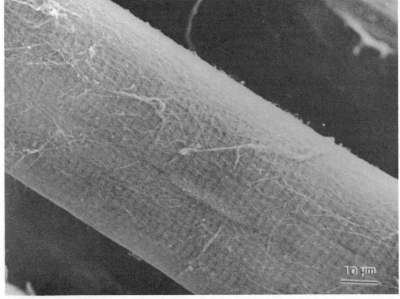

ability to be lengthened. The exact percentage that each contributes to the muscle's stiffness is not apparent. The extent to which the contractile elements contribute to muscle stiffness in the resting state appears to be related to the velocity of deformation. It also appears that the farther the muscle is stretched, the greater is the contribution of the noncontractile elements to the resistance to deformation. Although the therapist may not be able to change the resistance of muscle to deformation (which is provided by cross-bridge attachments in the contractile elements), the therapist does have the ability to modify and change the resistance provided by the passive connective elements. Before the therapist can affect the structures limiting JROM and MF (collagen and the contractile elements), the therapist must have a sound working knowledge of the physiology of each.

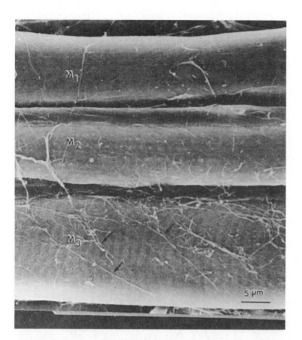

Figure 39-10. Fibrous connective tissue of muscle. Skeletal muscle fibers (M_1, M_2, M_3) appear as cylindrical units aligned in parallel bundles. Faint cross striations are visible along individual fibers. Coarse collagenous fibers of the endomysium run in various directions over and between muscle fibers (*arrows*). (Teased preparation of frog sartorius muscle fixed with tannic acid-OsO_4.) (Reprinted by permission of Ishikawa H, Sawada H, Yamada H: Surface and internal morphology of skeletal muscle. In Peachey LD, Adrian RH, Geiger SR (eds): Skeletal Muscle, p 2. Baltimore, American Physiological Society, 1983)

HOMEOSTASIS

Normal JROM and MF are necessary for optimal function. Connective tissue is a metabolically active substance that is undergoing constant change. The deformation of connective tissue, which is facilitated by motion, is necessary for homeostasis. The response of the tissue may be categorized as cellular modeling, ground substance and collagen response, and tissue response (Fig. 39-11).

CELLULAR MODELING

The stresses and forces imposed upon the tissues by motion throughout the range cause the fibroblasts to modulate collagen and GAG synthesis while enzymatic degradation removes collagen and GAG, which is no longer needed. The rate of turnover or change for GAG is much faster than for collagen.

GROUND SUBSTANCE AND COLLAGEN RESPONSE

The GAG synthesized by the fibroblasts binds with water, forming the ground substance, which in turn lubricates the collagen fibrils and minimizes excessive cross-linking by maintaining fibril distance. Motion precludes the development of anomalous cross-links. Stress and motion influence the deposition of newly formed collagen by orienting it along lines of tensile stress.

TISSUE RESPONSE

JROM and MF are maintained for the range through which the body part normally moves. The connective tissue maintains its integrity and strength, enabling it to resist appropriately the stresses imposed upon it.

MECHANICAL AND PHYSICAL PROPERTIES

Collagen exhibits various mechanical and physical properties when undergoing deformation. These properties allow it to respond to load and deformation appropriately, giving the tissue the ability to withstand high tensile stress. The three mechanical properties exhibited by collagen are elasticity, viscoelasticity, and plasticity. The physical properties exhibited are force relaxation, creep, and hysteresis.

MECHANICAL PROPERTIES

Elasticity is a springlike behavior through which elongation produced by tensile load is recovered after the load is removed. This property may be best symbolized by a spring (Fig. 39-12A).

Viscoelasticity is a viscous or fluidlike property that allows slow deformation with an imperfect recovery after the deforming force is

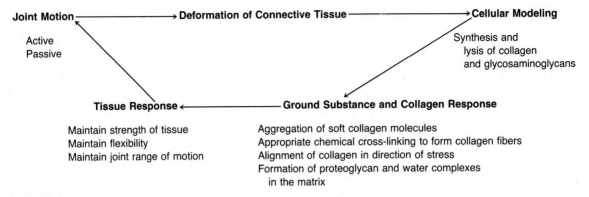

Figure 39-11. Periarticular connective tissue homeostasis. (Adapted by permission of Burkhardt S: Tissue healing with repair. Presented at National Athletic Trainers' Association Professional Preparation Conference, Nashville, TN, 1979)

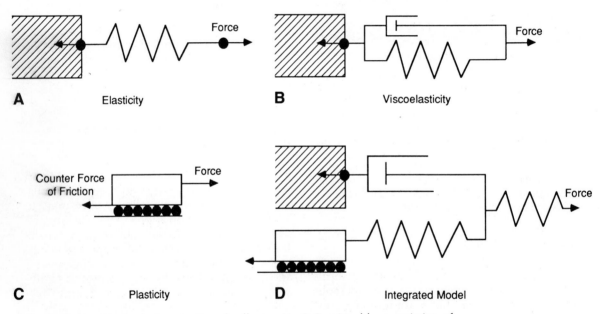

Figure 39-12. Mechanical properties of collagen. *(A–C)* Reprinted by permission of Viidik A: Functional properties of collagenous tissue. Rev Connect Tissue Res 6:144, 145, 149, 1973. *D:* Reprinted with permission from Frankel VH, Burstein AH: Orthopedic Biomechanics. Philadelphia, Lea & Febiger, 1970.)

removed. The recovery is the result of the elastic property, while the imperfection is the result of the viscous property. This change is not a permanent one. The property of viscoelasticity may be best symbolized by a spring and dashpot in parallel. The spring represents the elastic response and the dashpot represents the viscous response (Fig. 39-12B).

The final mechanical property is plasticity. With this property, residual or permanent change caused by deformation is maintained. Plastic change, which is difficult to achieve, may be best symbolized by the coulomb element of dry friction (Fig. 39-12C). The viscous properties of tissues permit permanent plastic deformation.

These mechanical properties do not occur separately in the tissues. All three properties are affected when the tissue is deformed (Fig. 39-12D).

PHYSICAL PROPERTIES

Butler and associates have extensively reviewed the physical properties of collagen. The physical properties exhibited by connective tissue are force relaxation, creep, and hysteresis. All three are time-dependent properties.

Force relaxation defines the decrease in the amount of force required to maintain a tissue at a set amount of displacement or deformation over time (Fig. 39-13A). The rate at which the force is applied will affect the resulting relaxation of the tissue. Generally speaking, the more rapid the rate of deformation, the larger the peak force and the greater the tissue's subsequent relaxation. Therefore, less force is required to maintain the tissue at a set displacement. One potential problem exists in attempting to influence the force relaxation response. The greater the velocity of deformation, the greater the chance of exceeding that tissue's ability to undergo viscoelastic and plastic change. If the capacities for viscoelastic and plastic change are exceeded, injury may occur.

In contrast to force relaxation, creep response is the ability of the tissue to deform over time while a constant force is being imposed upon it (Fig. 39-13B). This constant force causes the tissue to lengthen over time. The creep response allows viscoelastic and plastic change to occur in the tissue.

The final physical property of connective tissue to be discussed is hysteresis. The hysteresis response is the amount of relaxation a tissue has undergone during any single cycle of deformation and relaxation (Fig. 39-13C). It is an indication of the viscous property of the tissue.

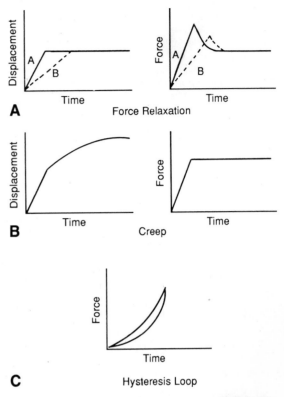

Figure 39-13. Physical properties of collagen. (Reprinted by permission of Butler DL, Grood ES, Noyes FR et al: Biomechanics of ligaments and tendons. Exercise and Sports Sciences Review 6:148, 150, 1979)

LOAD-DEFORMATION (STRESS-STRAIN) CURVE

The physical and mechanical properties of any tissue have a direct impact on the tissue's ability to tolerate load and to deform without a loss of integrity. The load-deformation curve for collagen presented in Figure 39-14 has been adapted from Butler and associates. To assist the reader in understanding the relationship of the physical and mechanical properties of collagen, the properties that are affected in each portion of the curve have been added to this drawing.

In Zone I, the "toe" region of the curve, the crimp structure or wavy pattern normally found in collagen fibrils changes to a more parallel arrangement. Little force is required to do

Figure 39-14. Load deformation curve. (Adapted by permission of Butler DL, Grood ES, Noyes FR et al: Biomechanics of ligaments and tendons. Exercise and Sports Sciences Review 6:145, 1979)

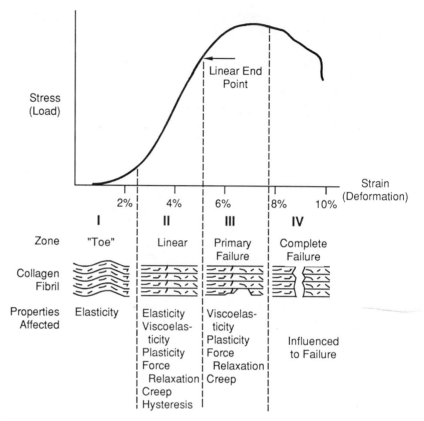

this; it is an elastic type of response. The greater the elongation in this region, the greater the stiffness and the force required to attain or maintain it. This region accounts for 1.5% to 4% of the total collagen elongation possible. Unloading the collagen within this region restores the crimp structure and resting length. The mechanical property of elasticity is affected in this portion of the curve.

In Zone II, the linear region, collagen has lost its crimp structure and is now parallel in its orientation. The load required to produce further deformation increases in a linear manner. (In resting muscle that is stretched passively, the greater the muscle length becomes, the greater the force required to hold that stretch.) All mechanical and physical properties of collagen are affected within this zone. The specific velocity at which force was applied, or the length of time that the force was applied, may

determine which specific property is affected. However, although all of these properties are time dependent, force relaxation is also influenced by the velocity of the deformation. When testing a group of collagen fibrils, the fibrils will tolerate a deformation of 2% to 5%. The end of the linear zone is characterized by the linear end point, which is the starting point for Zone III.

Zone III is the region of primary failure. Once the linear end point has been reached, isolated collagen fibrils begin to fail. Fibril failure occurs in an unpredictable manner. In this region, if the load has been applied too quickly, not allowing for viscoelastic and plastic change, the force relaxation response is affected in such a manner that the collagen fibril fails. Excessive viscoelastic and plastic change may cause collagen failure by allowing too much deformation by means of the creep response. Once the maximum tolerable load is reached, complete failure occurs when the collagen fibril has been deformed from 6% to 10% of its total resting length. The maximum strain at failure of collagen fiber bundles in human patellar tendon, lateral collateral ligament, anterior cruciate ligament, and posterior cruciate ligament has been demonstrated to range from 13% to 15%. The higher strain to failure of the group of collagen fibrils compared to the isolated fibril is thought to be a result of organization of the fiber bundles within the whole structure.

RESPONSES TO AGING, IMMOBILIZATION, AND REMOBILIZATION

AGING

Aging is a normal ongoing process of the human body. The principal concern regarding mobility of the joint with respect to the connective tissue structures is aging of the fibrous protein elements of collagen and elastin, because these make up the tendon, capsule, muscle, fascia, and aponeurosis. These elements influence the response of the tissue to stress, the amount of deformation possible, the ability of the tissue to return to its original length after deformation, and the method of transfer of force within the tissue.

During the aging process the total collagen content of tendon, capsule, and muscle along with collagen fibril diameter have been shown to increase, resulting in increased stability of the collagen fibril. The increased stability of the fibril is also a result of the maturation and development of stable and more complex intermolecular cross-links between the tropocollagen molecules. The increased maturation of these cross-links also increases the thermal stability of the collagen. Elastin shows an increase in the number of cross-links present and a decrease in the total number of elastin fibers.

Changes with aging are also evident in the ground substance. With increasing age, the components of the ground substance decrease. These decreases have been demonstrated in tendon and in muscle. The loss of these elements reduces the gel-fiber ratio found in the aging tissue. A high gel-fiber relationship assists in keeping the collagen fibrils separated. A loss of this ratio may allow some binding, which may assist in explaining the increase in stiffness with age (Table 39-5).

The physical properties of the crimp structure of the collagen fibril have also been shown to change with development and age. With increasing age, the wavelength of the crimp increases while the wave crimping angle decreases. Changes such as these allow the collagen fibril to reach the linear zone sooner, resulting in a steeper load-deformation curve. In clinical terms, reaching the linear zone and subsequently the linear end point sooner causes the tissue to reach its available limits of deformation sooner.

During the aging process the stiffness of a tissue, the passive resistance to deformation, may result in a loss of JROM (by means of capsular contracture) or a change in the static or dynamic flexibility of muscle, resulting in movement dysfunction.

Aging and JROM

General agreement exists that with the aging process, a tendency exists to lose JROM and MF.

Table 39-5. Age-Related Changes in Connective Tissue

INCREASED	DECREASED
Total collagen content	
Collagen fibril diameter	Water
Collagen cross-link maturation	Elastin
Collagen cross-link stability	Glycosaminoglycans
Number of elastic cross-links	

JROM changes occur not only with respect to age but also with respect to the specific joint. A comparison of the average male JROM values obtained by Walker and associates (ages 60 to 85 years) with those obtained by Boone and Azen (ages 0 to 19 years and 20 to 56 years) reveals that the ranges obtained decreased as age increased (Table 39-6). No studies currently in the literature make a similar comparison for females. Another excellent review of the JROM available at each joint, a classification of range in relation to age and sex, and techniques of measurement are provided by Wright.

Table 39-6. Comparison of Estimated Range of Motion as Males Age*

DEGREES OF MOTION	0–9 YR Mean	SD	20–54 YR Mean	SD	60–85 YR Mean	SD
Shoulder						
Abduction	185.4	3.6	182.7	9.0	155	22
Flexion	168.4	3.7	165.0	5.0	160	11
Extension	67.5	8.0	57.3	8.1	38	11
Medial rotation	70.5	4.5	67.1	4.1	59	16
Lateral rotation	108.0	7.2	99.6	7.6	76	13
Elbow						
Beginning flexion	0.8	3.5	0.3	2.7	6	5
Flexion	145.4	5.3	140.5	4.9	139	14
Forearm						
Pronation	76.7	4.8	75.0	5.3	68	9
Supination	83.1	3.4	81.1	4.0	83	11
Wrist						
Flexion	78.2	5.5	74.8	6.6	62	12
Extension	75.8	6.1	74.0	6.6	61	6
Radial deviation	21.7	4.0	21.1	4.0	20	6
Ulnar deviation	36.7	3.7	35.3	3.8	28	7
Hip						
Beginning flexion	3.5	4.3	0.7	2.1	11	3
Flexion	123.4	5.6	121.3	6.4	110	11
Abduction	51.7	8.8	40.5	6.0	23	9
Adduction	28.3	4.1	25.6	3.6	18	4
Medial rotation	50.3	6.1	44.4	4.3	22	6
Lateral rotation	50.5	6.1	44.2	4.8	32	6
Knee						
Beginning flexion	2.1	3.2	1.1	2.0	2	2
Flexion	143.8	5.1	141.2	5.3	131	4
Ankle						
Plantar flexion	58.2	6.1	54.3	5.9	29	7
Dorsi flexion	13.0	4.7	12.2	4.1	9	5

*0–19 yr, N = 53; 20–54 yr, N = 56; 60–85 yr, N = 30.

Aging and MF

Studies of MF utilize composite scores of an individual's ability to move through a range of motion in which a two-joint muscle (eg, the gastrocnemius) is stretched. MF has been demonstrated to decrease as children approach puberty, and then increase again (Kendall and Kendall; Hunter and associates). Upon reaching adulthood, it appears that both males and females gradually lose MF (Harris). However, even though MF decreases with age, research has demonstrated that it may be regained through the use of a specific exercise program.

According to Viidik

Connective tissues have a capacity to react to physical exercise by a retardation of the normal temporal changes. Moderate life-long training keeps the connective tissues "younger"; the retardation is achieved in the time period before maturity and in the years thereafter. The age changes seem to occur with the same speed in training as in sedentary individuals, all the time at a parallel but "younger" level.

Questions can be raised regarding whether certain age-associated changes seen in the make-up and physiology of connective tissue may be secondary to decreased physical stress.

In summary, age-related changes in the connective tissue result in a tendency to have a decreased range of motion. A loss of the normal gel-fiber ratio may result in an increased binding between collagen fibrils. The cross-links present also become more stable, causing a steeper load deformation curve and a tissue that is more resistant to deformation. As the primary clinician involved with movement dysfunction, the physical therapist is able to assist an aging population in maintaining optimal health, well-being, JROM, and MF.

IMMOBILIZATION

Many changes occur on the tissue level because of immobilization. Changes may be seen in both the joint and the muscle as a result of a lack of deformation of the connective tissue. Contracture of both muscle and capsule are responsible for restriction of motion. Changes in JROM may also be a result of proliferation of fibrofatty tissue within the joint space. Numerous investigations have been performed regarding the effect of rigid immobilization on the periarticular connective tissue (tendon, capsule, fascia, and associated capsular ligaments). These changes may be divided into those that happen on a cellular level, the response within the ground substance and collagen, and the response on a tissue level (Fig. 39-15). Clinically, it appears that the changes seen are not caused only by rigid immobilization from internal or external fixation, but will also take place if the joint does not move through a full normal range of motion that stretches periarticular connective tissue and muscle to its fullest extent.

Cellular Modeling

The total collagen content measured from immobilized periarticular connective tissue shows no significant change after nine weeks. These results would lead one to believe that no change occurs in the rate of synthesis of new collagen. However, investigation has demonstrated that an increase occurs in collagen turnover with immobilization, causing both increased synthesis and degradation (Amiel, 1982). These changes were shown in the medial collateral ligament and patellar tendon of rabbits. It is not known if other components of the periarticular connective tissue react differently. It is important to emphasize that a difference exists, because ligament is known to react differently from periarticular connective tissue under immobilization. With immobilization, ligament loses stiffness whereas periarticular connective tissue gains stiffness. The loss of ligamentous stiffness produces a weaker ligament, which is less able to tolerate stress imposed upon it.

The failure to exhibit a significant increase in collagen demonstrates that mechanisms more subtle than fibroplasia and scar formation are involved in the contracture process. No alteration occurs in the type of collagen produced during immobilization.

Ground Substance and Collagen Response

The response within the matrix or ground substance to immobilization is profound. The loss

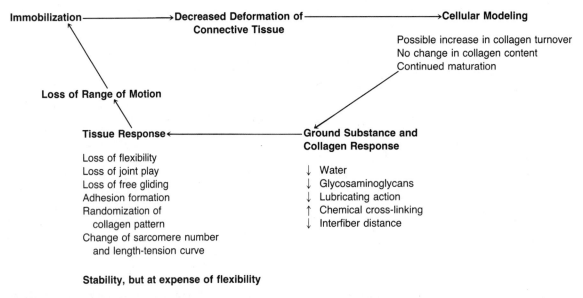

Figure 39-15. Changes caused by immobilization. (Adapted by permission of Burkhardt S: Tissue healing and repair. Presented at National Athletic Trainers' Association Professional Preparation Conference, Nashville, TN, 1979)

of GAG and water from the ground substance causes a change in the gel-fiber ratio and a decrease in the tissue's viscosity. This change allows a decrease in the lubrication action and the interfiber distance. The loss of GAG is significantly correlated to joint stiffness. The loss of this GAG buffer between collagen fibrils facilitates the synthesis of increased cross-links at strategic points between adjacent collagen fibrils (Figs. 39-16 and 39-17). As time passes, the cross-links become more stable and mature, providing more resistance to deformation. Therefore, it is important that motion take place to maintain the GAG buffer between collagen fibrils. The biochemical change in the gel-fiber ratio and the increased cross-links between fibrils affect the biomechanics of the tissue.

The biochemical and biomechanical changes described generally result in a qualitative change, *not* a quantitative change of the collagen structure within the connective tissue. The qualitative change in the collagen is attributable to a quantitative change in the number of cross-links.

Tissue Response

As time passes new collagen formation and accumulation, no matter how small, is important. Without motion, the fibril may be haphazardly laid down, interfering with proper joint mechanics and tissue deformation. This haphazard arrangement allows the formation of adhesions within the connective tissue. Fibrofatty proliferation may also take place in the joint recesses, interfering with motion.

One of the most profound changes on the tissue level is the change in muscle length. The changes that may occur with muscle shortening or lengthening have been researched by many authors. The works of the majority of these authors have been summarized well by Gossman and associates, who present the therapist with an organized synthesis of the literature as a basis for understanding length-associated changes in muscle and to assist in developing the rationale for preventing and correcting these length associated changes. The majority of the following information regarding anatomical changes of muscles immobilized in lengthened and shortened positions

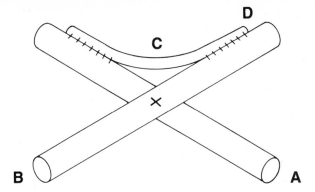

Figure 39-16. Intercept bending. (*A, B*) Preexisting fibers. (*C*) Newly synthesized fibril. (*D*) Cross-link as the fibril joins the fiber. (X) Nodal point where the fibers normally slide past one another freely. (Reprinted by permission of Akeson WH, Amiel D, Woo SLY: Immobility effects of synovial joints: The pathomechanics of joint contracture. Biorheology 17:95,

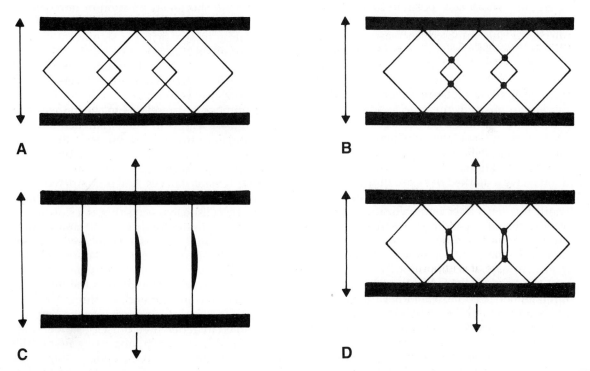

Figure 39-17. Restriction of excessive cross-linking. (*A*) Collagen fiber arrangement. (*B*) Collagen fiber cross-links. (*C*) Normal stretch. (*D*) Restricted stretch because of cross-link. (Reprinted by permission of Woo SLY, Matthews JV, Akeson WH: Connective tissue response to immobility: Correlative study of biomechanical and biochemical measurements of normal and immobilized adult rabbit knees. Arthritis Rheum 18: 262, 1975)

has been summarized from Gossman and associates.

Immobilization with Muscle Lengthened: Anatomical Changes

Animal studies indicate that muscle adapts to a lengthened position by increasing its number of sarcomeres. These new sarcomeres are formed at the end of the muscle fiber. The increase may occur as soon as within 24 hours of immobilization and is accompanied by a decrease in the length of the sarcomeres. When immobilization is discontinued, the muscles regain their "normal" sarcomere number and length. These changes in muscle length and the number of sarcomeres have been seen both with prolonged rigid immobilization and with muscles that continue to function while in the chronically shortened position (Kelsen and Wolanski, 1982). The adaptive response of muscle to the imposed increase in length seems to be related to age. In young animals it is not the muscle, but the tendon that elongates with immobilization in the lengthened position. In the adult there is no change in tendon length; instead, the muscle adapts by increasing the number of sarcomeres.

The chronology in which these events take place in immobilized muscle depends upon age. Animal studies have shown that infant rabbits have a marked decrease in muscle fiber length with a concomitant increase in tendon length five days after immobilization. During growth, the rate of addition of sarcomeres was lower in the immobilized limb than in the non-immobilized limb. During the next two weeks of growth and immobilization, there was an actual reduction in the number of sarcomeres in the immobilized muscle rather than a lower rate of addition. Concurrent with the decrease in the number of sarcomeres was an increase in sarcomere length. In other words, the muscle was adapting to meet its functional needs. The young rabbit demonstrates changes similar to the immature rabbit; however, these changes are slight. The adult rabbit shows no change in tendon or muscle length within the first five days of passive immobilization. In the adult, there is a significant increase in the number of sarcomeres and a decrease in the sarcomere length.

In summary, adult animal muscle adapts to a lengthened position by increasing its number of sarcomeres. Young animal muscle adapts by lengthening the tendon, which in effect places the muscle in a shortened position. This shortened position then causes a reduction in the number of sarcomeres.

Immobilization with Muscle Shortened: Anatomical Changes

Fixation of a muscle in a shortened position causes a decrease (up to 40%) in the number of sarcomeres. In conjunction with this, sarcomere length decreases. If immobilization is passive, the change in sarcomere number and length requires approximately five days to be seen. If the shortened position of immobilization is imposed by active means (electrical stimulation or spasticity), a significant change in the number of sarcomeres (up to 25%) may be noted in as little as 12 hours. The number and length of sarcomeres are recovered when immobilization is terminated. Change of sarcomere number is also related to age in the shortened muscle as it is in the lengthened muscle. In young mice there is a decrease in the rate of addition, whereas there is an absolute loss in the adult. The shortened muscles show steeper passive tension curves when compared with controls. These curves may be a reflection of connective tissue loss occurring at a slower rate than muscle tissue loss, resulting in a relative increase in connective tissue and a reduction in the extensibility of the muscle. Along with this relative increase in connective tissue, other investigators report an increase in the thickness of the perimysium and endomysium. An absolute proliferation of connective tissue has also been noted in denervated muscle (Sunderland, 1956). This proliferation, appearing first in the perimysium and then in the endomysium, was not present until after 29 days. During the initial period of denervation the essential reaction was atrophy of the muscle fibers, which would lead only to a relative, not an absolute, increase in the connective tissue.

All of the changes on a cellular, matrix, or

tissue level result in a loss of MF and JROM. These changes lead to movement dysfunction. If uncorrected, this movement dysfunction may lead to further immobilization, beginning a vicious, never-ending cycle for the patient.

REMOBILIZATION

The changes resulting from immobilization are reversible. The process of remobilization is summarized in Figure 39-18.

Cellular Modeling

Synthesis and lysis of collagen continue to occur while the production of GAG is stimulated by motion.

Ground Substance and Collagen Response

The ground substance, which lost components during immobilization, now regains these components. In turn, these gains return the gel-fiber ratio to normal, which increases the lubrication and interfiber distance of the collagen fibrils. The rate of recovery is faster than the rate at which fiber lubrication and interfiber distance were lost. The biochemical and biomechanical results show a good correlation: as

the components of the ground substance increase, the joint stiffness decreases.

Tissue Response

With motion, new collagen fibrils are now oriented along their lines of stress. Previously formed collagen fibrils are re-oriented along their proper lines of stress if they had been arranged in a haphazard manner. The correct length-tension relationship is reestablished by the addition or deletion of sarcomeres as appropriate. Because of these changes, JROM is increased and the joint mechanics return to normal. The vicious cycle is broken, and normal movement and function are restored.

THERAPEUTIC FACTORS AFFECTING CONNECTIVE TISSUE

The principal factors involved in the deformation of connective tissue are the amount, duration, and velocity of the applied force. The therapist may also use temperature and physical activity or exercise in a therapeutic manner to assist in the deformation of connective tissue.

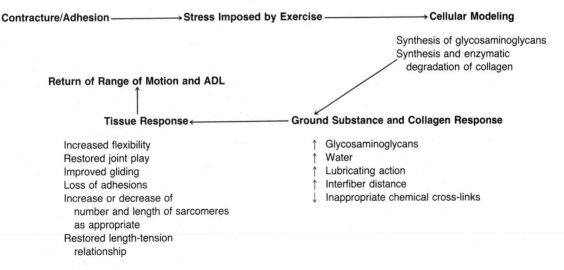

Figure 39-18. Remobilization. (Adapted by permission of Burkhardt S: Tissue healing and repair. Presented at National Athletic Trainers' Association Professional Preparation Conference, Nashville, TN, 1979)

TEMPERATURE

Temperature may have a profound effect on the physical and mechanical properties of collagen. Animal studies using in vitro preparations have demonstrated that the mechanical properties of collagen were temperature independent below a certain temperature (37°C in this animal model). Above this temperature, changes in the mechanical properties of tendon occur. The critical temperature at which the most profound changes can occur is 40°C.

Investigators have also explored the effects of therapeutic temperatures (which have an upper limit of 45°C) and load on the extensibility of collagen. All of these researchers have demonstrated that elevating the tissue temperature is beneficial when attempting to deform connective tissue.

When considering the effect temperature has on collagen, the therapist must keep in mind the following key points: (1) The amount of force required to attain or maintain a desired deformation decreases as temperature increases (Fig. 39-19); (2) the time required to deform collagen to the point of failure is inversely related to temperature (Fig. 39-20); (3) the higher the temperature, the greater the load collagen is able to tolerate prior to failure (Fig. 39-21); and (4) the higher the temperature, the greater the amount of deformation possible prior to failure (Fig. 39-22). Less damage occurs at higher tissue temperatures. Experimental observations attribute this fact to an enhanced ability of viscoelastic and plastic change to occur at higher temperatures. Heat alone in the absence of a deforming force will not cause a change in collagen deformation. A deforming force in the absence of heat will cause a change in collagen length.

Questions must now be raised regarding the amount of load to apply, the total time of load application, and whether it is best applied during or after the heating process. The greatest amount of residual change in the length occurs with the use of low-load, long-duration forces applied to the tissues while they are at their highest therapeutic temperatures. This type of loading is believed to have the greatest

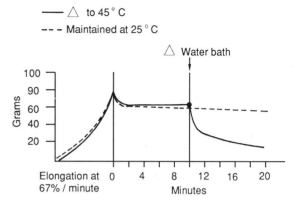

Figure 39-19. Effect of temperature on force relaxation response. Relaxation of tension in tendon (initial load, 73 g) at 25°C for 10 minutes and at 45°C for another 10 minutes. (Reprinted by permission of Lehmann JF, Masock AJ, Warren CG: Effect of therapeutic temperatures on tendon extensibility. Arch Phys Med Rehabil 51:484, 1970)

impact on the viscous elements of the collagen, compared to high-load, short-duration stress, which affects the elastic elements. A statistically greater amount of residual deformation ($p < 0.01$) has been reported in which the tissue temperature was elevated, the desired deformation was attained, and then that deformation was maintained while the tissue was cooled (Warren and associates, 1976).

Along with using therapeutic modalities to increase tissue temperature, intramuscular temperature may also be raised by active exercise (Fig. 39-23). Temperature increases to approximately 39°C from exercise are close to the critical temperature for collagen deformation, as discussed earlier. This increase in temperature has implications for designing a "warm-up" and flexibility program for any patient with movement dysfunction aggravated by a lack of JROM or MF.

The effect of temperature must also be considered relative to the innervation of the muscle-tendon unit. The sensitivity to tension varies among different golgi tendon organs (GTOs) and appears to be inversely correlated with the mechanical stiffness of the muscle-

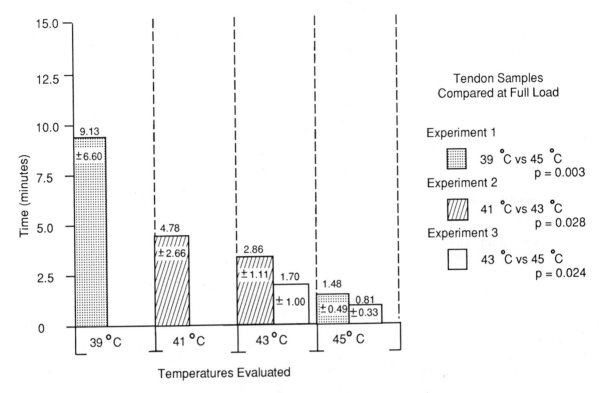

Figure 39-20. Effect of temperature on time of elongation to failure. Time to achieve 2.6% strain with treatment procedures using full load and comparing the temperatures of 39°C versus 45°C, 41°C versus 43°C, and 43°C versus 45°C. (Reprinted by permission of Lehmann JF, Koblanski JN: Elongation of rat tail tendon: Effect of load and temperature. Arch Phys Med Rehabil 52:467, 1971)

tendon unit in which it lies. The stiffer or less flexible the muscle-tendon unit, the less sensitive the GTO. Therefore, a tight or inflexible muscle will be more resistant to the recruitment and firing of the GTO. It is the strain or deformation of the GTO that is most important, not the amount of applied force. The sensitivity of the GTO to sustained stretch increased with increasing temperatures.

The combination of heat and stretching would appear to be the treatment of choice when an increase in the length of connective tissue is desired. This combination will allow the greatest deformation of the tissue using the lowest and safest deforming force possible. The time required to obtain change in the tissue

length would be shorter. This combination would maximize the amount of residual gain from elongation. The residual gain may also be enhanced by allowing the tissue to "cool" while in the elongated or deformed state.

Application of the principles of heat and deformation, just described for isolated tissue preparations, has also been explored with human subjects and demonstrates similar results.

It would appear that the application of cold would have the opposite effect of heat on connective tissue; however, according to Rigby and associates, no effect occurs on tendon below 37°C.

Prolonged application of ice has been

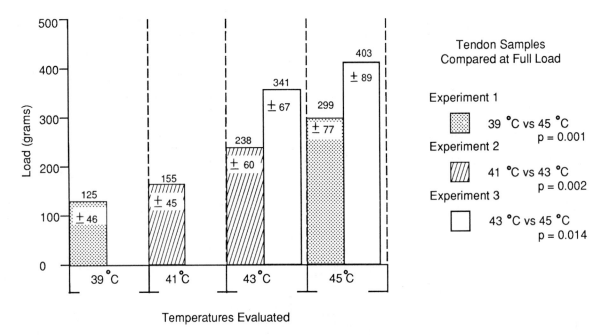
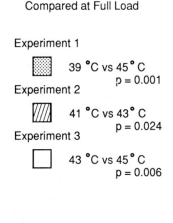

Figure 39-21. Effect of temperature on load to failure. Maximum load at rupture subsequent to treatment procedures incorporating the application of full load and temperatures compared at 39°C versus 45°C, 41°C versus 43°C, and 43°C versus 45°C. (Reprinted by permission of Lehmann JF, Koblanski JN: Elongation of rat tail tendon: Effect of load and temperature. Arch Phys Med Rehabil 52:468, 1971)

Figure 39-22. Effect of temperature on percent elongation to failure. Maximum strain at rupture subsequent to treatment procedures incorporating the application of full load and temperatures compared at 39°C versus 45°C, 41°C versus 43°C, and 43°C versus 45°C. (Reprinted by permission of Lehmann JF, Koblanski JN: Elongation of rat tail tendon: Effect of load and temperature. Arch Phys Med Rehabil 52:469, 1971)

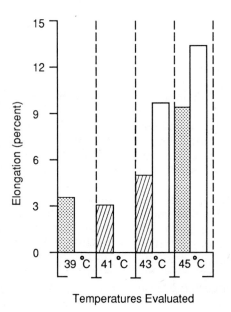

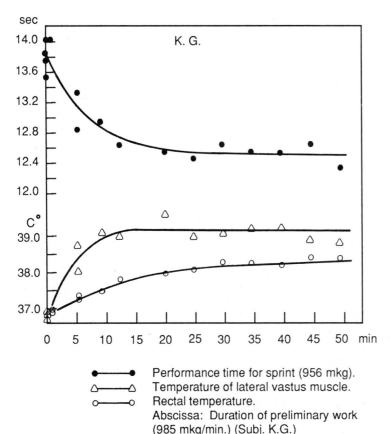

sec

14.0

13.6

13.2

12.8

12.4

12.0

K. G.

C°

39.0

38.0

37.0

0   5   10   15   20   25   30   35   40   45   50   min

●——● Performance time for sprint (956 mkg).
△——△ Temperature of lateral vastus muscle.
○——○ Rectal temperature.
Abscissa: Duration of preliminary work
(985 mkg/min.) (Subj. K.G.)

Figure 39-23. Effect of exercise on intramuscular temperature. (Reprinted by permission of Asmussen E, Boje E: Body temperature and capacity for work. Acta Physiol Scand 10:12, 1945)

shown to decrease spasticity. Therefore, perhaps the most beneficial use of cold would be to decrease the sensitivity of the muscle afferents and the contribution of the contractile elements to the resistance to deformation.

A cryostretching technique has been advocated by Knight. Cryostretching is used whenever a need exists to reduce low-grade muscle spasm. This type of spasm is often associated with muscle strains and postexercise muscle soreness. Cryostretching consists of cold application in conjunction with proprioceptive neuromuscular facilitation (PNF) stretching techniques.

Cold and static stretching are more effective than heat and static stretching in reducing muscle pain and electrical activity in injured muscle within 24 hours of injury. Application of cold at this time would appear to be appro-

priate to decrease pain and allow stretching to maintain the available pain-free range of motion. Once healing and scarring begin, it would appear that heat would be of greater value to increase the extensibility of the scar. This would allow the immature collagen fibrils to tolerate a greater amount of deformation without reinjury through enhanced viscoelastic and plastic change.

The brief application of cold cutaneous stimuli through the use of vapocoolants has been reported with differing results. Although the investigators used similar techniques, Halkovich and associates reported a significant increase in hamstring flexibility and resultant passive hip flexion ($p < 0.02$), whereas Newton ($p < 0.02$) and Kourey and associates ($p < 0.05$) did not. No precise conclusion is yet possible.

PHYSICAL ACTIVITY

In the years before World War II, resistive exercise was discouraged by many coaches, who reasoned that the athlete would become muscle-bound and lose flexibility. Over time, this myth has been disproved.

Exercise may have a positive effect on the strength, integrity, and organization of the collagen found in all types of connective tissue. Although the majority of these reports discuss changes in ligament, others discuss tendon and muscle.

The two critical goals of any JROM and MF program are to develop a tissue that will elongate over the required distance and that is strong enough to resist the forces placed upon it in order to minimize the chance of injury. A balance is required between tissue strength and extensibility.

The changes in the strength and stiffness of a tissue that has undergone elongation without a change in its integrity are summarized in Figure 39-24. No decrease is noted in the ability of this tissue to tolerate stress placed upon it. Because the tissue has longer fibers, it has less stiffness and is more easily deformable. These characteristics, which are an advantage in the muscle-tendon unit, could pose potential problems in other tissues (eg, ligament and joint capsule) that are the primary restraints to joint hypermobility.

Through a regular exercise program, an increase in collagenous strength and hypertrophy has been demonstrated in ligament and tendon. These changes are much more apparent after a ligament has been immobilized than in a "normal" ligament; however, speculation exists among noted authors that similar changes are possible in normal ligament (Akeson and associates, 1984). Tendon has also demonstrated an increase in strength and hypertrophy from exercise. The therapist must remember that these changes take several months. The effects of mobilization (movement) and immobilization on injured muscle in rats has been studied by Kvist and Jarvinen. With mobilization, scar formation and muscle

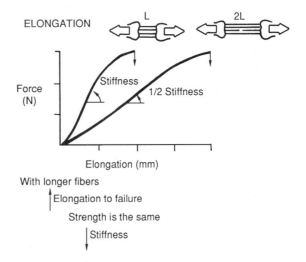

Figure 39-24. Effect of elongation on collagen. The influence of original length of tissue fibers on the shape of the load-deformation curve. (Reprinted by permission of Butler DL, Grood ES, Noyes FR et al: Biomechanics of ligaments and tendons. Exercise and Sports Sciences Review 6: 144, 1979)

regeneration were more rapid, the orientation of new muscle fibers was more parallel with surrounding fibers, and tensile properties of the muscle were greater. Again, because of the rate of turnover of collagen, it should be remembered that all of the potential changes in collagenous strength and hypertrophy take a period of many months.

The changes in connective tissue strength with hypertrophy of collagen fibers or with an increase in collagen mass are summarized in Figure 39-25. With hypertrophy of collagen or a broader collagen mass, the tissue is stronger. Although it does not lose ability to deform because of the increase in strength, it becomes stiffer and more resistant to deformation. Greater collagenous strength would be a benefit for all tissues, especially ligament, in order to avoid injury. The connective tissue in and around muscle must have strength, but it must also have the ability to elongate readily and easily; otherwise, dynamic flexibility is lost.

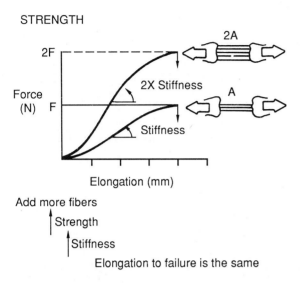

Figure 39-25. Effect of increased collagenous strength. The effects of increasing tissue cross-sectional area on the shape of the load-deformation curve. (Reprinted by permission of Butler DL, Grood ES, Noyes FR et al: Biomechanics of ligaments and tendons. Exercise and Sports Sciences Review 6: 144, 1979)

CLINICAL APPLICATIONS

The challenge to the physical therapist is to apply the information about the physiology of the connective tissues that permit or prohibit JROM and MF in the most efficient and safest manner. The therapist should consider the physiology of the connective tissue when utilizing manual therapy skills such as traction, mobilization, and manipulation for the joint, stretching exercises for various muscle groups, or new techniques such as myofascial release.

TRACTION, MOBILIZATION, AND MANIPULATION

This section is not intended to provide in-depth information regarding the use of manual therapy; instead, it presents considerations for the performance of manual therapy.

Passive movements of the articular surfaces of joints are used in the evaluation and treatment of movement dysfunction. Mobilization and manipulation are usually utilized to improve the motion of a hypomobile joint in order to relieve pain and improve function.

A therapeutic increase in the connective tissue temperature has been demonstrated to allow greater deformation of collagen in the most efficient and safest manner, while residual deformation may be enhanced by allowing the tissue to "cool" prior to removing the deforming force. If the goal is to increase joint play and motion, the therapist may use these considerations to advantage by increasing the tissue's temperature before performing traction or mobilization, and lowering the tissue temperature (if possible) before removing the deforming force. The appropriate use of therapeutic temperature will allow the therapist to use the smallest and safest load to obtain a change in connective tissue length. Use of an increased connective tissue temperature will also allow the tissues to tolerate a high load, if necessary, with less chance of causing trauma and thus initiating an inflammatory and reparative cycle. If the therapist desires to manipulate the joint or tear adhesions inhibiting joint motion, it would appear that reducing the temperature of the connective tissue and muscles surrounding the joint could be beneficial. Cooling the muscles surrounding the joint may increase the spindle threshold, thereby reducing the ability of the muscle to splint the joint. Cooling the connective tissue and adhesions reduces the percentage of elongation the adhesion must undergo and the force required to rupture the adhesion.

Grades of traction used in manual therapy have been presented by Kaltenborn, while grades of oscillation have been defined by Maitland (Table 39-7).

When using traction or oscillations, the therapist should have an appreciation of the physical and mechanical properties of collagen that are being affected and what portion of the load-deformation or stress-strain curve these techniques affect (Fig. 39-26).

Table 39-7. Traction and Oscillation Definitions

GRADE	DEFINITION
Traction	
I	No appreciable joint separation; nullify the compressive forces acting on the joint, due to muscle tension, cohesive forces between articular surfaces and atmospheric pressure. The joint is *loosened.*
II	"Slack is taken up" and the tissues surrounding the joint are *tightened.*
III	After the slack has been taken up, more traction force is applied and the tissues crossing the joint are *stretched.*
Oscillation	
I	Small amplitude near the starting position of the range
II	Large-amplitude movement that carries well into the range. It can occupy any part of the range that is free of stiffness or muscle spasm.
III	Large-amplitude movement that moves into stiffness or muscle spasm
IV	Small-amplitude movement stretching into stiffness or muscle spasm
V	Rapid movement performed at the limit of the range, going beyond the tissue's pathologic limit

Traction may be utilized in a sustained or intermittent manner when applied as a technique of manual therapy. Figure 39-26 depicts traction being applied as a sustained force. Grade I traction affects only Zone I or the "toe" zone of the load-deformation curve and the elastic property of the connective tissue. As the "slack is taken up" in Grade II traction, a greater number of physical and mechanical properties of the connective tissue are affected. The farther the therapist progresses toward reaching the tissue's pathologic limit, the greater the number of properties affected. With Grade III traction, once the pathologic limit of the tissue is reached and the tissue is placed on stretch, deformation may progress from the linear zone to the zone of primary failure or even to complete failure if the force or deformation are great enough. When traction is applied, the velocity of its application may have a profound affect on the tissue's force relaxation response. Too rapid an application may cause damage.

Passive oscillations of the joint affect the physical and mechanical properties of the tissues in a similar manner (Fig. 39-27). Grade I oscillations affect only the "toe" zone and the elastic response of the tissue. Grade II oscillations progress into the linear zone but do not reach the tissue's limit of deformation; therefore, only the physical properties of elasticity and viscoelasticity are affected. Only the mechanical property of hysteresis is affected because the tissue is allowed to return to its starting position and no deformation is maintained. Using Grade III oscillations, the linear zone of the load-deformation curve is affected. Because deformation is maintained over time during the course of the oscillations, the properties of plasticity, force relaxation, and creep may now be affected. Grade IV oscillations that are done at the end of the pathologic range in an effort to increase the JROM may exceed the linear end point of the tissue, and the tissue may be pushed into the zone of primary failure. In some cases this may be necessary to increase the JROM, but must always be done in as controlled a manner as possible in an effort to avoid excessive tissue trauma. Grade V oscillations or manipulations are used when it is necessary to tear an adhesion or restriction of the connective tissue. In this case the therapist is influencing the force relaxation response to the point of failure. The therapist should al-

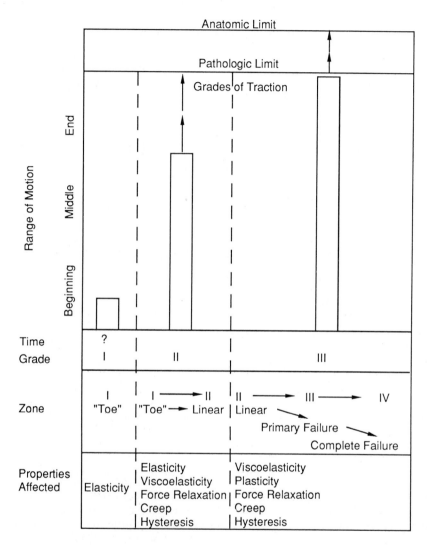

Figure 39-26. Mechanical and physical properties affected by traction.

always keep in mind the effect of velocity on the force relaxation response when using manual therapy.

STRETCHING EXERCISES

Enhanced flexibility achieved through stretching promotes greater compliance of the muscle-tendon unit. However, the therapist must determine the best method of stretching for each patient to gain the desired compliance.

Three methods of stretching are generally used in attempting to gain an increase in flexibility: static stretching, ballistic stretching, and stretching by means of various proprioceptive neuromuscular facilitation techniques.

Static stretching is a method in which a stationary position is held for a period of time, during which specified joints are locked into a position that places the muscles and connective tissues at their greatest possible length. Ballistic stretching involves quick motions

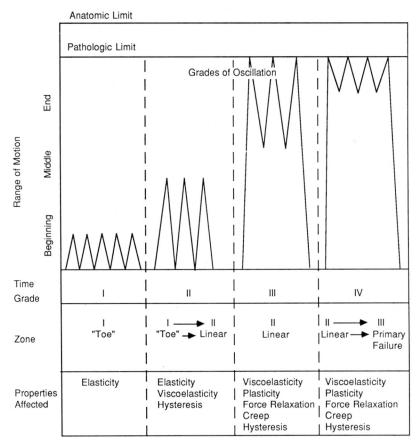

Figure 39-27. Mechanical and physical properties affected by mobilization.

characterized by bobbing or jerky movements imposed upon the muscles and connective tissue structures to be stretched. These movements are initiated by active contraction of the muscle groups that are antagonistic to those being stretched. Both methods have been equally effective in producing an increase in flexibility, but there are advantages and disadvantages to each.

Static stretching offers three distinct advantages: (1) less danger exists of exceeding the extensibility limits of the tissues involved; (2) energy requirements are lower; and (3) static stretching will not cause muscle soreness, and in fact may relieve it. These advantages are quite reasonable because connective tissue has a very high tensile resistance to a suddenly applied tension of short duration,

while demonstrating viscoelastic and plastic elongation when placed under prolonged mild tension. Static stretching may minimize any impact on the Ia and II spindle afferent fibers and maximize the impact on the GTO.

Most of the information previously presented would seem to support the concept that the therapist should never prescribe ballistic stretching. However, it is reasonable to question whether static work has been overdone at the expense of ballistic exercise. Some therapists would answer yes to this question, because ballistic stretching *is* appropriate to use with certain patients and in certain situations. It is the therapist's responsibility to determine which patients are appropriate for this type of program. The therapist can only make this judgment based on an understanding of the normal physiology and pathophysiology of the structures involved and an understanding of that particular patient and the activities in which he is involved. Any stretching program must be tailored to the individual patient. The program prescribed by the therapist for the athlete will be very different from that prescribed for the sedentary person or the geriatric patient with movement dysfunction.

Although ballistic stretching exercises may not be appropriate for the sedentary person or geriatric patient, they may be very appropriate for the athlete. If utilized appropriately, ballistic activities may play a vital role in the athlete's conditioning and training because athletic activities are predominantly ballistic in nature.

Early in the season, the athlete should predominantly use static stretching. The proportion of ballistic stretching to static stretching should be increased as the athlete's level of fitness and conditioning progresses. If ballistic stretching exercises are used, they should be preceded by static stretching and confined to a small range of motion, perhaps no more than 10% beyond the static range of motion. Ballistic stretching may be used to assist in the development of dynamic flexibility at the end of the athlete's available range.

The sedentary person and the geriatric patient do not use high-velocity activity in their daily lives; therefore, they do not need the high degree of dynamic flexibility required by the athlete. Static stretching exercises are more appropriate for this patient population in most instances.

The three techniques of proprioceptive neuromuscular facilitation (PNF) for increasing JROM and MF are the contract-relax (CR), hold-relax (HR), and contract-relax with agonist contraction (CRAC) techniques. These techniques seek to facilitate the GTO to inhibit the muscle in which it lies, and to use the principle of reciprocal inhibition.

Various authors and studies have concluded that PNF stretching techniques are effective in increasing flexibility. There appears to be no consensus regarding which is the single best technique. CRAC stretching has been shown to be significantly better than CR

stretching ($p<0.05$) (Moore and Hutton, 1980; Cornelius, 1984); CR was significantly better than HR ($p<0.05$) (Markos, 1979); and CR or HR was demonstrated to be significantly better than static or ballistic stretching ($p<0.05$) (Tanigawa, 1972; Prentice, 1983; Louden, 1985; Sady, 1982). Only Moore and Hutton have demonstrated no significant difference between static stretching and CRAC or CR stretching.

When considering the results of these studies, be aware that in most cases the amount of force used in stretching was not controlled. Only Moore and Hutton provided controlled stretching forces. The amount of force used to stretch with the CRAC, CR, and HR techniques may be greater than the force imposed by static or ballistic stretching, which may be a source of error in the studies.

However, a paradox exists in the literature. Although the premise behind stretching through the use of PNF techniques is to decrease the extrafusal muscle fiber activity, some research has shown the opposite to be true. Moore and Hutton have stated

> Recent experiments reveal that a static contraction preceding muscle stretch facilitates contractile activity through lingering after discharge in the afferent limb of the stretch reflex. Contrary to traditional views a muscle is initially more resistant to change in length after a static contraction.

Experimentally, Moore and Hutton then demonstrated that CR and CRAC conditions produce median values of 300% and 710% more hamstring activity, respectively, over static stretching electromyographic levels.

Within the same experiment the greatest change in the range of motion was seen with CRAC. CRAC also produced the greatest perception of discomfort. In an effort to explain the paradox of greater range of motion using CRAC over static stretching (although not to a significant level; $p<0.05$) despite a greater amount of EMG activity and perception of discomfort by the subject, Moore and Hutton hypothesized that in CRAC stretching the voluntary contraction of the antagonist to the muscle group being stretched masks discomfort and allows a greater stretch.

Once gained, MF must be maintained. How long a gain in flexibility will last after the cessation of a flexibility program remains unknown. However, it appears that once a flexibility program is stopped, the gain made will be lost over time. After a six-week flexibility training program using static, ballistic, or modified PNF stretching, Zebas and Rivera have demonstrated a significant increase in MF about the ankle, shoulder, hip, trunk, and neck. Significant gains occurred for all groups ($p<0.05$). After the cessation of a MF program a statistically significant loss ($p<0.05$) of MF occurred in all muscle groups after two weeks. A further gradual loss was measured at the end of four weeks. However, even with flexibility losses over a four-week cessation period, the amount of flexibility retained was greater than prior to the start of the stretching program.

Based upon the results of Wallin and associates, it appears that pursuing a flexibility program one time per week may be sufficient to maintain the flexibility gained, whereas engaging in a program three to five times per week will increase flexibility further.

In summary, static, ballistic, and PNF stretching techniques have been demonstrated to increase MF. Ballistic stretching may pose the greatest potential for microtraumatic injury. PNF stretching, although potentially the most effective, requires time and expertise, and may lead to discomfort for the patient. PNF stretching appears to be most valuable when the patient requires one-on-one intervention with the therapist. Static stretching may be done by the patient once he is properly instructed, and therefore may be the most desirable from the standpoint of results, time, expertise, and comfort. To improve flexibility, a stretching program should be pursued at least three times per week. To maintain flexibility gained, the patient should engage in the program at least one time per week. Once a stretching program is discontinued, the MF gained will gradually be lost.

STRETCHING SEQUENCE

The ultimate goal of any MF program is to increase the ability of the muscle to stretch through the necessary range of motion in the most efficient manner. Regardless of the type of patient for whom the therapist is developing a MF program, the *basic* components of the sequence are the same: (1) a general warm-up; (2) participation in an exercise or stretching program; and (3) a cool-down or postparticipation period. The number and complexity of each of these steps will vary with the individual patient, the type of activity in which he is involved, and the type of movement dysfunction. The following are suggestions for various patient populations.

The Athlete

The most efficient sequencing of five activities to improve the athlete's muscle flexibility are (1) general warm-up; (2) preparticipation stretching; (3) neuromuscular warm-up; (4) participation; and (5) postparticipation stretching. The time required for this sequence will differ depending upon the athlete and her specific needs.

General Warm-Up

As muscle contracts, heat is produced as a by-product and the intramuscular temperature increases. An increase in the intramuscular temperature should make stretching safer and more effective. The general warm-up should consist of repetitive, nonfatiguing exercise of the muscle groups to be stretched and should be approximately 10 to 15 minutes in duration to allow the increase in intramuscular temperature to occur. This exercise should occur in the athlete's readily available range of motion. The increase in intramuscular temperature from this activity will allow the tissue to deform with greater ease and minimize the chance of microtrauma. A secondary purpose may be to begin to condition the connective tissue and allow it to withstand the stress that will be imposed upon it. Examples for the runner would be cycling, a very brisk walk, or a very easy jog.

The effect of a warm-up period of cycling

on MF has been studied. Wilktorsson-Moller and associates have studied the effects of warm-up, massage, and stretching on lower extremity range of motion. Their data demonstrated a significant change after warming up only in dorsiflexion ($p<0.02$). A combination of warming up and stretching produced a significant change in hip, knee, and ankle range of motion ($p<0.02$–$p<0.001$). Hubley and co-workers have studied the effects of stationary cycling and static stretching on hip range of motion. They concluded that both static stretching and stationary cycling were equally effective for increasing hip range of motion and retaining the increase for a 15-minute period independent of activity. The authors did not evaluate the effect of stretching after warming up on a stationary cycle.

Massage may also prove to be beneficial during the general warm-up period; significant change has been reported for dorsiflexion and for the hamstrings following massage. No long-term carryover has been evident, however.

An initial cyclic phase or building-up process of deformation within the connective tissue's tolerable limits of deformation may be most efficient prior to the addition of a residual stationary stretch. This is the same analogy as has been proposed by Viidik. This process influences the hysteresis response and readily available elastic and viscoelastic deformation. After all of the readily available deformation is achieved, a stretch of long duration is required to increase the length of the tissues further by influencing the creep response. The athlete must exercise control in this phase to make sure the tissue's available amount of deformation is not exceeded, causing injury.

Preparticipation Stretching

Following warm-up and its concurrent increase in tissue temperature, slow, static stretching should be done. This slow, static stretching may decrease facilitation of the spindle afferents and assist in the facilitation of the GTO. Maintenance of the stretch will influence the viscoelastic and plastic properties of the connective tissue by influencing the tissue's creep response. After slow, static stretching, ballistic stretching (using a slowly progressing controlled velocity) may be done at the end of the athlete's available range of motion if indicated. Caution and control must be exercised with ballistic stretching to ensure that no microtraumatic injury occurs.

Neuromuscular Warm-up

The purpose of the neuromuscular warm-up is to begin to simulate the athlete's actual activity. The velocity of the activities chosen and the range of motion throughout which they are carried should be progressively increased over a series of repetitions. This progressive increase in velocity and range of motion will influence connective tissue (hysteresis and force relaxation responses) by further conditioning it to tolerate the stress to be imposed at the velocity and deformation necessary for training and competition. The repetition of activity at increasing velocities will also improve motor learning and skill necessary for competition.

It is important that this activity not be done until the tissues have gone through a general warm-up and preparticipation stretching program. The general warm-up and preparticipation stretching will assist in enabling the tissues to tolerate the stress imposed upon them during the neuromuscular warm-up. These activities will further increase the intramuscular temperature and the ability of the tissues to tolerate stress without injury.

During this stage the therapist may use PNF stretching techniques to assist the athlete in gaining flexibility.

Participation

The athlete is now ready to participate in the chosen activity. At this time, the highest intramuscular temperatures will be reached.

Postparticipation Stretching

After participation or training, the tissues are at their highest temperature. Slow stretching should again be done. Stretching at this time has two effects. First, it will assist in further improving flexibility. Second, postparticipation stretching will assist in decreasing or preventing muscle soreness commonly present after strenuous activity. When stretching after participation, the muscle or muscle groups to be affected should be maintained in an elongated position as the athlete "cools down." This static stretch may assist in maintaining the flexibility gained.

The Sedentary Patient and the Geriatric Patient

The programs that the therapist prescribes for sedentary or geriatric patients will be very similar. Both groups need good general static flexibility to minimize the amount of stress imposed upon the tissues during daily activities. Based upon their activity patterns, neither group has a great need for dynamic flexibility. The stretching sequence for these groups will be similar to that for the athlete, except that it is not usually necessary to include ballistic stretching or the neuromuscular warm-up phases.

General Warm-up

Just as for the athlete, the warm-up is an important preparation for any stretching activity that is to follow. The goals are the same, that is, to increase the intramuscular temperature and to obtain all of the readily available elastic and viscoelastic deformation that is possible through a cyclic process. As with the athlete, these activities are carried out in the readily available range of motion. The patient increases the range through which he is exercising as he sees fit. Modalities may be used as indicated to assist in increasing the tissue temperature; however, the progressive cyclic activity in which the patient participates must be accomplished. For the lower extremities, general exercise activity is appropriate, such as stationary cycling and walking. For the upper extremities, general exercise activity along with the use of an arm ergometer are appropriate. The key consideration in this phase is not to exceed the tissue's available deformation and cause injury.

Flexibility Exercises

For sedentary or geriatric patients, the flexibility exercises prescribed by the therapist usually consist of the activity in which the patient will be involved. Slow, static stretching should be prescribed for these patients, to be done on an independent basis. PNF stretching activities may be utilized by the therapist if one-on-one intervention is needed. Joint mobilization techniques should be used during this stage if indicated.

Cool Down

Following the stretching exercises and the treatment provided by the therapist, patients in this group may cool down by maintaining a position of stretch. The cool down may be further enhanced by the application of ice, if believed to be appropriate by the therapist. The ice may assist in the retention of deformation and may reduce any inflammatory response caused by the activity.

OTHER TECHNIQUES

The physical therapist should always be aware of the development of any technique that may help relieve the patient's movement dysfunction. For example, myofascial techniques have been presented to many therapists. The focus of treatment is the fascia of the body. The intent of the various myofascial techniques is to improve the ability of the fascia to deform and move within the body. With these techniques, the therapist may be able to reduce or eliminate a patient's pain, speed the healing process, and improve the patient's general function. To date, good clinical results have been reported when using these techniques with patients, although the exact reason for this success is uncertain at this time.

ANNOTATED BIBLIOGRAPHY

Adrian MJ: Flexibility in the aging adult. In Smith EL, Serfass RC (eds): Exercise and Aging: The Scientific Basis, pp 45–57. Hillsdale, NJ, Enslow, 1981

Akeson WH, Amiel D, Mechanic GL et al: Collagen cross linking alterations in joint contracture: Changes in reduceable cross links in periarticular connective tissue collagen after nine weeks of immobilization. Connect Tissue Res 5:15, 1977 (One of the first studies to examine the biochemical changes that take place with immobilization and demonstrate that a qualitative, not a quantitative, change takes place initially.)

Akeson WH, Woo SLY, Amiel D et al: The chemical basis of tissue repair: The biology of ligaments. In Hunter LY, Funk FJ (eds): Rehabilitation of the Injured Knee, pp. 93–148. St Louis, CV Mosby, 1984 (Excellent presentation and review of collagen and connective tissue physiology from a biomechanical, biochemical, and morphological basis. Concentration on ligament with some presentation related to tendon.)

The following references by Akeson, Amiel, and coauthors describe the anatomical, biomechanical, biochemical, and morphological changes that occur in collagen and connective tissue because of immobilization.

Akeson WH: An experimental study of joint stiffness. J Bone Joint Surg 43A:1022, 1961

Akeson WH, Amiel D, LaViolette D: The connective tissue responses to immobility: A study of the chondroitin-4 and chondroitin-6 sulfate and dermatan sulfate changes in periarticular connective tissue of control and immobilized knees of dogs. Clin Orthop 51:183, 1967

Akeson WH, Amiel D, LaViolette D et al: The connective tissue response to immobility: An accelerated aging response? Exp Geront 3:289, 1968

Akeson WH, Amiel D, Mechanic GL et al: Collagen crosslinking alterations in joint contractures: Changes in the reduceable crosslinks in periarticular connective tissue collagen after nine weeks of immobilization. Connect Tissue Res 5:15, 1977

Akeson WH, Amiel D, Woo SLY: Immobility effects of synovial joints: The pathomechanics of joint contracture. Biorheology 17:95, 1980

Akeson WH, Woo SLY, Amiel D et al: Rapid recovery from contracture in rabbit hindlimb. Clin Orthop 122:359, 1977

Akeson WH, Woo SLY, Amiel D et al: The connective tissue response to immobility: Biochemical changes in periarticular connective tissue of the immobilized rabbit knee. Clin Orthop 93:356, 1973

Amiel D, Akeson WH, Harwook FL et al: The effect of immobilization of the types of collagen synthesized in periarticular connective tissue. Connect Tissue Res 8:27, 1980

Amiel D, Frey C, Woo SLY et al: Value of hylauronic acid in the prevention of contracture formation. Clin Orthop 196:306, 1985

Amiel D, Woo SLY, Harwook FL et al: The effect of immobilization on collagen turnover in connective tissue: A biochemical-biomechanical correlation. Acta Orthop Scand 53:325, 1982

Asmussen E, Boje O: Body temperature and capacity for work. Acta Phys Scand 10:1, 1945 (Demonstrates how intramuscular temperature is increased by exercise.)

Balzas EA: Intracellular matrix of connective tissue. In Finch C, Hayflick L (eds): Handbook of the Biology of Aging, pp 222-240. New York, Van Nostrand Reinhold, 1977 (Describes changes in the physiology of connective tissue caused by the aging process.)

Banus MG, Zetlin AM: The relation of isometric tension to length of skeletal muscle. J Cellular Comp Physiol 12:403, 1938

Birari-Varga M, Biro T: Thermoanalytical investigation on the age related changes in articular cartilage, meniscus and tendon. Gerontol 17:2, 1971

Boone DC, Azen SP: Normal range of motion of joints in male subjects. J Bone Joint Surg 61A:756, 1979

Borg TK, Caufield JB: Morphology of connective tissue in skeletal muscle. Tissue Cell 12:197, 1980 (A discussion of types and functions of collagens associated specifically with muscle.)

Bronstein P: Structurally distinct collagen types. Ann Res Biochem 49:957, 1980 (A comprehensive basic science discussion of the synthesis and lysis of extracellular fibers [collagen and elastin], types of collagen and their distribution, and the physiology and role of the proteoglycans.)

Butler DL, Grood ES, Noyes FR et al: Biomechanics of ligaments and tendons. Exerc

Sports Sci Rev 6:126, 1979 (A classic reference with an excellent review of the literature and discussion of the physical properties of ligament and tendon.)

Butler DL, Kay MD, Stouffer DC: Comparison of material properties in fascicle-bone units from human patellar tendon and knee ligaments. J Biomech 19:425, 1986

Casella C: Tensile force in total striated muscle, isolated fiber and sarcolemma. Acta Phys Scandinav 21:380, 1951

Cecchi G, Griffiths PJ, Taylor S: The kinetics of cross bridge attachment and detachment studied by high frequency stiffness measurements. Adv Exp Med Biol 170:641, 1984

Ciullo J, Zarins B: Biomechanics of the musculotendinous unit: Relationship to athletic performance and injury. Clin Sports Med 2:71, 1983 (A discussion of musculotendinous injuries, considerations for their management, and their effect on athletic performance.)

Cornelius W, Jackson A: The effects of cryotherapy and PNF on hip extensor flexibility. Athletic Training 19:183, 1984

Crossman LJ, Chateauvert SR, Weisberg J: The effects of massage to the hamstring muscle group on range of motion. J Orthop Sports Phys Ther 6:168, 1984

Danielson CC: Thermal shrinkage of reconstituted collagen fibrils: Shrinkage characteristics upon in vitro maturation. Mech Aging Devel 15:269, 1981

deVries HA: Flexibility. In deVries HA: Physiology of Exercise for Physical Education and Athletics, 3rd ed, pp 462–472. Dubuque, IA, Wm. C. Brown, 1980 (A basic exercise physiology textbook. A well-written chapter on muscle flexibility and static/ballistic stretching is included. Recalculation of data presented by Johns and Wright on contribution of various tissues to limiting range of motion and flexibility.)

Dingle JT: The role of lysosomal enzymes in skeletal tissue. J Bone Joint Surg 55B:87, 1973

Enneking WF, Horowicz M: The intra-articular effects of immobilization on the human knee. J Bone Joint Surg 54A:973, 1972

Evans EB, Eggers GWN, Butler JK et al: Experimental immobilization and remobilization of rat knee joints. J Bone Joint Surg 42A:737, 1960

Fawcett DW: Textbook of Histology, 11th ed, pp 136–173 Philadelphia, WB Saunders, 1986 (Basic histology textbook with presentation and discussion of types of collagen associated with the various types of tissue.)

Frekany GA, Leslie DK: Effects of an exercise program on selected flexibility movements of senior citizens. Gerontologist 15:182, 1975

Fukami Y, Wilkinson RS: Responses on isolated golgi tendon response of the cat. J Physiol 265:673, 1977 (Presentation of the response of in vitro preparation of GTO to deformation and tension. Discussion of effect of temperature and tissue stiffness on GTO discharge.)

Gay S, Gay RE, Miller EJ: The collagens of the joint. Arthritis Rheum 23:937, 1980

Goldman YE, Simmons RM: Control of sarcomere length in skinned muscle fibers of rana temporaria during mechanical transients. J Physiol 350:497, 1984

Gossman MR, Sahrmann SA, Rose SJ: Review of length associated changes in muscle: Experimental evidence and clinical implications. Phys Ther 62:1799, 1982 (An excellent review of the anatomic changes that occur within muscle from immobilization and the clinical impact of these changes, which the physical therapist must consider during patient care.)

Halkovich LR, Personius WJ, Clamann HP et al: Effect of fluoromethane spray on passive hip flexion. Phys Ther 61:185, 1981

Hana H, Yamauro T, Takeda T: Experimental studies on connective tissue of capsular ligament. Acta Orthop Scand 47:473, 1976

Harris ML: Flexibility. Phys Ther 49:591, 1969

Henrickson AS, Fredricksson K, Persson I: The effect of heat and stretching on the range of hip motion. J Orthop Sports Phys Ther 6:110, 1984

Hill DK: Tension due to interaction between the sliding filaments in resting striated muscle: The effect of stimulation. J Physiol 199:637, 1968

Hubley CL, Kozey JW, Stanish WD: The effect of static stretching exercises and stationary cycling on range of motion at the hip joint. J Orthop Sports Phys Ther 6:104, 1984

Hunter SC, Etchison WC, Halpern BC: Standards and norms of fitness and flexibility in the high school athlete. Athletic Training 16:210, 1985

Ippolito E, Natoli PG, Postacchini F: Morphological, immunochemical and biochemical study of rabbit achilles tendon at various ages. J Bone Joint Surg 62A:583, 1980

Ishikawa H, Sawada H, Yamada E: Surface and internal morphology of skeletal muscle. In Peachey LD, Adrian RH, Geiger SR (eds): Skeletal Muscle, pp 1–22. Baltimore, American Physiological Society, 1983 (Presentation and discussion of microscopic anatomy of muscle epimysium, perimysium, and endomysium.)

Johns RJ, Wright V: Relative importance of various tissues in joint stiffness. J Appl Physiol 17:824, 1962 (A classic reference regarding the contribution of various joint tissues to joint stiffness and the limitation of range of motion. In vivo preparation using an animal model.)

Kakulas BA, Adams RD: Diseases of Muscle: Pathological Foundations of Clinical Myology, 4th ed, pp 3–60. Philadelphia, Harper & Row, 1985 (Textbook presentation of basic muscle histology and anatomy pertinent to this chapter. Excellent reference for muscle pathology.)

Kaltenborn FM: Mobilization of the Extremity Joints, 3rd ed, pp 23–25. Oslo, Olaf Norlis Bokhandel, 1980 (Classic textbook of Norwegian joint mobilization techniques. Defines grades of traction used during the application of manual techniques.)

Kastelic J, Galeski A, Baer E: The microcomposite structure of tendon. Connect Tissue Res 6:11, 1978 (Discussion of tendon structure from microscopic to macroscopic level. First presentation of composite structure of connective tissue structure from microfibril level to whole tissue level.)

Kastelic J, Palley I, Baer E: A structural model for tendon crimping. J Biomech 13:887, 1980

Kelley M: Effectiveness of cryotherapy technique on spasticity. Phys Ther 49:347, 1969

Kelsen SG, Wolanski T: Effect of elastase induced emphysema on diaphragm structure. Am Rev Respir Dis p. 208, 1982 (Demonstrates the changes that occur in muscle from lack of mobility.)

Kendall HO, Kendall FP: Normal flexibility according to age groups. J Bone Joint Surg 30A:690, 1948

Kleinman HK, Klebe RJ, Martin GR: Role of collagenous matrices in the adhesion and growth of cells. J Cell Biology 88:475, 1981

Knight KL: Cryotherapy: Theory, Technique and Physiology, pp 63–66. Chattanooga, TN, Chattanooga Corp, 1986

Kottke FJ, Pavley DJ, Ptak DA: The rationale for prolonged stretching for correction of shortening of connective tissue. Arch Phys Med Rehabil 47:345, 1966

Koury S, Mamary M, Kagan R et al: Effect of fluoromethane spray on hamstring extensibility during "contract-relax" and active stretching. Phys Ther 66:806, 1986

Kvist M, Jarvinen M: Clinical, histochemical and biomechanical features in repair of muscle and tendon injuries. Int J Sports Med 3:12, 1982

Lane J: Collagen and elastin. In Owen R, Goodfellow J, Bullough P (eds): Scientific Foundations of Orthopaedics and Traumatology, pp 30–35. Philadelphia, WB Saunders, 1980

Lehmann JF, Masock AJ, Warren CG et al: Effect of therapeutic temperatures on tendon extensibility. Arch Phys Med Rehabil 51:481, 1970

Leighton JR: Flexibility characteristics of males ten to eighteen years of age. Arch Phys Med Rehabil 37:494, 1956

Leighton JR: A study of the effect of progressive weight training on flexibility. J Assoc Phys Mental Rehabil 18:101, 1964

Leighton JR, Holmes D, Benson J et al: A study on the effectiveness of ten different methods of progressive resistive exercise on the development of strength, flexibility, girth and body weight. J Assoc Phys Mental Rehabil 21:78, 1967

Light N, Campion AE: Characterization of muscle epimysium, perimysium and endomysium collagens. Biochem J 249:1017, 1984 (Discusses type and function of collagens associated specifically with muscle.)

Louden KL, Bollier CE, Allison KA et al: Effects of two stretching methods on the flexibility and retention of flexibility at the ankle joint in runners. Phys Ther 65:698, 1985

Maitland GD: Vertebral Manipulation, 5th ed, pp 93–102. Boston, Butterworths, 1986 (This noted Australian author presents a grading and classification system for the use of oscillations during the application of manual techniques, along with their rationale.)

Markos PD: Ipsilateral and contralateral effects of proprioceptive neuromuscular facilitation techniques on hip motion and electromyographic activity. Phys Ther 59:1366, 1979

Mason T, Rigby BJ: Thermal transitions in collagen. Biochem Biophys Acta 66:448, 1963 (Presents basic science research regarding the effect of temperature on collagen extensibility)

Miglietta O: Electromyographic characteristics of clonus and influence of cold. Arch Phys Med Rehabil 45:508, 1976

Miller EJ: The collagens of the joint. In Sokolow L (ed): The Joints and Synovial Fluid, pp 205–242, 1978 (A comprehensive basic science discussion of the synthesis and lysis of extracellular fibers [collagen and elastin], types of collagen and their distribution, and the physiology and role of the proteoglycans.)

Mohan S, Radha E: Age related changes in muscle connective tissue: Acid mucopolysaccharides and structural glycoproteins. Exp Gerontol 16:385, 1981

Moore M, Hutton R: Electromyographic investigation of muscle stretching techniques. Med Sci Sports 12:322, 1980

Newton R: Effects of vapocoolants on passive hip flexion in healthy subjects. Phys Ther 65:1034, 1985

Nimni MC: The molecular organization of collagen and its role in determining the biophysical properties of connective tissue. Biorheology 17:51, 1980

Noyes FR, Trovik PJ, Hyde WB: Biomechanics of ligament failure: An analysis of immobilization, exercise and deconditioning effects in primates. J Bone Joint Surg 56A:1406, 1974

Olson JE, Stravino VD: A review of cryotherapy. Phys Ther 52:840, 1972

Peacock EE: Comparison of collagenous tissue surrounding normal and immobilized joints. Surg Forum 14:440, 1963

Peacock EE: Collagenolysis: The other side of the equation. World J Surg 4:297, 1980

Podalsky RJ, Schoenberg M: Force generation and shortening in skeletal muscle. In Peachey LD, Adrian RH, Geiger SR (eds): pp 173–174. Skeletal Muscle, Baltimore, American Physiological Society, 1983 (Presentation and discussion of muscle force generation and shortening characteristics. Discusses relationship between passive tension and muscle stiffness.)

Prentice WE: An electromyographic analysis of the effectiveness of heat or cold and stretching for inducing relaxation in an injured muscle. J Orthop Sports Phy Ther 3:133, 1982

Prentice WE: A comparison of static stretching and PNF stretching for improving hip joint flexibility. Athletic Training 18:56, 1983

Ramsey SW, Street S: The isometric length tension diagram of isolated skeletal muscle fibers of the frog. J Cellular Comp Physiol 15:11, 1940

The following references by Rigby and coauthors present basic science research regarding the effect of temperature on collagen extensibility.

Rigby BJ: The effect of mechanical extension upon the thermal stability of collagen. Biochem Biophys Acta 79:634, 1964

Rigby BJ, Hirai N, Spikes JD et al: The mechanical properties of rat tail tendon. J Gen Physiol 43:265, 1959

Rosenberg LC: Proteoglycans. In Owen R, Goodfellow J, Bullough F (eds): Scientific Foundations of Orthopaedics and Traumatology, pp 36–42. Philadelphia, WB Saunders, 1980

Sady SP, Wortman M, Blanke D: Flexibility training: Ballistic, static or proprioceptive neuromuscular facilitation? Arch Phys Med Rehabil 63:261, 1982

Saltin B, Hermansen L: Esophageal, rectal and muscle temperature during exercise. J Appl Physiol 21:1757, 1966 (Demonstrates how intramuscular temperature is increased by exercise.)

Sapega AA, Quedenfeld TC, Moyer RA et al: Biophysical isotope in range of motion exercises. Phys Sports Med 9:57, 1981 (The authors present a good, brief theoretical discussion of how the physiology of connective tissue relates to the gain or loss of range of motion. A suggestion for clinical intervention is given without data to prove its effectiveness.)

Schoenberg M, Brenner B, Chalovich JM et al: Cross bridge attachment in relaxed muscle. Adv Exp Med Biol 170:269, 1984

Sichel FJM: The relative elasticity of the sarcolemma and the entire skeletal muscle fiber. Am J Physiol 133:446-447, 1941.

Smith JR, Walker JM: Knee and elbow range of motion in healthy older individuals. Phys Occ Ther Geriat 2:31, 1983

Stolov WC, Fry LR, Riddell WM et al: Adhesive forces between muscle fibers and connective tissue in normal and denervated rat skeletal muscle. Arch Phys Med Rehabil 54:208, 1973

Stolov WC, Weilepp TG: Passive length tension relationships of intact muscle, epimysium and tendon in normal and denervated gastrocnemius of the rat. Arch Phys Med Rehabil 47:612, 1966

Stromberg DD, Weiderheilm CA: Viscoelastic description of a collagenous tissue in simple elongation. J Appl Physiol 26:857, 1969 (Description of viscoelastic tissue properties and anatomic make up of fascia.)

Sunderland S, Ray LJ: Denervation changes in mammalian striated muscle. J Neurol Neurosurg Psychiatry 13:159, 1956 (Demonstrates the changes that occur in muscle from lack of mobility.)

Tanigawa MC: Comparison of the hold-relax procedure and passive mobilization of increasing muscle length. Phys Ther 52:725, 1972

Tipton CM, Matthes RD, Maynard JA et al: The influence of physical activity on ligaments and tendons. Med Sci Sports Exerc 7:165, 1975

Tucker JE: Measurement of joint range of motion of older individuals. Unpublished Master's Thesis. Stanford, CA, Stanford University, 1964

Vialas AC, Tipton CM, Matthes RC et al: Physical activity and its influence on the repair process of medial collateral ligaments. Connect Tissue Res 9:25, 1981

Viidik A: Functional properties of collagenous tissue. Rev Connect Tissue Res 6:127, 1973 (A classic reference regarding the physiology and synthesis of collagenous tissues and their mechanical properties.)

Viidik A: Connective tissues: Possible implications of the temporal changes for the aging process. Mech Ageing Devel 9:267, 1979 (Presents changes that take place in the physiology of the connective tissue because of the aging process.)

Voss DE, Ionta MK, Myers GJ: Proprioceptive Neuromuscular Facilitation Patterns and Techniques, 3rd ed, pp xi–xviii. Philadelphia, Harper & Row, 1985 (This classic physical therapy textbook describes in detail the rationale and method of application for PNF stretching techniques.)

Walker JM, Sue D, Miles-Elkousy N, et al: Active mobility of the extremities in older subjects. Phys Ther 64:919-923, 1984.

Wallin D, Ekblom B, Grahn R, et al: Improvement of muscle flexibility, a comparison between two techniques. Am J Sports Med 13:263-268, 1985.

Warren CG, Lehmann JF, Koblanski JN: Elongation of rat tail tendon: Effect of load and temperature. Arch Phys Med Rehabil 52:465, 1971

Warren CG, Lehmann JF, Koblanski HN: Heat and stretch procedures: An evaluation using rat tail tendon. Arch Phys Med Rehabil 57:122, 1976

Wilktorsson-Moller M, Oberg B, Ekstrand J et al: Effects of warming up, massage, and stretching on range of motion and muscle strength in the lower extremity. Am J Sports Med 11:249, 1983

Wilmore JH, Parr RB, Girandola RN et al: Physiological alterations consequent to circuit weight training. Med Sci Sports Exerc 10:79, 1978

Wolf SL, Leibetter MD, Basajian JV: Effect of a specific cutaneous cold stimulus on single motor unit activity of gastrocnemius muscle in man. Am J Phys Med 55:177, 1976

Woo SLY, Ritter MA, Amiel D et al: The biomechanical and biochemical properties of swine tendons: Long-term effects of exercise on the digital extensors. Connect Tissue Res 7:177, 1980

Woo SLY, Matthew JV, Akesson WH: Connective tissue response to immobility: Correlative study of the biomechanical and biochemical measurements of normal and immobilized rabbit knees. Arthritis Rheum 18:257, 1975

Wright V (ed): Measurement of joint movement. Clin Rheum Dis 8:3, 1982

Zachazewski JE, Reischl SR: Flexibility for the runner: Specific program consideration. Topics Acute Care Trauma Rehab 1:9, 1986

Zebas CJ, Rivera ML: Retention of flexibility in selected joints after cessation of a stretching exercise program. Dotson CO, Humphrey JH (eds): In Exercise Physiology: Current Selected Research. New York, AMS Press, 1985

40 Improving Strength, Endurance, and Power

ROBERT MANGINE
TIMOTHY P. HECKMANN
VINCENT L. ELDRIDGE

The focus of this chapter is on muscle function and the development of strength, endurance, and power. Physical therapy is the cornerstone of treating muscle dysfunction, and reeducating this tissue is necessary before normal activity can be resumed. The factors underlying the treatment of muscle are the biomechanical aspects of muscle function, the neuromuscular interaction, the physiological aspects of muscle function, the effect of exercise on muscle, the effect of trauma and disuse on muscle, and the components of muscle rehabilitation. Once the physical therapist understands muscle and its function, most injuries or pathologies can be treated.

The musculoskeletal system is a two-part system composed of the muscles that form the movement system and the skeletal structures that form the lever system. These systems perform a wide range of functions, from static activity to high-velocity activity. Approximately 400 voluntary or skeletal muscles may account for up to 40% of the total body weight. When a muscle contracts to move the body lever, it accomplishes this activity by the strength that the muscle possesses. Muscle composition and the neuromuscular mechanism involved in muscle contraction will be reviewed before discussing muscle training programs.

MUSCLE COMPOSITION

The components of the gross structure of skeletal muscle are connective tissue, tendon, blood supply, nerve supply, and red and white muscle fibers. Several types of connective tissue help to bind skeletal muscle together. Each skeletal muscle is composed of thousands of muscle fibers. The sheath of tissue that surrounds each muscle fiber is called the endomysium. Muscle fibers are grouped together in bundles called fascicles. The fascicles, which contain various numbers of muscle fibers, are covered by a tissue called the perimysium. Encasing the entire muscle is another cover of connective tissue called the epimysium (Fig. 40-1).

A tendon has its own connective tissue, which is bound together at the end of skeletal muscle. The end of the tendon is then bound at its insertion to the outer covering of bone, called the periosteum. Tendon is composed of collagen fibers arranged in parallel, and is much stronger than the connective tissue of muscle. Thus, a tendon is able to withstand large forces that may be placed upon it by muscle. Often, those forces may exceed 1000 newtons of tension, which occurs at the patellar tendon during knee extension.

Skeletal muscle has a very large vascular network composed of both arteries and veins that run parallel to the muscle and form a complete system in and about the endomysium. This vast network allows for adequate clearing of the blood back to the heart to be reoxygenated before returning to the muscle. During high levels of activity, blood is shunted from the internal organs to the extremities for energy transportation and temperature regulation.

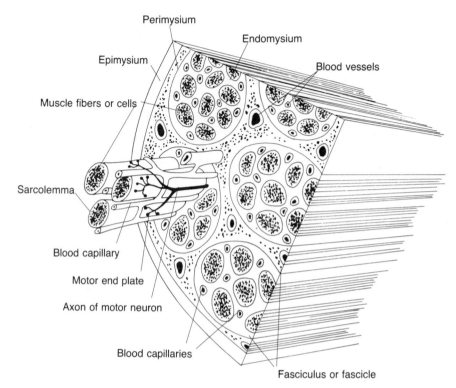

FIGURE 40-1. Relationship of connective tissue in skeletal muscle.

MICROSCOPIC MUSCLE STRUCTURE

A single muscle fiber observed under a light microscope has alternating light and dark striations. Inside the sarcolemma is the sarcoplasm, whose subcellular components are the nuclei, mitochondria, myoglobin, fat, glycogen, phosphocreatin, adenosine triphosphate (ATP), and hundreds of strands called myofibrils. The myofibrils are characterized by alternating light (I bands) and dark (A bands) areas (Fig. 40-2A). In the middle of each I band is a dark line called the Z line. Actin is located within the I bands and myosin within the A bands. The sarcomere length extends from one Z line to another and is anchored to the Z lines by actin. The Z lines adhere to the sarcolemma to provide stability to the entire structure in order to keep the actin filaments in alignment. The actin component also contains tropomyosin and troponin. The myosin filaments have tiny protein projections at the end, which extend

toward the actin filaments (see Fig. 40-2B). These projections are termed cross-bridges, and they serve to connect the units (see Fig. 40-2C).

SLIDING FILAMENT THEORY

The structural arrangement of the myofibril has led to the sliding filament theory. The sliding of one set of filaments (actin) over the other (myosin) shortens the muscle, which results in muscle contraction. This theory of muscle contraction can be broken down into five phases. The first is the rest phase, which is characterized by uncharged ATP cross-bridges and uncoupled actin and myosin (Fig. 40-3A). During this time, calcium is stored in the sarcoplasmic reticulum. The second is the excitation-coupling phase (see Fig. 40-3B). During this phase the nerve impulse causes calcium to be released. Calcium saturates troponin and "turns on" the actin. The ATP cross-bridges are then

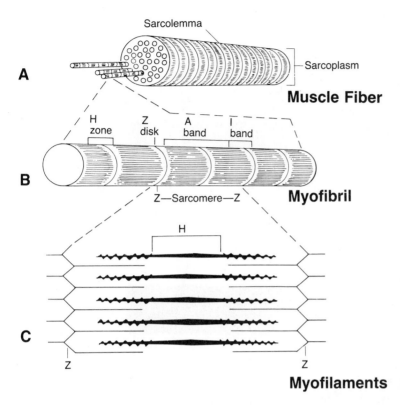

Figure 40-2. (*A*) A skeletal muscle fiber, showing the sarcoplasm surrounding the myofibrils. (*B*) A myofibril, the contractile unit of skeletal muscle, is composed of two protein filaments, actin and myosin. The I band contains only actin filaments. (*C*) The myosin filament projects toward the actin filament by means of cross-bridges. The H zone results from the absence of actin filaments.

charged, and the actin and myosin are coupled (actomyosin). The third is the contraction phase (see Fig. 40-3C). During this phase, the following occur: ATP is broken down into adenosine diphosphate (ADP) + inorganic phosphate (Pi) + energy, the energy surrounds the cross-bridges, the muscle shortens, and the actin slides over the myosin. The fourth phase is the recharging phase, which allows time for ATP resynthesis. The actin and myosin break down and are recycled (see Fig. 40-3D). The last is the relaxation phase. During this phase calcium is removed by the calcium pump, and the muscle returns to its resting state (see Fig. 40-3E).

NEUROMUSCULAR MECHANISMS

Skeletal muscle is innervated by two types of nerve fibers: efferent (motor) and afferent (sensory) fibers. Efferent nerves comprise approxi-

mately 60% of the nerves entering the muscle, whereas afferent fibers comprise the remaining approximately 40%. The efferent fibers are responsible for motor function in the form of muscle contraction. The afferent (sensory) fibers are responsible for the transmission of sensation, such as pain and position sense. A motor nerve fiber, also called an axon, is terminated at the neuromuscular junction, which is also called the motor end plate (Fig. 40-4). As a basis for understanding neuromuscular function, a description of the motor unit and the "all or none" principle follows.

THE MOTOR UNIT

The number of motor nerves entering a muscle varies widely. In addition, the number of muscle fibers greatly outnumbers the number of motor nerves. Because each fiber is innervated, the motor nerve must branch out to control each muscle fiber. Thus, a single motor nerve may innervate from 1 to 5 to 150 or more mus-

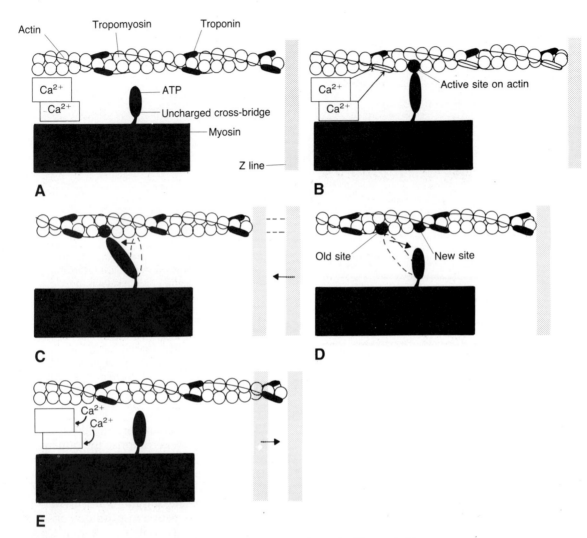

FIGURE 40-3. The sliding filament theory. (*A*) At rest, uncharged ATP cross-bridges are extended, actin and myosin are uncoupled, and calcium is stored in the reticulum. (*B*) During excitation-coupling, stimulation releases calcium, which then binds to troponin, "turning on" actin active sites; thus, actomyosin is formed. (*C*) During contraction, ATP is broken down, releasing energy that swivels the cross-bridges. Actin slides over the myosin, tension is developed, and the muscle shortens. (*D*) During recharging, ATP is resynthesized, and actin and myosin uncouple and are recycled. (*E*) When stimulation ceases, calcium is restored in the reticulum by the calcium pump, and the muscle relaxes. (Modified from Murray J, Weber A: The cooperative action of muscle proteins. Sci Am 230(2):58, 1974)

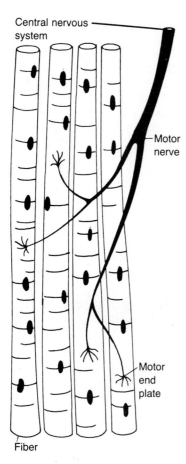

Central nervous system

Motor nerve

Motor end plate

Fiber

FIGURE 40-4. Motor unit of skeletal muscle. A single motor nerve in the central nervous system innervates several muscle fibers through the motor end plates. (Matthews DK, Fox EC: The Physiological Basis of Physical Education and Athletics, 2nd ed. Philadelphia, WB Saunders, 1976)

cle fibers. The motor unit is defined as an individual nerve fiber plus all the muscle fibers it innervates. The nerve fiber and muscle fibers function as a unit. The number of fibers innervated by a single nerve fiber within a muscle depends on the precision, accuracy, and coordination that is required of that particular muscle. For example, muscles about the eye may have one muscle fiber innervated by one nerve fiber, whereas a large muscle group such as the quadriceps may have 150 or more muscle fibers innervated by one nerve fiber.

"ALL OR NONE" PRINCIPLE

The all or none principle states that a nerve fiber will propagate the impulse completely or not at all regardless of the intensity of the stimulus. This principle holds true only for each muscle fiber or motor unit, not for the muscle as a whole. The muscle as a whole can function with gradual contraction, depending on how many motor units are fired.

STRENGTH

Muscular contraction generates an internal force that results in shortening (concentric), lengthening (eccentric), or no change in the muscle length (isometric). The tension that develops results in a force that is termed the muscle's strength. Muscle strength can vary greatly, depending on many factors in both the muscular and neural components.

Muscular strength traditionally has been tested by manual muscle testing (MMT) methods. These proved accurate and beneficial in the hands of many clinicians. The value of MMT in a wide range of pathological conditions and injuries is that it can supply baseline information before the initiation of care.

A second method of testing muscular strength is by isokinetic servomotor systems. The literature supports this method as valid and reliable in providing objective measurement of muscle performance. When using isokinetics to test strength, the velocity most commonly accepted is 60°/sec. This speed is used for slow-speed training methods. Other speeds often used in testing include 120°/sec, 180°/sec, and 300°/sec. Peak torque measurements for determining strength at these speeds correlate with other functional qualities, such as power and endurance.

PHYSIOLOGICAL EFFECTS OF STRENGTH TRAINING

Strength training will produce biomechanical changes (those occurring at the tissue level); systemic changes (those affecting the respiratory, circulatory, and oxygen transport systems); and other changes in body composition, blood chemistry, blood pressure, and adaptation to temperature changes. Three major biomechanical changes occur with strength training. They are aerobic changes, anaerobic changes, and relative changes in red and white fibers.

Aerobic Changes

The first aerobic change in skeletal muscle that occurs with training is an increase in myoglobin content. This response is specific to the particular muscle(s) involved in training. The main function of myoglobin is to aid the delivery of oxygen from the cell membrane to the mitochondria. Secondly, an increased oxidation of carbohydrates (glycogen) occurs, which increases the capacity to generate energy. This change is evidenced by an increase in the maximal oxygen consumption ($\dot{V}O_{2 \max}$). At a subcellular level, mitochondria increase in number and in size. An increase is also noted in the concentration of enzymes involved in the Kreb's cycle. As a result of training, the skeletal muscle is able to store more glycogen. Finally, an increased oxidation of fat occurs. Because fat serves as fuel during endurance activities involving prolonged submaximal work, increased oxidation results in less lactic acid buildup, and thus less fatigue.

Anaerobic Changes

The anaerobic changes that occur in skeletal muscle as a result of training include an increased capacity of the adenosine triphosphate-phosphocreatine (ATP-PC) system and an increased glycolytic capacity. Training increases the muscle storage of ATP and PC. In addition, key enzymes that are necessary to break down PC increase. These changes allow a rapid release of energy by the muscle cells for short durations of activity. The increased activity of the glycolytic enzymes helps to speed up the rate and quantity of glycogen broken down into lactic acid, thus improving performance in activities that require this energy system.

Fiber Changes

The relative changes that occur in red (slow-twitch) and white (fast-twitch) fibers include

three primary responses. First, the aerobic potential of skeletal muscle following training is increased equally in both red and white fibers. Second, the changes in glycolytic capacity are greater in white fibers because of the increased number of mitochondria in those fibers. Finally, a selective hypertrophy of both red and white fibers occurs, which is dependent on the kind of training or the sports activities performed.

Physiological changes are possible regardless of the type of training program, but sound physiological principles must be used to assure training success. The specific adaptation that is achieved in exercise programs is based on the imposed demand. This is known as the principle of specific adaptation to imposed demands (SAID principle).

STRENGTH TRAINING METHODS

Strengthening methods are used in therapeutic exercise. One must remember in rehabilitation that the physical therapist is reeducating injured or disused muscle tissue. Therefore, the literature available on normal muscle exercise may not necessarily apply.

The three most commonly used types of strengthening exercises are isometric, isotonic, and isokinetic. Even after the therapist selects the mode of exercise to be used, the intensity, frequency, overload principle, and duration must still be considered. Part of rehabilitation is to integrate multiple exercises to achieve the optimum result.

Isometric Strengthening

The word isometric can be broken down into its two components: iso (same or constant) and metric (length). This means that as the muscle is contracting, no resultant visible joint motion will occur. The movement that is seen is the increase in size of the muscle belly. The speed or velocity of angular displacement of the contraction is constant, and the external force applied to the muscle is greater than the internal force that the muscle can generate.

Many studies have addressed the parameters of isometric strengthening programs (ie, length of contraction, number of repetitions, and amount of tension generated). Early work by Hettinger and Muller (1953) helped to define some of the parameters. Ultimately, exercise programs must be based on the needs of the individual patient and must not be generalized programs. The minimum accepted length for holding an isometric exercise is between 6 and 10 seconds. Muscle contractions should exceed 70% of a maximum volitional contraction in order to build strength. Ten repetitions are required to increase static strength. The ideal number of repetitions in one set is between five and seven. However, for simplicity's sake, the patient may be instructed in the "rule of 10s": The contraction is held for 10 seconds, the contraction is repeated 10 times in one sitting, and 10 sets are performed each day. Table 40-1 provides an example of a basic isometric program for athletes.

An isometric strengthening program has several advantages. First, because no joint motion occurs during the contraction, isometrics can be used early in a rehabilitation program. This type of contraction may help to decrease the risk of irritating the joint, thereby minimizing any change in pain and swelling. Isometric exercise will help to improve static muscle strength, but it has little effect in maintaining the aerobic potential of the muscle. Isometrics also may help to delay the atrophy process after injury or surgery. Swelling may be decreased by the use of isometric contractions because the contractions act as a muscular pump to assist in fluid removal. Disuse is prevented and neural association is maintained through isometric muscular contractions, which stimulate the mechanoreceptor system in the joint capsule and surrounding ligaments. Isometric exercise does not require any additional equipment, may be performed anywhere easily, and need not consume a great amount of time. These last three points help to make isometric exercise programs instrumental in postinjury and postoperative exercise prescriptions (Fig. 40-5).

Table 40-1. Example of Basic Isometric Program for Athletes

CORE EXERCISES	JOINT AND EXERCISE ANGLE
Bench press	Elbow, 90°
Dead lift	Knee, 135°
Heel (toe) raises	Foot, 135°
Standing press	Elbow, 90°
Bent-knee sit-ups	Knee, 90°
Arm curls	Elbow, 90°
Upright rowing	Elbow, 135°

Program Considerations

Type: regular isometrics or functional isometrics

Frequency: 3–5 days per week

Duration: 4 weeks or more

Intensity: maximum

Duration of repetitions: 5–7 seconds

(Fox EL: Sports Physiology, 2nd ed, p 141, Table 7-3. Philadelphia, Saunders College Publishing, 1984. Modified from Hooks G: Weight Training in Athletics and Physical Education. Englewood Cliffs, NJ, Prentice-Hall, 1974.)

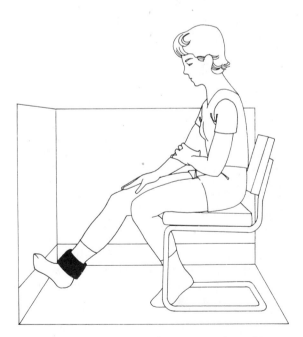

FIGURE 40-5. Patient performing a 45° quadriceps muscle contraction. This is done following the "rule of 10s": hold 10 seconds, perform 10 repetitions, do 10 sets a day.

However, isometric exercise programs have several disadvantages. Improvement in strength is fairly specific to the angle at which the exercise occurs. Some carryover appears to occur for approximately 10 to 15 degrees in each direction of the exercise angle. Thus, isometric exercises are limited in their ability to generate strength over a large range of motion. Therefore, when isometrics are employed in a rehabilitation program, multiple angle positions are important. A person's willingness to participate may determine the success of a program, and maintaining interest in isometric exercise for any length of time may be difficult. In addition, isometric exercises do not provide any eccentric or lengthening contractions. The last disadvantage to isometric exercise programs relates to a change in blood pressure that occurs with this type of regime. The Valsalva maneuver, which may occur with isometric exercises, increases intrathoracic pressure drastically. This increase in pressure causes both systolic and diastolic blood pressures to exceed normal values. Therefore, isometric exercise must be used with caution when a person has a history of hypertension or cardiac problems.

Isotonic Strengthening

The second means of strengthening muscle is through isotonic exercises. Initially, isotonic exercises may be performed with gravity-assisting weights. They proceed to gravity-resisting weights, and finally to the use of external weights. These patterns of exercise are commonly referred to as progressive resistive exercises (PRE). Isotonic contractions are categorized as (1) concentric contractions, which result in muscle shortening; and (2) eccentric exercises, which result in muscle lengthening (primarily contractions that are fighting gravity). Isotonic exercises imply that a fixed amount of resistance must be overcome by the muscle contraction in order for movement to occur (Fig. 40-6).

Isotonic training uses two methods of loading. The most common method is free weights using constant resistance, which involves a fixed amount of weight to be moved through a range of motion (ie, barbells, dumbbells, or vel-

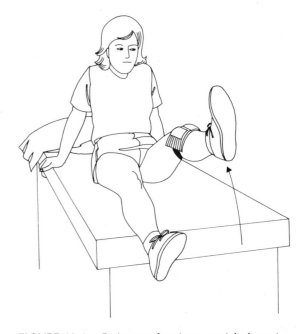

FIGURE 40-6. Patient performing a straight leg raise using a five-pound weight placed just below the knee to lower the forces on the knee. This activity requires an isotonic contraction of the rectus femoris muscle and an isometric contraction of the vastus muscles. When performing this exercise the therapist must consider load, placement of load, muscle function, and extreme modes.

cro cuff weights). A single-axis cable pulley system with constant resistance may also be used with this method. The second method is variable resistance isotonic training. Variable-resistance systems operate with a cam-shaped pulley system so that as the weight is lifted, the cable guide is lifted away from the rotating axis of the machine (eg, Eagle, Nautilus, Universal Gym, Hydra Fitness). By changing the cam position, the resistance varies through the range of motion.

Concentric exercise strengthening programs are the most common in rehabilitation. However, eccentric programs may be beneficial as part of postinjury and postsurgical strengthening programs. For example, after a knee injury, when a patient is unable to perform a straight leg raise, the leg may be lifted by the therapist or by a pulley system and the patient

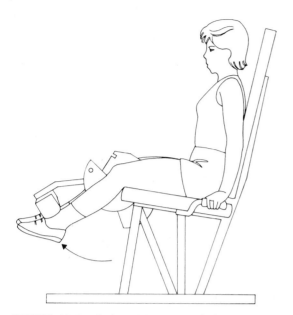

FIGURE 40-7. Patient using an Eagle leg extension machine that has the motion limited to prevent the last 30 degrees of extension, to protect the patellofemoral joint. The load is varied by altering the cam position. Both concentric and eccentric training can be accomplished using this device.

may take control of lowering it. In this case, the quadriceps muscles are contracting isometrically, and the iliopsoas muscle and the rectus femoris muscle are contracting eccentrically. However, this type of activity is not generally used for strengthening during a conditioning program. Even though the tension generated in the muscle is very high, side-effects (such as muscle soreness) make this program controversial. Probably the most functional strengthening program combines both concentric and eccentric contractions (Fig. 40-7).

Several types of isotonic training programs have been developed. One of the first and still most commonly used is the Delorme and Watkins (1948) method. They established the concept of repetition maximum (RM). The repetition maximum is the maximal amount of weight that can be lifted for 10 repetitions in one set before fatiguing. For each muscle group to be trained, three sets of 10 repetitions are used as follows: first set, 10 repetitions at one-half 10 RM; second set, 10 repetitions at three-quarters 10 RM; and third set, 10 repetitions at 10 RM. The ideal number of repetitions for strength gain is three sets of six, and the recommended training frequency is four times per week.

Similar to the Delorme technique is the Oxford program, which also uses the concept of repetition maximum; however, performance is in the reverse order. In the Oxford system, the first set is 10 repetitions at 10 RM; the second set is 10 repetitions at three-quarters 10 RM; and the third set is 10 repetitions at one-half 10 RM. Much disagreement exists about which of the isotonic programs is the most successful. The conclusion is that no one program will produce optimum strength in everyone. Agreement centers around the need for the use of the overload principle.

The overload principle is the physiological principle used in attempting to increase strength. The principle states that for strength to increase and for muscle hypertrophy to occur, the demands placed on the muscle must be greater than those normally incurred during activities of daily living. In addition, this change in resistance should be progressive and gradual. Table 40-2 outlines a basic isotonic weight training program for athletes.

In traditional strength training programs, it is accepted that the first 30% of muscle strength is the result of neuromuscular adaptation. However, for ongoing hypertrophy, the change is intermuscular. Thus, for maximal strengthening to occur, the resistance must be high with the number of repetitions low.

Utilizing isotonic exercise to gain strength has several advantages. This type of exercise is readily available to most persons, and the equipment is relatively inexpensive. Motivation consists of gradually increasing the amounts of weight (feedback or improvement). The overload principle may be used through a range of motion. Both concentric and eccentric contractions may be employed. Isotonic exercise programs may improve both strength and endurance. These programs allow the therapist to document the exercise progress objectively and allow for individualizing the program by

Table 40-2. Examples of Isotonic Weight-Training Programs for Athletes

MONDAY	WEDNESDAY	FRIDAY
Program One		
Squats	Same as Monday	Military press
Bench press		Bench press
Stiff-legged dead lift		Knee extension
Heel (toe) raises		Knee curls
Standing press		Scapular rowing
Bent-knee sit-ups		Tricep extension
Arm curls		Squats
Wrist curl or roller		Calf raises
Reverse wrist curl		Neck (flexion-side flexion)
		Chest press (adduction)
Program Two		
Bench press	Incline press	Military press
Power clean	Parallel bar dip	Bench press
Arm curl	Upright row	Knee extension
Pulldown—latissimus	Arm curl	Knee curls
machine	Shoulder shrug	Scapular rowing
Squat	Squat	Tricep extension
Pullover	Back hyperextension	Squats
Bent-knee sit-up	Wrist curl or roller	Calf raises
Heel (toe) raises	Reverse wrist curl	Neck (flexion-side flexion)
Wrist curl or roller		Chest press (adduction)
Reverse wrist curl		

Program Considerations

Frequency: 3 days a week
Duration: 6 weeks or more
Repetitions and load-first 2 weeks, 2 × 10 RM (sit-ups, 2 × 25): remaining weeks, 3 × 6 RM (sit-ups, 1 × 25 + 1 × maximum)
Rest between sets of exercise: 5–10 minutes

(Fox EL: Sports Physiology, 2nd ed, p 134, Table 7-1. Philadelphia, Saunders College Publishing, 1984. Modified from Hooks G: Weight Training in Athletics and Physical Education. Englewood Cliffs, NJ, Prentice-Hall, 1974; and O'Shea JP: Scientific Principles and Methods of Strength Fitness, 2nd ed. Reading, MA, Addison-Wesley, 1976.)

altering the sets, the repetitions, or the weights. Isotonic exercise also enhances the neurophysiological system.

However, many disadvantages are inherent in this type of exercise program. Isotonic exercises load the muscle at the weakest point of its range (that is, the amount of weight lifted is the amount that can be moved through the weakest point of the range). If the patient has pain during the exercise, safety is a concern because the weight must still be supported. Trauma can occur to the musculoskeletal system or to the joint itself if proper form and technique are not used. Momentum in the initial phase of the exercise may perform some of the work, thereby decreasing the overall work load. Isotonics do very little to develop quickness at functional speeds during activity. The problem that exists in all isotonic exercise performances is the speed of movement. The velocity of movement is accepted at 60°/sec when performed accurately; however, when initiating higher-speed exercise with a weight, a higher level of contraction is required. Thus, isotonic excercise cannot replicate exercise using accommodating resistance. These exercises are usually performed in planes of motion as opposed to patterns of motion, whereas motor activity employs both patterns and planes of movements. Another disadvantage to an isotonic exercise program is that it does little for aerobic development. Muscle soreness may also occur, especially with eccentric programs. Weight machines usually require large amounts of space and they are able to exercise only one muscle at a time. Isotonic exercise does not accommodate to either pain or fatigue during the range of motion. Evaluation of muscle performance in terms of work, power, and velocity using isotonic exercises is not possible at this time.

Isokinetic Strengthening

Isokinetic exercise provides another dimension to the concept of strength training. The term isokinetic means same speed, which indicates that the speed of the lever arm remains constant throughout the range of motion. The patient is unable to alter this speed. The resis-

tance offered by the machine is in direct proportion to the force offered by the patient throughout the range of motion of the exercise (Fig. 40-8).

Differences exist between isotonic and isokinetic exercises even though both employ exercise equipment. In isotonic exercise, the amount of resistance is fixed through the mechanical and physiological changes through the range. Therefore, maximal muscle tension and work are not achieved. Isokinetic exercise is also referred to as accommodating resistance exercise. The resistance changes, or accommodates, to the stronger and weaker points in the range of motion. Manual resistance exercise provided by the therapist uses the same principle; however, the equipment is able to be more objective.

In some respects, isokinetic strength train-

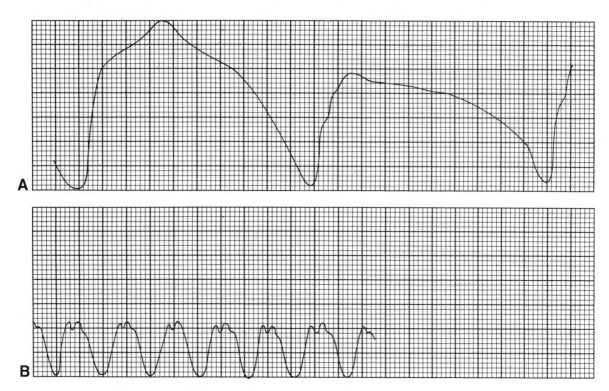

FIGURE 40-8. Resultant degrees in torque when performing a 300°/sec test (*A*) in comparison to a 60°/sec test. (*B*) With increasing speed, the ability to generate torque decreases.

ing programs are very similar to isotonic programs. It is suggested that the frequency of the program should be three times per week (every other day). Initially, the program should last approximately 6 to 12 weeks and then a maintenance program may be performed less frequently. Isokinetic exercise allows for training at variable speeds (ie, with the Cybex unit, 60°/sec, 120°/sec, 180°/sec, 240°/sec, and 300°/sec; with the Biodex unit, up to 450°/sec). According to Davies (1984), strength gains are specific to the speed of the exercise. Other studies suggest that some carryover occurs at other speeds. If one trains at the higher or faster velocity, some carryover (or increase) occurs at the lower or slower velocity. However, carryover does not occur from lower speeds to higher speeds, and does not occur in the smaller velocity range. Because functional activity occurs at different speeds, it is wise to train at various speeds (velocity spectrum training). This technique helps to train the muscle neurophysiologically. It has been demonstrated that the faster the speed of muscle contraction, the less the force that is generated (Fig. 40-9).

Isokinetic exercise has distinct advantages. It accommodates the resistance to changes in the mechanical and physiological properties of the muscle, as well as to the strong and weak points of the range of motion. Isokinetic exercise is also very safe. Patients will never have more resistance than they can handle, because the resistance offered is directly proportional to the force applied. Over the years, isokinetic exercise equipment has been shown to be both valid and reliable. Testing procedures and values have also been shown to be reliable (reproducible). Equipment currently available provides a permanent record of the patient's performance for record keeping. Isokinetic exercise permits training at multiple speeds to allow for training over a wide spectrum and, at high speed, to replicate functional performance. In addition, by working at faster speeds, isokinetic exercise develops power, decreases joint compressive forces, and enhances the neurophysiological system. A safety feature of only isokinetic exercise is that it allows for accommodation to both pain and fatigue (Fig. 40-10). Finally, isokinetic exercise permits objective measurement and allows supervision of submaximal and maximal programs and their progressions.

Isokinetic exercise also has its disadvantages. Isokinetic equipment is typically very costly, making it difficult for easy access by most patients. Isokinetic training programs are very popular in clinical treatment, but require constant patient follow up. From an evaluation standpoint, the interpretation of the data generated through testing requires highly trained personnel. When exercising more than one joint, the process is both time consuming and inconvenient. Lastly, some concern exists about the sensitivity of the equipment when testing and exercising large muscle groups (ie, hip and trunk).

STRENGTHENING PROGRAMS

Initiation of a muscle training program will be most effective if the following factors are taken into consideration: intensity, frequency, and duration of the training program; specificity of the training program; genetic factors; differences between the sexes; the mode of exercise used for training; and the maintenance of the training effects.

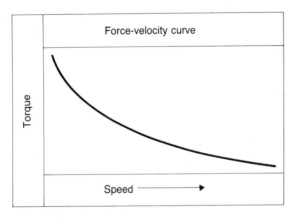

FIGURE 40-9. Force-velocity curve displays the relationship of speed and tension: the lower the force, the higher the speed of movement; the higher the force, the slower the speed of movement.

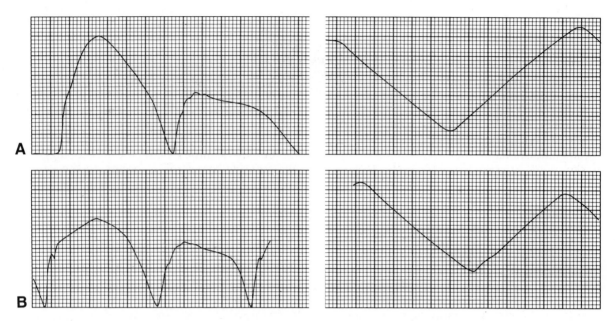

FIGURE 40-10. (*A*) Normal curve for a patient with an anterior cruciate ligament deficiency of the left knee. (*B*) Curve for pathological left knee with an anterior cruciate deficiency. Note significant loss of power (first 0.2 seconds of the graph) and overall strength.

Intensity, Frequency, and Duration

When establishing a strengthening program, one must keep certain principles in mind. For weight training, the overload principle must be incorporated (ie, a muscle must be loaded at higher than normal levels), and the overload must be progressive throughout the length of the program. Because smaller muscle groups fatigue more quickly, larger muscle groups should be exercised first, and exercise programs should be specific (ie, muscle groups used in an activity should be strengthened in a functional program). Isokinetic training principles are similar, but some differences should be noted: recommended training frequency is three times a week; the length of the training program should be a minimum of six weeks; exercise movements should simulate functional movements associated with the activity; training speeds should occur at a faster speed than that of the activity; for strength programs, three sets of 8 to 15 repetitions are recommended; and for endurance programs, a mini-

mum of three sets of 20 to 30 repetitions is suggested.

When the intensity of a training program increases, the physiological improvements are greater. However, the level of improvement is inversely proportional to the initial level of physical fitness. The level of gain is also greater in women then in men. Increases in training programs should be gradual in order to minimize the risk of injury and overuse syndromes. Excessive training is not uncommon and can lead to muscle breakdown.

Specificity

Training effects are specific to the type of exercise performed (eg, those trained on bicycle ergometer test better on the bicycle ergometer than they do on a treadmill). Furthermore, specific training patterns will result in only those muscles involved in the patterns being trained. Specificity of the training program is also relative to the adaptations seen in specific exercise modes and programs (eg, sprint programs versus endurance programs; bicycling programs versus swimming programs).

Genetic Considerations

The effects of training are generally not significantly affected by either age or gender. However, certain values seem to be determined by heredity, including maximal heart rate, lactic acid system capacity, $\dot{V}O_{2\,max}$, and most respiratory functions.

Gender Differences

When establishing a strengthening program, the differences between men and women must be considered. This is particularly important when initiating the program. The first difference is absolute strength. Men are generally considered to be stronger than women, but differences are based on particular muscle groups. If general muscle strength is considered, a 3:2 strength ratio of male:female is found. However, differences have been documented in both upper and lower extremities. For comparison, large differences exist in the chest, arms, and shoulders, but the smallest differences exist in the legs.

The second difference in strength relates to body size. Differences between the sexes decrease with respect to body size. Actually, leg strength per unit lean body mass is higher in women than in men. Lean body mass more closely approximates total muscle mass than does total body weight. Lean body mass is calculated by subtracting total fat weight from total body weight. In addition, the height of the person plays a small role in the difference in strength.

Strength as it relates to muscle size is another characteristic to be considered. Apparently, little difference exists between the sexes if one looks at strength in relation to the cross-sectional area of the muscle. When correlating this information to functional activity (eg., jumping) this theory holds true. Men and women are almost equal in jumping heights when the values are corrected for body size. Similarly, women may be slightly faster in sprinting activities when body size is taken into account.

Finally, the effects of training with weights for strength in a female population must be considered. Strength development in women can occur following a weight training program. There is little or no change in total body weight. However, a significant loss of relative and absolute body fat occurs, and a significant gain in lean body weight occurs. Although women do see significant changes in strength development, little evidence exists to suggest that muscle hypertrophy occurs to the same extent in women as it does in men. The male hormone testosterone regulates muscle hypertrophy. Therefore, women, under normal circumstances, will develop muscle toning, but not visible hypertrophy.

Mode of Exercise

Most noninjured or nondisabled persons will utilize one type of strength program, usually determined by accessibility of equipment. Someone who belongs to a spa or health club may use Nautilus, Universal Gym, or another type of exercise equipment. Very rarely will someone who lifts weights, either on machines or free weights, incorporate isometric exercises into the routine. However, in a rehabilitation program, a physical therapist may wish to utilize more than one form of exercise to accomplish different goals.

When establishing a treatment program, the following factors need to be considered: (1) protection of the injured area; (2) resting from stress, but not limiting function; (3) extent of the pain; (4) degree of swelling; (5) joint range of motion; (6) strength, power, and endurance; (7) flexibility; (8) the presence of mechanical dysfunction; (9) joint proprioception; (10) causative factors and whether they can be controlled; (11) provision of functional programs; and (12) whether assistive appliances (eg, tape, wraps, braces, orthotics) are indicated.

The progression of a program must be monitored, and both subjective and objective data should be reviewed when assessing the success of the program. Subjective data during reevaluation include the presence of pain, extent of swelling, and changes of function. Objective data include girth measurements, goniometric measurements, palpation, normal muscle testing, and isokinetic evaluations.

For a rehabilitation program, the progression of strengthening exercises may be as follows. Isometric exercise is usually utilized early because of its ability to protect the injured part. Submaximal isometric exercise is begun initially, and then the patient progresses to maximal isometric exercise. Multiple-angle isometric exercises are used, because carryover is only to about 10 to 15 degrees in each direction of the exercised angle. From this point, progression to the next level depends on access and availability of equipment. If isokinetic equipment is available, short-arc, submaximal isokinetic contractions are used. If equipment is not available, then short-arc, submaximal isotonic contractions are begun. The progression is to short-arc, maximal isotonic or isokinetic exercises. The final level involves full range-of-motion activities. Full-range, submaximal isotonic/isokinetic exercises are followed by full-range, maximal isotonic/isokinetic exercises. Many variables dictate the progression.

Many different programs have been developed for improvement in strength gains. A practical approach should be based on what equipment is available to the individual patient. The following principles should be followed in establishing a weight training program: (1) do not overload too fast; (2) strength training programs normally are performed three times per week; (3) performing one to three sets of six to ten repetitions has been shown to be advantageous; (4) exercise should be performed until fatigue; (5) only repetitions where good form and technique are used should be counted; (6) the form should be smooth and should allow for a momentary rest at the end of each repetition; (7) the weights should be worked through the full range of motion; (8) a specific training schedule should be established and it should be followed; (9) breathing is extremely important (inhale on lift, exhale on release); and (10) always warm up and cool down after strenuous weight workouts.

Two additional factors that should be examined when establishing a strengthening program are the particular activity in which a person participates, which will dictate the muscle groups to be strengthened, and the position the person plays, which will also influence training. Tables 40-3 and 40-4 show lists of sporting activities and weight exercises to help guide the development of a strengthening program. The tables also show a comparison of free weights, Universal Gym, and Nautilus, and what exercises and muscle groups are utilized. (Tables 40-1 and 40-2 show sample programs for isometric and isotonic exercises, which are common training programs for normal persons.)

Sport performance can definitely be associated with a weight training program. Both isometric and isotonic forms of strengthening programs have been shown to improve sport performance. However, progressive, resistive programs are generally considered to be superior. Secondly, the overload principle is extremely important for strengthening. Strenuous exercise is needed to get maximal results. Third, many studies have shown that increased strength aids the speed of movement. Lastly, specificity of training is a key to sports performance enhancement.

Maintenance

For a maintenance training program to be effective, the absolute minimum number of times per week a program should be completed is once. The studies to date show that at that level, some of the training effects may decrease slightly. Therefore, two times per week is prob-

Table 40-3. Sporting Activities

Backstroke	Hockey
Baseball	Hurdling
Basketball	Javelin
Breast stroke	Long jump
Butterfly	Pole vault
Discus and shot	Rowing
Distance run	Skiing
Football	Soccer
Freestyle	Sprinting
Golf	Tennis
Gymnastics	Wrestling
High jump	

Table 40-4. Suggested Weight Exercises for Various Sports Activities

SPORTS OR SPORTS ACTIVITY

Weight Exercise	Body Area	Backstroke	Baseball	Basketball	Breast stroke	Butterfly	Discus and shot	Distance run	Football	Freestyle	Golf	Gymnastics	High jump	Hockey	Hurdling	Javelin	Long jump	Pole vault	Rowing	Skiing	Soccer	Sprinting	Tennis	Wrestling
Arm curl	Upper and lower arm		✔	✔		✔	✔	✔		✔	✔	✔	✔				✔			✔	✔	✔	✔	✔
Back hyperextension	Lower back			✔			✔	✔		✔							✔	✔			✔		✔	
Bench press	Chest	✔	✔	✔	✔	✔	✔	✔	✔		✔						✔	✔				✔	✔	✔
Bent-arm pullover	Chest	✔	✔	✔	✔		✔	✔							✔	✔	✔	✔		✔				
Bent-knee sit-ups	Abdomen		✔	✔		✔	✔	✔		✔		✔	✔	✔	✔		✔	✔	✔				✔	✔
Bent-over rowing	Shoulder girdle						✔	✔						✔						✔				✔
Dumbbell swing	Lower back	✔	✔	✔	✔	✔	✔		✔		✔	✔		✔	✔				✔	✔	✔			
Good morning exercise	Lower back		✔			✔								✔					✔	✔		✔		✔
Heel (toe) raise	Lower leg			✔			✔	✔				✔		✔	✔									
Incline press	Upper arm	✔	✔			✔		✔		✔	✔	✔	✔	✔	✔	✔	✔		✔	✔			✔	
Knee (leg) extension	Upper leg	✔		✔		✔		✔				✔	✔	✔	✔	✔			✔	✔	✔			✔
Lateral arm raise	Shoulder	✔		✔							✔						✔						✔	
Leg curl	Upper legs			✔	✔	✔								✔	✔				✔		✔			
Leg raise	Trunk	✔			✔	✔				✔					✔									
Neck flexion and extension	Neck								✔					✔									✔	✔
Parallel bar dip	Shoulder, upper and lower arm								✔	✔	✔		✔						✔	✔	✔			✔
Power clean	Trunk, shoulder girdle		✔	✔	✔	✔	✔	✔	✔		✔		✔	✔	✔	✔	✔	✔		✔	✔			✔
Power snatch	Trunk, shoulder girdle										✔													
Press behind neck	Shoulder	✔				✔			✔															
Pulldown—lat machine	Shoulder girdle	✔		✔	✔	✔			✔			✔		✔	✔				✔	✔				✔
Reverse curl	Lower arm																						✔	
Reverse wrist curl	Forearm		✔	✔		✔		✔		✔	✔		✔		✔		✔		✔	✔			✔	✔
Shoulder shrug	Shoulder	✔							✔					✔		✔		✔		✔			✔	
Squat	Lower and upper back, upper legs	✔	✔	✔	✔	✔	✔	✔	✔	✔	✔	✔	✔	✔	✔	✔	✔	✔	✔	✔	✔	✔	✔	✔
Standing press	Shoulder, upper arms		✔	✔		✔		✔	✔	✔	✔				✔								✔	✔
Still-legged dead lift	Lower back			✔			✔	✔	✔	✔											✔		✔	
Straight-arm pullover	Chest		✔						✔								✔						✔	
Triceps extension	Shoulder, upper arm		✔	✔	✔			✔	✔			✔			✔	✔	✔	✔		✔			✔	
Upright rowing	Shoulder	✔	✔	✔			✔	✔	✔	✔	✔	✔							✔	✔	✔		✔	
Wrist curl or wrist roller	Forearm		✔	✔		✔		✔		✔	✔		✔		✔				✔	✔			✔	✔

(Fox EL: Sports Physiology, 2nd ed, pp 136–137, Table 7-2. Philadelphia, Saunders College Publishing, 1984. Modified from O'Shea JP: Scientific Principles and Methods of Strength Fitness, 2nd ed. Reading, MA, Addison-Wesley, 1976; and Hooks G: Weight Training in Athletics and Physical Education. Englewood Cliffs, NJ, Prentice-Hall, 1974.)

ably a much more efficient way of maintaining the improved effects of a training program.

ENDURANCE

Muscle endurance has been defined in various ways. Regardless of previous definitions, muscle endurance (or ability to resist fatigue) is ultimately a function of muscle strength. Specifically, muscle endurance is the ability of a given muscle or group of muscles to perform repeated contractions in an isometric, isotonic, or constant velocity form of exercise. Other definitions include the concepts of relative and absolute endurance. Relative endurance is the ability of a muscle to resist a decrease in its maximum peak torque capabilities during repetitive use. Absolute endurance is defined as the significant gain in total work performed.

Although an integral component of muscle performance, muscle endurance is often neglected in the literature and in the clinical environment, which usually focus on muscle strengthening. However, endurance is vital for complex daily tasks, for designated work requirements, and for participation in athletic or recreational events. As the duration or length of activity increases, the importance of muscle endurance becomes more obvious. This concept is pertinent for healthy persons engaging in activities to promote personal fitness. More importantly, the physical therapist must incorporate the concepts of muscle endurance into programs for persons who are disabled or injured from disease or trauma, or who have undergone a surgical procedure. The physical therapy program must be tailored to meet the specific needs of the individual patient, depending upon work, activity, or athletic requirements.

Endurance is measured by the rate of the decline of the slope in a regression line of a series of muscle contractions. Relative endurance may be measured by employing a load that represents a given percentage of a person's maximum voluntary contraction. In other words, relative endurance is the ability to lift a load that is "relative" to the maximum voluntary contraction for a given subject. Absolute endurance is measured by using the same load for all subjects regardless of maximum and voluntary contraction, and is assessed in terms of the significant gain in total work performed.

PHYSIOLOGICAL EFFECTS OF ENDURANCE TRAINING

The benefits derived from muscle endurance or low-resistance, high-repetition training depend upon muscle fiber typing, intramuscular circulation, enzymatic profiles, myoglobin stores, environmental conditions, state of training, and type of activity.

The physical therapist must be aware of the differences in physiological parameters for muscle strengthening and muscle endurance programs (Fig. 40-11). Muscle fibers are utilized selectively according to the level of work intensity. An increased depletion of slow-twitch muscle fiber glycogen stores is observed with submaximal exercise or low-resistance training as compared with an increased depletion of fast-twitch muscle fiber glycogen stores with high-resistance programs. Although con-

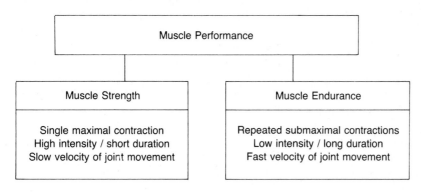

FIGURE 40-11. Continuum of muscular performance. Muscle performance is an interaction of strength and endurance. Rehabilitation protocols must account for both.

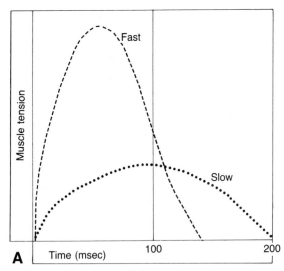

Biochemical Characteristic	Fiber Type	
	Red	White
Aerobic		
Myoglobin* content	High	Low
Fat content	High	Low
Mitochondrial content	High	Low
Oxidative enzyme levels	High	Low
Capillary density	High	Low
Anaerobic		
Glycogen content	Low	High
PC content	Low	High
Glycolytic enzyme levels	Low	High
Speed of contraction	Slow	Fast
Fatigue factor	Low	High

*Myoglobin is an oxygen-binding pigment similar to hemoglobin. It gives the red fiber its color.

FIGURE 40-12. The relationship between fast (IIa) and slow (I) fibers. (*A*) This graph displays the tension development variance. (*B*) Biochemical characteristics. (Matthews DK, Fox EC: The Physiological Basis of Physical Education and Athletics, 2nd ed. Philadelphia, WB Saunders, 1976)

troversial, endurance training has been shown to increase the surface area of primarily slow-twitch muscle fibers, but it also may increase the area of fast-twitch (type IIa) fibers. Fast-twitch fibers may be recruited during prolonged exercise as the slow-twitch fibers become fatigued (Fig. 40-12).

The ability to perform exercises depends on the activity of glycolytic enzymes and the Kreb's cycle enzymes. Costill (1979) has shown that elite long-distance runners had significantly increased levels of muscle succinate dehydrogenase (SDH) over middle-distance runners or untrained subjects. SDH activity is representative of the total number of mitochondria that facilitate the ability of the cell to oxidize fuels. This increase in SDH carbohydrates and fats provides the crucial fuels for muscle performance. Other adaptations that occur with muscle endurance training include an increase in the ratio of capillary to muscle fiber, an increase in myoglobin stores, and changes in anaerobic metabolism. Reduced muscle fiber size has also been reported as a result of endurance training in humans as well as animals. Smaller fibers would ultimately improve the

diffusion of oxygen and nutrients because of the shorter diffusion distances.

ENDURANCE TRAINING METHODS

Submaximal exercise and slow resistance training programs are well suited for improving muscle endurance. Specific programs used in the clinic must be designed to meet the requirements and needs for the individual patient. Emphasis for each program is based on the principle of specific adaptation to imposed demands (SAID): To observe specific changes caused by a specific activity in a group of muscles, the demands imposed must be just as specific. Such a program should focus on the following items: diagnosis, healing constraints, contributing medical factors, clinical evaluation (ie, swelling, pain), psychological factors, patient tolerance, and upper or lower extremity or total body involvement.

Muscle endurance programs typically focus on submaximal and repetitive exercises. Each program must consider functional capability; duration, frequency, and intensity of required activity; angular velocity of the joints (of the involved body part); and neuromuscular adaptation.

ENDURANCE PROGRAMS

One commonly used method for improving muscle endurance of the lower extremities is a regular or stationary bicycle. The stationary bicycle can be advantageous because of its versatility for a large cross section of diagnoses as well as its limitation of weight bearing and joint compressive forces. When evaluating a patient for possible use of the bicycle, one must consider cardiopulmonary, neuromuscular, and orthopaedic concerns. Initially, the bicycle should be used at a minimum resistance setting. The seat height must be adjusted according to orthopaedic considerations. Specific protocols for duration and frequency must be based on diagnosis as well as other factors mentioned previously. Each program should begin with a short session (ie, 5 to 10 minutes, one to two times per day) and progress according to patient tolerance and lack of symptoms. For most patients, progression should be targeted to increase intensity levels (relative to some maximal exercise and duration based on the SAID principle). It is vitally important to monitor the cardiopulmonary system closely when indicated (Fig. 40-13).

Swimming is another activity designed to improve muscle endurance. If swimming skills are adequate and a pool is accessible, swimming is advantageous to the general population as well as to orthopaedic and geriatric patients. Weight bearing and joint compressive forces can be controlled because of the buoyancy of water. A swimming program may begin with performance of specific exercises in the water, or sitting at the edge of the pool and kicking the legs in the water. The patient can progress to a kick board or float device, as well as to performing specific strokes (freestyle, backstroke, etc.). Again, the emphasis should be on time development, with gradual increase in the intensity of the specific exercise or stroke. Pool programs can also focus on walking and running (forwards and backwards) in waist- to chest-deep water to maximize functional patterns of training. The resistance of the water is constant and depends on effort, much like isokinetic methods of training.

Walking and running are also used to enhance muscle endurance. Careful consideration must be given to cardiopulmonary and orthopaedic concerns when recommending participation in running or jogging programs. Patients must be instructed individually, because the majority of patients are going to run

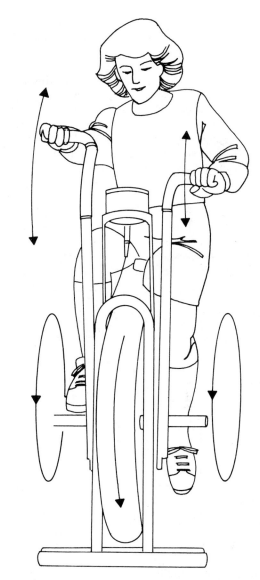

FIGURE 40-13. Patient performing on a bicycle to increase cardiovascular and muscular endurance. A slow, gradual buildup is important to avoid overuse injury.

or jog independently without supervision. Instructions should be specific, emphasizing functional progression and training geared toward the requirements of targeted sports and activities. Again, intensity must be controlled with emphasis on time development. Running is also advocated to enhance muscle endurance because most sport activities require it. Furthermore, running is very popular among patients. The individual program should be geared toward the specific needs of each sport.

Other methods of endurance training may incorporate the use of surgical tubing or any similar commercially available product. Emphasis is on submaximal resistance for a particular muscle or group of muscles. Three to five sets of 20 to 40 repetitions can be instituted as tolerated. In addition, the velocity of movement can be increased in accordance with the patient's tolerance. Application can be individualized to specific muscle groups as well as specific exercises (Fig. 40-14). Another technique that has been employed is walking against the resistance of surgical tubing or a rubber band type of material. Walking for short

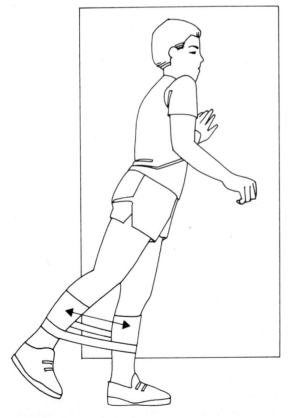

FIGURE 40-14. Surgical tubing may be incorporated into an exercise to train endurance.

distances offers low levels of resistance, which may be applied for short-duration activities. Proprioceptive neuromuscular facilitation techniques may also be of benefit with this type of exercise. Endurance may also be accomplished with the use of rowing machines, nordic tracks, and other mechanical devices that emphasize submaximal training over a prolonged period.

One last method of endurance resistance training is the use of an isokinetic (constant velocity) device, including velocity spectrum training. Thus, a range of angular velocities is preselected and the patient works throughout this range performing a set number of repetitions, or performing repetitions for a set period of time at each speed. The advantages of this type of exercise are numerous, but perhaps the most important is that it approximates the angular velocities that the joint experiences during normal daily and recreational activities. Each program should be specific to the joint(s) involved as well as to the sport that is being pursued. Higher-speed training (300°/sec to 450°/sec) has been found to be very useful in developing muscular endurance.*

Muscle endurance programs are vital for the rehabilitation process. Submaximal exercises or lower-resistance training programs may enhance muscular endurance. Clinical physical therapy programs should focus on individual evaluation along with specific activity requirements or desired performance levels. Direct application is based upon the SAID principle. Each program must be tailored and designed to meet the specific needs of the individual patient. Furthermore, these concepts should also be targeted toward normal, healthy populations for the prevention of injury.

POWER

Power is a multifaceted element of muscle performance that is often overlooked in rehabilitation. It is defined as the muscle's ability to produce a force through a range of motion in a given time. Thus, it is the rate at which the

*Robert Mangine, unpublished data.

muscle develops tension. It is also explained as the explosive capability of the muscle. A high proportion of white (fast-twitch) fibers are often found in persons displaying explosive speed.

POWER TRAINING METHODS

The methods of developing power are controversial, and are divided into two schools of thought. The first is based on the concept of initial low-speed, high-load training that increases the number of motor units firing at the time of contraction. As a greater number of units are recruited, the speed of contraction increases. Approximately six weeks of training will provide an increase in speed of contraction.

The second school of thought is based on the concept of speed-specific training effects. According to this concept, specific adaptation occurs with imposed demands and muscle change occurs in reference to the speed at which it is trained. This training is based on the SAID principle. Because power incorporates a time parameter and a rapid onset of movement, training should revolve around speed-specific effects. Therefore, training follows a low-resistance, high-speed, high-repetition protocol.

Although velocity spectrum training protocols are a common practice, high-speed training may result in a carryover into the low-speed testing ranges.

POWER PROGRAMS

Rehabilitation of speed as part of the exercise protocol is crucial for performing activities of daily living. An example of the necessity for speed-specific training is the knee, where tibial angular velocity in normal walking is approximately 270°/sec. It is often seen that slow-speed training (60°/sec) has no effect on high-speed function.

Power development must include high-velocity, high-repetition exercise protocols and must be incorporated into the programs for patients of all ages. Many functional exercises can be implemented by using rubber tubing or

rubber bands. The repetition level is high (20 to 50 repetitions) and the exercises are performed for three to five sets. High-speed movement is emphasized and careful supervision, especially in the presence of pathologic conditions of joints, is imperative (Fig. 40-15).

Another power program is a form of exer-

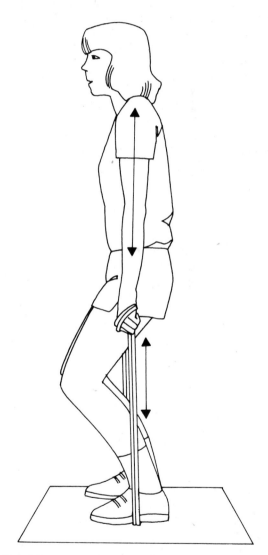

FIGURE 40-15. Patient performs a surgical tubing squat exercise at high speeds in a protected functional range of motion. The goal is to increase the patient's power.

cise termed plyometric training. The technique requires an eccentric contraction of a particular muscle group. Once the muscle has lengthened, a potential load of energy exists, which may be rapidly converted into kinetic energy by quick shortening of the muscle. An example of this type of exercise occurs in the lower extremity when a patient is required to jump from a platform to the floor, then rapidly return to the platform. The exercise is performed with a quick burst of movement to simulate functional speed and patterns. This exercise may be difficult and is usually implemented in the final stage of rehabilitation. Initially, a two-inch height and a low number of repetitions are attempted (eg, three sets of 15 repetitions are sufficient to start). A gradual increase in height, number of repetitions, and number of sets will occur based on the patient's activity level and functional needs.

Upper extremity plyometric exercises are also important and may be accomplished by using a heavy object, such as a medicine ball. The ball is thrown from patient to therapist using a rapid but safe technique. A variety of upper extremity positions, with or without trunk movements, may be used. Low numbers of repetitions and sets are performed initially, and are slowly increased to 30 to 40 repetitions for multiple sets (Fig. 40-16).

Power development may also employ isokinetic high-velocity training protocols. The program should start at 20 to 30 seconds of activity with midrange velocity and should slowly build to activity for 60 to 80 seconds. High-velocity interval training is the most func-

FIGURE 40-16. Polymetric training in the upper extremity. (A) A medicine ball is caught with the arms extended, and brought rapidly toward the body. (B) The ball is then quickly thrown forward, extending the arms.

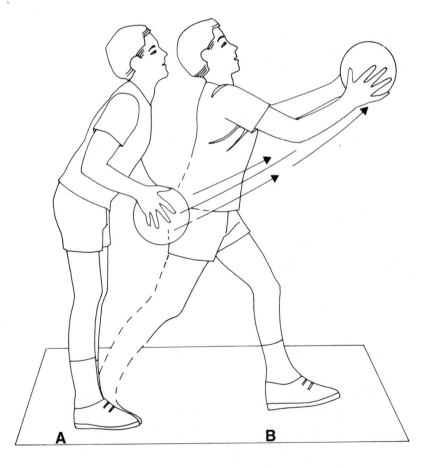

Table 40-5. Power/Interval Training Program*

	YARDS/REPETITIONS		YARDS/REPETITIONS
Week 1	20 × 16	**Week 4**	20 × 22
	40 × 12		40 × 18
	60 × 10		60 × 14
	80 × 8		80 × 12
Backwards	20 × 20	Backwards	40 × 15
Week 2	20 × 18	**Week 5**	20 × 22
	40 × 14		40 × 20
	60 × 12		60 × 15
	80 × 10		80 × 12
Backwards	20 × 25	Backwards	40 × 20
Week 3	20 × 20	**Week 6**	20 × 24
	40 × 15		40 × 20
	60 × 14		60 × 15
	80 × 12		80 × 12
Backwards	20 × 20	Backwards	40 × 25

*This example is a pre-season running program oriented toward aerobic increases using anaerobic training. Most sports are anaerobic in nature (short-burst sprints or movement and a brief recovery phase); therefore, a component of sprint training is essential, but prolonged bouts of work must be interjected to accomplish cardiovascular adaptation. The example here is used in soccer and was based on physical and performance assessments. A warm-up period is used prior to initiating the program.

tional program for power development. Interval training usually involves a work period of 30 seconds followed by 20 seconds of rest.

After midvelocity (120 to 180°/sec) exercise has been mastered, plyometric exercises may be initiated as part of the program. The final phase centers around sprint training with running for short distances of 40 to 60 yards. A high number of sprints may be used as a further method for speed training. The program involves a slow development over time. An example of a power/interval training program is seen in Table 40-5.

Power development is a stage of the rehabilitation process and is a necessary function for all rehabilitation programs. The program may vary among patients. Simple power exercises are initiated in the early phases of rehabilitation and are advanced to the use of interval sprinting as a final procedure before returning to full recreational or competitive activity.

Muscle rehabilitation programs must include the parameters of strength, endurance, and power. The therapist must consider both intrinsic and extrinsic factors involved in the exercise program. Careful implementation of exercise must not overly stress the patient, because irreversible joint damage can easily occur with pathologic conditions. The therapist must be ever aware of the findings of strength, endurance, and power studies to provide the most efficient mode of treatment for these patients.

ANNOTATED BIBLIOGRAPHY

Bandy WD, Eiland WG, McKitrick B: The Strength Compendium. Washington DC, Sports Physical Therapy Section of the American Physical Therapy Association, 1983

Basajian JV: Therapeutic Exercise, Student Edition. Baltimore, Williams & Wilkins, 1980

Costill DL: A scientific approach to distance running. Los Altos, CA, Track and Field News, 1979

Davies GJ: A Compendium of Isometrics in Clinical Usage. LaCross, Simon & Schuster, 1984

DeLorme T, Watkins A: Techniques of progressive resistance exercise. Arch Phys Med Rehabil 29:263, 1948

Fox EL: Sports Physiology, 2nd ed. Philadelphia, Saunders College Publishing, 1984

Hettinger T, Muller E: Muskelleistung and Muskeltraining. Arbeitsphysiol 5:111, 1953

Hooks G: Weight Training in Athletics and Physical Education. Englewood Cliffs, NJ, Prentice-Hall, 1974

Kisner CB, Allen LC: Therapeutic Exercise. Columbus, The Ohio State University Physical Therapy Division, 1979

Matthews DK, Fox EC: The Physiological Basis of Physical Education and Athletics, 2nd ed. Philadelphia, WB Saunders, 1976

Murray J, Weber A: The cooperative action of muscle proteins. Sci Am 230(2):58, 1974

O'Shea JP: Scientific Principles and Methods of Strength Fitness, 2nd ed. Reading, MA, Addison-Wesley, 1976

41

Enhancing Cardiopulmonary Function

CATHERINE M. E. CERTO

The management of cardiac and pulmonary patients has drastically changed over the last several decades. From the 1930s until the late 1960s patients' activity levels were severely limited. These restrictions formerly placed on all patients recovering from either a cardiac or a pulmonary insult are currently viewed as excessive. It is now believed that a far more aggressive approach is not only safe but is more likely to facilitate the patient's return to an active and productive life-style. The established practices of cardiac and pulmonary rehabilitation have succeeded in lowering mortality and recurrence rates. Although the data from large-scale controlled investigations are still incomplete, considerable objective information suggests that exercise rehabilitation programs result in improved physical, physiologic, and psychological well-being of cardiac and pulmonary patients.

These programs of rehabilitation emphasize the same basic essentials:

1. Early and repeated graded exercise testing to establish functional capacity to use as a baseline for recommending or prescribing exercises during the recovery and to use as an indication of the need for pharmacological or surgical intervention;
2. Individually prescribed graded training programs; and
3. A team approach to address the wide spectrum needs of these patients.

This chapter will focus on the physiologic rationale for training of cardiac and pulmonary patients, the principles of exercise prescription, and the special considerations for each of these populations.

PROGRESSIVE ACTIVITY PROGRAMS

THE PHYSIOLOGIC RATIONALE FOR EXERCISE TRAINING

The exercise training session has become the cornerstone for cardiac and pulmonary rehabilitation programs. The rationale for this emphasis is the result of the fact that these programs lead to improved functional capacity, reduce risk factors for recurrent cardiac or pulmonary insults, and have a favorable influence on the psychological functioning of these patients. Selection of the proper intervention tool necessitates careful consideration of the pathophysiologic mechanisms that limit exercise capacity and that may differ as a function of the underlying disease and its manifestations.

Aerobic capacity (maximal oxygen uptake) reflects the maximal rate at which oxygen can be utilized. Endurance-type exercise enhances aerobic capacity and is the principal objective for exercise intervention. The effect of training on aerobic capacity is a result of changes in musculoskeletal and cardiovascular mechanisms. The most important of these changes are increased cardiac output and increased tissue utilization of oxygen. Ventilation capacity and lung diffusion capacity are not limiting factors for coronary patients, but are limiting factors for patients with significant obstructive disease.

In addition to the improved physiologic parameters, aerobic exercise training has been shown to improve the quality of life. For both cardiac and pulmonary patients exercise training has been shown to improve their *joie de vivre* or zest for life. This improvement is seen through an increase in patients' ability to tolerate activities of daily living, a decrease in fear of exercise, an increased tolerance of dyspnea, a decrease in anxiety, and an improved adjustment to disability.

Aerobic Training in Patients with Coronary Artery Disease

Most studies demonstrate that the hemodynamic changes consistent with a training effect can be achieved during submaximal levels of activity in patients with coronary artery disease. These beneficial effects of exercise include significant lowering of heart rate and systolic blood pressure, which are the major determinants of myocardial oxygen demand. An increased threshold for angina is documentation of training-induced benefits in this population. However, controversy still exists over whether central or peripheral factors dominate in limiting aerobic capacity in patients with coronary artery disease. As a group, coronary patients have a statistically significant reduction in maximal oxygen uptake ($\dot{V}O_{2\,max}$) compared to normal persons. $\dot{V}O_{2\,max}$ in coronary patients, as in normal persons, depends on two components: the cardiac output (delivery) and the arteriovenous oxygen difference ($A\text{-}\dot{V}O_2$) (extraction). Clausen (1981) found that various comparative studies between normal and coronary subjects demonstrated no differences in $A\text{-}\dot{V}O_2$ difference, because $A\text{-}\dot{V}O_2$ difference is a function of peripheral vascular and metabolic factors. Thus, the basis for quantitative reduction in $\dot{V}O_{2\,max}$ in coronary disease resides in the impairment of left ventricular function that limits augmentation of stroke volume and cardiac output. Subjects with coronary disease tend to have lower stroke volumes (SV_{max}), lower heart rates (HR_{max}) and lower peak levels of maximal $\dot{V}O_2$ when compared to normal

subjects. At any given submaximal $\dot{V}O_2$, the contribution of cardiac output is significantly lower in patients with coronary disease, while $A\text{-}\dot{V}O_2$ differences tend to be higher in these same patients when compared with normal subjects. Therefore, the characteristic finding during exercise in subjects with coronary disease is a greater reliance on peripheral oxygen extractive factors than on central delivery mechanisms to sustain oxygen uptake during exercise. The limits of exercise tolerance differ in patients with varying degrees of coronary dysfunction. Thus, the mechanisms by which training improves maximum exercise capacity may also differ among individuals.

Aerobic Training in Patients with Chronic Pulmonary Disease

Aerobic capacity in patients with chronic obstructive pulmonary disease (COPD) may be limited by symptoms of breathlessness, related to reduced ventilatory capacity or respiratory muscle fatigue or both, at work loads requiring less than maximal attainable cardiac output. Therefore, aerobic exercise appears not to improve the indices of pulmonary function. Belman and Wasserman (1982) have shown that those pulmonary programs that employ exercise as a treatment demonstrate the increased ability of the patient to exercise with a reduction in oxygen consumption. The reasons postulated for this change are decreased sensitivity to dyspnea, decreased oxygen cost of breathing, and increased peripheral oxygen utilization attributable to an increased peripheral blood flow. Nicholas and colleagues (1970) suggested that improved motivation and willingness to tolerate dyspnea, rather than true physiologic adaptations, could account for training-induced improvements in such patients.

Another approach to improving exercise capacity while reducing symptoms of breathlessness during exercise in patients with lung disease has involved the training of the respiratory muscles. The rationale for this approach is based upon the fact that the aerobic capacity of these muscles independently contributes to ventilatory and aerobic exercise capacity. Stubbing and associates (1980) found that the requirements of the respiratory muscles during exercise in normal subjects represented only a small proportion of the total $\dot{V}O_2$, and therefore were not a limiting factor in exercise performance. They further demonstrated that in patients with airway disease, a disproportionate increase in ventilation was observed at a given work load. This exponential increase in ventilation leads to a greater metabolic requirement of the respiratory muscles, leaving a lesser reserve for working skeletal muscle. The literature supports the improved exercise performance with respiratory muscle training in patients with chronic airway disease.

In summary, aerobic exercise training may substantially improve the exercise capacity and the quality of life in patients with a variety of cardiac and pulmonary disorders. Attention to the symptomatic and physiologic limits of exercise capacity facilitates formulating the appropriate exercise prescription for each patient, and therefore may optimize the results of aerobic exercise training.

PRINCIPLES OF EXERCISE PRESCRIPTIONS

The exercise prescription is the cornerstone of any exercise program. The prescription should include frequency, intensity, duration, type of exercise, and progression of activity. These principles of exercise are applicable to the development of exercise programs for persons of any age or functional capacity whether in the absence or presence of disease. The major differences in prescribing programs for specific populations are how the principles of frequency, intensity, duration, and rate of progression are adjusted to meet individual needs.

The safety of an exercise prescription for an individual patient is best determined from objective measurements of fitness, including observations of heart rate (HR), electrocardiographic tracing (ECG), blood pressure (BP), and functional capabilities obtained from a graded exercise test (GXT). The subsequent

overall objective of the treatment program is to enhance the cardiovascular efficiency, flexibility, muscular strength, and endurance of the participant.

The American College of Sports Medicine has made the following recommendations for developing exercise programs for asymptomatic adults:

- *Frequency of conditioning:* minimum of three times a week up to five days per week
- *Intensity of conditioning:* physical activity of 65% to 95% of maximum heart rate or 50% to 85% of maximal oxygen uptake
- *Duration of conditioning:* 15 to 60 minutes of continuous or discontinuous aerobic activity. Duration is dependent on the intensity of activity prescribed.
- *Type of activity:* any activity that uses large muscle mass, can be maintained for a period of time, and is rhythmical and aerobic in nature, ie, brisk walking, swimming, jogging, bicycling. Small muscle activity may be used as an adjunct to any exercise program with proper application.
- *Rate of progression:* progression of the exercise conditioning program is dependent on the individual patient's functional capacity, health status, age, and needs or goals. The endurance or aerobic phase of the exercise prescription has three stages of progression: initial, improvement, and maintenance.

FREQUENCY OF EXERCISE SESSION

The frequency of exercise is dependent upon intensity and duration. The intensity of exercise may be prescribed by METS (metabolic equivalents). According to the American College of Sports Medicine, MET is a multiple of the resting rate of O_2 consumption ($\dot{V}O_2$ rest). One MET represents the approximate rate of O_2 consumption of a seated person at rest ($\dot{V}O_2$ rest) and is approximately 3.5 mL/O_2/kg/min. It has been established that three to five times a week is sufficient to improve and maintain functional capacity. For some cardiopulmonary patients whose post-acute status of functional capacities are less than 3 METS, sessions of five minutes several times per day are best. For persons with capacities between 3 and 5 METS, one to two daily sessions are advisable. Participants with capacities of 5 to 8 METS should exercise at least three to five times per week.

INTENSITY OF EXERCISE SESSION

The most difficult problem in designing an exercise program is the establishment of the appropriate exercise intensity. Initial monitoring of the subject is essential to ensure that the intensity prescribed is not exceeded. The intensity must assure that the proper percentage of functional capacity prescribed for any given person is maintained for the aerobic period. For instance, a well-trained athlete may be able to maintain 80% of functional capacity for over two hours, whereas a poorly conditioned person could maintain 80% of functional capacity for just a few minutes.

The average conditioning intensity for asymptomatic persons is between 60% and 70% of functional capacity. For patients with cardiac disease who have a low functional capacity, the intensity may be prescribed at 40% of functional capacity. For patients with pulmonary disease the intensity may be prescribed at as low as 20% to 40% of functional capacity. The intensity of exercise may be prescribed by one of three methods: heart rate, METS, or rating of perceived exertion (RPE). These methods will be described later in the chapter.

DURATION OF EXERCISE SESSION

The aerobic period of training should be at least 20 to 30 minutes long. This length of time is related to the intensity prescribed (60% to 70% of $\dot{V}o_2$). Very fit persons are able to exercise for longer periods at higher intensities. Persons with low functional capacities should exercise at lower percentages of functional capacity for shorter durations. The duration and intensity of exercise for patients with cardiac and pulmonary disease are dependent upon the time since the incident. Because intensity levels of the activities are usually so low, they may be performed three to four times per day for 5 to 10 minutes each session. As the intensity increases, the length of each session will also increase but the frequency per day will decrease. Duration-intensity level should be modified when the patient's functional capacity increases and when physiologic adaptation to exercise occurs. For the patient with cardiac and pulmonary disease, the increase and adaptation can be interpreted to occur when the patient perceives the intensity to be easier, when the heart rate is lower for the same exercise intensity, or when the symptoms appear at a higher exercise intensity or not at all for the same intensity.

Although the aerobic portion of any exercise program is critical, sufficient time must be allotted for the warm-up and cool-down periods. The warm-up period should be anywhere from 5 to 15 minutes of slow yet progressive exercises that prepare the patient for the more strenuous activity of the aerobic period. The beneficial effects of warming up have been well documented. For most patients with cardiac or pulmonary disease who have not exercised for a long time, proper warm-up activities will reduce the incidence of musculoskeletal injuries. This particular group is usually overweight and sedentary. They generally have poor abdominal musculature and very weak low back muscles. Therefore, a few extra minutes of careful instructions and more supervision time are essential for these persons. If care is not given, they may injure themselves early in the program, causing pain, frustration, and setback. Eventually such patients loose enthusiasm and may drop out of the program.

The cool-down period usually consists of low-level activities that allow time for the heart rate and blood pressure to return to near pre-exercise levels. If vigorous exercises are stopped quickly, the blood tends to pool in the veins of the lower extremities, which places an increased burden on the heart and eventually the brain. Maintaining adequate circulation also enhances the removal of metabolic waste and will lessen the development of muscle soreness usually seen after exercise.

RATE OF PROGRESSION

The physiologic effects of exercise that usually indicate a need for alteration of the exercise prescription are lowered heart rate and blood pressure for a given intensity, a lower RPE value for a given intensity, or the absence of symptoms for a given intensity.

For most persons, the conditioning effect of exercise allows them to increase the exercise intensity performed per session. As a conditioning effect occurs, adjustments of the prescription for physically active persons can be made with little fear of risk. However, modifying an exercise prescription for sedentary, older, or symptomatic patients necessitates more caution. For these persons, the degree of risk involved in exercise is a function of the interaction of age, functional capacity, and symptoms and severity of the disease. Initially the exercise intensity should be set at approximately 1 MET lower than the established training intensity. Target heart rates used in conjunction with signs and symptoms will be the best objective and subjective indicators for adjusting the exercise prescription. Therefore, no magic formula exists for establishing an exercise prescription. The principles of exercise serve as guidelines, and careful adjustments of these will assist in the individual determination of the subject's training level. The exercise prescription will need constant monitoring initially and frequent revisions as the patient's ability to complete the exercise improves.

EXERCISE PRESCRIPTION

The American College of Sports Medicine identifies three methods used to establish an exercise prescription. They are exercise prescription by heart rate, by METS, and by perceived exertion.

Exercise Prescription by Heart Rate

In order to prescribe exercise by heart rate, the patient's maximal heart rate must be estab-

lished. The maximal heart rate, which is normally established by graded exercise testing, is the highest rate achieved at the highest exercise intensity achieved. When exercise testing is not possible, an estimate of maximal heart rate is achieved by subtracting the person's age from 220 (eg, $220-50=170$) for lower-extremity activity and subtracting age and 11 from 220 (eg, $220-50-11=159$) for upper-extremity activity. This maximal heart rate is then multiplied by a given percentage of functional capacity (usually 60% to 70%) to determine the "target" heart rate.

Maximal heart rate	170
Conditioning intensity	x 0.60
(% of HR)	102 beats per minute

Therefore, 90 beats per minute would be the target heart rate for training for this person.

A second method commonly used to determine target heart rate is by factoring in the resting heart rate. The difference between the maximal and resting heart rate is determined, then multiplied by the percentage of functional capacity desired for training, and finally the resting rate is added to that number.

Maximal heart rate	170
Resting heart rate	− 70
	100
Conditioning intensity	
(percent of HR range)	× 0.70
	70
Resting heart rate	
Target heart rate	+ 70
	140

Exercise Prescription by METS

The intensity of exercise may be prescribed by METS. If a patient, through exercise stress testing, is identified as having an 8-MET capacity, the prescription for exercise can be determined by multiplying the MET capacity by the percentage of functional capacity best identified for training of that person.

$$8 \text{ METS} \times 70\% \text{ (or } 0.70) = 5.6 \text{ METS}$$

Thus, this person may select activities for training that are known to require energy expenditure at the desired MET level. Many texts provide the mean and ranges for MET requirements of common activities.

Exercise Prescription by Perceived Exertion

The rating of perceived exertion (RPE) scale (Fig. 41-1) has been shown to be of benefit in evaluating a subject's response to exercise. This numerical scale is designed to estimate a person's subjective response to exertion. Studies show that a strong correlation exists between heart rate and perception of exertion, such that the RPE increases linearly with heart rate in response to a given intensity of exercise. For this reason, the RPE is frequently used as a means of establishing actual heart rate response to exercise. During the last decade the clinical application of RPE in patients with cardiac and pulmonary disorders has significantly increased. Pandolf (1983) demonstrated that the maximal capacity can be predicted equally as well with RPE and heart rate. His finding suggests that the use of a combination of RPE and HR is more accurate in predicting maximal exercise capacity than either the separate use of perceived exertion or heart rate.

Borg Scale

6.
7. Very very light
8.
9. Very light
10.
11. Light
12.
13. Somewhat hard
14.
15. Hard
16.
17. Very hard
18.
19. Very very hard
20.

Figure 41-1. Scale of perceived exertion. (After Borg GAV: Perceived exertion: A note on history and methods. Med Sci Sports 5:90, 1973)

Pollock (1986) suggested that RPE ratings of 12 and 13 correspond to approximately 60% and 70% of functional capacity, which is the level of exercise intensity most commonly recommended for training. Studies have also shown that the physiologic changes that occur with training are in concert with the reduction in the perception of effort for a given exercise intensity.

Gutmann (1981) showed that patients with coronary insufficiency or myocardial infarction, or both, have consistently higher RPEs for a given heart rate than a group of age-matched controls. With training, however, the RPE was normalized and the linear relationship with heart rate maintained. The initially high RPE values were believed to reflect a lower maximum capacity or qualitative differences in perception (eg, pain, shortness of breath). Therefore, a combination of physiologic and psychological factors may account for a proportionately greater amount of the variance in the RPE response early in the rehabilitative process.

The use of the RPE with the anaerobic threshold (AT) may provide a more useful physiologic basis for exercise prescription than the use of the percent of $\dot{V}O_{2\,max}$ or target heart rate. Initially, during a progressive exercise the rate of pulmonary minute ventilation (VE) will increase linearly with increments in work rate. Eventually, however, there will be an exercise intensity at which VE will increase nonlinearly. This exercise level at which VE abruptly increases is called the anaerobic threshold. At this level of exercise the onset of metabolic acidosis can be detected in one of several ways: (1) an increase in blood lactic acid; (2) a corresponding decrease in blood pH and bicarbonate; (3) an increase in respiratory exchange ratio (R); and (4) a deviation from linearity in the relationship between oxygen consumption and ventilation (Wasserman, 1964). The anaerobic threshold or ventilation threshold can be detected by graphing VE and $\dot{V}O_2$. The point where ventilation deviates from its linear relationship with oxygen consumption is the anaerobic threshold. The anaerobic threshold plays an important role both in sports and in clinical medicine. Many cardiopulmonary exercise laboratories include the measurement of anaerobic threshold as part of their standard evaluation. For cardiopulmonary patients, the anaerobic threshold is thought to be a direct measurement of exercise intensity at which the cardiovascular system fails in its ability to supply O_2 to the tissue. Therefore, use of the anaerobic threshold in an exercise prescription is a good indicator of performance.

The onset of the anaerobic threshold normally occurs between 55% and 65% of the maximal oxygen uptake. It is also known that a rating of 12 to 13 corresponds to approximately 60% to 70% of maximal heart rate reserve. The mean RPE at the anaerobic threshold has been documented to correspond to a rating of 13 on the RPE scale. According to patients, exercise at this level is perceived to be "somewhat hard." Thus, the exercise intensity corresponding to the anaerobic threshold can be prescribed reasonably well by telling patients to work at an intensity that they perceive to be "somewhat hard."

Pharmacologic agents now provide the foundation for the medical management of cardiopulmonary disease. Various drugs may affect exercise performance by altering the myocardial response to exercise, the peak physical exercise capacity, the exercise electrocardiogram, the heart rate, and the blood pressure responses. The beta blockers and the calcium-channel blockers are two of the most popular drugs. For patients taking these medications, an exercise prescription based on target heart rate alone is ineffective in evaluating the level of exercise intensity performed in relation to the heart rate response. For this reason, the RPE is frequently used for patients taking beta or calcium-channel blockers as a means of estimating actual heart rate response to exercise.

Lastly, even though heart rate is the best tool available for monitoring exercise performance, patients should not become obsessed with constantly stopping to take the heart rate. Therefore, the use of the RPE scale allows a patient to concentrate more on how a particular intensity of exercise feels, yet have some assurance that he is within his target heart rate.

This ability to use the Borg scale will also make it easier for patients to monitor environmental influences on exercise performance. For instance, on a very hot, humid day, a patient whose usual exercise intensity is perceived as "somewhat hard" (13) may feel "very hard" (15). The subject will then reduce the intensity of the exercise until he perceives the work load to be "somewhat hard."

EXERCISE PRESCRIPTION FOR SPECIAL POPULATIONS

EXERCISE PRESCRIPTION FOR PATIENTS WITH CORONARY HEART DISEASE

In recent years, exercise programs in the form of cardiac rehabilitation have become a widely accepted mode of treatment for patients with coronary heart disease. Cardiac rehabilitation is divided into several phases (Fig. 41-2). Phase I is the period of inpatient management from the acute onset to hospital discharge; Phase II is the active rehabilitation period from home to outpatient hospital-based programs including initial "life-style alterations"; and Phase III is the long-term supervised conditioning and maintenance program, usually conducted in a community center.

The physiologic as well as the psychological limitations imposed by coronary disease necessitates that the exercise prescription at each of the phases be individualized. Emphasis should be placed on developing realistic goals for recovery that are consistent with the limitations imposed by the disease. Attention to the symptoms and physiologic limitations at each of the stages of convalescence is imperative. During the initial stages setting the proper intensity and duration is critical (Table 41-1). Limitations as a result of signs, symptoms, medication changes, orthopedic problems, or neuromuscular problems can influence progression. No magic formula exists for establishing an individual patient's exercise prescription. Close monitoring of the patient's responses to the prescription along with target heart rate and RPE responses will assist in establishing a safe and effective program.

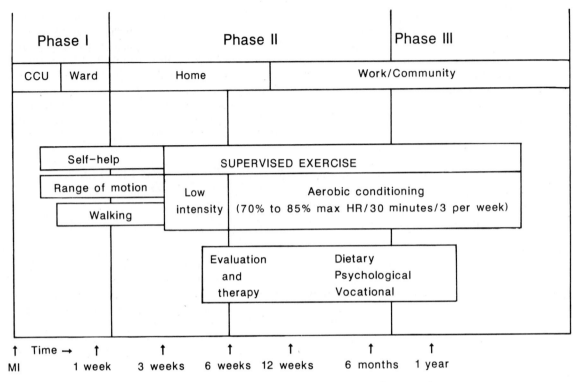

Figure 41-2. Rehabilitation following myocardial infarction: an integrated approach. (Reproduced by permission from Wagner E, Williams RS: Rehabilitation after myocardial infarctions. In Andreoli KG, Zipes DP, Wallace AG et al (eds): Comprehensive Cardiac Care, 6th ed, p 400. St Louis, 1987, The CV Mosby Co)

Table 41-1. Guidelines for Exercise Prescription for Cardiac Patients as Recommended and Practiced at Mount Sinai Medical Center, Milwaukee, WI*

PRESCRIPTION	PHASE I (INPATIENT PROGRAM)	PHASE II (DISCHARGE TO 3 MONTHS)	PHASE III (>3 MONTHS)	HEALTHY ADULTS
Frequency	2–3 times/day	1–2 times/day	3–5 times/week	3–5 times/week
Intensity	MI: RHR + 20 CABS: RHR + 20	MI: RHR + [†], RPE 13 CABS: RHR + 20[†], RPE 13	70%–85% max HR reserve	60%–90% max HR reserve
Duration	MI: 5–20 min CABS: 10–30 min	MI: 20–60 min CABS: 20–60 min	30–60 min	15–60 min
Mode/activity	ROM, TDM, bike, 1 flight of stairs	ROM, TDM (walk, walk-jog), bike, arm erg, wgt trg	Walk, bike, jog, swim, cal, wgt trg, endurance sports	Walk, jog, run, bike, swim, endurance sports, wgt trg, cal

*Symbols and abbreviations: MI, myocardial infarction patient; CABS, coronary artery bypass graft surgery patient; HR, heart rate (beats/minute); RHR, standing resting heart rate; ROM, range-of-motion exercise; TDM, treadmill; arm erg, arm ergometer; cal, calisthenics; wgt trg, weight training; RPE, rating of perceived exertion.

[†]After 6–8 weeks after the surgery or event, a symptom-limited exercise test is performed. Heart rate intensity is then based on 70% of the maximum heart rate reserve.

(Pollock ML, Schmidt D: Heart Disease and Rehabilitation, Chap. 25. New York, John Wiley & Sons, copyright © 1986. Reprinted by permission of John Wiley & Sons, Inc.)

Phase I Inpatient Exercise Programs

The objectives of Phase I of rehabilitation are to provide low levels of exercise to prevent the hazards of bed rest, reduce orthostatic hypertension, and maintain joint mobility. Exercise begins in the coronary care unit and consists of low-level active exercises starting in the supine position, progressing to sitting, and eventually to standing. Progressive ambulation and (lastly) stair climbing are an integral part of the inpatient exercise program. Sessions may be as short as 5 to 10 minutes. During this initial critical period after a myocardial infarction, activities are prescribed at a low level between 1 and 3 METS to allow for proper myocardial healing. Subsequently, in the progressive coronary care stage, exercise intensity is gradually increased to 5 METS. Prior to discharge a low-level, symptom-limited graded exercise test is performed. The purpose of this test is to evaluate functional capacity and symptom-limited heart rate in an effort to establish a proper exercise intensity for the next phase of cardiac rehabilitation. Table 41-2 outlines a progressive program for patients with myocardial infarction, and Table 41-3 outlines a program for patients with coronary artery bypass graft. Patient education is an integral part of each phase of rehabilitation. The framework of this educational process begins early in Phase I with individual instructions on identifying and modifying reversible risk factors for the progression of coronary artery disease. Most cardiac rehabilitation programs use the exercise portion of the program as the core, with the educational efforts embellishing the exercise prescription.

Phase II Outpatient Exercise Programs

Phase II usually begins after discharge from the hospital. The objectives of this phase are to begin to improve the functional capacity, to promote early return to normal activity, and to promote positive life-style changes. During this period the patient's functional capacities may vary from 4 to 6 METS. For patients with functional capacities above 5 METS, the heart rate and RPE method of prescription should be used. Frequency of sessions should be three times a week. Duration should increase from 5 to 15 minutes and progress to 30 minutes. As functional capacity improves, intensity can be gradually increased. Anginal patterns, frequent changes in medication, and minor bone and joint stiffness may influence the exercise prescription. Table 41-4 describes a 12-step walking program that can be used initially during this phase for patients who have had either a myocardial infarction or a coronary artery bypass graft. The patient progresses from step to step as tolerated. Later in the Phase II stage, some patients may be capable of jogging. Table 41-5 outlines a progressive walk-jog program for these patients.

Phase III Community-Based Programs

Patients in Phase III may have participated in inpatient and outpatient hospital-based programs, or they may enter this phase with no prior involvement in an organized program. Depending upon the facilities and the personnel, patients with varying levels of cardiac and pulmonary problems may participate. As a rule, three to six months have elapsed since the incident, and patients have the following: clinically stable or decreasing angina; medically controlled arrhythmias during exercise; a knowledge of signs and symptoms; an established exercise prescription; an ability to self-regulate their exercise; and a minimal functional capacity of 6 METS. Table 41-6 shows a 16-step walk-jog program for patients in a Phase III program. The objectives of this phase are maintenance of function, compliance with an exercise program, and risk factor education and modification. Depending on the complexity of the patient profile, this phase may last for several months. Patients often remain in a program of this nature for up to one year in an effort to achieve initial goals and establish compliance.

SPECIAL CONSIDERATIONS FOR EXERCISE PRESCRIPTION

Special considerations for exercise prescription are given to patients with the following: angina, a pacemaker, chronic ventricular failure, systemic hypertension, and peripheral

(*Text continues on p. 779.*)

Table 41-2. Inpatient Myocardial Infarction Cardiac Rehabilitation Program

STEP/DATE	CARDIAC REHABILITATION/ PHYSICAL THERAPY	WARD ACTIVITY	PATIENT EDUCATION
1 1.5 METs ____/____/____	Ward Rx: Passive ROM to major joints, active ankle exercises, 5 repetitions; deep breathing (supine) twice a day.	1. Bed rest. 2. May feed self.	Orient to CCU. Orientation to exercise component of rehabilitation program.
2 1.5 METs ____/____/____	Ward Rx: Active-assistive ROM to major muscle groups, active ankle exercises, 5 repetitions; deep breathing (supine/sitting) twice a day	1 Feeding self. 2. Partial AM care (washing hands and face, brushing teeth in bed). 3. Bedside commode.	Answer patient and family questions regarding progress, procedures, reason for activity limitation. Explain perceived exertion (RPE).
3 1.5 METs ____/____/____	Ward Rx: Active ROM to major muscle groups, active ankle exercises, five repetitions; (sitting) twice a day.	1. Begin sitting in chair for short periods as tolerated 2 times a day. 2. Bathing self. 3. Bedside commode.	
4 1.5 METs ____/____/____	Ward Rx: Active exercises—shoulder: flexion, abduction; elbow flexion; hip flexion; knee extension; toe raises; ankle exercises; 5 repetitions; breathing (standing) twice a day.	1. Bathroom privileges. 2. Sitting in chair 3 times a day. 3. Up in chair for meals. 4. Bathing self, dressing, combing hair (sitting).	
5 1.5–2 METs ____/____/____	Ward Rx: Active exercises–shoulder: flexion, abduction, circumduction; elbow flexion; trunk lateral flexion; hip: flexion, abduction; knee extension; toe raises; ankle exercises; 5 repetitions (standing); twice a day. Monitored ambulation of 100–200 ft, twice a day, with physician approval.	1. Bathroom privileges. 2. Up as tolerated in room. 3. Stand at sink to shave and comb hair. 4. Bathe self and dress. 5. Up in chair as tolerated.	Answer patient and family questions. Orient to ICCU phase of recovery. Present discharge booklet and other printed material (AHA). Encourage patient and family to attend group classes or do 1-to-1 sessions.
6 1.5–2 METs ____/____/____	Ward Rx: Standing— Exercises outlined in step 5, 5–10 repetitions; once daily. Monitored ambulation for 5 min (440 ft).	1. Continue ward activity from step 5. 2. Increase ambulation up to 440 ft with assistance if appropriate, two times per day.	Instruction in pulse taking and rationale. Explain value of exercise. Present T-shirt and activity log.

Table 41-2. (continued)

STEP/DATE	CARDIAC REHABILITATION/ PHYSICAL THERAPY	WARD ACTIVITY	PATIENT EDUCATION
___/___/___	Exercise Center: Transport to Inpatient Exercise Center (IEC) for monitored ROM/strengthening exercises from step 5, 5–10 repetitions; leg stretching (posterior thigh muscles, gastrocnemius), 10 repetitions; treadmill and/or bicycle 5 min; and stair climbing (2–4 stairs) with physician approval.	3. Walk short distance in hall or room.	
7 1.5–2.5 METs ___/___/___	Ward Rx: Standing— Exercises from step 5 with 1-lb weight each extremity, 5–10 repetitions; once daily. Monitored ambulation for 5–10 min (440–1100 ft)	1. Continue ward activity from step 6. 2. Sit up in chair most of the day. 3. Increased ambulation up to 1100 ft daily.	Begin discharge instructions with patient and family when appropriate. Encourage group class attendance or offer 1-to-1 as needed.
___/___/___	Exercise Center: Transport to IEC for monitored ROM/strengthening exercises from step 6 with 1-lb weight each extremity, 5–10 repetitions; leg stretching, 10 repetitions; treadmill and/or bicycle 5–10 min; and stair climbing (4–8 stairs).		
8 1.5–2.5 METs ___/___/___	Ward Rx: Standing— Exercises from step 5 with 1-lb weight each extremity, 10 repetitions; once daily. Monitored ambulation for 10 min (up to 1980 ft) if appropriate.	1. Continue ward activity from step 7. 2. Increase ambulation up to 1980 ft daily.	
___/___/___	Exercise Center: Ambulate to IEC for monitored ROM/strengthening exercises from step 6 with 1-lb weight each extremity, 10 repetitions; leg stretching, 10 repetitions; treadmill and/or bicycle 10–20 min; and stair climbing (10–12 stairs).		

continued

Table 41-2. (continued)

STEP/DATE	CARDIAC REHABILITATION/ PHYSICAL THERAPY	WARD ACTIVITY	PATIENT EDUCATION
9 1.5–2.5 METs ____/____/____	Ward Rx: Standing— Exercises from step 5 with 2-lb weight each extremity, 10 repetitions; once daily. Monitored ambulation if appropriate.	1. Up as tolerated in room. 2. Increase ambulation up to 2640 ft daily.	Begin instruction in home exercise program. Initiate referral to phase II if appropriate. Explain predischarge graded exercise test (PDGXT) and upper limit heart rate.
____/____/____	Exercise Center: Ambulate to IEC for monitored ROM/strengthening exercises from step 6 with 2-lb weight each extremity, 10 repetitions; leg stretching, 10 repetitions; treadmill and/or bicycle 20–25 min; and stair climbing (12–14 stairs).		
10 1.5-3 METs ____/____/____	Ward Rx: Exercises from step 5 with 2-lb weight each extremity, 10 repetitions; once daily. Monitored ambulation if appropriate.	1. Up as tolerated in room. 2. Increase ambulation up to 3300 ft daily.	
____/____/____	Exercise Center: Ambulate to IEC for monitored ROM/strengthening exercises from step 6 with 2-lb weight each extremity, 10 repetitions; leg stretching, 10 repetitions; treadmill and/or bicycle 25–30 min, and stair climbing (14–15 stairs).		

(Pollock ML, Schmidt D: Heart Disease and Rehabilitation, Chap. 25. New York, John Wiley & Sons, copyright © 1986. Reprinted by permission of John Wiley & Sons, Inc.)

Table 41-3. Inpatient Coronary Artery Bypass Patient Rehabilitation Program*

STEP/DATE	CARDIAC REHABILITATION/PHYSICAL THERAPY	WARD ACTIVITY†	PATIENT EDUCATION
1 1.5 METs ___/___/___	AM Ward Rx: Sitting with feet supported—active assistive to active ROM to major muscle groups, active ankle exercises, active scapular elevation/depression, retraction/protraction, 3–5 repetitions; deep breathing. Monitored ambulation of 100 ft as tolerated. PM Ward Rx: Sitting with feet supported—Active ROM to major muscle groups, 5 repetitions; deep breathing. Monitored ambulation 100–200 ft with assistance as tolerated.	1. Begin sitting in chair (when stable) several times/day for 10–30 min. 2. May ambulate 100–200 ft with assistance, 1–2 times daily.	Orient to CVICU. Reinforce purpose of physical therapy and deep breathing exercises. Orient to exercise component of rehabilitation program. Answer patient and family questions regarding progress.
2 1.5 METs ___/___/___	Ward Rx: Sitting—repeat exercises from step 1 and increase repetitions to 5–10; deep breathing twice a day. Monitored ambulation of 200 ft with assistance as tolerated (stress correct posture) twice a day.	Continue activities from step 1.	Continue above.
3 1.5-2 METs ___/___/___	Ward Rx: Standing—Begin active upper extremity and trunk exercises bilaterally without resistance (shoulder: flexion, abduction, internal/external rotation, hyperextension, circumduction backward; elbow flexion; trunk: lateral flexion, rotation), knee extension (if appropriate); ankle exercises; 5–10 repetitions; twice a day. Monitored ambulation of 300 ft twice a day.	Increase ambulation to 300 ft or approximately 3 corridor lengths at slow pace with assistance twice a day.	Begin pulse-taking instruction when appropriate and explain RPE scale. Answer questions of patient and family. Reorient patient and family to ICCU. Encourage family attendance at group classes.
4 1.5–2 METs ___/___/___	Ward Rx: Standing—Active exercises from step 3, 10–15 repetions; twice a day.	Increase ambulation to 500 ft at slow pace with assistance twice a day.	

*Heart rates, blood pressures, and comments are recorded on the Inpatient Data Record or Exercise Log.
†Ward activity, activities performed alone, with family, or primary nurse.
(Pollock ML, Schmidt D: Heart Disease and Rehabilitation, Chap. 25. New York, John Wiley & Sons, copyright © 1986. Reprinted by permission of John Wiley & Sons, Inc.)

continued

Table 41-3. (continued)

STEP/DATE	CARDIAC REHABILITATION/PHYSICAL THERAPY	WARD ACTIVITY†	PATIENT EDUCATION
5 1.2–2.5 METs ____/____/____ ____/____/____	Monitored ambulation of 424 ft twice a day. Ward Rx: Standing—Active exercises from step 3, 15 repetitions; once daily. Monitored ambulation for 5–10 min (424–848 ft) as tolerated. Exercise Center: Walk to Inpatient Exercise Center (IEC) for monitored ROM/strengthening exercises from step 3, 15 repetitions; leg stretching (posterior thigh muscles, gastrocnemius), 10 repetitions; treadmill or bicycle 5–10 min (refer to treadmill/bicycle protocol) with physician approval.	1. Increase ambulation up to 3 laps (up to 1320 ft) daily as tolerated. 2. Begin participating in daily (ADL) and personal care as tolerated. 3. Encourage chair sitting with legs elevated.	Orient to IEC. Continue instruction in pulse taking and use of RPE scale. Explain value of exercise. Present T-shirt and activity log.
6 1.5–2.5 METs ____/____/____ ____/____/____	Ward Rx: Standing—Active exercises from step 3 with 1-lb weight each upper extremity, 15 repetitions; once daily. Monitored ambulation for 10–15 min (up to 1980 ft) if appropriate. Exercise Center: Walk to IEC for monitored ROM/strengthening exercises from step 5 with 1-lb weight each upper extremity, 15 repetitions; leg stretching, 10 repetitions; treadmill and/or bicycle 15–20 min; and stair climbing (6–12 stairs) with assistance.	1. Increase ambulation up to 1980 ft daily. 2. Encourage independence in ADL. 3. Encourage chair sitting with legs elevated.	Give discharge booklet and general discharge instructions to patient and family. Encourage group class attendance. Individual instruction by physical therapist, nutritionist, pharmacist.
7 2–3 METs ____/____/____ ____/____/____	Ward Rx: Standing—Active exercises from step 3 with 1-lb weight each upper extremity, 15 repetitions; once daily. Monitored ambulation for 15–20 min (up to 3300 ft) if appropriate. Exercise Center: Walk to IEC for monitored ROM/strengthening exercises from step 5 with 1-lb weight each upper extremity, 15 repetitions; leg stretching, 10 repetitions; treadmill and/or bicycle 20–30 min; and stair climbing (up to 14 stairs) with assistance.	1. Continue activities from step 6. 2. Increase ambulation up to 3300 ft daily.	Discuss referral to phase II program if appropriate.

Table 41-3. (continued)

STEP/DATE	CARDIAC REHABILITATION/PHYSICAL THERAPY	WARD ACTIVITY†	PATIENT EDUCATION
8 2–3 METS ___/___/___ ___/___/___	Ward Rx: Standing—Exercises from step 3 with 2-lb weight each upper extremity, 15 repetitions; once daily. Monitored ambulation if appropriate. Exercise Center: Walk to IEC for monitored ROM/strengthening exercise from step 5 with 2-lb weight each upper extremity; 15 repetitions; leg stretching, 10 repetitions; treadmill and/or bicycle 20–30 min; and stair climbing (up to 16 stairs).	1. Continue activities from step 7. 2. Increase ambulation up to 3746 ft daily.	Reinforce prior teaching. Explain PDGXT and upper limit heart rate. Continue with possible referral to phase II.
9 2–3 METs ___/___/___ ___/___/___	Ward Rx: Standing—Exercises from step 3 with 2-lb weight each upper extremity, 15 repetitions; once daily. Monitored ambulation if appropriate. Exercise Center: Walk to IEC for monitored ROM/strengthening exercises from step 5 with 2-lb weight each upper extremity, 15 repetitions; leg stretching, 10 repetitions; treadmill and/or bicycle 20–30 min; and stair climbing (up to 18 stairs).	1. Continue activities from step 8. 2. Increase ambulation up 5060 ft daily.	Finalize discharge instructions. Complete referral to phase II.
10 2–3 METs ___/___/___ ___/___/___	Ward Rx: Standing—Exercises from step 3 with 3-lb weight each upper extremity, 15 repetitions; once daily. Monitored ambulation if appropriate. Exercise Center: Walk to IEC for monitored ROM/strengthening exercises from step 5 with 3-lb weight each upper extremity, 15 repetitions; leg stretching, 10 repetitions; treadmill and/or bicycle 20–30 min; and stair climbing (up to 24 stairs). A predischarge graded exercise test (PDGXT) is recommended at this time.	1. Continue activities from step 9. 2. Increase ambulation up to 5936 ft daily.	

*Heart rates, blood pressures, and comments are recorded on the Inpatient Data Record or Exercise Log.
†Ward activity, activities performed alone, with family, or primary nurse.
(Pollock ML, Schmidt D: Heart Disease and Rehabilitation, Chap. 25. New York, John Wiley & Sons, copyright © 1986. Reprinted by permission of John Wiley & Sons, Inc.)

Table 41-4. Twelve-Step Walking Program for Outpatients

FUNCTIONAL CAPACITY (METs)	STEP	SPEED (MPH)	ELEVATION (%)	DURATION (MIN)	METs	ENERGY EXPENDITURE (kcal/min)
5 METs	1	1.5	0	20–30	2.0	2.0
	2	2.0	0	20–30	2.0	2.5
5–8 METs	3	2.0	0	5	2.0	2.5
		2.5	0	40–60	2.5	3.0
	4	2.5	0	5	2.5	3.0
		3.0	0	40–60	3.0	3.7
8 METs	5	3.0	0	5	3.0	3.7
		3.5	0	40–60	3.5	4.2
	6	3.0	0	5	3.0	3.7
		3.5	0 (1 min)	40–60	3.5	4.2
		3.5	2.5 (4 min)		4.2	5.9
	7	3.0	0	5	3.0	3.7
		3.5	0 (1 min)	40–60	3.5	4.2
		3.5	2.5 (6 min)		4.2	5.9
	8	3.0	0	5	3.0	3.7
		3.5	0 (1 min)	40–60	3.5	4.2
		3.5	2.5 (10 min)		4.2	5.9
	9	3.0	0	5	3.0	3.7
		3.5	0 (1 min)	40–60	3.5	4.2
		3.5	2.5 (14 min)		4.2	5.9
	10	3.0	0	5	3.0	3.7
		3.5	2.5	40–60	4.2	5.9
	11	3.0	0	5	3.0	3.7
		3.5	0 (1 min)	40–60	3.5	4.2
		3.5	5.0 (1 min)		6.9	7.5
	12	3.0	0	5	3.0	3.7
		3.5	0 (1 min)	40–60	3.5	4.2
		3.5	5.0 (2 min)		6.9	7.5

(Pollock ML, Schmidt D: Heart Disease and Rehabilitation, Chap. 25. New York, John Wiley & Sons, copyright © 1986. Reprinted by permission of John Wiley & Sons, Inc.)

Table 41-5. Five-Step Walk-Jog Program for Outpatients

STEP	SPEED (MPH)	ELEVATION (%)	DURATION (MIN)	METs	METs (AVERAGE/WORKOUT)	ENERGY EXPENDITURE (kcal/min)
1	3.0	0	5			3.7
	3.0 (1 min)	0		3.0		3.7
	5.5 (1 min)	0	30–40	8.3	6.5	12.0
2	3.0	0	5			3.7
	3.0 (1 min)	0		3.0		3.7
	5.5 (2 min)	0	30–40	8.3	7.24	12.0
3	3.0	0	5			3.7
	3.0 (1 min)	0		3.0		3.7
	5.5 (4 min)	0	30–40	8.3	7.5	12.0
4	3.0	0	5			3.7
	3.0 (1 min)	0		3.0		3.7
	5.5 (7 min)	0	30–40	8.3	7.7	12.0
5	3.0	0	5			3.7
	3.0 (1 min)	0		3.0		3.7
	5.5 (10 min)	0	30–40	8.3	7.8	12.0

Table 41-6. Sixteen-Step Walk and Walk-Jog Program for Cardiac Patients in Phase III (Community-Based or Home) Exercise Program

FUNCTIONAL CAPACITY (METs)	STEP	SPEED* (MPH)	DURATION (MIN)	METs	METs (AVERAGE/WORKOUT)	ENERGY EXPENDITURE (kcal/min)
5 METs	1	2.5	30–60	2.5	2.5	3.0
	2	3.0	30–60	3.0	3.0	3.7
	3	3.25	30–60	3.25	3.25	4.0
5–8 METs	4	3.5	30–60	3.5	3.5	4.2
	5	3.75	30–60	4.0	4.0	4.9
	6	4.0	30–60	4.6	4.6	5.5
8 METs	7	3.75 (2 min)	30–45	4.0	4.6	4.9
		5.0 (30 sec)		6.9		8.3
	8	3.75 (2 min)	30–45	4.0	5.0	4.9
		5.0 (1 min)		6.9		8.3
	9	3.75 (2 min)	30–45	4.0	5.5	4.9
		5.0 (2 min)		6.9		8.3
	10	3.75 (1 min)	30–45	4.0	6.0	4.9
		5.0 (2 min)		6.9		8.3
	11	3.75 (1 min)	30–45	4.0	6.3	4.9
		5.0 (4 min)		6.9		8.3
	12	3.75 (1 min)	30–45	4.0	6.5	4.9
		5.0 (6 min)		6.9		8.3
	13	3.75 (1 min)	30–45	4.0	6.6	4.9
		5.0 (8 min)		6.9		8.3
	14	3.75 (1 min)	30–45	4.0	6.6	4.9
		5.0 (10 min)		6.9		8.3
	15	3.75 (1 min)	30–45	4.0	7.9	4.9
		5.5 (10 min		8.3		10.1
	16	3.75 (1 min)	30–45	4.0	8.0	4.9
		5.5 (12 min)		8.3		10.1

*Two lines denote interval training; for example, in step 7, the patient will alternate 2 minutes of walking at 3.75 mph with 30 seconds of jogging at 5.0 mph.

(Pollock ML, Schmidt D: Heart Disease and Rehabilitation, Chap. 25. New York, John Wiley & Sons, copyright © 1986. Reprinted by permission of John Wiley & Sons, Inc.)

vascular disease. Each of these diagnoses requires an understanding of the underlying pathophysiology in order to establish an exercise program that is safe and effective. Each of these complications in itself is problematic, yet many patients have more than one of these underlying diagnoses.

Angina Pectoris

Many participants in rehabilitation programs have angina pectoris as a daily complication. Patients with stable angina are excellent candidates for exercise programs. The goal of physical conditioning for the patient with angina is to increase the amount of exercise performed before the onset of limiting angina. Patients must first be able to identify if the pain is true ischemic pain or musculoskeletal pain. With repeated episodes of angina associated with exertion, anxiety, and the like patients soon begin to distinguish the difference. Secondly, or concurrently, the patient must identify the location of the symptom. Often patients believe that anginal pain is crushing on the left side of the chest. However, it is known that anginal pain can be located in the area of the substernum, jaw, teeth, throat, interscapular area, elbow, arm, wrist, or epigastric area.

The anginal scale (Fig. 41-3) is beneficial in teaching patients to grade their anginal symptoms during exercise as well as assisting them in determining the proper exercise intensity to improve functional capacity. During the exercise session, angina intensities should not exceed a level of five on the scale. If discomfort exceeds a rating of six, exercise should stop. If pain is not resolved, nitroglycerin should be administered.

Anginal Scale

1. None at all
2. Extremely light
3. Very light
4. Quite light
5. Not so light, rather strong
6. Strong
7. Very strong
8. Extremely strong
9. Unbearable

Figure 41-3. Grading of anginal symptoms during exercise. (American College of Sports Medicine: Guidelines for Graded Exercise Testing and Exercise Prescription. London, Henry Kempton Publishers, 1980)

Many patients with angina experience the onset of symptoms with very low levels of exercise. Therefore, exercise intensity for these patients should be set just below the angina threshold. As conditioning occurs, the onset of angina will appear at higher levels of exercise intensity. Many patients use nitroglycerin either before or during exercise as a means of sustaining the aerobic period of exercise for a longer time. In some instances patients may be identified as having a phenomenon called "walk-through angina." These patients describe the onset of pain at low levels of exercise that disappears with further increments of exercise intensity. Terminating the exercise session for such patients at the onset of pain would retard the ability to improve functional capacity. However, care should be taken in identifying and monitoring these patients during the aerobic phase of their exercise prescription.

Many patients with angina are also pharmacologically managed by beta blockers or calcium-channel blockers. For these patients exercise prescription based on heart rate is ineffective; however, accurate exercise intensity levels can be prescribed if the Borg scale is used in conjunction with the angina scale.

The exercise session for patients with angina should begin with a prolonged warm-up period. This period allows for vasodilation in the skeletal muscles and prepares the cardiac muscle for the aerobic phase. Patients with severe angina may benefit from intermittent exercise until sufficient stamina for sustained exercise is achieved. Proper breathing while exercising is critical for all persons, but especially for patients with angina. Patients who tend to hold their breath while exercising produce a valsalva maneuver, which causes an increase in intrathoracic pressure and may bring angina to a threshold with very little activity. When the discomfort gets to the level of five or six on the angina scale, the exercise intensity should be decreased until the discomfort subsides. Once the patient feels recovered, the exercise intensity can be resumed. As training occurs, patients will begin to exercise for longer durations before having to decrease the intensity. Concomitantly, the recovery periods will be shorter and shorter. The cool-down period should be gradual and prolonged. Patients should feel totally recovered before adjourning to the locker room. Prolonged bouts of angina during exercise that do not subside with a reduction in activity or by the use of nitroglycerin should receive immediate medical attention.

Patients with Pacemakers

Patients who have rhythm disturbances or conduction aberrations are often treated with pacemakers. Exercise prescription for these patients requires a knowledge of the individual's heart rate, blood pressure, and symptom response to exercise. An understanding of the conduction disturbance and the pacemaker type and programming are also important.

The specific problem posed by pacemakers during exercise is the rate-emitted response to increased activity. Exercise prescription should be based on the results of a graded exercise test along with blood pressure levels and the RPE response to increments of exercise intensity. Patients with pacemakers can engage in most training activities appropriate for their functional capacity and underlying heart disease. Care should be taken to avoid excessive arm and shoulder movements. The American College of Sports Medicine (ACSM) guidelines for exercise prescription may be followed for these patients. Intensity should be monitored by using systolic blood pressure response as a guideline.

Chronic Ventricular Failure

Patients with chronic ventricular failure are often severely limited by shortness of breath, angina, and fatigue. These symptoms are largely the result of elevated pulmonary venous pressure, inadequate rise in cardiac output during exercise, and reduced vasodilating capacity in the active extremities. Although these patients are often poor candidates for exercise programs, training may improve skeletal muscle adaptation, may reduce cardiac output requirements for any given level of work, and thereby improve $\dot{V}O_2$ at submaximal levels. However, the potential benefits and role of exercise training in management of patients with chronic congestive failure is still conflicting. What is known, is that peripheral deconditioning and severe limitation of activity is detrimental to functional capacity. Therefore, very low-level intermittent activity is prescribed for these patients. The training effect on heart rate, blood pressure, and subjective improvement in function can be seen. The best monitoring tool for these patients besides ECG telemetry is blood pressure measurement. For most of these patients, the resting levels of the systolic and diastolic pressures are increased. As they begin to exercise and systolic pressure increases, a concomitant increase occurs in diastolic pressure in an effort to assist with the increase in work demand. However, if as the exercise continues the diastolic pressure begins to fall, this is a definite sign that the failing ventricle is unable to keep up with the exercise intensity.

Systemic Hypertension

The effect of exercise training on the management of systemic hypertension is a function of the severity of the cardiac and vascular disease. For patients with mild hypertension, exercise has been shown to reduce heart rate, cardiac output, and blood pressure both at rest and during exercise. However, when formulating the prescription of exercise for these patients, care must be taken to avoid the generation of high and potentially harmful systemic arterial pressure during exercise. It should be kept in mind that mean arterial pressure increases during both dynamic and isometric exercise; however, during dynamic exercise a rise in systolic blood pressure will occur, whereas during isometric exercise a concomitant increase in diastolic pressure will also occur.

Today, most hypertensive patients are managed with pharmacological agents. Many of these drugs may alter the acute and chronic response to exercise; therefore, it is imperative to be familiar with the physiological alterations produced by these agents when prescribing exercise for patients with hypertension.

Peripheral Vascular Disease

Patients with significant peripheral vascular disease (PVD) are at a much higher risk of having associated coronary and cerebral vascular disease than those without peripheral impairment. The aerobic capacity of the exercising limbs of these patients may be limited by fixed obstruction in the arterial circulation of the exercising extremity rather than by the reduced regional vasodilatory capacity or the inability to augment cardiac output. For these patients, the obstruction manifests itself in the form of claudication pain. Aerobic activity for these patients cannot be maintained for long periods. Short intervals of intense exercise for 10 to 20 minutes, followed by lower levels of activity, are usually achievable. Activities should include walking, stationary bicycling, or pool activities. The beneficial effects of training on the exercise capacity of PVD patients may be limited by the development of claudication pain at low levels of exercise intensity. Studies have shown that for these patients, upper-extremity exercises concomitant with leg work (rowing) serve as a good adjunct to training.

EXERCISE PRESCRIPTION FOR PATIENTS WITH PULMONARY DISEASE

Exercise programs in the form of pulmonary rehabilitation have become a widely accepted mode of treatment for patients with pulmonary dysfunction. Although the phases of pulmonary rehabilitation are not defined in precisely the same manner as cardiac rehabilitation, the intent is inherently similar in terms of progression, education, and life-style alterations. The inpatient phase, Phase I, of pulmonary rehabilitation is commonly referred to as chest physical therapy. The patients in this phase are usually acutely ill with documented pulmonary disease or with pulmonary complications caused by disease, trauma or surgery. Phase II is the active rehabilitation period, which may begin prior to discharge and continue through the home program phase. This phase usually includes exercises coordinated with breathing exercises and a moderate walking program. Phase III is the outpatient rehabilitation phase, which includes supervised conditioning and maintenance, education, and life-style alterations.

Management of the patient with pulmonary disease requires an understanding of the pathophysiology of the disease, the psychological impact of symptoms and limitations, as well as the effectiveness of the treatments prescribed. To facilitate the resolution of pulmonary problems, most physical therapy treatments are performed to improve ventilation and increase oxygenation; decrease oxygen consumption; improve secretion clearance; and maximize exercise tolerance for the patient with either acute or chronic pulmonary disease. Limitations as a result of acute exacerbations can significantly influence progression. Close monitoring of patients' shortness of breath, heart rate, pallor, or RPE responses will assist in establishing a safe and effective program.

Phase I Inpatient Exercise Programs

Patients in Phase I are generally recovering from a pulmonary insult or pulmonary complication and may be initially intubated and ventilated.

Positioning techniques and breathing exercises are the two therapeutic exercises administered during this time to increase ventilation and oxygenation. Research indicates that pos-

tural changes (prone, supine, lateral) may alleviate dyspnea while physiologically improving arterial oxygenation. Breathing exercises appear to influence the rate, depth, and distribution of ventilation or the muscular activity associated with breathing. The breathing exercise most commonly prescribed is diaphragmatic breathing.

Diaphragmatic breathing exercises appear to enhance diaphragmatic descent during inspiration and diaphragmatic ascent during expiration. If done properly, these exercises alleviate dyspnea, reduce the work of breathing, and improve ventilation and oxygenation. As patients become more stable they are gradually taught a program of bronchopulmonary hygiene that includes postural drainage, percussion, vibration, shaking, and coughing. If done correctly and consistently, successful clearance of secretions can be maintained. This is the primary goal or objective during this phase.

Preoperative and postoperative chest physical therapy services have become a routine adjunct to surgical management. Any patient undergoing surgery that requires general anesthesia is at risk for postoperative complications. Anesthesia, surgery, pain, and trauma interfere with normal breathing patterns and cause a decrease in respiratory drive, a depressed cough reflex, and an increase in mucus pooling. Patients with documented cardiac or pulmonary disease as well as those whose conditions affect pulmonary reserves are at the greatest risk of pulmonary complications after surgery. For these patients, the physiological effects of inactivity (bed rest) postoperatively may cause a decrease in efficiency of the use of oxygen, muscle weakness, and an increased energy expenditure for a given activity. The goals of preoperative and postoperative physical therapy are as follows: (1) promote pulmonary hygiene; (2) maintain range of motion; (3) prevent venous stasis; (4) modify pain; and (5) provide patient education in an effort to decrease anxiety.

Preoperative patient assessments include chart review, patient interview, and physical assessment. The physical assessment includes observation, palpation, auscultation, percussion, and range of motion. A standard postoperative treatment is demonstrated with the patient. Rolling, positioning for bronchial drainage, percussion, vibration, and splinted coughing are practiced.

Postoperative patient assessment will determine the aggressiveness needed to achieve pulmonary hygiene. This assessment can be performed when it has been determined that the patient is stable enough to tolerate treatment.

No formula exists for treating postoperative pulmonary patients. Treatments may be very short or last up to an hour. It may be very aggressive, involving many chest physical therapy modalities or it may include only breathing exercises. These factors are determined by thorough assessment, patient tolerance, or hospital protocol.

Phase II Outpatient Programs

Phase II is the active rehabilitative period, which may begin prior to discharge and continue at home as a home program. During this period, in addition to bronchopulmonary hygiene, patients are learning how to deal with dyspnea on exertion. Most patients refrain from activity out of fear and discomfort. However, continued inactivity will further decrease exercise tolerance. During exercise, the work of breathing in pulmonary patients constitutes a major portion of oxygen consumption. Patients are instructed in relaxation exercises that will reduce general body work. Once patients have mastered relaxation exercises in a sitting or supine position, they proceed to performing these activities while standing and eventually while ambulating. The forward-leaning posture position for sitting, standing, and walking is also recommended in conjunction with relaxation exercises to reduce work. A moderate walking program (such as the one outlined in Table 41-4) gives the patient the opportunity to coordinate exercise with breathing exercises. Lastly, patients are shown how to apply the above principles in an effort to modify their activities of daily living (ADL) and eventually the work environment. For instance, if patients become dyspneic while standing and shaving, a forward seated position on a high seat will eliminate the unnecessary work done to stand erect.

Phase III Pulmonary Rehabilitation

Phase III of pulmonary rehabilitation continues to encourage a comprehensive multidisciplinary program. The exercise component is only one segment of the total program and is based upon the results of the pulmonary stress test and goals related to functional improvement. Prior to commencing an exercise program, efforts should be made to improve airway clearance. Postural drainage and positioning to clear secretions are useful for patients with chronic obstructive pulmonary disease (COPD) followed by coughing and huffing. Positioning, vigorous percussion, deep breathing, and shaking for 10 minutes may adequately clear the airways for effective ventilation yet does not tax the patient so as to impede the aerobic period.

Supportive Oxygen Use

The use of supportive oxygen with exercise continues to be conflicting for pulmonary patients. Studies have demonstrated that with supplemental oxygen greater exercise intensities and durations are performed with lower respiratory rate, exercise minute ventilation, and $\dot{V}O_2$. However, other studies refute these findings. The issue of concern here is how low the levels of oxygen saturation should be before supplementary oxygen is required. Consensus does exist in that when the desaturation is below 85%, supplemental oxygen is commonly used during exercise with COPD patients.

SPECIAL CONSIDERATIONS FOR EXERCISE PRESCRIPTION

The exercise prescription must be individualized in accordance with the patient's degree of respiratory dysfunction. The most difficult parameter to establish for these patients is the exercise intensity. The American College of Sports Medicine (ACSM) guidelines for healthy persons recommend training intensity at levels of approximately 60% of functional capacity. However, as a result of impaired ventilatory capacity, most pulmonary patients are not able to train at intensities even close to anaerobic threshold. Therefore, intensities as low as 20% to 40% of $\dot{V}O_{2\ max}$ may be prescribed. Prescriptions based on heart rate or perceived exertion are viable options for these patients. Belman and Wasserman (1982) have described the mechanisms by which patients with pulmonary disease appear to achieve higher heart rates with low levels of exercise. Therefore, symptom-limited heart rate can easily be used along with frequency and duration for establishing a safe and effective prescription for training. For pulmonary patients who can only achieve one to two minutes of the aerobic intensity, intermittent exercise with gradual lengthening of the aerobic period is effective. The frequency for this minimal level of activity may be prescribed four times a day. As the length of the aerobic period increases, then the frequency may be decreased. The mode of activity used for training should be identified by the patient because compliance is highly dependent upon the patient's selection.

Warm-up and cool-down periods are essential for any exercise regimen. For this group of patients, rhythmic upper-extremity exercises along with trunk rotation will improve thoracic mobility. These exercises coordinated with controlled relaxation of the shoulder girdle are essential. Reasonable goals of exercise training in such patients include (1) decrease in breathlessness and therefore an improved tolerance of low-level exercise; and (2) prevention of the physiologic hazards of inactivity. A study by Nicholas and co-workers (1970) suggested that improved motivation and willingness to tolerate dyspnea, rather than true physiologic adaptations, accounted for training-induced improvement in these patients. Another approach to reducing the symptom of breathlessness in pulmonary patients has been the attempt to train respiratory muscles aerobically. This theory is based on the fact that the aerobic capacity of the ventilatory muscles independently contributes to limited ventilatory and aerobic exercise capacity. Stubbing (1980) explains that in normal subjects the requirement of the respiratory muscles during exercise represents only a small portion of the total $\dot{V}O_2$ and is not a factor that limits exercise performance. However, in patients with airway disease a disproportionate increase occurs in ventilation at a given work load. Therefore, the greater metabolic requirement of the respiratory muscles accounts for a proportionately larger total $\dot{V}O_2$, thus leaving a smaller reserve for the working skeletal muscle of the limbs. This finding suggests that patients improve functionally by using trained ventilatory muscles to counterbalance the increased work of breathing, resulting in a decrease in the frequency of exacerbation and decompensation. Further investigation of the role of respiratory muscle training is necessary.

Additional special considerations for exercise prescription are given to patients with the following: pulmonary hypertension, cystic fibrosis, COPD, exercise-induced asthma, and congestive heart failure.

Each of these diagnoses requires an understanding of the underlying pathophysiology to establish an exercise program that is safe and effective. Each of these complications in itself is problematic, yet many patients have both pulmonary and cardiac complications in combination with other underlying diagnoses.

Pulmonary Hypertension

Patients with known pulmonary hypertension or those whose arterial tension is less than or equal to 50 mm Hg at rest generally require oxygen supplementation for initial testing and subsequent training. For these patients, reduction of oxygen demand is the key to successful endurance improvement. Strategies for reduction of oxygen demand may include reduction in the work of breathing through breathing exercises, postural alterations to reduce accessory movements that may cause increased oxygen demands, and relaxation exercises that may help to eliminate work extraneous to the prescribed activity. The exercise session should begin with prolonged warm-up in order to allow the patient to slowly accommodate to the increase in oxygen demand. Concentration on breathing exercises while exercising will assist with the periods of dyspnea. Dyspnea is not a reason for stopping exercise. Cutting back on the exercise intensity while concentrating on breathing exercises and relaxation will help the dyspnea to dissipate. Conditioning occurs very slowly in the pulmonary patient, and the onset of dyspnea is not delayed with improved functional capacity, as angina onset is delayed in conditioning with coronary patients.

Cystic Fibrosis

The chronic pulmonary dysfunction in cystic fibrosis (CF) is related to increased secretion of abnormally viscous mucus, impaired mucociliary transport resulting in airway obstruction, overinflation, and infection. This disease requires postural drainage and breathing exercises. The frequency of these treatments is dependent upon the pulmonary involvement. Physical activities such as swimming and jogging are appropriate for these patients. Warm-up and cool-down sessions should include slow rhythmic stretching that includes the trunk musculature. The aerobic period should be kept at moderate intensities so as to keep periods of dyspnea at a minimum. Research has shown that physical activity designed to improve exercise tolerance helps patients with CF to mobilize secretions as well as improve body image.

Chronic Obstructive Pulmonary Disease

Patients with mild to moderate COPD may improve exercise capacity with an intermittent walk/jog or jogging program without producing significant hypoxia or arrhythmias. The warm-up sessions should include rhythmic bending and stretching exercises, trunk twisting, and side bends. Initially, the aerobic period should use progressive walking on the treadmill. The treadmill allows speed and elevation to be used for increasing exercise intensity while monitoring heart rate and oxygen saturation. For patients with moderate to severe COPD, a bicycle ergometer should be used to improve functional capacity. The ergometer allows for total body support, thereby

reducing oxygen consumption while training. Warm-up for these patients should include alternating upper-extremity exercise with walking in place. Supplemental oxygen may be used in an effort to sustain the activities long enough to obtain a mild training effect. Saturation measured by ear oximetry and heart rate should be monitored throughout the session.

Exercise-Induced Asthma

Exercise-induced asthma (EIA) or exercise-induced bronchoconstriction (EIB) develops after strenuous exercise in patients with asthma or hay fever. Exercise-induced asthma usually occurs after five to eight minutes of exercise, depending on the type of exercise. Medications prescribed for EIA include corticosteroids, mediator release inhibitors, sympathomimetics, and bronchodilators. The dosage depends upon the individual patient, the activity level, and the type of activity. Training programs for asthmatics should include good warm-up and cool-down periods consisting of stretching, flexibility, and breathing exercises. Initially, the aerobic phase should consist of intermittent activities of five-minutes' duration. It is not uncommon for some asthmatics to experience a temporary increase in wheezing episodes when starting a program. Recent findings have demonstrated that the severity of bronchoconstriction following exercise is decreased if the air is humidified.

Congestive Heart Failure

Patients with significant congestive heart failure should not receive bronchial drainage in the Trendelenburg position. Experience has shown that these persons have increased respiratory distress and cardiac arrhythmias while reclining with the head lower than the feet. This position increases venous return to the failing heart and can produce an increased amount of pulmonary edema. Patients with congestive heart failure should be treated in the horizontal position rather than in the Trendelenburg position. After their cardiac status improves, they can often tolerate the standard bronchial drainage positions.

ANNOTATED BIBLIOGRAPHY

American College of Sports Medicine: Guidelines for Graded Exercise Testing and Exercise Prescription. London, Henry Kempton, 1980 (An excellent handbook on the principles of exercise prescription by the field's leading investigators.)

Andreoli K, Fowkes F, Zipes D et al: Comprehensive Cardiac Care: A Text for Nurses, Physicians, and Other Health Practitioners. St Louis, CV Mosby, 1987 (A thorough overview of all aspects of cardiac care for health professionals.)

Belman MJ, Wasserman K: Exercise training and testing in patients with chronic obstructive pulmonary disease. American Thoracic Society 10(2):38, 1982 (Landmark study of the effect and role of exercise and testing in the management of pulmonary disease patients.)

Casciari R, Fairshtu R, Harrison A: Effects of breathing retraining in patients with chronic obstructive pulmonary disease. Chest 79(4):393, 1981 (A descriptive study of the effects of external load on respiratory muscle training. Results support ventilatory muscle training.)

Clausen J: Circulatory adjustments to dynamic exercise and effect of physical training in normal subjects and in patients with coronary artery disease. Prog Cardiovasc Dis 18:459, 1976 (A classic study demonstrating the hemodynamic effects of exercise on normal persons and cardiac patients.)

Fardy PS, Bennett JL, Reitz NL et al: Cardiac Rehabilitation. St Louis, CV Mosby, 1980 (A classic and well-done handbook on cardiac rehabilitation.)

Gutman MC, Squires RW, Pollock ML et al: Perceived exertion heart-rate relationship during exercise testing and training in cardiac patients. J Cardiac Rehabil 1:52, 1981 (A well-designed study demonstrating the use of perceived exertion in exercise testing as well as training.)

Nicholas J, Gilbert R, Auchincloss J: Evaluation of exercise therapy program for patients with chronic obstructive pulmonary disease. Am Rev Respir Dis 102:1, 1970 (A study that evaluates both the physiological and psychological adaptations of training in pulmonary disease.)

Pandolf KB: Advances in the study and application of perceived exertion. In Terjung RL (ed): Exercise Sports Science Review, Vol II, pp 118–158. Philadelphia, The Franklin Institute Press, 1983 (Historical perspective as well as a current update of the applicability of perceived exertion in exercise testing and training.)

Pollock ML, Schmidt D: Heart Disease and Rehabilitation. New York, John Wiley & Sons, 1986 (Sample cardiac rehabilitation programs for Phase I, II, and III as well as documentation of the interchangeability of RPE ratings and percentages of $\dot{V}O_2$.)

Stubbing D, Pengelly L, Morse J et al: Pulmonary mechanics during exercise in subjects with chronic obstruction. J Appl Physiol 49:511, 1980 (A comparison of requirements of the respiratory muscles during exercise in normal subjects versus COPD patients.)

Wasserman K, McElory MB: Detecting threshold of anaerobic metabolism. Am J Cardiol 14:844, 1964 (A useful and well-documented methodology for measuring the physiological parameter of anaerobic threshold.)

42

Interventions in Cardiac and Cardiopulmonary Transplants

H. STEVEN SADOWSKY

Physical therapists are active participants in the rehabilitation of cardiac and cardiopulmonary transplant patients. The purpose of this chapter is to provide physical therapists with information about the terminology, pathophysiology, medications, and procedures most commonly encountered in the care of cardiac and cardiopulmonary transplant patients.

CANDIDACY CRITERIA

The primary criterion for a patient to receive a cardiac or cardiopulmonary transplantation is the presence of end-stage disease commensurate with the Class IV criteria of the New York Heart Association classification of cardiac disability and an estimated prognosis for survival limited to weeks or months. The disease process cannot be remedied by other standard forms of medical or surgical treatment. Specific criteria for cardiac transplantation recipients are presented in Table 42-1. The additional criteria for cardiopulmonary transplantation are presented in Table 42-2.

OPERATIVE PROCEDURES

CARDIAC TRANSPLANTATION

The donor heart is removed through a midline sternotomy by first ligating and dividing the superior vena cava (SVC) immediately below the entrance of the azygos vein and then ligating and dividing the inferior vena cava (IVC).

Table 42-1. Candidacy Criteria for Cardiac Transplantation

1. Age less than 50 years
2. Pulmonary artery mean pressure less than 40 mm Hg
3. Pulmonary vascular resistance less than 10 Wood units
4. No severe renal or hepatic dysfunction secondary to cardiac decompensation
5. No evidence of active infection
6. No evidence of recent or unresolved pulmonary infarction
7. No diabetes mellitus requiring insulin control
8. No active peptic-ulcer disease
9. Ability to comply with the protocol

(Sadowsky HS, Rohrkemper KF, Quon SYM: Rehabilitation of Cardiac and Cardiopulmonary Recipients: An Introduction for Physical and Occupational Therapists, 3rd ed, p 1. Stanford, CA, Stanford University Hospital, 1986. Used with permission.)

Table 42-2. Candidacy Criteria for Cardiopulmonary Transplantation

1. Close size matching of recipient and donor (to approximate lung volumes)
2. Clear chest roentgenogram
3. PaO_2 greater than 400 mm Hg on 100% oxygen
4. Good lung compliance (peak inspiratory pressure less than 25 cm H_2O, at normal tidal volume)
5. Pulmonary secretions are not grossly infected

(Sadowsky HS, Rohrkemper KF, Quon SYM: Rehabilitation of Cardiac and Cardiopulmonary Recipients: An Introduction for Physical and Occupational Therapists, 3rd ed, p 1. Stanford, CA, Stanford University Hospital, 1986. Used with permission.)

The aorta is transected at the origin of the innominate artery and the pulmonary artery is transected at its bifurcation. The pulmonary veins are divided individually at their pericardial reflections. The dissected heart is immersed in saline at 3° to 4°C.

Following median sternotomy and central cannulation of the vena cavae and the aorta, the recipient is placed on the cardiopulmonary bypass machine. The aorta is crossed-clamped and the great vessels are divided at the commissures of the semilunar valves. The atria are transected above their atrioventricular grooves, but posterior to the atrial appendages, and the recipient's heart is removed.

The donor left atrium is opened via connecting incisions through the pulmonary veins and anastomosed to the recipient's left atrial remnant. After ligation of the donor's superior vena cava, the right atrium is anastomosed, starting from the lower end of the interatrial septum. Donor and recipient aortas are then joined. Finally, the pulmonary arteries are anastomosed (Fig. 42-1). The patient is weaned from the cardiopulmonary bypass machine after initiation of an isoproterenol infusion to keep the heart rate between 100 and 110 beats per minute (chronotropic and inotropic effects of isoproterenol increase cardiac output). Two

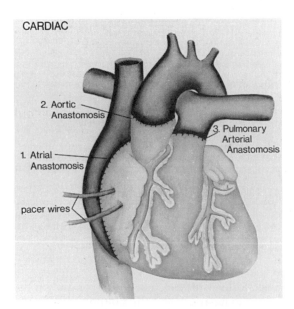

Figure 42-1. The transplanted heart *(light)* following anastomosis to the recipient's atrial remnant and great vessels *(dark)*. Atrial pacing wires are shown in the right atrium.

temporary pacing wires are placed in the right atrium, and the chest is then closed with mediastinal drainage tubes in place.

CARDIOPULMONARY TRANSPLANTATION

The donor heart and lungs are removed through a median sternotomy by dissecting the vena cavae and aorta as for a cardiac transplantation. The trachea is transected above the carina and the heart/lung bloc is placed in saline at 3° to 4°C.

The recipient is placed on the cardiopulmonary bypass machine following sternotomy and pericardectomy. The phrenic nerves are preserved. The heart is removed, leaving a portion of the posterior right atrium in place. Prior to its division, the left bronchus is stapled to minimize the risk of contaminating the surgical field. The left lung is then excised and removed. Following removal of the right lung, remnants of the pulmonary artery are eliminated with the exception of a small segment left in place in the region of the ductus ligament to preserve recurrent laryngeal nerve function. Finally, the trachea is exposed in the midline and divided just above the carina; remnants of the main bronchi are then removed.

Transplantation is started with the anastomosis of the donor and recipient tracheae. Then, the ascending aortae are joined and the right atria are anastomosed (Fig. 42-2).

COMPLICATIONS

Infection accounts for the majority of post-transplantation deaths (60%), followed by acute rejection (18%), atherosclerosis (11%), and malignancy (5%) (Sadowsky, Rohrkemper, and Quon). The most serious infections are bacterial and/or fungal pulmonary infections (lung involvement has been present in 65% of all infectious complications).

Just as blood cells are "typed" to prevent the recipient's reaction to the donor's cells, tissues are also typed to help prevent graft rejection. More than 25 HLA antigens (considered to be the most important antigens that can

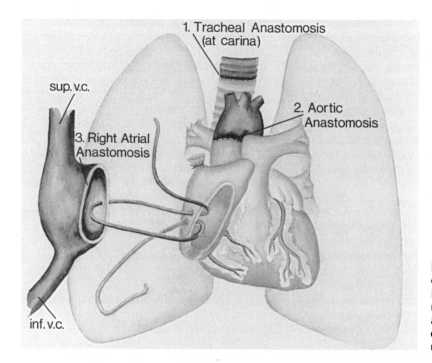

Figure 42-2. Transplantation of the heart-lung bloc. Following tracheal and aortic anastomosis, the donor (*light*) right atrium is sutured to the recipient's (*dark*) right atrial remnant.

cause rejection) have been identified. However, the specific genes responsible for them can only code for four of the antigens in any one person. By determining the genetic locus of these antigens in the sera of the donor and recipient, tissues can be matched for compatibility. Because there are so many possibilities, however, exact matching is almost impossible. Fortunately, not all of the HLA antigens are severely antigenic (Guyton). Cardiac transplant recipients have a high risk of developing accelerated graft atherosclerosis, particularly when graft donors are older than 35 years, or if a mismatch of human lymphocyte antigen has occurred at the A2 locus (Bieber and co-workers).

Long-term immunosuppressive therapy has been associated with lymphoproliferative malignancy (Penn). Lymphoma seems most likely to develop in patients with idiopathic cardiomyopathy, especially if the patient is younger than 20 years.

A large percentage of transplant recipients develop significant hypertension as a result of their cyclosporine regimen.

SURVIVAL STATISTICS

One-year survival rates have dramatically improved since the onset of the clinical transplantation program, primarily due to improved survival during the first three postoperative months. For the 28 children (under 18 years old) who have received transplants at Stanford University Medical Center, one-year survival has been 96%. Five-year survival rates have improved from 18% to approximately 60%. When compared to a six-month survival rate of less than 5% for patients selected for transplantation but for whom no donor organ became available, the therapeutic efficacy of cardiac transplantation is undeniable. Furthermore, in a study of transplant recipients (at least six months postoperatively), 89% of the recipients indicated a good to excellent quality of life (Lough).

IMMUNOSUPPRESSION

In addition to damaging the myocardial cell wall, it is believed that immune injury to the intima of the coronary arteries results in the aggregation and activation of platelets, promoting the proliferation and migration of myointimal cells through the elastic lamina, thus facilitating lipid deposition (Fig. 42-3). Therefore, transplant patients require vigorous pharmacological therapy to prevent graft rejection and atherosclerotic changes. Although other agents may be used at specific times in the immunosuppressive regimen, the primary immunosuppressants are cyclosporine, prednisone, and azathioprine.

IMMUNOSUPPRESSIVE AGENTS

1. *Cyclosporine* is a fungal metabolite that inhibits T-lymphocyte activity. It is taken by mouth in water, juice, or chocolate milk at 12-hour intervals. Known side-effects include tremoring, headache, hypertension, swelling and tenderness of the gums, diarrhea (related to the olive oil base), kidney or liver dysfunction, hirsutism, development of fibrous tissue in the breasts, increased susceptibility to viral infection, and malignant tumors.

2. *Prednisone* is a glucocorticoid substance that increases protein catabolism, thus decreasing the use of amino acids for protein synthesis and converting them to glucose. The resultant elevation of blood glucose levels triggers insulin release and induces lipogenesis and fat redistribution. Prednisone interferes with histamine synthesis, thus increasing capillary permeability in response to tissue trauma, and inhibits the release of proteolytic enzymes by stabilizing cell membranes. By inhibiting ACTH release, prednisone suppresses adrenocortical activity and antagonizes the effects of vitamin D in calcium absorption. The side-effects are usually dose and duration dependent and may include: euphoria, insomnia, hypertension, congestive heart failure, cataracts, peptic ulcer, increased appetite, gastrointestinal irritability, hypokalemia, hyperglycemia, carbohydrate intolerance, acne, delayed wound healing, muscle weakness, hirsutism, and adrenal insufficiency.

   Withdrawal symptoms may include fatigue, arthralgia, dizziness, depression, fever, and fainting.

3. *Azathioprine* (Imuran) interferes with normal utilization of purine by the cell, thus inhibiting DNA synthesis. Dosage is dependent upon white blood cell count. The side-effects may include: leukopenia, bone marrow suppression, nausea, vomiting, anorexia, mouth ulceration, jaundice, hepatotoxicity, rash, arthralgia, and muscle wasting.

4. *Prednisolone,* an analogue of hydrocortisone, is given intravenously during episodes of acute rejection to augment immunosuppression (see *Prednisone* for actions and possible side-effects).

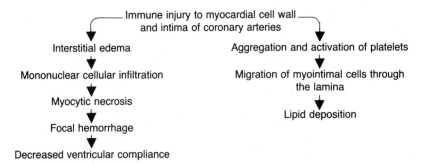

Figure 42-3. Cascade of events leading to graft rejection or atherosclerosis as a result of immune injury to the transplanted heart. (Reprinted by permission of Department of Physical and Occupational Therapy, Stanford University Hospital, Stanford, CA)

5. *Antithymocyte globulin* (ATG) suppresses peripheral blood T-helper cells and total T cells. ATG of equine origin may be given intravenously for the first week postoperatively depending on the particular immunosuppression regimen to which the patient is assigned. During episodes of severe rejection or in the first three postoperative days for heart-lung recipients, ATG of rabbit origin may be given intravenously or by intramuscular injection into the quadriceps muscle. The side-effects may include erythema and swelling around the injection site, leg pain and cramps, and flu-like aching in the joints.

6. *Orthoclone OKT3* (Muromonab-CD3) is believed to react with and block the function of a dalton molecule that is located in T-cell membranes and associated with antigen recognition and signal transduction. It has also been shown to block the generation and function of T-effector cells, thus blocking all known T cell functions. Limited data regarding retreatment with Orthoclone OKT3 are available, but detectable antibodies to this agent have been found in most patients and this could limit its efficacy for readministration.

REJECTION

Generally, four grades of rejection exist (Sadowsky, Rohrkemper, and Quon). These are no rejection, mild rejection, moderate rejection with myocyte necrosis, and severe rejection with myocyte necrosis and hemorrhage.

Mild or moderate rejection is unassociated with any reliable clinical symptomatology. Severe rejection was historically heralded by reduced work capacity, a decrease in myocardial voltage on the electrocardiogram, and the development of an atrial gallop rhythm. However, these clinical signs may be masked or absent in patients treated with cyclosporine. Therefore, a transvenous right ventricular endomyocardial biopsy must be performed to diagnose and confirm the severity of graft rejection.

In most cases, mild rejection is not treated, but observed closely and followed by rebiopsy in three to four days. Moderate and severe rejection are usually treated initially with a daily intravenous infusion of steroids for three days. Rebiopsy is performed one to two days after the final dose. If indicated by the results of the biopsy, a second pulsed course of steroids is given.

If rejection is very severe, or is unremitting to steroid therapy, ATG is given by intramuscular injection or by intravenous infusion. Physical therapists provide therapeutic ultrasound treatments following intramuscular ATG injections. Ultrasound is given for its phonophoretic effect and for symptomatic relief of pain associated with localized muscle spasm due to an inflammatory reaction at the site of ATG injection.

GENERAL PHARMACOLOGICAL REGIMEN

Antihypertensives, diuretics, and a few miscellaneous medications are prescribed to counteract the untoward reactions to immunotherapy. The most often used pharmacologic agents are listed below.

ANTIHYPERTENSIVES

1. *Prazosin hydrochloride* (Minipress) relaxes the arteriolar and venous smooth muscle. The side-effects may' include: dizziness, headache, drowsiness, depression, palpitations, orthostatic hypotension, blurred vision, dry mouth, nausea, vomiting, diarrhea, and constipation.

2. *Methyldopa* (Aldomet) alters the sympathetic outflow by stimulating the alpha adrenergic receptors of the vascular smooth muscle. The side-effects may include hemolytic anemia, headache, sedation, weakness, dizziness, reduced mental activity, bradycardia, myocarditis, edema, weight gain, orthostatic hypotension, dry mouth, nasal stuffiness, diarrhea, and hepatic necrosis.

3. *Captopril* inhibits angiotensin-converting enzyme, thus preventing pulmonary conversion of angiotensin I to angiotensin II. The side-effects may include leukopenia, agranulocytosis, dizziness, fainting, tachycardia, hypotension, loss of taste, renal failure, proteinuria, anorexia, and rash.

DIURETICS

1. *Hydrochlorothiazide* inhibits sodium reabsorption in the ascending part of Henle's loop. The side-effects may include agranulocytosis, aplastic anemia, dehydration, orthostatic hypotension, nausea, anorexia, hepatic encephalopathy, hypokalemia, hyperglycemia, hyperuricemia (asymptomatic), dilutional fluid/electrolyte imbalances, dermatitis, photosensitivity, and rash.
2. *Furosemide* (Lasix) inhibits reabsorption of sodium and chloride at the proximal portion of the ascending part of Henle's loop. The side-effects may include agranulocytosis, dehydration, orthostatic hypotension, transient deafness (associated with too rapid an infusion), abdominal discomfort, hypokalemia, hypochloremic alkalosis, dilutional electrolyte/fluid imbalances, and dermatitis.
3. *Mannitol* increases the osmotic pressure of the glomerular filtrate, inhibiting reabsorption of water and electrolytes. The side-effects may include rebound increase in intracranial pressure, headache, angina-like chest pain, tachycardia, plasma volume expansion (transient), blurred vision, rhinitis, thirst, nausea, vomiting, urinary retention, fluid/electrolyte imbalances, and cellular dehydration.

MISCELLANEOUS

1. *Dipyridamole* (Persantin) inhibits platelet binding and adhesion. The side-effects may include headache, dizziness, weakness, hypotension, fainting, nausea, vomiting, diarrhea, and rash.
2. *Docusate sodium* (Colace) softens the stool by reducing the surface tension of the interfacing liquid contents in the bowel. The side-effects may include throat irritation, bitter taste, abdominal cramping, and diarrhea.
3. *Potassium chloride* (K-Lor, Slow-K) replaces potassium in cases of hypokalemia. The side-effects, which may be attributable to a resultant hyperkalemia, include paresthesias, confusion, weakness, peripheral vascular collapse, cardiac arrhythmia, ECG changes (prolonged PR interval, wide QRS complex, ST segment depression), nausea, vomiting, abdominal pain, diarrhea, oliguria, pallor, and cold skin.
4. *Calcium carbonate* (Titralac) elevates gastric *p*H, reduces pepsin activity, strengthens the gastric mucosal barrier, and increases esophageal sphincter tone. The side-effects may include constipation, nausea, flatulence, and hypercalcemia.
5. *Nystatin* (Mycostatin) acts as an antifungal antibiotic by altering cell permeability and allowing leakage of intracellular contents (probably by binding to sterols in the fungal cell membrane). The side-effects may include diarrhea, nausea, and vomiting.

EXERCISE RESPONSE OF THE DENERVATED HEART

On the ECG, the transplant recipient exhibits two P waves. One is produced by the recipient's sinoatrial node; the other by the donor's sinoatrial node. The recipient's sinoatrial node increases its rate of depolarization normally in anticipation of exertion, but this increase is unassociated with a QRS complex because the depolarization wave is not conducted across the scar line of the anastomosis. The donor sinoatrial node is responsible for the ensuing QRS complex, but, because it lacks innervation, does not produce anticipatory changes in heart rate in response to sudden increases in demand.

Isometric exercise is known to increase systemic blood pressure in normal adults independently of the size of the muscle mass

Table 42-3. Postoperative Activity End-Point Guidelines

The following guidelines are suggested end points to continued activity. They are quite broad, and must, therefore, not become dictates that usurp your clinical judgments.

1. Resting heart rate greater than 120 beats per minute (bpm), or unusual heart rate increase (ie, greater than 20 to 30 bpm increase over baseline)
2. Systolic blood pressure increase greater than 40 mm Hg, or a decrease of more than 15 mm Hg from baseline
3. Rate–pressure product (heart rate × systolic blood pressure) increase of more than 800 to 1200 units over baseline
4. Dyspnea index greater than level 3

Dyspnea Index

Level 0: No shortness of breath; can count to 15 (takes about 8 sec) without taking a breath in the sequence

Level 1: Mild shortness of breath; can count to 15, but must take one breath in the sequence; continue activity at this intensity

Level 2: Moderate shortness of breath; needs two breaths to count to 15; this is the desired level of activity intensity

Level 3: Definite shortness of breath; must take three breaths in the sequence of counting to 15; use breathing control techniques

Level 4: Severe shortness of breath; unable to count or speak; cease activity

If the patient completes the sequence at any level by rushing to complete the sequence, add a plus (+) to the level.

5. ST segment depression or elevation of more than 1 mm
6. Vertigo
7. Claudication
8. Excessive fatigue
9. Increase in rales, or acquisition of a previously absent third heart sound (S_3)
10. Other abnormal symptoms

(Sadowsky HS, Rohrkemper KF, Quon SYM: Rehabilitation of Cardiac and Cardiopulmonary Recipients: An Introduction for Physical and Occupational Therapists, 3rd ed, Appendix I. Stanford, CA, Stanford University Hospital, 1986. Used with permission.)

involved or the amount of work being performed. This increase in pressure is proportional to the intensity of the contraction (percent of maximal voluntary contraction [MVC]). Sustained contractions (greater than 15% MVC) result in reflex increases in heart rate, in arterial vasoconstriction in nonexercising muscle, and in cardiac output with minimal change in stroke volume (Longhurst and Mitchell).

Although no concomitant increase in heart rate occurs during isometric exercise, cardiac transplant recipients exhibit a blood pressure response similar to that of normals. The increase in blood pressure is most likely attributable to the total peripheral resistance rather than to any increase in the cardiac output (Savin and co-workers).

Since transplant recipients lack immediate cardioacceleratory sympathetic stimulation, they exhibit an impaired chronotropic ability to respond to sudden increases in work. Consequently, on-demand increases in cardiac output are attributable to augmented preload and the Frank–Starling mechanism. Later in exercise, cardiac output increases in response to a combination of chronotropic and inotropic influences associated with rising levels of circulating catecholamines (Pope and associates, Savin and co-workers).

In comparison with normals, transplant recipients exhibit a more gradual, linear diminution in heart rate following exercise. A greater anaerobic contribution to work output is reflected in a higher respiratory exchange ratio, a higher minute ventilation, a wider arterial-venous oxygen difference, a higher peak lactate level, and a lower volume of oxygen consumption at any given work load.

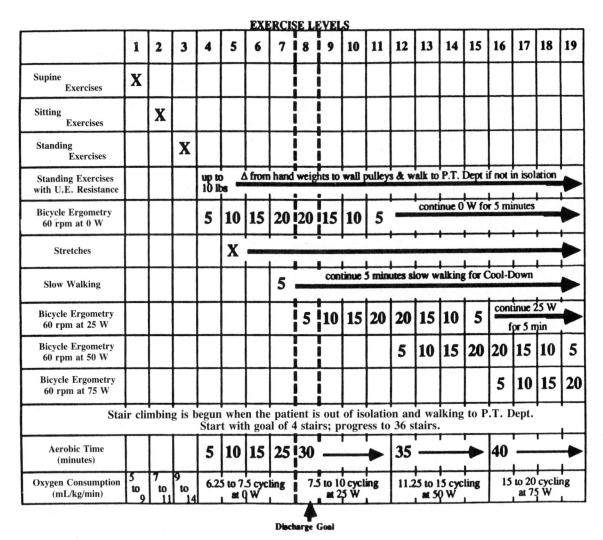

EXERCISE LEVELS

	1	2	3	4	5	6	7	8	9	10	11	12	13	14	15	16	17	18	19
Supine Exercises	X																		
Sitting Exercises		X																	
Standing Exercises			X																
Standing Exercises with U.E. Resistance				up to 10 lbs	Δ from hand weights to wall pulleys & walk to P.T. Dept if not in isolation ⟶														
Bicycle Ergometry 60 rpm at 0 W				5	10	15	20	20	15	10	5	continue 0 W for 5 minutes ⟶							
Stretches					X	⟶													
Slow Walking							5	continue 5 minutes slow walking for Cool-Down ⟶											
Bicycle Ergometry 60 rpm at 25 W								5	10	15	20	20	15	10	5	continue 25 W for 5 min ⟶			
Bicycle Ergometry 60 rpm at 50 W												5	10	15	20	20	15	10	5
Bicycle Ergometry 60 rpm at 75 W																5	10	15	20
Stair climbing is begun when the patient is out of isolation and walking to P.T. Dept. Start with goal of 4 stairs; progress to 36 stairs.																			
Aerobic Time (minutes)				5	10	15	25	30 ⟶				35 ⟶				40 ⟶			
Oxygen Consumption (mL/kg/min)	5 to 9	7 to 11	9 to 14	6.25 to 7.5 cycling at 0 W				7.5 to 10 cycling at 25 W				11.25 to 15 cycling at 50 W				15 to 20 cycling at 75 W			

Discharge Goal

Figure 42-4. Cardiac and cardiopulmonary transplant recipient exercise protocol. (Sadowsky HS, Rohrkemper KF, Quon SYM: Rehabilitation of Cardiac and Cardiopulmonary Recipients: An Introduction for Physical and Occupational Therapists, 3rd ed, Appendix J. Stanford, CA, Stanford University Hospital, 1986. Used with permission.)

EXERCISE REGIMEN

Cardiac and cardiopulmonary transplant recipients progress through a series of discontinuous and continuous exercises beginning on the first postoperative day, following extubation. Their programs differ only in the rate of progression. Work-rate progression is determined on the basis of clinical and laboratory indications so as not to overstress the oxygen transport system. A guideline for determining patient tolerance to activity based on clinical symptomatology is presented in Table 42-3. The patient is expected to repeat the exercise regimen once daily on his own, and to report to the physical therapy department once daily for progression under the therapist's guidance. A typical patient at Stanford University starts physical therapy after extubation on the first postoperative day, beginning with active-assistive supine exercises of all the extremities. Progression to active standing exercises involving the major joints and muscle groups is usually accomplished by the third postoperative day. Upper extremity resistance is then added at the therapist's discretion. Because the patient is still in protective isolation, bicycle ergometry serves as the primary mode for aerobic exercise and is usually begun by the fifth or sixth postoperative day. The protocol for exercise progression used at Stanford is presented in Figure 42-4. (One should not interpret the exercise levels as the activity to be performed on a particular postoperative day.) The average length of hospitalization for heart and heart-lung recipients is 38 days (Sadowsky and co-workers). At time of discharge from the hospital, the patient is provided with discharge activity guidelines.

ANNOTATED BIBLIOGRAPHY

Bieber CP, Hunt SA, Schwinn DA et al: Complications in long-term survivors of cardiac transplantation. Transplant Proc 8:207, 1981 (A discussion of the development and prevalence of complications seen in cardiac transplant recipients.)

Committee on Exercise, American Heart Association: Exercise Testing and Training of Apparently Healthy Individuals: A Handbook for Physicians. American Heart Association, Dallas, TX, 1976 (A guide for the use of exercise tests and the prescription of exercise for persons exhibiting no symptoms of cardiovascular disease.)

Guyton AC: Textbook of Medical Physiology, 5th ed, pp 88–98. Philadelphia, WB Saunders, 1976 (A discussion of immune reactions, antigens, and blood and tissue typing.)

Longhurst JC, Mitchell JH: Reflex control of the circulation by efferents from skeletal muscle. In Guyton AC, Young DB (eds): International Review of Physiology III, pp 125–148. Baltimore, University Park Press, 1979 (A discussion of the normal control mechanisms of circulation in skeletal muscle.)

Lough ME: Life satisfaction following heart transplantation. Presented at Cardiac Transplantation at Stanford, Stanford, CA, February 8, 1985 (A report on the results of a survey of transplant recipients regarding their satisfaction with their postoperative life-styles.)

Penn I: Malignant lymphomas on organ transplant recipients. Transplant Proc 13:207, 1981. (A discussion of the prevalence of lymphoproliferative disease and the factors that may predispose transplant recipients to develop it.)

Pope SE, Stinson EB, Daughters GT et al: Exercise response of the denervated heart in long-term cardiac transplant recipients. Am J Cardiol 46:213, 1980 (A report of the cardiovascular changes resulting from dynamic exercise performed by cardiac transplant recipients.)

Sadowsky HS, Rohrkemper KF, Quon SYM: Rehabilitation of Cardiac and Cardiopulmonary Recipients: An Introduction for Physical and Occupational Therapists, 3rd ed. Stanford, CA, Stanford University Hospital, 1986 (A description of the selection criteria, operative procedures, and postoperative care of cardiac and cardiopulmonary transplant recipients.)

Savin WM, Alderman EL, Haskell WL et al: Left ventricular response to isometric exercise in patients with denervated and innervated hearts. Circulation 61(5):897, 1980 (A comparison of the effects of isometric exercise on the cardiovascular systems of patients with denervated and normally innervated hearts.)

Savin WM, Haskell WL, Schroeder JS et al: Cardiorespiratory responses of cardiac transplant patients to graded, symptom-limited exercise. Circulation 62(1):55, 1980 (A report of the cardiovascular and pulmonary function changes seen as a result of the performance of low-level exercise stress tests by cardiac transplant recipients.)

43 Neurological Training and Retraining

ELIZABETH H. LITTELL

Inexperienced physical therapists sometimes consider treatment of the patient with abnormality and dysfunction of the central nervous system as complex and frustrating. Therapists with more experience in this area are more apt to describe it as challenging and extremely rewarding. This chapter is addressed to therapists who are still at the stage of concern over their ability to interact effectively with the patient with a central nervous system disorder. Physical therapy for patients with neurological problems or dysfunction is still an area in which personal opinion concerning treatment, usually expressed by adherence to various "schools" of treatment, predominates. In this chapter I will address the basic principles of treatment of neurologic patients, the historical background to the several schools of neurologic treatment, and basic techniques that the therapist can use to provide effective treatment.

At the outset the therapist must remember that all therapy for patients with neurological problems or dysfunction is predicated on two major assumptions: (1) damaged or incorrectly developed central nervous systems retain the capability of modifying their function through learning processes, and (2) a certain amount of redundancy exists in the central nervous system such that the function of missing structures can be assumed more or less adequately by other neural systems. Patient evaluation is directed at determining not only to what extent limitations exist, but also to what extent the assumptions underlying treatment are valid for any given patient. For some types of dysfunction these assumptions have only limited validity, given the current ability to restore structure and thereby function in the central nervous system. In such cases, therapy should be addressed more properly to adaptation to the dysfunction than to its correction.

BASIC PRINCIPLES

All of the approaches to treatment of the patient with central nervous system dysfunction stress direct patient-therapist interaction, even when mechanical modalities and non-therapist assistants have also been incorporated. Therapists are using their "educated" central nervous system to communicate with and support the activities of the damaged central nervous system of the patient. This may sound mysterious, but it is probably the reason why some therapists have been so successful in therapeutic interaction with patients. The ability to "tune in" to the patient can be learned through theory and experience, but to a certain extent it is an innate ability that some therapists possess to a very high degree. In this chapter, I will show you what opportunities exist for patient-therapist interaction, and give some guidelines for how to emphasize such interaction for the benefit of the patient.

A second common principle is the use of sequential ordering of treatment. In all the methods that have been proposed, a sequence in which therapeutic activities can be introduced most beneficially has been clearly stated. Two primary sequences have been used most frequently: (1) normal maturational sequences of sensory-motor behavior, and (2) the sequence of return of motor function following stroke. The first sequence has been most widely applied with the greatest number of variations. The variability is not surprising considering the number of subsequences that can be described in the category of normal sensory-motor development. The sequence that will be referred to most frequently here is the normal sensory-motor development progression emphasized by Rood, but others will also be discussed as appropriate to certain types of patient problems.

A third commonality among all approaches to therapy for the patient with a neurological problem is that of using principles of learning as a basis for treatment application and progression. This is seen primarily in the extensive use of repetition of appropriate sensory-motor behavior, both in a single session and over a number of sessions. Other essential aspects of learning theory are also applied, such as careful structuring of the environment, graded difficulty of tasks, constant evaluation of progress, and detailed setting of attainable objectives. Adherence to these principles can make treatment successful and satisfying for both the patient and the therapist, if only because the steps necessary for success are realistic, and success itself is clearly defined and agreed upon by all participants.

The enormous variability evident in physical therapy for these patients springs in great part from these three common principles. Reliance on direct patient-therapist interaction as a basis for developing treatment techniques and theories inevitably led to differences both in what the therapist was doing and in the rationale for treatment. Different ways of handling patients led to differences in their observed responses. These led in turn to differences in opinion concerning the most appropriate and effective handling or interaction methods to use. Emphasis on the importance of following

a sequence of development of sensory-motor function has also led to variation, because so many different possible sequences exist that depend largely on the types of patients most commonly treated. A final factor that has led to variability, rather than uniformity, in treatment methods is dependence on a variety of theoretical interpretations of how the human central nervous system works. Development of a school of treatment consists of a series of interactions between individual clinical experience and theoretical interpretation of results by many therapists over several years. Enormous changes in our understanding of the function and structure of the central nervous system have occurred during the development of the current schools of thought about physical therapy for patients with neurological problems; therefore, it is not surprising that differences in opinion are more common than agreement.

HISTORICAL BACKGROUND

Five therapists—Jean Ayers, Berta Bobath, Signe Brunnstrom, Margaret Knott, and Margaret Rood—have been instrumental over the past 40 to 50 years in developing highly effective theory-based treatment approaches for the patient with dysfunction of the central nervous system. Each of these therapists, working alone or in collaboration with a physician, has integrated her personal clinical experience based on various types of patients with the currently available theoretical interpretation of neural function. The expansion of experimental knowledge in neuroscience in the past 10 to 15 years has also set the stage for precise clinical testing of the theories of each school of treatment, which will almost certainly lead to greater integration of the ideas developed by each school and its adherents.

Jean Ayers, an occupational therapist, has worked extensively with the application of vestibular stimulation to patients, most commonly children, who have a variety of neurological dysfunctions ranging from cerebral palsy to learning disabilities and attentional disorders. She has emphasized the necessity for integrating structured and ordered sensory experiences with desired motor behaviors, creating the approach termed *sensory integration therapy*. She is well known for stressing the importance of spatial and body image integration and left-right communication within the central nervous system for the development of normal motor and normal cognitive function. In recent years, she has been involved in intensive clinical testing of her hypotheses concerning the importance of vestibular sensation on motor and cognitive function.

Berta Bobath, a physical therapist, has collaborated with her husband Karel Bobath, a neurologist, in developing an approach to treatment of the neurologic patient that is based extensively on the importance of developing normal muscle tone as a preparation for normal movement patterns. Her initial work focused on children with cerebral palsy. Not surprisingly, she emphasized the sequence of normal sensory-motor reflex development. She subsequently expanded her work to adult patients with neurological dysfunction. One of her primary treatment goals has been the use of postures and movement patterns to inhibit maladaptive and dysfunctional motor behavior and to release normal motor patterns. Bobath's theories have been expanded into the approach known as *neurodevelopmental treatment* (NDT). The process of this school of treatment is as follows:

- inhibition of abnormal behavior or postures through positioning and the use of specific movement patterns,
- facilitation of normal sensory-motor behavior by using the normal movements released by the prior inhibition process, and
- reinforcement of inhibition of abnormal behavior by the repeated use and development of the released normal movements.

As a result of this process, treatment under this approach very definitely stresses being "in tune" with the patient during treatment.

Signe Brunnstrom, a physical therapist, initiated her theories of treatment while working primarily with adult patients who had suffered a stroke. She based her approach on a combination of very precise observation of the sequential changes in motor function that typically occurred following stroke and an understanding of the reflex function of the nervous system then current (during the first half of this century). Her suggestions for therapy emphasize eliciting motor behavior in the sequence in which it would normally occur following stroke, which is not the same as the sequence of normal maturation. The limitation of this approach has been both a blessing and a curse for therapists. Her extremely detailed and accurate observations have provided one of the best available resources for understanding motor recovery from stroke, but her insistence on using the stroke recovery sequence as the basis of advancing the patient's progress has limited the applicability of much of her work to stroke patients only. In general, her approach is not applicable to children or to brain-injured adults. However, her description of basic reflex behaviors can be used to understand the sensory-motor function of these patients, and some of the techniques she developed are appropriate to treating a variety of sensory-motor problems.

Margaret Knott, a physical therapist working with the physiatrist Herman Kabat and later with the physical therapist Dorothy Voss, developed the treatment approach known as *proprioceptive neuromuscular facilitation* (PNF). Initially, the main emphasis of PNF treatment was on the use of carefully applied and timed proprioceptive stimuli to elicit and improve motor activity. Additional tactile, visual, and auditory stimuli were centered around the basic use of proprioceptive stimuli. Originally, this treatment method depended only minimally on any particular developmental or recovery sequence, emphasizing instead a sequence of refining motor behavior that moved from proximal to distal portions of the extremities or the trunk. Voss later added motor activities in a normal maturational sequence. Of all the treatment schools discussed in this chapter, only this one finds major applicability beyond the field of physical therapy for patients with neurological dysfunction. Because of its primary emphasis on active motor behavior and on strengthening of motor activity, this approach can be extremely useful whenever muscle weakness is a problem. This same emphasis requires careful use of PNF with patients who are minimally capable of producing normal movement, so that abnormal motor patterns are not reinforced.

With a background in both occupational and physical therapy, Margaret Rood worked extensively from a theoretical understanding of the importance of system and organism integration for the production of normal sensory-motor behavior. Unfortunately, many therapists find her published work extremely difficult to adapt to clinical practice. However, later therapists, including Shirley Stockmeyer, Margot Heiniger, and Shirley Randolph, have helped to make her theories more understandable. Rood was one of the first therapists to emphasize the importance of the *sensory* half of sensory-motor behavior. She used a wide variety of stimuli, many of them tactile, as a means of access to the patient's central nervous system. She also strongly emphasized the importance of autonomic function as a basis for normal sensory-motor behavior at a time when most therapists were scarcely aware that this was a factor worth considering. Rood used a developmental sequence, primarily stressing the progression from postural adjustment to postural maintenance ("hold" or "co-contraction" patterns) and eventually to distal goal-directed movement on the basis of proximal stability.

APPROACHES TO TREATMENT

As can be seen from the previous discussion, at least five different approaches could be used with the neurologic patient. Each has merit, and any may be successful with a given patient provided the therapist is competent in using that particular approach. However, it is not necessary to be an expert in any one approach to be able to provide some benefit to the patient. No matter which particular technique the therapist is using, four broad categories need to be addressed during treatment:

1. Establishment and maintenance of focused interaction with the patient;
2. Use of appropriate and effective sensory input related to movement;
3. Establishment of the ability of the patient to move and support movement; and
4. Optimal integration of patient function with the process of living in society.

INTERACTION WITH THE PATIENT

As therapists, we rapidly become used to establishing a framework of interaction with our patients that resembles normal business or social interaction in that it depends primarily on verbalization for exchanging of ideas. It also maintains a certain "distance" between the patient and the therapist. The type of interaction necessary with the neurologic patient is both more embracing and more focused than this general social pattern. The intent is to become, as a patient-therapist pair, mutual extensions of each other's central nervous system. In order for this to occur, several aspects of interaction need to be addressed:

1. State of arousal of the patient. In order for the therapist to interact with the patient, the patient must be able to respond to the stimuli that the therapist presents. If you are treating a person with a spinal cord injury, this initial consideration may be no problem. However, if you are treating a person with a closed head injury, state of arousal may be the point at which you will have to start working on interaction.
2. Ability of the patient to focus attention on an individual stimulus. At many points during treatment, you will find it essential to focus the patient's attention on particular events or stimuli. As treatment progresses, attention may be withdrawn from the details of sensory-motor behavior, but initially it is necessary to be able to direct and hold attention specifically.
3. Ability of the patient to use sensation in a meaningful way. The patient must be able

to receive, perceive, and integrate the stimuli you are using as an aid to producing motor activity.

Although these abilities have been considered primarily for the patient, the therapist must also display these behaviors during therapy! Think, for example, of the ineffectiveness of the therapy when the therapist is providing passive range of motion to a comatose patient while carrying on a conversation with another person in the room. In this instance, the therapist is not attending to the stimuli provided by the patient.

Generating Arousal

A wide variety of stimulus modalities may be needed to produce arousal. The intent is to determine stimuli to which the patient will respond, preferably consistently. Appropriate stimuli include any that are normally very meaningful on a basic level to humans in general or to the particular patient. Protopathic stimuli (those related to survival and not highly discriminated) and special sense stimuli are generally useful. Some possibilities are listed in Table 43-1. Two and occasionally more stimuli may be presented simultaneously. For example, odor and taste are natural combinations. Tactile and pressure stimuli may be combined with auditory and visual stimuli, or auditory stimuli may be combined with taste or odor stimuli. Combinations should be done so that the stimuli provided interact in a way that would normally serve to focus attention on one of the stimuli used. There should not be a conflict between stimuli. For example, apply tactile stimulation to the patient's arm while saying, "Look at your arm."

Stimulus intensity does not necessarily have to be very great, particularly if the localization of the stimulus is precise. This is particularly true of stimuli applied to the face, especially in the mouth or perioral region. Stimuli should be repeated a number of times before concluding that they are ineffective. Generally speaking, the frequency of stimulation should be low. When arousal and general responsiveness are a problem, response latencies to any stimulus may be very long. Stimulus frequency

can be increased once a response has been elicited. At this point, the therapist must become very responsive to the patient's motor activity, and must modify intensity and frequency of stimulation so as to maintain and, if possible, increase the motor activity. For example, if you have increased arousal by repetitive use of the patient's name, the patient's attention may be focused by changing to simple statements, such as "hello," "good morning," or "I am going to work with you." Continued repetition of the patient's name is decreasingly likely to enhance attention. Introduction of more complex statements will also decrease attention.

Focusing Attention

Learning of sensory-motor behavior is probably not possible unless attention is focused on the particular activity during the learning process. The attention that is indicated is not necessarily conscious attention to individual components of a given motor behavior, but the internal "attention" of the sensory-motor system to all relevant sensory and efference (internal feedback) information related to the activity being performed. With the neurologic patient, therapy is predominantly a learning process, so the ability to attend to it is essential. Treatment approaches that enhance attention include:

- Decreasing or eliminating competing stimuli in the environment or within the patient;
- Choosing a stimulus or sensory-motor activity that is meaningful to the patient;
- Increasing stimulus intensity (but not to the level where it becomes noxious or generates an aversive response);
- Providing slight variation over time in the stimulus to limit adaptation or habituation;
- Adding selected associated stimuli that enhance the meaning of the relevant stimulus (eg, using a vocal command to move at the same time as providing a proprioceptive stimulus that will elicit movement).

When working with a patient for whom focused attention is a problem, it is advisable to keep the periods of time during which atten-

Table 43-1. Stimuli that Alter State of Arousal*

STIMULUS	LOCATION
Stimuli that Increase Arousal	
Nondiscriminatory Stimuli	
Brief, light tactile stimulation	Face, particularly perioral region
	Palms of hands
	Soles of feet
	Abdomen
Brief temperature stimulation (warm or cold)	Face, particularly perioral region
	Palms of hands
	Soles of feet
	Abdomen
Deep pressure	Face
	Over any muscle; can be directed towards desired location of motion
Special Sense Stimuli	
Sound—use precise sounds, particularly meaningful words (eg, names); sounds may need to be of a quality or intensity that would provoke a startle response in a normally aroused person	
Voice—use lively, excited, commanding tones	
Odors—use intense odors that are likely to have pleasant meaning to the patient; or, odors that would produce an aversive response in the normally aroused person	
Taste—use pleasant and intense tastes (be cautious when introducing substances to the mouth of a patient who cannot swallow safely)	
Proprioceptive Stimuli	
Upright position—tonic stimulation of static receptors of the labyrinth	
Passive movement—repetitive phasic stimulation of muscle, joint, and skin proprioceptors	
Stimuli that Decrease Arousal	
Inverted tonic labyrinthine reflex (see Table 43-3)	
Special Sense Stimuli	
Voice—use soothing, quiet, friendly tones	

*See Table 43-2 for stimuli that affect general alpha motor neuron excitability; these stimuli also generally affect arousal in the same direction in which they affect excitability.

tion is to be focused on a particular activity relatively brief. The intent is to complete the attended activity successfully without losing attention. From the therapist's point of view, attention is also important. If you find your attention wandering from the activity at hand, it is time to change activities before you lose communication with the patient.

Meaningful Use of Stimuli

Stimulus information that is sensed, that is, entered into the central nervous system, can be used for initiating or sustaining reflex motor behaviors of varying complexity, depending on the extent to which the sensory information is distributed within the central nervous system. If stimulus information in a particular modality or location cannot be sensed, it is of no use to the therapist in generating any type of motor behavior. In such a case, alternative modalities or locations must be utilized. In order for stimulus information to be perceived and used as a basis for cortically directed motor behavior (usually "voluntary"), the information must (1) reach the cortex and (2) be integrated correctly with additional sensory and ongoing cortical information. Problems related to lack of perception of stimulus information may be evident as sensory neglect syndromes. The patient may be capable of moving the affected part of the body, but does not move voluntarily because of the lack of sensory awareness of the body part. Sensory neglect can often cause a patient to become "one sided" and to use body parts only on the unaffected side of the body midline. Depending on the extent of loss of perception, this problem may be overcome by using alternate sensory modalities to provide information. Or, the patient does use body parts for movement, but restricts movement to only the space of which he is aware. In this case movement into the neglected space may assist the patient in reintegrating sensory information from that space. As examples:

- A patient with sensory neglect of an extremity resulting from loss of perception of tactile or proprioceptive information can substitute visual guidance to initiate active use. For example, tell the patient, "*Look* at your hand; lift it towards your other hand."
- A patient with sensory neglect of part of the visual field can be taught to use head and extremity movements into that region of space such that objects there are brought into the functioning visual field.

The therapist should be aware, however, that such alternatives remain at the conscious level, and therefore cannot completely replace loss of normal sensory perception.

When the patient perceives stimulus information in all modalities, but cannot use this information concurrently to produce normal motor behavior, a problem exists in integration of sensory information. Distorted perception of one or more of the relevant sensations may be part of the difficulty. In this situation, the therapist should first emphasize development of motor behavior using the sensory information that is handled most normally by the patient. Introduction of additional disruptive sensation should be avoided. Abnormally perceived or poorly integrated sensory information should be introduced gradually into simple sensory-motor acts that are well integrated. A return to completely normal use of multiple interactive sensations is more the exception than the rule. The patient will frequently have to be assisted in adapting to an altered sensory environment.

An additional problem with the use of sensation involves the patient's positive acceptance of the particular stimulus. The therapist should always determine whether the patient will accept or have a positive response to tactile and thermal stimuli, particularly cold stimuli and tactile stimuli in specific locations. Tactile defensiveness indicates a predominance of avoidance behavior over exploratory behavior, probably as a result of frontal lobe activity that has not been adequately integrated with parietal lobe activity. Defensive responses may be limited to stimulation only on certain regions of the skin surface or may be more generally evident. Repeated tactile stimulation over the relevant areas to promote habituation and the addition of deep pressure stimuli in these areas can help to overcome tactile defensiveness. The therapist should also make sure that the apparent tactile defensiveness is not due to activation of pain pathways by normally nonpainful stimuli (a type of dysesthesia). In that case, repeated stimulation will only aggravate the problem.

Problems in interacting and communicating with the patient using meaningful stimuli are a constant during all phases of therapy, although the details may change at different times. While the therapist is working on achieving optimal movement, the requirements for effective interaction will be continually present.

MOVEMENT AND SUPPORT OF MOVEMENT

Three major considerations exist when addressing movement and its support:

1. The ability of the body as a whole to support the energy expenditure of movement;
2. The ability of the central nervous system to program appropriate muscle "readiness" or "stiffness" to support the desired type of motor activity (classically discussed under the topic of skeletal muscle tone, either general or local); and
3. The ability of the central nervous system to produce appropriate motor "hold" or "move" patterns using relevant sensory information before, during, and after the motor activity.

The second and third considerations are typically addressed sequentially, either in the overall treatment program or during individual treatment sessions. The first consideration, which essentially deals with the patient's ability to maintain homeostasis during exercise, must be addressed concurrently with the other two. Therapy for the neurologic patient, to a very real extent, can be seen as an exercise training program.

Energy Support for Movement

Two aspects of appropriate energy support can be considered. First, the physical therapist should be aware of the patient's overall fitness level. Many neurologic patients will be in a relatively deconditioned or unconditioned state, so therapy will have to address conditioning as well as return of normal sensory-motor function. Ideally, relatively aggressive therapy would be started early to prevent deconditioning from occurring, but this is not always possible. The care team may not be aware of the potential problems of deconditioning or more often, additional medical complications may limit the possibilities for active therapy. Patients of any age who have been chronically limited in motor function will need a gradual build-up in physical intensity of therapy sessions. As a result of interaction between the sense of effort in producing a motor act and the autonomic behavior that leads to systemic support, what may appear to the therapist as very limited motor activity may be inducing major changes in autonomic function. The cardiorespiratory parameters that would be monitored during any other type of training program should also be monitored for these patients.

The other aspect of energy support for movement involves the availability of normal neural control mechanisms that regulate cardiorespiratory (and other system) responses to motor activity. Therapists have developed very few techniques for correcting problems in neural control of energy availability. Rood and to a certain extent Ayers have addressed the interaction between autonomic activity and muscle tone. In general, not enough attention has been directed toward improving impaired autonomic system regulation other than by considering the fitness training aspects of therapy. For comparison, this is rather like directing one's attention to strengthening exercises for a muscle "weakened" by loss of normal central neural control while ignoring the neurological problems that caused the decrease in function. If homeostatic regulation appears to be a significant problem with a patient, the following approaches might be tried. They have been neither proven nor disproven to be consistently clinically successful, so careful cardiorespiratory monitoring of the patient should be a part of the treatment.

1. Repeated presentation of a stimulus that stresses the cardiorespiratory system. This approach essentially assumes that the neural control for cardiorespiratory responses is intact or nearly so, and simply needs to be strenghtened by training. An example would be standing a patient daily as a means of increasing normal baroreceptor reflex responses.
2. Concurrent presentation of additional stimuli that would tend to elicit similar or supportive autonomic responses to those desired. Generalized thermal stimulation could be added as a means of adjusting

blood flow patterns during motor activity.

3. Increasing the cognitive and emotional preparation for motor activity. Autonomic support systems and skeletal motor pathways for movement are activated concurrently during preparation for movement. Increasing the preparatory stimuli and perhaps providing greater emphasis on the emotional aspects of the anticipated movement may facilitate autonomic system involvement.

4. Utilizing biofeedback to help the patient become more aware of autonomic behavior, thus facilitating control of that behavior. This would be an effective approach primarily with relatively isolated problems where autonomic motor control pathways are available, but are not being normally activated because of lack of appropriate sensory integration. As with any use of biofeedback, the patient must be able to receive and integrate appropriately the feedback signal.

Additional therapeutic techniques that may be used to modify and enhance autonomic adjustment to therapy will be considered when the problem of adjusting general muscle "tone" is addressed, because many stimuli appear to affect both systems in an interactive way.

Skeletal Muscle Readiness for Movement

Treatment approaches can be used to adjust muscle tone either generally throughout the body or within specific muscle groups. The concept of muscle tone has many different descriptions and definitions. For the purposes of this chapter, "tone" refers to the observed ability of the motor system to prepare a muscle or group of muscles for specific types and patterns of movement and to support movement while it is occurring. On a physiological basis, tone thus refers to the ability of the motor system to alter the probability of exciting alpha motor neurons and their related interneurons through a number of means. Of major importance is the ability to modulate activation of gamma motor neurons and to enhance input

from muscle receptors, specifically muscle spindles and Golgi tendon organs. Therefore, when considering treatment addressed at modifying tone, techniques that interact with these neural systems more or less directly will be analyzed. Inappropriate alpha motor neuron excitability is such a universal problem with the neurologic patient that a wide variety of treatment techniques have been developed for dealing with the difficulties presented. The basic, and experimentally established, assumption behind addressing alpha motor neuron excitability early and continually in treatment is that normal motor behavior cannot occur on the basis of inappropriate excitability.

General alpha motor neuron excitability is developed through the activity of a number of neural systems, including predominantly the reticular system in relation to its arousal functions, the vestibular system, and the proprioceptive system of the neck. The latter two systems operate on alpha motor neuron excitability through the responses described as tonic labyrinthine and tonic neck reflexes. The reticular system is the pathway for transmitting arousal states to the skeletal muscles and to internal organs. For this reason, stimuli and manipulations that affect one output of the system (either somatomotor or autonomic) are likely to affect the other in parallel. Stimuli that can be used to modify general alpha motor neuron excitability as well as autonomic behavior through the reticular system are outlined in Table 43-2. The stimuli that increase excitability generally tend to activate the sympathetic portion of the autonomic nervous system, leading to systemic changes such as increased heart rate, increased myocardial contractility, and increased ventilation. Central effects of these stimuli include increased general arousal. The patient may become more ready to attend to specific stimuli. However, the therapist should be aware that an excess of stimuli tending to increase general alpha motor neuron excitability may decrease the ability of the patient to focus attention.

The therapist should also consider the emotional status of the patient when working

Table 43-2. Techniques for Modifying General Alpha Motor Neuron Excitability Through Reticular System Intermediation

TO INCREASE EXCITABILITY	TO DECREASE EXCITABILITY
Modalities	
Varied and unfamiliar	Limited and familiar
Varied stimulus qualities within a given modality	Limited variation in stimulus quality
Intensity	
Extremes of intensity (near the threshold or near maximum tolerance level)	Moderate, consistent intensity with limited variation
Timing	
Irregular frequency of application, nonrhythmical or with a strong rhythm, rapid	Rhythmical, relatively slow frequency of application
Examples	
Bright lighting	Dim lighting
Varied, bright colors	Limited, "quiet" colors
Variety of visual stimuli	Limited number of visual stimuli
Variety of tactile textures	Limited texture variation
Lively music	Quiet music
Cold skin stimulation	Neutral warmth to the skin
Rapid, large-range passive movement	Slow passive movement through full range
Varied phasic vestibular stimulation (eg, vigorous swinging, rotation, varied head movements)*	Slow, repetitive vestibular stimulation (eg, rocking, gentle swinging)

*Caution must always be used with vigorous vestibular stimulation because the threshold for aversive responses (such as nausea) can be quite close to the level of stimulus needed for appropriate arousal responses.

to improve general alpha motor neuron excitability. Positive states of mind, anger, and sometimes fear tend to provide a generalized increase in excitability, but negative states of mind tend to be inhibitory. Emotional states can affect excitability in specific patterns. Consider the postures assumed when one is angry, fearful, or joyful. Generally speaking, the therapist would not want to elicit negative states, but can find establishment of positive emotional states beneficial to normalization of excitability. Careful use of voice quality can modify emotional status and thus have an important effect on general alpha motor neuron

excitability. A number of therapeutic approaches such as Feldenkrais, Body Work, Touch for Health, Rolfing, and others emphasize the reciprocal relationship between mental status and skeletal motor activity. Because of their attention to the close interaction among these systems, such therapeutic approaches can be effective in treating problems that appear to be resistant to other more classical interventions. In general, therapists working with neurologic patients may benefit from learning some of these techniques and applying their concepts in treatment. Not only can they be helpful in adjusting alpha motor neuron excitability, but they can also be used in establishing effective communication with the patient.

Tonic labyrinthine and neck reflexes may be used to elicit specific patterns of general alpha motor neuron excitability. Often, a more positive approach is to avoid placing the patient in positions in which these tonic reflexes will dominate motor behavior and thus inhibit variability. For example, if a patient demonstrates excessive extension, one therapeutic approach to modifying alpha motor neuron excitability would be to position the patient prone as a means of inhibiting extension and facilitating more balanced activity between flexor and extensor muscles. Alternatively, the posture that elicits excessive activity may be slightly modified at key points, or the patient may be positioned in a neutral posture between extremes of reflex-inducing positions. Key points are typically axial joints such as the neck, or proximal extremity joints such as the shoulder or hip. Very distal extremity joints can also function as key points for influencing excitability. For example, wrist and finger extension and forearm pronation can be used to assist inhibition of generalized flexor activity of the entire upper extremity. The patient either may be positioned in reflex inhibitory postures or may be moved with passive or active-assisted movement in inhibitory patterns that incorporate these postures. Such use of "reflex-inhibiting postures" was suggested early by Bobath and was later modified to provide a more active approach with the use of "reflex-inhibiting patterns." Use of tonic reflexes to modify alpha motor neuron excitability is outlined in Table 43-3. Examples of key points are given in Table 43-4.

Specific approaches for modifying alpha motor neuron excitability for individual muscles or functional muscle groups have proliferated over the past half century. Appropriate sensory modalities to use are those through which the therapist can have a limited and more or less direct effect on gamma activation patterns and muscle sense utilization in the muscles under concern. Primary modalities

thus include proprioception and tactile sensation. Stimuli that evoke responses with relatively long latency and persistence, such as tonic postural reflexes, are more useful in modifying alpha motor neuron excitability than stimuli such as deep tendon reflexes, which evoke a more rapid and short-lived response. The latter stimuli may be of more use in eliciting a brief motion than in adjusting excitability. When stimuli that elicit brief responses are used, they must be followed rapidly with additional stimuli to reinforce and "capture" the movement. Table 43-5 summarizes proprioceptive and tactile stimuli that may be used to produce local changes in muscle activity.

Some controversy has developed over the use of existing dominant tonic patterns as a means of eliciting movement. Brunnstrom seemed to describe reliance on normally occurring and sequentially developing patterns of alpha motor neuron excitability (flexor and extensor synergies) as a basis from which to generate movement in the hemiplegic patient. Bobath, on the other hand, insisted that abnormal tonic patterns should be interrupted whenever possible, and certainly not used as a basis for eliciting movement. Closer examination of Brunnstrom's work suggests that the differences may not be as great as they appear. Although Brunnstrom did allow the patient to move in synergistic patterns, she did not emphasize these patterns, but continually used stimuli that would help the patient to build more normal movement out of the synergy pattern ("breaking up of synergies"). No satisfactory experimental evidence exists that either approach is superior for all types of patients.

Because the therapist can only apply few stimuli in limited locations at any given time, a sequence of normalizing alpha motor neuron excitability is necessary. First, adjust general excitability with attendant alterations (prior or subsequent) in posture. Then, direct attention to adjusting excitability throughout an extremity by working with proximal muscles or distal "key" muscles. A full description of such techniques can be found in Bobath or NDT writings in particular, as well as in discussions of man-

Table 43-3. Use of Tonic Reflexes to Modify General Alpha Motor Neuron Excitability

DESIRED CHANGE	POSITION USED	REFLEX INVOLVED
Decreased general extension in trunk and extremities	Prone, or Supine, neck flexed, or Side lying	Tonic labyrinthine, or Tonic labyrinthine *inhibited*
Decreased general flexion in trunk and extremities	Supine, or Side lying	Tonic labyrinthine, or Tonic labyrinthine *inhibited*
Decreased extension in upper extremities	Moderate neck flexion	Symmetrical tonic neck (used or inhibited, depending on range of flexion)
Decreased flexion in lower extremities	Moderate neck flexion	Symmetrical tonic neck (used or inhibited)
Decreased flexion in upper extremities	Moderate neck extension	Symmetrical tonic neck (used or inhibited)
Decreased extension in lower extremities	Moderate neck extension	Symmetrical tonic neck (used or inhibited)
Decreased extension in upper and lower extremity of one side	Neck rotation away from extended extremities, or Neck in midline	Asymmetrical tonic neck Asymmetrical tonic neck *inhibited*
Decreased flexion in upper and lower extremity of one side	Neck rotation toward flexed extremities, or Neck in midline	Asymmetrical tonic neck Asymmetrical tonic neck *inhibited*
Increased extension of neck, trunk, and proximal joints of extremities	Prone, sitting or kneeling, head lower than heart	Inverted tonic labyrinthine*
Flexible availability of trunk flexion and extension ("normalization" of increased or decreased trunk muscle tone)	Rotation of trunk segmentally in any position	No specific reflex used

*Inverted tonic labyrinthine position is also useful for decreasing arousal.

Table 43-4. Use of Key Points to Modify Alpha Motor Neuron Excitability (Examples)

LOCATION OF KEY POINT	POSITION	EFFECT
Shoulder	Humeral external rotation Flexion to just above mid-range Scapular adduction	Decreased flexion tone of upper extremity Trunk and neck extension
Wrist	Wrist extension Forearm pronation	Decreased flexion tone of upper extremity
Hand	Thumb abduction and extension	Decreased flexion tone of upper extremity
Hip	Femoral external rotation Extension	Decreased flexion tone of lower extremity

Table 43-5. Tonic and Phasic Stimuli Used to Modify Local Alpha Motor Neuron Excitability

STIMULUS	RESPONSE
Tonic Stimuli	
Tonic vibration over muscle belly or tendon	Increase in excitability in vibrated muscle; decrease in excitability in antagonist muscle
Prolonged variable stretch of muscle (tonic stretch reflex)	Increase in excitability in stretched muscle; decrease in excitability in antagonist muscle*
Prolonged intense stretch of muscle at end of available range (clasp-knife reflex)	Increase in excitability of antagonist muscle; decrease in excitability of stretched muscle*
Sustained pressure over muscle belly (or tendon)	Decrease in excitability of muscle stimulated; increase in excitability of antagonist muscle
Prolonged cooling of skin and underlying muscle	Decrease in excitability of underlying muscle[†]
Joint compression[‡] of weight-bearing joints with less than normal body weight	Decrease in excitability of muscles crossing joint
Joint compression of weight-bearing joints with normal or greater body weight	Increase in excitability of muscles crossing joint
Joint traction	Increase in excitability of flexor muscles crossing joint (traction in the hand may elicit increased excitability in both flexors and extensors)
Phasic Stimuli	
Rapid stretch of muscle (phasic stretch reflex)	Increase in excitability in the stretched muscle; decrease in excitability in antagonist muscle
Rapid rubbing of the skin over a muscle	Increase in excitability in the underlying muscle[§]
Repeated light touch to the skin over a muscle (light tapping, mild pinching)	Increase in excitability in the underlying muscle[§]
Brief application of cold to skin over a muscle	Increase in excitability in the underlying muscle[§]

*The effects of tonic stretch are very range dependent. Stretch within the mid-range of the muscle, especially when it is variable, is more likely to produce a tonic stretch reflex. Stretch at the extreme lengthened range of the muscle may produce either a phasic stretch reflex (which may become repetitive if stretch is maintained and if alpha motor neuron excitation is high) or a clasp knife reflex (sudden release of stretch muscle activity) if significant tension is sensed by the Golgi tendon organs. The clasp-knife reflex has limited therapeutic application.

[†]Prolonged cooling by icing may have a long-latency excitatory rebound effect.

[‡]Joint compression will have varying effects on muscles crossing the joint depending on the normal weight-bearing status of the joint and on the amount of compression force used relative to the normal compression force generated by gravity acting on proximal body mass.

[§]Tactile and temperature stimuli applied briefly can elicit varying responses depending on both the location of stimulation and the patient's acceptance of that stimulus. Application of either stimulus may elicit a generalized flexor withdrawal response of the stimulated extremity, regardless of the location of stimulation on the extremity. Repetitively applied brief tactile stimuli may also produce long-latency responses that are generally excitatory to the underlying muscle.

aging tone by several other therapists (including Rood, Knott, and Brunnstrom). Additional techniques that modify alpha motor neuron excitability are discussed later in conjunction with elicitation of specific movement patterns. Anytime a particular type of movement is occurring, associated alterations in alpha motor neuron excitability will also be taking place; therefore, certain types of movements and the stimuli used to elicit them are also useful in adjusting excitability.

Movement Patterns

Four classes of movement exist that develop more or less sequentially, but that are used concurrently in the mature person with an intact central nervous system. They can be described as three classes of "move" patterns and one class of "hold" patterns. The first class of movement patterns, which develops earliest, includes all of the basic movement reflexes or responses that adjust body or body part posture in response to a variety of environmental stimuli. Hold patterns involve muscle co-contraction, which permits joint stabilization and maintenance of posture. These patterns are refined after the basic postural movements have developed. The final two classes of movement patterns include locomotor movement and specific goal-directed or fractionated movement. These classes are typically initiated and directed to a large extent by voluntary control, although many movements in these categories may become highly automatic and stereotyped with learning. Locomotion and fractionated movement are developed on the basis of postural adjustment and postural maintenance patterns. Components of the control systems of both of these earlier movement classes are used in the production of locomotion and frac-

tionated movement. Hold patterns correspond generally to the "heavy work" patterns described by Rood. Fractionated movements correspond to her "light work" patterns. In the process of refining motor behavior, the therapist must sequentially develop or integrate these classes of movement.

Basic postural reflex or response movement patterns can be elicited by (1) inhibiting tonic postures, which in turn are inhibitory to the desired (or any) movement, and (2) using stimuli that would normally elicit the desired movement responses. The process of inhibiting tonic postures has already been discussed with the topic of normalizing general alpha motor neuron excitability. Table 43-6 lists the normally used phasic reflexes that elicit pos-

TABLE 43-6. Phasic Posture-Adjusting Reflexes

REFLEX OR RESPONSE NAME	STIMULUS	MOTOR RESPONSE
Spinal Movement Reflexes		
Phasic stretch	Quick stretch of muscle or tendon	Contraction of stretched muscle, relaxation of antagonist; synergist muscles may participate
Withdrawal	Noxious stimulus; light touch or quick temperature stimulus	Flexor withdrawal of stimulated extremity, extension of opposite extremity; occasionally withdrawal into extension if flexor surface is site of stimulation
Righting Reflexes		
Optical righting	Visual stimulus normally oriented with respect to gravity	Adjustment of neck to bring face vertical and eyes horizontal*
Labyrinthine	Phasic or tonic stimulation of labyrinth	Readjustment of head position to bring face vertical and eyes horizontal
Neck	Rotation of head on body	Readjustment of body to regain straight alignment of head and body
Body	Rotation within trunk or between head and trunk	Sequential segmental readjustment of body and extremities to regain straight alignment
Vestibulo-ocular[†]	Tonic or phasic stimulation of labyrinth	Nystagmus (in response to phasic stimulation) or deviation of gaze (in response to tonic stimulation)

*If the vertical stimulus is not normally oriented with respect to gravity, or is not perceived as being normally oriented, the postural adjustment will be such as to bring the plane of the eyes perpendicular to the perceived vertical. In many persons, eye rotation is normally substituted for neck flexion in achieving optimal conjugate eye positioning.

[†]Although the vestibulo-ocular reflex is not typically classed as a righting reflex, it does serve to bring one body part (the eyes) into alignment as a result of stimulation through a proprioceptive special sense.

continued

TABLE 43-6. Phasic Posture-Adjusting Reflexes (continued)

REFLEX OR RESPONSE NAME	STIMULUS	MOTOR RESPONSE
Balance Responses		
Equilibrium responses	Displacement of the body in any direction beyond the balance point from any position	Abduction and extension of the extremities opposite the direction of displacement, protective extension of extremities in the direction of displacement; righting of head and trunk with trunk becoming convex in the direction of displacement
Protective extension	Rapid downward and away from midline displacement of the body and head	Extension of both upper extremities
Hopping	Displacement from standing in any direction	Righting of head and trunk; rapid hopping of lower extremities in direction of displacement
Placing and Support Reactions		
Placing	Pressure on dorsum of foot or hand	Flexion, followed by extension, of the extremity to bring foot (or hand) on top of stimulating surface
Positive support	Repeated pressure against sole of foot in upright position	Extension of lower extremities, righting of head and trunk
Negative support	Sustained pressure against sole of foot in upright position	Flexion of lower extremities, trunk, and neck
Orienting Responses		
Rooting reflex	Light tactile stimulation in perioral region	Moving of head in direction of stimulus; opening of mouth
Auditory orienting	Any attended sound	Adjustment of neck to bring eyes facing sound, with subsequent righting of body[++]
Tactile orienting	Any attended tactile sensation	Adjustment of neck to bring eyes to focus on the stimulus, with subsequent righting of body
Manual orienting	Tactile stimulation of the hand	Adjustment of hand posture to prepare for grasp or manipulation of stimulating object

[++]If the patient has a discrepancy in auditory function between the two ears, auditory orienting will bring the head into position to equalize *perceived* input to the two ears.

tural adjustment movements. The intensity of response elicited will depend on the intensity of the stimulus used and the speed of its application. Repetition of the stimulus has variable value, depending on the nature of the response being elicited and the state of arousal and attention of the patient. The very simple phasic stretch reflex can usually be repeated extensively without development of habituation. Righting and equilibrium responses may habituate in some patients, but rarely to the point of extinction. The most complex responses, such as the orienting responses that depend on stimulus novelty, will habituate with repetition in many (though not all) patients. The orienting responses depend on the ability of the patient to attend to the stimulus; thus, a novel stimulus is more likely to produce attention and orientation.

When both stimulus and response are phasic or transient events, the movement elicited will not be sustained unless either the stimulus is sustained (which is not always possible) or additional supportive stimuli are rapidly provided. The most typical stimulus used as a follow up after eliciting postural movement (and other types of muscle activation as well) is resistance. Resistance to an existing isotonic contraction introduces an error signal into the motor control system, which in turn elicits additional activation of the resisted muscle. If the discrepancy between intended and actual movement is great enough, synergistic muscles will also be activated (radiation response). This mechanism for activating muscles works best if the patient is intending to exert voluntary control over the movement or is actually doing so. The error signal generated by resistance essentially concerns the difference between intended force or effort required to produce the desired movement and actual movement required. If no intended signal is present, there is nothing with which to compare the actual state of the muscle. However, because resistance to movement of itself can be a stimulus eliciting contraction, this technique is also of benefit in the absence of voluntary initiation of movement.

Additional supportive stimuli that may be used in the process of "capturing" a movement response include brief, carefully timed vocal commands (as in PNF), quick stretch of the active muscle (a form of using resistance), visual observation of the movement by the patient, and tactile stimulation over the active muscle. Clearly, effective use of these additional stimuli is extremely dependent on timing because the initial activation is of short duration.

Although use of these basic environment-response patterns can elicit specific motor patterns, in many patients they dominate motor activity to the extent that normal hold patterns of co-contraction and normal fractionated movement patterns cannot be generated or exist only as ineffective modifications of the basic response movements. In many of these situations the dominating movement pattern may be elicited by very mild stimuli or by stimuli that would not normally evoke the pattern. In these cases therapy must be directed at first inhibiting and then integrating these basic movements. Three possibilities exist for inhibiting basic reflex movement patterns: (1) applying stimuli to elicit opposite or alternative movement patterns; (2) applying stimuli that directly inhibit the undesired pattern; and (3) habituating the undesired pattern (stimulus desensitization). Often, the first two approaches can be combined. The concept of using reflex inhibiting patterns of movement, as developed by Bobath, is an excellent example of applying stimuli that inhibit an undesired pattern. The stimuli in this case consist of both movement out of the undesired pattern and tactile and proprioceptive stimulation at points that can influence the entire pattern of movement. The desired movement is controlled by handling at "key" points from which sensory information can affect activity in a large number of muscles. Details on how to use this particular approach can be found in articles by Bobath and by later NDT therapists.

Habituation occurs with the repeated application of relevant stimuli. As noted previously, some basic movement patterns are more amenable to the habituation process than others. Stimuli are most effective for habituation if they have the characteristics of monotony: similarity of intensity and quality, and regularity of timing. Stimuli of moderate intensity are typically most effective, although high intensity may be necessary in some cases (eg, for deep pressure stimuli). When intensity is close to threshold, the stimuli are apt to be perceived as variable as a result of slight variations in threshold for the response, and they are therefore not as useful for habituation.

Resistance to isotonic movement was described earlier as means of capturing or sustaining the movement response to a phasic stimulus. The rationale for using resistance was that it elicited the detection of error between initial move commands and the result of those commands. The response was an increase in activation that spread beyond the muscles initially involved to include their synergists. This process of "radiation" can be used extensively both to increase activation of groups of muscles in a resisted pattern of movement (as is done in PNF) and to elicit action in originally inactive muscles not directly associated with the resisted movement (as was suggested by Brunnstrom). Associated patterns used by Brunnstrom consist of mirror-image activation in the upper extremities (eg, flexion elicits flexion) and antagonist pattern activation in the lower extremities. However, in cases where the patient has movement predominated by stereotyped patterns, strong resistance is likely to elicit these patterns rather than more controllable movements. For this reason some therapists, particularly Bobath, have suggested avoiding the use of strong resistance until the patient has developed the ability to produce controlled fractionated movement patterns.

Hold Patterns

Co-contraction or stabilization patterns are developed on the basis of normal (or relatively normal) alpha motor neuron excitability and the existence of postural movement patterns. Hold patterns of muscle activation should not be confused with the relatively immobile postures seen in patients in whom abnormal general alpha motor neuron excitability predominates. Hold patterns may appear similar to the pathological condition of rigidity, in which an excess of inflexible activation is produced that limits expression of any type of movement pattern. During a normal hold contraction the muscle is relatively stiff, but is still flexible. Movement is permitted but deviations from the desired joint position are minimized by the existing pattern of gamma motor neuron excitation and muscle sense enhancement. Hold patterns maintain joints in mid-range positions in resistance to disturbing forces that would tend to move the joint towards the end of range in any particular direction. Hold patterns

are most typically expressed in axial and proximal extremity joints and are usually developed in a proximal to distal progression. In the lower extremity, hold patterns at the ankle appear to be of major importance for maintenance of upright posture or stance, and central motor control is directed primarily towards ankle rather than hip or knee co-contraction. In the hands and feet, hold patterns are less important, although because of the requirements of stance, they may exist in the feet. Stimuli useful in eliciting hold patterns are predominantly proprioceptive and of moderate to high intensity. Stimuli should be applied while the joint is in the mid-range of movement. Appropriate stimuli are listed in Table 43-7.

Production of hold patterns is particularly difficult in patients with disrupted timing of skeletal motor activation, such as in cerebellar dysfunction or other disorders that produce ataxia. The therapeutic approaches already indicated may be used with these patients to produce a relatively rigid fixation of a joint, which is not the same as the adaptable stabilization produced during a normal "hold." Unfortunately, the central nervous system does not appear to have other pathways to substitute for the timing circuits in the cerebellum. Use of alternative stimuli as an aid in supplying timing cues is usually not successful because of unacceptably long latency times between such stimuli and an appropriate motor response. Integration of cognitive stimuli for timing and their expression in motor behavior through cortical circuits is a lengthy process. With this in mind, the therapist would need to supply auxiliary timing cues in advance of the appropriate time. Similar timing problems affect the production of locomotion and fractionated movements. Timing usually is not as much of a problem in the production of postural adjustment movements, partly because smoothness of activation of muscles and accuracy of joint location is not as important for such movements.

Locomotion

Locomotion basically combines rhythmic alternating flexion and extension movements of op-

Table 43-7. Stimuli for Eliciting Hold Routines

STIMULUS	SOURCE
Joint compression (Rood)* (with force equal to or greater than body weight, see Table 43-5)	Manual pressure applied on both sides of the joint (may be intermittent or continuous, usually of high intensity) Gravity
Tapping (Bobath)	Brief passive movement of proximal body parts such that gravity produces a quick stretch of one set of muscles (frequently done in all relevant directions from mid-range)
Resistance (Knott)	Rhythmic stabilization—requests for active movement with resistance to the movement sufficient to allow only an isometric contraction in alternating directions from mid-range

*Names in parentheses indicate therapists who have described use of the technique in detail.

posite extremities with rotation of the trunk and neck. Although locomotor movements are very stereotyped in normal persons, they do not completely follow the patterns of any basic postural adjustment response. Key considerations in developing or regaining locomotion include (1) the ability to activate opposite extremities in an alternating pattern; (2) smooth and rhythmic shifts in use of opposite extremities; and (3) integration of trunk and neck rotation with flexion and extension patterns of the extremities. Programs for developing locomotion can begin with rhythmic weight shifting in any position in which the patient has functional trunk control. As the ability to maintain posture improves, the positions used can progress from those providing extensive postural support, such as sitting, to those providing less support, such as kneeling or standing. Alternating extremity flexion and extension movements can be combined with trunk rotation, as is seen in many PNF patterns. Eventually these PNF patterns must be modified, because locomotion does not involve flexion or extension of all joints in an extremity at the same time. Shoulders and hips can be used as key contact points for controlling weight shifts, extremity movement, and trunk rotation. Occasionally, the head may be used as a contact point for controlling rotation throughout the body axis. Tactile and proprioceptive stimulation must be timed to enhance the rhythmicity of the alternating movements produced.

Fractionated Movements

The category of fractionated or goal-directed movement includes movements that are voluntarily initiated and that occur on the basis of appropriate postural adjustment of the body. They usually require stabilization of proximal joints. Because of the voluntary nature of this movement, the patient must be actively involved in eliciting and sustaining it, even when reflex responses are also used as a means of initiating movement. Interaction between the therapist and patient must therefore be at a conscious level for both, even if the communication required is not verbal. Fractionated movements are elicited by using commands that engage the patient's will to move. Such commands may be verbal (eg, "Now, move!"), visual (eg, offering an object as a target for reaching or tracking), auditory but nonverbal (eg, presenting a sound for reaching or tracking), or tactile (eg, using a tactile stimulus as a target or goal). Commands may be offered individually or in supportive combinations. When the ability to activate the muscle voluntarily is limited, additional stimuli, usually tactile and proprioceptive, may be used to elicit initial reflex muscle activation. These stimuli would be very similar to phasic stimuli used as a means of increasing local alpha motor neuron excitability (refer to Table 43-5). Following initiation of the movement, additional proprioceptive or tactile stimuli may be used to enhance the activity, for example, resistance to the movement, or tactile guiding in the required direction of movement. Both techniques are used extensively in the manual contacts of PNF.

Fractionated movements may show deficiencies in speed of execution, accuracy of execution, or range. Difficulty in moving from slow to rapid, ballistic type movement is best addressed by starting with slow movements against resistance and gradually increasing the speed and decreasing the resistance. This progression mimics the normal progression of learning ballistic movements. In patients with timing disorders it may not be possible to reach the level of producing an accurate and rapid ballistic movement. When accurate execution of movement is a problem, a useful progression is to work from slow, small movements to more rapid and larger movements. Often, when difficulties exist in either speed or accuracy, the patient will try to overcome the difficulty by increasing co-contraction of all muscles involved in the movement. This increased activity in turn can produce alterations of excitability (hypertonicity) or co-contraction (rigidity), depending on the particular motor control patterns available to the patient. The therapist must be aware of the development of such changes in motor behavior and be prepared to counter them by (1) not requiring execution of fractionated movement well beyond the capability of the patient and (2) reapplying techniques that will reduce general excitability. Difficulty in producing the desired range of motion may be attributable to alterations in basal ganglia function through which scaling of movement patterns occurs. Alterations may be either in the direction of abnormally large (as seen in hemiballismus and some types of chorea) or abnormally small (as in parkinsonism) ranges of motion. Reflex inhibiting patterns may be useful in reducing excessively large movements. Elicitation of postural movements may be necessary to overcome excessive reduction in movement range.

Motor Planning

Treatment of the patient who is capable of producing near-normal or normal movement but who does not routinely do so is one of the most challenging areas of therapy. One cause of lack of movement in patients with an apparently intact motor system is sensory neglect, which has already been addressed. The other two causes of absence of movement or illogical use of motor capabilities are loss of motor drive and dyspraxia. All three problems may appear as indifference or simple lack of motivation or of intelligence on the part of the patient.

Absence of movement because of loss of motor drive is probably the result of damage to the limbic portions of the cortex, which affects all internally generated movements. The patient may be capable of perceiving accurately both internal and external signals that would normally lead to initiation of motor behavior. Direct specific commands may elicit movement. Two adaptive approaches are possible to such a problem: (1) provide external cues and commands to elicit the desired movement, and (2) provide a learning process through which the patient reintegrates movement-generating meaning with appropriate internal (rather than external or command) signals. Effectiveness of either approach may be very limited. Use of external cueing for movement will typically remain necessary because the limbic meaning-generating system, like the cerebellar timing system, is too unique and complex to admit easy substitution.

Dyspraxia (in the extreme case, apraxia) is a class of movement disorders in which elements of sequential or complex movements can be performed normally or almost normally, but the logic necessary to create normal ordering of these elements is lacking. The dysfunction is the result of damage to the parietal and to a certain extent frontal lobes. As one might expect, there are as many discrete varieties of dyspraxia as there are types of sensory-motor integration performed in these areas of the brain. Motor function may be affected globally or for only certain types of motor behavior or groups of muscles (such as in oro-facial dyspraxia). Specific therapeutic approaches to the problem must be used for each particular type of dyspraxia. In general, recognizing that the problem is one of loss of motor logic or planning, any therapeutic technique should incorporate meaningful external logic cues. Such cues should be simple, highly ordered, and consistent over time. (Imagine the first time you tried to tie a specific knot. You knew the desired end result, and you had the sensory-motor ability to make all the required moves, but you could not smoothly, if at all, produce the desired end result. If you were provided with a simple diagram ilustrating the sequence of moves required, you could then perform the complete action.) Another useful, general approach for therapy of dyspraxia involves placing the desired movement sequence in a context that is meaningful and familiar to the patient. This approach is essentially another way of providing meaningful cues for performance. For additional suggestions on approaches to specific types of dyspraxia, refer to the bibliography.

With each of these problems of cortical-level movement production, it is essential to recognize that the patient is usually not demented, willfully difficult to treat, or unmotivated. In many cases, particularly with dyspraxia, the patient will feel as baffled and frustrated as the therapist, if not more so, and will sincerely appreciate means of adapting to or correcting the problem. Patience, repetition, and very careful structuring of the learning-therapeutic environment are essential for success in treatment.

USE OF EQUIPMENT IN THERAPY

Adjuncts to hands-on therapy for neurologic patients fall into the following categories:

1. Aids for positioning the patient (either the whole body or individual parts);

2. Nonmanual stimulation tools:
3. Sensory aids for the therapist or patient to enhance discrimination of motor behavior.

These adjuncts to manual contact and visual and auditory observation are useful because the therapist cannot always do all of the following: make manual contact with all the desired locations at the same time; maintain contact or interaction with the patient over a sufficiently long time; provide, through the therapist's own motor behavior, adequate stimulation for the patient; and adequately discriminate the relevant motor behavior (also true for the patient). Because equipment cannot, for the most part, be described as "smart" (ie, it cannot change its characteristics or mode of interaction with the patient when the patient's behavior changes), it should not be relied upon as a substitute for routine direct therapist-patient interaction. Equipment will be used most effectively when the therapist and patient both view it as an extension of the therapist-patient interaction.

EQUIPMENT FOR POSITIONING

Positioning equipment can function either in a static or dynamic mode and can be used to adjust position or movement either for the whole body or for individual body parts. Useful aids for positioning or guiding movement of the whole body are listed in Table 43-8, and include balls, foam shapes, equilibrium boards, swings, molded or structurally modified furniture, standing frames, and ordinary furniture. In the static mode these structures are used to establish and maintain a given posi-

Table 43-8. Equipment Used for Whole-Body Positioning

EQUIPMENT FOR STATIC POSITIONING	EQUIPMENT FOR DYNAMIC POSITIONING
Molded or structurally adapted furniture	Large ball
Regular furniture (functionally adapted to the needs of the patient)	Large foam shapes, eg, wedges, cylinders
Standing frame (for normal or prone standing)	Equilibrium board
Large foam shapes, eg, wedges, cylinders	Rotation board or stool
	Swing (upright or prone positioning)
	Rocking chair

tion, thus freeing the therapist for more detailed and dynamic interaction with the patient, or to provide a means to extend the benefits of certain positions beyond the therapy session. When this equipment is used for extended periods, precautions must be taken to ensure that its static nature does not become a negative factor as a result of dynamic changes in the patient's posture. Enforced extended maintenance of any given static posture, such as might be provided by molded furniture, a standing frame, or even foam shapes, does not provide normal variation in tactile and proprioceptive information to the central nervous system. Therefore, static devices should be designed either to provide for a range of appropriate movement and posture adjustment while maintaining a general posture, or they should be used for limited time spans. (Imagine, for example, that you are forced to maintain for an hour, without moving, exactly the same position in a comfortable chair. Probably long before the end of that time, you would be aware of generalized and specific discomfort. This sensation of discomfort is the result of both stimulation that has become noxious and interpretation by the central nervous system of the normal, but abnormally prolonged, sensation as a strong signal requiring you to move. Similar changes in sensory input almost certainly occur for the patient with relatively intact sensation who is required to maintain a constant position over time.) Another reason, of course, for permitting some movement flexibility during static positioning is to maintain homeostasis, particularly of circulatory function, in the positioned parts of the body as well as in the body as a whole.

During therapy sessions some of the same types of equipment listed in Table 43-8 can be used to provide dynamic postural stimulation for the patient. Balls, foam shapes, swings, and equilibrium boards are examples of equipment used for dynamic positioning. By supporting the body weight of the patient, this equipment permits the therapist to supply dynamic stimulation, particularly to the vestibular system, with minimal effort and maximal control of the movement and the patient's po-

sition. Use of equipment for this purpose has been described in particular detail by Ayers and NDT therapists and to a certain extent by Rood. Ayers has also described the use of specialized "furniture" or environmental shapes to form therapeutic environments through which the patient moves in structured ways that are said to enhance vestibular sensory integration and spatial-motor skills. Because these adjuncts to therapy will supply tactile and proprioceptive sensation, the therapist needs to be aware of the effects of this sensory information on the motor activity of the patient and adjust it as needed to inhibit or facilitate specific alpha motor neuron excitability and motor behavior.

Equipment that can provide control of parts of the patient's body consists primarily of casts and braces (orthoses), which can be used either to provide static support and control for specific joints or dynamic control of movement. Static orthoses may serve the function of support primarily, as would be the case with lower extremity locked braces. As a result of the necessary skin contact of such orthoses and the position they impose on joints and their associated muscles, these orthoses will also provide tonic tactile and proprioceptive stimulation to the body part. This stimulation should be adjusted so that it does not elicit unwanted changes in alpha motor neuron excitability. By the same reasoning, the positioning achieved and the contact of the brace or cast may be used to provide desired inhibitory or facilitatory sensation to the body part. For example, positioning of the ankles and toes and establishment of specific contact points with the feet can be very important in facilitating either stance or movement of the entire lower extremity. Dynamic orthoses permit movement within the controlled joints and usually assist the movement by providing either facilitation through sensory stimulation or assistance through mechanical forces. Because of their interaction with phasic stretch reflexes, dynamic orthoses must be designed with particular care when they are to be used on a body part in which abnormal alpha motor neuron excitability exists. Details on manufacture and application of specific static and dynamic orthoses can be found in texts dealing specifically with orthotics.

NONMANUAL STIMULI

Many occasions occur when the therapist cannot, by manual contact alone, supply the quality, diversity, frequency, or intensity of tactile or proprioceptive stimulation necessary to produce the desired change in alpha motor neuron excitability or movement. In such cases, additional tools may be used very effectively for stimulation. These tools can be grouped by their primary action on tactile receptors, thermal receptors, or proprioceptors or by their direct action on sensory neurons. Some stimulation tools such as vibrators, will activate more than one sensory modality. Examples of tools falling into these categories are listed in Table 43-9. In addition to these tools, orthoses and casts may be used to provide sustained tactile and proprioceptive stimulation. Several stimulating tools or materials may be used in combination or with manual contact to enhance certain motor responses (eg, ice and phasic stretch could be combined to elicit muscle contraction). Combining stimuli can be more effective than providing them in isolation, but should not be attempted until the therapist is familiar with the use of each stimulus alone.

Functional Electrical Stimulation

Direct electrical stimulation of either peripheral nerves or of selected portions of the central nervous system is being increasingly used both as a temporary, therapeutic technique and as a long-term supportive technique. Electrical stimulation of peripheral nerves can be used either to activate sensory fibers, most specifically Ia fibers from primary spindle endings, or alpha motor neurons. When sensory fibers are activated, the intent is to substitute this neural activity for afferent activity produced by ordinary stimulation. By this means both phasic reflex responses and more persistent "learned" alterations in tonic behavior may be elicited in the central nervous system at both spinal cord and higher levels. Both types of responses can serve as adjuncts to support desired locomotor and goal-directed movements. Of course, stimulation of alpha motor neurons causes direct activation of the innervated muscles for the period of time that the stimulus is present. Such direct activation is not usually implicated in producing persistent changes in central neural behavior, although repeated use of this type of stimulation over time may assist the patient in learning certain patterns of motor activity, just as providing manual assistance to the movement may.

Peripheral nerve stimulation has been used predominantly in producing or assisting locomotor movements that are phasic, relatively stereotyped, and repetitive, and that can function adequately without ongoing feedback modification (the stimulation tends to override feedback commands). A prime example of such use is in functional electrical stimulation-assisted gait for patients following stroke or spinal cord injury. In this situation, the physical therapist is both an evaluator who determines the appropriateness of potential applications of the technology and the precise location and effective stimulus parameters and an instructor who teaches the patient and any necessary care providers how to use the device.

Real limitations on the use of peripheral nerve stimulation exist. Unresolved problems still exist in the equipment, particularly concerning electrode placement, skin tolerance for the electrodes, and production of consistent effects from fixed stimulus parameters. Limits exist in the number of muscles or muscle groups and in the types of movement patterns that can be effectively activated in this way. As indicated above, movements produced by peripheral stimulation tend to be stereotyped. As yet, the problems of permitting flexibility and sensitivity to sensory information in the stimulating system have not been adequately resolved. Additionally, the production of normal co-contraction by electrical stimulation is very difficult. Significant advantages offered by peripheral nerve stimulation include the production of more nearly normal movement locally than can be achieved with orthoses and the

Table 43-9. Examples of Stimulation Tools

CATEGORY/EXAMPLE	USE
Tactile Stimulation	
Brush, fine hair	Facilitate movement and increase excitability in underlying muscles when moved rapidly over the skin; may produce an aversive response; may produce an excessive increase in excitability with a relatively long latency
Materials of varied texture	Enhance discriminatory touch and manual orientation responses
Light vibration (75–125 Hz)	Increase excitability and facilitate movement in underlying muscles (frequencies less than 75 Hz may be inhibitory; frequencies greater than 125 Hz may be noxious and may damage tissue)
Cotton ball or similar material	Lightly touching the skin will either elicit orienting movements or aversive movements depending on the predominant state of the cortex
Proprioceptive Stimulation	
Vibration over tendons or muscle bellies	Increase excitability and enhance movement of vibrated muscle (tonic vibration reflex);use same frequencies as for tactile stimulation
Orthokinetic cuff (combined modalities)	Part applying constant pressure over a tendon (proprioception) decreases excitability in related muscle; part applying varying touch stimulation enhances movement in underlying muscles
Sand or similar material	Applies tonic pressure stimulus to body part immersed and moving in the sand; decreases excitability in related muscles (related tactile stimulation may enhance orienting and exploratory movement)
Thermal Stimulation	
Ice	See Table 43-5
Neutral warmth	See Table 43-2
Electrical Stimulation of Peripheral Nerves*	
Low frequency, threshold intensity stimulation	Selective activation of large-diameter myelinated fibers, primarily from primary spindle endings in nerves from muscle or mixed nerves; elicits H reflex[†]
Low frequency (less than 30 Hz), intensity supramaximal for H reflex	Direct but not selective activation of alpha motor neurons[††]

*Electrical stimulation for purposes of management of pain (TENS) is discussed elsewhere in this text.

[†]Due to the very specific nature of the stimulus, fibers activated and the reflex response produced are not identical to the fibers activated and the response produced in a phasic stretch or deep tendon reflex.

[††]Activation of additional sensory fibers may produce variable and not always predictable results depending on the nerve stimulated, stimulus parameters, and ongoing sensory-motor status of the patient.

enhancement of homeostasis within the muscles thus activated. Complex stimulation systems are viewed as adjuncts to the use of more conventional orthoses for support and control of movement in the neurologic patient.

Electrodes implanted in the central nervous system are also used to direct and modulate sensory-motor behavior. The two sites used for such stimulation are the spinal cord and the cerebellum. Spinal cord stimulation has been used predominantly as a means of modifying general alpha motor neuron excitability in patients with spinal cord injury. Stimulation of the dorsal portion of the spinal cord acts primarily through its effect on ascending discriminatory touch and proprioceptive sensation in the dorsal columns and spinocerebellar tracts. Electrodes placed ventrally may act either through interaction with nondiscriminatory modalities in the lateral cord or with descending information, particularly in pathways that carry tonic commands (eg, reticulospinal, tectospinal, vestibulospinal). Ventral stimulation may also directly affect ventral horn interneurons or motor neurons. Spinal stimulation is typically sustained rather than applied periodically.

Cerebellar stimulation has been used as a means of increasing the overall level of activity of the cerebellum. Relatively precise electrode localization is possible with the technique, but there is still a great deal to be learned concerning the functional value of stimulating different regions of the cerebellum. As might be expected, cerebellar stimulation is used primarily on patients with ataxia or timing difficulties in the production of movement. Technical difficulties in the use of implanted central neural stimulators are predominantly the result of shifts in electrode location. Functionally, difficulties may arise as a result of alterations in neural response to the constant stimulation. As an evaluator, the therapist is involved in determining the availability of ascending and descending spinal pathways and cerebellar circuits. The functional value of consistently altering general alpha motor neuron excitability and motor coordination must also be assessed. Following electrode implanation, the

therapist assists the patient in learning to use the altered motor control now available.

Augmented Sensory Information

In some situations, information concerning motor activity that is available by direct observation (visual, auditory, tactile, or proprioceptive) is inadequately precise to permit control of the activity by either the patient or the therapist. In such cases, devices to augment the available sensory information, specifically biofeedback devices, may be useful. They are of particular value when the motor behavior under consideration is produced by the autonomic rather than the skeletal motor system, because sensory information concerning the behavior is typically not available at the conscious level. Biofeedback uses electrical sensing of some relevant parameters of the behavior to be controlled and transduces the electrical signal into a mode that can be easily sensed by the patient and therapist. Signaling modes include visual, auditory, and tactile. For the neurologic patient, the signaling mode is chosen on the basis of availability of sensory modalities in the patient's central nervous system and relevance of the sensory modality to the behavior to be modified. The second consideration is often ignored (usually because of equipment limitations), but can be an important factor in the efficiency of the system. Sensory augmentation through biofeedback techniques is valuable when the intent is to clarify sensory information and to focus the patient's attention on the particular motor function being monitored. Biofeedback can be combined with other sensory stimulation aimed at facilitating the required motor activity.

INVOLVEMENT OF THE PATIENT'S CAREPROVIDERS

Therapy sessions with neurologic patients are very intense (not necessarily the same thing as very stressful) both for the therapist and the patient. Partly for this reason, and also for reasons of sheer practicality, you cannot expect to provide therapy to an individual patient for more than one to two hours a day. For the rest of the time the patient will not be in *your* therapeutic environment, but in a variety of other settings. In order for therapy to be most effective, it must be designed both to carry over into these other environments and to be compatible with them. Several principles will help in extending your therapeutic efforts.

1. When appropriate, use therapeutic approaches that are known to have long-lasting effects. For example, some mechanisms for modifying general alpha motor neuron excitability, such as positioning, are effective only during application and for a short time thereafter, whereas others, such as neutral warmth, can be effective for an hour or longer.
2. Use adjuncts to manual contact. Orthoses will inhibit unwanted sensory-motor behavior through the tactile and proprioceptive input they provide (eg, inhibitory casting). Functional electrical stimulation will reinforce the sensory input given in therapy.
3. Whenever possible, teach the patient stimulation and movement behaviors that he can easily do correctly, and that will assist in consolidating learning which has occurred in therapy.
4. Teach all careproviders how to assist the patient in ways that will reinforce or at least not negate the gains made in therapy.
5. Be aware of the physical, psychological, and social framework of the environments in which the patient actually spends most of his time and adapt treatment, teaching, and goals for the patient accordingly.

The therapist-careprovider-environment interaction is extremely important. On the one hand, careproviders must be included in the therapy process in many ways. They can provide essential information on the patient's environment and past and current sensory-motor behavior that may not be clear from the patient-therapist interaction, no matter how good it is. They are also, depending on the patient's level of independence, an essential means of extending your therapeutic efforts. On the other hand, do not expect or require careproviders, particularly if they are family members, to become surrogate or alternative neurologic therapists. The intense therapist-patient interaction that ideally occurs during therapy cannot easily be extended beyond the usual time for therapy, and it is quite unlike most family interactions. This is not to say that family members cannot provide supportive therapy or that they may not become better at many aspects of patient handling than the therapist.

ORGANIZATION OF TREATMENT

So many problems and so many possible treatment approaches to each problem need to be addressed with the neurologic patient that the relatively inexperienced therapist may find initiating treatment difficult because of the extensive decision making required! This final section, with the accompanying diagram in Figure 43-1, is intended to provide some guidelines for decision making that will help the therapist both in initiating and in continuing neurologic therapy. You will note throughout that treatment and evaluation are congruent and interactive aspects of therapy.

Where to start? As the King said in *Alice*: "Begin at the beginning and go on till you get to the end. Then stop." This advice is useful, but like most logic it is good only if the terms "beginning" and "end" are adequately defined. The initial patient evaluation will have been performed making some assumptions about treatment progression; if the therapist assumes that treatment will progress according to a normal maturational sequence, then the evaluation will seek to determine where the patient currently is along that sequence. If the initial evaluation has not been performed with treatment progression already in mind, then the first requirement will be to perform an evaluation that supplies information relevant to the desired treatment progression. If the treatment sequence used as a basis for evaluation is complex, as is the normal maturational sequence,

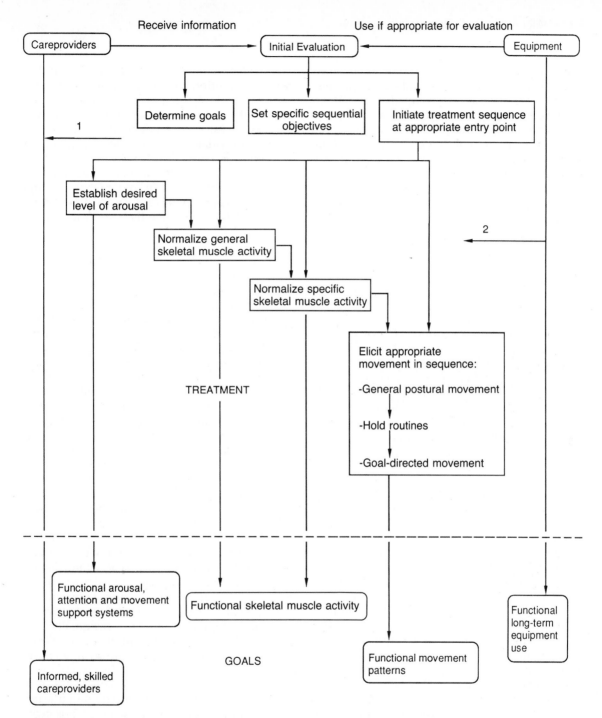

Figure 43-1. General flow diagram illustrating the steps in treating the neurologic patient. Evaluation continues throughout treatment; the process of receiving appropriate information from careproviders thus will continue throughout the therapy process. Instruction of careproviders, as indicated by arrow *1*, also is an ongoing process. Use of equipment as indicated by arrow *2*, either for evaluation or for therapy, should occur when appropriate. The final goals of therapy are indicated at the end of the process.

the evaluation will also determine congruence in behavior among different subsequences (eg, if feeding behavior is developed to the same level as eye-hand coordination). The following guidelines assume that the therapist will be following a maturational sequence similar to that used as a basis for discussion of treatment approaches in this chapter. The guidelines assume that the patient can progress within or between treatment sessions from one level of activity to the next. In many cases, such progression will not occur or will occur very slowly, and the therapist will have to repeat the work from the beginning at each treatment session.

Initially, determine the level of arousal of the patient and adjust the environment, if possible, by choosing a treatment setting to develop and support the desired arousal and attention level during each treatment session. After the first session(s) with the patient, this adjustment of the environment can be done before the treatment session in anticipation of the expected needs of the patient. Unfortunately, technology has not yet advanced to the stage where interactive adjustments of environmental factors can occur easily within a therapy session.

Having established the desired level of arousal, concentrate on general alpha motor neuron excitability, particularly *if* this has not been adjusted appropriately while manipulating arousal. Local adjustment of alpha motor neuron excitability can then be addressed. Because of the interactive nature of excitability and movement, the process of adjusting excitability can be combined to a certain extent with the process of eliciting desired movement or hold patterns of activity depending on the ability of the therapist to attend to both processes simultaneously. Integrating therapy to the point where both excitability and movement are affected simultaneously in an appropriate way is not always easy for the inexperienced therapist; therefore, when necessary these two components of therapy should be addressed separately. As indicated earlier in the chapter, movement should be developed sequentially, starting with general postural movements,

then adding hold routines, and concluding with locomotion or goal-directed movement. Normal general alpha motor neuron excitability must be maintained as much as possible while working on movement patterns. In addition, appropriate levels of arousal and general homeostatic support function must be maintained because these facilitate production of normal sensory-motor behavior. If at any time control of earlier levels is lost, treatment must return to the level at which control is available.

The therapist must be prepared to repeat therapeutic approaches many times to permit learning to occur, but the repetition should always include some variation and some attempt to progress slightly beyond the previous level. As is true of normal development, progression of the neurologic patient should not require perfection of one level of behavior before initiating the next higher one. Progression can occur as soon as a given level of behavior can be elicited and maintained without constant stimulation from the therapist and conscious attention by the patient. Activities occurring in any given level will, as a general rule, facilitate greater control over the prior level so long as advancement is not too rapid.

Use of equipment should be limited in the early stages of therapy unless the therapist is particularly familiar with a given piece of equipment. Equipment can limit therapy as well as enhance it (eg, if a therapy ball is available you are more likely to use it, even if its use may not be totally appropriate). Perhaps more importantly, equipment comes between the therapist and the patient, and if used too early may limit the development of maximally productive therapist-patient interaction. When equipment is introduced a limited number and variety of pieces should be added at any given time, and the patient (and therapist) should be given adequate time to develop therapeutic use of the equipment. Changing types of equipment radically from one treatment session to the next will limit learning of therapeutic use of the equipment. However, this does not mean that use of a particular piece of equipment must be continued if its initial introduction has produced definitely disruptive responses in the patient.

Interaction with careproviders should begin with the initial evaluation and continue throughout therapy. It is important that the therapist use careproviders, as well as the patient, as constant sources of information about progress and problems. Instruction of careproviders in skills that will assist the patient and enhance therapy should also occur continuously and gradually; postponing instruction until treatment is nearly completed will significantly decrease its effectiveness. Use principles of learning with the careproviders just as you do with the patient; in particular, give them adequate time to practice skills and seek answers to their questions. Learning how to do unfamiliar skills correctly takes time.

Determining the appropriate end point for treatment of the neurologic patient is at least as difficult as determining the starting point. No standardized "end points" are generally available, and terms such as "maximum benefit" have so many possible interpretations as to be of little guidance on their own. Figure 43-1 illustrates end points of functional availability of various sensory-motor behaviors. "Functional" here means a style of sensory-motor behavior that will permit the patient to interact effectively, but not necessarily normally, with his environment. The concept of functional behavior is useful to predict the treatment end point, but the goal of function may not always be obtained in each type of behavior. Treatment end point can be set pragmatically by determining that the patient has reached a plateau at which the withdrawal of therapy will neither limit the likelihood for progression nor increase the probability of deterioration.

CONCLUSION

The therapist needs to consider the following key points in order to provide effective treatment of the neurologic patient:

1. Establishment of a close patient-therapist interaction through which the capabilities of the therapist's central nervous system can correct and enhance the patient's capabilities.
2. Progression of therapy according to a consistent sequence of sensory-motor behavior relevant to the individual patient.
3. Selection of stimuli from the wide range of possible stimuli that will be appropriate to the patient and to the progression sequence chosen.
4. Involvement of careproviders at all stages of therapy.
5. Application of principles of learning when dealing with both the patient and careproviders.
6. Realistic determination of goals and end point for treatment in accordance with the functional needs and capabilities of both the patient and careproviders.

Within this general framework the therapist should feel free to experiment and gain experience in using the wide variety of approaches currently available in therapy for the patient with neurological dysfunction.

ANNOTATED BIBLIOGRAPHY

The following books provide detailed information about specific schools of therapy, including both theoretical background and description of evaluative and treatment procedures. Little current information is available on Rood per se, partly because many of her ideas have become incorporated in other approaches to therapy. Ayers has published extensively; the interested reader can use the text reference here as a starting point. Current information on Bobath therapy, or NDT, is predominantly in journal articles rather than texts.

Ayers AJ: The Development of Sensory Integrative Theory and Practice. Dubuque, IA, Kendal/Hunt, 1974

Bobath B: Motor Development in the Different Types of Cerebral Palsy. New York, William Heinemann, 1975

Bobath B: Adult Hemiplegia: Evaluation and Treatment, 2nd ed. London, William Heinemann, 1979

Bobath K: A Neurophysiological Basis for the Treatment of Cerebral Palsy. New York, William Heinemann, 1975

Brunnstrom S: Movement Therapy in Hemiplegia. New York, Harper & Row, 1970

Northwestern University Special Therapeutic Exercise Project (NUSTEP): An exploratory and analytical survey of therapeutic exercise. Am J Phys Med 46(1), 1967 (Collection of now classical descriptions of therapeutic approaches of Bobath, Brunnstrom, Knott, and Rood. This text is out of print, but worth the effort to search out.)

Voss DE, Ionta MK, Myers BJ: Proprioceptive Neuromuscular Facilitation, 3rd ed. Philadelphia, JB Lippincott, 1985

The books listed below carry recent information on various treatment techniques for different types of neurologic problems.

Miller N: Dyspraxia and Its Management. Rockville, MD, Aspen Systems, 1986 (Current, thorough discussion of the various types of dyspraxia. Describes each type, its probable causes, and specific suggestions for therapy aimed at either recovery or adaptation.)

Umphred DA (ed): Neurological Rehabilitation. St Louis, CV Mosby, 1985 (Separate chapters in this text supply detailed descriptions of treatment techniques and rationales for all types of neurologic patients the therapist is likely to see. Excellent current supplement for either the detailed texts dealing with specific therapeutic approaches or for the NUSTEP manual cited above.)

The theoretical basis for treatment of neurologic patients has received attention in other chapters of this text. Listed below is an additional reference text that supplies a very thorough rationale for neurologic therapy with numerous suggestions for application of neurologic principles in therapy.

Brooks VB: The Neural Basis of Motor Control. New York, Oxford University Press, 1986

44 Balance and Coordination Training

CAROLYN A. CRUTCHFIELD
ANNE SHUMWAY-COOK
FAY B. HORAK

Physical therapists often divide balance and coordination tasks and skills into particular categories for protocols of assessment and treatment. The term "coordination" usually brings to mind some specific fine motor task, such as the finger-to-nose test, manipulating nuts and bolts, or the old familiar heel-to-shin test. Our concept of balance is similarly restricted and narrowly defined. It is envisioned that someone without balance simply falls easily, is dizzy, or demonstrates shaky or ataxic movements. Clinical tests for balance are generally limited to having the patient stand on one leg with eyes open and eyes shut, or telling him not to allow the clinician to push him over, while disturbing his equilibrium by pushing his trunk or by rocking a tiltboard.

It is clear that "balance" and "coordination" are terms that have never had satisfactory clinical definitions. From a more universal perspective, coordination may be considered the essence of movement; indeed, it may cover all aspects of movement, including balance. From a biological perspective, coordination may be defined as the function that constrains the body's limitless degrees of freedom into a single, efficient, functional unit. Coordination is required for the exquisite performance of fine motor skills, such as playing the piano or performing gymnastic routines. In a global sense, coordination is required for postural control, making it possible to stand, walk, run, jump, perform occupational tasks, cook, clean house, care for children, and perform the infinite array of movements encountered in everyday tasks.

If all movements, including balance, have aspects of coordination, then dysfunction in any type of musculoskeletal movement could result in some dysfunction in coordination. Balance, like coordination, is an essential part of movement and skill. Balance is the ability to maintain equilibrium; that is, it is the ability to maintain the center of body mass over the base of support.

For example, if normal walking is considered to be a perfectly timed sequence of muscle activity that occurs in response to both internal and external forces, then it is easy to consider walking as a task requiring coordination as well as balance. If the ankle is sprained, however, altered joint kinematics and the presence of pain change the pattern of muscle activity. A dysfunction in coordination has occurred, producing a movement dysfunction that is recognized as a characteristic limp. A dysfunction in balance has occurred because the body's center of mass may be displaced over the uninvolved leg such that the center of body mass lies closer to its limits of stability. In this case, the problem is easily localized in the clinical assessment, and effective treatment is undertaken to help heal the tissue disruptions and diminish the pain. The result after healing is a restored balance and a coordinated gait pattern.

Movements are often divided into two

main categories: gross movements and fine movements. Gross movements include such activities as posture, balance, and extremity movements that involve large muscle groups (eg, creeping, standing, running, and throwing a ball). Fine movements usually involve small muscle groups, in particular, the manipulation of objects with the hands. These activities require dexterity and in some measure are under cortical control. Parameters of fine movements that can be assessed are speed, control, accuracy, and reaction time.

In testing coordination, the therapist should attempt to assess the integration of sensory and motor systems in the performance of movements. One of the greatest needs in physical therapy is to reduce normal activities to components that can be assessed and treated. However, very often the activity or component that is evaluated and treated actually has no real relationship to the difficulty at hand.

An example of such a problem is the use of manual muscle testing. No correlations have been made with manual muscle test grades and the ability of the patient to function. Possibly, the reason is that the conditions required of muscle testing are not always those required for function. Manual muscle testing requires isolated joint movement and isolated muscle action. Most tests are of a non-weight-bearing nature in which the distal part of the extremity is free while the proximal part holds against external resistance. A function the patient may not be able to perform could require a weight-bearing posture and a diagonal pattern of movement, which involves multiple joints and muscle groups in a harmonious pattern.

What does it mean to have good or normal balance and coordination? How is it measured? What causes dysfunction in balance and coordination? What can be done to rehabilitate the patient who has such a dysfunction?

SYSTEMS MODEL OF MOTOR CONTROL

How human movement is viewed depends upon the theory of motor control that is be-

lieved to best explain such movement. Therefore, before discussing assessment and treatment techniques it is necessary to explore the neurophysiologic substrata of balance and coordination that is related to the systems theory of motor control, which we espouse. The systems theory of motor control was first offered by Bernstein (1896–1966) and other Russian physiologists. Many theories of motor control abound, and some have been presented in other chapters.

Information related to this theory has been expanded and applied by such researchers as Nashner, Shumway-Cook, Horak, and others. Four assumptions underlying the systems theory as we have adapted it to postural control are listed below.

1. Subsystems interact in a circular network.
2. All movements are organized around behavioral objectives.
3. Basic units of movement are preprogrammed synergies.
4. Intersensory interaction for postural orientation is flexible and context dependent.

CIRCULAR NETWORK OF SUBSYSTEMS

The traditional clinical approach to evaluating balance and coordination in the neurologic patient in the western culture is based on a reflex approach or hierarchical approach grounded in research by Sherrington, Magnus, and Jackson. The reflex model, and its extension the hierarchical model of postural control, assume that subsystems of movement are arranged hierarchically, with such systems as muscular, visual, joint, and vestibular reflex loops controlled at the lowest level. The reflex model presumes that the "higher" centers must dominate "lower" centers in order for skilled movement to emerge.

In clinical practice, therapists following the reflex model or hierarchical model will attempt to integrate primitive or "low-level" reflex activity while attempting to get the equilibrium or "high-level" reflexes to take over the patient's motor function. It is often assumed that the presence of the former prevents the emergence of the latter.

Unlike the reflex and hierarchical models, the systems model assumes that sensorimotor subsystems underlying postural control relate to each other within a circular network. In the systems model, no higher and lower arrangement exists between the subsystems. The vestibular, visual, and somatosensory systems, for instance, interact in a flexible manner for postural orientation depending upon what goals the movement is to accomplish and what the conditions are in the environment. Each subsystem may be dominant at different times. For example, as the type or quality of the surface on which we are standing changes, these qualities will be registered by the somatosensory system. If the information in the visual field changes, the visual system will register such changes. The subsystem presenting the most accurate information at the moment will dominate and ultimately determine the appropriate motor response.

GOAL-ORIENTED MOVEMENTS

All movements are goal oriented, that is, they are used to accomplish some behavioral objective. A major goal of postural control is to keep the center of gravity over the base of support. If the goal is not accomplished, responses are modified until the goal is accomplished. Modification of responses requires active participation by the subject and knowledge of the results of subsequent movements.

Therapists who rely on the systems model will strive to facilitate all the different components of movement and integrate them so that a variety of movements are possible. In this manner learning and fine-tuning of movements will result. Such a variety is necessary for the patient to respond to environmental conditions and to achieve the goals the movement is meant to accomplish.

PREPROGRAMMED SYNERGIES

The basic units of movement in the systems model are preprogrammed packages of muscle activity, or synergies. A synergy consists of a particular group of muscles that have been linked together in a certain sequence. The timing of muscle activation within a synergy is consistent and precise to ensure that each muscle in the synergy is activated in the proper order and at the proper time. This packaging of muscle groups greatly simplifies the way in which the nervous system will access a motor reaction in response to sensory input. Rather than having to decide which muscles to include and in what order they should be activated, the brain need only determine which synergy must be used and how strong or large it must be.

Nashner, Horak, and their associates produced a series of elegant research projects that identified postural synergies or strategies. Subjects stood on a platform that would suddenly perturb their balance by translating them forward or backward. This translation produces a perturbation similar to having a rug pulled from under you. A relatively small backward translation, or pull of the rug, causes the person to fall forward (forward sway). Most subjects responded to a backward translation by contracting the gastrocnemius, hamstring, and the paraspinal muscles in that order to counteract or correct the forward sway. If the subjects were perturbed by a forward translation or pull, the usual result was the contraction of the tibialis anterior, quadriceps, and abdominal muscles in that order to correct the resultant backward sway.

These responses to forward and backward perturbations, which began distally with the ankle musculature, constitute the ankle synergy or strategy. The forward and backward pendular movement that results from activation of the ankle synergy is identical to what we know as postural sway (Fig. 44-1).

In further experiments, ankle movements were reduced by having subjects stand crosswise on a beam attached to the platform. A narrow beam under the feet does not provide sufficient surface for the subject to press against in order to produce effective counterforces. To minimize sway and return the body's center of mass to within the supporting base of the feet, the supporting surface must be large and firm enough to produce a counterforce to the muscular contraction that causes ankle movement.

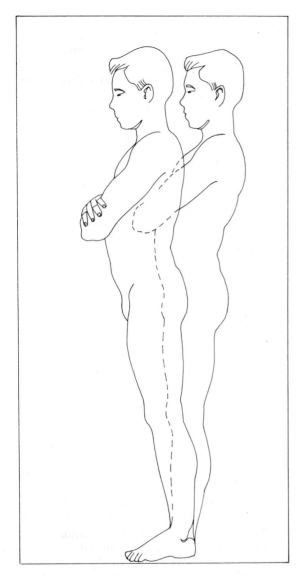

Figure 44-1. Forward and backward sway of the ankle synergy.

When subjects were perturbed while standing on a narrow beam, different muscle packages were activated. When the platform was translated backward, the subject swayed forward and the abdominal and quadriceps muscles were activated, to return the center of mass back over the feet. Conversely, a forward translation produced a backward sway, and the paraspinal and hamstring muscles were activated. These responses are referred to as the hip synergy. It is important to note that the same direction of perturbation reverses the sequence of muscular activity in the hip synergy from proximal to distal, compared with the distal to proximal activity in the ankle synergy. Very little ankle activity was present during the hip synergy (Fig. 44-2). The nervous system then is provided with various strategies for postural reactions to accomplish the goal of equilibrium.

When the perturbation or disturbance to equilibrium is relatively small and the supporting surface is adequate, the ankle synergy is the primary strategy used to maintain balance. When the subject is given a perturbation that is too large to be controlled by the ankle synergy, or if the supporting surface is not adequate for the production of the ankle synergy, the hip synergy will usually be elicited. If the center of gravity is displaced far enough, the person will take a step forward or backward, which may be referred to as a stepping strategy. The interaction of these synergies in response to sensory input elicited in environmental contexts is the essence of coordinated movements for balance.

MULTIPLE ROLES OF SENSORY INFORMATION

In the systems model, balance and coordination are dynamic integrative functions that use multiple sensory inputs. The systems model requires that motor output be flexible, adaptable, and responsive to changes in the environment. Sensory systems interact with motor systems at all levels, ensuring environmental adaptation. The response to a particular stimulus depends upon the environmental context in which it is presented. The same stimulus may produce different responses in different contexts.

Sensory information assumes multiple roles in the control of movement. Sensory cues may trigger a postural response. Sensory cues containing essential information about the en-

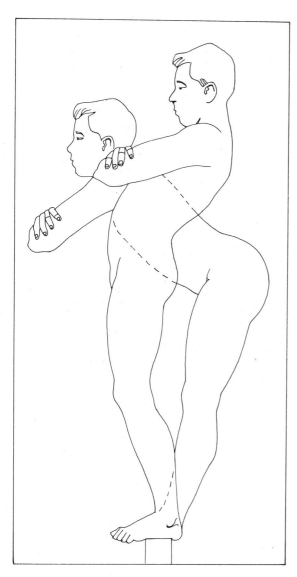

Figure 44-2. The hip synergy.

The use of multiple senses in postural control preserves freedom of movement while retaining effective automatic stabilization for the maintenance of balance. The nervous system uses three sensory inputs for postural orientation. These senses include vision (for object-to-object orientation), vestibular input (self-to-earth orientation), proprioception (self-to-self orientation), and exteroception (self-to-object orientation). The last two are often referred to collectively as somatosensory inputs.

The organization of redundant sensory cues is a complex process. The nervous system must determine which senses are giving useful information and which are giving conflicting information about the environment and the body's relationship to it. This information is necessary for the nervous system to determine the position of the center of mass in relation to gravity and to determine the nature of the supporting surface on which the body stands, sits, or lies. Once the correct information is determined, the motor system will select the appropriate package or synergy that will move the center of mass to equilibrium.

Postural control depends upon the redundant inputs from the visual, somatosensory, and vestibular systems. The visual system registers movements of objects in the environment and our movements within the environment. It is possible, however, for our eyes to deceive us. Have you ever been sitting in a train, bus, or car and when the adjacent object (such as another train) moved, you suddenly felt that you were moving? In this case the visual system was not relaying correct information about your movement in relation to gravity.

The nature of the supporting surface on which you are standing, walking, sitting, or lying is registered by somatosensory inputs from muscle spindles and joint and cutaneous receptors. These receptors tell us whether the supporting surface is slick, rocky, soft, hard, and so forth. These receptors also provide information to assist the nervous system in judging self-to-self information, such as the position of the various joints of each limb in relation to each other.

The vestibular system registers the posi-

vironment may be used when learning new movements or when fine-tuning movements. Physical therapists who base their treatments on the systems model will provide a variety of experiences for their patients to help them respond to environmental demands, keep them flexible, and increase their functional capacity.

tion and movements of our bodies relative to gravity. It has been suggested that the role of the vestibular system in balance is to act as a reference system, resolving intersensory conflicts that arise when other sensory systems fail to convey correct information. Thus, in the moving train example, when the eyes tricked you into believing that you were moving, the somatosensory system was relaying information to the contrary. The vestibular system helps resolve the conflict between these two senses. Once the conflict has been resolved, you quickly know that you were not moving, but that the train adjacent to you was moving. Such intersensory conflicts are frequently encountered in everyday functioning. If we cannot resolve these conflicts rapidly, inappropriate motor responses will occur and movement dysfunction results.

Nashner (1982) developed a moving platform protocol that tested the interaction of senses for postural control by systematically controlling the availability of sensory cues for postural orientation. Sensory inputs were eliminated, or alternatively subjects were provided inaccurate orientation information. Body sway was measured under six conditions (Table 44-1). In condition 1, the subject was standing quietly. In condition 2, he was standing and blindfolded so that vision could be eliminated. A box with a visual pattern surrounded the subject in condition 3. The box moved as the subject swayed and, therefore, the eyes failed to register the movement. Because the body was actually moving, the visual system was presenting inaccurate information concerning sway to the central mechanisms. So, in condition 3 an intersensory conflict existed between the visual system and the receptors registering motion in the ankles. The vestibular system resolved this conflict, and with all three of these conditions the normal subjects swayed very little. As might be expected, a slightly greater sway was evident in condition 3.

In condition 4, the platform on which the subject was standing was rotated in conjunction with the body sway. Thus, in the usual circumstance, if the body swayed forward the ankles would be in relative dorsiflexion and the joint receptors and muscle spindles would register this movement. In the experimental condition, however, the platform rotated into plantarflexion in concert with the forward inclination of the body such that the relative dorsiflexion did not occur. The net effect of this situation was that the joint and muscle receptors failed to register movement at the ankle although body movement was clearly taking place. Normal subjects had a significantly greater sway in condition 4 than in the first three conditions.

The greatest sway occurred in the fifth and sixth conditions. In condition 5, the subject was blindfolded to eliminate vision and the platform was rotated to provide inaccurate support surface information. Condition 6 combined the rotating platform and the visual box so that the subject received inaccurate information from both the somatosensory and the visual systems.

Two conclusions were suggested from these experiments. First, we rely most heavily

Table 44-1. Sensory Conditions for Systematically Evaluating Intersensory Interaction

CONDITION	ACTIVITY
1	Standing quietly, eyes open
2	Standing, eyes blindfolded
3	Standing, with visual box surrounding subject, eyes open
4	Standing, platform rotates with body sway
5	Standing, rotating platform, eyes blindfolded
6	Standing, rotating platform, visual box surrounding subject

on our somatosensory systems for orientation for postural control. Second, the greatest sway is produced when both somatosensory and visual information is removed or is inaccurate for postural control, leaving vestibular inputs to mediate balance.

Once the normal responses to the experimental conditions were established, subjects who had vestibular system disorders were put through the same protocol (Black and Nashner, 1985). It was surprising to discover that subjects with reduced vestibular function did not sway more than normal subjects in the first two conditions, which duplicate the Romberg test. Yet the Romberg test has been accepted for many years as the basic evaluation procedure to detect problems with balance and, more specifically, abnormal vestibular function. Because the subjects still had accurate information about the support surface from the somatosensory system, they fared quite well.

PREPARATORY ACTIVITY WITHIN POSTURAL CONTROL

Horak and co-workers (1984) demonstrated that voluntary movements are coupled with anticipatory postural activity. Electromyographic recordings on subjects who did a rapid flexion movement of the arm showed activity in the legs and trunk that preceded deltoid muscle activation for arm movement. Thus, preparatory postural adjustments are important in reducing disequilibrium associated with a rapid coordinated movement.

A close observation of some simple movements will disclose muscle activation and possibly weight shifts that precede a potentially destabilizing voluntary movement. Individuals who have deficits in the ability to perform the preparatory set or shift will also have dysfunction of the attempted voluntary movement.

DIFFERENTIAL EXAMINATION FOR DISORDERS OF BALANCE AND COORDINATION

Differential tests now used to evaluate coordination and balance have many flaws (Horak).

As noted earlier, the Romberg test, which consists of standing with eyes open and eyes closed on one or both legs, fails to detect disequilibrium in subjects who have vestibular dysfunction and who do, indeed, have disequilibrium. If a subject is asked to walk a balance beam with heel-to-toe patterns, as may be done in certain tests of balance, the ankle synergy is effectively eliminated because of biomechanical limitations at the ankle and loss of medial-lateral stability. The resulting use of the hip synergy by the subject may be graded as a failure because the movements are rather large and may be considered ungainly, even though the movement pattern is appropriate in this circumstance. Most of the balance test results are measured and the norm obtained by recording the time a particular position can be held or whether a task is completed within a certain time.

Although the body may assume an unlimited number of positions and still remain in equilibrium, in most positions only a few degrees of sway are possible if the subject is to remain in equilibrium and not fall or change to another position. This limitation in postural range of motion makes it difficult to detect critical postural adjustments with simple observation alone.

During standard balance tests, sensory conditions are not systematically changed or eliminated by altering the visual surroundings or the nature of the supporting surface. However, systematic variations are necessary to determine which senses the subject can rely on for postural orientation. Further, these tests do not evaluate conditions that require different prepackaged synergies or strategies for postural movement (Shumway-Cook and Horak, 1986). Often evaluation of balance is attempted by using a tiltboard or a ball to disturb the patient's center of gravity. Other types of balance disturbances that are used include perturbing the subject by pushing against the trunk with the command "Don't let me push you over." Most often large perturbations are given. The result we expect is not always clear. If we cannot push the patient over, did he pass? What is his score if he falls over but catches himself with a protective reaction?

Useful and practical equipment for the clinical assessment of postural control is not available. Expensive and highly complex computerized force platforms and motion analysis machines can provide accurate center of mass positions and kinematic analyses of motion, but the relationship between these measures and the clinical assessment of balance function is unclear.

Further compounding the problem of assessment is the requirement for as objective a measure as possible. Simple descriptions of movements and postures are not sufficiently reliable for baseline or treatment progression measures. Neither do these descriptions separate or divide posture control into basic functional components. Knowledge of the parts or components of posture control is necessary to break down the analysis and determine the problems that produce a dysfunctional movement or posture.

Horak has proposed some methods for clinical assessment of balance. Tools and devices used in this assessment are familiar to all physical therapists, and include postural grids and plumb lines. Scales can be developed to measure results. Stopwatches provide accurate time recordings. Video recorders and Polaroid photographs will allow more accurate analysis and permanent recording of results.

These and other such tools combined with a systematic analysis should yield measurable results. Most importantly, the results should be of clinical relevance. Three important neurophysiological components of postural control requiring assessment have been described: biomechanical, movement strategies, and sensory organization (Horak).

EVALUATION OF BIOMECHANICAL COMPONENTS OF BALANCE

The integrity of the musculoskeletal system should be evaluated first in a patient with balance disorders to determine the effect of musculoskeletal limitations on postural control. The presence of pain, alterations in joint range of motion, or alterations in muscle strength or length may produce dysfunction in balance. The therapist must differentiate between problems caused by a normal central nervous system acting on an abnormal biomechanical structure, or dysfunction caused by an abnormal central nervous system acting on a normal biomechanical structure, or possible combinations of the two.

Evaluation of joint range of motion is essential. If joints that are involved in the posture or movement of interest are restricted or lack accessory motions, the posture itself will be altered. Postures and movements that occur in the presence of muscle weakness may be similar to those that result when joint motion is limited.

The presence of pain will affect the quantity and quality of movement because normal movement cannot be superimposed over pain. Movement altered by pain may become habitual and persist even after the pain has disappeared. The therapist should attempt to gather sufficient patient history concerning pain to judge whether such conditions could have existed that may explain or contribute to the circumstances at the present.

Muscle weaknesses, imbalances in muscle length or strength, and lack of muscular endurance will affect the quality of movement as well as the type and maintenance of posture. Remember, however, that manual muscle tests may not provide a functional measure of strength. This is particularly true of postural weight-bearing patterns. It may be more useful to devise a measure for the muscle in a functional mode. For example, the gluteus medius muscle may be better evaluated by standing on one leg and attempting to raise the pelvis on the opposite side. Quadriceps muscles may be better evaluated during semi-squats or other such functionally related activities.

EVALUATION OF MOTOR COMPONENTS OF POSTURAL CONTROL

Evaluation of Movement Strategies

The basic strategies that are used when anterior-posterior perturbations are encountered are the ankle and hip synergies described earlier. It is possible to evaluate these synergies without expensive equipment. Muscles may be palpated during perturbations to determine whether they have been activated. Additionally, as you become familiar with the appearance of the synergies, it becomes possible to see the substitution of one synergy for another or alterations in the synergies. Grids drawn on the wall or printed on transparent plastic can provide background for visual or photographic measurements.

The type of synergy that will be elicited by perturbation will depend upon the type of support surface on which the patient will be standing and the intensity of the perturbation. A small perturbation will not move the center of mass very far and can be countered with an ankle synergy if the support surface is firm and wide enough to provide counterforces to ankle rotation.

How the perturbation is presented is of critical importance. If you say "Don't let me move you," the subject will set most of the involved musculature to prevent being moved. This rigid response is not usually helpful when attempting to assess the subject's ability to recover from a perturbation. It is better to instruct the subject, "Let me move you but try not to fall." With these instructions the therapist will more likely elicit an ankle synergy, if one is present, with a relatively small perturbation.

Larger and more rapid perturbations usually elicit a hip synergy. In addition, if the supporting surface does not resist ankle rotational forces sufficiently to shift the center of mass, a hip synergy will result. To test whether the hip synergy is present, the patient may stand crosswise on a narrow balance beam and a perturbation may be provided if necessary to disturb the center of gravity. Positions that do not allow both ankles to produce an ankle synergy effectively may also be used. Examples of such positions include having the subject use a heel-to-toe stance or stand on one foot. This activity can be done lengthwise on a balance beam or simply on the floor. The largest and fastest perturbations may result in a stepping strategy.

It is important to change systematically the speed and intensity of the perturbations in con-

junction with alterations in the supporting surface. Both expected and unexpected perturbations should be experienced and evaluated. A routine or protocol should be developed for your clinic that makes it easy to evaluate the movements and record the results as objectively as possible. The routine also should require a minimum of time.

When abnormalities are present, the therapist should attempt to answer the following questions: (1) Do the abnormalities lie within the synergies themselves? If the patient has disorders of timing, sequencing, or scaling his responses, you will want to pinpoint them so proper treatment can be applied following evaluation. (2) Does the patient have a limited number of strategies that can be elicited? (3) Although the patient has a full repertoire of strategies available, does he use them inappropriately? For example, a subject may have a hip synergy that can be elicited, but he consistently falls from the beam because the hip synergy is not elicited in that instance.

Evaluation of Anticipatory Postural Adjustments

As noted previously, many movements are preceded by a corresponding postural set. Preparatory postural adjustments may be analyzed through careful observation of movements that will potentially disturb balance.

It is preferable to define preparatory activity associated with movement in normal persons first. Palpate muscles to confirm activity if an electromyograph is not available. Then compare these results with your patient when he is asked to perform the movement. Does the weight shift occur? Are the correct muscles activated? If the correct muscles are activated, but the preparatory motion is ineffective, most likely the onset of muscle activation is delayed.

Evaluation of Active Versus Imposed Weight Shifts and Active Movement

The ability to perform active weight shifts in both standing and sitting may be assessed by having the patient shift weight in all directions (forward, backward, and side to side). The quality of these movements should be noted. What are the limits or boundaries of stability? These boundaries are described by determining how large the active sway in each direction may be and still maintain stability. These weight shifts may be measured with a grid or plumb line. Most likely some observations of normal persons will help in learning to determine the extent of abnormality in a patient.

Weight shifts in a variety of positions can be imposed upon the patient by using a tiltboard. The tilt imposed should be varied and not usually large and rapid. Each postural position is stable within only a few degrees. A protective reaction is elicited only when the patient's center of mass exceeds the base of support, forcing the patient to use the arms to prevent a fall. A scale may be developed to measure how many degrees of tilt can be imposed in which the subject maintains equilibrium (Fig. 44-3).

EVALUATION OF SENSORY ORGANIZATION FOR POSTURAL ORIENTATION

Shumway-Cook and Horak (1986) have described a clinical approach to assessing the effect of sensory interaction on balance. The Clinical Test for Sensory Interaction in Balance (CTSIB) helps to identify which sense an individual relies on for postural orientation. Additionally, it allows the therapist to test a patient's ability to solve intersensory conflicts without depending on sophisticated and expensive machinery.

The patient may be tested using the six sensory conditions described previously. The box used to present inaccurate visual information may be fabricated from a Japanese lantern following instructions given by Shumway-Cook and Horak (1986). The basic principle is to devise a box or globe that can be placed over the patient's head and suspended in such a manner that the hood or globe moves when the head moves (Fig. 44-4). The inside of the device should contain lines or patterns for visual stimulation and fixation. The globe must be large enough to place the visual stimulation a reasonable distance from the eyes so that focusing may occur. A helmet with adjustable straps, a dental headband, or similar mechanisms may be used to suspend the device from the head.

The principle of the rotating platform may

Figure 44-3. An example of a grid that can be made for measuring degrees of tilt.

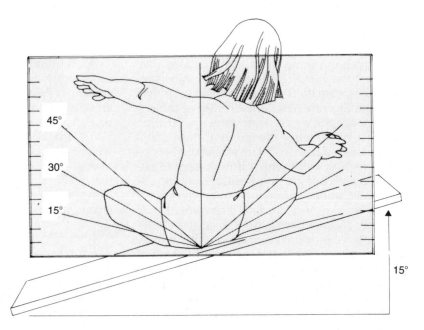

45°

30°

15°

15°

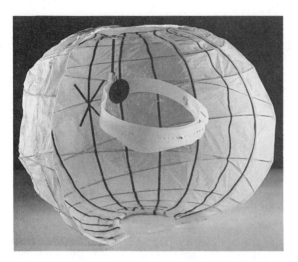

Figure 44-4. Visual-conflict dome worn by patient to produce inaccurate visual orientation during balance testing. (Shumway-Cook A, Horak FB: Assessing the influence of sensory interaction on balance. Phys Ther 10:1548, 1986. Reprinted with permission of the American Physical Therapy Association.)

be accomplished by having the subject stand on a relatively unstable or compliant surface, such as a piece of dense foam. This material allows the ankle joint to rotate and prevents the somatosensory systems from relaying accurate information regarding vertical orientation from the ankle joints and the skin (Fig. 44-5).

A rotating platform as described above can also be made of a combination of compliant materials. The bottom layer should consist of dense foam, the middle layer of a less dense foam, and the top layer of a very compliant foam (such as Pudgie foam). With these combinations the foot will sink rapidly and the ankle will actually rotate farther before counterforces can occur. This situation will produce more inaccurate somatosensory feedback than will a single layer of dense, less compliant foam. Experiment and see what works best for you.

To measure the amount of sway that occurs from the various conditions, a grid or plumb line may be used. Video recording or Polaroid photographs are the most useful methods of permanent recording for accurate analysis. A stopwatch may be used to measure the time the subject can maintain the position without moving the feet or arms or deviating from the erect position. Subjects should be able to maintain the position for 60 seconds in each of three trials. Instructions to the patient must be clear and standardized so that they are the same for all patients.

The Validity of Nystagmus Tests and Other Tests

Vestibular dysfunction has been suggested as a contributing factor in sensory-motor dysfunction of patients with such disparate diagnoses as spastic cerebral palsy, developmental delays, learning disabilities, and Down syndrome. As a result, considerable resources within physical and occupational therapy are directed toward the diagnosis and treatment of vestibular dysfunction.

Many clinical tests exist that are assumed to be valid for identifying vestibular dysfunction, including the postrotatory nystagmus test, Romberg tests, and the ability to assume a prone extended posture. Recent research suggests that these tests do not measure what they are purported to measure. As mentioned previously, the Romberg tests are not sensitive tests of vestibular function. In addition, motor skills often used to assess vestibular function, such as the prone extension tests, do not correlate with the presence or absence of vestibular function. Many sensory and motor components contribute to motor skills; therefore, they cannot be used as indicators of *vestibular* function alone.

The most common clinical approach to evaluating the vestibular system is visual observation of the duration of post-rotatory nystagmus. However, several methodological problems are associated with this approach. Visual observation is often inaccurate. Electronystagmography can be used for more objective recording of eye movement responses to rotation. Additionally, nystagmus testing should be performed in the dark with the head restrained to rule out both visual-vestibular and cervical-vestibular interactions.

Finally, nystagmus tests measure the integrity of the horizontal semicircular canals.

VISUAL CONDITIONS

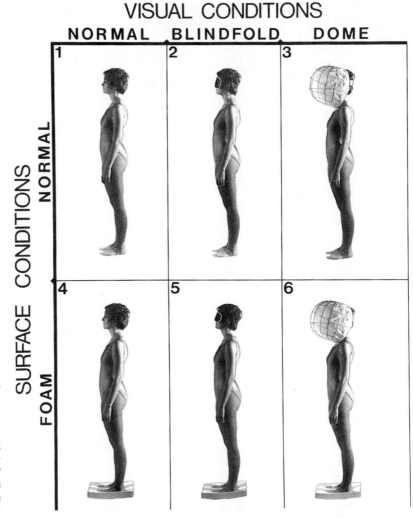

Figure 44-5. The sequence of six sensory conditions for testing the ability to resolve intersensory conflicts. (Shumway-Cook A, Horak FB: Assessing the influence of sensory interaction on balance. Phys Ther 10:1549, 1986. Reprinted with permission of the American Physical Therapy Association.)

Correlation between nystagmus testing and posturography tests, which assess primarily vertical otolithic function, is poor.

Current evidence suggests that vestibulo-ocular reflex (VOR) function is relatively independent of vestibulo-spinal function underlying postural control. Hence, one cannot necessarily infer vestibular-based postural dysfunction from VOR testing.

Horak and co-workers evaluated the vestibular function in hearing-impaired children and learning-disabled children 7 to 12 years of age. Balance and coordination problems have

been reported previously in both groups. A common assumption by many therapists holds that vestibular dysfunction underlies balance and coordination problems. However, evidence for peripheral vestibular abnormalities as a cause for coordination problems is poor. These researchers found that while many children who had hearing impairments had abnormal VOR function, most children failed to show deficiencies in motor performance other than balance, as measured by the Bruininks-Oseretsky Test of Motor Proficiency. In contrast, the majority of children with learning disorders had normal VOR function, yet showed significant deficiencies in motor performance.

This study casts doubt on the assumed relationship between peripheral vestibular dysfunction, as measured by VOR tests, and motor deficiencies. Disorders of balance and coordination may result from problems with other peripheral sensory systems or motor systems as well as from the vestibular dysfunction. Patients with central nervous system lesions who do not have peripheral sensory abnormalities may still have marked movement dysfunction in balance and coordination. CNS lesions may affect the integration of information from a variety of sensory inputs. Thus, movement dysfunction may result from inadequate central integrating functions rather than disease or disorders of the receptors themselves.

Examination of Disorders in Nonequilibrium Coordination

Traditional views of coordination in motor skills do not incorporate concepts of balance or equilibrium that have been described above. Traditional nonequilibrium tests of coordination usually involve fine motor skills and assess movement capabilities in several modes. Ac-cording to O'Sullivan and co-workers (1981), some of these modes are (1) reciprocal motion, which tests the ability to reverse movement from agonist to antagonist; (2) synergy, or muscle groups acting together; and (3) accuracy, or the ability to gauge or judge distance.

The Bruininks-Oseretsky Test of Motor Proficiency (Bruininks, 1978) is probably the most complete test with established norms for certain aspects of motor proficiency in children 7 to 14 years of age. The test includes items for strength and balance; however, the most useful and detailed parts of the exam relate primarily to fine motor skills or tests of nonequilibrium coordination.

Many simple tests of fine motor coordination have long been used for clinical evaluation (Table 44-2). The familiar finger-to-nose, finger-to-finger, and finger opposition tests can be used to evaluate reciprocal motion, synergy, and accuracy. Other reciprocal motion tests include rapid pronation and supination of the forearm, patting the hand rhythmically on the knee or a table, and tapping the foot. Pointing activities and throwing or kicking a ball are useful for examining synergy and accuracy. More precise accuracy tests include drawing a circle and tracing a figure eight with the foot.

Table 44-2. Coordination Tests and Parameters Evaluated

MOVEMENT	RECIPROCAL MOTION	SYNERGY	ACCURACY
Finger to nose	x	x	x
Finger to finger	x	x	x
Finger opposition	x		
Pronation-supination	x		
Patting (hand)	x		
Heel-knee-toe	x	x	x
Tapping (foot)	x		
Pointing		x	x
Past pointing		x	x
Toe to examiner's finger			x
Throwing a ball		x	x
Kicking a ball		x	x
Drawing a circle			x
Figure eight with foot			x

Measures usually consist of the amount of time (in seconds) that a position may be held or how many times a certain number of repetitions may be completed. On occasion, the number of correct repetitions may be a more useful measure. To pass a given part of the test, accuracy must also be determined. In the finger-to-nose test, for instance, the patient must accurately touch the nose in addition to any time elements considered.

When circles are drawn or mazes solved, it is useful to provide borders around the circle or maze and count errors when the borders are violated. Again, these procedures are timed. Other timed dexterity tests that may be used are putting small items in a box, putting washers on pegs, or putting removable pegs into a pegboard. Various designs may be copied on the pegboard by inserting the pegs in a particular pattern, although cognitive processes may be more important than coordination in such a procedure.

Scores of quality may be developed, such as 2 points for the movement performed normally, 1 point if performed with inaccuracies or difficulties, and 0 if the movement cannot be performed. Other divisions may be made to suit your purposes.

ACTIVITIES FOR TREATING DISORDERS OF BALANCE AND COORDINATION

Using a systems approach to assessing components of abnormal postural control enhances the breadth of treatment techniques that may be used to resolve balance problems. A rich array of treatment procedures and possibilities resides in the evaluation procedures themselves. Most, if not all, of the methods and mechanisms used to evaluate balance and coordination must be repeated and practiced for treatment effects. For example, if your patient has difficulty with the portion of the balance examination in which sensory conflicts are tested by standing on a foam pad, practicing standing on the foam pad itself would certainly constitute a reasonable treatment procedure.

Disorders of balance and coordination are present in patients with many kinds of diagnoses, including upper motor neuron lesions. The reasons for such dysfunction in movements and postures are multiple and varied. If patients are evaluated systematically and if the underlying neurophysiologic mechanisms are understood, appropriate treatment procedures will be developed.

The activities presented first in the section on General Exercises are a graded series of exercises for balance, using various methods for changing the sensory conditions. You begin with the very simplest postures and movements and progress to more complex balance and movement skills. Practicing simple active weight shifts in gradually increasing ranges is appropriate for a patient beginning remediation of balance deficits. As the patient improves, availability of sensory cues during practice of balance should be systematically altered. As the patient masters relatively simple postures and movements, the same sensory conditions can be used for such complex movements as walking, more complex balance activities, and so forth. For instance, once a patient can stand, perform weight shifts, and do spiral diagonal trunk movements on a foam pad, have her walk on a foam mattress or floor mat.

All of these activities should be useful for achieving control of problems of muscular scaling, timing, and sequencing. Following the section on General Exercises, some ideas concerning specific problems that were evaluated in the section on Differential Examination will be presented. These include disorders of movement strategies, anticipatory postural adjustments, and sensory organization.

An important concept in treating patients with movement dysfunction is that a wide variety of experiences should be provided. Aspects of the treatment program such as amplitude, duration, direction, intensity, and speed should be varied. Patients must experience different kinds of supporting surfaces. The patient who can function on a tile floor in your clinic most likely will continue to have difficulty at home on carpet. These conditions must be a part of the patient's experience during the training regimen.

GENERAL EXERCISES FOR BALANCE AND POSTURAL CONTROL

The exercises begin with the simplest and progress onward. Every exercise described can be modified further by altering the visual cues available to the patient. This alteration may be done by diminishing visual input with dark glasses, or by removing vision by closing the eyes or blindfolding the patient. Visual inaccuracies may be presented with the hood or globe.

At any point the therapist may provide perturbations to increase the difficulty level and change conditions. Remember to tell the patient, "Let me move you but try not to fall." Perturbations should be graded in intensity and presented in a variety of directions and to different parts of the body.

Sitting

It may be necessary to begin treatment under stable conditions by using the sitting position. The patient should sit on the edge of a chair, maintaining good alignment, and do simple weight shifts from right to left and forward and backward. These should be done while attempting to enlarge the area of the weight shift and continuing to maintain stability. Change the visual cues and add perturbations.

More complex balance activities will require sufficient postural control to perform movements that have a much greater range than the weight shifts performed in simpler activities. Again, it will be useful to do these activities by varying the visual cues and providing perturbations. In sitting, more complex activities may begin with trunk rotations. Proprioceptive neuromuscular facilitation (PNF) activities in diagonal rotational patterns can be used. Include the head in the movements. Add the arms so that reaching up and back to the left occurs with reversal of motion down and forward to the right. These PNF activities are commonly called "lifts and chops." If the patient has difficulty keeping the arms together, a medium-sized ball or similar object may be held in the hands.

More complicated routines may be developed. The patient may sit on a Swiss gymnastics ball rather than the rigid chair. This change in supporting surface requires new and additional postural adjustments to perform the activities. In addition, the therapist may impart a wide range of postural demands by simply manipulating the ball. An infinite variety of activities may be devised for use with the gymnastics ball for sitting as well as for prone and supine trunk-supported activities. These exercises may incorporate various alterations in the visual feedback that the patient experiences.

Standing

Activities that were used to evaluate standing balance make useful treatment programs. For beginning balance activities, the goal is to keep the body in good alignment while systematically changing the conditions of the exercises. Activities should be performed while changing visual cues and providing perturbations.

The first level of difficulty includes weight shifts performed in standing. These may be voluntary postural sway-type movements. The patient should shift forward and backward and side to side, attempting to enlarge the area of the sway and still maintain stability so that the vertical can be reassumed appropriately.

Shifting the body mass should be practiced while maintaining vertical alignment with changes in the support surface. Have the patient stand on the toes and on the heels. Another variation would be to stand on one foot and then the other. Standing on the foam platform that was made for sensory conflict testing will provide another challenge for postural adjustments. This condition may be varied by having the patient stand on the foam with one foot and then the other. Standing on the heels and then on the toes while on the foam platform should be tried. The patient can stand on a tiltboard to provide an unstable base of support. The therapist may shift the tiltboard laterally and forward and backward, or the patient may impart the tilt to the board by voluntarily shifting body weight in the desired direction.

Put the visual globe or hood that is used during testing on the patient's head. All of the weight shifts and perturbations can then be repeated under these conditions. The foam platform and the visual globe or hood should be combined to provide a challenging and complex condition for these activities.

This material provides an adequate list of suggestions and examples of methods for varying the sensory conditions and postural requirements to develop standing balance and postural set. With a knowledge of the postural mechanism and a little imagination and practice, an infinite variety of activities to expand on those presented may be developed.

To gain control of larger movements and more complex activities, some patients must begin with simple rocking of the weight forward and backward, as if to take a step. The patient progresses to forward and backward stepping, and then walking. More complicated activities include movements of the head and neck. The upper extremities may be added as in forward and upward reaching. Spiral diagonal PNF patterns may be used to incorporate rotation in the trunk. For example, the patient should lift both arms up and back to the left, following with the eyes and head, and then rotate down and forward to the right side. During the latter movement, the knees are bent and the movement is followed with the head.

More Complex Movement Activities

Many familiar "developmental" movements and activities are useful in working with patients who have movement dysfunction. These movements provide a variety of experiences as well as a range in difficulty relative to the number of weight-bearing joints and demands upon particular muscular patterns of activity. Rolling over, moving from prone or supine into sitting, kneeling, creeping, and walking, and crossover walking or braiding are good examples of complex activities. Obstacle courses, balance beam walking, marching, and walking on the commands of "start" and "stop" provide other avenues of variety and difficulty for practice and improvement.

Activities that demand and develop total body coordination and balance include swimming, skipping, jumping, hopping, hopscotch, and jumping rope. Dancing and activities with music and rhythm are useful.

At the highest level of demand for patients who are ready are organized games, which may be modified for particular purposes as necessary. Wallyball, volleyball, hopscotch, dodge ball, croquet, miniature golf, roller-skating, and bicycling are but a few examples of pleasurable recreational activities that provide social interaction and require balance, agility, and coordination of all body parts. Obviously, patients must have the necessary postural control to perform these activities. Practicing inappropriate movements under the stressful demands of such recreational activities would hinder progress and produce frustration.

POSSIBLE ACTIVITIES FOR SELECTED PROBLEMS

Biomechanical Factors

Any abnormalities in joint range of motion, muscle strength, and other non-neural components of balance must be corrected first. As mentioned earlier, these conditions may be the sole cause of or may contribute to abnormalities in equilibrium.

Improper Motor Strategies

Certain patients may not be able to access certain synergies. Patients with vestibular loss, for instance, usually do not exhibit a hip synergy. The ankle synergy is often not an available choice for patients who have diminished or absent somatosensory input.

Methods that might be used to facilitate an ankle synergy include many of the standing weight-shift activities listed in the section on General Exercises. In the beginning it may be necessary to keep the range of sway small and controlled. Graded perturbations should begin with only slight amplitudes and slow speeds.

Initially, more stable surfaces that are broad and noncompliant will be required. Begin on a wood, tile, or concrete floor. Progressions would include less compliant surfaces, such as carpet, and then perhaps floor mats. The objective of this progression would be to elicit the ankle synergy under progressively more difficult conditions. When the supporting surface becomes so noncompliant that an ankle synergy could not be effective, the limits for eliciting this synergy have been exceeded.

One clue, of course, that the patient has no ankle synergy is that the response to all postural demands, including slight perturbations, is a hip synergy. If this response occurs, the therapist may stabilize the hips manually with compression and resistance. Such techniques should decrease the movements at the hip. If these movements are suppressed, the patient may gain an appreciation for smaller arcs of sway and begin to gain some control of movement at the ankle. Another position in which it is biomechanically difficult to use the hip synergy is a squat. Rocking back and forth in a squat position should require ankle activity. Standing on an incline may also help to force activity at the ankle.

Progression may include varying visual cues, as described in the section on General Exercise. Although the patient may not have difficulty resolving intersensory conflicts, the increased demand that is required when vision is altered should provide a further progression of difficulty for eliciting the ankle synergy.

Sensory stimuli may be offered under a number of circumstances. Specific muscles in the synergy can be facilitated with vibration or other sensory stimuli. Approximation through the ankle may be useful to enhance sensory feedback through the joints and bottom of the feet to aid the patient in awareness. Somatosensory input through the skin may be increased if the patient is barefooted.

For patients who lack a hip synergy, activities that limit the effectiveness of ankle rotation are likely to be the best choices because they would force the patient to use a hip synergy. Standing on a balance beam, either forward or sideways, will minimize the usefulness of the ankle synergy and should be helpful in developing the hip synergy. Tandem walking with a heel-toe alignment, walking on a rail, and standing on one foot require the hip

synergy to maintain equilibrium. Any position or activity that favors the hip synergy may be used to try to elicit it.

The patient must know what the objectives of the exercises are and what the expected result will be. With this knowledge and cognitive awareness of the body and its movements, it should be easier for the patient to learn the correct responses. With repetition and variation in demand, the automatic nature of the responses will develop. Practice and experience in many different contexts will result in adaptability to the environment.

Some patients will have disorders within a synergy. For example, some patients with spastic hemiplegia have been shown to have a reversal of muscle activation within a synergy rather than having or accessing the incorrect synergy. Disorders within synergies will be more difficult to treat than problems with accessing synergies. Although palpation can confirm muscle contraction, it is not likely to be sensitive enough to determine a few milliseconds difference in the onset of contractions. Instead, you must rely upon your knowledge of the correct order of muscle activity in the synergy that you wish to facilitate. Using this knowledge, try to induce muscle activity in the correct order with vibration, tapping, and other facilitatory input while eliciting weight shifts, performing perturbations, and so forth.

If the equipment is available, a biofeedback machine and an electrical stimulator can be rigged to produce stimulation to the desired muscle when some other muscle or a switch has been activated. This immediate feedback with a stimulus strong enough to cause a muscle contraction may be effective in eventually changing the sequence.

Lack of Anticipatory or Preparatory Postural Adjustments

Your patient may not be capable of rapid movements or may become unstable when reaching for an object. As discussed in the section on Differential Examination, the prerequisites to these movements are the anticipatory adjustments. If the preparatory activities are missing or delayed, you must attempt to facilitate them.

The first step is to break the movements down into the weight shifts involved, which will simplify the movements and restrict them to the desired ones. Many of the activities listed in the general exercises may be useful. Hand weights, ankle weights, medicine balls, and similar devices may be useful in accentuating body shifts in preparation for a movement such as raising an arm to the side or holding or throwing a medicine ball.

Use your hands to provide feedback for the desired movement. Mirrors and grids may help the patient get a feeling for what is necessary. Do weight shifts in sitting first, and then move to standing. Practice and repetition with a variety of conditions are required. Vary the visual and somatosensory feedback as well by having the patient close her eyes or do the shifts on different surfaces. The patient needs to understand what should occur, for instance, that she should automatically shift her weight backward if she is to lift an object forward. Stimulate required muscles if desired by vibrating, touching, icing, or using electrical stimulation or biofeedback.

Sensory Organization Problems
Patients with balance and coordination disorders may be dependent upon one particular sensory system for stability. Many patients do not have the ability to resolve intersensory conflicts. When incorrect or confusing visual or somatosensory information is present, staggering, falling, or abnormal movements may occur.

For patients who depend heavily upon visual information, it will be necessary to increase their reliance on somatosensory and vestibular input. These patients will need experience and practice with most of the activities listed in the general exercises. Most likely it will be necessary to begin with weight shifts after vision has been eliminated by closing the eyes or blindfolding the patient. If the activities are too difficult, visual cues should be diminished with dark glasses rather than eliminated. Using blinders might help to decrease the input from

peripheral vision to narrow the scope of visual information. Patients can progress to more and more complex positions and movements with visual alterations.

Other patients may not be able to resolve intersensory conflicts. The same movements and positions can be used with conditions of inaccurate visual and somatosensory input. The patient can stand, do weight shifts, produce dynamic movements, and walk on uneven surfaces, sand, foam, carpet, floor mats, or other surfaces. All of these should be done with alterations in visual cueing by using blindfolds and the visual hood or globe that was made for assessing responses to visual conflicts.

ACTIVITIES FOR TREATING DEFICITS IN NONEQUILIBRIUM COORDINATION

Suggestions have already been made concerning total body coordination activities that involve balance and equilibrium. In this section the activities for developing nonequilibrium coordination or fine motor skills will be presented.

Many of the activities used to evaluate finger dexterity and eye-hand coordination can be used for treatment programs. Repetition of some standard activities may be useful: finger to nose, finger to finger, heel to knee, sliding heel down shin to toe, rapid alternating movements in pronation and supination, tapping feet alternately while making circles with fingers, tapping foot and finger on the same side and on opposite sides in synchrony, and rapid opposition of the thumb to fingers.

Catching, throwing, and kicking a ball are good for developing fine motor skills. Balls used may range from tiny rubber ones to tennis balls to basketballs or beach balls. Games such as pin-the-tail-on-the-donkey are useful for developing dexterity as well as a sense of direction.

Pen and pencil activities might include drawing vertical lines with the left hand and crosses with the right simultaneously, drawing circles, and tracing mazes. Cutting with scissors, placing small items into a small box or into two small boxes with both hands, and moving pegs on a pegboard are all good exercises for dexterity.

The twisting motion involved in using a screwing motion is a difficult task to perform because the hands do opposite motions simultaneously. This activity may be practiced by putting nuts on bolts of various sizes. For children, toys are available that require screwing motions.

Activities of daily living that require eye-hand coordination and fine motor skills are tying shoes, brushing the hair, and applying eye make up. Many other activities will come to mind as you consider everyday actions most of us are required to make. If a large variety of activities are presented and practiced, the patient will have a greater opportunity for fully regaining impaired functions.

ANNOTATED BIBLIOGRAPHY

Black FO, Nashner LM: Postural control in four classes of vestibular abnormalities. In Igarashi M, Black FO (eds): Vestibular and Visual Control on Posture and Locomotor Equilibrium. Basel, S Karger, 1985 (Describes the response of patients with vestibular deficits to situations in which sensory information is removed or confused.)

Bruininks RH: Bruininks-Oseretsky test of motor proficiency: Examiners manual. Circle Pines, MN, American Guidance Service, 1978 (This is a normed examination for motor performance. It has been normed on children.)

Horak FB: Clinical measurement of postural control in adults. Phys Ther, to be published (Presents systematic approach to evaluating postural control in the clinic setting without expensive equipment.)

Horak FB, Esselman P, Anderson ME et al: The effects of movement velocity, mass displaced and task certainty on associated postural adjustments made by normal and hemiplegic individuals. J Neurol Neurosurg Psychiatry 47:1020, 1984 (Experiments on preparatory and anticipatory postural adjustments for movement.)

Horak FB, Shumway-Cook A, Crowe TK et al: Vestibular function and motor proficiency in hearing impaired and learning-disabled children. Dev Med Child Neurol, to be published (A classic work that refutes the concept that movement dysfunction has a relationship with peripheral vestibular deficits in the learning disabled, or that all children need an intact peripheral vestibular system to develop appropriate motor skills.)

Nashner LM: Adaptation of human movement to altered environments. Trends in Neuroscience 5:351, 1982 (Discusses the various senses and their contribution to the control of posture.)

Nashner LM, Woollacott M: The organization of rapid postural adjustments of standing humans: An experimental conceptual model. In Talbot RE, Humphrey DR (eds): Posture and Movement: Perspectives for Integrating Neurophysiological Research on Sensorimotor Systems, pp 243–257. New York, Raven Press, 1979 (Describes the typical synergies produced as a response to surface perturbations.)

O'Sullivan SB, Cullen KE, Schmitz TJ: Physical Rehabilitation: Evaluation and Treatment Procedures, pp 27–35. Philadelphia, FA Davis, 1980 (A review of coordination skills and evaluation procedures.)

Shumway-Cook A, Horak FB: Assessing the influence of sensory interaction on balance. Phys Ther 66:1548, 1986 (Shows how to construct a visual helmet and how to assess the six visual and surface conditions for sensory integration.)

Shumway-Cook A, Woollacott MH: Dynamics of postural control in the child with Down Syndrome. Phys Ther 65:1315, 1985 (Dispels the belief that Down syndrome problems relate to hypotonia.)

45 Physical Agents: Heat and Cold Modalities

SUSAN L. WHITNEY

It is likely that our prehistoric ancestors used thermal agents for the treatment of pain and dysfunction. Perhaps they found that the water of a hot spring could soothe the aches and pains developed during a hard day of hunting and gathering. Modern humans still find comfort and relaxation in a hot tub, whirlpool bath, or hot shower, and the health care community has employed a variety of techniques for heating body tissue. These have ranged from heated objects to burn tissue (the cautery), to various conductive forms, to ever-expanding technology to produce heat artificially.

The clinical decision-making process about using these modalities must keep pace with the therapeutic choices contemporary physical therapy provides. Specifically, the therapist needs a basic understanding of the physical properties of thermal energy, as well as the physiological effects of an exchange of heat between the body and the modality. This knowledge is then incorporated with the therapist's skill to measure response to treatment and is further enhanced by experience with similar patients and treatments. Failure to maintain a balance between scientific base and empirical observation results in either treatment regimens that lack solid physiological foundation or ones that do not allow for individual variation. This chapter will provide the therapist with an appropriate background to assist in selecting thermal modalities appropriate to the patient.

HEAT TRANSFER

Like all other sources of kinetic energy, thermal therapeutic agents obey the second law of thermodynamics, which states that all heat transfer takes place from a hotter object towards a colder one. Heat may be added to the body (eg, with a moist heating pad), or removed from the body (eg, by applying ice). A sufficient temperature difference between the agent and the body and a sufficient duration of application must exist for a therapeutic effect to occur. These factors will vary somewhat with the physical properties of the different modalities (eg, the difference in the specific heat of substances such as water, paraffin, and the cellulose particles used in Fluidotherapy). Variations in technique of application and the area of the body to which the agent is applied also affect the degree of response. Body tissues function most effectively between 36°C and 38°C (Duffield). Temperatures of 45°C and above will cause tissue damage, whereas temperatures in the extremities under 18°C will cause pain, although function can be maintained at even lower temperatures.*

The relationship between temperature and tissue function can be summarized by the Arndt-Schultz principle, which states that an optimum amount of energy is absorbed per

*See Appendix: Celsius–Fahrenheit Conversion for an explanation of how to convert from one scale to another. Briefly, 9/5 degrees Celsius + 32 = degrees Fahrenheit; 5/9 (F − 32) = degrees Celsius.

unit of time that will stimulate normal function in tissue. Any amount below this level will result in no therapeutic effect, whereas an excessive amount will cause damage. The law also applies to the withdrawal of heat from the body by cold application.

There are five types of heat transfer. *Conduction* is the transfer that results when two objects are in direct contact with one another (ie, hot or cold pack). *Convection* occurs when a liquid or gas moves past a body part (ie, Fluidotherapy). *Evaporation* involves the change in state of a liquid to a gas with a resultant cooling (ie, vapor coolant spray). *Conversion* of one form of energy to heat occurs with ultrasound. *Radiation* involves the transmission and absorption of electromagnetic waves (ie, microwave diathermy). Thermal agents that transfer heat by means of the first three methods will be discussed in this chapter.

Several factors influence the therapist's choice of method of heat transfer, including (1) body part to be treated (considering area and contour of the segment); (2) depth of target tissue to be treated; (3) ease of application, especially if the treatment is to be continued at home by the patient; (4) ability to perform exercise while the modality is being applied; (5) duration of the treatment; and (6) expense of purchase, operation, and maintenance of the modality. With the variety of more sophisticated modalities available on the market, one must have a critical eye to determine whether newer truly is better. Historically, the use of modalities tends to be cyclical in nature, as evidenced by the resurgence of electrical stimulation, iontophoresis, and phonophoresis. The therapist must continue to review the literature as claims of therapeutic success are either supported or refuted by unbiased research.

THERMOREGULATION BY THE BODY

Although the human body functions best between 36°C and 38°C, this temperature is certainly not uniform throughout the body. Rectal temperature, which is considered normal core temperature for scientific study, is somewhat higher. Conversely, skin temperature of the head and torso (33.3°C) is lower than the core, and gradually decreases distally. Skeletal muscles at rest show a similar pattern, although the temperature of muscle is higher than that of the skin. A normal daily fluctuation also occurs, with body temperatures lower in the morning and higher in the afternoon. However, the fluctuation is small relative to the normal temperature, and a steady state is maintained.

The maintenance of the steady state is achieved through both physiological means and conscious efforts. When one is consciously aware of environmental temperature changes, one adjusts behavior by changing clothes or by voluntary body movement. The basic human need for comfort serves as motivation for controlling temperature. Along with conscious activity, involuntary responses assist in the delicate balance between heat production and heat elimination in both rest and exercise. At rest, heat is produced by the internal organs and brain through the metabolism of carbohydrates, fats, and proteins. This heat is transferred from the core to the outer tissues by a conductive process through muscle and fat and by a convective process through the bloodstream. When muscles work, their metabolism increases and becomes a source of heat production. Shivering is an involuntary muscle response to generalized cooling in which the body attempts to prevent severe changes in body temperature.

In addition to metabolic mechanisms, temperature is regulated by vasomotor controls and by the sweating mechanism. Generally speaking, when the body is exposed to cold, vasoconstriction occurs in the periphery to prevent convective heat loss as the superficial circulation is exposed to the cooler environment. Muscle and fat will insulate the body from significant conduction loss, and core temperature can be maintained (provided, of course, that the exposure to cold is neither too severe nor of too long a duration to cause hypothermia). When the body is exposed to a warmer environment or produces more heat in exercise, vasodilation occurs to transfer heat from the body. To assist in the process the sweat glands secrete water, which evaporates on the surface of the skin and cools the body. As the environmental temperature increases, the sweating process becomes more and more important, eventually taking over as the primary method of heat loss when the skin and environment are the same temperature or when the body is exercising vigorously. Neural regulation of these processes occurs through the sympathetic nervous system with much of the integration in the hypothalamus. Through this mechanism a number of physiological changes occur in several body systems. They are summarized in Tables 45-1 and 45-2.

Table 45-1. Generalized Effects of Heat Exposure

Cardiovascular

Vasodilation of skin vessels
Increased cardiac output
Decreased stroke volume
Decreased blood pressure
Increased pulse rate (initial decrease possible)
Increased capillary permeability
Increased removal of metabolites

Respiratory

Increased rate
Possible increased alkalinity of blood

Skin

Increased temperature (tissue damage if over 45° C)
Increased sweating

Internal Organs

Decreased interstitial blood flow and motility
Decreased gastric secretion and motility
Decreased renal blood flow and urinary output

Neuromuscular

Decreased pain
Decreased muscle activity
Decreased blood flow to muscle at rest

Basal Metabolic Rate (BMR)

Increased

Table 45-2. Generalized Effects of Cold Exposure

Cardiovascular

Vasoconstriction of skin vessels
Increased arterial blood pressure
Decreased venous blood pressure
Decreased heat rate
Increased cardiac output
Increased stroke volume

Respiratory

Decreased rate
Increased tidal volume

Skin

Decreased temperature
Decreased sweating

Internal Organs

Increased intestinal blood flow and motility
Increased gastric secretion and motility

Neuromuscular

Shivering

Basal Metabolic Rate (BMR)

Decreased

EXPOSURE TO THERMAL AGENTS

Applications of therapeutic thermal agents are usually localized to a specific body area experiencing injury or dysfunction. For the most part, generalized or consensual effects are limited; however, on numerous occasions the therapist must be cognizant of these effects. A patient receiving multiple local applications of heat (for example, a patient with rheumatic disease involving several large joints) must be monitored to prevent problems such as heat exhaustion. Hydrotherapy, which requires immersion of the body or the injured part, requires similar considerations. Because of its high specific heat, water is able to transmit more heat for each degree of temperature change than any other substance. The body, with its high water content, also has a high specific heat, which allows the body to store heat without a sudden increase in body temperature. However, as more of the body is immersed in warm water, less of the body surface is available from which evaporative cooling can take place. A simple rule of thumb governing the use of modalities such as the whirlpool would be that as more of the body is immersed, the temperature of the water should be decreased. If a therapeutic pool with a controlled warm temperature is involved, patients at risk for heat-related illness should have limited exposure, either by decreasing the time in the pool or limiting the degree of body immersion.

PHYSIOLOGICAL EFFECTS OF LOCAL HEAT

For a heat application to be therapeutic, the amount of thermal energy transferred to the target tissue must be sufficient to stimulate normal function without damaging tissue. Generally speaking, a temperature between 40°C and 45°C in the tissue is considered effective for treatment. Factors such as rate of temperature rise and duration of time that the tissue is in the therapeutic range also must be considered. Because an increase in blood flow is a primary response to heat application, a slower rise in temperature will be offset by the continual recirculation of cooler blood to the area. Temperatures slightly lower than 40°C will result in some mild, mostly superficial, effects.

Local heating effects may be classified as follows: (1) effects resulting from direct physical or chemical changes in tissue brought about by increased temperature of the tissue, and (2) effects mediated indirectly through neural or circulatory mechanisms. The total net physiological effect results from the simultaneous function of both direct and indirect means.

EFFECTS OF HEAT ON BLOOD FLOW

A discussion of the effects of local heat application usually begins by describing the increase in blood flow that results from vasodilation of superficial blood vessels. The blood vessels of the skin are the primary means by which heat is dissipated, and this heat dissipation is achieved neurologically either through a spinal reflex or through axon reflexes coming from branches arising from the receptor neuron. In addition, vasodilation is facilitated by chemical mediation through such substances as histamine and prostaglandins, which are the chemical means through which the inflammatory process takes place. Capillary permeability is also increased by the heat, and edema may result.

Although the effects of heat on cutaneous blood flow are significant, the effects on deeper tissues are not as pronounced or as well understood. Little or no change occurs in muscle with heat application. The effects of heat on joint blood flow and temperature is not completely understood, and conflicting reports exist. Some research suggests that a decrease in joint temperature occurs with heat application (and an increase occurs with cold application).

Application of heat may also enhance local blood flow during exercise. Both factors added together will produce a greater increase in blood flow than either factor alone. It is important to remember that the increased metabolic demands of exercise stimulate the increased blood flow in muscle tissue.

EFFECTS OF HEAT ON METABOLISM

Cell function (ie, metabolism) will increase with an increase in temperature, providing that the temperature increase does not cause tissue damage (following the Arndt-Schultz principle). Thus, an increase in metabolism within the thermally tolerable range will greatly aid the healing process, especially when accompanied by an increase in blood flow to enhance the removal of waste products. However, of importance is the fact that if heat is applied too early in the acute inflammatory process, it will cause vascular congestion and will delay resolution of inflammation by increasing metabolism, waste product formation, and edema.

Although acute inflammatory processes

are adversely affected by the application of heat modalities, these agents can be valuable in chronic inflammatory conditions. The stimulation of metabolism and vascular changes can enhance normal function of the tissues involved.

EFFECTS OF HEAT ON CONNECTIVE TISSUE

Collagen fibers, which are found in connective tissue such as muscle and tendon, have among their properties the ability to deform and elongate when a stretch is applied. Additionally, the viscosity of collagen allows it to remain at a slightly greater length after the stretch is removed, within limits determined by the tissue's elasticity. Heat applied while a stretch is given will enhance the viscous properties and relax the normal elastic properties. This results in an increase in the ability of the collagen to retain its elongation, provided that the stretch is slow and steady. The best results are obtained if heat is applied during the stretch, *and* if the stretch is maintained until cooling occurs after the heat is removed. Stretching only *after* heat application does not yield the same results. Clinically, these principles must be applied more consistently when the goal is to increase range of motion and decrease joint contractures. Often, patients receiving heat modalities are put in a position of comfort, which means that the target joints are in a resting or slack position during the treatment. For example, the arthritic patient with knee flexion contractures is often positioned supine in slight knee flexion, with hot packs above and below the knee. Perhaps better results would be obtained if the patient were to lie prone, with the hot pack placed posteriorly over the knee to try to increase the knee range of motion.

Additionally, heat application can benefit patients who have a primary inflammatory disease of joints (eg, rheumatoid arthritis) in which the normal viscoelastic properties are disrupted. Several studies have demonstrated that elastic stiffness of the joint structures can be decreased with heat application. Subsequently, the patient's subjective complaints of joint stiffness are reduced, which can enhance the performance of exercise or activities of daily living.

EFFECTS OF HEAT ON NEUROMUSCULAR STRUCTURES

The subjective feeling of reduction of pain probably formed the basis for the initial therapeutic use of heat. Ironically, understanding of the mechanism behind this observation is still not well documented, partly because the receptors and fibers that mediate the sensation of heat in the therapeutic range have not been identified. Extremes of heat and cold, as with other noxious stimuli, travel over A delta and C fibers. Additional study has suggested the presence of polymodal nerve endings, which are able to respond to thermal, mechanical, and chemical stimuli. However, the apparent role of these high-threshold receptors is to serve as a warning mechanism against possible tissue damage. Therapeutic temperature ranges probably stimulate some unidentified type of unencapsulated endings, and the information then travels through A delta and C fibers; however, this hypothesis is not proven.

What remains is the clinical observation that heat decreases pain. Several hypotheses attempt to explain this phenomenon. One type of nerve fiber is known to inhibit presynaptically fibers of the same type in the spinal cord. If A delta and C fibers mediate thermal input, then pain, which also travels through these fibers, may be inhibited through this mechanism. If this hypothesis is true, then the effect of decreased pain will last only while the stimulus of increased temperature is present. Indeed, recall how many times a patient has stated, "It feels good while it's on, but once the heat is off, the pain returns."

Another possible explanation for pain relief with heat application concerns effects on the pain-spasm cycle. Pain arising from soft tissue injury or dysfunction can result in a tonic muscle contraction (ie, spasm). An increase in temperature of the secondary (II) muscle spindle afferents will cause a decrease in discharge of these afferents, thus tending to decrease alpha motoneuron firing. In addition, heating of the IB fibers from the Golgi tendon organ (GTO) causes an increase in their firing. The IB fibers, which are also inhibitory to the alpha motoneurons, would combine with the decrease of II activity to decrease muscle spasm. If the decrease of spasm is great enough, the pain-spasm cycle will be broken, resulting in a decrease in pain. This presupposes that the heat penetrated enough to increase the temperature of the spindle and GTO. Most superficial heat modalities are unable to do this, but they are able to decrease gamma efferent discharge, thereby indirectly decreasing alpha motoneuron activity.

One other possible mechanism of pain relief is indirectly through metabolic and circulatory means. Heat application can improve cell function. Thus, an increase in local blood flow will aid removal of waste products thereby eliminating chemical irritants that can cause pain.

In addition to the effects of heat on pain and spasm, an increase in muscle temperature may also cause a decrease in that muscle's strength and endurance. This decrease was found in studies using shortwave diathermy and whirlpool.

PHYSIOLOGICAL EFFECTS OF LOCAL COLD APPLICATION

Cold application (cryotherapy) removes heat from the body, resulting in a decrease in temperature of body tissue. As with thermal modalities, the temperature differential between the cold application and the body must be sufficient to cause heat transfer. The modality must be applied for a sufficient length of time and must remain at a cold enough temperature for that period without warming to an ineffective temperature. (Chemically activated cold packs often warm too quickly to be effective.) The area of the body cooled also is a factor.

Cryotherapy also demonstrates circulatory, metabolic, connective tissue, and neuromuscular effects. Many of the effects are opposite to those of heat; some are comparable, but are believed to work through different physiological mechanisms. Knowledge of the mechanisms of cryotherapy is not complete.

One advantage of conductive cooling agents over their thermal counterparts is that temperature changes can occur in deeper tissue while cold is applied. Although most heat from a hot pack is carried away by the superficial circulation with little or no temperature change in the underlying tissues, these same tissues experience a slow, gradual decrease in temperature when cold is applied. The reason for this observation is that the warmer subcutaneous tissues lose heat to the cooler skin. This process continues even after the modality is removed, until the areas rewarm to the pretreatment levels. (Rewarming may take several hours, depending on the modality used and posttreatment activity, eg, if exercise is performed afterward, rewarming occurs more quickly.)

EFFECTS OF COLD ON BLOOD FLOW AND INFLAMMATION

As heat causes vasodilation, cold application results in reflex vasoconstriction of the cutaneous blood vessels, which is accomplished through the sympathetic nervous system. In addition, the decrease in temperature causes direct smooth muscle contraction, which tends to constrict blood vessels. An increase in the viscosity of the blood combined with vasodilation will result in an overall decrease in blood flow. Some studies have shown that joint blood flow decreases with cold application, but conflicting results exist in the research performed on the effects of cold on intraarticular temperature. Both decreases and increases in joint temperatures have been reported in different studies.

If the tissue temperature reaches 10°C or lower (usually as a result of application lasting over 30 minutes in clinical practice), a reflex vasodilation may occur. This phenomenon, known as the Hunting reaction, tends to be cyclical and is believed to result from an axon reflex. The function of the Hunting reaction is to prevent tissue damage from excessive cold. Although the idea of cold-induced vasodilation is not new and is accepted by most clinicians, it is not without controversy. Knight (1985) goes to great lengths to dispute the existence of the Hunting phenomenon; however, most treatment protocols (including those Knight utilizes) suggest ice application of 30 minutes at a time.

The choice of cold is universally accepted in acute injury as a result of the observation that edema is reduced by the cold. However, research verification of this result is limited. Most studies did not use clinically accepted treatment protocols, and looked primarily at the amount of edema and not the inflammatory exudates. Clearly, further studies are needed that more realistically reflect the clinical uses of cryotherapy.

EFFECTS OF COLD ON METABOLISM

Cooling of human tissue will decrease the metabolic activity of the cells that make up the tissue. Because of this reduction, the energy requirements and oxygen consumption of cells will be decreased. Some authors suggest that this reduction may be the most important effect of cryotherapy in an acute injury. Decreased metabolism means that tissues can function even when the circulation is compromised by acute injury, either by physical tears of blood vessels or resultant edema and vascular congestion. The decreased metabolism will tend to prevent secondary tissue damage, thus allow healing to take place in a shorter time. Indeed, surgeons are now exploring the use of cooling to reduce the effects of surgical injury and to maintain tissue integrity during complex procedures.

An additional benefit to cold application is a decrease in enzyme activity. Enzymes that may cause tissue destruction may be inhibited by cold; thus, another mechanism exists by which tissue damage is lessened in acute injury.

EFFECTS OF COLD ON CONNECTIVE TISSUE

Cold is not the treatment of choice in reducing joint contractures and improving tissue extensibility. Cooling will tend to increase tissue viscosity, and consequently will increase the resistance to movement. Thus, the patient will report an increase in stiffness after cold application. Heat application is much more appropriate, especially when a stretch is to be applied to the joint and muscle.

EFFECTS OF COLD ON NEUROMUSCULAR STRUCTURES

Cold can decrease pain in several ways. Cold, like heat, may act as a counterirritant that pre-synaptically inhibits pain stimuli. A mechanism unique to cryotherapy is the reduction of nerve conduction velocity (especially in small myelinated fibers). The increased impedance to conduction will also tend to result in decreased pain. Cold also tends to decrease synaptic transmission, thus slowing conduction further. (This effect should be noted as another reason to guard against prolonged application, as cases of neurapraxia and axonotmesis have been recorded.) In addition, cryotherapy may indirectly affect pain in the acute stages of injury by preventing secondary tissue injury.

Cryotherapy may also benefit the neurological patient with spasticity. Several studies have shown a decrease in the Achille's tendon jerk and a decrease in clonus in both humans and cats (Lehman and co-workers; Michlovitz). At the same time, the H reflex response was observed to increase, suggesting that the cold facilitated the alpha motoneuron while decreasing the activity of the gamma efferent, and thus decreasing muscle spindle sensitivity. These findings were based on the assumption that a decrease in intramuscular temperature occurred. However, other results suggest evidence of reflex activity occurring through cutaneous afferents when skin cooling occurs. This reflex also tends to decrease tendon jerk response. The difficulty remains in predicting what the response will be, because several mechanisms have been suggested. From available studies and from empirical evidence, therapists may assume that cold is an effective adjunct to treatment of inappropriate muscle activity. How effective is a question that remains for further basic and clinical research.

Cold may also influence muscle strength and endurance. Short-term cold application may facilitate muscle function through reflex activity mediated by cutaneous afferents (eg, Rood's quick icing technique). The results of decreasing intramuscular temperature are varied, and are open to interpretation because different measures of muscle function have been used. Several studies found an increase in twitch tension with cooling, whereas others found a decrease. Grip strength can be decreased during and immediately after cooling, but may increase over and above retest levels after several hours. Still other studies found increased strength after ice massage. Muscle endurance tends to decrease after cooling below 27°C but with cooling to 27°C normal function can be maintained. However, performance of skilled motor tasks may be decreased by cold. Thus, if cold can reduce spasticity in the neurologically involved patient (not an absolute certainty by any means), then teaching a motor task after application of cold may be difficult.

INDICATIONS FOR USE OF THERMAL AGENTS

The effects of local heat and cold application discussed previously are compared and contrasted in Table 45-3. A brief review of how these modalities fit into the sequence of treatment of injury, from acute to subacute to chronic, will aid in clinical choices.

Cold causes vasoconstriction and decreased tissue metabolism, which prevents secondary injury; thus, it is the treatment of choice in the acute stages of injury. Additionally, the cold will help to reduce pain, and along with compression and elevation appears to retard the formation of edema. As healing proceeds (usually after 24 to 72 hours), heat may be applied gradually to promote vasodilation to increase blood flow to the injured area thus, providing nutrients and removing waste products. An increase in tissue metabolism can speed repair. Pain can be relieved through counterirritation or through decreased muscle spasm. However, care should be taken that heat is not started too early, because increased bleeding and swelling may result, thus prolonging the inflammatory process. Contrast baths may provide a bridge between acute and subacute stages.

Heat is used in chronic problems to stimulate a small-scale acute inflammatory reaction which may promote normal tissue function. Furthermore, heat can be used with stretching exercises to increase the effects of the stretch and increase range of motion. Cold may be used in this stage after exercise if the exercise increases pain and swelling.

Table 45-3. Comparison of Local Heat and Cold Application

HEAT	COLD
Circulation	
Vasodilation	Vasoconstriction
Increased blood flow	Decreased blood flow
Increased edema	Decreased edema
Metabolism	
Increased	Decreased
Connective Tissue	
Decreased viscosity	Increased viscosity
Increased ability to stretch	Decreased ability to stretch
Decreased stiffness	Increased stiffness
*Pain**	
Decreased	Decreased, after an initial increase
Neuromuscular	
Decreased muscle spasm	Decreased spasticity
Decreased muscle strength	Increased or decreased strength
Decreased endurance	Decreased endurance
	Decreased skilled motor tasks

*Both heat and cold may increase pain if application causes tissue damage.

CONTRAINDICATIONS AND PRECAUTIONS FOR USE OF THERMAL AGENTS

Application of thermal agents is not indicated for patients who have impaired sensation to heat or cold. Thus, sensation should be tested at the initial assessment. In addition, disruptions in circulation from peripheral vascular disease, venous insufficiency, or vasculitis may limit the use of thermal agents. The predisposition for tissue damage is high because the vasculature is not able to adapt to the changes in temperature. Care should also be taken with patients who have cardiorespiratory problems, especially if the application is to a large area or to multiple areas.

Heat should not be used in the acute stage of injury or whenever fever or any acute inflammatory process is present. Heat may cause metastasis of malignancies and should be used very cautiously if at all with a patient who has cancer. (However, if in the judgment of the clinician, a terminal cancer patient would benefit from the palliative use of heat, it may be used.)

Cold should not be used after 48 hours on open wounds or over peripheral nerves that are regenerating. Care should be taken to avoid prolonged cold exposure over areas where nerves or nerve trunks are fairly superficial (eg, the axillary area). Some patients may display hypersensitivities to cold, including cold urticaria (hives), cold erythema, purpura, or Reynaud's phenomenon and other vasospastic disorders.

HYDROTHERAPY: AN OVERVIEW

Hydrotherapy (the external use of water in the treatment of disease) has been used for centuries because it is inexpensive, it is readily available, and the temperature is easy to regulate. Hydrotherapy is derived from the Greek words *hydro* (water) and *therapia* (healing). In the era of Hippocrates (460–375 BC), contrast baths were used for treatment. Hippocrates's students studied hydrotherapy and recommended it for people with rheumatism, jaundice, and pneumonia. Cold was recommended for fractures and dislocations.

The people of the Roman empire used water for various purposes. They used cool water, tepid baths, hot baths, and rooms with moist air for their general well-being. Through the ages, people have used water for healing, including what currently are called moist air, whirlpools, and contrast baths.

Body water makes up a large percentage of body weight. In adult males the amount varies from 50% to 73% and in adult females it usually ranges from 44% to 65%. The variation occurs because of the percentage of body fat, which is greater in females than in males. The differences in body fat are important for the ability of the body to float or sink in water. The body's water serves as a heat reservoir. Warm water has a soothing effect on people and promotes relaxation. In physical therapy, water is often used to promote healing of injured tissue because it aids in increasing blood flow to an injured area.

Water therapy is amazingly versatile. It can be used over a localized area (eg, the finger) or over portions of the body (eg, by immersion in a Hubbard tank). The temperature can be regulated from cold to warm or even hot, depending on the desired therapeutic effects. Therapeutic temperature ranges are listed in Table 45-4. Water, compared with other ordinary fluids, is an extremely good heat conductor.

Water without dissolved ions is a poor electrical conductor. Normal tap water has enough dissolved ions to make it a conductor of electricity by increasing its resistance. This fact is especially important for electrical safety in a hydrotherapy or pool area. Without grounding the outlet or without using ground-fault circuits, electrocution is possible if wiring is faulty or the clinician is careless (Fig. 45-1). In its pure form, water has a pH of 7.0, which means it is neither a base nor an acid, and thus is the perfect liquid.

PHYSICAL LAWS OF WATER

The physical laws and properties of water—refraction, Pascal's law, buoyancy, Newton's

Table 45-4. Temperature Ranges for Whirlpool Treatments

	TEMPERATURE RANGE (°C [°F])	
Very cold	1–13	(35–55)
Cold	13–18	(55–65)
Cool	18–26	(65–80)
Tepid	26–32	(80–92)
Neutral	33–35	(92–96)
Warm	35–37	(96–99)
Hot	37–40	(99–104)
Very hot	40–43	(104–110)

law of cooling, Archimedes' principle, specific gravity, viscosity, turbulence, and humidity—are important considerations for any type of water therapy.

Refraction is very important in treating patients safely. Refraction is the change in the angle of incidence each time light passes through a new medium. Air and water are the two media in treatment. When the therapist is looking at the patient's limbs in water, the limbs are not where they appear to be as a result of refraction. Refraction can be very dangerous if the patient has poor proprioception and the therapist is inattentive. The patient must be carefully guarded to avoid a fall when exiting from the whirlpool. Therapeutic pool steps need to be marked at the edges because it is very difficult to gauge depth. By following the edge markers, chances of falling are lessened.

Pascal's law states that fluid pressure is exerted equally on all surfaces at rest at a given depth, and therefore is very important to the physical therapist and the recreational scuba diver. As the water gets deeper, pressure increases. Pascal's law is the principle on which Jobst pressure garments were based. Immersion in deep water decreases swelling, which has to do with the pressure gradient that water itself has created. Therefore, it is ideal to place a patient with swelling at the deep end of a pool to decrease the swelling further and assist the venous pumping. If the patient's vital capacity is low (less than 1.5 L), care must be taken when fully immersing the chest.

Buoyancy is a force experienced as an upward thrust on the body and is in the opposite direction as the force of gravity. Buoyancy will assist movement as the limb is moved towards the surface of the water. Use of a longer lever

Figure 45-1. This type of ground fault circuit is optimum for all treatment areas, especially if there is water in the area.

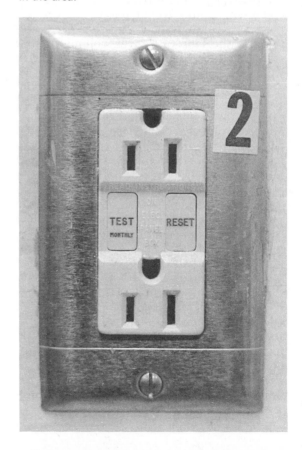

arm will also increase the effects of buoyancy. Therefore, if the patient has a weak shoulder muscle, he should initially raise the arm to the surface with the elbow fully extended and the wrist in neutral. As the shoulder muscle gets stronger, the lever arm may be shortened to increase its strength.

Newton's law of cooling states that the rate of cooling of a person in a given time is proportional to the difference in temperature between the environment and the body. This principle is also important for hydrotherapy areas and pools. If a large difference exists between the patient's temperature and the environment, the patient's rate of cooling will be accelerated. This is particularly important for patients with rheumatoid arthritis. Significant changes from warm to cold temperature will often cause these patients to become very stiff. Usually, the objective of pool therapy or hydrotherapy is to relieve stiffness and pain, so it would defeat the treatment's entire purpose if the room or water temperature were too low.

Specific gravity or relative density is defined as the ratio of a given volume of substance to the mass of the same volume of water. The specific gravity of water is 1. An object with specific gravity of more than 1 will sink. Logs that may weigh a ton or more can float because their specific gravity is less than 1. Humans are precariously close to having a specific gravity of greater than 1 (specific gravity 0.95). Thus, when a human is floating and inhales air, the body rises; when the air is exhaled, the body will sink. In addition, adipose tissue weighs less than muscle; thus, the person with a high adipose content can float more easily than a more muscular person. Often, muscular people can float in salt water because the specific gravity of water increases when salt is dissolved in it.

Archimedes' principle states that when a body is entirely or partially immersed in a fluid at rest, it experiences an upward thrust equal to the weight of the fluid at rest. This principle is important in determining whether a person or object will float. If the object's specific gravity is 1, it will float just below the water surface. A human with air in the lungs has a specific grav-ity of 0.95, which means that he can float. If too much of the body is exposed or is out of the water, the human will sink, because there is not enough water to support the body. Because of this phenomenon, therapists working with patients in the supine position often use floats around the ankles or pelvis to aid in floating.

Viscosity is the friction that occurs between molecules of a liquid and causes resistance to the liquid flow. Liquids that have a high viscosity flow slowly. If the liquid has a low viscosity, it flows quickly. Water has a low viscosity and can flow quickly, resulting in turbulence. Raising the temperature of water decreases its viscosity, making it flow even faster. Turbulence is the irregular movement of fluid, with the creation of eddies. Turbulence can be created by a mechanical agitator or by fast movement in the water. You can increase the difficulty of an exercise by increasing the turbulence of the fluid, which can easily be accomplished by moving more quickly.

Surface tension is a force exerted between the surface molecules of water. The tension exerts only a slight force, but with very weak muscles it might be easier to work just below the surface.

Humidity is important with hydrotherapy. Hydrotherapy areas are often very warm. If the air temperature and humidity are high, the body has great difficulty losing heat. Most hydrotherapy areas have at least a 50% humidity level. As the humidity and air temperature increase, evaporation of sweat becomes increasingly difficult. Sweating is the body's mechanism for maintaining a relatively constant temperature. Without the ability to sweat, the patient may develop a heat illness (heat exhaustion or heat stroke). If a patient's thermoregulation is not working well, care should be exercised in immersion. As immersion increases, a patient has less ability to sweat. For example, one group of patients susceptible to heat illness are those with spinal cord injuries who can sweat only above the level of the lesion. The thermoregulatory mechanism of a patient with C4 quadriplegia would be extremely stressed in a Hubbard tank with a warm water temperature that is located in a room with high humidity and high temperature. If maintained for too long, such conditions could be life threatening.

PHYSIOLOGICAL EFFECTS OF WATER

The effects of hydrotherapy are similar to the physiological effects of heat (Fig. 45-2). One of the specific effects of water is that during immersion the arterioles and capillaries dilate, resulting in a decrease in blood pressure and a decrease in peripheral resistance. This can cause fainting especially if large portions of the body are immersed. Care must be taken to guard the patient closely when first removing him from the water. Another physiological effect specifically related to water therapy is that often the patient feels tired after having a large portion of the body immersed.

POOL THERAPY

ADVANTAGES

Therapeutic pools used for physical therapy have many advantages. Patients who are afraid to fall and who are afraid of breaking bones generally enjoy pool therapy because they can move and exercise freely without fear of injury. The pool may provide aerobic fitness exercise. Running in deep water is an excellent exercise and can be used for patients of all ages. However, patients with cardiac disease would have to be careful because the pool may be too stressful to the cardiovascular system.

Active assistive exercises may be easily performed in the pool and may encourage patients who are very weak. The patient's treatment may be progressed in the pool by increasing the speed of the activity, increasing the number of repetitions, changing the length of the lever arm, moving from more to less stabi-

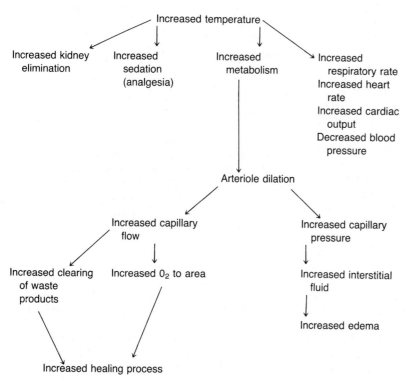

Figure 45-2. Physiological effects of hydrotherapy.

lization, and using small to larger floats to resist movement.

The pool depth may significantly affect the percentage of weight bearing on a limb. At pool depths of 60 in, the percentage of weight bearing may vary from 5% to 12% of the patient's body weight. This fact has significant implications for patients who should be partial weight bearing, but who are unable to understand the concept of partial weight bearing.

Some typical goals of pool therapy are to promote relaxation, increase circulation, increase range of motion and strength, improve ambulation, improve coordination, and improve psychological well-being. Patients usually enjoy water therapy.

DISADVANTAGES

Pool therapy is an extremely effective modality, but it does have some drawbacks. The pool may occasionally become contaminated with fecal bacteria and would need to be drained and cleaned thoroughly. The possibility always exists that a patient may fall, especially while entering and exiting from the pool, so great care should be exercised. One reason a patient may fall is because capillary vasodilation occurs in the water, which may decrease blood pressure and cause the patient to faint on exiting from the pool. The patient might also fall if it is difficult to see the steps because of reflection and refraction. The water provides an excellent media for exercise, but it does make stabilization and isolation of the body parts difficult. The patient may even start to float away from you. Another thing to consider with movement in water is the timing or temporal sequencing of the task. The correct timing of the movement in retraining may be important, but may be very difficult to assess if the exercise is being performed under water.

The chlorine added to most pools to combat the growth of algae and *E. coli* bacteria may cause skin irritation. The chemicals and pool maintenance can be very expensive, so the pool must be adequately utilized to make it cost efficient. Many therapeutic pools are also open in the evening or weekends to disabled swimmers or arthritis groups.

Finally, the most dangerous thing that can occur in a pool is drowning. All pools should have an emergency plan to remove patients from the water quickly. A seizure, transient ischemic attack, or cardiac arrest can cause havoc without a well-designed emergency exit plan.

EQUIPMENT

Optimally, a rail should surround the perimeter of the pool to allow the patient to stabilize himself while performing exercises (Fig. 45-3). Chairs or stools that can be put under water are valuable, and should be heavy enough to stay at the bottom of the pool. Lead or buckshot may be inserted into the tubing to make it more stable. Any object put in the pool should be frequently checked for rust.

Floats should be available. Life preservers are worn by patients who do not feel secure in the water. Rings and rubber tubes (floats) can be used to help secure the patient, and horseshoe-shaped cushions can support the head. Any of these devices will make the patient feel more secure.

Wooden paddles are used to increase the resistance of the water by increasing the surface area in which the hand must move. The same principle is true in giving a patient fins or flippers. Floating toys and balls give an added dimension to the pool program. Patients with rheumatoid arthritis often develop shoulder range-of-motion limitations. A group game of volleyball may help to regain some range of motion. Exercise that is fun is much nicer for the physical therapist and the patient.

It is best if the patient supplies his own bathing suit and sandals. However, hydrotherapy departments should also be equipped with disposable swim suits.

ENVIRONMENT

Air temperature, water temperature, and ventilation are important in a hydrotherapy area. The air temperature should be between 19°C and 24°C, which is usually a comfortable temperature for the patient on entering and exiting the pool. Water temperature may vary between 33°C and 36°C, depending on what patients are

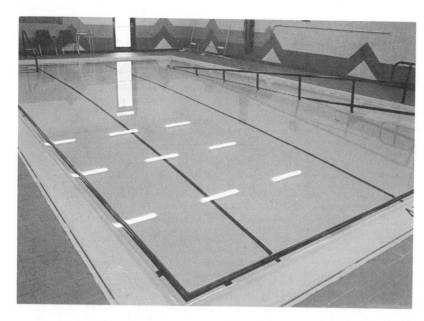

Figure 45-3. A therapeutic pool. Note the stairs, ramp, and rails surrounding the pool for adequate support.

using the pool. Patients who have osteoarthritis and rheumatoid arthritis usually enjoy higher water temperatures. Water at this temperature, with a high humidity, feels like a warm bath. The relative humidity should be between 50% and 65%. Upon entering a pool area, it should feel like a very warm and humid summer day. When a pool is being designed, drafts should be avoided and fans or air conditioning should be installed so that the pool area does not become too warm. The high humidity, warm air, and high water temperature combine to make pool therapy exhausting for the physical therapist. Dressing rooms, showers, and a resting place for patients and staff should be available in the immediate pool area.

HYGIENE

Samples of the pool water should be taken at regular intervals to make sure that the water is not contaminated. The samples should also be taken at different times of the day. Chlorine or bromine is often used in pools to maintain the pH level between 7.2 and 7.8. A pH of 7.5 is optimal.

Foot hygiene is also important. Patients or therapists with infected feet should not enter the pool, and walking without shoes should be discouraged. Rinsing the feet in fungicide kept in a shallow bucket or trough may be helpful before entering the pool. However, care must be taken to avoid spilling the fungicide because it might cause nose or eye irritation to people in the pool. Patients must shower before entering the pool. All pools should have a good filter system and scum traps at the water level.

CONTRAINDICATIONS AND PRECAUTIONS

A patient who has bowel incontinence should not enter the pool. However, if a paraplegic or quadriplegic patient is on a regular bowel program, he should be allowed to attend pool therapy. Patients with urinary tract infections, tinea pedis, plantar warts, respiratory problems, severe epilepsy, unstable blood pressure (high or low), or open wounds that could not be covered with a waterproof barrier should not be allowed in a therapeutic pool. Suicidal patients also should not be allowed in a pool.

WHIRLPOOL THERAPY

A whirlpool is defined as a bath of water that is agitated by an electric turbine. Many sizes and types of therapeutic whirlpools are available. Newer whirlpools are made of a plastic material; however, most are still made of stainless steel. Whirlpools can either increase or decrease heat to an area depending on the water temperature chosen. Whirlpools transmit energy primarily by means of conduction. With a warm or cool whirlpool, the therapeutic effects are similar to those of heat or cold (See Tables 45-1 and 45-2).

TREATMENT TIME AND TEMPERATURES

Most whirlpool treatments are for 20 to 30 minutes. When the patient is almost fully immersed or the water is very warm, the time may need to be shortened. If the water is cool and the patient is fully immersed, treatment time should also be decreased. If the patient is being fully immersed, the temperature should not exceed 37.8°C. With chronic conditions, the temperature range should be between 37.2°C and 40°C. The best treatment temperature for a patient who has an open wound, cardiac condition, or peripheral vascular disease would be a neutral or warm temperature from 33.3°C to 37.2°C. In patients without circulatory or nervous system disorders, temperatures within the therapeutic range may be used.

SAFETY CONSIDERATIONS

The most basic safety consideration while using hydrotherapy is never to leave the patient alone. It only takes a few seconds for a patient to slip or slide into the water. The patient must be secured in some way with a belt or strap. Just because the patient appears to be adequately strapped in does not mean that the therapist or aide should leave the area. Someone should be in the hydrotherapy area at all times.

If using a Hoyer lift to transport the patient into a walking tank, pool, or Hubbard tank (Fig. 45-4), the attachments should be checked for safety and should not be tangled. A life preserver for some patients may make them more comfortable. Restrictive clothing should be removed, but respect for the patient's privacy and modesty should be maintained. Some whirlpools have hydraulic lifts that can raise and lower the patient into the tank (Fig. 45-5).

The temperature should be checked prior to immersing the body part. The area to be treated should be inspected before immersion so that the treatment can be evaluated. Edema, color, size of wounds, skin temperature, and sensation should be noted. A timer should be

Figure 45-4. A Hubbard tank with its overhead lift and two agitators.

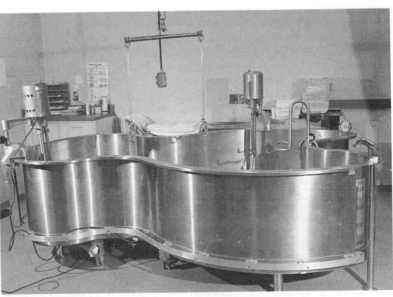

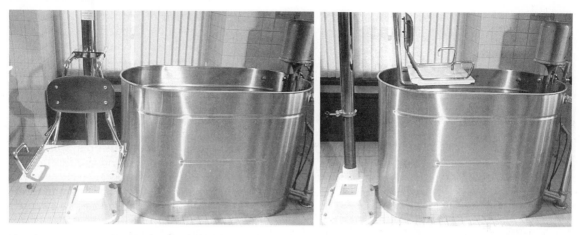

Figure 45-5. *(A)* A highboy whirlpool with the seat outside the tank. *(B)* A highboy whirlpool with the seat inside the tank.

set so that the patient gets the maximum benefit.

The pressure on the agitator and the direction of the flow should be adjusted according to the patient's needs. Some patients cannot tolerate the agitator being directed toward the body. Angling it off the side of the tank is most appropriate for this type of patient. The agitator can also be adjusted to increase or decrease its force. The aeration value can also affect the movement of the water. With the aeration value completely open, greater turbulence occurs; thus, for the patient with a very sensitive limb, the aeration and agitation will have to be carefully adjusted to obtain maximal benefit. Patients with a pressure sore may need the debriding effects of a powerful agitator force, but may not be able to tolerate it. Angling of the agitator still allows for significant turbulence. The agitator should be faced away from the patient when first immersed, then the force should be gradually increased, and finally the agitator should be slowly angled towards the patient.

Hydrotherapy is commonly used to loosen dressings, and then continued for the agitation effects. When loosening and removing dressings, the operator must be careful to remove all of the dressing from the water. If some dressing remains, it may be sucked into the agitator and can clog it, or it can cause infections to spread because it may become lodged in the actuator. Patient gowns also should be kept away from the agitator.

The agitator should never be turned on when the bath is empty. The turbine is cooled by the circulating water and will overheat and malfunction without water in the system. The small hole towards the bottom of the shaft of the agitator must be at least 5 cm (2 in) below the water line or the machine will overheat (Fig. 45-6). The other important safety consideration is that the patient should not stick clothes, fingers, or toes in the turbine ejector, which may injure the patient or damage the machine.

The height of the agitator may be adjusted depending on the patient's problem. This adjustment should never be done when the patient's limb is under the agitator. The agitator is usually held in place by a suspension bracket. It is important to adjust the height of the agitator to treat the body part most effectively.

CARE

Cleaning whirlpool tanks and turbines can be an arduous task. Each clinic has its own protocol for cleaning. Some hospital personnel will pick up the turbines and place them in a bucket

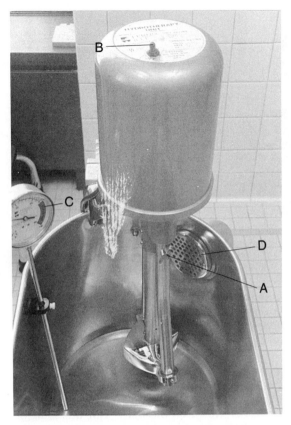

Figure 45-6. Whirlpool agitator. *(A)* Wing nut that adjusts aeration; *(B)* On-off switch; *(C)* temperature gauge; and *(D)* the overflow drain.

with a cleaning solution so that the turbine gets fully clean. Cleaning the unit is particularly difficult if patients have open wounds or infectious conditions. Strong cleaning agents are often used to try to kill the contaminants after someone with an infection has been in the whirlpool. Green soap, bleach, Cydex, alcohol, PhisoHex, and povidone-iodine (Betadine) are often used as cleaners. All should be used with caution around patients, and the instructions on the bottles should be carefully read to make sure that they are safe. When open wounds are treated in a whirlpool, some departments may empty the whirlpool, soak the whirlpool with a cleaning solution and steaming water, agitate it for 5 to 10 minutes, and finally rinse the tank out.

With the advent of acquired immunodeficiency syndrome, most departments are cleaning their whirlpools with bleach as a preventive measure to destroy the virus. This procedure should be done after any patient with an open wound has had a whirlpool treatment.

Cultures should be performed routinely to make sure that no infectious agents are present in the tanks. Most facilities have the cultures performed monthly. The cultures should be taken from the turbine, around the thermometer, and around the drain because these areas are frequent sources of cross contamination. Sometimes water out of the tap can be a source of infection. Water supplies may have *Staphylococcus* organisms and thus the whirlpool would not be the source of the problem. It is important to know what is normally in the water supply. If the culture comes back positive, it is advisable to observe how the whirlpools are being cleaned and, if necessary, to try another cleaning agent. All whirlpools need to be carefully scrubbed around the turbine, thermometer, drain, and along the seams.

ADVANTAGES

An advantage of a whirlpool treatment is that patients can be positioned securely and comfortably. They usually feel relaxed and enjoy the treatment. The water allows more effort-free movement because of the effect of buoyancy. Patients who have very weak muscles are often able to move them in water, which can provide a significant psychological boost.

The agitation of the whirlpool is also extremely helpful to debride or clean the skin. After cast removal, patients are often put into a whirlpool to remove the dead skin. The warm water also will help the patient to regain range of motion.

DEBRIDEMENT

Debridement of wounds in whirlpools is very effective. Often, the dressings need to be soaked off first in the water if they are adherent in order to decrease pain. Some dressings are applied so that the dressing sticks to the wound, and therefore, just removing the dressing is a form of debridement. The whirlpool aids in loosening the necrotic tissue, and makes it much easier to remove.

In many physical therapy clinics, the physical therapist performs the debridement using a sterile debridement kit. It is extremely important to maintain faultless sterile technique so that no cross infections occur. Care must also be used when redressing the wound. Medications may have to be applied and certain procedures may need to be followed for redressing the area. In some facilities, the patient's wound is dressed with a sterile towel and the patient is sent up to his room where the nursing staff applies the new dressing.

Many burn tanks do not have seams, which can significantly decrease the possibility of the spread of an infection (Fig. 45-7). Some Hubbard tanks and whirlpools have specifically designed plastic liners that fit into the tank so that the patient's body will not come in contact with the unit. These liners are often used with patients who have burns.

Because whirlpools are made of stainless steel, they may rust unless the stainless steel is dried between uses. The whirlpools do not look clean when rusted, and some patients

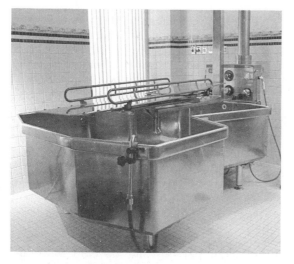

Figure 45-7. This specialized burn tank has seamless sides to decrease the chance of cross contamination.

may refuse the treatment. Because all whirlpools are expensive, especially if they are mounted in the floor, the extra care necessary to prevent rust is worth the effort.

THERAPEUTIC HEAT

FLUIDOTHERAPY

Fluidotherapy is a modality that was developed by an engineer in the early 1970s and was used first clinically in 1976 (Borrell and coworkers). It is a dry heat modality that consists of solid cellulose particles suspended in air (Fig. 45-8). Units come in different sizes. Some can heat only the hand or foot. Others require the patient to lie on the unit for the low back area. The turbulence of the gas-solid mixture provides thermal contact with objects that are immersed in the medium. It has been referred to as a "dry whirlpool," and it heats by convection (Valenza and co-workers). Upon looking inside the machine, it appears to be a boiling liquid. The medium has a uniform temperature throughout and because of the turbulence, excellent skin contact is achieved. The machine has a 250-W heater and a 300-W auxiliary heater that sterilizes the particles. No danger exists of the patient touching any of the heating elements.

The machine must be turned on before patient use because it needs to warm up. The machine has temperature, duration, and agitation controls. Treatment temperatures will range from 43.3°C to 50.5°C. Many patients will not be able to tolerate temperatures greater than 49°C. No established guidelines exist for what temperature is most appropriate for various pathological conditions. With the lower extremities, especially the feet, caution must be exercised to avoid tissue damage. The feet generally are treated at a lower temperature than the upper extremities. As with all therapeutic modalities, the greater the temperature tolerated without tissue damage, the greater the physiological effect.

The patient should be positioned comfortably for the treatment. Potential benefits of flu-

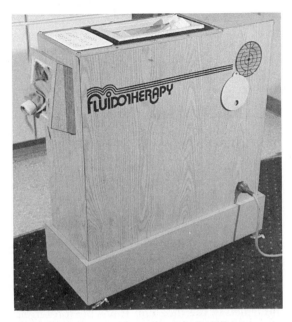

Figure 45-8. An upper extremity Fluidotherapy machine. The extremity can be inserted from the top or from the front of the machine, and is then secured by a Velcro strap.

idotherapy are as follows: (1) the patient is able to exercise without great difficulty; (2) the machine does not have to be cleaned after each use; (3) it has a massaging effect; (4) it may provide some pressure against the skin; (5) the particles may serve as a counterirritant; (6) it increases blood flow to the treated tissue; (7) it has good conductance and can be tolerated at relatively high temperatures as compared with water; (8) it can be used with metal implants; and (9) the pressure fluctuations within the machine may aid in decreasing edema in the area. The treatment time will vary depending on the condition, but usually is between 15 and 20 minutes.

Patients with rheumatoid arthritis, osteoarthritis, silastic joint replacements, wounds, sprains and strains, and even amputations have been treated successfully with Fluidotherapy. It has been used to promote relaxation, increase blood flow to an area, and decrease pain.

If an open wound exists, a dressing over the area is recommended and the patient should be treated using a low temperature setting. Fluidotherapy should not be used immediately after injury or insult to the tissues, because it will only aggravate these conditions. The increase in blood flow to the area will enhance wound healing without the danger of infection. Some therapists will use a sterile rubber glove over the hand to provide protection to the open skin area. An increase in treatment temperature would then be indicated for the heat to penetrate through the rubber. The use of fluidotherapy for subacute and chronic problems is increasing.

PARAFFIN

Paraffin is a conductive form of superficial heat that is often used for heating uneven body surfaces. The paraffin liquid consists of melted wax and mineral oil. The ratio is usually seven parts paraffin to one part mineral oil. Paraffin can be bought in most grocery stores for use in the paraffin unit in the clinic, or it can be purchased premixed with the mineral oil. Paraffin is a solid at room temperature. It is essential to add the mineral oil, or the wax will melt at a temperature that is too warm for the therapeutic range.

The paraffin's melting point is lowered by adding the mineral oil, and its specific heat is then between 0.5 and 0.65, which is much less than water (specific heat = 1). The lower specific heat allows paraffin to be applied directly to normal skin without burning.

Most patients enjoy the paraffin application. The paraffin insulates the body part and maintains the heat well. Patients appreciate the warmth of the paraffin and the moisturizing effect of the mineral oil. The paraffin also has the advantage of providing heat over the entire surface area. Paraffin is good for distal extremities, and is very easy to adapt for home use.

Using paraffin has some disadvantages. A few patients are very sensitive to the heat produced from paraffin and develop mottling. Mottling is prevalent with paraffin use, and is extremely common in people who have fair skin or who react strongly to ultraviolet rays of the sun. Patients have to remain still to get the greatest benefit from the insulating properties of paraffin. Thus, for small children or patients who cannot follow directions, paraffin is probably not the treatment of choice. The other disadvantage of paraffin is that it can easily fall to the floor during removal, and may make the floor slippery.

Paraffin is most commonly used for subacute or chronic inflammatory or traumatic conditions such as bursitis, joint stiffness, tenosynovitis, osteoarthritis, and rheumatoid arthritis. Contraindications for paraffin include all those for heat. New scars, open wounds, active infections, peripheral vascular disease, debilitating conditions, and peripheral nerve injuries are potential contraindications for paraffin.

Application

Dip and Wrap Method

Three types of paraffin application are used in physical therapy. The most common is the dip and wrap or glove technique (Fig. 45-9), which

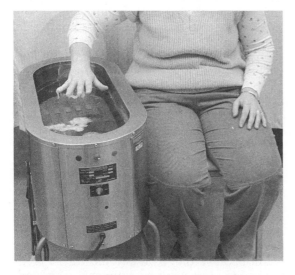

Figure 45-9. Paraffin application using the dip and wrap method. The patient will dip 8 to 12 times, and then the extremity will be covered with a plastic bag and a towel for insulation.

gives the lowest rise in tissue temperature. It is common because it does not require the use of the machine, other than the initial application time. The patient must be instructed in certain safety considerations prior to immersion in the paraffin. The patient must have washed the body part and removed all jewelry, and the skin of the extremity must be inspected. If immersing the hand, the fingers must be spread in a comfortable position that can be maintained during the dipping and later while wrapped in a towel. The patient also should be careful not to touch the bottom of the machine because it may be very hot. The temperature of the paraffin as measured by the thermometer must be between 52°C and 53°C. If it is below 51.7°C, the paraffin will start to solidify; above 52.8°C, the paraffin may burn the patient who is very sensitive to heat. Patients can tolerate an upper extremity bath up to 58°C (Griffin and Karselis). Lower temperatures should be used for the lower extremity. Because the foot is farther from the heart, it is more difficult for the foot to dissipate the heat.

Most paraffin applications last 20 minutes. If a patient is unable to tolerate a 20-minute treatment, the time should be adjusted according to individual needs.

An advantage of the paraffin dip and wrap method is that it allows the therapist to elevate the body part after the paraffin has been applied. As with other methods, the skin becomes moist, supple, and hyperemic. Massage to the distal extremity can be done easily after the paraffin application.

After all the safety precautions have been checked, the actual procedure is as follows. The patient is instructed to spread either the fingers or toes and lower the extremity into the unit. The patient removes the extremity from the wax after about five seconds, and is instructed not to move the extremity. If the wax cracks, it no longer insulates the skin, and the new wax lies next to skin that is already warmer than the pretreatment temperature. Because of this, patients may complain of burning and may not be able to tolerate the treatment. Usually the patient lowers the extremity 8 to 12 times into the paraffin unit. The dip and wrap method produces an initial rapid increase in skin temperature, but produces little change in subcutaneous and muscle temperatures. The dip and wrap method is the most commonly used method in the home.

Immersion

The immersion method entails placing the body part in the paraffin bath and leaving it there for 15 to 20 minutes. This treatment usually feels very warm to the patient, and many patients cannot tolerate the tissue temperature rise. Another potential problem is that occasionally the hot wax may penetrate the glove either distally (through the cracks in the wax) or proximally (by the extremity being immersed farther into the wax). This penetration may result in a burning sensation, and the patient often has to discontinue the treatment. Mottling frequently occurs with this method. However, patients who can tolerate large amounts of heat prefer the immersion method. The immersion technique gives the highest tissue temperature rise.

For most patients, only one extremity at a time can be immersed in the paraffin because of the way the paraffin baths are built.

Dip and Immerse

The last type of paraffin application is the dip and immerse method, which combines the two methods. It involves dipping the extremity into the paraffin, removing it until the wax becomes dull (about five seconds), and then immersing the body part. This method is warmer to the patient than the dip and wrap method, but is cooler than the immersion technique.

Some therapists paint paraffin on proximal joints with a brush for pain relief.

Paraffin is an easy modality to use. It relieves pain, relaxes the distal muscles, and often increases range of motion when the treatment is followed by exercises. Fluidotherapy, hydrotherapy, and paraffin are compared in Table 45-5.

MOIST AIR UNITS

Moist air units are not commonly used because they are large and expensive. The patient is placed on a padded plinth, and a large, rectangular, stainless steel unit with a U-shaped cutout is rolled over the patient's trunk. The rectangular unit contains the heating device, which heats primarily by means of convection. The patient may be positioned either prone, sidelying, or supine. The purpose of the moist air treatment is to increase the local temperature by providing a saturated moist atmosphere to the area treated. The patient develops significant hyperemia in the area treated, and the treatment may cause a 5- to 10-degree increase in the distal skin temperature. Significant sweating occurs as the water-soaked warm air is blown over the patient.

The water tank must be filled with about 2.5 gal of warm water, and the unit must be preheated. The usual temperature of the water for treatment is about 46.1°C. When it reaches 54.4°C or greater, even with normal subjects, significant mottling can occur. When the temperature has reached the preset level, the pilot light will go off. The patient is then appropriately positioned, and the U-shaped unit is rolled into position. A gown is the most appropriate attire for the patient because clothing will be soaked. Curtains over the U-shaped hole must be tucked in to maintain the moist-air environment. If the curtains are not tucked properly, the patient will feel a draft.

The part of the patient's body that is not in the unit must not be heavily covered. The patient must be able to dissipate heat, because the goal of the treatment is not to increase the core temperature significantly. Most patients are treated for 30 minutes with the unit. If the unit suddenly turns off during the treatment, fuses for the motor or the heating element may need to be replaced. After the treatment, the unit needs to be wiped off.

Patients who will particularly benefit from moist air units are those with rheumatoid arthritis, osteoarthritis, and back pain. It is important that the treatment area be relatively warm because they will become chilled from the sudden temperature difference. There are two problems with the unit: the U-shaped hood cannot be removed, so the plinth can only be used for moist air treatments; and the table is slightly longer than a regular plinth. An

Table 45-5. Advantages and Disadvantages of Using Fluidotherapy, Paraffin, and Hydrotherapy

HYDROTHERAPY	PARAFFIN	FLUIDOTHERAPY
Patient Comfort		
If the patient is immersed, he may float and not be well stabilized with a typical arm or leg tank. Patient is comfortable.	Dip and wrap is comfortable. With immersion, patient may be in an awkward position.	It can be very comfortable with proper positioning.
Wound Healing		
Excellent for wound healing, especially with hydrotherapy and then debridement.	Would not be used with an open wound.	Aids in wound healing; if the area is open, it should be covered with a sterile dressing and immersed.
Cost and Maintenance		
The machines and operation can be very costly, especially if immersing large body parts. With all machines, cleaning time is needed before the next use.	The paraffin machine is fairly expensive depending on the size, but is inexpensive to operate. Replacement paraffin is inexpensive. The machine doesn't have to be cleaned after each use.	The fluidotherapy units are expensive, but do not require any clean-up time and rarely need any additional particles.
Intra-articular Temperature Rise		
Whirlpool at 38.8°C delivers the least heat (Borrell et al, 1980).	Paraffin dip and wrap method provided a temperature rise above whirlpool and less than fluidotherapy (Borrell et al, 1980).	Fluidotherapy at 47.8°C gives the highest intra-articular tissue temperature increase (Borrell et al, 1980).

advantage is that patients enjoy the treatment, often fall asleep during treatment, and often feel symptomatic relief.

COMMERCIAL HOT PACKS

Commercial hot packs are a conductive type of superficial moist heat. Most patients find that these heating packs are comfortable and relieve pain. The outer covering of the pack is canvas. Inside is a silicon dioxide (SiO_2) gel, which holds water well. When used for the first time, they swell to several times their dry size. The pack will not leak unless the canvas fabric is ruptured. If the pack inadvertently touches the heating unit, it may scorch, causing the gel to leak and cloud the surrounding water.

The local application of hot packs will produce all of the effects of heat (see Table 45-1). Patients usually enjoy the moist heat, especially when positioned properly. Adequate support of the limbs and comfort are important for effective treatment.

The temperature of the hot pack unit is set anywhere between 65°C and 90°C. Care must be taken when reaching into the unit for the heating pack. Most departments have tongs available to remove the heating pack from the hot water. The hot pack should be drained of excess water before being placed on towels or in a hot-pack cover. If the towels become wet, the heat can be transferred to the patient too quickly, resulting in a burn. In addition, if the patient lies on the hot pack without extra toweling, the heat may be transferred too quickly and could result in a burn. The patient initially becomes hyperemic, and then mottling occurs, which may be caused by paralysis of the arterioles in the dilated state. When mottling occurs, areas of hyperemia are noted, and white areas that appear ischemic are also observed. Temporary paralysis of the blood vessels may occur in the ischemic area. If this continues without heat removal, permanent skin damage may occur. Therefore, it is imperative that the therapist or support personnel remain in the area during a hot pack application. Patients commonly complain of the hot pack being too hot, in which case extra toweling will have to be applied. A hot pack burn can cause permanent skin discoloration.

In some physical therapy departments, patients are never allowed to lie on the moist heat. However, with proper toweling, this position can be valuable because some patients cannot tolerate the weight of the hot pack. The patient with back pain who is comfortable in flexion then can lie on the moist heat. The weight of the hot pack in the prone position is advantageous for the patient whose back pain is centralized with extension. Hot packs do become cooler during the treatment, so the risk of burns to the tissue becomes less with time. Therefore, with proper toweling and supervision, a patient can lie on a hot pack.

The advantages of hot packs are that they are inexpensive and reusable, they cool over time, and multiple areas can be treated effectively. If too many hot packs are required, a Hubbard tank treatment or pool therapy should be considered.

Hot packs are used frequently for the treatment of contractures and subacute and chronic inflammatory conditions; to promote relaxation; and to decrease the electrical resistance of the skin before the use of electrical stimulation.

Some precautions are necessary when using hot packs. A patient with decreased or no sensation should not have hot packs applied because of the possibility of a burn. Therefore, the integrity of the anterolateral system (lateral spinothalmic tract) in the spinal cord must be assessed by means of hot and cold sensation testing before applying the hot pack. Acute inflammatory conditions will be aggravated by the application of heat, so hot packs should be avoided. Skin infections on the patient's body may be spread by the hot pack application, and possibly to other persons, if proper care is not taken. A patient with a malignancy that may metastasize should not receive hot packs, although I believe that hot packs can and should be used as a palliative measure for the patient with terminal cancer who needs relief of pain.

Patients who are very young or extremely old may have difficulty dissipating the heat, so caution should be exercised with the application of a hot pack. With peripheral vascular disease, extreme caution should be used because direct application of heat over the area of decreased circulation may cause a burn. Consensual heating may be the most effective treatment for patients with decreased circulation. If the patient has ischemic pain in the foot, heat may be applied at the knee or back to try to increase the distal circulation in the patient with compromised distal blood flow. It is very important to assess the popliteal and femoral pulses to be sure that the proximal circulation is not compromised as well.

If the patient has edema, hot pack application may only increase it. Hot packs should not be applied within the first 24 to 48 hours after an injury, because doing so will increase the swelling. If the patient is confused or has claustrophobia, hot packs may not be the treatment of choice.

The moist heat causes a temperature rise in local tissue, and the tissue will reach its highest point about eight minutes after the application (Lehmann and co-workers). A hot pack does not significantly heat the muscle layer because of the insulating properties of adipose. Because the moist heat pack starts to cool after 20 to 30 minutes, most clinicians apply the hot packs for 20 minutes.

Hot packs are frequently used for patients with rheumatoid and osteoarthritis. Horvath and Hollander (1949) found that with the use of hot packs on the knees of patients with rheumatoid arthritis, a decrease in intra-articular temperature occurred. The decrease in temperature is called "reflex cooling" and has been widely disputed in the literature. Mainardi and colleagues (1979) used electric mitts for 30 minutes, twice daily for two years on 17 symmetrically involved rheumatoid arthritis patients. One hand was a control and the other received the heat. They saw a rapid rise in joint temperature and saw no acceleration of the rheumatoid arthritis in the treated hand. Subjectively, the patients reported positive results but no change was noted in grip strength, swelling, and tenderness. The treatment did not slow down or hasten the progress of the disease as measured by roentgenograms. Harris and McCroskery (1974) have even stated that with rheumatoid arthritis the increase in joint temperature may cause the cartilage to break down. More conclusive studies remain to be reported on the use of heat with the arthritic patient.

Cold is often used to treat patients with rheumatoid arthritis and osteoarthritis. Hecht and co-workers (1983) used heat or cold in treating patients who have had total knee replacements. After 10 treatment sessions, no difference in passive range of motion was noted except that the cold treatment group had decreased girth. Traditionally moist heat has been chosen because the patients feel better with the heat. If swelling is a problem the study by Hecht and colleagues (1983) supports the use of ice until the swelling resolves.

Before application of the hot pack, the patient's skin should be inspected and pain and temperature sensation must be assessed. During the first treatment session, the skin should be checked during and after the treatment to ensure patient safety. Six to eight layers of toweling are needed to cover the hot pack. The thickness of the toweling may need to vary during the day, especially with frequent use. The hot packs should rewarm about 15 to 30 minutes before reuse. In the morning, the hot packs are much warmer, so extra toweling is required for the first use. Commercial hot-pack covers are available, but must also be covered by toweling to avoid burns and to prevent the spread of infections.

The patient must realize that the guiding principle is not "the more heat I tolerate, the better I'll get." They should experience a mild sensation of warmth. Patients may be disturbed when they do not feel the heat right away, and should be told that it will take a few minutes for the heat to penetrate through the toweling.

Different sizes of hot packs are commercially available. The standard size is 10 by 12 in, a back pack is 12 by 20 in, and a neck pack is 18 by 4 to 6 in. Other sizes are available, but these are the most commonly used. The hot pack should conform to the body part, and the patient should be covered with a sheet to avoid chilling. The patient must have a call button or a bell so that he can get assistance if the hot pack becomes too warm.

Hot packs are used frequently in physical therapy and are a valuable adjunct to treatment. They are reasonably priced and can be used effectively to promote relaxation, to help to gain range of motion after the application, and to help to decrease pain in the local area treated.

ELECTRIC HEATING PAD

Most commercial electric heating pads maintain their temperature during use and often have different levels of intensity. They are a conductive form of heat and can be bought in most stores. These heating pads can cause burns because patients tend to fall asleep and the heat continues to penetrate the tissues. Some of the newer electric heating pads can be preset to turn off at a specific time, which makes them much safer for home use. Some electric heating pads are available that try to mimic the effects of hot packs. They either run water through a machine and into the heating unit next to the patient, or they provide for a pocket where a moist sponge-like material is inserted within the heating pad.

Care must be taken to avoid any electrical hazards. The electrical wiring, the plugs, and the cord must be checked frequently for safety, breakage, or fraying. Three-prong plugs with a ground are imperative for clinic use. Ideally, the electric heating pad should be plugged into a ground fault interrupter, which causes the power to the unit to be shut off when greater than 6 mA of leakage occurs. Therefore, if an electrical problem occurs in the heating pad, the patient would not be injured. These principles are valuable to remember with any electrical equipment used in physical therapy. It is important to check the safety of the heating pads periodically.

The electric heating pads relieve pain and promote relaxation, especially for the patient who cannot tolerate the weight of a hot pack. Many patients with rheumatoid arthritis use electric mitts at home. If the patient has chosen to use an electric heating pad at home instead of a hot pack, it is important to have a family member bring it into the clinic so that the therapist can do a safety check.

WET VERSUS DRY HEAT

Wet heat produces a greater rise in tissue temperature compared with dry heat at a similar temperature (Abramson and co-workers). At higher temperatures, wet heat cannot be tolerated as well as dry heat. Most therapists choose between wet and dry heating based on patient preference.

CONTRAST BATHS

Contrast baths were used during the time of the Roman empire. Contrast baths may decrease joint pain and stiffness, and may improve the peripheral blood flow. The alternating hot and cold baths provide vasodilation and vasoconstriction of the local blood vessels.

Many therapists will use cold initially after an acute injury, then progress to contrast baths to promote circulation and remove the metabolites, and later use heat. The contrast baths help to reduce the edema in the subacute stage. Contrast baths are effective in improving circulation to pressure sores as long as the temperatures are not too extreme. Sinus headaches may be relieved by means of a shunting of the blood supply from the head with the application of contrast baths to the hands or the feet. Patients with rheumatoid arthritis feel a decrease in pain and joint stiffness after contrast bath application.

Contraindications and precautions are similar to those for cold application. Care should be taken with malignancies because the hyperemia may increase the blood flow and cause the malignant cells to spread. If a patient has cardiac instability, respiratory instability, or a tendency to hemorrhage, the treatment should not be used (Hayes).

The patient must be positioned comfortably (Fig. 45-10). The feet or hands are most commonly treated, and it is possible to treat both feet or both hands simultaneously.

The temperatures for the hot and cold bath will vary depending on the patient's condition. The warm bath temperature range should be between 35°C and 43°C. The cold bath temperature should be between 13°C and 18°C. If the patient cannot tolerate extreme temperature changes and the therapist still believes contrast baths will be effective, the therapist may choose the upper cold temperature range and the lower warm water range. Patients with vascular disorders and some with rheumatoid arthritis may not be able to handle large temperature differences. A candy thermometer or dairy thermometer will measure the temperature accurately. A patient should never be im-

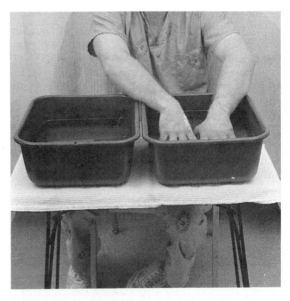

Figure 45-10. Setup for a contrast bath. The patient is fairly comfortable during treatment.

mersed without the water temperature being checked first.

If more warm water needs to be added later in the treatment to maintain a stable temperature, the patient's body part should be removed from the bath to avoid a burn. If the patient has an open skin lesion, a disinfectant should be added to the water and the bath should be thoroughly cleaned between uses.

The time of the treatment varies, and timers may be helpful. Some therapists will keep the patient in the warm water for 10 minutes, then cold water for one minute, hot for four minutes, alternating cold and hot baths and ending in the hot bath. Others may immerse the body part for three to five minutes in the warm water, and then one minute in the cold water, ending in the warm water. The treatment time will vary from 20 to 30 minutes. Contrast baths are an inexpensive and easy method for improving circulation, decreasing pain, and decreasing joint stiffness. With proper instruction, the patient can perform the program at home.

THERAPEUTIC COLD

COLD PACKS

Cold packs of various sizes are commercially available as canvas- or vinyl-covered silica gel. They usually are kept in a refrigeration unit to keep them cool. The optimum temperature for the cold pack is between -5°C and 0°C. Cold packs are reusable and must be cleaned between uses. They do not decrease the skin temperature nearly as quickly as ice bags, but can be tolerated better by patients who do not like cold therapy. They can easily mold to the body part and are relatively light. They do not break open easily, as ice bags do, and maintain their cool temperature for 20 to 30 minutes. After removal from the patient, they should be refrozen for at least two hours before the next patient use. Most cold packs are applied on top of the body part. It would be unusual for the patient to lie on top of the cold pack.

Many therapists apply a wet towel to the skin surface first, then apply the cold pack and cover the area with dry towels or a sheet to insulate the area. Depending on what the patient can tolerate, either a warm or cold towel may be used. The cold from the pack will penetrate much more effectively with a cold towel. Cold packs are usually applied for about 20 minutes and are most commonly used for acute inflammation, acute or subacute trauma, to decrease edema, and to decrease pain.

Commercial cold packs are available and contain chemicals that become cool when squeezed. These packs are expensive, can be used only once, and do not get very cold. When ice is not available, they may be helpful, but ice is always preferable to these commercial packs. They may cause a chemical skin burn if they open accidentally. Most are used only for emergency first aid.

For home and office use, some physical therapists will make their own cold packs by mixing ice chips or crushed ice with alcohol in a 2:1 mixture in a sealed bag. These packs can be reused, are inexpensive, and do not freeze into a solid mass of ice. It feels like an ice slush and can be molded nicely to a body part. They need to be kept in a freezer, and the cold will last for at least 20 minutes.

ICE BAGS

Ice bags are used in physical therapy to decrease pain and decrease inflammation. It is best if the ice bags are made of crushed or chipped ice, because they will conform much better to the body part. It is easiest to put the ice in a plastic bag, close it, and then apply a wet towel next to the patient's skin. The towel can be warm or cold. Physical therapists working with athletes whose skin sensation and circulatory system are intact will actually apply the ice bag directly to the skin. This method should be avoided in patients with circulatory problems because their tissue could develop frostbite. Usually ice bag treatment times range from 10 to 20 minutes. Ice bags are particularly helpful for the patient who has had surgery to decrease swelling and pain in the area. Sensation over a surgical scar must be carefully checked, because some degree of sensory loss is not uncommon in this area.

ICE MASSAGE

Ice massage is used clinically to decrease pain in a localized area. It is simple, inexpensive, and an easily accessible modality. The indications and contraindications for cold are included in the effects of heat and cold. Ice massage is often applied over a bursa, tendon, muscle, or over small areas of muscle spasm to decrease pain and increase function. The easiest way to apply the ice massage is by freezing a wax or styrofoam cup of water with a wooden tongue depressor or popsicle stick in the middle so that the person applying the ice will not get cold. Ice cubes can also be used.

During application, a towel is used to wipe water seepage from the treated area, because excess water will be cold and may make the patient uncomfortable. The ice massage is applied by making small overlapping circles. An area of 10 by 15 cm can be treated in 5 to 10 minutes. If a larger area is involved, ice massage is not the treatment of choice. The treatment usually takes between 5 and 10 minutes for the area to have a decrease in sensation. The patient will usually experience cold, burning, aching, and then numbness. When the therapist can touch the area and the patient is unable to feel the touch, the treatment is completed. The ice massage produces analgesia and may continue to do so for 3 to 5 minutes after treatment. To take maximum advantage of the analgesic effect, exercise or stretching should be done immediately after treatment. This treatment can be done by reliable patients at home, and written instructions must be given to ensure that the patient uses the modality safely.

ICE SLUSH AND ICE TOWELS

Ice towels are often used to try to decrease spasm or spasticity in either a relatively large or small area. They are used with fairly good success on the athlete to decrease cramps in the gastrocnemius muscle. Ice slush baths are used with neurological patients to decrease excessive muscle activity and to improve volitional control. With the ice slush bath, the extremity is immersed for about 3 to 5 seconds and then removed from the bath.

With the ice towel treatment, the towel may be on the body part for 45 seconds to 4 or 5 minutes, depending on when the towels start to rewarm. It is best to use shaved or crushed ice because it will melt rapidly. Cubed ice will often stick to the towel and make areas of uneven skin contact. If the therapist is to apply these for 5 to 10 minutes, it is advisable to use rubber gloves. The towels are immersed in cold fluid and the ice bath. The towels must be wrung out and then applied to the specific body area. It may take 5 to 10 minutes for anesthesia to occur. Many physical therapists will use a hold-relax technique during the towel application to try to increase range of motion. If the patient is having a cramp in his gastrocnemius muscle group, it may be helpful while the area is cooled to ask for a maximal contraction of the dorsiflexors to use the principle of reciprocal innervation. A passive stretch can also be applied during ice towel application. By decreasing spasm or spasticity, range of motion may be regained and pain may be decreased.

COMPRESSIVE CRYOTHERAPY

Compressive pumps are available that provide external pressure plus cooled water to an extremity to decrease swelling in an area and to prevent loss of function. These machines apply intermittent pressure to try to increase the interstitial pressure and pump fluid back into the venous system. At least two types of units are commercially available. The larger machines have a refrigeration unit that cools the water. Smaller, portable units use ice to maintain the proper temperature.

Starkey (1976) used ice, elevation, and compression with high school athletes and also ice, elevation, and intermittent compression. After a 30-minute treatment, the ice, elevation, and intermittent compression was more effective in decreasing edema. This finding has implications for all physical therapists who work with acute injuries. If edema can be kept to a minimum, the patient can return to full function more rapidly.

Pressure values for the arm should be about 40 to 60 mm Hg, and for the lower extremity approximately 60 to 80 mm Hg. The pressure setting should never exceed the diastolic pressure. The maximum pressure may be determined by taking the patient's blood pressure and subtracting 10 from the diastolic pressure. This measurement avoids guessing and prevents the patient from experiencing tingling, numbness, or a pulsation below the unit, all of which indicate that the pressure is too high.

Usually the time on-off ratio is 3:1. The treatment time with a compressive cryotherapy machine will vary, but it usually lasts 10 to 15 minutes. With some of the larger units, two limbs may be treated simultaneously. The therapist must watch the temperature on the machine when using two appliances because the cooled water may warm significantly.

Ice, elevation, compression, and rest are important for any new injury. These machines have been used with sprains, strains, contusions, and for reducing edema in acute injuries. Athletes usually can handle the compression and cold therapy. Patients with circulatory problems would have extreme difficulty tolerating this treatment.

VAPOCOOLANT SPRAYS

The most common type of vapocoolant spray used in physical therapy is fluoromethane, which is a mixture of two flurocarbons. The liquid is contained in a bottle. The spray removes heat from the skin and underlying tissues and feels like a cool jet stream of fluid on the skin. It is nonflammable, nonexplosive, and nontoxic, but has the ability to freeze the skin if held over one area for more than six seconds. Ethyl chloride was the first type of vapocoolant spray used. It is flammable and explosive, can be a fire hazard, and is not supposed to be inhaled; thus, it is rarely used in physical therapy.

The pioneering work in the use of a cold spray treatment was done by Travell (1983). She used the vapocoolant spray for myofascial dysfunction. Travell called her technique "stretch and spray," whereas in most of the physical therapy literature, it is called spray and stretch. She identified localized areas of pain as trigger points. A myofascial trigger point is a hyperirritable localized area of a muscle or fascia that, with compression, may cause referred pain. Some trigger points may be painful only to palpation, whereas others hurt and may refer pain without ever touching the skin. In physical therapy a trigger point may also have been called a "muscle knot." The most common areas for trigger points are the back, shoulder girdle, neck, and muscles of mastication. Travell believes that a muscle that contains a trigger point is shortened and weak and that the trigger point may have occurred initially because of a muscle strain or chronic overload. Patients with trigger points may have a multitude of diagnoses, including idiopathic myalgia, fibrositis, and myofascitis.

These trigger points are most commonly seen in a person's middle years, and are more common in women than in men. They may cause pain, which may range from minimal to severe radiating pain with autonomic changes. Travell believes that in a trigger point area circulation is decreased, metabolites are increased, and a sensitization of the nerves occurs. By spraying the skin the cutaneous afferents are stimulated, thus decreasing the gamma motoneuron firing. This change in muscle spindle sensitivity may allow for greater stretching. Once greater range of motion is achieved, an increase may occur in blood supply to the area and ischemic pain may decrease.

These painful trigger points are treated with a multitude of therapeutic agents including spray and stretch, ice massage, ice bags, moist heat, the neuroprobe, ultrasound, and massage. Spray and stretch is easy to apply and is very economical in terms of patient time, therapist time, and cost. Depending on the location of the problem, the patient may be able to do the spray and stretch treatment at home after careful instructions.

Spray and stretch is commonly used to increase range of motion and decrease pain. The muscle being stretched must be stabilized at either its insertion or origin (Fig. 45-11). Overly aggressive stretching may decrease range of motion and increase pain. Demonstrate the cold spray first on yourself to decrease the patient's anxiety, and then apply it to a nonpainful area so that the patient will relax. Care should be taken to avoid the eyes and to avoid inhaling the vapors. To judge the effectiveness of the treatment, measurements are essential before and after treatment. In physical therapy laboratories, on subjects with nonpathological muscles, I have seen up to 20-degree increases in range of motion with straight leg raising. With patients, the increases are usually less dramatic but are quantifiable.

Spray and stretch in physical therapy is used for the treatment of trigger points, subacute or chronic sprains or strains, bee stings, and calf cramps. The goals of spray and stretch include increasing range of motion, decreasing muscle spasm, and decreasing local, referred, or chronic pain. The bottle should be held upside down at a 30-degree angle to the surface, and the spray should be applied parallel to the fibers of the muscle. The bottle is held 45 cm (18 in) from the body part, and the spray should move at a speed of 10 cm/sec (4 in/sec). The parallel sweeps should move in one direction, and the skin overlying the muscle should be exposed to the spray two to three times. If more spray and stretch is indicated, the body part must be rewarmed to avoid injuring the skin. Often a hot pack is applied, and then the sequence of spraying and stretching can be repeated with the goal of regaining full range of motion. The entire muscle should be sprayed. If the spray is applied too close to the skin or too many times, muscle cooling may occur.

If possible, between each spray, you would like the patient to achieve an even greater stretch. After maximal range of motion has been achieved, it is best to do active exercise to maintain the newly gained motion. Travell has stated that whether you to go from origin to insertion or vice versa is based on the patient's response. When spraying a trigger point with a reference area of pain, Travell advocates traveling parallel to the direction of the muscle fibers with the trigger point, then moving towards the area of referred pain.

If the patient is very sensitive to the cold spray, it is possible to move the spray closer to the patient, move the spray faster, or to use a finer nozzle. Moving the spray closer to the patient makes it feel warmer. In addition, by moving the spray faster, the coolant is in touch with the skin for a shorter period of time. With a finer nozzle, less coolant is released in a given

Figure 45-11. Spray and stretch technique for the upper trapezius muscle. A stretch is applied to the muscle at the same time as the spray application.

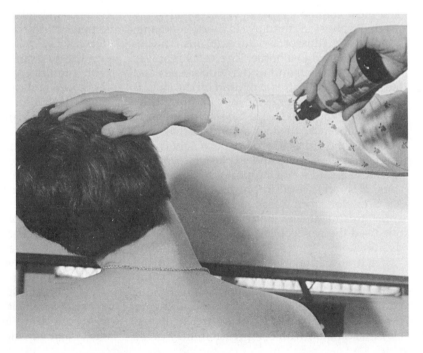

amount of time. These three factors may be especially important for the patient who does not tolerate cold well, yet who would benefit significantly from the modality. The patient may be disturbed by the white tracings (lines) that remain on the skin after application, which are from sebum being dissolved from the pores. If spray and stretch is used frequently, any lanolin-based cream will replace the oils.

The vapocoolant spray treatment can be augmented by warm showers, stretching, and postural exercises. While working on an increase in range of motion and a decrease in pain, preventive measures should be taught, such as good body mechanics, relaxation exercises, proper posture, stretching, and strengthening exercises to avoid potential problems. The physical therapist must not only treat the problem, but also try to influence the cause of the dysfunction. There are important considerations for choosing any cold modality. Table 45-6 reviews a few factors that should be considered when deciding which modality is most appropriate for various patient conditions.

Table 45-6. Different Modes of Cold Application

MODE	EFFECT ON RANGE OF MOTION	COST AND MAINTENANCE	TREATS A LARGE AREA?	DECREASES SWELLING?	TREATMENT TIME
Cold pack	May decrease ROM after cold application.	Relatively inexpensive	It could but care must be taken not to produce hypothermia.	Yes	About 15–20 min
Ice bag	May decrease ROM after cold application.	Inexpensive	No	Yes	About 15-20 min
Ice massage	By decreasing pain in localized area, may increase or decrease ROM.	Inexpensive	No	Yes	Until the area becomes numb—usually 5–10 min for a small area (larger area takes longer).
Ice towel	Will usually decrease ROM after application.	Inexpensive	Yes	Yes, but it is only effective for a short period of time.	3–5 min, and then starts to lose effectiveness
Cryopressure	May increase ROM because there is less edema.	More expensive—the smaller portable units are less expensive but the large units are very expensive.	Yes	Yes	Anywhere from 10–20 min (some treat for much longer periods of time).
Evaporative coolants	More increase in ROM after application when stretch is applied.	Inexpensive	Not usually (the treatment is usually localized to a small area).	No	3–5 min for the actual application

APPENDIX: CELSIUS–FAHRENHEIT CONVERSION

Most texts use the Celsius scale. If it is necessary to convert from Celsius to Fahrenheit, use the following formula:

⅘ degrees Celsius + 32 = degrees Fahrenheit

In reading owner's manuals for machines, it is very important to know which temperature scale is being used. For example, if the whirlpool temperature gauge was set at 36°C and the therapist wanted to convert it to degrees Fahrenheit, the calculation would be as follows:

⅘ × 36 + 32 = degrees Fahrenheit

Therefore, 36°C is equal to 96.8°F. To convert to Celsius from Fahrenheit, use the following formula:

⅝ (F − 32) = degrees Celsius

So, if you wanted to convert 95°F to Celsius, you would calculate as follows:

⅝ (95 - 32) = degrees Celsius

Therefore, 95°F is equal to 35°C.

ANNOTATED BIBLIOGRAPHY

Abramson DI, Tuck S, Lee SW et al: Comparison of Wet and Dry Heat in Raising Temperature of Tissues. Arch Phys Med Rehabil 48:654, 1967 (The authors compared wet and dry heat. They found that moist heat may penetrate slightly deeper, but dry heat increased the skin temperature more effectively.)

Borrell RM, Henley EJ et al: Fluidotherapy: Evaluation of a new heat modality. Arch Phys Med Rehabil 58:69, 1977 (The authors reported on a heat modality called Fluidotherapy. They compared the heat absorption in the hand with paraffin, whirlpool, and Fluidotherapy. The hand absorbed the greatest heat with Fluidotherapy.)

Borrell RM, Parker R et al: Comparison of in vivo temperatures produced by hydrotherapy, paraffin wax treatment, and Fluidotherapy. Phys Ther 60(10):1273, 1980 (The authors compared in vivo intra-articular finger temperatures when the subjects received a whirlpool, paraffin, and Fluidotherapy. They found that the least intra-articular temperature rise was with the whirlpool, a greater rise with the paraffin, and highest rise with Fluidotherapy.)

Duffield MN (ed): Exercise in Water, 2nd ed. London, Bailliere Tindall, 1976 (This book contains an excellent overview of pool therapy and exercise programs for the disabled.)

Griffin JE, Karselis TC: Physical Agents for Physical Therapists, 2nd ed. Springfield, IL, Charles C Thomas, 1982 (A very comprehensive book on therapeutic agents, light, and electricity used in physical therapy.)

Harris ED, McCroskery PA: Influence of temperature and fibril stability on degradation of cartilage collagen by rheumatoid synovial collagenase. N Engl J Med 290:1, 1974 (The authors found a three to four times increase in human cartilage degradation when the joint temperature was increased from 33°C to 36°C. This increase in intra-articular temperature is commonly seen with rheumatoid arthritis.)

Hayes KW: Manual for Physical Agents, 3rd ed. Chicago, Northwestern University Medical School Program in Physical Therapy, 1984 (An excellent guide on how to perform most of the physical agents and some of the electrical modalities used in current physical therapy practice.)

Hecht PJ, Bachmann S, Booth RE et al: Effects of thermal therapy on rehabilitation after total knee arthroplasty. Clin Orthop 178:198, 1983 (The authors studied 36 osteoarthritic patients who had total knee replacements. One group received just exercise, and the other two received either exercise and heat or exercise and cold therapy. There were no significant changes except that cold decreased swelling and may decrease pain in some patients.)

Horvath SM, Hollander JL: Intra-articular temperature as measure of joint reaction. J Clin Invest 28:469, 1949 (The authors studied rheumatoid arthritic knees and found that the intra-articular joint temperature correlated with the patient's disease process.)

Knight KL: Cryotherapy: Theory, Technique, and Physiology. Chattanooga Corp, Education Division, 1985

Lehmann JF, Silverman DR et al: Temperature

distributions in the human thigh produced by infrared, hot pack and microwave applications. Arch Phys Med Rehabil 47:291, 1966 (The authors found that in the human thigh the greatest tissue temperature rise occurred with moist heat at eight minutes post-application. The moist heat did not penetrate to the muscle layer.)

Lehmann JF (ed): Therapeutic Heat and Cold, 3rd ed. Baltimore, Williams & Wilkins, 1982

Mainardi CL, Walter JM, Spiegel PK et al: Rheumatoid arthritis: Failure of daily heat therapy to affect its progression. Arch Phys Med Rehabil 60:390, 1979 (Seventeen rheumatoid arthritics applied heat to one hand two times daily for two years. The authors found symptomatic relief, but no changes in swelling, tenderness, grip strength, and no changes on x-ray films.)

Michlovitz SL: Thermal Agents in Rehabilitation. Philadelphia, FA Davis, 1986

Starkey JA: Treatment of ankle sprains by simultaneous use of intermittent compression and ice packs. Am J Sports Med 4:142, 1976 (The author compared the treatment of ice, elastic wrap compression, and elevation with mechanical compression, cold, and elevation. Those receiving the mechanical pressure returned to activity sooner.)

Travell JG, Simons DG: Myofascial Pain and Dysfunction: The Trigger Point Manual. Baltimore, Williams & Wilkins, 1983 (This is the most comprehensive book available on the use of spray and stretch and the use of injections to decrease pain in trigger point areas.)

Valenza J, Rossi C, Parker R et al: A clinical study of a new heat modality: Fluidotherapy. J Am Podiatry Assoc 69(7):440, 1979 (The authors describe the uses of Fluidotherapy, some of the physiologic changes, and review a few clinical case studies.)

46

Physical Agents: Electrical, Sonic, and Radiant Modalities

JOSEPH KAHN

Heat, cold, light, sound, mechanics, and electricity are included in the array of available modalities for the clinician. Therapeutic applications of known principles of physics comprise a considerable sector in the use of these modalities in the practice of physical therapy. Thus, the physics, physiology, indications, contraindications, and recommended procedures for each of the following modalities will be discussed: shortwave diathermy, microthermy, ultrasound, phonophoresis, iontophoresis, electrical stimulation, transcutaneous electrical nerve stimulation, infrared, ultraviolet, and the cold laser.

ELECTROTHERAPEUTIC MODALITIES

Because the body's systems operate on an electrochemical basis, electrochemical procedures may be used to treat malfunctions. This section will deal with electrotherapeutic modalities. Electrotherapeutic modalities traditionally have been classified by frequency differentiation. However, modern concepts in physics demand a more definitive differentiation. (For example, ultrasound is high in the frequency range but is not electrical in nature.) Thus, each modality is looked at in a more comprehensive manner, including parameters and concepts that include, but are not limited to, frequency. For many years, I have separated the modalities into the following two groups: those using electrical current to produce various effects (eg,

heat, sound, physical, and chemical changes from radiation and light in the form of the cold laser); and those involving application of electrical current to the body for specifically designed results (eg, analgesia, muscle contraction, healing enhancement, and ionic transfer). In both categories, modalities are based upon electrophysical concepts, have characteristic biological and physiological effects, and are indicated for clinical application according to these effects.

HIGH-FREQUENCY CURRENTS

Shortwave Diathermy and Microthermy

High-frequency currents produce heat deep within the tissues by induction. The two types of applications used for high-frequency currents are condenser-type electrodes and induction drums. The condenser-type electrodes utilize two applicators separated by air or the patient. The induction drums contain field-producing coils and are most commonly used for the purpose of heating. Induction drums are far more common today than the traditional condenser pads and pancake (induction) coils (Fig. 46-1). Tissues within the induction field of the drum oscillate at the same frequencies as the diathermy unit. This rapid oscillation, measured in megacycles (Mc), results in heating deep within the tissues. Superficial tissues do not ordinarily become heated. Here, the principles of physics dictate that the density of the tissues involved determines the amount of heat produced locally. Muscle tissue, with a high

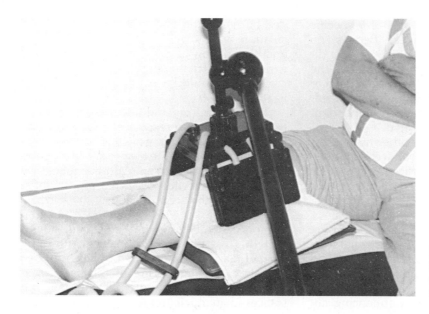

Figure 46-1. Shortwave diathermy, using the induction drum technique, for internal derangement of the knee.

water content, will generally become warmer than the surrounding tissues. Dissipation of the heat produced will depend upon transfer of the heat by the circulating blood to distant areas, the radiating effect on nearby tissues, and the attenuation as a result of the contact conduction to cooler adjacent tissues. Shortwave diathermy is recommended whenever heat is required in deeper tissues without surface heating. Pelvic, thoracic, and sinus and aural cavities are excellent targets for this type of heating. Joints, too, are prime subjects for high-frequency heating techniques because even intervening osseous tissues (eg, patella) will not insulate the underlying tissues from the penetrating effects of diathermy. Large muscle groups (eg, quadriceps) will respond well to diathermy because the muscles have a high water content. Fatty tissues do not become heated with diathermy, although microthermy does seem to be absorbed to a greater degree in fatty layers (Wadsworth). Microthermy is more concentrated and effective when fewer intervening layers of fatty tissue exists, because the radiation is more readily absorbed in fatty tissue.

The basic differences between diathermy and microthermy lie in the methods producing radiations, frequency-wavelength relationships along the electromagnetic spectrum, penetrating qualities, and absorptive characteristics. Generally speaking, diathermy at 7-, 11-, or 22-m wavelengths will produce mild, volumetric heating, whereas microthermy at 10 to 12.5 cm tends to concentrate the heating in a smaller region. In either case, the penetration will be relative to the density and type of tissues within the field (Wadsworth).

Shortwave diathermy produces heat by means of high-frequency oscillations obtained with high voltages and channeled through treatment drums, pads, or coils by means of insulated cables. The patient is placed within the circuit and the high-frequency field is "tuned" to the unit's output, much like a radio is "tuned" to the broadcasting studio's output.

With microthermy, the higher frequency/shorter wavelength radiation is obtained from an electronic device called a magnetron. Here, the acceleration of electrons within a disk-like, perforated iron core provides the extremely high frequencies needed for microwave transmission to the tissues. These higher-frequency transmissions are focused and "beamed" into the tissues from varying distances through specially designed treatment "heads" for specific targets and anatomical variances. Because no tuning is required, the radiation may be directed at the target area according to the instructions found with each treatment head or director. The heat produced is highly localized, with penetration and absorption dependent upon the specific tissues targeted.

Both diathermy and microthermy are utilized in physical therapy to produce heat in tissues deeper than the superficial layers. The most common targets for high-frequency currents have been the joints, the deep muscles, the pelvic region, the thoracic cavity, and sinus and inner ear conditions. Nonacute arthritis, deep myositis, nonspecific pelvic inflammation, bronchitis, otitis media, sinusitis, and prostatitis are among the many conditions effectively treated with high-frequency currents. Diathermy has been useful in enhancing absorption of iontophoretically and phonophoretically introduced substances to deeper levels. This enhancement is thought to be based upon the known capillary expansion that occurs with heat, although no references are to be found for this procedure. Clinically, however, effects have been found to be greatly enhanced by the application of diathermy following either iontophoresis or phonophoresis (Kahn, 1985).

Because manufacturers differ widely in the number, type, and arrangement of controls, adherence is suggested to recommended procedures, dosages, and operations for each unit. Automatic controls for power *or* tuning are commonly found today, thus eliminating the dual control method found with older equipment. With the older units, power settings would be leveled at a minimal stage during the *tuning* operation. When the patient was properly tuned, indicated by the highest reading on the meter outside of the danger zone, the power was then readjusted to comfort levels for the remainder of the treatment time. With the newer, automated equipment, the power is preset by the manufacturer or selector switches. Similarly, the tuning may be self adjusting by a feedback circuit in the induction drum(s). Overheating is an ever-present danger; burns should be avoided by sufficient insulation with towels over bony prominences and elimination of cable-skin contacts. Hotter is not better! Treatment with diathermy or microthermy should be at tolerable, comfortable heating levels.

Both diathermy and microthermy are contraindicated in the presence of acute inflammation, hemorrhage, or growing tumors. With acute inflammation, the tissues are already red, hot, painful, and swollen. Additional heat will add to the congestion by increasing the influx of blood into the area. Obviously, hemorrhage will be increased with the added circulation. Tumors generally favor heat and circulation for growth. (Investigations into the benefits of hyperthermia with cancerous growths indicate a limitation to the favoring of the heat by tumors.) Furthermore, internal metallic substances demand extreme caution with these modalities, if not prohibition. Although the metal will not become hot enough to produce damage, the presence of tissue-metal interfaces provides areas of trapped heat with little opportunity for dissipation of the heat produced, and subsequently can lead to deep-seated burns. High-frequency apparatus should not be used in the presence of a pacemaker, because of the high frequency's effect on the frequency-sensitive components of the pacemaker. Caution is suggested with pregnant patients because vasomotor shifts and circulatory changes may affect the fetal circulation. Hypotensive patients may have their low blood pressure driven even lower by the vasodilation produced by deep heat. Patients with severe cardiac involvement also may be adversely affected by sudden shifts in circulation and demands upon the heart.

Microthermy is not recommended around the eyes or testicles because of the hypersensitivity of these structures. Manufacturers' warnings and recommendations should be heeded concerning additional precautions. The federal government provides excellent source material and guides for both diathermy and microthermy equipment (US DHHS, 1981).

Used wisely and competently, shortwave

diathermy and microthermy should be valuable adjuncts to all other modalities and procedures in physical therapy practice.

ELECTRICAL STIMULATION

Electrical stimulation (ES) has been utilized for more than 100 years in the laboratory and in the clinic. The control of treatment parameters, however, has been expanded in an effort to produce better results with less discomfort. Today, clinicians may select and adapt frequencies, pulse durations, intensities, and other parameters for individualized regimens. Currently, the equipment available to practitioners offers documentation of progress and monitoring of patient conformity to the prescribed procedures at home.

However, certain facts remain unchanged through these many years, and serve as respected guidelines for practitioners. These are as follows.

1. Normally innervated musculature responds readily to both alternating current (AC) and direct current (DC) stimulation.
2. In the presence of reaction of degeneration (RD) to the nerve, the ability to respond to AC is lost.
3. Continuous DC by itself will not elicit contractions from normally innervated or denervated musculature. The body readily accommodates to a continuous flow of current. Muscles react best to a changing current flow, such as with the "make and break" of the flow or a change in direction (polarity). Continuous DC is primarily used for iontophoresis, which is a process of introducing chemical substances into the body and where muscle contraction is not desired (see Iontophoresis). With DC, the negative pole has been found to produce the greater stimulation, most probably because of the sodium hydroxide (NaOH) produced at the cathode. Consequently, the negative-pole electrode is usually recommended as the stimulating electrode (Shriber).

4. Stimulation of denervated musculature must utilize an *interrupted DC* with a sufficiently long duration, because denervated musculature requires a longer duration (ie, wider pulse width) for stimulation than normally innervated musculature. Studies involving chronaxie and strength-duration curves document this phenomenon. Chronaxie, which measures the duration necessary to obtain minimal reactions at specified intensities, indicates that most normal muscles will respond to durations of less than 1 msec. Conversely strength-duration curve testing indicates the necessity for higher intensities to produce contractions when the durations are short. Both of these clinical tests have lost popularity in favor of the more complex electromyograph (EMG). Very few generators with an interrupted DC mode are now available to clinicians. When this modality is indicated, a continuous DC waveform is interrupted by the physical therapist using a hand-held interruptor key electrode. This hand method technique has the advantage of a longer duration because of the relatively slow finger movement when compared with the faster electronically timed pulses (Fig. 46-2).
5. Continuous AC with a frequency of at least 50 c/sec (Hz) may be utilized to tetanize musculature to obtain relaxation of spasm.
6. Surged modes of AC are believed to stimulate slow-twitch fibers because peak intensities are reached over a brief period of delay, whereas pulsed or interrupted modes of AC are believed to stimulate fast-twitch fibers because peak intensities are reached almost instantaneously. Work in England indicates the possibility of transformation of fast-and slow-twitch fibers to their opposites by superimposed differential frequency stimulation to the appropriate nerves (Jones). This process is known as a "biogenetic engineering" among researchers. Clinicians must decide which type of fibers are in need of stimulation and

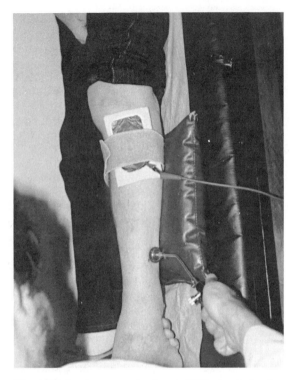

Figure 46-2. Interrupted galvanic (DC) stimulation for peroneal dysfunction. Here, the indifferent electrode (positive) is placed at the proximal portion of the nerve neural pathway, while the stimulating electrode (negative) is moved along the peripheral distribution of the nerve.

design a treatment plan accordingly (Fig. 46-3).

7. An optimum frequency for general stimulation has been found to be between 80 and 100 Hz. Most standard low-volt equipment has available frequencies in this range. In addition, interferential current equipment provides 80 to 100 Hz as the net frequency. The approximation of this frequency to the traditional tetanizing frequency of 50 to 60 Hz is not coincidental. Lower frequencies would not provide a smooth tetanic contraction; higher frequencies would necessitate high intensities, which could be irritating to the patient.

8. Equipment operating with less than 100 V is generally termed "low volt"; that operat-

ing with up to 500 V is currently termed "high-volt galvanic." The use of the term "galvanic" means the current is not a pure DC, but rather is an interrupted current with a twin spiked waveform and in some cases, a negligible but present negative component. Although supposedly polarized, the differential polarity is too small to be effective for either ion transfer or denervation stimulation. Some polar effects may be assumed at the electrode surface-skin contact interface. These effects may be useful in the management of edema because the permeability of membranes is involved, which is a phenomenon known to be responsive to polarity characteristics. High-volt techniques usually require at

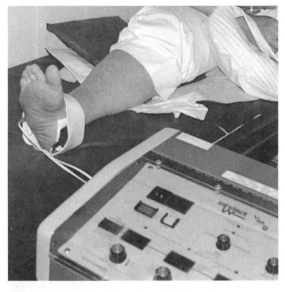

Figure 46-3. Transarthral electrode placements at the ankle to ensure stimulation around the entire joint. Current will flow along the first moist layer around the joint rather than traverse the highly resistant tissues between the electrodes. A high frequency (100 Hz) would be used for fast-twitch fiber stimulation, and a lower rate (4 Hz) would be selected for slow twitch fiber stimulation. Because muscles contain unequal distributions of *both* types of fibers, frequency may be changed during treatment to accommodate both targets.

least *three* electrodes, with one serving as a reference or indifferent electrode.

9. High-volt galvanic stimulation utilizes the deeper penetration of higher-frequency (or shorter-wave length) currents in the low microseconds range to eliminate discomfort by bypassing the superficial sensory nerve endings in the skin (Alon). However, the shorter duration requires the considerably higher voltages offered by these units (strength-duration curve phenomenon) which, in turn, tends to *increase* skin sensation. Patient reaction has been varied with this equipment (Fig. 46-4) (Alon). The "Russian stimulation" apparatus refers to units offering frequencies in the mid-range of 2400 to 2500 Hz. These mid-range frequencies may offer deeper penetration, but do so at the price of increased voltages, as previously noted. Because these mid-range frequencies are too rapid to produce contractions, the base frequencies must be pulsed (eg, 1 to 120 Hz) in order to elicit muscular contractions.

10. Interferential current stimulation utilizes medium-frequency currents of approximately 4000 Hz and 4100 Hz (varies with manufacturers), which are crossed subcutaneously by selected electrode placements. The resulting interferential pattern cancels out the difference in frequencies and leaves the balance to be usually in the optimal 80 to 100-Hz range. The characteristics of the medium-high frequencies (80 to 100 Hz) make these infrared frequencies penetrate to a tissue level considerably deeper than if administered with surface electrodes at the same range using standard low-volt apparatus. The phenomenon of increased penetration with increased frequencies (or shorter wavelengths) is a standard principle of physics. Most interferential units offer a "sweep" mode in addition to individual frequency selectors, which allow a sweep across several frequencies in an effort to stimulate as many frequency-differentiated fibers as possible. Because denervated musculature requires longer-duration stimulation, the lower frequency-longer wavelengths (durations) apparently recruit the injured fibers to a greater extent than higher frequency-shorter wavelengths. This phenomenon suggests that the interferential apparatus has the possibility of being a diagnostic tool because of the differential frequency responses between normal and abnormal musculature. Several manufacturers of interferential current apparatus also offer vacuum suction electrode devices to pro-

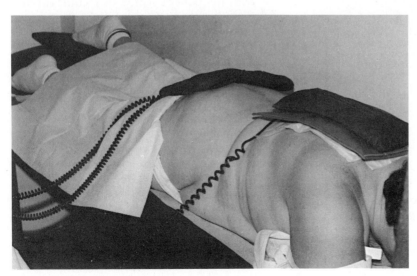

Figure 46-4. High-voltage galvanic stimulation. The two active pads are placed bilaterally on the gluteal muscles and the indifferent pad is placed on the dorsal spine. A moist towel is inserted under the larger pad for greater skin contact and decreased resistance.

vide increased skin contact and electrical transmission, the efficacy of which in providing improved transmission has not yet been demonstrated clinically. Interferential techniques require the use of *four* electrodes in a crossed pattern (Fig. 46-5).

Many manufacturers of transcutaneous electrical nerve stimulation (TENS) devices also offer electrical stimulation (ES) units similar in size and operation; however, they are considerably more expensive. These units generally offer stimulating currents in the biphasic category with additional parameters for modification of waveform (eg, time on/off; rate of rise time-reciprocal or synchronous patterns; surged-pulsed regimens; and percentage of power selection). These units are battery operated and portable, and are therefore valuable for home-care practitioners; for bedside, nursing home, or housebound patients; and, in some cases, for athletic (locker room) administration. The advantage of multiple daily use by the patient makes these units ideal adjuncts to physical therapy care (Fig. 46-6).

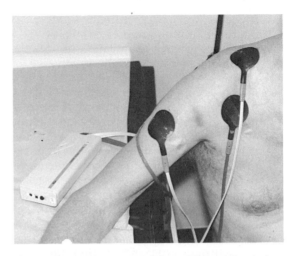

Figure 46-6. Programmed low-voltage stimulation. The crossed-pattern electrode placement is *not* interferential because all four electrodes carry the same frequency. Current is amplified at the crossing point by reinforcement of the waveform.

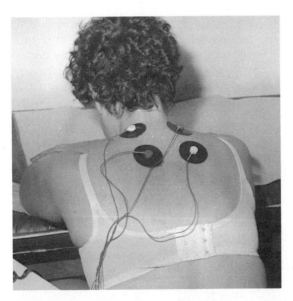

Figure 46-5. Interferential current stimulation. The electrodes are arranged in a crossed pattern over the dorsal cervical spine.

Electrical stimulation is designed to

1. offer total fiber response (recruitment) as compared to the normal less than total fiber response of untrained muscles during active exercise (Kahn, 1987; Benton and co-workers);
2. provide relatively weight-free exercises with the patient seated or recumbent during stimulation (Kahn, 1987; Benton and co-workers);
3. increase circulation by means of the pumping action of muscles upon the vessels (Kahn, 1987; Benton and co-workers);
4. increase phagocytosis (Kahn, 1987; Benton and co-workers);
5. produce mild heating (Joule's law) with all of the benefits accrued from increased temperatures within the tissues (Kahn, 1985);
6. increase the production of beta-endorphins, leading to analgesia (Mannheimer);
7. serve as an osteogenic stimulant in certain circumstances (eg, nonunited fracture management) based upon the piezoelectrical qualities of human bone (Kahn, 1985; 1987); and

8. enhance open wound healing (see discussion of TENS) (Kahn, 1985; 1987).

Electrical stimulation is indicated for muscles requiring assistance for relaxation (spasm), for exercise (disuse atrophy, weakness, paralysis, and training), for pain (secondary to the above), and as an adjunct to the healing processes of the body (ie, nonunited fractures or open wounds).

Contraindications for electrical stimulation are few. It is not recommended (1) in the presence of active hemorrhage, because the pumping motion of stimulated muscles would tend to increase blood flow and exacerbate the hemorrhage; (2) at spontaneous fracture sites where undesired movements may increase stress on weakened bone; (3) in patients with severe cardiac arrhythmias where additional stress with increased circulation would be undesired; (4) in patients with phlebitis where the danger of embolism is ever present; and (5) in certain instances when a pacemaker is present (ie, higher frequencies could disrupt the operation of older types of pacemakers).

Selection of specific parameters, electrode placements, and other essentials of competent and effective administration of electrical stimulation are found in the manuals and texts in the annotated bibliography.

The administration of ES for the treatment of idiopathic scoliosis is an excellent example of the utilization of this modality with specific parameters and electrode placement. Patients use the ES units for eight hours during sleep to contract stretched muscles on the convexity of the curve. Often, this procedure eliminates the need for 23-hours-a-day bracing. Parameter selection generally calls for a medium pulse width of 200 to 300 μsec and a low frequency ranging from 20 to 50 Hz. Intensities are usually sufficient to produce visible contractions of the target muscles at tolerable levels for the patient, because stimulation must allow sleep. The duty cycle ranges are from three to six seconds on and three to six seconds off. Electrode placements vary: Early protocols placed electrodes paravertebrally; current techniques place the electrodes along the lateral rib cage. Results with both techniques have been excellent.

TRANSCUTANEOUS ELECTRICAL NERVE STIMULATION

One special type of electrical stimulation is designed to modify pain. Transcutaneous electrical nerve stimulation (TENS) is specifically oriented to the stimulation of nerve fibers known to be involved with transmitting signals to the brain that are interpreted by the thalamus as pain. Although electrodes are placed on the surface of the skin and electrical impulses are transmitted transcutaneously, the particular waveforms used with TENS equipment are targeted to be received by large-diameter, myelinated A fibers, which are reserved for proprioceptive transmission. These particular fibers are sensitive to biphasic waveforms (ie, waveforms with both positive and negative phases) or monophasic wave forms with a noncontinuous or interrupted form. Continuous or noninterrupted wave forms are generally transmitted by means of the small, unmyelinated C fibers, which are known to carry painful stimuli. In A fibers, transmission is believed to be about 30 m/sec, whereas C fiber transmission is considerably slower, at about 3 m/sec. Therefore, the TENS units produce a phasic output designed to stimulate only A fibers and not C or motor fibers.

Effective TENS administration usually does not involve muscle contraction, although some practitioners claim success with visible contraction elicited (Mannheimer). Transmission from both A and C fibers travels along the mixed nerve pathways and enters the spinal cord through the posterior horn's substantia gelatinosa, where specialized T cells process the incoming messages. Here, the two separate circuits are differentiated by the biophysical operations within these cells. A gating mechanism takes over and allows only one or the other transmission to pass through. The Gate Theory postulated by Wall and Melzack has become the foundation of electrical pain control. If transmission along A fibers is predominant, the pain signal that is sent along the C fibers is inhibited at the T cell and does not enter the ascending tracts to the thalamus. On the other hand, should the input along C fibers outweigh that along A fibers, pain will be manifested. Therefore, the basis of the Gate Theory is to overload the fibers with A-type stimulation, and thus successfully block incoming C transmission at the "gate" in the posterior horn. The TENS apparatus provides this selective stimulation to A fibers.

One may then ask the following question: Why does the analgesia last even after the TENS stimulation is stopped? The latest theory is based upon the concept of the body's own pain killers, beta endorphins, which are produced by the pituitary gland and have a role in pain modification. Pain serves as a stimulant to the body to increase production of endorphins to combat pain. Researchers have found that electrical stimulation, not necessarily painful, to the surface of the skin will also stimulate endorphin production (Mannheimer). Currently, the issue of differential frequency values in endorphin enhancement is being studied. Reports have indicated increased analgesia, believed to be endorphin related, to *low-frequency* stimulation (ie, 1 to 10 Hz). How-

ever, other research has not found this increased analgesia.

Electrode placement is an important factor, but is relatively simple. Trigger points, acupuncture points, and nerve roots are utilized for electrode placements by most practitioners. Charts are available from most manufacturers showing recommended placement sites. For a handy reference the following placements are suggested: nerve root (dermatome); point of pain; acupuncture point distal to the point of pain; and acupuncture point proximal to the point of pain. Several other placement techniques are found in texts and manuals for TENS practice (Kahn, 1985; 1987), including transarthral, interferential (crossed) patterns, and other placements identified for specific types of patients or conditions (eg, the obstetrical patient, the postsurgical patient, TMJ, and other dental applications (Fig. 46-7).

Parameters

Frequency (rate), or the numbers of pulses per second (pps) of the phasic input bears heavily upon the success of treatment. The higher frequencies (ie, 80 to 120 Hz) have generally been found to produce good analgesia with acute

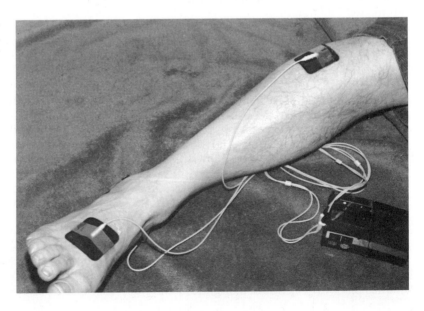

Figure 46-7. TENS applied for pain control in reflex sympathetic dystrophy of the lower extremity.

conditions. The lower frequencies (ie, 1 to 10 Hz) are apparently more effective with chronic conditions, often with a delayed onset of relief, but producing longer-lasting relief than with the higher frequencies (Mannheimer). The skilled clinician determines the optimum settings for each patient and for each stage of the condition being treated.

Duration or pulse width, ranging from 50 to 400 msec in most current equipment, determines the actual amount of energy delivered to the tissues during treatment. The wider the width, the more energy delivered. The sensation of increased strength is apparent when the pulse is widened even though the intensity remains constant. A medium pulse width (ie, 150 msec) has been found to be the optimum duration for most patients; however, adjustment in *either* direction must be made if needed (Kahn, 1987).

Intensity (amplitude) will vary with each patient and each condition. One preferred technique is to maintain the minimum amperage so that patients barely feel the tingle of the current. Another technique is to maintain a stronger milliamperage, sometimes eliciting muscle contraction. As an advocate of the Arndt-Schultz law, I favor the *least* stimulation to produce the most profound effect. The operating amperage claimed by manufacturers for their products will vary considerably [up to 80 milliamperes (mA)] but what actually matters is the amount reaching the patient, not what is registered on a milliammeter or oscilloscope. If TENS administration is painful, the clinician is defeated before starting.

Modulation offers the clinician a valuable weapon against accommodation. The patient will accommodate readily to stimulating current, especially those with prolonged application. By modulating or varying the current form periodically, the accommodation is delayed and in some cases prevented completely. This delayed accommodation is usually accomplished by a 10% variation in the frequency or a similar variation in the pulse width. Amplitude modulation is not commonly offered, because preset intensities should be maintained for adequate stimulation.

Pulse or burst parameters in TENS units provide the clinician with "packages" of stimuli consisting of multiple stimuli within bursts or pulses. This mode offers a more *phasic* input and is a muscle as well as a neural stimulant with proper electrode placements (ie, motor points). With electrodes placed at motor points and the unit in the burst mode, increased amplitude will generally produce visible muscle contractions, thus adding to the versatility of the standard TENS apparatus. This procedure is most useful when treating pain *and* muscular weakness or paresis-paralysis (eg, "foot drop" or "wrist drop" with peripheral neuropathies). For foot drop, electrodes are placed at the fibular head and the anterolateral aspect of the supralateral malleolar area. For wrist drop, electrodes are placed at the lateral epicondylar region and the extensor surface of the forearm at the wrist. Visible contractions should be elicited, at patient tolerance, coincidental with the frequency of the burst mode.

Obstetrical TENS

TENS has been found to be of value in controlling the discomfort of labor and delivery. Several references may be found in the literature claiming success with similar techniques and protocols (Kahn, 1987). Proximally placed electrodes at the T8-L1 paravertebral sites are activated in the morning on the day of imminent delivery to provide overall dorsolumbar level analgesia. Distally placed electrodes at L5-sacral paravertebral sites are activated only during labor contractions. At the second stage of labor, the distal electrodes are removed to the anterior abdominal surface, in a V pattern suprapubically. Again, these are activated during contractions. The TENS parameters are generally those used for acute pain (ie, high rate, medium pulse width, and intensities at patient's level of tolerance).

With cesarean section deliveries, as with other surgical procedures, postoperative incisional pain may be controlled with electrode placements parallel to the scar or at appropriate acupuncture points (Mannheimer; Kahn, 1985, 1987).

TENS has also been found effective in controlling the nausea of morning sickness during the early stages of pregnancy. Electrodes are placed at the right acromioclavicular tip and right "hoku" point (an Oriental term for the dorsal web space between thumb and forefinger). Parameters are for acute pain: high rate, medium width, and minimal intensity. Thirty minutes each morning usually provides satisfactory control. It should be noted that this technique is, strangely, not effective if electrodes are placed on the left side (Kahn, 1985).

Nonunited Fracture Management

Many references to the use of electrical stimulation to enhance osteogenesis may be found in the literature. Constant and low-frequency pulsed DC and AC, as well as high-frequency modes, have been reported to be effective (Kahn, 1985). Experience has been favorable with standard TENS units utilizing traditional compensated monophasic or biphasic waveforms. Low intensities in the microampere range are suggested, with the TENS electrodes separated sufficiently for attenuation through the intervening tissues. With plaster casts in position, this separation is obvious. With no cast in place, electrode placement becomes the choice of the practitioner according to the fracture site and personal experience. The "sandwich" technique, the crossed-pattern technique, and variations of either may be considered. The parameters are highest rate (80 to 120 Hz), widest pulse widths (300 μsec), and the lowest intensities (lowest on the available scale). The application of the TENS should be for one hour, four times daily. The presence of infection or osteotomies (or both) delays, minimizes, and even prevents osteogenic enhancement (Fig. 46-8).

Other Uses

Recent reports indicate TENS as an effective modality in the control of pain with temporomandibular joint (TMJ) dysfunction and other dental conditions. Electrode placements are usually at the TMJ involved (unilateral or bilateral) and at the corresponding hoku sites. The parameters are set for acute pain: high rate and medium widths (Kahn, 1985, 1987).

TENS has also been found to be an effective modality for many podiatric conditions.

The full value of TENS as an analgesic agent remains to be evaluated with additional clinical investigations.

IONTOPHORESIS

Probably the most underutilized, misunderstood, and underestimated modality in electrotherapy is iontophoresis. The concept of introducing chemical substances into the body with direct current is neither new or extraordinary. The professional literature contains many references to *ionic* transfer for medical purposes dating back to the late 1800s (Abramowitsch). Most of the adverse criticism attempting to discredit this procedure has been from the clinical viewpoint, because the physics and chemistry involved are basic and are theoretically sound. Competent administration of iontophoresis in accordance with basic theoretical principles demonstrates the efficacy of this complex, yet effective, modality. The technique appears to make the difference between success and failure.

Iontophoresis is the introduction of chemical substances into the body for therapeutic purposes by means of a direct current. Ionizable substances (ie, acids, bases, salts) are ionized or broken up into the ionic components of their molecular structures by the passage of direct current through the solution or ointment-mixture containing these molecules. Because of the polarity involved with DC, a differential reaction occurs at the positive- and negative-pole electrodes. Following the basic law in physics of "like poles repel," the positive pole will repel only positively charged ions and radicals and the negative pole will repel only negatively charged ions and radicals. Therefore, the clinician must be aware of the polarity of the ion to be administered and then must place the source substance under the appropriate electrode. Ions are obtained from aqueous solutions, ointments, and creams containing the desired ions and radicals. Some of the more common of these are magnesium (+) ions from magnesium sulfate (Epsom Salt) solution; mecholyl (+) from mecholyl (chloride)

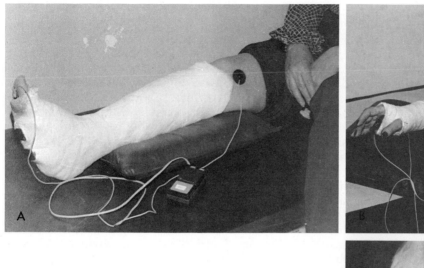

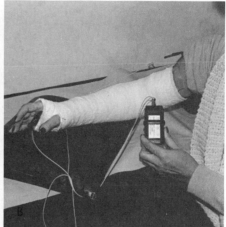

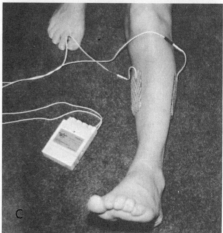

Figure 46-8. Application of TENS to enhance osteogenesis. *(A)* A casted nonunited fracture of the fibula. *(B)* Placement within the cast for a nonunited fracture of the forearm. *(C)* A mid-shaft fibular nonunited fracture with no cast. Self-adherent gel electrodes are used.

ointment; hydrocortisone (+) from hydrocortisone (chloride or oxide) ointments; zinc (+) from zinc oxide ointment; copper (+) from copper sulfate solution; calcium (+) from calcium chloride; lithium (+) from lithium carbonate or chloride; acetate (−) radicals from acetic acid; salicylate (−) from methyl salicylate; chlorine (−) from sodium chloride; and lidocaine (+) from a glycol ointment. Others may be found in appropriate texts and manuals (Kahn, 1987).

Effective techniques require placement of "like" poles in approximation. A positively charged ion must be placed under the positive electrode; a negatively charged ion must be placed under the negative electrode. If the ionic source is an aqueous solution, it is recommended that a low percentage concentration be utilized to facilitate dissociation (eg, 2% to 5% only). If the source is an ointment, lower percentages will also aid in proper transportation of ions (eg, 1% to 5%).

Electrode pads or towels should be soaked thoroughly in the source solutions. Ointments should be massaged into the target tissue prior to placement of water-soaked electrodes.

The negative electrode should always be larger than the positive—at least twice the size, if possible. Traditional texts and manuals have recommended that the indifferent electrode always be the larger one in order to "direct" the current. However, electrons flow in the same direction, *from negative to positive*, regardless of the electrode size. (Many standard texts refer to the flow of "current" from positive to negative. Although this is an accepted viewpoint from a literal standpoint, it is not technically correct (Karselis). Therefore, the electrons' *direction* of flow will not be altered by electrode size, but will be *shaped* by the size and placement of electrodes. The negative-pole electrode has a high concentration of hydrogen ions that will produce a strong sodium hydroxide (NaOH) formation at the electrode surface, which is quite irritating to the skin. The mild hydrochloric acid reaction at the oxygen-rich positive-pole electrode is minimally irritating. Therefore, to minimize the NaOH irritation at the negative-pole electrode, the square area of the electrode is increased in order to reduce the current density at any one point. High current density produces irritation, burns, and the like. Consequently, it is suggested that the negative electrode be the larger one even when it is the active electrode (ie, the electrode used to repel ions into the tissues).

The term "active electrode" usually indicates the electrode at which the ions are driven into the tissues; the indifferent or inactive electrode is simply a "ground" electrode offering a vector for the flow of current. These terms lose their significance when *double iontophoresis* is administered (ie, ions are driven into the tissues under both electrodes, at separated sites on the body, each with opposite polarity). Neither is an "indifferent" electrode because both are active electrodes.

Current intensity is recommended to be at 5 mA or less for all treatments. It is very likely that many of the early failures with iontophoresis were the result of concentrations that were too high or intensities that were beyond 5 mA. Intensities of 1 mA per square centimeter of electrode surface had been suggested, which would bring the average treatment intensity to well over 30 mA—more than enough to produce poor results *and* burns. The basic simple existing formula for iontophoresis (also called ion transfer) is

$I \times T \times ECE$ = grams introduced
I = intensity (amperes)
T = time (hours)
ECE = electrochemical equivalent (standardization quantities found in chemical texts)

These are, of course, reduced to milliamperes, minutes, and milligrams by appropriate mathematical operations.

Of note is the fact that the percentage of the source is *not* a factor; no advantage is obtained with high concentrations for ionic transfer. The intensity-time relationship is the key factor. An example of the use of magnesium sulfate for iontophoresis would be as follows:

Example: Magnesium sulfate iontophoresis, 30 minutes at 5 mA
0.005 mA $\times 0.5$ hours $\times 0.115$ ECE
magnesium = 0.0002875 g (0.2875 mg)

In this example, 0.2875 mg of magnesium will be introduced into the tissues with a treatment of 30 minutes, at 5 mA intensity. The same amount would be transferred if the treatment were for one hour at 0.0025 mA.

Intensities are adjusted to variations in skin resistances (ie, fair, dry skin, freckles, and the like) that affect the transmission of electric current as a result of high resistance, and consequently affect the ionic introduction. Current is always turned on and off slowly to avoid neuromuscular stimulation. The "make or break" phenomenon responsible for muscular contractions may be avoided by strict adherence to this rule.

Only continuous, direct current (often referred to as galvanic current) will produce clinically effective therapeutic iontophoresis. Oscillations, perturbations and interruptions in the waveform will diminish, minimize, and (most often) negate ion transfer. Many of the current models of high-voltage galvanic neuromuscular stimulation equipment have been erroneously used for this purpose with poor results. These units are designed to produce a twin-spiked, interrupted waveform of extremely short duration (ie, microamperage, which is totally unsuited to iontophoresis based upon the intensity-time relationship) (Alon). Any model of low-volt apparatus offering a continuous, ripple-free DC waveform and a meter or digital readout for monitoring is suitable for this procedure. The pathophysiological targets for ion transfer with appropriate therapeutic ions include pain (lidocaine); inflammation (hydrocortisone, salicylate); edema (mecholyl, hyaluronidase, salicylate); ischemia (magnesium, mecholyl, iodine); muscle spasm (magnesium, calcium); fungi (copper), calcific deposits (acetate); gouty tophi (lithium); scars and keloids (chlorine, iodine, acetate); and hyperhidrosis (tap water) (Figs. 46-9 and 46-10).

Because of the probability of mutual repulsion detracting from the intended vectors, it is not advised to place two chemicals under the electrode simultaneously, even if they bear the same polarity. An exception to this would be the use of the substance "Iodex with methyl salicylate," which is a commercially available mixture of iodine and salicylate, both negative ions, in a common base.

Burns are to be avoided. Metal-skin contacts are the most common causes of burns with DC. Careful placements of electrodes and constant monitoring during treatment are mandatory if burns are to be prevented. Well-soaked electrodes or thoroughly moistened towel padding are essential to avoid dry areas that lead to high-resistance burns. Except when treating open lesions, abraded, open, and raw skin areas should be avoided, as should be pimples, scratches, or other denuded areas. Freckles are unusually sensitive to electric current because they offer very high resistance to current, and are often the site of burns. Minimal current intensities, size differential between positive and negative electrode, and constant milliammeter monitoring are mandatory. Prevention is the best way to manage burns. If they occur, burns are treated as ordinary lesions with an antibiotic dressing, reassurance, and patience, because they take time to heal.

Contraindications for iontophoresis are similar to those for any patient with a history of allergic reactions or sensitivities to the chemicals used (eg, iodine if seafood hyperreactions; metals if bracelets, medals, or jewelry hyperreactions). Careful history taking is essential to success.

Treatment times range from 10 minutes to 45 minutes, depending upon the condition and the anatomical sites for application. Administration of iontophoreisis twice or three times per week is acceptable, with daily treatment occasionally indicated. Iontophoresis, like other modalities, is rarely administered as the sole treatment, but is generally combined with adjunctive procedures to complete a total approach regimen (eg, diathermy, electrical stimulation, manual procedures).

Specific techniques with individual conditions are explained and discussed in manuals

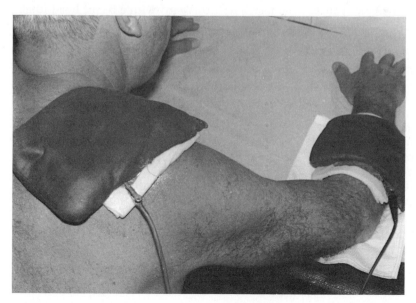

Figure 46-9. Iontophoresis with hydrocortisone or mecholyl is applied for a shoulder condition. The indifferent electrode is placed on the forearm. Note the paper towel/aluminum foil electrodes, alligator clips, and the size difference of the electrodes. The negative electrode is the larger one, as suggested in the text.

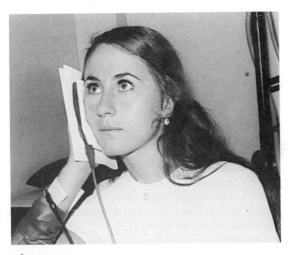

Figure 46-10. Hydrocortisone iontophoresis for Bell's palsy is applied prior to traditional electrical stimulation.

and texts recommended in the Annotated Bibliography.

ULTRASOUND

Technically speaking, ultrasound is *not* electrotherapy. Sound waves are not electrical; however, their behavior suggests many electrical qualities and traditionally ultrasonic procedures have been categorized with electrotherapy. Unlike electromagnetic radiation, sound waves require a medium for transmission. Air itself is a very poor conduction medium for sound wave transmission; hence, physical therapists use water, mineral oil, and specially designed coupling gels to assure sufficient transmission of the therapeutic sound waves.

Standard commercial current parameters of 110 V, 60 Hz AC are transformed into higher voltages (ie, 500 V) within the ultrasound units. This higher voltage is utilized to increase the frequency from 60 Hz to 1 million hertz (MHz). Federal regulations, at this writing, limit physical therapists to ultrasound units with 0.7 to 1.0 MHz frequencies. Several manufacturers are now promoting the use of higher-frequency units, although no official

notification of any changes in the regulations has been given (US DHHS, 1985).

The 1 MHz frequency is then imposed upon a piezoelectrical crystal (ie, PZT [lead-zirconium-titanate], quartz, or other suitable substance). The piezoelectrical qualities of these substances transform the electrical impulses into mechanical oscillations *at the same frequency* as the electrical stimulus. The piezoelectrical phenomenon is a reversible process. When the crystalline structure in a piezoelectrical substance, including human bone, is deformed or otherwise structurally disturbed, an electrical current will be generated proportional to the deforming force's frequency and intensity. The oscillating crystal cemented to the metallic or plastic faceplate of the transducer (soundhead) transmits the oscillation by means of the faceplate through the coupling gel to the patient's skin. Penetration is reported to be as deep as 4 cm; however, attenuation through differential tissues and distances will alter and reduce effective penetration (Wadsworth).

Power required for ultrasound ranges from 0.5 to 2.0 W/cm^2. Total wattage will depend upon the size of the transducer heads. They are generally of 5.0 or 10.0 cm^2. A total wattage of 5 W has been found to be optimal for clinical applications (Kahn, 1987). Therefore, for each soundhead: 0.5 W/cm^2 with a 10 cm^2 head totals 5 W; 1.0 W/cm^2 with a 5 cm^2 head totals 5 W.

Recommended treatment times are offered by most manufacturers. I have found 2 to 4 minutes of ultrasound administered twice or three times weekly to be an effective dosage for most conditions. When administered under water, the timing is increased to 6 to 8 minutes, because the dispersion and resistance of the water obviously reduces the driving force of the wave front.

The techniques of administration consist of slowly moving the soundhead in a circular pattern over the area to be treated while simultaneously advancing along a lineal track so as to cover a larger area. Texts and manufacturers usually suggest sounding of dermatome nerve roots in addition to the target zone, because neural tissue apparently transmits sound waves well. One to two minutes for each nerve root is recommended (Kahn, 1985).

When the treatment is administered under water, it is highly recommended by all manufacturers and qualified sources that the whirlpool tank or other metallic receptacles *not* be used for this purpose (personal communications with the Burdick Corp [1977] and the Birtcher Corp [1975]). Fiberglass or plastic receptacles should be used. Placement of the transducer under water may be either adjacent to and directed *at* the target site, or at a slight distance from and parallel to the target site, thus allowing the sound wave front to be dispersed and reflected, reverberating from the walls of the receptacle. With this second technique, treatment time must be extended to 6 to 8 minutes to allow sufficient time for the reflected-attentuated waves to affect the tissues. Specially designed handles are used with subaqueous techniques so that the clinician's hands are not submerged during treatment for lengths of time. Repeated underwater exposure of the hands during many daily treatments could lead to overexposure and consequent problems for the therapist.

The physiological effects of ultrasound have traditionally been divided into four phases: mechanical, chemical, biological, and thermal (Wadsworth; Shriber). The first three are so closely linked that they will be combined for explanation.

The oscillations at 1 MHz vibrate the tissues rapidly enough to disrupt loose or weakened molecular bondings. This phenomenon softens scar tissue, has a sclerolytic effect on collagenous fibers, and speeds up chemical reactions similar to "shaking the test tube" in the chemistry laboratory. Extremely high dosages, which are *not* used in physical therapeutic applications, can cause permanent changes (damage) to tissues by the "cavitation" effect or collapsing of existing molecular structures. The permeability of membranes is favorably affected because of both the mechanical oscillation and the mild heating produced by the ultrasound energy. A more valuable and often underestimated biological effect is the ability for ultrasound energy properly applied to increase the extensibility factor in tendons. Thus, a direct and practical application exists in the management of muscular spasm.

Last, but certainly not least in importance, is the thermal effect of ultrasound. Some still consider it a deep heating mechanism (Griffin). However, many clinicians, including this author, consider ultrasound *primarily* as a mechanical modality rather than a heating modality. Heat is produced with absorption of ultrasound energy; however, this heat is confined to circumscribed areas under the transducer head at the time of sonation. In addition, most heat is produced at interfaces where little or no heat dissipation occurs because it is confined in the interface between tissue layers. When this heat buildup is trapped beneath the periosteum, a transformation or "shearing" of the usually longitudinal waveform of ultrasound to the transverse form found with electromagnetic radiation takes place. Within the confines of the subperiosteal interface the ultrasonic beam is refracted, passing through the differential tissue media, back and forth between the surfaces of the bone and periosteum. With no egress for the heat to dissipate, a periosteal burn may ensue as a consequence of this "shearing" effect. Ultrasound is of little value in the attempt to heat large volumes of tissues (eg, muscles and joints), and may be helpful only in limited regions when indicated. The controversy still exists between adherents of the ultrasound/heat and ultrasound/mechanical concepts.

Ultrasound is indicated primarily for tight or spasmodic musculature, tendons, and the like. It has also been found helpful as an analgesic when the discomfort is based upon spasm, adhesions, and scar tissue. The nonthermal effects have also been reported to be valuable in the management of sinusitis and TMJ. Underwater techniques are of great assistance in the management of disorders at bony prominences and anatomically inaccessible locations, such as the elbow, wrists, fingers, ankles, and toes.

The following are the contraindications for ultrasound. (1) Sounding is not recommended of the eye, of growing epiphyses, of bony prominences with the manual technique, of the pregnant uterus, of areas prone to hemorrhage, and of hyposensitive areas. (2) The use of high-frequency apparatus in the presence of an implanted pacemaker is not recommended. (3) Ultrasound in areas of implanted metallic fixation is also questionable, because the sound waves may tend to concentrate in and about the metal-tissue interfaces rather than the target areas. Heat buildup there could be a problem. Rapid oscillations from the ultrasound energy may also present problems in the cements used with joint replacements. (4) Sounding at the carotid artery region should be avoided. (5) Finally, the prohibition regarding sounding of the spine has been questioned in the face of the advice to sound the nerve roots—actually the spinal cord. What has probably been meant all along is to avoid "bouncing" the soundhead over the spinous processes during sounding of the back musculature. The proximity of the periosteum of the spinous process could lead to periosteal burn, described earlier, if not discomfort for the patient.

PHONOPHORESIS

Similar to iontophoresis in concept, but differing in the physical chemistry involved, phonophoresis provides the clinician with the ability to introduce *molecules* into the tissues by means of the energy of the sound wave front. This procedure is in contrast to the *ions* introduced with DC. With phonophoresis, the body must then break down the molecules into the appropriate ions and radicals for recombination and function within the body systems. Some practitioners claim more immediate effects with ultrasound when compared with iontophoresis; however, this claim may be the result of the more rapid absorption of substances because of the increased permeability of the membranes produced by the ultrasound (Kleinkort and Wood). Claims for deep penetration of the molecules are questionable, because molecular sizes preclude penetration more than a millimeter or two through intervening tissues even though the ultrasound may penetrate several centimeters.

Several of the molecules utilized for pho-

nophoresis are identical to those ion sources used with iontophoresis: mecholyl, hydrocortisone, salicylates, iodine, lidocaine, and zinc. These are all in ointment or cream form. Ointment is preferred because creams may contain preservatives irritating to the skin. Again, the controversy over high or low percentage exists. I prefer the lower 1% to 5% while other clinicians use 10% compounds. Comparative studies are not conclusive. Phonophoresis is *not* administered under water because the dispersion of the chemicals would be too great. The attenuation of the wave front strength would be diminished sufficiently to preclude effective penetrative force of the ultrasound.

The technique for phonophoresis involves massaging the appropriate ointment into the target area. The standard transmission gel is applied, and then the ultrasound is administered at the recommended (usual) dosages (ie, 2 to 5 minutes at a total 5W). It is not necessary to increase the wattage with phonophoresis. Recommended treatment frequency is twice or three times weekly (Fig. 46-11).

Contraindications depend upon patient sensitivities or allergies to the substances introduced, similar to those for iontophoresis.

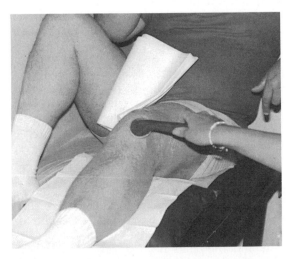

Figure 46-11. Ultrasound/phonophoresis with mecholyl ointment is used on the knee to stimulate vasodilation.

Ultrasound and phonophoresis are effective modalities for physical therapy. Ultrasound is most effective in the management of spasm and of shortened muscle-tendon tissues. When pain is involved, the addition of molecular introduction by means of phonophoretic techniques is recommended. Molecular substances effective in the management of ischemia, inflammation, congestion and delayed-healing wounds are available.

ULTRASOUND AND ELECTRICAL STIMULATION

The combination of ultrasound with electrical stimulation is a common modality. No references exist for the rationale and advantage of this combined technique. Whether the saving of time and the convenience for the practitioner are sufficient rationales for this procedure remains to be seen. Each modality *separately* has been proven effective. If and why they are more or less effective in combination has yet to be reported. Electrical stimulation causes muscles to *contract,* whereas ultrasound is an effective muscle *relaxant.* Can both be effective if administered simultaneously? An electrical stimulation treatment takes about 20 minutes or more; ultrasound, only 2 to 5 minutes. It is difficult to conceive of either achieving its goal in the differential time allotments. Some have suggested the combination is best accomplished with "pulsing" the ultrasound (ie, automatically having the energy "on" and "off") about 60 times per second so that a longer treatment time may be given without unwanted heat buildup. If and when indicated or requested, several units are available that can offer this combined modality, and the request should not be based upon a trade name.

RADIATION

Electromagnetic radiation as it is emitted by the sun provides a wide array of frequencies/wavelengths for the physical therapist. Each band within the spectrum has specific physiological effects when utilized for therapeutic purposes. Three of these bands are of interest to the practitioner, although a fourth—the visible spectrum (7700 to 3900 Å)—is constantly around and is involved with all three. (Current literature uses the nanometer unit in place of the traditional angstrom unit with an adjustment of one decimal place, so that the visible spectrum is 770 to 390 nm). Infrared, ultraviolet, and the cold laser make up the full span of therapeutic radiation currently used in physical therapy. The infrared and ultraviolet bands bracket the familiar ROYGBIV (red, orange, yellow, green, blue, indigo, and violet) color separation of the visible spectrum. The cold laser used in physical therapy utilizes a helium-neon source whose spectrum lies within the red section of the visible band at 632.8 nm. Infrared lasers whose spectrum is at 904 nm (well within the infrared band of 770 nm and approximately 12,010 nm) are also available to clinicians.

INFRARED

Just beyond the red end of the visible band is the infrared spectrum. Radiation in this region is absorbed by the body as heat. The absorption level is thought to be at approximately 3 mm, at which depth superficial nerve endings and small capillaries benefit from the thermal effects of the radiation. Blood vessels carry the absorbed heat into the general circulation, which accounts for the rise in temperature with exposure to infrared radiation. All of the physiological benefits from the heat are found with infrared, including (1) temperature rise; (2) increased circulation; (3) vasodilation; (4) mild analgesia; (5) increased phagocytosis; (6) increased metabolic processes; and (7) increased permeability of tissue membranes.

The hyperemia produced by infrared radiation is transient, diffuse often described as "mottled," and disappears within 30 to 45 minutes following exposure. Infrared is indicated whenever mild, superficial heating is required for any of the physiological reasons mentioned previously.

The contraindications are few and include the following: (1) presence or danger of hemorrhage; (2) desensitized areas; (3) acute inflammation; and (4) certain dermatological inflammatory conditions.

Infrared is available to the clinician in two main forms: luminous and nonluminous sources. Luminous sources are the familiar conical bulbs, which are adaptable to most standard electrical sockets. These are found in white, amber, or red depending upon the manufacturer. The slight difference in wavelengths is insignificant and does not readily affect the efficiency of these bulbs. (My preference has always been for the red because that is the closest in spectral position to the actual infrared band.) These bulbs may be used with a variety of reflectors for clinical convenience (Fig. 46-12).

The nonluminous sources include bimetallic burners or coiled wires similar to household toasters. Although these glow when heated to functional capacity, they are still considered nonluminous. An example of traditional non-

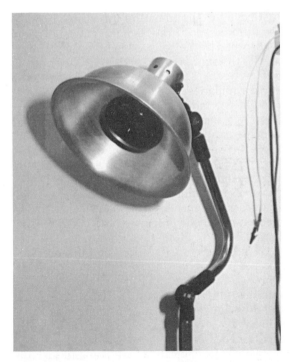

Figure 46-12. The typical infrared lamp contains a 250 W ruby-red luminous bulb in the reflector.

luminous heating would be a household radiator or an ordinary heating pad. The larger, clinical lamps with bimetallic burners produce great, but invisible, heat and should be monitored at all times.

Radiation in the infrared band is subject to the laws of radiation physics (ie, inverse square and cosine laws). Dosages and techniques of administration are based upon these guidelines. The inverse square law states that the intensity of radiation varies inversely with the square of the distance from the source ($I = 1/d^2$). An example would be the *ninefold decrease* in intensity when the distance is *increased by one third*. Conversely, if the distance were *decreased*, the intensity would *increase* as the square of the distance.

The cosine law states that the intensity of radiation will fall off relative to the angle at which the radiation strikes the surface of the target. Maximum intensity will be found with the angle of incidence at 90 degrees (perpendicular) with decreases proportional to the cosine of the angle of incidence ($I = \cos A$).

Treatment techniques usually indicate distances of 24 to 36 inches from the skin for 10 to 30 minutes. Some caution is advised for the eyes because the heat may dry out the normally moist film over the eyes. However, no danger of corneal damage exists as it does with ultraviolet or laser. Infrared is often used as an adjunct to other modalities during treatment sessions.

ULTRAVIOLET

At the opposite end of the visible spectrum, the ultraviolet wavelengths range from 390 nm down to approximately 15 nm. Like infrared, this band is invisible. However, unlike infrared, ultraviolet has a profound physiological effect upon body tissues. Absorbed at less than 1 mm in depth, the *chemical* effects of these wavelengths are therapeutically valuable. Steroid metabolism has long been known to be stimulated by ultraviolet radiation; vasomotor responses have been enhanced; bacteriocidal qualities have been noted; and an anti-rachitic effect has been traditionally assigned to these wavelengths (Wadsworth).

The absorption levels range from 0.3 mm to 0.5 mm in the far band (ie, 290 to 180 nm) and from 0.1 mm to 0.3 mm in the near band (ie, 400 to 290 nm). (Far and near bands are so termed according to their position relative to the visible spectrum.)

The physiological effects vary with wavelengths and include the following: 250 to 300 nm, erythema; 300 to 400 nm, pigmentation changes; 240 to 300 nm, anti-rachitic; and 360 to 390 nm are used with photosensitizing medication in the PUVA technique of ultraviolet radiation for psoriasis (PUVA stands for *p*hotosensitization with *u*ltraviolet in the *A* band, 360 to 390 nm).

The degree of erythema depends upon several factors: (1) patient sensitivity; (2) intensity of radiation; (3) distance from radiation source; (4) angulation of radiation; (5) duration of exposure; and (6) skin texture, with flexor surfaces more sensitive than extensor surfaces, and blonds and redheads more sensitive than brunettes. Children should receive half-dosages.

The erythema produced by ultraviolet radiation is totally different from that produced by infrared. The effect of infrared is purely *physical*, whereas the ultraviolet erythema is actually a *chemical* change in the tissues and is therefore more profound, longer lasting, and therapeutically advantageous.

Ultraviolet radiation is indicated in the following: (1) dermatological conditions, including alopecia, dermatitis, furunculosis, herpes zoster and simplex, impetigo, lupus vulgaris, pityriasis rosea, ringworm, and acne; (2) calcium-phosphorous diseases; (3) some forms of nonpulmonary tuberculosis; (4) some upper respiratory manifestations; (5) osteomyelitis; and (6) more commonly local ulcerations and open lesions.

Probably one of the most common targets for ultraviolet radiation is psoriasis (Fig. 46-13). Traditional regimens call for application of a crude coal tar ointment prior to radiation. Known as the Göeckerman technique, this procedure is still favored by clinicians especially in Europe. More recently clinical trials with ordinary white petrolatum instead of the coal tar preparation have proven to be at least as effective as the coal tar without the odor and expense associated with the tar (Kahn, 1985).

PUVA, as mentioned previously, utilizes the special wavelengths in the 360 to 390 nm band ("black light"). Ordinarily, the human body will not absorb this band even though these wavelengths are extremely effective in the management of psoriasis. Therefore, a photosensitizing agent is ingested before exposure to enhance absorption and utilization of this radiation. Patients are warned to avoid exposure to sunlight for several hours after ingest-

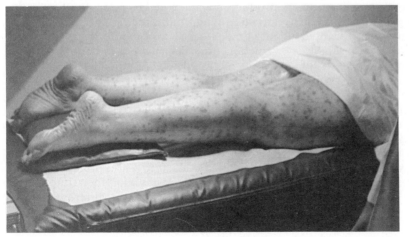

Figure 46-13. Ultraviolet radiation administered for psoriasis.

ing the medication, similar to the precautions for acne preparations using similar photosensitizing agents. Exposures with the PUVA procedure are much shorter than with standard ultraviolet radiation and are measured in seconds rather than minutes in most cases. Monitoring of the patient's blood chemistry is also advised, because the ingested agents have been known to cause blood changes. Consultation with the attending dermatologist is necessary with all patients undergoing PUVA procedure.

The contraindications to ultraviolet radiation are (1) active pulmonary tuberculosis; (2) severe cardiac involvements; (3) lupus erythematosus; (4) acute diabetes; and (5) skin disturbances in the acute phases.

Because the cornea absorbs all wavelengths beyond 295 nm, special care should be taken when radiating in the vicinity of the eyes. The eyes should be covered at all times. Treatments must be timed to the second. The physical therapist should not leave the room during exposure and should wear protective goggles to avoid reflected radiation from walls, sheets, and the like.

Determining ultraviolet dosages usually involves obtaining the minimal erythemal dosage (MED) for each patient prior to the institution of regular treatments. The MED represents the minimal exposure with only a faint "pinking" of the target tissues 24 hours following exposure. Test strips for MED determination may be made from ordinary cardboard or other common opaque materials, with openings for selected exposures of varying durations while shielding the rest of the patient from unwanted exposure. Exposures may begin with 30 seconds and may be increased by five seconds for each subsequent exposure until the proper MED is determined for the patient. The MED is then used as a basis for future treatments with 5- to 10-second increments each visit. Traditional "sunburn" dosages should be avoided to prevent unwanted peeling over target zones. Newly denuded skin will necessitate a redetermination of the MED. Increments should be discontinued in the event of sunburn or peeling or both.

When treating conditions involving systemic manifestations (eg, psoriasis), it is strongly recommended to use *total body exposure* to obtain maximum absorption even though lesions may appear in localized areas. To manage equal exposures for the total body surface, the patient may be treated in four stages with equal dosages: upper back, lower posterior extremities, upper chest and face, and lower anterior extremities. When "quartering" the patient, as just indicated, the untreated areas must be draped with sheets. Prominent landmarks on the anterior surfaces (breasts, ribs, protruding abdomen, anterior iliac spines) should be protected with white petrolatum or mineral oil as needed. The dosages for ultraviolet radiation administration include suberythemal dosages (SED), minimal erythemal dosages (MED), first degree erythemal dosages (1ED), second degree erythemal dosages (2ED), and third degree erythemal dosages (3ED). SEDs are suggested with the PUVA technique. These dosages may be administered daily if indicated.

MEDs were explained previously. These dosages may be administered daily or every other day. 1EDs produce a typical "sunburn" with itching and some exfoliation (peeling). These dosages may be administered two to three days apart. 2EDs produce a more pronounced burning, peeling, and discomfort. These dosages may be administered two weeks apart. 3EDs are administered only locally and produce edema and blistering for tissue destruction when indicated. A specialized apparatus that is used for open lesions, tissue destruction, and the like emits radiation in the far bands for intensified erythemas. These Kromeyer lamps are compact portable units, which are air or liquid cooled and have orificial attachments for penetrating wounds and mucous membrane targets. This type of radiation is also used to irradiate blood in specialized equipment. These units often have detachable filters available for the 350 to 400 nm band (Wood's light), which are useful for their fluorescent effect on microorganisms in differential diagnosis in dermatology.

Phototherapy is a procedure involving ultraviolet radiation in small dosages and limited wavelengths for newborn nurseries to aid in the prevention of jaundice in neonatal infants. Although physical therapists are not directly involved with this procedure, it is prudent for clinicians to be aware of and familiar with the rationale for this application of ultraviolet radiation. The distance from lamp to patient should be about 30 to 36 inches, with the lamp at a 90-degree angle to the surface to obtain maximum intensity, as per the cosine law.

Ultraviolet equipment is usually classified as either "hot" quartz or "cold" quartz (Fig. 46-14). The hot quartz lamps produce ultraviolet radiation through vaporization of mercury in a quartz tube. Incidental heat is produced simultaneously, which, although not therapeutic, is sufficient to warrant care by the clinician regarding contact burns. Cold quartz lamps obtain ultraviolet radiation in a similar way. However, the tubing is coiled helically, is narrower, and does not produce as much heat, probably as a result of the cooling effect of circulating air between the tubing coils. The main difference is the range of wavelengths with each. Hot quartz lamps *generally* emit ultraviolet radiation in a wide spectrum, often from 180

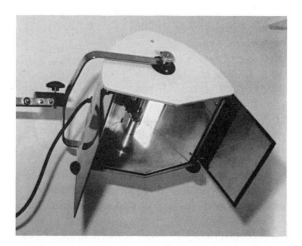

Figure 46-14. Traditional clinical hot quartz ultraviolet lamp with the "barn doors" open for treatment.

nm through 400 nm, rivaling the sun. In this manner both bands B and A are available. (The B band is the spectrum minus the 360 to 390 nm section.) Cold quartz lamps generally emit radiation in the shorter, far band, and tend to produce a more intense erythema. Both types of lamps or tubes should be cleaned periodically with carbon tetrachloride to prevent filtration of therapeutic radiation by dirt, dust, and grease. Both types of lamps should be thoroughly preheated prior to treatment.

COLD LASER

Laser is literally *l*ight *a*mplification by *s*timulated *e*mission of *r*adiation. Although cold lasers are available in the 904-nm band (infrared), this section will be concerned only with the helium-neon cold laser in the 632.8-nm band.

A mixture of helium and neon gases is stimulated electrically to emit radiation in the 632.8-nm band. This radiation is transmitted along an optic fiber to a probe tip, where it is administered to the target tissues. This mechanical phase is the practical demonstration of the physical phenomena associated with incandescent substances emitting characteristic, identifiable radiation. This procedure is useful in astronomy and astrophysics, enabling scientists in both fields to identify chemical properties of materials at great distances or at submicroscopic sizes.

Laser light is completely different from ordinary light. Three characteristic qualities differentiate laser light from ordinary light.

1. *Monochromaticity.* All radiation emitted from the HeNe mixture is in the same spectral band of 632.8 nm. Ordinary light is composed of all wavelengths from 390 nm through 770 nm, the visible spectrum of red, orange, yellow, green, blue, indigo, and violet (ROYGBIV).
2. *Coherence.* All radiation from a single laser source has identical waveforms. This phenomenon leads to reinforcement and amplification because of the conformity of troughs and crests. Ordinary light consists

of a conglomeration of multiple waveforms of the various wavelengths in the visible spectrum.

3. *Nondivergence.* Laser emissions are unidirectional, with negligible divergence even at great distances. An ordinary light source emits radiation in all directions.

These three characteristics make laser light different from all other light. It is not usually accepted that light has power, but it does, although minimal. The laser, because of the amplification, is considerably more intense than ordinary light. Current models of the cold laser are rated at 1 mW, which is about the same intensity as a 60-W household light bulb held several inches from the skin. When administered in the pulsed mode, some of the available power is lost, and the laser operates at approximately 50% efficiency, or at 0.5 mW. Units with 5 mW of available power are being considered for clinical use.

Research has indicated that the 632.8-nm wavelength is ideal for therapeutic purposes because of its unique quality of penetrating the cell membrane. Stimulation is to the *intracellular* components (eg, mitochondria) responsible for metabolic changes. RNA, DNA, and other substances vital to growth and repair have been cited in the literature as being involved with laser radiation at that level.

The physiological effects of the HeNe 632.8-nm cold laser are some minimal heating and local dehydration, both of which are reversible. Overdosage may lead to protein coagulation, thermolysis, and evaporation, none of which should occur with prescribed dosages and recommended techniques.

Currently, the primary use of the cold laser is to enhance healing of open lesions (Fig. 46-15). Administration of the cold laser to open wounds, ulcerations, decubiti, and incisions has proven successful. References appeared in the professional literature at the early stage of development of this modality (Kleinkort, 1982).

Exposure of only 90 seconds per square centimeter of wound surface is apparently an

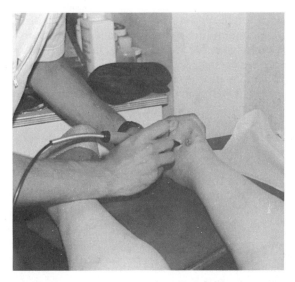

Figure 46-15. Helium/neon (632.8 nm) cold laser is administered to an open lesion on the foot to enhance healing.

optimal dosage (Kleinkort, 1982; Kahn, 1985, 1987). Administration is three times weekly or even daily if indicated with the probe tip 1 to 2 mm from the surface. A new lesion will require the beam in a continuous mode, whereas chronic wounds may respond better to a pulsed mode of 10 to 20 pps. A possible justification of this protocol may be the same rationale as with TENS in the slow-rate mode, in that production of endorphins and other chemicals are enhanced to a greater extent than with high-rate modes. My clinical experience with this procedure has shown moderate-to-excellent success with most lesions, with the exception of the lesion where active infection is present. Pus and drainage apparently preclude laser intervention, much the same as with electrical stimulation for nonunited fractures (see discussion of TENS).

When used for pain management, the cold laser simply becomes another stimulating modality at precise points on the body: trigger points; nerve roots; acupuncture points; and pain sites.

For pain control techniques, the probe tip

is in direct contact with the target point(s). Recommended dosage is 15 to 30 seconds per point. For acute pain, the laser should be in the continuous or high-rate mode (80 pps). For chronic conditions, a lower rate is suggested (10 to 20 pps). Six to eight points usually are sufficient to provide rapid relief. The duration of analgesia varies with individual patients, from several minutes to several hours.

Because light does have power and can stimulate tissues, it becomes another noninvasive alternative to narcotic dependency for analgesia. Additional physiological benefits from the cold laser are being studied, and include paresthesia modification, circulatory enhancement, increasing ranges of motion, and dental applications.

No reported side-effects or untoward reactions to the cold laser have been reported. *Direct lasing of the eye is contraindicated.* The traditional precautions for pregnancy, cardiac involvement, and small children apply to the cold laser as with all other modalities. Clinicians must also ascertain that patients are *not* ingesting photosensitizing medication for any condition (related to the target condition or not), because this could seriously affect the results and may possibly lead to overabsorption.

ANNOTATED BIBLIOGRAPHY

Abramowitsch D, Neousskine B: Treatment by Iontophoresis. New York, Grune & Stratton, 1946 (Unfortunately out of print, this is the best of the earlier monographs on iontophoresis, including history and technical data.)

Alon G: High Voltage Stimulation. Chattanooga, TN, Chattanooga Corp, 1984 (A comprehensive approach to electrical stimulation, emphasizing high-voltage galvanic parameters and applications.)

Benton LA, Baker LL, Bowman BR et al: Functional Electrical Stimulation. Downey, CA, Rancho Los Amigos Hospital, 1980 (Well-illustrated manual of clinically applied electrical stimulation, with several contributing authors.)

Griffin J: Physiological effects of ultrasonic energy as it is used clinically. JAPTA 46(1): 18, 1966 (A comprehensive report on therapeutic ultrasound as it was known at that time.)

Jones R: Research Reports (England). Neurotech Corp, 85 Flagship Dr, Suite A, N Andover, MA 01845 (Fascinating studies involving the alteration of fiber properties by differential frequency stimulation.)

Kahn J: Clinical Electrotherapy, 4th ed. Syosset, NY, Joseph Kahn, 1985 (A popular clinical manual for electrotherapeutic modalities; for students and practitioners.)

Kahn J: Principles and Practice of Electrotherapy. New York, Churchill Livingstone, 1987 (A new text covering the physics and techniques of all electrical modalities discussed in this chapter.)

Karselis T: Descriptive Medical Electronics and Instrumentation. Charles B Slack, Thorofare, NJ, 1973 (An excellent technical reference covering the basic electrophysics of clinical modalities.)

Kleinkort J, Foley RA: Laser Clinical Management 2(4):30, 1982 (One of the early American articles outlining the characteristics and clinical aspects of the cold laser.)

Kleinkort J, Wood F: Phonophoresis with 1% vs 10% hydrocortisone. Phys Ther 55:1320, 1975 (An interesting report offering clinical evidence of effective introduction of hydrocortisone by phonophoresis.)

Mannheimer J, Lampe G: TENS. Philadelphia, FA Davis, 1984 (A comprehensive volume covering the background, technical aspects, and clinical applications of TENS.)

Melzack R, Wall PD: Pain mechanisms: A new theory. Science 150:971, Nov. 1965 (A 20th century classic on pain theory that generated research on pain measurement and treatment.)

Shriber WJ: A Manual of Electrotherapy, 4th ed. Philadelphia, Lea & Febiger, 1981 (A traditional electrotherapy course text with minimal clinical coverage, but good for basics.)

US Dept of Health and Human Services: Assessment Report Series. Rockville, MD, Shortwave Diathermy, 1:16, 1981 (An overall presentation of higher-frequency modalities from the viewpoints of regulations, standards, and administration.)

US Dept of Health and Human Services: The Ultrasonic Equipment Standard. Rockville, MD, HHS Publication FDA 85-8240, July 1985 (An excellent publication describing and discussing ultrasound as a physical therapy modality.)

Wadsworth H, Chanmugam A: Electrophysical Agents in Physiotherapy. New South Wales, Australia, Science Press, 1980 (A general electrotherapy text, with unusually good coverage of the infrared and ultraviolet modalities.)

47 Mechanical Agents: Traction

H. DUANE SAUNDERS

The various types of spinal traction and their effects, indications and contraindications for use, and effective spinal traction techniques will be discussed in this chapter.

When used appropriately and correctly, traction is claimed by numerous authors to be an effective and beneficial method of treatment (Cyriax; Gupta and Ramarao; Harris; Hood and Chrisman; Judovich, 1952, 1955).

EFFECTS OF SPINAL TRACTION

Correctly performed, spinal traction can produce many positive effects. Among these are distraction or separation of the vertebral bodies, a combination of distraction and gliding of the facet joints, tensing of ligamentous structures of the spinal segment, widening of the intervertebral foramen, straightening of spinal curves, and stretching of the spinal musculature.

The relative degree of flexion or extension of the spine during traction determines which of these effects is most pronounced. For example, greater separation of the intervertebral foramen is accomplished with the spine in a flexed position during traction treatment, whereas greater separation of the disk space is achieved with the spine in a neutral position.

Figures and portions of the text are copied with permission from Saunders HD: Evaluation, Treatment and Prevention of Musculoskeletal Disorders, New edition. Minneapolis, Educational Opportunities, 1985.

TYPES OF SPINAL TRACTION

CONTINUOUS TRACTION

Continuous spinal traction can be applied for as long as several hours at a time. This extensive duration requires that only small amounts of weight be used, since the patient's skin cannot tolerate prolonged traction at high poundages. Thus, it is generally accepted that, when applied to the lumbar spine, this form of traction is ineffective in achieving separation of the vertebrae (Judovich, 1955).

SUSTAINED (STATIC) MECHANICAL TRACTION

Sustained traction involves application of a constant amount of traction for periods varying from a few minutes to one-half hour. The shorter duration is usually coupled with heavier weight. Sustained lumbar traction is most effective if a split table is used to reduce friction. The traction source can be either hanging weights or a mechanical device specially made to produce the traction force. Mechanical devices must maintain constant tension. In other words, as the patient relaxes during treatment, the desired amount of traction must be maintained automatically to compensate for the slack that develops. This method is most widely used in Europe, and much of the European literature describes various applications of sustained traction.

INTERMITTENT MECHANICAL TRACTION

Intermittent traction utilizes a mechanical device that alternately applies and releases traction every few seconds. When applied to the lumbar area, a split table is utilized to reduce friction. This is probably the most popular form of traction currently used in the United States.

MANUAL TRACTION

In this technique, the therapist grasps the patient and manually applies a traction force. Manual traction is usually applied for a few seconds, but it can be applied as a sudden, quick thrust. This hands-on traction allows the therapist literally to feel the patient's reaction. Sometimes it is more difficult for the patient to relax during manual traction than during mechanical traction because the exact amount of force that will be applied cannot be anticipated.

POSITIONAL TRACTION

The patient is placed in various positions, using pillows, blocks, or sandbags to effect a longitudinal pull on the spinal structures. Positional traction usually incorporates lateral bending and only one side of the spinal segment is affected.

AUTOTRACTION (LUMBAR)

A special traction bench composed of two sections that can be individually angled and rotated is used with autotraction. Patients apply the traction by pulling with their own arms, and they can alter the direction of the traction as treatment progresses. Treatment sessions can last one hour or longer and are supervised by a clinician (Natchev).

GRAVITY LUMBAR TRACTION

With gravity lumbar traction, the lower border and the circumference of the rib cage are anchored by a specially made vest secured to the top of the bed. The patient is placed on a circular bed or specially made table that is tilted into a vertical or nearly vertical position. In this position the free weight of the legs and hips (about 40% of the body weight) exerts a traction force on the lumbar spine by gravity (Burton).

Two other types of gravity traction have become very popular recently through commercial efforts. One technique utilizes special boots that attach to the subject's ankles. The patient is then able to suspend himself from a frame into a fully inverted position. The other technique involves a device in which the patient is supported on the anterior thighs and is able to hang inverted in a hip and knee flexed position. Both techniques will achieve a traction force of approximately 50% of the total body weight on the lumbar spine. An excellent study by Kane showed significant separation of both the anterior and posterior margins of the lumbar vertebral bodies at all levels as well as increased dimension of the intervertebral foramina using the inversion boot method. However, these techniques are not without some risks (Kane).

INDICATIONS FOR SPINAL TRACTION

HERNIATED NUCLEUS PULPOSUS WITH DISK PROTRUSION

Spinal traction is indicated for the treatment of herniated nucleus pulposus (HNP) with disk protrusion (Cyriax; Gupta and Ramarao; Hood and Chrisman; Judovich, 1952, 1955; Parsons and Cummings). Evidence exists that a disk protrusion can indeed be reduced and spinal nerve root compression symptoms relieved with the application of spinal traction. Using epidurography, Mathews studied patients thought to have lumbar disk protrusion. By applying sustained traction forces of 120 pounds for 20 minutes, he showed that the protrusions were flattened and that the contrast material was drawn into the disk spaces. He also found recurrence of the bulging defects (Mathews). Gupta and Ramarao also used epidurography to demonstrate reductions of lumbar disk protrusions in 11 of 14 patients treated with 60 to 80 pounds of weight. The weight was applied for intermittent periods every three to four hours for 10 to 15 days. They also found definite clinical improvement in those patients in whom defects were reduced (Gupta and Ramarao). Studies such as these show that traction can indeed separate lumbar vertebrae and lead to decreased pressure at the disk space with a resulting suction force. In addition, material can be drawn from the epidural space into the disk space. Similarly, it may be concluded that any anatomical correction produced is unstable. Thus, if patients are not carefully treated with a total management regimen, traction alone is not likely to be successful.

As with all conservative treatment approaches for disk protrusion, patient education and a gradual, cautious return to activities are necessary if the traction is to be successful. Patients may need the support of a lumbosacral corset or a modified Taylor or chairback brace. Extension principles also are often important in helping to reduce herniation and to maintain the correction once it has been achieved. Positions and activities that increase intradiscal pressure (eg, forward bending and sitting in lumbar flexion) should be avoided.

DEGENERATIVE DISK JOINT DISEASE

The argument is often raised that, although traction can cause separation and widening of the intervertebral foramen and intervertebral disk space, the effect will only be temporary. It is true that the separation shown on x-ray films will disappear at least partially soon after traction has been discontinued. If traction is applied to a patient with a narrowed intervertebral foramen or one who has osteophyte or ligamentous encroachment, the disk space and intervertebral foramen will not be restored to their original size and structure. The relief experienced by these patients after the traction treatment must be explained from another basis. Many persons have osteophytes and/or

narrowing of the disk space and intervertebral foramen without signs and symptoms of spinal nerve root impingement. Often, patients in whom the degenerative changes have obviously been present for some time will have a sudden onset of symptoms related to a certain activity or position. A very fine line must exist between cases in which encroachment on the spinal nerve root occurs and those cases in which it does not occur. The traction treatment must, in some manner, move, separate, or realign the segment in such a way as to relieve the impingement.

JOINT STIFFNESS/HYPOMOBILITY

Traction may be regarded as a form of mobilization because it involves the passive movement of joints by mechanical or manual means. Any condition of joint dysfunction (joint hypomobility) may respond favorably to traction. One argument against using traction for mobilization is that it is nonspecific and simultaneously affects several joints. However, when traction is applied to a series of spinal segments, each segment in that series receives an equal amount of traction. If that amount is sufficient to mobilize the segment, it is irrelevant that other segments are also receiving the same amount of traction unless, of course, traction is contraindicated for those other segments. If this is the case, a more specific technique of joint mobilization should be selected.

CONTRAINDICATIONS FOR SPINAL TRACTION

Traction is contraindicated in structural disease secondary to tumor or infection, in patients with vascular compromise, and in any condition for which movement is contraindicated.

Precautions for traction include conditions such as acute strains, sprains, and inflammation that would be aggravated by traction. Traction applied to patients with joint instability of the spine may cause further strain. Other relative contraindications may include pregnancy, osteoporosis, hiatal hernia, and claustrophobia.

MECHANICAL LUMBAR TRACTION TECHNIQUE

The following points are essential to the administration of therapeutically effective lumbar traction.

1. The traction force must be great enough to effect a structural change (movement) at the spinal segment. Judovich advocated a force equal to one-half of the patient's body weight on a friction-free surface as a minimum necessary for producing therapeutic effects in the lumbar spine (Judovich, 1955).
2. A split table is necessary to eliminate friction.
3. Patients must be able to relax.
4. The use of a heavy duty, non-slip traction harness is essential. If patients do not feel secure, they will almost certainly remain tense during treatment. An effective one-size-fits-all heavy duty lumbar traction harness is illustrated in Figure 47-1. This harness is lined with a vinyl material that causes it to adhere to the patient's skin, thus eliminating the slipping that is common with cotton-lined belts. Both the pelvic and thoracic pads should be placed next to the patient's skin. The pelvic harness should be secured to the patient first. It is properly positioned when the top web belt

crosses approximately at the umbilical level. The thoracic pads should be positioned so that they lie on the lateral-inferior chest wall. The thoracic pads are in proper position when both web belts are below the xiphoid process and are actually positioned and held on the inferior rim of the eighth, ninth, and tenth ribs. When properly positioned, the pelvic and thoracic belts will overlap slightly.
5. All of the slack in the harnesses must be taken up before the split table is released. It is a good idea to begin the treatment with progressively stronger pulls, with the split table in a locked position. After two or three progressions, the split table can be released during a rest phase if intermittent traction is being used. If sustained traction is being used, the table can be released, always avoiding a sudden jerk. This release may be accomplished by holding or blocking the movement of the table top as the mechanism is released, then gradually letting the table separate.
6. The patient position (prone or supine) and the amount of flexion or extension used will depend upon the disorder being treated and the comfort of the patient. In my experience, disk herniation with protrusion is effectively treated with the patient lying prone, with a slightly flattened to normal lordosis. Joint hypomobility and

Figure 47-1. Supine lumbar traction technique with the lumbar spine in a flexed position. Note the heavy-duty, non-slip harness and split, friction-free table.

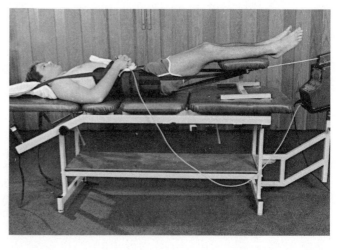

degenerate disk disease are usually treated more effectively with the patient lying supine and the lumbar spine in a straight (flattened) position.

A postural component is often involved with disorders of the lumbar spine. Initially, traction treatments may have to be administered in positions that accommodate the patient's position, but as progress is achieved, the treatment should be given in positions that encourage the return to normal posture. For example, most patients suffering disk herniation with protrusion will have a flattened lumbar lordosis and will be limited in spinal extension. One of the treatment goals will be to return this patient to normal posture. Although it may be impossible to place the patient in a position of normal lordosis initially, the therapist will want to work in that direction as treatment progresses.

When applying lumbar traction in the supine position it is best to remember that it is not necessarily the position of the legs or the rope angle to the table that controls the amount of lumbar flexion. The choice of pelvic harness is probably the most important determinant of the amount of spinal flexion achieved (see Fig. 47-1).

Lumbar traction can be administered effectively in the prone position as well as in the supine position. When using prone traction, the amount of lumbar flexion can be controlled with pillows under the pelvis and, as mentioned above, by using the correct pelvic harness. If the therapist wishes to apply lumbar traction with the spine in normal lordosis, the prone position is probably best. The harness should be positioned with an anterolateral pull. The patient lies flat on the table and the rope angle to the table is varied to control the exact amount of lordosis (Fig. 47-2).

Prone traction can be especially effective for the patient who has moderate to severe pain and muscle guarding. The patient can be positioned prone for modality treatments and the traction can follow without moving the patient. Another advantage of prone traction is that the therapist can palpate the interspinous spaces to ascertain the amount of movement that is taking place during the treatment (Fig. 47-3).

7. The traction mode (sustained or intermittent) selected will depend on the disorder being treated and the comfort of the patient. Disk protrusions are usually treated more effectively with sustained traction or with long hold-rest periods (60 seconds hold, 20 seconds rest) of intermittent traction, whereas joint stiffness and degenerative disk disease usually respond to shorter hold-rest periods of intermittent traction.

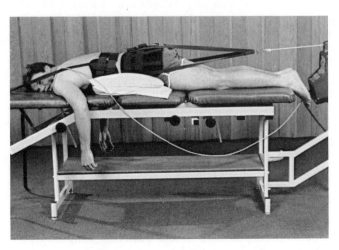

Figure 47-2. Prone lumbar traction technique with a posterolateral pull and a pillow under the hips. This technique allows for prone traction to be done in various degrees of flexion, depending upon the number of pillows used.

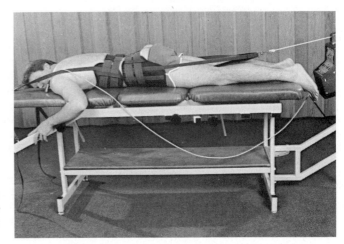

Figure 47-3. Prone lumbar traction with an anterolateral pull. This technique enables the treatment to be given with the lumbar spine in normal lordosis.

8. When disk protrusion is treated with spinal traction, the treatment time should be short. As the disk space is widened, the intradisk pressure is decreased. This anatomical change has a beneficial effect and, at least in my opinion, explains the demonstration by Mathews of movement of contrast medium into the disk space. It seems that this decrease in pressure will be maintained only for a short time, since osmotic forces will soon equalize pressure to that of the surrounding tissue. If equalization does occur, the suction effect on the protrusion is lost. Theoretically, an increase in intradisk pressure with respect to the surrounding tissue might result when the traction is released. Consequently, the patient may experience a sharp increase in pain after treatment. I have not observed this adverse reaction in intermittent treatments of less than 10 minutes and sustained treatments of less than eight minutes. Often, the first treatment is only three to five minutes long.

THREE-DIMENSIONAL LUMBAR TRACTION

Postural changes accompany many of the spinal disorders treated by physical therapists. It is sometimes difficult to determine if the abnormal posture is the result of the pathological disorder, or if the postural change is the cause of the disorder. However, regardless of this relationship, return to normal posture is always one of the treatment goals. For example, the patient with herniated nucleus pulposus with disk protrusion often has a flattened lumbar spine and a lateral scoliosis. One of the goals of treatment should be to return this patient to normal posture. However, this normal posture is not always possible initially in the course of treatment, and attempts to straighten the lateral scoliosis or restore the lordosis often cause an increase in the peripheral signs and symptoms and a general worsening of the condition. When this is the case, traction is often the treatment of choice if it can be administered in such a way that the patient's flexed and laterally shifted posture is not disturbed. As discussed previously, the initial treatment is often given in the prone position with pillows under the lumbar spine to maintain flexion. The harness strap from the convex side of the scoliosis is hooked to the traction source. Thus, the traction treatment is given without disturbing the patient's postural position. On subsequent treatments, the amount of flexion and the amount of unilateral pull are lessened as the patient is gradually worked back into a normal postural position.

A three-dimensional traction table may offer an advantage to this method of treatment in that the table can be positioned initially to accommodate to the patient's abnormal posture; as the traction force is being given, the table can be adjusted gradually to return the patient toward the normal posture. Since three-dimensional traction tables have only been available commercially for a short time, clinical experience with them is limited. I believe that they may offer considerable advantage, especially in the ease and convenience of administering treatment (Fig. 47-4).

CERVICAL TRACTION TECHNIQUE

Many of the comments concerning lumbar traction technique are equally appropriate for cervical traction. In addition, the following points are essential.

1. The first question that should be resolved concerning cervical traction technique is seated versus supine positioning. Although both positions are commonly used, research reveals that the supine position is superior (Harris; Saunders).

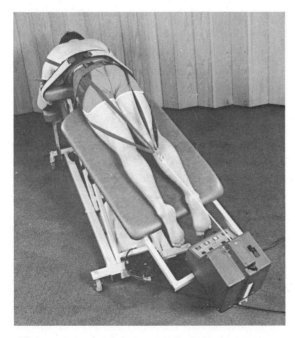

Figure 47-4. Three-dimensional mechanical traction. The table may be positioned initially to accommodate the patient's abnormal posture. As the traction force is being given, the table can be adjusted to correct the patient's posture. Note that the traction device moves with the lower section of the table.

2. The angle of the rope to the table is not the only factor influencing the correct amount of flexion or extension that must be considered. In fact, it is probably less important than the choice of head halters or cervical traction devices. The most satisfactory choices seem to be those that position the head in a neutral position, enabling the pull to be exerted to a greater degree at the occiput than at the chin.
3. Many studies have been made to determine the amount of cervical traction force necessary to cause separation. Consensus is that 20 to 30 pounds is the minimum necessary to achieve separation (Saunders).
4. It is also of interest that some researchers have found compression or narrowing of the joint space with application of cervical traction. This narrowing is often attributed to muscle guarding and to the patient's inability to relax during traction. These findings are most common when patients are seated (Saunders).
5. When receiving traction the patient must feel secure and must be able to relax. The force of the traction must not cause pain to the extent that the patient cannot relax. The use of modalities preceding the traction treatment may be helpful in this regard. Patient comfort should be considered when making a choice between intermittent or sustained cervical traction, since either can be effective.
6. Treatment time should be relatively short (5 to 10 minutes) when treating a herniated nucleus pulposus protrusion. Times can be increased slightly for other conditions. Patient comfort should always be the primary consideration when determining duration of treatment.

THE SAUNDERS CERVICAL TRACTION DEVICE

Conventional cervical traction methods utilize head halters that fit under the chin anteriorly and on the occipital bone posteriorly. A common problem encountered in administering cervical traction is aggravation of the temporomandibular joints because of the force applied

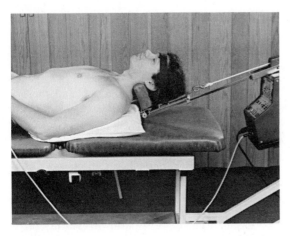

Figure 47-5. The Saunders Cervical Traction Device does not contact the jaw. This eliminates many of the problems associated with conventional cervical traction head halters. (This device is marketed by the Chattanooga Corporation.)

at the chin. The exact amount of force on the chin depends upon the design and adjustment of the head halter, the direction (flexion or extension) of the traction force, and the amount of the traction force. Nevertheless, even when the utmost care is taken to minimize the force on the chin, often sufficient force exists to cause an undesirable effect on the temporomandibular joints.

The cervical traction device shown in Figure 47-5 does not contact the chin or place any force on the temporomandibular joints. The Saunders Cervical Traction Device meets all of the general requirements for application of cervical traction. It can be utilized in the optimal range of head and neck positions with any amount of force and duration (intermittent or sustained.) The most favorable patient position (supine) is used, and no encroachment occurs upon the chin and temporomandibular joints (Saunders).

ANNOTATED BIBLIOGRAPHY

Burton C: Low Back Pain, 2nd ed. Philadelphia, JB Lippincott, 1980 (Discusses gravity lumber reduction traction treatment.)

Cyriax J: The treatment of lumbar disk lesions. Br Med J 2:1434, 1950 (Traction and extension exercises to treat herniated nucleus pulposus.)

Gupta R, Ramarao S: Epidurography in reduction of lumbar disc prolapse by traction. Arch Phys Med Rehabil 59:322, 1978 (Traction and extension exercise designed to treat herniated nucleus pulposus.)

Harris P: Cervical traction: Review of literature and treatment guidelines. Phys Ther 57:910, 1977 (Discusses use of traction to treat cervical disorders.)

Hood L, Chrisman D: Intermittent pelvic traction in the treatment of the ruptured intervertebral disc. J Am Phys Ther Assoc 48:21, 1968 (Case studies on the treatment of herniated nucleus pulposus with lumbar traction.)

Judovich B: Herniated cervical disc. Am J Surg 84:649, 1952 (Traction used to treat cervical disk syndrome.)

Judovich B: Lumbar Traction Therapy. JAMA 159:549, 1955 (Outlines lumbar traction technique.)

Kane M: Effects of gravity-facilitated traction on intervertebral dimensions of the lumbar spine. Master's Thesis. US Army-Baylor University Program in Physical Therapy, Academy of Health Sciences, Fort Sam Houston, Texas, 1983 (Study to determine the effect of inversion traction on lumbar disk space.)

Mathews J: Dynamic discography: A study of lumbar traction. Ann Phys Med 9:275, 1968 (A study showing the effectiveness of traction in reducing lumbar disk protrusion.)

Natchev E: A Manual on Auto-Traction Treatment for Low Back Pain. Stockholm, Natchev, 1984 (Autotraction indications and technique.)

Parsons W, Cummings J: Mechanical traction in the lumbar disc syndrome. Can Med Assoc J 77:7, 1957 (Study discussing the effectiveness of lumbar traction and extension exercises.)

Saunders H: Evaluation, Treatment and Prevention of Musculoskeletal Disorders. Minneapolis, Educational Opportunities, 1985 (Detailed review of indications for lumbar and cervical traction. Description of cervical and lumbar traction techniques.)

48 Mechanical Agents: External Compression

CORINNE ELLINGHAM

Daily activities, good nutrition, and planned exercise are the natural ways of maintaining proper fluid balance in living tissue. The rhythmic action of muscle contraction promotes venous and lymphatic movement in a centripetal direction toward the heart, ensuring healthy tissue. If interruption or damage to the vascular system or other soft tissue should occur, then the delicate balance of proper fluid is altered. The problems that might result are edema, vascular insufficiency, or deep vein thrombosis.

Proven techniques of external compression are an accepted way of preventing or relieving the problems mentioned above that occur when fluid balance in living tissue is affected. Excess fluid contained in the interstitial spaces is normally encouraged to return through the circulatory system but can be assisted by various forms of external compression.

PHYSICAL THERAPY AND THE MANAGEMENT OF EDEMA

Edema may result from inadequate or obstructed lymphatic vessels that may develop after the removal of upper extremity lymph nodes in radical mastectomies or from collapsed malfunctioning lymphatics in the lower extremities. Other causes include varicose veins, venous stasis, leg ulcers, dermatitis, postoperative phlebitis, chronic and acute venous insufficiency, improper fitting of casts, or injury. The degree of involvement may vary from minimal (not disrupting normal functioning) to maximal (interfering with dressing and other everyday activities).

Successful management of edema depends on four critical factors: early diagnosis of the underlying pathology, professional treatment, anticipation and management of complications, and education aimed at the prevention of recurrences (Nelson). Physical therapists have a direct role in the treatment of edema and its complications and in patient education. The physical therapist can also promote appropriate problem recognition and education and can prevent future complications by encouraging physicians routinely to refer patients with lymphedema-associated conditions for early evaluation and treatment.

Treatment goals include reduction of edema and pain, increased range of motion, objective and subjective measurement of change, and patient care. These goals are approached with patient-centered treatment programs that may include any or all of the following modalities: taping, elastic support bandaging, intermittent compression, gradient support, massage, and exercise.

While many treatment centers still advocate a conservative approach, I advocate the successful management of lymphedema with a strong program of precise and continuous evaluation, early and vigorous treatment, and thorough and individualized patient education.

TAPING

Therapeutic taping is applied to splint soft tissue. The success of the taping is dependent upon the judgment of the therapist and the proper application of the bandage.

The two basic considerations for taping pertain to the type of injury and the function of the tape. One must first consider the site and nature of the injury and the circulation in this area before selecting the taping to be applied. Various techniques will have different effects on the tissue. The next consideration requires a determination of the function of the taping. The taping may be designed to protect the part, to prevent or reduce edema, to support the part, to restrict or limit motion, or to provide needed heat.

The principles of good taping techniques include the following:

1. Do not apply directly to the wound.
2. Move from distal to proximal on the extremity.
3. Apply the greatest pressure distally.
4. Leave a small portion of the distal extremity exposed, so that change in skin color and temperature can be monitored. Interference with the circulation is cause for immediate removal and retaping.
5. Do not allow the two skin surfaces to come into contact with each other; place gauze or cotton between the two surfaces for protection.
6. Position the part for function and comfort; the appropriate position of the body or body segment should remain constant throughout the taping session.
7. Apply the tape with even pressure.
8. Wash the area with neutral soap and dry thoroughly, if possible.
9. Protect wounds or abraded areas.
10. Do not leave tape on for extended periods of time (four or five hours).
11. The width of the tape selected depends on the size of the part.
12. If underwrap is needed to protect the skin because of the presence of hair, realize that the strength of the taping procedure is somewhat jeopardized.

ELASTIC SUPPORT BANDAGING

The elastic bandage provides temporary external support. It can be used for short-term prevention or treatment of edema. The support bandage will also facilitate the return of the skin to its normal length.

Two types of elastic bandages are manufactured: the bandage with the rubber-wrapped thread woven longitudinally into it, and the bandage whose elastic properties are solely the result of the twist and weave of the cotton fibers making up the fabric. The rubber-wrapped thread type bandage is most effective in treating edema because it holds its elastic property over time. Elastic bandages come in widths of 2, 3, 4, and 6 inches and are 5, 10, and 15 yards in length, depending on the manufacturer.

The laundering care of the elastic bandage is important. Bandages should be laundered by hand with a neutral soap and rinsed well, using warm water and two or three separate rinses. The bandages are best dried by placing them flat on a bath towel on a level surface. Two methods of bandaging are commonly used, the spiral and the figure-eight wrap. The figure-eight method has been shown to provide more even pressure with significantly less change in volume. The figure-eight method takes a little longer to apply and uses a greater length of bandage, but is more effective in preventing edema, particularly in the lower extremity (Whitmore and colleagues).

INTERMITTENT COMPRESSION

Intermittent compression reduces venous stasis and peripheral edema by applying intermittent pressure to the skin and underlying tissue, thus causing an increase in interstitial pressure and the movement of lymphatic fluid back into the venous system. At the initial evaluation, the patient's history is taken to determine if contraindications (such as congestive heart failure, thrombophlebitis, and pulmonary edema) exist to external compressive therapy.

Next, both extremities, involved and uninvolved, are visually examined and palpated for tissue quality, skin temperature, redness, tenderness, and other signs of complications. If inflammation is suspected, therapy is withheld until the physician is notified and the possible inflammation treated. An edematous extremity will feel firm and the skin will appear stretched and shiny. With treatment the skin should become soft and supple.

Evaluative measurements, taken initially and with each subsequent visit, include the following: serial circumferences, volume, range of motion, muscle strength, sensation, and blood pressure.

At the first visit, serial circumferences are taken of both the involved and uninvolved extremity; thereafter the involved extremity is measured at each visit and the uninvolved periodically.

The upper extremity should be measured at the following sites: metacarpal phalangeal area; wrist; one third of the distance between the wrist and the olecranon process; two thirds of the distance between the wrist and the olecranon process; olecranon process; one third of the distance between the olecranon process and the axilla; and two thirds of the distance between the olecranon process and the axilla. The lower extremity should be measured at the following sites: metatarsal phalangeal area; ankle; one third of the distance between the ankle and the head of the fibula; two thirds of the distance between the ankle and the head of the fibula; head of the fibula; one third of the distance between head of the fibula and the greater trochanter; and two thirds of the distance between the head of the fibula and the greater trochanter.

To ensure consistent circumference measurements, the same therapist should measure the extremity before and after treatment, using a slight indentation of the tissue if tension on the tape is appropriate.

Initially, with external compression therapy, the distal circumferences will decrease and the proximal circumferences will increase. In time, as fluid is pumped from the extremity, the proximal circumferences can also be expected to decrease. Studies show the areas of measurable difference to be greatest in the mid-forearm in the upper extremity and the ankle

and calf in the lower extremity.

Volume is measured by water and air displacement using a clear plastic, graduated cylinder into which the involved extremity will fit. The graduated cylinder is filled with enough tepid water to produce overflow when the extremity is submerged, and the amount of water in the large graduated cylinder is recorded. The patient is positioned beside the graduated cylinder, facing the drain (Fig. 48-1). For upper extremities, the arm is submerged until the third finger touches the bottom. If the extremity is too long for the graduated cylinder, the fingers are flexed and the arm is submerged to the metacarpal phalangeal joints. For lower extremities, the foot should rest flat on the bottom of the cylinder. If the extremity does not reach the bottom, clear plastic blocks are placed in the graduated cylinder until they can be touched. The volume of the extremity is determined by measuring the amount of water displaced from the original amount in the graduated cylinder.

Pressure application begins distally and then slowly spreads up the extremity to encourage the flow of lymph and venous fluids in a centripetal direction. Some intermittent compression units apply equal pressure to the entire area. This external pressure must be greater than the internal hydrostatic pressure exerted by edematous tissues.

Mechanical compression units apply pressure through a pneumatic "sleeve" that is made of washable neoprene/nylon and comes in a variety of lengths for both upper and lower extremities. A sleeve may cover part or all of the extremity. To select the best sleeve for the patient, the length of the involved area and the proximal circumference are measured. The pneumatic sleeve should cover the entire involved area.

The mechanical compression units vary in complexity from lightweight home models designed to treat one extremity to complex institutional models capable of treating four extremities at a time, with each connection pressurized as necessary.

Compression devices for edema use short durations of high pressure and multiple com-

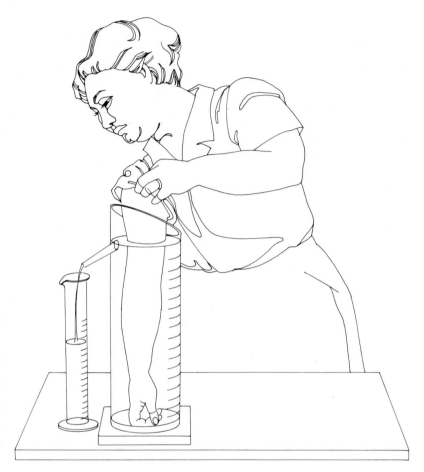

Figure 48-1. A large, clear plastic graduated cylinder used for volumetric measurement of an edematous upper extremity. It is designed with the slope in the back so it fits the contour of the shoulder joint. There should be some overflow when the whole arm is positioned in the cylinder. The principle of water and air displacement is applied in volume measurement.

partment compression. To produce a milking effect on the extremity, the device employs a series of overlapping compartments that apply sequential compression in a centripetal direction. The rationale for multicompartment compression is that of moving pressure from distal to proximal areas. For external compression treatment, the patient is made comfortable, usually in the supine position. Restrictive clothing and jewelry should be removed. The extremity is covered entirely with stockinette to prevent skin abrasion and for hygienic purposes. Then the extremity is elevated to enhance the return of fluid. As illustrated in Figure 48-2, a padded wooden wedge the width of the extremity can be used to support the extremity at a 45-degree angle with the arm and

external appliance in 20 to 70 degrees of abduction. This elevated and abducted position facilitates the removal of fluid and ensures the patient's comfort.

Three variables must be considered when using a compression unit: amount of pressure, cycle of on-to-off, and duration of treatment. If the patient's response to treatment is not satisfactory, it may be necessary to adjust one or more of these variables.

The pressure on all mechanical pumps is calibrated in millimeters of mercury (mm Hg). The amount of pressure used is determined by the patient's blood pressure. The initial setting should be 80 mm Hg, or 20 mm Hg below the patient's systolic pressure. For example, if the patient's blood pressure is 120/80, the initial

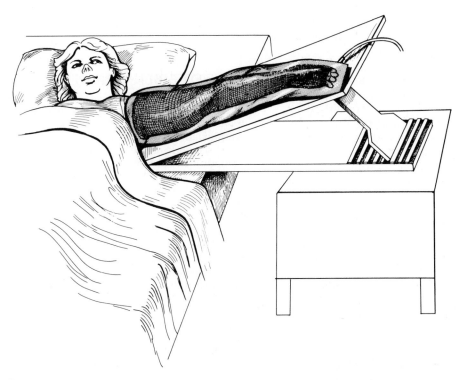

Figure 48-2. A versatile wooden extremity elevator. The elevation can be changed easily to meet the patient's needs. The arm is covered entirely with cotton stockinette, and then the correctly fitted pneumatic appliance is put on. The arm may be positioned either in a neutral or thumb-up position. The wooden elevator and the extremity are positioned in 20 to 70 degrees of abduction and not more than 45 degrees of forward flexion to facilitate the movement of lymphedema from the extremity during external mechanical compression.

pressure setting will be 80 mm Hg and may eventually be increased to 100 mm Hg or 20 mm Hg less than the systolic pressure. To be most effective, the amount of pressure must be equal to or greater than the patient's diastolic pressure. If a unit has multiple compartments, the distal pressure setting is the greatest and the pressure decreases from compartment to compartment proximally along the extremity.

The pressure cycle, if adjustable, should be set so that pressure is "on" longer than it is "off." For a one-minute cycle, the machine should be on for 45 seconds and off for 15 seconds—a 3:1 ratio.

The duration of the initial treatment may be dictated by the patient's tolerance of the pressure and the severity of the edema. Patients with lymphedema may require two to six hours of intermittent compression that may be divided between morning and afternoon.

GRADIENT SUPPORT

Gradient support garments provide compressive therapy when the patient is not receiving intermittent compression. The garments are designed so that support is greatest at the distal end and decreases gradually as the support nears the proximal end of the extremity. The Dacron-core elastic garments are custom-made for the patient's support needs. Elastic net or elastic bandage can be used temporarily until a gradient support garment is available. A figure-eight wrap is recommended (Whitmore and co-workers).

The patient should be fitted for a gradient support garment early in treatment and the garment should fit well. Patients are often fitted for their *first* gradient support garment before the edema has subsided and then are refitted when therapy has achieved its optimal results. If worn on a regular basis, gradient supports will last two to three months.

The patient should be measured for a gradient support garment when the swelling is at the minimum, usually in the morning or after the patient has rested. The manufacturer's directions should be followed. When measuring, the straps or ribs of the measurement tape must run perpendicular to the spine of the tape. Commercial, over-the-counter garments are also available at less cost but are not as satisfactory as custom-fitted garments.

MASSAGE

Massage may be used to reduce hard, nonpliable edema, adhesions in the underlying tissues, or to reduce excessive edema in the hand. The massage technique most often used is effleurage or a gentle stroking in a centripetal direction. Edematous tissue must be massaged with extreme care to avoid stretching, scratching, or bruising the skin. Massage is most effective when used in conjunction with other forms of external compression.

EXERCISE

A combination of isometric exercise and elastic bandaging is an effective way to produce a milking action. Exercise programs must be individualized according to the patient's needs. These programs usually consist of range-of-motion movements, performed in an antigravity position to enhance functional use of the extremity and to enhance venous return.

PATIENT EDUCATION

As appropriate, instructions should be given concerning the management of edema treatment at home, including the care of equipment, hygiene and skin care, antigravity positioning, defined exercises, and reasons for follow-up care.

ANNOTATED BIBLIOGRAPHY

MacCaughey AM: A comprehensive physical therapy program for the postmastectomy lymphedema patient. Literature distributed with scientific exhibit, American Physical Therapy Association Conference, Chicago, June 30–July 5, 1968 (Discusses the formation of lymphedema and the general management as viewed by a physical therapist using a variety of approaches. The pamphlet is well organized and suggests a progressive approach to the problem of lymphedema.)

Nelson, PA: Recent advances in treatment of lymphedema of the extremities. Geriatrics 21:162, 1966 (Details a program of treatment of infection, rehabilitation of the shoulder function, use of elastic sleeve, and skin care. A follow-up study of 223 patients with postmastectomy lymphedema is presented along with the patient's comments and the positive findings for 78% of the patients.)

Richmand DM, O'Donnell TF, Zelikovski A: Sequential pneumatic compression of lymphedema. Arch Surg 120:1116, 1985 (Study of a device that uses a sequential milking pattern of pressure for short duration and high pressure in the treatment of 27 patients. Indications are that the device will reduce lymphedema rapidly and safely.)

Salzman EM, Davies GC: Prophylaxis of venous thromboembolism. Ann Surg 191:207, 1980 (Describes the prophylactic use of low-dose heparin or external pneumatic compression (EPC). Results are positive impression of the effect of using EPC in treating pulmonary embolism as an alternative to using heparin.)

Whitmore JJ, Burt MM et al: Bandaging the lower extremity to control swelling: Figure-8 versus spiral technique. Arch Phys Med Rehab, October, 487, 1972 (Presents the results of treating 10 subjects using three conditions: no wrap, figure-eight wrap, and spiral wrap. Results show the figure-eight wrap was almost twice as effective as the other two approaches. Advantages and disadvantages of the two bandaging methods are discussed in the management of lower extremity edema.)

49 Mechanical Agents: Cardiovascular and Pulmonary Aids

H. STEVEN SADOWSKY

Physical therapists employ many techniques to promote bronchial hygiene, to improve breathing efficiency, and to improve cardiopulmonary reserve. In the acute care setting, patients may be so ill that they have little or no cardiopulmonary reserve and the maintenance of homeostasis can account for almost all of their energy expenditure. To optimize the planning and implementation of therapeutic programs, it is necessary for the physical therapist to have an understanding of the information derived from numerous monitoring and assessment devices or procedures.

Pressure-recording, volume-collecting, or flow-sensing instruments are commonly used to measure the physiological variables that may indicate a patient's level of homeostasis. Such devices consist of some or all of the following basic components: (1) a transducer or device to detect the event; (2) an amplifier to increase the magnitude of the signal from the transducer; and (3) a recording instrument or meter to display the resultant signal. The monitoring equipment used in many acute care or critical care settings relates information about a patient's blood pressures, cardiac electroconductivity, fluid balance, oxygenation status, or metabolic demand. This information, in conjunction with a diagnosis and other pertinent patient information, may be quite useful to the therapist in assessing a patient's responses to a treatment or in choosing a particular intervention.

HEMODYNAMIC MONITORING

ARTERIAL PRESSURES

Arterial blood pressure is the result of the rate of flow of blood (cardiac output) through and against the resistance of the circulatory system (systemic vascular resistance). In the acutely ill patient with cardiopulmonary disease, a low stroke volume and excessive peripheral vasoconstriction may make Korotkoff's sounds impossible to hear. Therefore, rather than a blood pressure cuff, an intra-arterial pressure monitoring device is used to measure systolic, diastolic, and mean pressures.

The systolic blood pressure (the maximum systolic left ventricular pressure) reflects the compliance of the large arteries and the total peripheral resistance. In the normal adult, systolic pressure is usually about 120 mm Hg. However, systolic blood pressure also normally increases with age. The systolic blood pressure should be expected to increase with exertion, normally increasing linearly (7 to 8 mm Hg per metabolic equivalent) as the intensity of activity increases. If the systolic blood pressure falls or fails to increase as the work load increases, one may assume that the functional reserve capacity of the heart has been exceeded. It is also considered unsafe if the systolic blood pressure exceeds 225 to 230 mm Hg. If these situations should develop, activity should be curtailed or terminated.

The diastolic blood pressure is the lowest point of declining pressure resulting from the runoff of blood from the proximal aorta to the peripheral vessels, and reflects the velocity of the runoff and the elasticity of the arterial system. The duration of the diastolic period of the cardiac cycle is directly related to the rate; thus, the longer the period of diastole, the greater the fall of the diastolic pressure. The diastolic blood pressure is normally about 80 mm Hg, though it increases somewhat with the aging process. The diastolic blood pressure does not change much during repetitive, rhythmic activities involving the lower extremities, such as bicycling, walking, or running. However, during upper extremity exercise or isometric exercise involving any muscle group, the diastolic blood pressure normally increases. Nonetheless, activity should be curtailed or halted if the diastolic blood pressure exceeds 130 mm Hg.

The mean arterial pressure (MAP) is the average pressure tending to push blood through the circulatory system. It reflects the tissue perfusion pressure. The mean arterial pressure is closer to the diastolic than the systolic pressure because the duration of diastole is greater than that of systole. The mean arterial pressure is not, therefore, a true arithmetical mean of systolic and diastolic pressures. The normal mean arterial pressure varies from 70 to 110 mm Hg and is useful clinically because it yields one number that relates to cardiac output and the systemic vascular resistance. A mean arterial pressure of less than 60 mm Hg would indicate an inadequate tissue perfusion pressure.

VENOUS PRESSURES

Blood from all the systemic veins returns to the right atrium of the heart, and for this reason the pressure in the right atrium is often called the central venous pressure (CVP). The normal central venous pressure is less than 5 mm Hg. The central venous pressure is measured by means of a catheter introduced percutaneously into one of several suitable veins (internal jugular, subclavian, or medial basilic). The catheter is positioned in the midsuperior vena cava and permits measurement of right atrial pressure. Measurement of the central venous pressure is most useful for monitoring blood volume and the adequacy of central venous return. However, by measuring the oxygen saturation of the blood in the right atrium, reasonable estimates of cardiac output or oxygen consumption may be calculated (more accurate measurement of venous oxygen saturation is obtained from the mixed venous blood in the pulmonary artery).

The flow-directed, balloon-tipped catheter permits acquisition of information regarding pulmonary artery oxygenation and pressures on the right side of the heart. Oxygen samples may be used to assist in the diagnosis of intracardiac shunts or in the calculation of cardiac output or oxygen consumption values. Evaluation of pressures on the right side of the heart permits assessment and diagnosis of the degree of specific chamber or valvular pathologic conditions and indirectly reflects left ventricular function.

The left ventricular end-diastolic pressure (LVEDP) is the primary indicator of left ventricular performance and reflects the compliance of the ventricle. The pressures in the left ventricle and in the left atrium (in the absence of mitral valve pathology) are equal at the end of diastole because the mitral valve is still open. Because no valves exist in the pulmonary venous system, the pressures in the pulmonary veins, pulmonary capillaries, and the pulmonary artery are also equal at the end of diastole. Thus, the pulmonary artery end-diastolic (PAD) pressure is equal to the left ventricular end-diastolic pressure (normally less than 12 mm Hg) in the absence of pathologic conditions. However, when the pulmonary vascular resistance (PVR) is elevated (eg, with pulmonary embolism, hypoxia, chronic lung disease, or other dead-space producing disorders), the pulmonary artery pressure, not the left ventricular end-diastolic pressure, will reflect the high pulmonary vascular resistance. In such situations, the pulmonary capillary wedge pressure (PCWP; normally less than 12 mm Hg) should be monitored. It is important that patients are not engaged in treatment when the catheter is in the "wedge" position because of the potential for pulmonary arterial rupture. Furthermore, the level of the transducer, in relation to the heart, must be kept in mind when interpreting the pressure readings, because the patient's position changes with activity. Table 49-1 summarizes normal pressures for the right and left sides of the heart.

CARDIAC OUTPUT

The amount of blood ejected with each contraction of the heart is called the stroke volume (SV). The amount of blood pumped by the heart per unit time is termed the cardiac output (CO). Unless an intracardiac shunt is present, the output of both the right and left ventricles is essentially the same. The normal resting cardiac output is 4 to 8 L/min and the normal stroke volume ranges from 60 to 130 ml. Cardiac output normally increases as activity increases. However, pathological conditions can greatly affect cardiac output and impinge upon a patient's homeostatic tolerance.

The clinical determination of cardiac output is generally made by the thermodilution method. A cold bolus of saline is injected into the right atrium by means of the proximal lumen of a flow-directed, thermal-sensitive catheter; the resultant temperature change is sensed by a thermistor in the tip of a catheter located in the pulmonary artery. A temperature-time curve is constructed, and the cardiac output is calculated (Forrester). The mean stroke volume is calculated by dividing the cardiac output by the ventricular rate over a specific period of time. Diseases such as an arterial-venous fistula, anoxia, and Paget's disease may ultimately decrease the peripheral vascular resistance and increase cardiac output by means of an increased venous return to the heart. Conversely, conditions that result in decreased blood volume will reduce the venous return to the heart, yielding a decrease in cardiac output.

Unfortunately, simple cardiac output measurements do not take into account an individual patient's specific needs with respect to actual body size. For this reason the cardiac output per square meter of body surface area, the cardiac index, is often reported. The normal cardiac index for adults is approximately 3.0 L/min/m.^{2} A cardiac index less than 2.2 L/min/m^2 is considered diagnostic of cardiogenic shock (Schroeder and Dalie). Cardiogenic shock is a condition in which the blood supply to the tissues of the body is insufficient because of inadequate cardiac output.

ELECTROCARDIOGRAM

The electrocardiogram (ECG) is a graphic representation of the electrical activity of the heart. An electrocardiographic tracing demonstrates depolarization and repolarization of the atria and ventricles, although atrial repolarization is masked by ventricular depolarization.

ECG paper is divided into many squares. Each small square is 1 mm on a side; each larger square is 5 mm on a side (Fig. 49-1). Time is measured on the horizontal plane. Each small square represents 0.04 second in time; each larger square represents 0.2 second in time. Voltage is measured vertically. The ECG machine is calibrated so that 1 mV is equal to two large squares (10 mm). The single vertical lines along the edge of most ECG papers are 3 inches apart, representing 3-second intervals.

Table 49-1. Normal Cardiovascular Pressures

RA$_m$ Pressure*	2–6 mm Hg
RV Pressures	
Systolic	20–30 mm Hg
End-diastolic	<5 mm Hg
PA Pressures	
Systolic	20–30 mm Hg
Diastolic	<12 mmHg
Mean	<20 mm Hg
Mean PCW pressure	4–12 mm Hg
LA$_m$ Pressure*	<12 mm Hg
LV Pressures	
Systolic	<150 mm Hg
End-diastolic	<10 mm Hg
Aortic pressures	
Systolic	<150 mm Hg
Diastolic	<90 mmHg

*Mean values

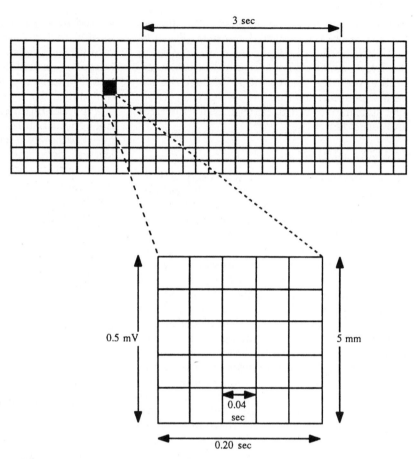

Figure 49-1. ECG paper displays time on the horizontal axis and electrical voltage on the vertical axis.

Electrocardiograms are valuable in the diagnosis of cardiac disease because they permit analysis of disturbances in the electroconductive system of the heart. Specific mechanical events are associated with the electrical changes depicted on an electrocardiogram. However, it cannot always be assumed that a mechanical event results from an electrical event (electromechanical dissociation).

The position of the positive (recording) electrode in relation to the spread of the electrical impulse is referred to as the "lead." By convention, there are 12 electrocardiographic leads: Three standard limb leads, three augmented limb leads, and six precordial leads. The shape of the waveform produced by the electrical activity of the heart is determined by which lead is being monitored. Therefore, al-

though a normal tracing from each lead will have the same basic components, the shape of the tracing is different for each lead. The isoelectric line, or baseline, running the length of the tracing, results when there is no electrical activity or when electrical forces negate each other. An upright deflection on the tracing indicates that the electrical impulse is moving predominantly toward the positive electrode, whereas a downward deflection indicates movement away from the positive electrode. The normal ECG tracing is composed of a P wave, a QRS complex, and a T wave (Fig. 49-2).

The P wave results from the depolarization of the atria. Normally not longer than 0.11 second in duration, the P wave indicates the conduction time for atrial depolarization. In nor-

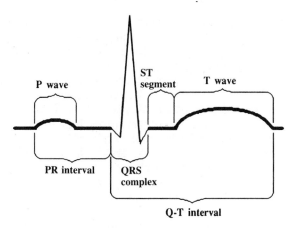

Figure 49-2. The components of a normal ECG tracing. Tracings are normally made at a paper feeding speed of 25 mm/sec.

mal atria, the P wave is not more than 3 mm in height. The PR interval, representing the time from the beginning of atrial activation to the beginning of ventricular activation, results from the depolarization of the atria and the "holding" of the impulse by the atrioventricular node. The PR interval is normally between 0.12 and 0.20 second in duration.

The QRS complex results from the depolarization of the ventricles. The QRS complex normally lasts between 0.06 and 0.10 second, and represents the conduction time for ventricular depolarization. After a P wave, the next upward deflection on the tracing is called an R wave. A downward deflection before the R wave is called a Q wave; a downward deflection after the R wave is called an S wave. In some instances there may be more than one upward deflection on a tracing after the P wave. Additional upward deflections are called R prime waves (R'). If there is no upward deflection at all, the downward deflection is called a QS complex.

The T wave represents the repolarization process in the ventricles. The Q-T interval is indicative of the refractory period of the heart. Although the Q-T interval varies with the heart rate, at normal rates it is less than half the preceding R to R interval. The atrial or ventricular rhythms are said to be regular if the P to P or R

to R intervals are equal (±1 small square), and irregular if they are not. To calculate heart rate, use one of the following formulas.

1. When the rhythm is regular:
   a. Count the number of large squares between two R waves and divide into 300;
   b. Measure the time between two R waves and divide into 60; or
   c. Count the number of small squares between R waves or P waves and divide into 1500.
2. When the rhythm is irregular, count the number of cycles in a six-second strip, and multiply by 10 (Conover).

OXYGEN ADMINISTRATION DEVICES

Physical therapists working with patients with cardiopulmonary disease come into contact with supplemental oxygen delivery systems. The portable systems (eg, cylinders or liquid oxygen canisters that permit oxygen to accompany a patient away from the bedside) will be considered, and not the hospital bulk delivery system that directs oxygen to an outlet at the patient's bedside.

The storage of medical gases in cylinders has been common since the 1890s. When full, the contents of an oxygen cylinder exert about 2200 psi of pressure. Though cylinders vary in size, the physical therapist is most likely to encounter D or E sizes. These cylinders are green, or sometimes green and white, and are labeled "Oxygen." When full, D cylinders contain approximately 356 L of oxygen and E cylinders contain approximately 622 L of oxygen. A valve reduces the high pressures from the gas to a lower working pressure, usually 50 psi. The outlet from the reducing valve is then connected to a flowmeter, which controls and indicates flow.

Portable liquid oxygen systems are in common use outside the hospital setting. The oxygen stored in these systems is under much greater pressure than cylinders, and therefore a liquid oxygen system has a greater capacity with a lower weight. Liquid oxygen systems are similar to cylinders in that they utilize reducing valves and flowmeters, although most have a nipple adapter built in to the valve for direct connection to an oxygen administration device.

The gases used for therapeutic purposes are often stored with all water vapor removed, that is, 100% dry. The lack of humidity could be irritating to the mucosa of the pulmonary passageways. At low flow rates (less than 4 L/min) humidification of the gases may not be necessary. At flow rates of less than 10 L/min simple humidifiers may be used to add sufficient humidity to make the gas comfortable. When the upper airway is bypassed (for example, when the patient has a tracheostomy tube in place or is intubated), the gas must be heated to increase its capacity to carry water vapor. Heated humidifiers are often used when flow rates exceed 10 L/min or when the upper airway is bypassed. Aerosolized water is another means by which medical gases may be humidified. Aerosols are produced by nebulizers, of which there are many types.

Oxygen administration devices include nasal cannulas, masks, tents, hoods, and incubators. The *nasal cannula* is used with low oxygen flow rates between 1 and 6 L/min. A nasal cannula does not permit precise control of the amount of oxygen (referred to as the fraction of inspired oxygen [Fio_2] that is delivered to a patient. Table 49-2 presents approximate inspired oxygen equivalents for nasal cannula flow rates, assuming that the patient's respiratory rate and pattern are normal. Whether a humidifier is used in conjunction with a nasal cannula may depend upon the preference of

the individual physician. However, at flows exceeding 3 L/min the nasal mucosa may become dried and irritated with sustained use of nonhumidified gas.

The delivery of an accurate and consistent Fio_2 requires that the flow of gas be sufficient to exceed the patient's peak inspiratory flow demand, which generally requires higher flow rates than can be tolerably achieved by nasal cannula. Therefore, masks are used. The *simple mask* is designed to provide a flow of gas into a face piece that fits over the patient's nose and mouth. Some simple masks also include a diluter to add room air, and thus increase the total gas flow as the oxygen flows into the mask. Depending on the amount of air added, the oxygen percentages that can be delivered through a simple mask range from 35% to 55% with oxygen flow rates of 6 to 10 L/min (for adults). Several different types of masks are used for administering medical gases. Two dilution-type mask systems frequently encountered in the clinical setting are the *aerosal mask* and the *Venturi mask*. The aerosol mask was originally designed for the administration of aerosols. However, these masks are widely used for the administration of precisely controlled percentages of oxygen with high gas flows. The Venturi mask also delivers a precise percentage of oxygen while providing a greater flow of gas to a patient. Oxygen flow rates for Venturi masks vary depending upon the Fio_2 desired, and these masks may or may not be humidified.

In the pediatric setting, oxygen *tents, hoods,* or *incubators* are frequently used. With tents, the Fio_2 attained depends upon the incoming gas flow, the canopy volume, and the degree to which the tent is sealed. Tents generally envelope the patient's upper torso or entire body. Continuous oxygen monitoring is necessary because patient care requires entering the tent, and therefore alters the Fio_2. Ice reservoirs are often incorporated for temperature control. Oxygen hoods, small plastic enclosures placed over just the patient's head, permit nursing care without hindering oxygen therapy. Incubators are used for similar reasons as tents, but

Table 49-2. Approximate Percent Oxygen with Nasal Cannula at Different Flow Rates

FLOW RATE (L/MIN)	Fio_2
1	0.24
2	0.28
3	0.32
4	0.36
5	0.40

generally warm rather than cool the environment.

INSPIRATORY POSITIVE-PRESSURE DEVICES

This section is an introduction to the concepts and machinery used in the implementation of physical therapy in the respiratory care setting.

By convention, the terms "mechanical ventilation" or "mechanical ventilator" refer to the use of positive-pressure ventilators. Mechanical ventilation may range from the relatively simple intermittent augmentation of a patient's spontaneous inspiratory efforts to the complete control and maintenance of the ventilatory status of an apneic patient.

The intermittent augmentation of a patient's spontaneous inspiratory efforts has for many years been called intermittent positive-pressure breathing (IPPB). Historically, IPPB has a definite connotation, referring to the short-term treatment procedure by which a patient is provided inspiratory positive pressure, usually for the purpose of administering aerosolized medications. The long-term mechanical support of a patient's ventilatory status is often called intermittent positive-pressure ventilation (IPPV). Many machines are commercially available for IPPB or IPPV.

Whether with regard to IPPB or IPPV, the equipment connecting the patient to the machinery is called the *circuit*. The circuit generally consists of tubing and valves that attach either to a mask or mouthpiece, or directly to an endotracheal or tracheostomy tube. In the performance of various bronchial hygiene procedures or simply to facilitate positioning for patient comfort, the circuit may need to be disconnected from the patient. Disconnection may involve the simple removal of a mask or mouthpiece as would be done with the termination of an IPPB treatment or may involve the disengagement of the circuit from an endotracheal or tracheostomy tube in conjunction with hyperoxygenation. This latter effort necessitates stabilization of the endotracheal or tracheostomy tube while the circuit is removed, taking care to assure that the patient is not inadvertently extubated, and then manually ventilating the patient with a resuscitation bag (discussed later).

Mechanical ventilation is frequently associated with a veritable alphabet soup of terms for the description of airway maneuvers used in the augmentation or control of a patient's ventilatory status. These include the following: inspiratory hold, a maneuver in which either the preset pressure or predetermined volume is reached and held for some period of time; positive end-expiratory pressure (PEEP), a threshold-like resistance applied after exhalation, which permits the circuit pressure to drop to a set level above atmospheric pressure; expiratory retard, an orificial resistance applied to exhalation whereby the circuit pressure is permitted to drop slowly to atmospheric as the expiratory gas flow ceases; constant positive airway pressure (CPAP), the application of an elevated baseline pressure (greater than atmospheric) from which a patient spontaneously breathes; controlled ventilation, the provision of positive-pressure breaths at a set rate without patient participation; assist-control ventilation, the provision of positive-pressure breaths at a set rate unless the patient triggers the machine by creating a negative inspiratory force less than the threshold pressure set on the machine, in which case the machine delivers a positive-pressure breath at the rate established by the patient's efforts; intermittent mandatory ventilation (IMV) or synchronized intermittent mandatory ventilation (SIMV), the provision to the patient of a source of gas from which he may spontaneously breathe, while the ventilator intermittently provides positive-pressure breaths that may or may not be synchronized with any spontaneous efforts.

INCENTIVE SPIROMETRY AND INSPIRATORY RESISTANCE DEVICES

Approximately six to nine times an hour, the normal adult takes a deep inhalation, or sigh, that approaches the total lung capacity. In a pattern of shallow breathing, without periodic deep breaths, yawns, or sighs, a gradual alveolar collapse develops. If not corrected or reversed, this collapse can lead to gross atelectasis. Trauma, disease, and surgical procedures all contribute to such abnormal patterns of breathing. For example, a patient may avoid a prolonged inspiratory effort because of incisional pain or muscle weakness. Therefore, prophylactic breathing exercises with sustained maximal inspiratory efforts may be indicated.

The incentive spirometer is designed to provide the patient with visual input while he performs sustained maximal inspiratory maneuvers. It is hoped that this visual input encourages the patient to use the unit and to work toward increasing his maximal inspiratory effort. Although the patient is encouraged to use the incentive spirometer independently, the device should not be placed at the patient's bedside without first providing proper instruction for its use. Several brands of incentive spirometers are commercially available (McPherson).

Physical therapists are unique in their ability to assess and intervene in the rehabilitation of unused muscles. While it is easy to see the atrophy of arm or leg muscles following the removal of a plaster cast and to appreciate that the prolonged disuse of these muscles may predispose them to weakness and rapid fatigue, too often this same association is not made with reference to the respiratory muscles following prolonged mechanical ventilatory support. A fundamental principle of exercise training is to work a muscle to the point of fatigue and then allow it to rest. This principle should be just as applicable to the respiratory muscles of weaning patients as to arm or leg muscles of athletes.

In a study on respiratory muscle strengthening and endurance training, subjects utilized 3 to 5-second maximal inspiratory and expiratory maneuvers at 20% increments over their vital capacity ranges for strength training, and ventilation to exhaustion three to five times daily for endurance training. Strength trainers increased maximal pressures by 55%; endurance trainers increased their ability to sustain hyperpnea from 81% to 96% of their pretraining maximal voluntary ventilation (largest volume that can be breathed per minute by voluntary effort [MVV] while increasing their MVV by 14% (Leith and Bradley). An eight-week regimen of 30 minutes of daily inspiratory resistance training also revealed a 21.5% increase in mean maximal inspiratory force (MIF) (Gross and co-workers).

BEDSIDE PULMONARY FUNCTION AND CLINICAL MONITORING DEVICES

Physical therapy interventions for respiratory patients are designed to promote bronchial hygiene, improve breathing efficiency, or promote physical reconditioning. To this end, the therapists involved may need to perform bedside pulmonary function testing or monitoring to ascertain treatment efficacy. Table 49-3 lists some of the data that may be collected at the bedside using relatively small and portable volume-collecting or flow-sensing devices. Additional tests may be performed at the bedside, but they require more sophisticated equipment. Particularly with respect to weaning from mechanical ventilation, bedside spirometry or pulmonary function testing is indispensable. Several parameters, reflecting oxygenation status, ventilatory mechanics, respiratory muscle strength, and ventilatory demand, may be predictive of weaning success (Pierson; Hodgkin and co-workers).

Table 49-3. Pulmonary Function Data Readily Obtainable at the Bedside

Tidal volume (V_t)
Respiratory frequency (f)
Minute ventilation (V)
Vital capacity (VC), nonforced or timed
Forced vital capacity (FVC)
Forced expiratory volume per unit time (FEV_t)
Peak expiratory flow (PEF)
Maximal inspiratory force (MIF)

Oxygenation may be inferred from several clinically obtainable measurements. An acceptable arterial oxygen saturation (Sao_2) and arterial oxygen pressure (Pao_2) with an $Fio_2 \leq 0.5$ is often cited as a criterion guideline preparatory to weaning attempts, as long as the Pao_2/Fio_2 ratio is greater than 200 mm Hg (Jung). The literature on oxygenation criteria for weaning generally predates the widespread use of positive end-expiratory pressure (PEEP) in the treatment of adult respiratory distress syndrome, but a PEEP ≤ 7.5 cm H_2O is desirable prior to the initiation of weaning.

Ventilatory mechanics are probably best inferred in most cases by the inspiratory capacity (IC). A tidal volume of at least 5 mL/kg and a static system compliance greater than 30 mL/cm H_2O may be predictive of weaning success (Pierson; Jung).

Ability to meet ventilatory demand may be inferred from expiratory minute ventilation ($\dot{V}_E$), dead space to tidal volume ratio (VD/V_t), and CO_2 production ($\dot{V}CO_2$). A $\dot{V}_E$ less than 10 L/min, for a $PaCO_2$ of 40 mm Hg, is one parameter highly predictive of weaning success (Sahn and Lakshminarayan).

Monitoring of the respiratory muscles is important because these are the only skeletal muscles upon which life is dependent, and they deal primarily in terms of elastic and resistive loads. For the respiratory muscles, the force-length and force-velocity relationships are inferred from measurements of pressure (force developed, divided by surface area over which it acts), changes in volume (implying changes in length), and flow rate of volume change (implying velocity). Thus, respiratory muscle strength may be inferred from the maximal inspiratory force, inspiratory capacity or vital capacity, peak flow rate, or forced expiratory volume in one second (FEV_1).

OTHER MECHANICAL DEVICES

Some of the equipment used by the physical therapist in the respiratory care setting is not readily classified into the previously discussed categories. This type of equipment includes mechanical percussors, manual resuscitators, and negative-pressure ventilators.

MECHANICAL PERCUSSORS

The modalities of percussion and vibration, as employed in the performance of a bronchial hygiene regimen, constitute a significant portion of the treatment time. Judiciously applied, these modalities have been shown to augment the mobilization and elimination of excessive secretions. Yet, as many therapists can attest, these techniques can be difficult to learn and can be quite fatiguing if not properly performed. Electrically or pneumatically powered mechanical percussors are commerically available to ameliorate these difficulties. However, the efficacy of these mechanical adjuncts are as highly dependent upon their proper use as the manual techniques. Although it may be true that these devices conserve the therapist's energy, they eliminate an often overlooked and underrated nonverbal communication system between therapist and patient—touch.

MANUAL RESUSCITATORS

In some instances the therapist must disconnect the patient from the mechanical ventilator for a prolonged period of time. In such instances, the patient will require ventilatory assistance with a manual resuscitator. Several manufacturers produce manual resuscitators, and the valve systems are unique to each. Manual resuscitators use self-inflating bags, which, when compressed, deliver a volume of gas to the patient by means of one-way valves (Fig. 49-3). When compressed, gas flow from the bag enters the valve and pushes the diaphragms against the exhalation ports. The flow of gas then opens the inhalation valve, permitting gas to flow to the patient. When flow from the bag ceases and exhalation begins, exhaled gas from the patient pushes the inhalation valve closed and opens the diaphragms, allowing gas to flow out the exhalation ports. The bag intake port may be fitted with an oxygen reservoir system for the delivery of oxygen-enriched breaths.

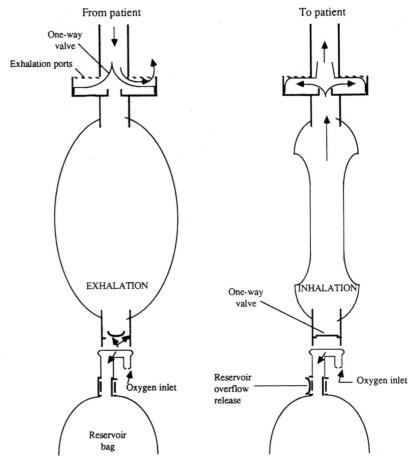

From patient

One-way valve

Exhalation ports

EXHALATION

To patient

INHALATION

One-way valve

Reservoir overflow release

Oxygen inlet

Oxygen inlet

Reservoir bag

Figure 49-3. Schematic representation of a typical manual resuscitation bag showing gas flow and valves on inhalation and exhalation. An oxygen reservoir system may be added to increase the available fraction of inspired oxygen delivered with each breath.

NEGATIVE-PRESSURE VENTILATORS

Finally, mention should be made of a negative-pressure ventilator—the cuirass. Basically, the cuirass is a rigid shell that encloses the patient's anterior thorax so that subatmospheric pressure can be exerted within the shell. A vacuum cleaner-like pump generates the negative pressure. The shells are usually custom made for each patient, although prefabricated shells are available. The cuirass is probably not more widely used because (1) it tends to be noisy, (2) provision of patient care may be hampered, and (3) regulation of inspiratory/expiratory ratios is difficult. However, these units are useful for providing augmentation to spontaneously breathing patients with weakened respiratory musculature. Additionally, ventilatory mechanics are more physiologic than with positive-pressure machines, and many patients do not require a tracheostomy.

ANNOTATED BIBLIOGRAPHY

Conover MB: Understanding Electrocardiography, 3rd ed. St Louis, CV Mosby, 1980 (Provides an introduction to the understanding and interpretation of electrocardiograms.)

Forrester JS: Thermodilution cardiac output determination with a single flow-directed catheter. Am Heart J 83:303, 1972 (Describes the use and benefits of the thermodilution technique used in the clinical determination of cardiac output.)

Gross D, Riley E, Grossino A et al: Influence of resistive training on respiratory muscle strength and endurance in quadriplegia. Am Rev Respir Dis 117:343 (suppl), 1978 (Describes the results of a ventilatory muscle training program for a patient population.)

Leith DE, Bradley M: Ventilatory muscle strength and endurance training. J Appl Physiol 41:508, 1976 (The classic paper describing the use of ventilatory muscle training.)

McPherson SP: Respiratory Therapy Equipment, 3rd ed. St Louis, CV Mosby, 1985 (Describes the equipment used in respiratory care.)

Schroeder JS, Dalie EK: Techniques in Bedside Monitoring, ed 2. St Louis, MO, CV Mosby Co, 1981. (Describes hemodynamic monitoring and its use in the care of critically ill patients.)

The following sources discuss some of the parameters used in determining a patient's suitability for weaning from mechanical ventilatory assistance.

Hodgkin JE, Gray LS, Burton GG: Techniques of ventilator weaning. In Burton GG, Hodgkin JE (eds): Respiratory Care, 2nd ed, pp 648–655. Philadelphia, JB Lippincott, 1984

Jung RC: Weaning criteria for patients on mechanical respiratory assistance. West J Med 131:49, 1979

Pierson DJ: Weaning from mechanical ventilation in acute respiratory failure: Concepts, indications, and techniques. Resp Care 28:646, 1983

Sahn SA, Lakshminarayan S: Bedside criteria for discontinuation of mechanical ventilation. Chest 63:1002, 1973

50 Manual Techniques

GARVICE G. NICHOLSON
RICHARD A. CLENDANIEL

INTRODUCTION

To quote Grieve, some form of manual treatment has been around as long as pain itself. Hippocrates (*ca* 460 to 380 BC) described treatments comparable to our manual techniques of today. He spoke of rubbing and movement and stipulated it must be done gently and in a range that is not painful. Hippocrates' suggestions sound similar to those of Robert Maigne and Geoffrey Maitland, two authorities of manipulative therapy. However, the fact that manual techniques have stood the test of time has not ensured their acceptance throughout the health care delivery system. Unfortunately, such valuable treatments as massage and manipulation have been viewed with skepticism. In the case of massage, its widespread use outside of organized health care has perhaps diluted its reputation for therapeutic value. Although this may also apply to manipulative therapy of the joints, animosity between organized medicine and practitioners of manipulation is perhaps the more likely reason for lack of acceptance.

"Hands-on" methods have been a part of physical therapy since its inception and still occupy a major role in the treatment of pain and movement dysfunction. No substitute exists for skillful and confident handling as a means of reassuring patients that they are in the hands of a caring and capable practitioner. This in and of itself may be a powerful "therapeutic weapon" and when applied in a knowl-

edgeable and prudent manner, enhances the chances for a successful outcome.

The intent of this chapter is to present a variety of manual techniques commonly used by the physical therapist. It is well beyond the scope of one chapter to provide a comprehensive treatment of each classification; indeed, volumes have been written on each. The reader should also recognize that varying amounts of disciplined practice in the clinic may be necessary before one can effectively administer certain of the techniques. The reader is encouraged to integrate related material in other chapters of this book and to use the suggested supplemental references when more depth is needed. Before proceeding to specific procedures, some general considerations are presented that apply to all of the techniques in varying degrees.

VASCULAR CONSIDERATIONS

Virtually all cells in the body are dependent on consistency in their milieu for normal function. The capillary pools must be able to deliver fresh oxygenated blood to the extracellular fluid and to remove waste products that accumulate. The low-pressure venous and lymphatic vessels are more susceptible to compression and impaired flow as a result of distortions in the myofascial compartments. Therefore, movement dysfunction may have a serious impact on a person's overall health because of resultant changes in the extracellular fluid. Specific bodily regions may directly impair vascular function when somatic dysfunction is present. For example, scalene muscle spasm associated with cervical spine dysfunction will compromise the subclavian artery. Manual techniques (such as massage) to facilitate venous return, passive stretching of contractured muscles, and mobilization of hypomobile joints have obvious implications in the improvement of overall health.

MECHANICAL CONSIDERATIONS

In cases of recent injury to the musculoskeletal tissues, the healing process is strongly influenced by the forces that are applied to the tissues. Carefully applied passive movements may influence the collagen formation so that a strong mobile scar is formed that allows greater function and is resistant to reinjury. Early mobilization may also prevent adherence to adjacent tissues, for example, a collateral ligament sprain may produce adherence to the underlying capsular tissue and periosteum. In chronic disorders, considerable pain may result from adaptively shortened structures as a result of excessive deformation activating the nociceptors. Thus, joints have less pain-free range for everyday postures and functional movements, and adjacent regions become overstressed attempting to compensate.

A frequently asked question is "What is the advantage of passive movement over active movement? Aren't we creating dependence of the patient on the therapist?" Many examples may be used to justify passive movement as a vital part of a treatment program. Consider a patient with a frozen shoulder, that is, glenohumeral adhesive capsulitis. These patients develop a compensatory movement pattern that involves overuse of the scapulothoracic muscles and disuse of the scapulohumeral muscles. Left untreated, the patient may continue this compensatory movement pattern indefinitely. However, specific mobilization techniques for the glenohumeral joint and appropriate exercises are often effective in alleviating the problem. Additionally, during the acute and subacute stages of soft tissue lesions, pain and protective muscle guarding may prevent active

function. For reasons already discussed, carefully applied passive movement may be helpful in relieving pain and muscle guarding, thus avoiding complicating sequelae.

NEUROLOGIC CONSIDERATIONS

The sophistication of the human nervous system is probably unequaled in all of nature. The body is under the constant control of voluntary and involuntary neural mechanisms. Applied neurophysiology has long been incorporated into the treatment approaches of physical therapists dealing with patients with upper motor neuron lesions. Physical therapists also have recognized the importance of applied neurophysiology in dealing with peripheral musculoskeletal problems. In addition to the traditional neurological testing of motor, sensory, and reflex functions, we submit that careful palpatory examination is invaluable in monitoring the body's response to both internal and external stimuli. The ability to detect alterations in muscle activity and other tissue texture abnormalities provides essential direction in treatment selection and assessment of the results.

Optimal neuromusculoskeletal function depends on afferent information being transmitted from the receptors in the various tissues. Postural and kinesthetic information arises from mechanoreceptor activity in the capsules and ligaments of joints, muscle spindle and golgi tendon receptors, periosteum of bone, and skin and adipose tissues. In addition, within these tissues are nociceptive receptors that are activated by abnormal amounts of mechanical or chemical stimuli. Of interest to the physical therapist is that the amount of nociceptive transmission reaching the central nervous system (ie, the perception of pain) is inversely related to the amount of activity in the faster conducting proprioceptive systems. Wyke has proposed that pain relief afforded by massage, manipulation, vibration, or movement in general is related to this inhibitory function of the mechanoreceptors. Conversely, in cases of reduced mobility, as with muscle spasm or aging, the potential for pain inhibition that occurs with normal functioning is greatly reduced. The implication of manual techniques activating pain-inhibiting mechanisms is obvious; however, in cases of high irritability it may be quite a challenge to select a technique that is tolerable, yet effective.

JOINT MOBILIZATION TECHNIQUES

A wide variation exists in terminology and conceptualization of manipulative procedures and their proposed effects. For example, physical therapists may use mobilization, articulation, or manipulation to treat joint dysfunction. Osteopaths use muscle energy techniques or manipulation to correct somatic dysfunction. Chiropractors adjust vertebral subluxations. Cyriax manipulates or applies traction to the spine to reduce intervertebral disk derangements. Mennell manipulates to restore normal joint play. Each of these disciplines or approaches represents quite a great amount of variation in how treatments are actually applied. A definitive description of the "manipulable lesion" has yet to be agreed upon, rendering each manipulation or mobilization a trial with its effectiveness appropriately judged by a careful assessment of the patient's signs and symptoms. The information to follow is from many "schools of thought." The illustrated procedures are those we have found to be safe and effective in our practice, which deals primarily with outpatient musculoskeletal problems.

Some general principles that apply for the safe and effective use of mobilization are as follows:

1. The patient must be relaxed in order to test and treat the joint adequately.
2. The patient must be balanced. This principle applies to sitting and recumbent positions.
3. The therapist should hold or maintain contact with the patient in an area immediately adjacent to the part being treated.
4. One part should be held stable while the other is moved on it. Belts or sandbags may be required to assist in stabilization.
5. Never push into pain or spasm unless it is clearly a "stretch pain" (eg, tight hamstrings that are not irritable).
6. Use the minimum amount of force necessary to achieve a release or adequate improvement in motion.
7. Select salient examination findings to reassess after each treatment. Correlate the effect of treatment on these findings and on the symptoms.

The spectrum of techniques available to the skilled therapist allows manual intervention even in the presence of some serious illnesses. What would be an absolute contraindication for a high velocity or forceful technique may be a precaution for a grade I or grade II oscillation. Certain conditions are absolute contraindications to manual treatment: malignancy or bone disease of the area to be treated; active inflammatory or infectious arthritis; central nervous system signs; and fracture. Regional contraindications include vertebral artery involvement, cauda equina compression, and instability of the craniovertebral unit. Relative contraindications or precautions include severe pain or irritability, hypermobility, muscle spasm, pregnancy, excessive steroid use, neurologic signs, rheumatic diseases, osteoporosis, spondylolisthesis, history of malignancy, anticoagulant medications, and recent surgery.

EXTREMITY MOBILIZATION TECHNIQUES

Glenohumeral Joint

Distraction (Fig. 50-1)
PATIENT: Supine with humerus slightly flexed and abducted. Right hand is at therapist's left side.
THERAPIST: Standing at right side of patient. Right hand grasps medial proximal humerus. Left hand stabilizes distal lateral humerus.
PROCEDURE: Therapist turns body counterclockwise to move humeral head laterally away from glenoid fossa.
Comments: An effective trial treatment producing a general capsular stretch, often the only movement tolerated in irritable lesions. Small adjustments in rotation may be necessary to get the desired movement.

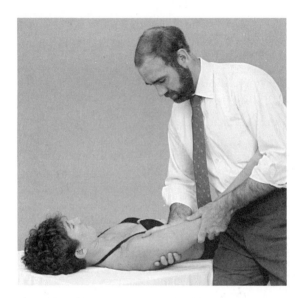

Figure 50-1. Glenohumeral joint distraction.

Posterior Glide of Humerus (Fig. 50-2)
PATIENT: Same as for distraction.

THERAPIST: Same as for distraction except that right hand is now placed over the proximal anterior humerus.

PROCEDURE: Therapist leans forward and allows body weight to glide humerus posteriorly.

Anterior Glide of Humerus (Fig. 50-3)
PATIENT: Same as for distraction.

THERAPIST: Same as for distraction except that right hand grasps proximal posterior humerus.

PROCEDURE: The humerus is lifted anteriorly.
Comments: It may be necessary to stabilize the scapula with a belt if stronger stretching is desired. Or, the prone position may be used for better scapular stabilization.

Inferior Glide (Fig. 50-4)
PATIENT: Supine with right humerus abducted 70 to 90 degrees.

THERAPIST: Standing at right side of patient. Right hand grasps distal medial humerus. Heel of left hand contacts proximal lateral humerus just below greater tuberosity.

PROCEDURE: Therapist shifts body from left to right and glides humerus inferiorly.
Comments: Inferior glide is often the most restricted accessory motion in cases of severe stiffness. It may be necessary to work in other directions that are less restricted during the initial sessions.

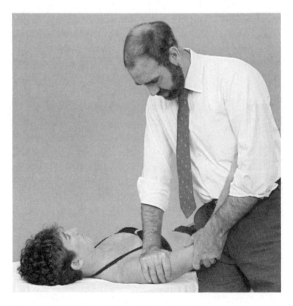

Figure 50-2. Posterior glide of humerus.

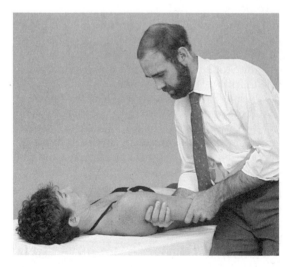

Figure 50-3. Anterior glide of humerus.

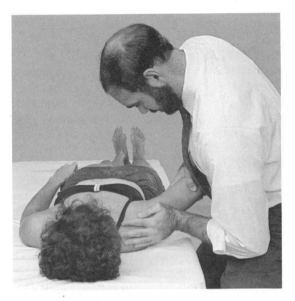

Figure 50-4. Inferior glide of humerus.

Scapulothoracic Joint

Distraction (Fig. 50-5)

PATIENT: Lying on left side at edge of table with body contacting therapist.

THERAPIST: Standing in front of patient. Right hand grasps superior vertebral border of right scapula. Left hand grasps inferior vertebral border of scapula.

PROCEDURE: Very slowly, therapist leans on patient's right arm to adduct the scapula while simultaneously working the fingers under the costal surface.

Comments: The winging or distractive motion is a vital movement for reaching behind the back. Often, the rhomboid or trapezius muscles are tender, necessitating much patience and gentleness. Fingernails should be trimmed for this technique.

Upward Rotation of Scapula (Fig. 50-6)

PATIENT: Same as for distraction except the right arm is abducted, resting on therapist's right forearm.

THERAPIST: Right hand grasps superior scapula while left hand holds inferior angle.

PROCEDURE: Therapist pulls up with hand while right hand allows shoulder girdle to move farther into abduction.

Comments: The scapula may be moved in virtually any direction from this position, depending on the restriction to be treated.

Sternoclavicular Joint

Inferior Glide of Clavicle (Fig. 50-7)

PATIENT: Supine with arms resting on table.

THERAPIST: Standing at head of patient. Pads of both thumbs contact medial superior surface of left clavicle.

PROCEDURE: Therapist pushes the clavicle inferiorly.

Comments: Oscillating movements are generally more effective at this joint.

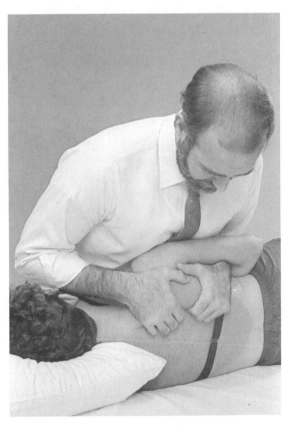

Figure 50-5. Scapulothoracic distraction.

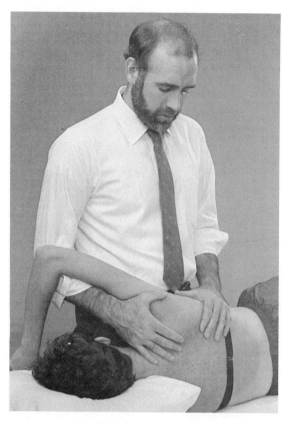

Figure 50-6. Upward rotation of scapula.

Inferior Glide of Clavicle: Alternate Method, Isometric Technique (Fig. 50-8)

PATIENT: Supine with shoulder hyperextended about 10 degrees, elbow fully extended with forearm off edge of table.

THERAPIST: Right hand grasps proximal anterior humerus and lifts the shoulder girdle into some protraction. Left hand holds distal anterior forearm.

PROCEDURE: Patient is instructed to lift the upper limb straight up against the unyielding resistance given by the therapist's left hand. An isometric contraction of the subclavius muscle is produced, and moves the clavicle inferiorly.

Comments: Superior subluxation of the clavicle may result from tightness of the sternocleidomastoid muscle. Such tightness is common in

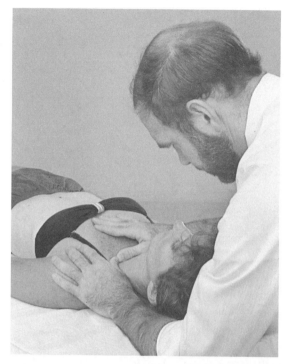

Figure 50-7. Inferior glide of clavicle.

patients with forward head postural problems. Stretching of the sternocleidomastoid may be accomplished by sidebending the cervical spine away from and rotating it toward the

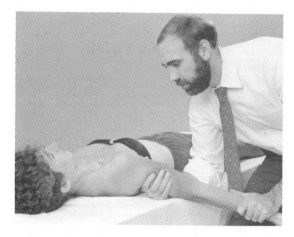

Figure 50-8. Inferior glide of clavicle using isometric technique.

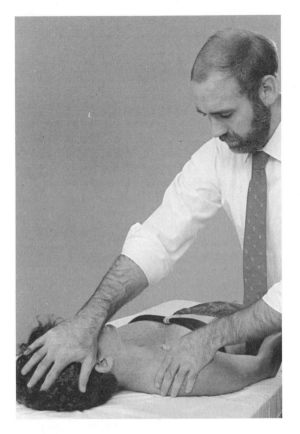

Figure 50-9. Superior glide of clavicle using isometric technique.

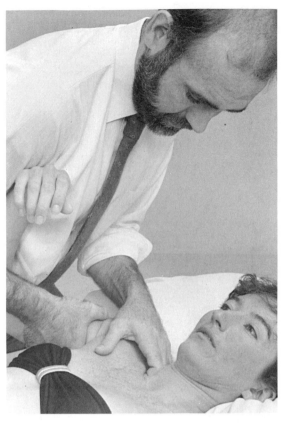

Figure 50-10. Anterior glide of clavicle showing soft tissue technique for supraclavicular area.

tightened side while the clavicle is held down.

Superior Glide of Clavicle: Isometric Technique (Fig. 50-9)

PATIENT: Supine with cervical spine in approximately 20 degrees of left lateral flexion.

THERAPIST: Standing at right side of patient with right hand contacting right side of head. Left thumb contacts inferior medial surface of the right clavicle.

PROCEDURE: Patient is instructed to move the head to the right against the unyielding resistance provided by therapist's right hand. An isometric contraction of the sternocleidomastoid muscle is produced, pulling the clavicle superiorly. The therapist's left thumb assists by guiding the clavicle superiorly.

Anterior Glide of Clavicle: Soft Tissue Technique for Supraclavicular Area (Fig. 50-10)

PATIENT: Supine with right arm slightly flexed and abducted.

THERAPIST: Standing at patient's right side with right hand holding proximal medial humerus. Left hand is positioned with fingers contacting superior posterior clavicular shaft.

PROCEDURE: Shoulder girdle is moved in a circular rhythmic fashion in the sagittal plane while the left fingers are gently moved under the clavicle.

Comments: Exquisite tenderness is common, and gentleness is stressed. Often this movement is a helpful adjunctive treatment in cases of thoracic outlet syndrome.

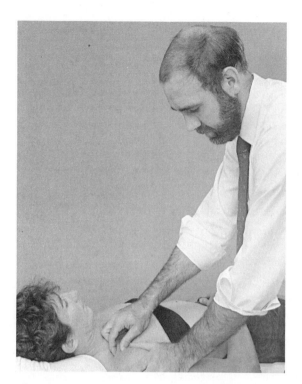

Figure 50-11. Anterior-posterior glide of clavicle.

Acromioclavicular Joint

Anterior-Posterior Glide (Fig. 50-11)
PATIENT: Supine with forearm resting on abdomen.

THERAPIST: Standing at patient's right side, with right hand grasping lateral clavicular shaft with pads of thumb and fingers. Left hand holds proximal humerus.

PROCEDURE: Right hand moves clavicle back and forth while left hand stabilizes shoulder girdle.

Humeroulnar Joint

Distraction (Fig. 50-12)
PATIENT: Supine with left elbow flexed about 90 degrees and forearm resting on therapist's shoulder. Distal humerus rests on a firm pad.

THERAPIST: Seated at patient's left side with hands clasped around proximal forearm.

PROCEDURE: Therapist pulls in a distal posterior direction, producing distraction of the ulnar and humeral surfaces.
Comments: In conditions of traumatic arthritis, a concurrent myositis involving the brachialis muscle may complicate improvement in function. In such cases, vigorous stretching should be avoided; however, gentle distraction as described may be helpful.

Radiohumeral Joint

Longitudinal Distraction (Fig. 50-13)
PATIENT: Supine with left elbow flexed about 60 degrees.

THERAPIST: Standing at patient's left side with left hand stabilizing at distal anterior humerus. Right hand holds distal radius in neutral pronation-supination.

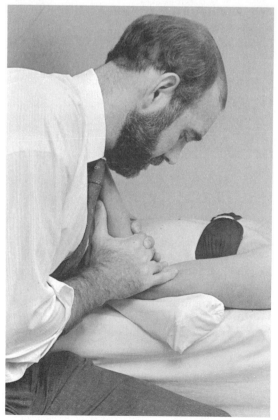

Figure 50-12. Distraction of humeroulnar joint.

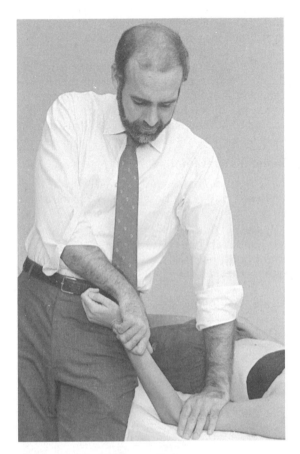

Figure 50-13. Radiohumeral distraction.

PROCEDURE: Therapist pulls upward in line with shaft of radius.

Posterior-Anterior Glide of Radial Head (Fig. 50-14)

PATIENT: Supine with left elbow flexed, forearm supinated.

THERAPIST: Standing at left side of patient, left hand holds distal forearm in supination. Right thumb contacts posterolateral surface of radial head.

PROCEDURE: Therapist moves radial head anteriorly by adducting his right arm and simultaneously supinating the patient's forearm, transmitting the force to the thumb contact.

Comments: The tissue about the radial head is often quite tender. It is essential that the pres-

sure not come from the thumb flexors, because this creates discomfort for the patient and impairs the therapist's ability to feel the motion.

Anterior-Posterior Glide of Radial Head (Fig. 50-15)

PATIENT: Supine with left elbow flexed.

THERAPIST: Standing at patient's left side, both hands hold proximal forearm with thumbs against anterior surface of radial head.

PROCEDURE: Radial head is moved posteriorly by an ulnar deviation of both hands.

Inferior Radioulnar Joint

Supination (Fig. 50-16)

PATIENT: Supine with forearm supinated (if possible).

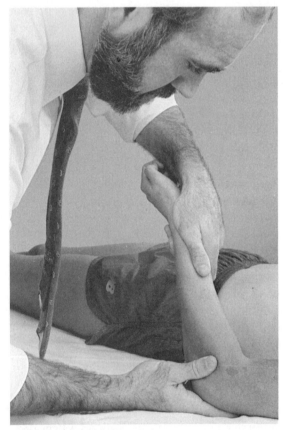

Figure 50-14. Posterior-anterior glide of radial head.

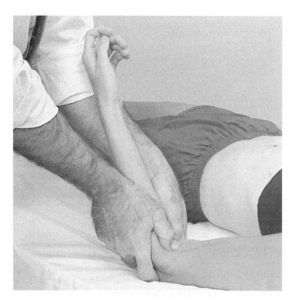

Figure 50-15. Anterior-posterior glide of radial head.

THERAPIST: Therapist holds left distal forearm so that the left thenar eminence stabilizes the anterior surface of the ulna while the right thenar eminence contacts the anterior radius.

PROCEDURE: Therapist's left hand moves radius posteriorly in supination.

Pronation
PROCEDURE: Patient's forearm is placed in the pronated position. Therapist now contacts the dorsal radius with the left thenar eminence while stabilizing the distal ulna with the right hand.

Wrist

Longitudinal Distraction of Carpal Joints (Fig. 50-17)
PATIENT: Supine with wrist in slight flexion.

THERAPIST: Standing at patient's left side with right hand holding distal carpal row and left hand holding distal forearm.

PROCEDURE: Therapist pulls his hands in opposite directions to produce a longitudinal movement of the hand and wrist. It is necessary to "bunch" the skin toward the wrist so the stretch will not be impeded by the skin. Dorsal glide to facilitate flexion and volar glide

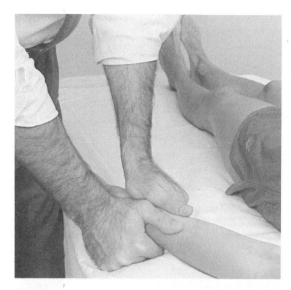

Figure 50-16. Supination of radioulnar joint.

to facilitate extension may also be done from this position. It is often necessary to mobilize the individual carpal bones. Refer to Maitland and Kaltenborn for an explanation of these techniques.

Fingers
The metacarpophalangeal (MCP) and interphalangeal (IP) joints can all be treated accord-

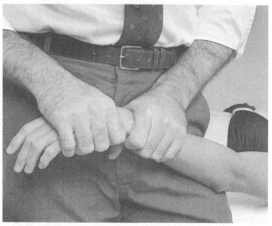

Figure 50-17. Longitudinal distraction of carpal joints.

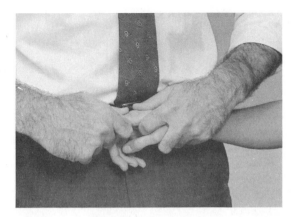

Figure 50-18. Distraction of metacarpophalangeal joint.

ing to the same principles. All of them involve a concave mobile surface on a convex proximal surface. The gliding motions to be described subsequently will all be in the same direction as the osteokinematic motion of the phalanges (eg, flexion of the MCP joint involves a volar glide of the proximal phalanx on the metacarpal). The MCP joints have greater ranges of physiologic and accessory motion than do the IP joints.

Distraction of Right Index Metacarpophalangeal Joint (Fig. 50-18)
PATIENT: Seated.

THERAPIST: Holds right hand of patient supported against his abdomen. Therapist's left thumb and index finger hold metacarpal while right thumb and index finger hold proximal phalanx.

PROCEDURE: Therapist pulls proximal phalanx distally to distract the MCP joint surfaces.
Comments: Dorsal glide to facilitate extension or volar glide to facilitate flexion is also done from this position.

Hip

Distraction: Neutral Position (Fig. 50-19)
PATIENT: Supine with right hip slightly flexed, abducted, and externally rotated.

THERAPIST: Standing. Right hand holds around right medial malleolus and calcaneous. Left hand holds around distal lateral leg.

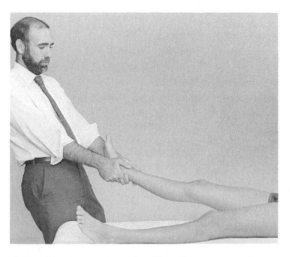

Figure 50-19. Distraction of hip joint in neutral position.

PROCEDURE: Therapist leans backward, pulling along long axis of femur.
Comments: It may be necessary to use a padded belt in the groin to stabilize the pelvis.

Distraction: Flexed Position (Fig. 50-20)
PATIENT: Supine with hip and knee flexed, foot flat on table.

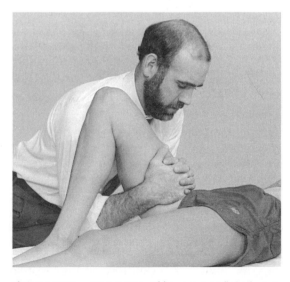

Figure 50-20. Distraction of hip joint in flexed position.

THERAPIST: Crouches at patient's right side and clasps hands around proximal medial thigh.

PROCEDURE: Therapist leans backward, pulling in a lateral inferior direction.

Flexion-Adduction with Compression (Fig. 50-21)

PATIENT: Supine with hip flexed to about 90 degrees and knee fully flexed.

THERAPIST: Standing at patient's right side, hands clasped over anterior knee.

PROCEDURE: Therapist begins by allowing body weight to compress through long axis of the femur. Then the hip is taken into adduction until resistance is felt. The hip is moved 30 to 50

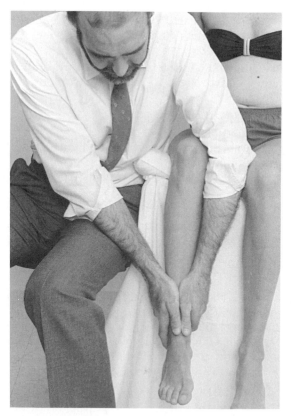

Figure 50-22. Distraction of knee joint.

degrees farther into flexion while adduction and compression are maintained.

Comments: As a test, the movement should be compared to the contralateral side to establish whether the symptoms are reproduced or if there is just routine discomfort. If used as a treatment, the therapist attempts to identify a small arc of pain or stiffness in the tested range of movement. Once the arc is identified, the therapist may rock back and forth over it as if trying to smooth it out. This technique should not be used with irritable joints where pain is the predominant factor.

Knee (Tibiofemoral)

Distraction (Fig. 50-22)

PATIENT: Seated on treatment table with firm pad under distal femur.

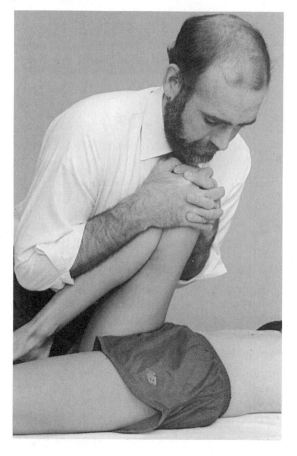

Figure 50-21. Flexion-adduction with compression of hip.

THERAPIST: Seated on low stool to patient's right side. Both hands grasp distal leg just above malleoli.

PROCEDURE: Therapist leans forward and allows body weight to pull downward on the leg.

Anterior Glide of Tibia: Flexed Position (Fig. 50-23)

PATIENT: Supine with left hip and knee flexed, foot flat on table.

THERAPIST: Seated on top of patient's left foot. Both hands grasp proximal leg just below knee.

PROCEDURE: Therapist leans back, pulling the tibia anteriorly.

Posterior Glide of Tibia

PATIENT: Same position as anterior glide of tibia.

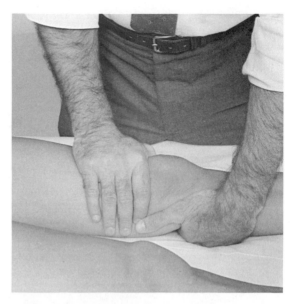

Figure 50-24. Posterior glide of femur, extended position.

THERAPIST: Same position as anterior glide of tibia.

PROCEDURE: Therapist leans forward, pushing tibia posteriorly.

Posterior Glide of Femur: Extended Position (Fig. 50-24)

PATIENT: Supine with hip and knee extended.

THERAPIST: Standing at left side of patient. Right hand contacts anterior distal femur while left hand stabilizes under proximal posterior femur.

PROCEDURE: Femur is pushed posteriorly as therapist leans down, allowing body weight to transmit force through the upper limb.

Comments: This technique is effective for restoring terminal knee extension.

Internal Rotation of Tibia (Fig. 50-25)

PATIENT: Supine with left hip and knee flexed.

THERAPIST: Standing at patient's left side. Left hand holds under calcaneous. Right arm and forearm contact medial surface of patient's leg, and patient's thigh is secured against the right side. Right hand is holding around the fifth

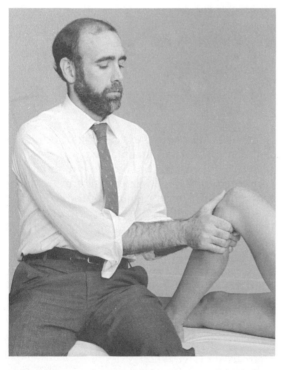

Figure 50-23. Anterior glide of tibia, flexed position.

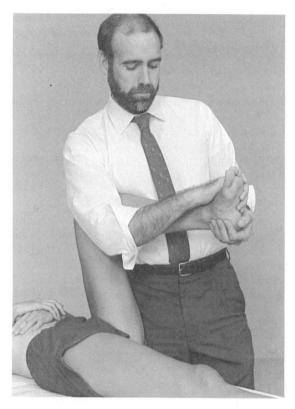

Figure 50-25. Internal rotation of tibia.

metatarsal and dorsum of foot and the left hand holds under the calcaneous.

PROCEDURE: The tibia is rotated internally by the right hand moving medially and the left hand pulling laterally.

External Rotation of Tibia

PATIENT: Same as internal rotation of tibia.

THERAPIST: Same as internal rotation of tibia, except the right hand now holds the medial side of the foot.

PROCEDURE: External tibial rotation is produced by the right hand moving the foot laterally while the left hand moves the calcaneous medially.

Patellofemoral Joint

Inferior Glide of Patella (Fig. 50-26)
PATIENT: Supine.

THERAPIST: Standing at patient's left side, ulnar side of right hand contacts superior pole of patella. Left hand is placed over patella.

PROCEDURE: Therapist glides patella distally with right hand. Left hand is used to guide the patella, and can be used to add compression if indicated.

Comments: The articulation between the patella and femur is critical for normal function of the knee. Dysfunctions may severely impair eccentric and concentric function of the quadriceps muscle or, in the case of hypomobility, may restrict knee flexion. For more detail about variations in this technique and guidelines for adding compression, refer to *Peripheral Manipulation* by Maitland.

Superior Tibiofibular Joint

Anterior-Posterior Movement of Fibula (Fig. 50-27)
PATIENT: Supine with right hip and knee flexed, foot flat on table.

THERAPIST: Seated on top of patient's foot facing patient. Right hand stabilizes proximal tibia medially while left thumb and fingers hold proximal fibula.

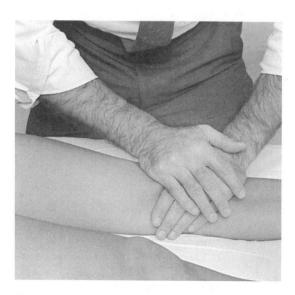

Figure 50-26. Inferior glide of patella.

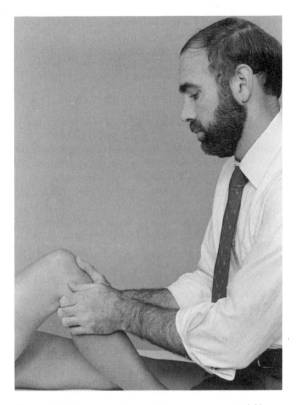

Figure 50-27. Anterior-posterior movement of fibula.

PROCEDURE: The fibula may be moved anteriorly or posteriorly, depending on the direction of restriction.

Comments: Dysfunctions at the superior tibiofibular joint commonly cause symptoms distally in the leg or ankle rather then proximally. It is helpful to compare the position of the fibular head bilaterally in determining which direction to move it. Usually, it feels stiff in both directions when dysfunction is present.

Inferior Tibiofibular Joint
Posterior Glide of Fibula (Fig. 50-28)
PATIENT: Supine.

THERAPIST: Standing at patient's feet facing patient, left thenar eminence contacts anterior surface of right lateral malleolus. Left hand holds medial malleolus.

PROCEDURE: Left hand pushes lateral malleolus posteriorly while right hand stabilizes medial malleolus.

Anterior Glide of Fibula (Fig. 50-29)
PATIENT: Prone with feet off end of table.

THERAPIST: Standing at patient's feet, right thenar eminence contacts posterior surface of right lateral malleolus. Left hand stabilizes around medial malleolus.

PROCEDURE: Therapist pushes lateral malleolus anteriorly.

Talocrural Joint

The ankle mortice allows for dorsiflexion and plantarflexion movements of the foot. Mechanically speaking, the wider anterior surface of the talus must glide posteriorly within the inferior tibiofibular joint during dorsiflexion and anteriorly during plantar flexion. The preceding techniques for treatment of the inferior tibiofibular joint are usually required in conjunction with those following.

Distraction (Fig. 50-30)
PATIENT: Supine with right thigh against therapist's iliac crest, knee flexed with leg in therapist's lap.

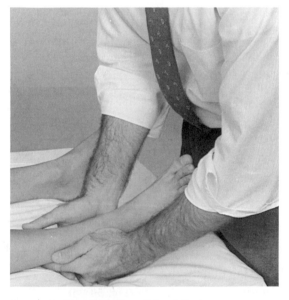

Figure 50-28. Posterior glide of fibula.

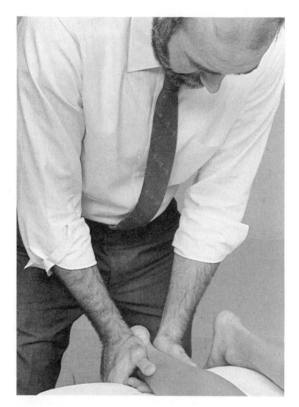

Figure 50-29. Anterior glide of fibula.

THERAPIST: Sitting with back to patient, web space of right hand contacts dorsum of foot. Web space of left hand contacts posteriorly on calcaneous. Thumbs should meet just below medial malleolus.

PROCEDURE: Direction of force is distal, resulting in distraction to both the talocrural and subtalar joints.

Posterior Glide of Talus (Fig. 50-31)

PATIENT: Supine with right foot off end of table.

THERAPIST: Standing at patient's right side, left hand stabilizes around distal medial leg. Right hand contacts dorsum of foot with web space over neck of talus.

PROCEDURE: Therapist leans forward, using body weight to push talus posteriorly.

Posterior Glide of Tibia (Anterior Movement of Talus) (Fig. 50-32)

PATIENT: Supine with right knee flexed enough to allow inferior surface of the calcaneus to contact the table, yet ankle should be plantarflexed.

THERAPIST: Right hand stabilizes around medial side of the forefoot. Left hand contacts anterior surface of tibia.

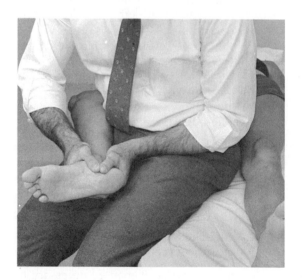

Figure 50-30. Distraction of talocrural joint.

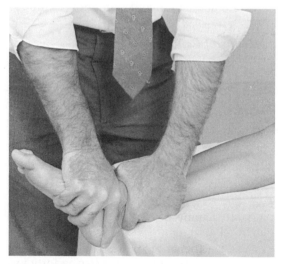

Figure 50-31. Posterior glide of talus.

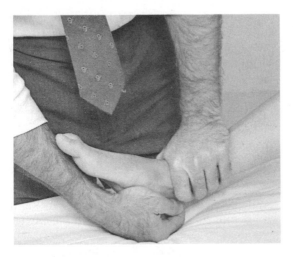

Figure 50-32. Posterior glide of tibia.

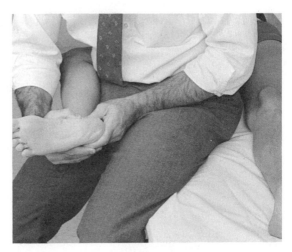

Figure 50-33. Inversion of calcaneus.

PROCEDURE: Left hand pushes tibia posteriorly.

Subtalar Joint

The subtalar joint is a complex articulation between the talus, calcaneus, and navicular bones. The joint allows for inversion of the foot, which is a combined motion of plantarflexion, adduction, and supination of the calcaneus. Conversely, eversion combines dorsiflexion, abduction, and pronation of the calcaneus.

Inversion of Calcaneus (Fig. 50-33)
PATIENT: Same position as for distraction of talocrural joint.
THERAPIST: Same as for distraction, except index fingers now move distally on calcaneus and thumbs move proximally to serve as a fulcrum just under medial malleolus.
PROCEDURE: Therapist moves calcaneus medially by radially deviating the wrists and pushing up with the index fingers.

Eversion
PATIENT: Same position as for distraction of talocrural joint.
THERAPIST: Same position as for distraction, except index fingers are moved superiorly just under lateral malleolus to serve as a fulcrum.

PROCEDURE: Therapist pushes down with thumbs by ulnarly deviating at the wrists to move the calcaneus laterally.
Comments: This technique stretches the very strong deltoid ligament. A substantial amount of force sustained for several seconds repetitively may be necessary in cases of hypomobility.

General Inversion of the Foot (Fig. 50-34)
PATIENT: Supine with left foot off end of table.
THERAPIST: Seated at end of table. Left hand stabilizes distal leg while right hand grasps around lateral side of foot with fingers dorsally over metatarsals.
PROCEDURE: Therapist twists the foot medially into inversion or supination.

General Eversion of the Foot (Fig. 50-35)
PATIENT: Same as for inversion.
THERAPIST: Same as for inversion, except that the right hand now stabilizes the distal leg while the left hand grasps around the medial side of the foot.
PROCEDURE: The left hand twists the foot into eversion or pronation.

As with the wrist, it may be necessary to treat the individual bones of the forefoot and

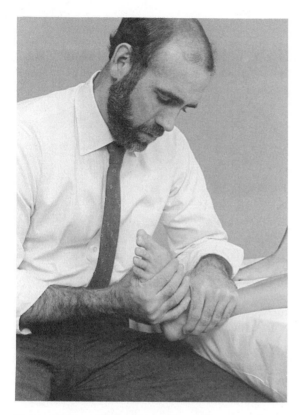

Figure 50-34.   General inversion of foot.

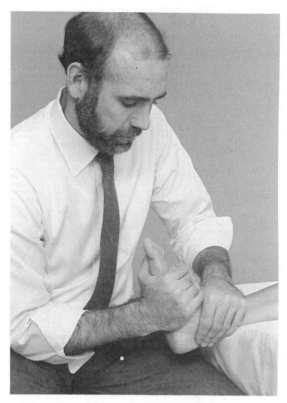

Figure 50-35.   General eversion of foot.

midfoot with specific techniques. The reader is referred to *Manual Therapy for the Extremity Joints* by Kalterborn for the details of these procedures. The same principles for mobilizing the fingers may be applied to the toes. They all involve a concave mobile surface on a convex proximal surface. The gliding motions are in the same direction as the osteokinematic motion of the phalanges. During the motions of flexion and extension, the proximal phalanx glides plantarward and dorsally, respectively.

SPINAL MOBILIZATION TECHNIQUES

Cervical Spine

Cervical Sidegliding Test (Fig. 50-36)

PATIENT: Supine with head and neck supported in a slight amount of flexion.

THERAPIST: Sitting or standing at head of patient. Pads of index fingers contact articular pil-

lars of segment posterolaterally and remaining fingers and palms support under temporo-occipital area. Abdomen supports top of patient's head.

PROCEDURE: This technique is used to test segments C2 to C6. The superior segments are tested first. The C2-3 joint is located by identifying the large C2 spinous process just below the suboccipital space and then moving the index fingers laterally to contact the articular pillar. The therapist now shifts his body from right to left, translating the head and neck to the left, which creates right sidebending at the level of the right palpating finger. The motion is then repeated in the opposite direction for comparison. The next segment is then tested by moving both fingers approximately one finger width caudally.

Comments: Some therapists prefer to maintain the head stationary against the abdomen and

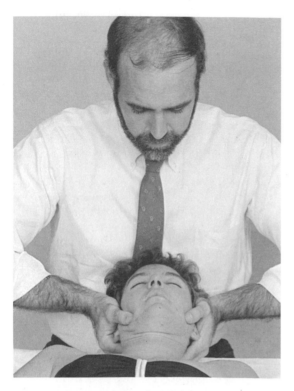

Figure 50-36. Cervical sidegliding test.

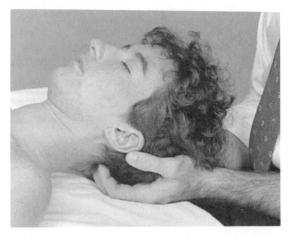

Figure 50-37. Inhibitive traction.

perform the translation with arm movement. This creates a more pure sidebending at each level. The test can also be modified by placing the neck in more flexion or extension which assists in determining the direction of the joint restriction. The test should be done slowly and assessed visually as well as by palpation. Care should be taken not to contact the articular pillar too far laterally, because this creates discomfort and makes patient relaxation difficult.

Inhibitive Traction (Fig. 50-37)
PATIENT: Supine.

THERAPIST: Seated at head of patient with radial three fingers of both hands contacting the suboccipital space. The fingers should be flexed at the IP joints to be oriented perpendicularly to the posterior arch of C1. The palms of the hands are initially supporting under the occiput.

PROCEDURE: As the posterior cervical muscles relax, the fingers sink deeper toward the posterior arch of C1. The therapist's shoulders are very slowly abducted so as to remove the palmar support from the occiput and create more pressure on the fingers. When the tissues are completely relaxed, the fingers may be slowly flexed to distract the cranium from the upper cervical segments. Optimal time is usually two to five minutes.

Comments: This procedure is effective in relaxing the posterior cervical muscles. It may be used as a preparatory treatment for other mobilization procedures. In addition, it may give considerable relief in cases of occipital headaches.

Cervical Manual Traction (Fig. 50-38)
PATIENT: Supine.

THERAPIST: Standing or sitting, right hand cups around chin with forearm against right side of face. Left hand holds around occiput.

PROCEDURE: Therapist leans backward, pulling with both hands.

Comments: The traction force may be applied statically, holding for several minutes, or intermittently, depending on the intent. For example, acute pain of nerve root irritation may be best treated with gentle static traction, whereas chronic stiffness may respond to more vigorous intermittent forces. Continual assessment

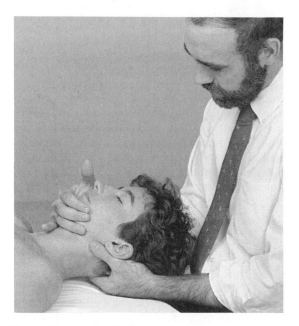

Figure 50-38. Cervical manual traction.

Cervical General Rotation (Fig. 50-39)

PATIENT: Supine.

THERAPIST: Standing or sitting, right hand cups around chin with forearm against right side of face. Left hand holds around occiput.

PROCEDURE: The head and neck are turned toward the side of the hand holding the patient's chin.

Comments: The difficulty in this technique is in maintaining the rotation on a vertical axis and not allowing lateral flexion or translation to occur. This rotation on a vertical axis is essential because specific areas of locking may result when both lateral flexion and rotation are introduced. The rotational movement may be applied as an oscillation at various amplitudes within the range or as a slow stretch directly into the barrier. In cases of high irritability where pain is the dominant feature, it is best to rotate in the nonpainful direction or within the pain-free part of the range.

and reassessment of the symptoms and signs should be done, especially in the initial sessions. Even though many consider traction the safest form of passive treatment, some patients do not tolerate it well during their irritable stages. Posttraumatic cases with segmental hypermobilities may respond adversely to traction in the early stages of healing.

The traction may be made more specific by altering the angle of neck flexion. If a particular problem segment can be identified, then it should be positioned near its neutral range of flexion-extension. Generally, the upper cervical segments OA-C2 are best treated near neutral or 0 degrees of flexion, the middle segments C3-6 in approximately 30 degrees of flexion, and the lower segments C7-T3 in 40 degrees to maximal cervical flexion. A palpating finger is placed between the spinous processes of the dysfunctional segment while the traction force is applied and released to determine the angle of flexion when the most separation occurs. Greater specificity can also be obtained by moving the right hand distally to encircle the top half of the dysfunctional segment.

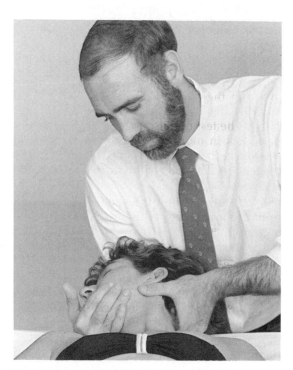

Figure 50-39. Cervical general rotation.

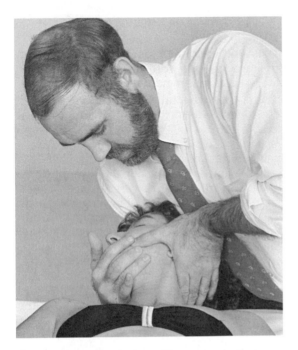

Figure 50-40. Cervical specific rotation in flexion.

Cervical Specific Rotation in Flexion (Fig. 50-40)

The intent of this technique is to move the left articular facet of the superior part of the segment superiorly and anteriorly.

PATIENT: Supine.

THERAPIST: Standing or sitting at head of patient. Right hand cradles chin as for general rotation technique. Left index finger contacts the left articular pillar of the superior part of the segment.

PROCEDURE: The neck is taken first into flexion until motion arrives at the desired segmental level. Right rotation is then added until the barrier is engaged. A small amount of traction is added with the right hand while the left hand glides the joint up and forward. It is critical to keep the cervical spine on the vertical axis to avoid locking. The technique is best done slowly, holding each stretch several seconds.

Cervical Rotation in Extension (Fig. 50-41)

PATIENT: Supine with head off end of table.

THERAPIST: Sitting or standing at end of table. Right hand holds right occipital region. Left index finger contacts the left articular pillar of the segment to be mobilized.

PROCEDURE: The head and neck are carefully extended until motion arrives at the desired segmental level, then left lateral flexion and rotation are added until the barrier is engaged. The therapist now begins a combined movement of left rotation, lateral flexion, and extension. The motion should be done rhythmically and slowly, with the left hand being the primary mobilizing force.

Comments: The intent is to glide the left articular facet of the segment posteriorly and inferiorly. The technique is a particularly effective soft tissue technique as well. The movement should be avoided if it causes an increase in peripheral upper limb symptoms, as with ipsilateral nerve root lesions. The patient should also be examined for signs and symptoms of vertebral artery involvement before applying this procedure.

Cervical Dorsal Glide (Fig. 50-42)

This technique results in a combined motion of forward bending the upper and midcervical spine while backward bending the lower cervi-

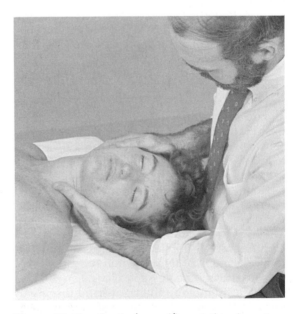

Figure 50-41. Cervical specific rotation in extension.

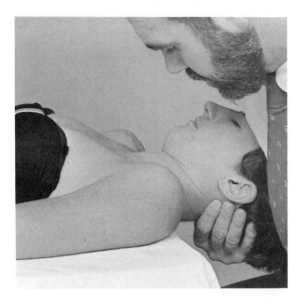

Figure 50-42. Cervical dorsal glide.

cal and upper thoracic segments. It is the same motion that patients perform actively as a corrective exercise for the forward head posture. It is often a helpful adjunct to the active exercise.

PATIENT: Supine with head off end of table. The edge of the table should meet the spine just below the segment to be mobilized or at the apex of the local kyphosis if present.

THERAPIST: Sitting at end of table or standing. Right hand is placed under occiput while the right pectoral region contacts the patient's forehead.

PROCEDURE: With head held firmly between the hand and shoulder, the therapist leans forward and maintains the patient's face parallel to his or her body. The movement is a translation of the head and neck posteriorly.

Cervical Accessory Movement Techniques

Maitland (1986) has described a series of short lever techniques to examine and treat the various spinal regions. The accessory movement techniques employ direct contact with the posterior elements of a vertebra. In the cervical spine the spinous process may be contacted and the vertebra moved in a posterior to anterior direction (central posterior-anterior pressure), or the lateral portion of the lamina may be contacted (unilateral posterior-anterior movement) and moved asymmetrically. Usually a central technique is employed for symptoms that are in the midline or are evenly distributed to both sides. Unilateral techniques are employed for unilateral symptoms, usually applied as an oscillation directly to the side of the symptoms or where hypomobility is detected. It is important that the force and amplitude of the treatment movements be less than that which reproduces the symptoms or muscle guarding. Usually a sense of release is felt by the therapist during the application of these techniques. Mechanically speaking, posterior-anterior movements result in some degree of extension and are contraindicated in the case of nerve root lesions with peripheral pain on extension.

Short lever accessory movement techniques widen the spectrum considerably with regard to the use of manual techniques for irritable lesions or where a great amount of caution is required. With such gentle forces, therapists are able to intervene in cases where tissues are weakened (eg, osteoporosis). Another advantage is being able to sense the local response of the tissues during treatment with palpation contacts so close to the joint.

Unilateral Posterior Anterior Movement (C1-C6) (Fig. 50-43)

PATIENT: Prone, hands cupped under forehead. Patient must be comfortable, with neck and shoulders relaxed. Sometimes it is necessary to place pillows in the axilla. The cervical spine should be approximately in its neutral position.

THERAPIST: Standing at head of patient, thumbs placed back to back, tip contacts posterior articular pillar.

PROCEDURE: Therapist moves the vertebra anteriorly by leaning forward, allowing body weight to transmit force through the arms to the thumbs. The intrinsic muscles in the hand must not be held tense, or else sensitivity is lost and patient discomfort results.

Comments: Oscillating movements at 2 to 3 c/sec are generally recommended.

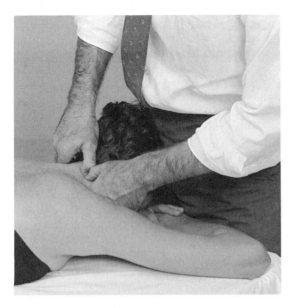

Figure 50-43. Cervical unilateral posterior-anterior movement.

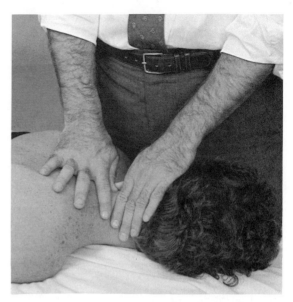

Figure 50-44. Cervical thoracic transverse movement.

Transverse Movement C7-T3 (Fig. 50-44)

In the region of the cervicothoracic junction, the spinous processes are long and easily accessible. Effective unilateral pressures may be used in this relatively less mobile area. Although relatively little mobility exists in the upper thoracic segments, what is available is critical for normal posturing of the head and neck. Upper thoracic stiffness results in excessive stress in the lower and midcervical segments.

PATIENT: Prone. May position neck in neutral as for unilateral posterior-anterior pressures or many turn head toward the side to which therapist is standing.

THERAPIST: Standing at left side of patient, right thumb pad contacts the left side of the spinous process. Thumb is held down in groove between the transverse process and spinous process by pressure from adjacent index fingers. The left thumb contacts the dorsal surface of the right thumb.

PROCEDURE: Pressure is directed transversely, moving the spinous process from left to right.

Comments: Usually, it is recommended that the therapist push toward the side of the symptoms initially to rotate the vertebra opposite to the side of the pain. Of course, if treating a specific mobility restriction that is not irritable, one would use a direct technique to free the restriction. One may also enhance the specificity of this technique by stabilizing the adjacent superior or inferior segment with one thumb directed in the opposite direction to the mobilizing thumb.

Thoracic Spine

Thoracic Manual Traction (Fig. 50-45)

PATIENT: Sitting on a stool with arms crossed on top of each other, hands on shoulders, and elbows pointing downward.

THERAPIST: Standing behind patient, clasps fingers under patient's elbows.

PROCEDURE: Patient is to relax and allow head to rest against therapist's chest. Therapist lifts up by extending hips and knees.

Comments: It is helpful to have the patient inhale. This will extend the thoracic area and the therapist can take up the slack. As the patient exhales, more distractive force will result. Also,

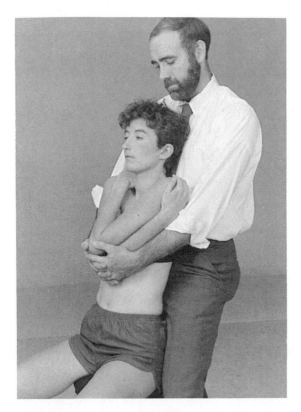

Figure 50-45.   Thoracic manual traction.

the amount of flexion or extension can be altered by having the patient slump more or less.

Thoracic General Flexion (Fig. 50-46)

PATIENT: Same position as for manual traction. Patient's feet should be flat on floor with knees separated so that she feels balanced.

THERAPIST: Standing at right side of the patient, right forearm is over top of patient's arms and right hand holds patient's left arm. Left hand contacts spine below the segment to be mobilized.

PROCEDURE: Patient is instructed to slump until motion arrives at the appropriate level. Left hand stabilizes with anterior inferior pressure while therapist leans to the right, stretching into further flexion.

Comments: It is helpful to have the patient exhale during the stretch phase.

Thoracic Extension (Fig. 50-47)

PATIENT: Sitting on stool, feet flat on floor, and arms crossed. The patient is leaning forward, resting on the therapist's right thigh; patient's ischial tuberosities must be securely on stool.

THERAPIST: Right foot up on stool with thigh supporting patient's upper body weight. Right hand holds patient's left upper arm and left thenar eminence contacts over segment to be treated.

PROCEDURE: Therapist moves patient into extension by translating his body to the right while increasing the posterior anterior pressure of the left hand. It is again helpful to have the patient exhale during the movement phase.

Thoracic Lateral Flexion (Fig. 50-48)

The example shows lateral flexion to the right.

PATIENT: Same position as for extension, except the patient will start in less extension if the treatment is performed in neutral.

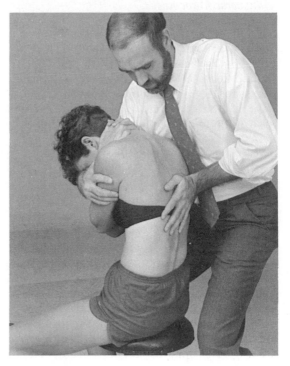

Figure 50-46.   Thoracic general flexion.

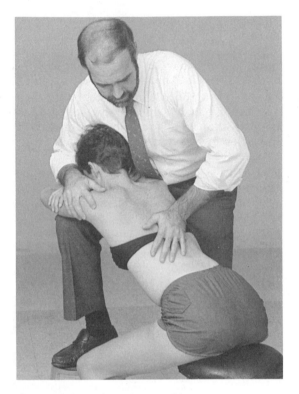

Figure 50-47. Thoracic extension.

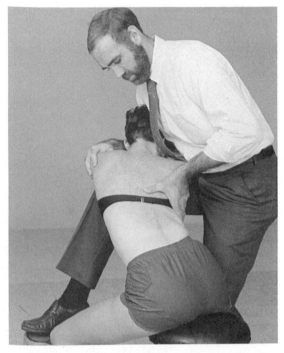

Figure 50-48. Thoracic lateral flexion.

THERAPIST: Same position as for extension, except that the left thumb will be against the right side of the spinous process *below* the level to be mobilized.

PROCEDURE: Therapist allows his left hip and knee to flex, pulling the patient into right lateral flexion while the left thumb stabilizes against the lower part of the segment.

Thoracic Rotation and Lateral Flexion (Fig. 50-49)

When treating neutral group dysfunctions, the coupled rotation and sidebending restrictions are in opposite directions. This is obvious in scoliosis by the observation that the rib hump is on the side of the convexity. The example shown is for a left thoracic convexity with restricted left lateral flexion and right rotation.

PATIENT: Sitting on stool, feet flat on floor, and hands clasped behind neck.

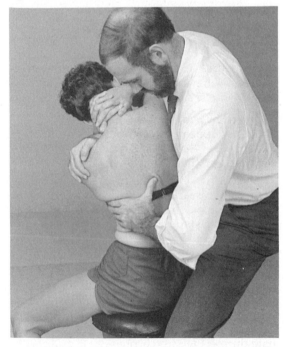

Figure 50-49. Thoracic rotation and lateral flexion.

THERAPIST: Stands to right side behind patient. Places right arm so that it is *under* the patient's right arm yet over the left holding onto the top of the left shoulder. Left thumb stabilizes at the apex of the convexity.

PROCEDURE: The trunk is kept in neutral flexion and extension. The patient is instructed to allow the left shoulder to drop down, increasing left lateral flexion, and to let the right shoulder move back, increasing right rotation. The therapist may now stretch further into left lateral flexion by lifting up or into more right rotation by turning his body clockwise. In addition, a combined motion may be performed by simultaneously increasing the sidebending and rotation components. It may also be helpful to use respiration, increasing the stretch during the exhalation phase. Another adaptation is to use isometric contractions of the antagonistic muscles, then taking the patient farther into the range. (See later discussion of muscle energy procedures.)

Thoracic Accessory Movement Techniques

Central Posterior-Anterior Pressure (Fig. 50-50)

PATIENT: Prone, close to the edge of the table near therapist.

THERAPIST: Standing to either side of patient, cephalic hand contacts spinous process with ulnar volar surface just anterior to pisiform bone. Caudal hand reinforces over the cephalic hand.

PROCEDURE: Therapist needs to position himself directly over the patient. This allows the therapist to extend the elbows and use body weight to move the vertebra anteriorly.

Comments: Treatment movements may be gentle oscillations for the treatment of pain or a progressive stretch as the patient exhales.

Thoracic Diagonal Transverse Process Technique (Fig. 50-51)

In the midthoracic spine, the spinous processes are arranged like tiles on a roof, angled such that their tips are one half to one full level below the transverse processes. Rotational accessory movement techniques can best be done by contacting the transverse processes, which

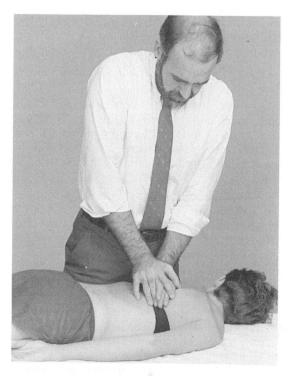

Figure 50-50. Thoracic central posterior-anterior movement.

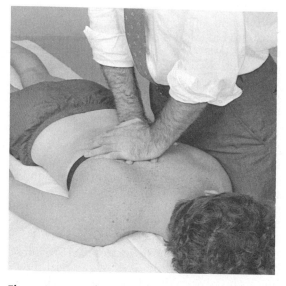

Figure 50-51. Thoracic diagonal transverse process technique.

are prominent, although concealed beneath the longissimus thoracis muscle. In the following example, T6 will be mobilized in left rotation.

PATIENT: Prone, close to edge of table toward therapist.

THERAPIST: Standing at left side of patient, right index finger contacts the left T6 transverse process and right long finger contacts the right T7 transverse process. The ulnar side of the left hand is placed over the fingers of right hand.

PROCEDURE: The therapist is positioned over the patient with elbows extended so that body weight will transmit an anteriorly directed force through the left hand on the spine. T6 and T7 are rotated in opposite directions, resulting in a left rotation of T6.

Comments: Positional asymmetry and tissue texture abnormalities are helpful in determining the problem segment. The treatment movement can be a rhythmic oscillation or a progressive stretch as the patient exhales. Care should be taken not to let the finger contacts wander too far laterally because unnecessary stress may be placed on the costotransverse and costovertebral joints.

Lumbar Spine

The movements of flexion, extension, lateral flexion, and rotation may be tested passively as illustrated in Figures 50-52 to 50-55. The intent of these tests is to identify the segments that are either hypomobile or hypermobile and thereby direct the therapist in treatment planning. The following examples illustrate passive mobility testing.

Lumbar Flexion Test (Fig. 50-52)

PATIENT: Sidelying with hips and knees flexed, knees slightly off edge of table.

THERAPIST: Stands facing patient, holding distal posterior leg with right hand. Either index or long finger of left hand is in lumbar interspace to be tested. Patient's knees must be securely in therapist's groin.

PROCEDURE: Therapist locates L5-S1 interspace. Motion is introduced by therapist moving his body from right to left, repeatedly flexing and extending hips in the range of the seg-

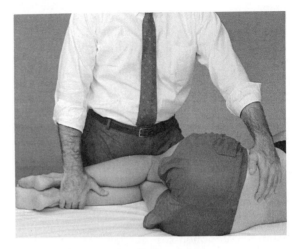

Figure 50-52. Lumbar flexion test.

ment to be tested. Therapist assesses the amount of flexion by feeling the degree of separation that occurs between the spinous processes. The more hip flexion that is introduced, the more cephalad will be the motion in the spine because motion is progressing from caudad to cephalad.

Lumbar Extension Test (Fig. 50-53)

PATIENT: Sidelying with right hip extended, knee flexed to about 90 degrees.

THERAPIST: Standing facing patient, holding under left thigh and leg with right forearm, left hand stabilized spine and palpates lumbar interspace.

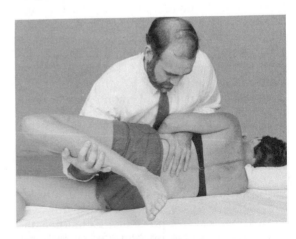

Figure 50-53. Lumbar extension test.

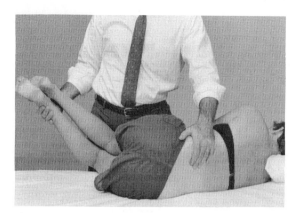

Figure 50-54. Lumbar lateral flexion test.

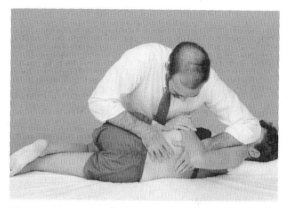

Figure 50-55. Lumbar rotation test.

PROCEDURE: Motion is introduced by extending the patient's left hip. The greater the hip extension, the more cephalic the motion that occurs in the spine.

Comments: This test can be a very strenous one for the therapist. It is critical for the therapist to get close to the patient and bend at the knees rather than at the waist.

Lumbar Lateral Flexion Test (Fig. 50-54)
The example shows left lateral flexion.

PATIENT: Sidelying with hips and knees flexed.

THERAPIST: Standing facing patient. Right hand grasps both lower legs distally and anteriorly. Left hand palpates the interspace on the left side toward which the sidebending occurs.

PROCEDURE: Motion is introduced by moving the legs up and down. The higher the legs are raised, the more cephalad the motion progresses.

Lumbar Rotation Test (Fig. 50-55)
The example shows testing left rotation.

PATIENT: Sidelying with right hip and knee slightly flexed. Left hip and knee flexed so that left foot can rest in right popliteal space. Right shoulder forward so that patient is not lying on it.

THERAPIST: Stands facing patient and leans forward. Left forearm contacts patient's left anterior shoulder. Right forearm stabilizes pelvis,

and right index or long finger palpates lower side to the right of interspace tested.

PROCEDURE: Motion is introduced by therapist pushing patient's left shoulder backward while feeling motion between the spinous processes with the right palpating finger. The farther the shoulder is moved backward, the more caudal will be the motion occurring in the spine.

Comments: Rotation is difficult to palpate because of the small range of motion available and the sequencing. Sequencing is best defined by the following example: When testing the L2 segment, the intent is to feel the L2 spinous process move down to the right before the L3 spinous moves. This small excursion only occurs at one precise interval in the range of movement.

Lumbar treatment techniques are illustrated in the following examples.

Lumbar Flexion (Fig. 50-56)
Mobilization to increase flexion at L4 will be explained in the following example.

PATIENT: Sidelying according to preference (right sidelying is shown). Right shoulder is pulled forward until rotation occurs above the level to be treated, in this case, until L3 has rotated to the left on L4. The uppermost thigh is placed in the therapist's groin.

THERAPIST: Left forearm stabilizes along left shoulder and left rib cage with the left index and long finger holding the L4 spinous process. The right arm and forearm encircle the

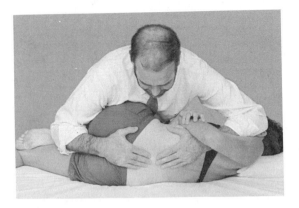

Figure 50-56. Lumbar flexion.

pelvis and the right hand holds the sacrum and L5.

PROCEDURE: Flexion is introduced by the therapist moving his right upper limb and body as a unit from his right to left while stabilizing with the left hand.

Comments: This reasonably specific technique involves locking the cephalic spinal segments in left rotation. It should be confirmed that the patient can tolerate flexion and rotation before performing this technique.

Lumbar Extension (Fig. 50-57)
Extension may be performed as was shown in the testing procedure, or as follows.

PATIENT: Right sidelying position as described for flexion, except that the right hip is brought into hyperextension. The left hip is in slight flexion and the left knee is flexed.

THERAPIST: Left forearm stabilizes along left shoulder and rib cage and left hand contacts the spinous process of the segment to be treated. Heel of right hand contacts left ischial tuberosity, and the right forearm is directed in a superior and slightly posterior direction.

PROCEDURE: Extension of the spine is introduced by anteriorly tilting the pelvis with the right hand as it pushes superiorly and posteriorly.

Lumbar Lateral Flexion (Fig. 50-58)
The example explains lateral flexion to the right of L4.

PATIENT: Right sidelying position with hips and knees flexed to 90 degrees. Right shoulder is pulled forward until rotation occurs at L3. (Care should be taken to avoid rotating too far because this will decrease the available motion at L4. Rotating in this direction, however, has the dual advantage of increasing the available right lateral flexion movement in the spine by moving the shoulder out of the way.) As much of the patient's femur as possible should be on the table and still allow the patient's legs to drop off the table. This avoids the table edge cutting into the lower thigh.

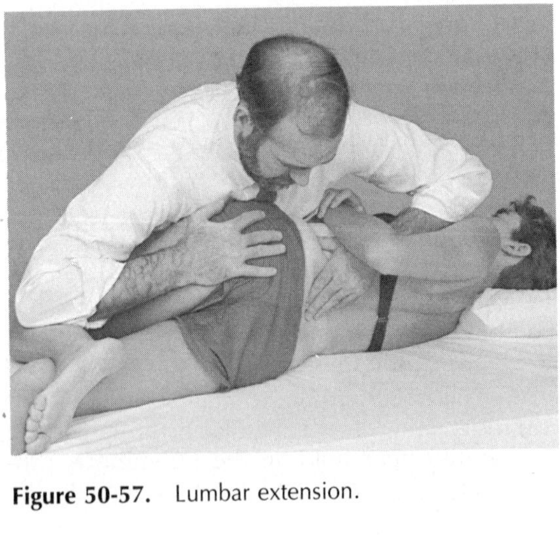

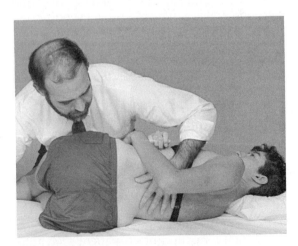

Figure 50-57. Lumbar extension.

Figure 50-58. Lumbar lateral flexion.

THERAPIST: Left forearm stabilizes along left rib cage and left thumb holds the spinous process of the segment to be treated (L4), while right hand lowers patient's feet toward floor until motion occurs at the desired level.

PROCEDURE: A right lateral flexion stretch is produced by stabilizing with the left thumb while the right hand pushes the feet farther down. It is also helpful to use muscle energy or isometric techniques from this position. (See guidelines for isometric techniques later in this chapter.) Patients with painful hips will not tolerate this well.

Lumbar Rotation (Fig. 50-59)

The example explains rotation of L4 to the left.

PATIENT: Right sidelying position. Left hip and knee are flexed until motion occurs below level to be treated (L5). Right shoulder is pulled anteriorly until rotation arrives *above* the level to be treated (L3). Now the "slack" is taken out above and below the desired segment (L4).

THERAPIST: Left forearm contacts anterior left shoulder of patient and left thumb is on the top side of the L4 spinous process. Right forearm contacts the left superior lateral buttock just behind the greater trochanter, and right fingers hold the underside of the L5 spinous process.

PROCEDURE: The right forearm and hand provide the mobilizing force by pulling the pelvis

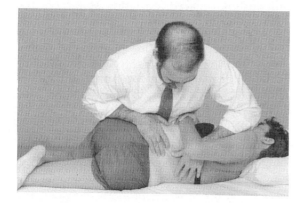

Figure 50-59.   Lumbar rotation.

anteriorly while the right fingers pull L5 into a right rotation, which amounts to a left rotation of L4. The segments above are stabilized by the therapist's left forearm and thumb pushing down on L4.

Comments: Rotation is a very effective treatment in many lumbar conditions but can also be harmful if used indiscriminately. It must be remembered that rotation amounts to compression, and conditions such as irritable disk lesions may be worsened with it. This technique is effective for segments T10 to L5 but will vary according to the location of the segment. To localize the treatment to the lower thoracic spine, a considerable amount of hip flexion with less thoracic rotation would be used. Conversely, lower lumbar lesions require less hip flexion but greater rotation to get "down to" the level. It is helpful to use respiration, exhaling during the stretch phase. Gentle beginning or midrange oscillations may be used in more irritable situations. Isometric or muscle energy forces may also be employed (see guidelines later in this chapter).

Lumbar Accessory Movement Techniques

Lumbar Central Posterior-Anterior Movement (Fig. 50-60)

PATIENT: Prone, close to side of table toward therapist.

THERAPIST: Standing at side of patient, with ulnar side of cephalic hand contacting spinous process of the segment to be mobilized or tested. The ulnar contact is just distal to the pisiform bone. Caudal hand reinforces over the mobilizing hand, as shown.

PROCEDURE: Therapist positions himself over the patient so that body weight can produce an anteriorly directed movement.

Comments: A useful treatment for promoting lumbar extension or for central or symmetrically distributed symptoms.

Lumbar Unilateral Posterior-Anterior Movement (Fig. 50-61)

PATIENT: Prone.

THERAPIST: Standing to left side of patient. Ulnar side of left hand contacts segment to be treated. Right hand holds around the right lateral pelvis.

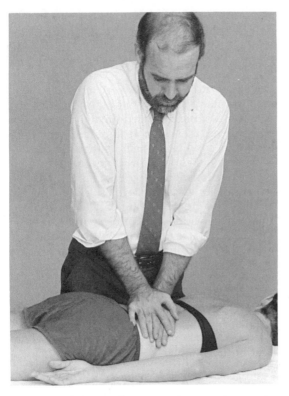

Figure 50-60. Lumbar central posterior-anterior movement.

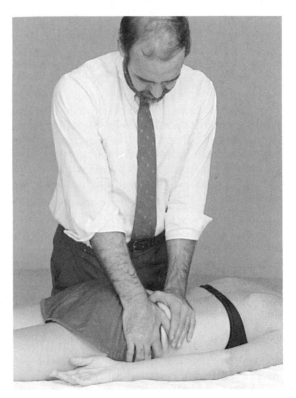

Figure 50-61. Lumbar unilateral posterior-anterior movement.

PROCEDURE: Right hand takes up slack by lifting right side of pelvis until rotation occurs at desired level. Therapist now leans forward, with left arm moving segment into a left rotation.

Comments: This technique also is effective for the soft tissue when applied to the side of the hyperactive paraspinal muscles.

Sacroiliac Joint

The sacroiliac is a complex articulation between the sacrum and pelvis. Motion at this articulation is also complicated by the many potential axes. For this discussion we shall only consider anterior or posterior rotation of the innominates on the sacrum. To examine for sacroiliac dysfunction, one must palpate the bony prominences on the pelvis and compare right and left for symmetry. The anterior superior iliac spines, posterior superior iliac spines, iliac crests, pubic tubercles, and ischial tuberosities may be palpated. It is essential to compare the anterior findings with the posterior findings. For example, a superiorly displaced anterior superior iliac spine would correlate with an inferiorly displaced posterior spine on the same side if the innominate were rotated posteriorly. Motion tests should also be done. We prefer to use the standing and sitting flexion tests. During these tests, the patient bends forward at the waist while the examiner palpates the movement of the posterior superior iliac spines. Normally, there should be a symmetrical movement of the posterior superior iliac spine on each side as the spine flexes and the pelvis rolls forward. If dysfunction is present, one side will move sooner and farther on the side of the dysfunction, probably because the sacrum is not moving properly between the innominates and pulls one side along with it.

The following techniques are used to treat either an anterior or posterior innominate. These dysfunctions are generally described according to the positional findings, although restricted motion is implied; for example, an anterior innominate implies restricted posterior rotation.

Posterior Rotation (Fig. 50-62)

The example illustrates a left anterior innominate.

PATIENT: Right sidelying position. If no lumbar problems exist, the spine may be extended and rotated to increase specificity. The right hip should be extended (slightly more than shown in the illustration). Left hip and knee are flexed, with knee supported on the therapist's abdomen.

THERAPIST: Stands facing patient. Right hand contacts ischial tuberosity with right forearm directed superiorly and anteriorly. Left hand contacts anterior superior iliac spine with forearm directed posteriorly and inferiorly. Forearms and hands are now positioned to produce a force couple resulting in posterior rotation of the left innominate.

PROCEDURE: Therapist pushes with each hand while slightly moving body from his right to left in order to flex the patient's hip, assisting the innominate movement.

Anterior Rotation (Fig. 50-63)

Rotation of a right posterior innominate is shown.

PATIENT: Prone with left leg off table, left foot on floor or stool. The intent of having the leg off the table is to increase the specificity by creating opposing counterforces. Flexion of the lumbar spine and posterior rotation of the opposite side of the pelvis accentuates the anterior rotation on the right.

THERAPIST: Standing in close contact to support the patient's pelvis. Right hand holds under the right anterior thigh and brings the hip into slight adduction. Left hand is over the left posterior iliac crest; preferably, elbow is extended.

PROCEDURE: Anterior rotation is produced by simultaneously pushing down with the left

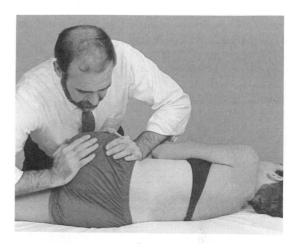

Figure 50-62. Posterior innominate rotation.

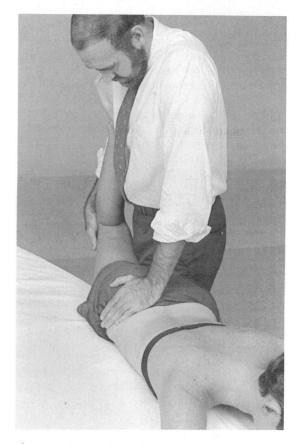

Figure 50-63. Anterior innominate rotation.

hand and pulling up with the right hand to hyperextend the hip. It may be helpful to work with the patient's respiration or to use isometric (muscle energy) forces (see guidelines discussed later in this chapter).

Comments: Sacroiliac dysfunctions are a common finding in postural problems. Resolution generally requires a correction of muscle imbalances in the trunk and lower limbs.

ISOMETRIC TECHNIQUES (MUSCLE ENERGY)

Isometric or muscle energy techniques refer to a specific form of manual treatment that involves precise positioning by the therapist and controlled voluntary muscular contraction by the patient. Some practitioners refer to them as "patient cooperation techniques" because they require concentration and effort by the patient. These procedures may be used to mobilize restricted joints and to lengthen or strengthen muscles. Although isometric techniques share some features with the "hold-relax" methods of proprioceptive neuromuscular facilitation, important differences must be considered for mobilization of the spinal joints: (1) positioning of the patient is determined by the direction of the joint restriction in all three planes of movement; (2) precise localization of forces to engage the restrictive barrier (for a discussion of barriers, see Chapter 19) directly seems to be critical for a successful result; and (3) the contractile forces generated by the patient are generally submaximal, because strong efforts usually result in cocontraction of agonist and antagonist muscles, and strong efforts also make maintenance of localization difficult.

Other guidelines for the successful application of isometric procedures are as follows: (1) the patient must be balanced; (2) the therapist's counterforce must be unyielding; and (3) both the therapist and patient should relax after each contraction, before the barrier is relocalized.

Palpatory examination procedures for isometric techniques are different from those commonly employed for spinal joint mobilization. The primary difference is a visual assessment of transverse process levels at different points in the sagittal plane range of motion. A good method of conceptualizing the application of palpation findings is with regard to the gliding motion of the facet joints during flexion and extension. During flexion at any spinal segment (with the exception of the atlanto-occipital, sacroiliac, and sacrococcygeal joints), the inferior facets of the superior part of the segment slide superiorly and anteriorly during flexion, and inferiorly and posteriorly during extension.

Because most dysfunctions are unilateral (or at least asymmetrical), palpation findings will change when subjected to the flexed or extended positions. For example, Figure 50-64 shows a vertebral segment that is restricted in right rotation, right lateral flexion, and extension. Or possibly, it is positionally flexed, left rotated, and left laterally flexed. Mechanically speaking, this vertebral segment may assume an asymmetrical position in neutral with the left transverse process more prominent than the right. If the spine were now extended, the left transverse process could become even more prominent posteriorly because the left side is free to move posteriorly but the right is not. Conversely, they are both free to move forward so that the asymmetrical findings may disappear in flexion.

Examining for transverse process levels in this manner is difficult for some to accept. The depth of the transverse processes in the lumbar region requires sensitivity and practice for the therapist to develop confidence and profi-

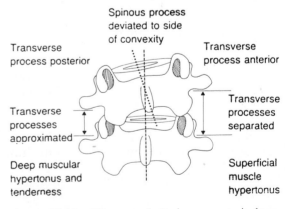

Figure 50-64. Diagram of single-segment dysfunction.

ciency with the technique. The test requires visual as well as tactile perceptiveness. It has the advantage of greater reliability for teaching purposes. The findings do not change as readily as they do with traditional passive mobility tests, which become a treatment when examiners are repeatedly comparing findings. On the other hand, palpation does not assess the quality of the movement abnormality, only that dysfunction is present. It is often advisable to use passive physiological or passive accessory motion tests, or both, in conjunction with visual tests when confirming segmental findings. One should also remember to correlate all three criteria for determining segmental dysfunction: asymmetry of position, range of motion, and tissue texture abnormalities.

The following illustrations explain the examination procedures specific to the applied isometric technique.

Checking Transverse Process Levels in Neutral (Lumbar Spine)

PATIENT: Prone, lumbar spine in neutral position.

THERAPIST: Standing to side of patient that allows dominant eye to be over spine (eg, if therapist's right eye is dominant, then he would stand to the left side of the patient). Thumbs are positioned over transverse processes of the segment.

PROCEDURE: Slow pressure is applied by the thumbs, allowing them to sink to the level of the transverse process. Equal pressure is determined by comparison of blanching under nails. The level of each thumb in the transverse plane is visualized. After visualization, posterior-anterior pressure may be applied to each side, noting resistance to the movement.

Checking Transverse Process Levels in the Extended Position (Fig. 50-65)

PATIENT: Prone, up on elbows with chin in hands.

THERAPIST: Same position as for neutral testing.

PROCEDURE: Same as for neutral. Therapist notes if neutral asymmetries increase or decrease, or if new levels of dysfunction appear.

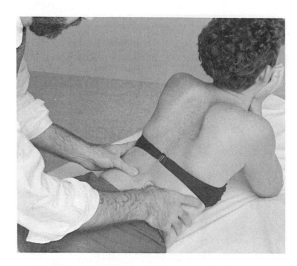

Figure 50-65. Checking transverse process levels in extension.

Checking Transverse Process Levels in Flexion (Fig. 50-66)

PATIENT: Kneeling with hips, knees, and spine fully flexed. Elbows and head rest on pillows to relax paraspinal musculature.

THERAPIST: Stands to left side and behind patient. The contact points for thumbs are the same as in neutral testing.

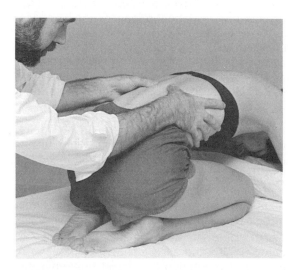

Figure 50-66. Checking transverse process levels in flexion.

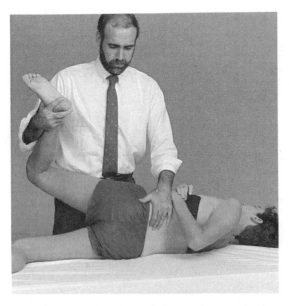

Figure 50-67. Isometric technique to increase lumbar extension, left rotation, and left lateral flexion.

PROCEDURE: Therapist notes levels of thumbs and occurrence of changes, as in the hyperextended position.

The treatment application using the findings of the transverse process examination involves positioning the patient to engage the barrier in all three planes. The following example will explain a method for treatment of a lumbar segment that is positionally flexed, sidebent right, and rotated right (Fig. 50-67). Such a segment would be restricted in extension, sidebending left, and rotation left.

PATIENT: Lying on the right side or the side of the posterior transverse process. Right hip is extended in order to place the spine in generalized extension.

THERAPIST: Standing, facing patient. Right hand holds left leg while left hand palpates the interspace of the restricted segment.

PROCEDURE: Therapist pulls right arm of patient forward and allows patient to move into maximal left rotation. Therapist now engages left sidebending barrier by raising the left

lower limb. The barrier is now engaged in all three planes. Patient is now instructed to pull the left leg down toward the table with approximately one third of her strength, while the therapist provides *unyielding* resistance with the right hand. After approximately seven seconds of isometric contraction, *both* the therapist and the patient must relax. The position is now adjusted by raising the leg to increase the sidebending and extension by bringing the hip into extension. This process is repeated approximately three times, and the transverse process levels and the active movements of the patient are reexamined.

Comments: If a release is not obtained after the first three repetitions, then repeat the procedure again. Sometimes it is effective to resist the isometric contractions in other planes of movement (eg, having the patient push the left shoulder forward to release the rotational restriction). The strength of the isometric contractions may need to be adjusted according to the segmental level to be treated. In order to reach high lumbar or low thoracic segments, greater force is usually necessary than for the lower lumbar segments. Precise localization of the barrier is critical. Novice therapists frequently go beyond the barrier engagement, especially with major motion restrictions. The resistance to the patient's contractions must be unyielding. The isometric contractions should not be anywhere close to maximal effort because this will cause cocontraction of antagonistic muscles, and may not release. These techniques are quite efficient and effective with relatively little force on the part of the therapist. Perhaps the fact that all three planes of motion are treated enhances the effect. However, they often make the patient quite sore for 24 to 48 hours after treatment. Following these treatments with grade II oscillations in one of the planes of movement often reduces the soreness.

The following example will explain a technique to release a lumbar segment that is extended, sidebent left, and rotated left (ie, restricted in flexion, sidebending right, and rotation right) (Fig. 50-68).

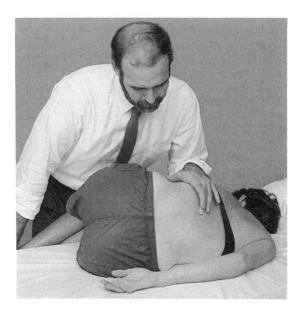

Figure 50-68. Isometric technique to increase lumbar flexion, right rotation, and right lateral flexion.

PATIENT: Patient lies on the right side, or opposite the side of the posterior transverse process. The chest is turned down toward the table and close enough to the edge to allow the legs to drop down. The hips are flexed enough to flex the lumbar spine.

THERAPIST: Stands facing patient. Left hand palpates lumbar segment, while right hand holds feet.

PROCEDURE: The feet are lowered until the sidebending barrier is engaged. The patient is instructed to raise her feet up toward the ceiling with approximately one third to one half of her strength, while the therapist provides unyielding resistance. After about a seven-second hold, both patient and therapist relax and the barrier is then adjusted. First the legs are lowered farther to adjust the sidebending, and then the hips are flexed farther to increase the lumbar flexion. The process is repeated three times and the patient is reexamined.

Comments: See comments for previous technique.

SOFT TISSUE MOBILIZATION

Soft tissue mobilization is a treatment technique to normalize the general mobility of muscles, tendons, ligaments, and fascia; and to decrease excessive muscle activity. With neuromusculoskeletal dysfunctions, one often finds limited mobility between the various fascial layers, between fascia and bone, and within the muscle. This limited mobility within the soft tissues may be the result of scars, microtrauma, overuse, traumatic accidents, or habitual patterns of use. For normal mobility and optimum function to occur, these specific soft tissue restrictions need to be alleviated. Examination of soft tissue mobility involves several procedures: assessment of the mobility of the skin and superficial fascia over deeper structures, the ability of the soft tissues to move around bony landmarks, the general mobility of soft tissues over surrounding tissues, and the mobility of muscle tissue. In the following section, the examination techniques for the different steps and treatment techniques for specific structures will be described.

SKIN AND SUPERFICIAL FASCIA MOBILITY

Examination of the skin and superficial fascia includes evaluation of the mobility of these tissues over the underlying structures. These superficial restrictions must be treated initially, otherwise the treatment of deeper structures will be painful and inefficient. The first examination technique is skin rolling, which evaluates the ability of the skin to be raised from the underlying structures. This technique is performed over the length of a muscle or bone.

PATIENT: The patient should be positioned so that the area to be examined is well exposed and easily accessible to the therapist. The patient should also be positioned to facilitate relaxation; all body parts should be adequately supported.

THERAPIST: The therapist places both hands on the area to be treated with the radial border of the thumbs resting on the patient. The distal phalanges of the index fingers are also placed on the skin.

PROCEDURE: The therapist "pinches" the skin between the index fingers and thumbs. This "pinch" is not painful, and is actually just lifting the skin from the underlying structures. While holding the skin between the thumbs and index fingers, the therapist places the distal phalanx of the middle fingers on the patient's skin in line with the thumbs and index fingers. As the therapist gently grabs the skin with the middle fingers, the index fingers are removed from the skin and the thumbs are pushed towards the middle fingers. Now while the skin is held between the thumbs and middle fingers, the distal phalanges of the index fingers are placed on the skin, beyond the middle fingers. As the skin is grabbed with the index fingers, the middle fingers are removed and the thumbs are gently pushed towards the index fingers. This process is repeated until the skin in the area has been examined. If the skin is not mobile over the underlying structures, the therapist will have difficulty in lifting the skin. Often as the therapist attempts to roll the restricted skin, the skin will appear dimpled, like an orange peel.

Similarly, the skin gliding test is also performed over the length of a muscle or bone. However, in this technique the skin is not lifted from the deeper structures; rather, the ability of the skin to slide in multiple directions over the deeper structures is tested. Not only is the location of the restriction identified, but the direction of the restriction is also determined. Because this technique is a superficial one, the pressures applied through the contact points are minimal. An example of this technique in the cervical region follows (Fig. 50-69).

PATIENT: Supine, with the head supported by the therapist's left hand. To examine the right anterolateral tissues, the patient's cervical spine is slightly flexed and rotated to the left.

THERAPIST: The therapist uses the distal phalanx of the index finger or middle finger for the examination. The chosen contact point is placed on the skin to be evaluated.

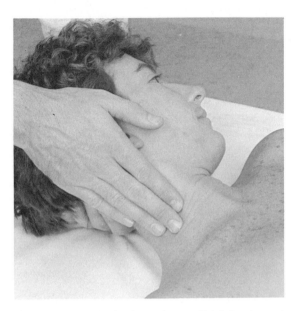

Figure 50-69. Evaluation of superficial fascia and skin.

PROCEDURE: Apply light pressure with the digit, and push the digit along the skin. The motion is performed slowly enough so that the skin can deform around the digit. If performed too quickly, the digit will skip over the skin. As the finger moves through the skin and superficial fascia, the ability of the skin to deform around the digit is assessed. In areas where the skin does not easily move over the underlying structures, a more detailed examination is conducted. Once these areas of limited mobility are identified, an imaginary clock is "drawn" over the region, with 12 o'clock being cephalad and 6 o'clock being caudad. The therapist places a finger on the restriction, and then gently deforms the skin in the directions identified by the clock. At this point the therapist is assessing the mobility and end-feel of the soft tissues. When the specific direction of the restriction is determined, the therapist can treat the restriction. When the restriction has been alleviated, the examination of the superficial tissues can continue.

Treatment of these superficial restrictions may be done in several different ways, de-

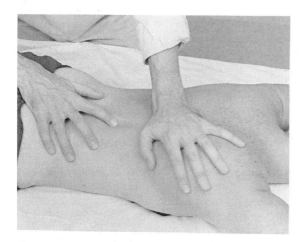

Figure 50-70. Treatment of superficial restrictions by placing the tissues under tension.

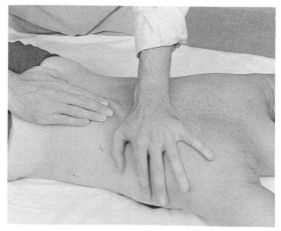

Figure 50-71. Treatment of superficial restrictions with a spiral technique.

pending upon the severity of the restriction and the acuteness of the condition.

PATIENT: Unchanged from the position assumed for the examination of the superficial tissues.

THERAPIST: Same as during the examination procedure, with the digit on the restricted skin.

The following technique can be used in situations where the restriction is not too severe and the patient's condition is not acute (Fig. 50-70).

THERAPIST: Again using the imaginary clock, the therapist places the other hand "six hours" from the direction of the restriction. For example, if the restriction is at 7 o'clock, then the other hand would be placed at 1 o'clock.

PROCEDURE: The contacting digit stretches the skin in the direction of the restriction until resistance is felt. At that point, the other hand pulls the skin in the direction opposite to the restriction. Therefore, the restricted skin is pulled past the contacting finger by the pressure of the other hand. This pressure is maintained until the restriction releases. Once the release is felt, the area is reassessed and the examination procedure continues.

If the patient has an acute condition in this area, the stretch applied in the previous tech-

nique may exacerbate the symptoms. In this instance, the following technique may be employed.

THERAPIST: The therapist places the other hand in the direction of the restriction (in this example, at 7 o'clock) several inches from the actual restriction.

PROCEDURE: The contacting digit again stretches the skin in the direction of the restriction. As in the previous case, the other hand pulls the skin in the direction opposite to the restriction. As a result of the orientation of the therapist's hands, the skin by the restriction is now placed on slack. The contacting digit then applies slow pressure in the direction of the restriction, until the release is felt. Again the area is reassessed, and the examination proceeds.

If the superficial restriction is severe and the previous techniques do not effect an adequate release, then the following unlocking spiral technique may be used (Fig. 50-71).

THERAPIST: Hand placement is similar to the hand placement in the initial treatment technique. However, another finger may be placed on the skin for additional support.

PROCEDURE: After the contacting digit has stretched the skin to the point of resistance and the other hand has placed an additional stretch on the tissues, the contacting digit applies further stress to the restriction by forming a circular motion. This circular motion will be in either a clockwise or counterclockwise direction, whichever motion produces the most stress to the restriction. The pressure is maintained until the restriction releases. After reassessment, the examination is continued.

Two methods of detecting and three methods of treating superficial fascial restrictions have been described. The following examination and treatment methods for deeper structures are similar to the techniques for superficial restrictions. The deeper tissues will be examined for restrictions, and then the tissues will be treated according to the direction of restrictions. The main differences between the techniques are the contact surfaces and the amount of pressure that is used.

SOFT TISSUE MOBILITY AROUND BONY PROMINENCES

The next step in the examination procedure is assessment of the mobility of soft tissues around bony prominences. Various contact surfaces can be used depending upon the depth of the tissue and the area to be treated. Common contact surfaces include the distal phalanx of the thumb or first two fingers, the proximal interphalangeal joints, and the elbow. The examination procedure is performed by deforming the tissues along the length of the bony prominence. The initial stroke is carried out at a superficial level, with subsequent strokes performed at deeper levels. When restrictions are detected, the specific direction of the restriction is assessed by the clock method described previously. Examination and treatment techniques for the spinous processes, ribs, and iliac crests will be described.

A common site for soft tissue restrictions associated with spinal dysfunction is between the spinous processes and paravertebral musculature. Assessment of these restrictions is easily done with either the distal phalanx or proximal interphalangeal joint contact points.

PATIENT: Prone, with all body parts appropriately supported.

THERAPIST: Stands on either side of the patient, because the region can be easily reached from either side. When using the distal phalanx contact surface, usually either the thumb, index finger, or middle finger is used. The digit is placed just lateral to the spinous process, so that a portion of the digit is in contact with the side of the spinous process.

PROCEDURE: Starting with light pressure, the distal phalanx is drawn along the spinous processes to check the mobility of the soft tissues around these bony prominences. When restricted mobility is identified, the specific direction of the restriction is determined by deforming the tissue in multiple directions, as was done with the superficial tissues. When the specific restriction has been identified, the therapist can go ahead and treat this area. After the restriction has been alleviated, the therapist can proceed with the examination. When the superficial layer has been examined, the therapist repeats the procedure using more pressure, which permits assessment of the mobility of deeper tissues.

To treat these soft tissue limitations, the therapist can use techniques similar to those for the treatment of skin restrictions. With the distal phalanx contact point, the therapist can treat the tissues by placing them on stretch, by shortening the tissues around the lesion, or by using a spiral technique. An example of treating the tissues by placing them on stretch follows.

PATIENT: Prone, with all body parts appropriately supported.

THERAPIST: When the specific restriction has been identified, the therapist will place the other hand "six hours" from the direction of the restriction. As described previously (see Fig. 50-70), the therapist's right index finger is placed along the spinous process with the force being directed towards 6 o'clock (the direction of the restriction). The therapist's other hand is placed superior to the right hand, at the 12 o'clock position.

PROCEDURE: The contacting digit stretches the skin in the direction of the restriction (6 o'clock) until resistance is felt. At that point, the left hand pulls the skin in the direction opposite to the restriction (12 o'clock). Therefore, the restricted tissue is pulled past the contacting finger by the pressure exerted from the left hand. This pressure is maintained until the restriction releases. Once the release is felt, the area is reassessed and the examination continues.

The other method for assessing the soft tissue mobility around the spinous processes uses the proximal interphalangeal joints of the fingers as the contact surface. This technique is a more general one than the previously described method, but it is effective in the examination and treatment of the deeper layers. The therapist must concentrate on the layer of tissue that is being examined or treated with this technique. A common error is to proceed to deeper layers without having cleared the more superficial layers. If this error is made, a hard band, which does not release, will be palpable while examining the deeper layer. This often aggravates the patient's symptoms (Fig. 50-72).

PATIENT: Same position as for the previous technique.

THERAPIST: Stands at the side of the area to be treated. The therapist makes a loose fist with

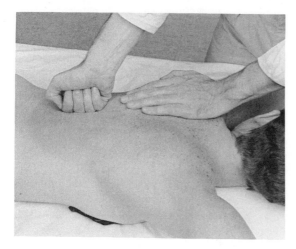

Figure 50-72. Examination and treatment of deeper fascia using the PIPs.

the examining hand and places the dorsal aspect of the proximal interphalangeal joints on the skin adjacent to the spinous process.

PROCEDURE: Directing the pressure inferiorly and anteriorly, the therapist pushes his hand along the spinous processes. When a restriction is identified, the specific direction of the limitation can be determined by deforming the tissue in multiple directions. After this restriction has been treated, the therapist can continue with the examination procedure.

The treatment technique using the proximal interphalangeal joints follows the same principles outlined for the previous techniques, where the tissues are placed on stretch (see Fig. 50-72).

PATIENT: The patient's position is unchanged.

THERAPIST: The therapist will maintain one hand at the restriction, while the other hand is placed "six hours" from the contact surface. In the figure, the therapist's right hand is placed at 6 o'clock and the left hand is placed at 12 o'clock.

PROCEDURE: The therapist applies pressure with the right hand to the soft tissue in the direction of limitation until resistance is felt. The surrounding tissues are placed on stretch by pulling the tissues towards 12 o'clock with the left hand. This pressure is maintained until the restriction releases around the right hand. Once the restriction is released, the therapist reassesses the involved tissue and then continues with the examination.

Commonly, the intercostal soft tissues become restricted from either traditional musculoskeletal dysfunctions or following pulmonary problems. These soft tissue restrictions can lead to limited rib mobility and decreased pulmonary function. Soft tissue massage techniques are an effective method of restoring costal mobility. Examination and treatment of the intercostal tissues is performed with either the distal phalanx of the first, second, or third digit. Care must be taken in treating this region in osteoporotic patients.

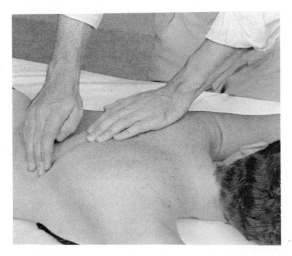

Figure 50-73. Examination and treatment of intercostal restrictions.

PATIENT: Either prone or supine, depending on which aspect of the rib cage is being examined. In Figure 50-73, the patient is prone so that the posterior rib cage can be examined.

THERAPIST: Stands on either side of the patient. The contact point is placed in the intercostal space, just lateral to the vertebral column.

PROCEDURE: Starting with light pressure in order to examine the superficial structures, the finger is pushed laterally along the intercostal space. The examination movement is carried laterally to approximately the mid-axillary line. In the region of the scapula, the examination is performed from vertebral column to scapula and from the scapula laterally. This stroke may be repeated several times at each tissue depth, so that the borders of the ribs as well as the intercostal tissues will be examined. When a restriction is located, the specific direction of restriction is identified using the imaginary clock described earlier. When the specific restriction is treated, the examination is continued.

The treatment of intercostal restrictions is similar to the treatment techniques described previously (see Fig. 50-73).

PATIENT: Same position as for the examination.

THERAPIST: Position is unchanged.

PROCEDURE: The contacting finger deforms the soft tissues in the direction of the restriction until resistance is palpated. Depending on the severity of the symptoms, the other hand either places the tissues on stretch or slack. In the figure, the therapist's left hand is placed "six hours" from the direction of the restriction in order to stretch the involved tissue. The restricted tissue is allowed to deform gradually around the contacting finger.

A more general technique for treating intercostal restrictions is depicted in Figure 50-74.

PATIENT: Lying on the uninvolved side, with the arm on the involved side abducted.

THERAPIST: Stands facing the patient. One arm cradles the the patient's abducted arm with the hand grasping the axilla. The web space between the thumb and first finger of the other hand is placed on the superior border of the lower rib involved in the restriction.

PROCEDURE: By pushing the rib inferiorly with one hand and elevating the shoulder girdle

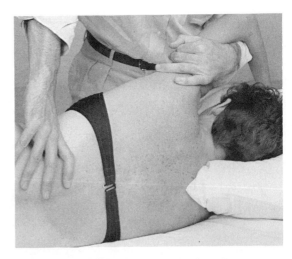

Figure 50-74. General treatment technique for intercostal restrictions.

with the other hand, the therapist applies a stretch to the intercostal soft tissues. The stretch is maintained until a gradual release of the tissues is felt. This process is repeated at all the involved levels.

Another common area of soft tissue restrictions is along the crest of the ilium. These restrictions are especially prevalent in patients with lumbosacral dysfunctions. The examination and treatment of these restrictions can be performed with the phalanges or proximal interphalangeal joints (PIPs). However, as a result of the extent and depth of these restrictions, using a partially flexed elbow is often an effective technique (Fig. 50-75).

PATIENT: Prone.

THERAPIST: Stands facing the patient, and places the partially flexed elbow at the medial aspect of the iliac crest.

PROCEDURES: Starting superficially with light pressure, the elbow is pushed along the iliac crest to approximately the mid-axillary line. When restrictions to mobility are palpated, the specific restriction can be determined using the imaginary clock. After the restriction is treated, the examination of this area continues at deeper tissue levels.

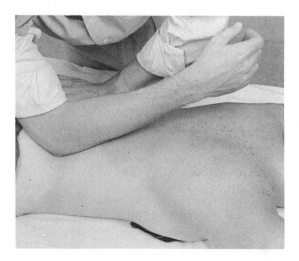

Figure 50-75. Treatment of soft tissue restrictions along the iliac crest.

Treatment of the restriction may also be performed with the elbow.

PROCEDURE: To treat the specific restriction, the elbow would stretch the tissue until resistance to deformity is felt. Then the other hand would apply a stretch of the tissue in the opposite direction. When the restriction releases, the examination process would continue.

An alternative method of treatment is to identify only the level of the restriction and to treat the restriction in the direction of the iliac crest.

PROCEDURE: In this instance, the therapist's elbow will follow the contours of the iliac crest, treating the most superficial limitations first. When a restriction is identified, gradual pressure will be applied to the involved tissue along the iliac crest. As the restriction gradually releases, the examination along the crest would continue.

MUSCLE TISSUE MOBILITY

The final aspect of the examination and treatment scheme is to identify restrictions within and between the muscles themselves, or the assessment of muscle play. Similar to joint play, muscle play is defined as the accessory motions of the individual muscles (Johnson). A muscle under normal conditions should be able to move independently from surrounding tissues and should be pliable when it is manually deformed. Abnormal muscle play is characterized by a lack of elasticity and by resistance to deformation when outside pressure is applied. Both specific and general examination and treatment techniques for the erector spinae and hamstring muscle groups will be described.

PATIENT: Prone.

THERAPIST: Stands at the side of the patient. To examine the erector spinae muscle group, the therapist places either the fingertips or the pads of the thumbs against the border of the muscle belly (Fig. 50-76).

PROCEDURE: Starting at the most superficial level, the therapist gently deforms the muscle tissue by pressing the contact points against

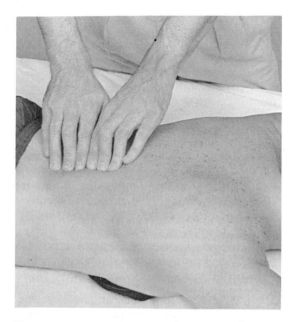

Figure 50-76. Examination and treatment of muscle play using a perpendicular stroke.

the border of the muscle. When the excursion limit of the muscle is reached, the pressure on the tissue is released. As this process is repeated along the length of the muscle, the end-feel of the tissue is noted. Normal end-feel has an elastic quality. The examiner should detect free mobility and then a gradual increase in tension. At the extremes of this motion, the muscle should still feel pliable. If limited mobility or decreased elasticity is noted, the examiner should determine the direction of the restriction, as was done with the superficial fascia restrictions. After identifying the restriction, the therapist will treat the dysfunction. When the entire length of the muscle has been examined and treated, the therapist will repeat this process at the next deepest layer of muscle.

To examine the hamstring musculature, similar perpendicular techniques may be used along the lengths of the specific muscles. Because these muscles run parallel to each other, it is also important to assess their ability to slide past each other. This assessment is performed by a technique that is done along the borders of

these muscles parallel to their long axes (Fig. 50-77).

PATIENT: Prone, with legs well supported.

THERAPIST: The therapist identifies the borders of the individual muscles through palpation. Either the tips of the fingers or the thumb may be used as a contact point. This contact surface is placed at the proximal end of the hamstring muscle group at the border between two muscles.

PROCEDURE: Starting with light pressure to examine the superficial tissues, the therapist slides the finger along the border of the muscle. The therapist gradually increases the pressure on subsequent strokes to examine the deeper layers. The muscle bellies should separate easily under the pressure of the therapist's fingers. Inability of the muscles to separate indicates restricted mobility between the fascial coverings of adjacent muscles. As with the previous techniques, when a restriction is identified, it is treated. After treatment of the restriction, the examination continues along the length of the muscles.

Treatment of muscular restrictions may be done with either specific or general techniques. The specific techniques are performed in a direction either perpendicular or parallel to the

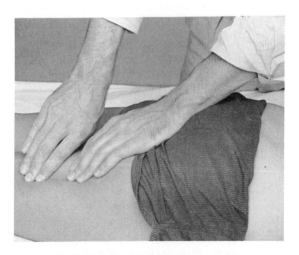

Figure 50-77. Examination and treatment of muscle play using a parallel technique.

long axis of the muscle. In addition, the perpendicular techniques may be performed in either an oscillatory fashion or with a sustained stretch. The specific techniques will be discussed first, followed by an explanation of the general techniques.

Treatment of decreased play in the erector spinae muscles may be performed with a perpendicular technique. The contact surfaces are the same as used in the examination technique for this area (see Fig. 50-76).

PATIENT: Prone, in a comfortable position.

THERAPIST: Stands at the patient's side. The hands are placed on the patient's back so that the fingertips or thumbs can apply pressure in the direction of the restriction.

PROCEDURE: The therapist must apply enough pressure in an anterior direction to localize the treatment at the desired tissue depth. To use an oscillatory technique the therapist will repeatedly deform the muscle to the point of tension in the direction of the restriction. This technique is done in a rhythmical fashion at a rate of several cycles per second. Care must be taken to continue the treatment at the desired tissue depth.

In order to treat these restrictions with a sustained pressure technique one hand is used to apply the pressure to the involved tissue while the other is used to stretch the tissue.

PATIENT: Prone, in a comfortable position.

THERAPIST: Stands to the side of the patient. The contact surface, either the fingertips or thumb of one hand, is placed on the involved erector spinae muscles in the direction of the restriction. The other hand is placed at an angle of 180 degrees from the direction of the restriction.

PROCEDURE: Using the contact surface, the therapist deforms the tissue to the point of tension in the direction of the restriction and at the desired depth. The other hand applies a counterstretch to the tissues away from the restriction. The therapist maintains the pressure until the involved muscular restriction gives way. This technique is the same one that was performed for the superficial fascia.

These perpendicular techniques may be used on any muscular restriction. To perform the parallel technique, the same contact points are used as for the examination process. As an example of this process, treatment of the hamstrings muscle group will be described (see Fig. 50-77).

PATIENT: Prone with legs well supported.

THERAPIST: Stands to the side of the patient, facing the patient's feet. Using the fingertips or thumb of one hand, the restriction is located. While this hand position is maintained, the other hand is placed proximal to the contact hand on the patient's leg.

PROCEDURE: The second hand applies a stretch to the patient's hamstrings away from the contact point. This stretch is maintained until the soft tissue restriction is released.

The general techniques are used to treat restrictions of greater magnitude. The aim of the treatment is to deform the muscles so that they will be forced to spread out. These techniques incorporate the examination stroke along with the treatment. The contact points for the general techniques are usually larger body areas such as the dorsal surface of the proximal phalanges, the elbow, or the forearm. An example of the technique for the erector spinae muscle will be described first, followed by a description of a technique for the hamstring muscle group (Fig. 50-78).

PATIENT: Sits on a stool, with the feet flat on the floor.

THERAPIST: Stands behind the patient. The contact surface is the dorsal aspect of the proximal phalanges of the fingers on both hands. The hands are placed paravertebrally at the cervicothoracic junction.

PROCEDURE: Applying slight pressure anteriorly and inferiorly, the therapist instructs the patient to flex forward slowly. This flexion should proceed only to the level of the therapist's hands. As the therapist slides the hands inferiorly, the patient slowly flexes forward in time with the therapist's motion. While the therapist's hands are moving inferiorly, the muscle tissue is being deformed. At the same

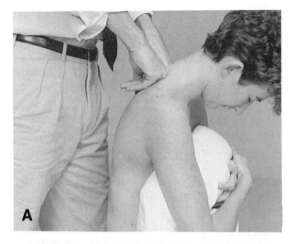

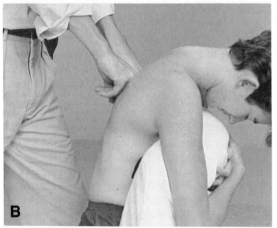

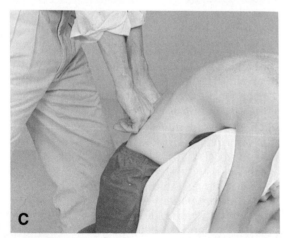

time, the tissue is evaluated for restricted muscle play. If such a restriction is found, the progression of the motion is slowed until the restriction is released. The stroke is finished when the therapist reaches the level of the sacrum and the patient is fully flexed. It is important that the therapist and patient time this technique so that the patient does not flex below the level of the therapist's hands.

A similar general technique may be used when treating a large restriction in the hamstring muscle group (Fig. 50-79).

PATIENT: Prone, with the legs well supported.

THERAPIST: Standing at the patient's side. The ulnar borders of the forearms are used as the contact surfaces. One arm is placed at the level of the ischial tuberosity or the proximal edge of the restriction. The other forearm is placed just distal to the first arm.

PROCEDURE: The therapist stabilizes the tissues to be treated with his more proximal arm. He then applies pressure anteriorly and inferiorly with his more distal arm to deform the tissues. Maintaining this pressure, he gradually slides his arm along the length of the hamstring muscle group. As with the prior tech-

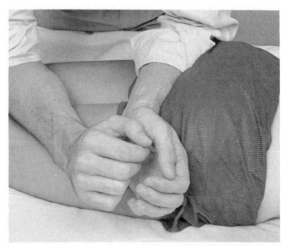

Figure 50-78. General examination and treatment technique for paraspinal musculature: (*A*) starting position, (*B*) mid-range, and (*C*) finishing position.

Figure 50-79. General treatment technique for muscular restrictions.

nique, this stroke includes some evaluation. If decreased muscle play is identified, the progression of the stroke is decreased until the restriction is released. This stroke may be performed at subsequently deeper layers by increasing the anterior pressure.

EXAMINATION AND TREATMENT OF INVOLUNTARY MUSCLE ACTIVITY (SPASMS)

Perpendicular strumming is a technique used for evaluation of muscle play and for the treatment of increased muscle contraction. The technique employs either specific contacts, such as the thumbs, or general contacts, such as the distal phalanges of the fingers. The selection of contact points depends upon the size of the muscle to be treated. With the contact points along the border of the muscle belly and the force directed perpendicular to the long axis of the muscle, the therapist will deform the tissue by pushing into the muscle belly and allowing the edge of the muscle to pass back beneath the contact points. This technique can be performed either unilaterally or bilaterally. In the unilateral technique, the fingers remain on the lateral border of the musculature and oscillate only the lateral border of the muscle belly. The bilateral technique requires that contact be made on both borders of the muscle belly. An example of this technique applied to the lumbar spine follows (Fig. 50-80).

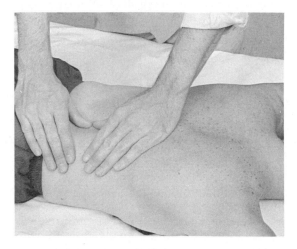

Figure 50-80. Perpendicular strumming to erector spinae muscles.

PATIENT: Prone, with appropriate support.

THERAPIST: Stands on either side of the patient. In this case, where the contralateral side is being treated, the therapist's thumbs would be placed on the medial border of the muscle and the fingertips would be placed on the lateral border.

PROCEDURE: The therapist deforms the muscle laterally with the thumbs, after the medial border has slipped beneath the thumbs, the therapist deforms the muscle medially with the fingers. It is important to maintain a consistent rhythm with this technique and to move the contact surfaces proximally and distally over the muscle belly. To use this technique as an examination tool, the therapist would assess the muscle play as the strumming along the length of the muscle is performed. Areas that revealed decreased play would be examined more closely using the more specific examination techniques.

The perpendicular strumming may also be used in the treatment of involuntarily increased muscle activity or spasm.

PROCEDURE: Once the area of increased activity has been identified, the strumming can be applied over this area. With the treatment technique, the strumming is conducted along the muscle belly until the tone has decreased. The frequency and amplitude of the strumming should be large enough so that the rest of the patient's body oscillates during the treatment.

Alternate methods of treating localized regions of increased muscle activity are sustained pressure techniques. The perpendicular strumming techniques should be used in the treatment of larger regions of increased activity, but the sustained pressure techniques are more specific and should be applied to discrete areas. The body part used to apply the pressure will vary, depending on the size and depth of the area to be treated. Small, superficial regions can be treated with the pad of the thumb or finger, whereas deeper and slightly larger regions may require the use of the tips of all fingers or the elbow. The actual application of the sustained pressure should be with an amount of pressure just less than that which will further increase muscle contraction. As the pressure is maintained by the therapist, the patient's muscle should relax. With relaxation of the muscle the therapist can apply the pressure at a deeper level by allowing the contact surface to sink through the relaxed muscle. This basic technique can be applied with various modifications to increase its effectiveness. Some of these options are as follows: sustained pressure with oscillation of adjacent body parts, sustained pressure with imagery or visualization, sustained pressure with "localized" breathing, and sustained pressure with localized muscle contraction.

One particularly effective application of this technique is with treatment of the psoas muscle. The psoas muscle commonly has localized hyperactivity. This increased activity of the psoas muscle may be the result of lumbosacral dysfunctions, spondylolysis, or postural shortening of the muscle (Fig. 50-81).

PATIENT: Supine, with the hips and knees flexed. This position may be attained by having the patient's feet flat on the plinth, or by placing the legs up on a stool.

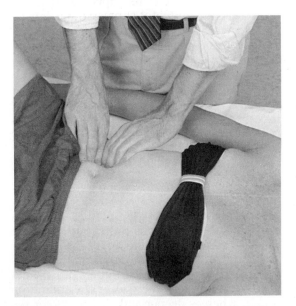

Figure 50-81. Sustained pressure to psoas muscle.

THERAPIST: Standing to the side of the patient on the side to be treated. The fingertips of both hands are placed just lateral to the border of the rectus abdominis muscle at the level of, or just inferior to, the umbilicus.

PROCEDURE: With the patient's abdominal muscles relaxed, the therapist will gently press the fingers posteriorly until the anterior surface of the psoas muscle is contacted. The psoas can be identified by palpation of the muscle belly while the patient gently flexes the ipsilateral hip. If the therapist feels a pulsing sensation, he should move his fingertips laterally to avoid applying sustained pressure to the abdominal aorta. While palpating along the psoas muscle, the therapist may locate regions of increased muscle activity, or the patient may identify areas of tenderness. These regions should be treated with the sustained pressure technique, following the guidelines mentioned previously. The sustained pressure technique to the psoas muscle may be effectively combined with gentle contractions of the muscle.

Comments: Following treatment, the psoas muscle should be less painful to palpation, and it should display a greater resting length.

TRANSVERSE FRICTION MASSAGE

Transverse friction massage is a specific massage technique advocated by Cyriax. It is designed to increase the mobility and deformability of soft tissues. The tissue changes associated with the inflammatory process and with fatigue stress often result in a proliferation of collagen fibers. The excess collagen fibers usually are arranged in a fashion that does not follow the lines of normal stress. This altered alignment may limit the mobility of the repaired tissue over the surrounding tissues, or it may decrease the extensibility of the repaired tissue. Either situation will cause increased stresses to the healing tissue, which will result in further microtrauma, pain, and collagen proliferation.

In general terms, the technique involves applying pressure to the involved tissue with either the pad of the thumb, index finger, or long finger. Then a small-amplitude rubbing motion is applied to the lesioned tissue in a direction perpendicular to the normal orientation of the fibers. Because the amplitude of the stroke is small and the treated tissues are often deep structures, a lubricant is not used.

The patient should be positioned so that the area to be treated is well exposed and the tissue to be treated is under minimal tension. This position is accomplished by placing joints in the loose-packed position if capsular or ligamentous structures are to be treated and by placing muscles in the shortened position if muscles or tendons are to be treated. In addition, the region to be treated should be adequately supported to limit the tension produced by postural muscles. The only exception to this rule is in treating restrictions between tendons and their synovial sheaths. In this instance the muscle should be placed in a lengthened position to stabilize the tendon so that the sheath can be mobilized with the massage.

Once the patient has been adequately positioned, the therapist should be positioned so that the transverse friction massage may be applied to the involved area. To reduce the therapist's muscle tension and to increase personal comfort, the proximal portion of the arm used in treatment should be stabilized and supported. The pad of the finger used in treatment should be placed over the involved area while the rest of the hand lightly grasps the treated region to increase stability. If either the index or long finger is used, the distal phalanx of the other finger can be placed on the distal phalanx of the treating finger. This positioning will enable the therapist to apply more pressure without applying too much stress to the distal interphalangeal joints (DIP) of the fingers.

The initial strokes should be conducted with enough pressure to move the patient's skin along with the therapist's finger, which will reduce the friction between the skin and finger. Friction between the finger and skin, from either too little pressure or too large an amplitude, will cause skin irritation, blistering, and discomfort. The stroking should occur at a rate of 2 to 3 c/sec. Initial mild tenderness is not uncommon, and these initial symptoms should

dissipate within the first two minutes of treatment. After the two minutes of light transverse friction massage, if the initial tenderness has subsided, the amount of pressure should be increased. However, if the symptoms have not subsided, the treatment is terminated and the therapist should reassess the amount of pressure that was applied to the tissue. With the increasing pressure, the depth of the treatment increases. Again, the patient may experience some initial tenderness with the increased depth of treatment. If these symptoms decrease within two minutes of treatment, then the pressure can be increased again. The initial treatment should last approximately five to six minutes. At the end of treatment, the patient's signs and symptoms should be reassessed. If the treatment was effective, an improvement should occur in either the resisted tests or the joint play tests. During subsequent treatments, the depth and duration of the massage can be increased according to the behavior of the signs and symptoms. At the final stages of treatment, the friction massage may last from 10 to 15 minutes. As with other treatment strategies, a successful treatment should result in a decrease in pain and an improvement in active and passive movements. Specific treatment techniques for the right supraspinatus tendon and the coronary ligaments of the right medial meniscus will be described in detail below (Fig. 50-82).

PATIENT: Seated comfortably with the affected arm supported. The support can be applied through either the arm of the chair or properly positioned pillows. The shoulder is placed in either a neutral position or in a slight amount of extension to bring the tendon anterior to the acromion.

THERAPIST: Standing posterior to the patient on the side of the lesion. The pad of the treating finger of the left hand is placed over the tendon, between the acromion and greater tubercle of the humerus. The finger is oriented in an anterior-posterior direction, which is perpendicular to the fibers of the supraspinatus tendon. The rest of the treatment hand lightly grasps the patient's shoulder to stabilize the humerus. The therapist's right hand grasps the

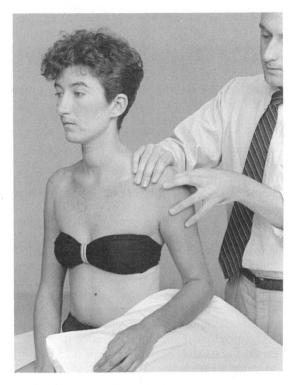

Figure 50-82. Transverse friction massage to supraspinatus tendon.

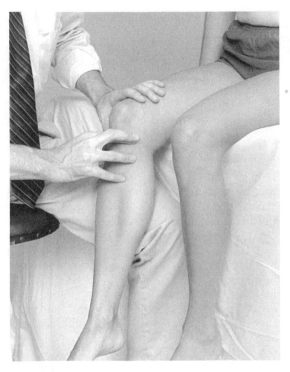

Figure 50-83. Transverse friction massage to coronary ligaments of the meniscus.

patient's shoulder girdle from the superior aspect to provide further stability.

PROCEDURE: Pressure is applied to the tendon through the treating finger, and small-amplitude oscillations are performed in an anterior and posterior direction. The usual sequence of increasing pressure at two-minute intervals is observed. Following treatment, resisted shoulder abduction should be less symptomatic.

Following trauma to the knee, scarring of the coronary ligaments of the meniscus or deep capsular ligaments often occurs. This scarring results in decreased mobility of the meniscus and painful motion of the involved knee. Transverse friction massage to this area often relieves the pain and hypomobility (Fig. 50-83).

PATIENT: To perform this technique on the right medial coronary ligament of the menis-

cus, the patient is seated on the plinth with the knees flexed over the edge.

THERAPIST: Seated on a stool facing the patient, so that the right hand can be placed on the medial joint line. Either the index finger or middle finger, backed by the other finger, is placed on the medial joint line over the scarred tissue. The fingers are pressed laterally into the joint and inferiorly so that the pad of the finger is oriented towards the medial tibial plateau. The rest of the digits of the right hand are placed on the lower leg. The left hand grasps the lateral aspect of the knee to stabilize the joint during treatment.

PROCEDURE: The fingers move in an anterior and posterior direction with the pressure directed inferiorly and laterally. As with the other transverse friction techniques, the initial pressure should be light, and depending upon the signs and symptoms, the subsequent pressures are increased gradually. Following the treatment, the knee should have a greater range of motion with less pain.

The specific techniques described above can be applied to any tendon or ligament that is accessible through the skin. The connective tissue to be treated will display limited mobility and extensibility. If the tissue is a tendon, the isometric resisted tests to the muscle and passive motion in the opposite direction will be painful. If the connective tissue is noncontractile, stressing the structure will reproduce the symptoms. Transverse friction massage in a direction perpendicular to the normal orientation of the connective tissue fibers may improve both the mobility and circulation of the involved structure. After treatment, the mobility of the structure should be increased and stressing the structure should be less painful.

SHIATSU/ACUPRESSURE

Shiatsu is an ancient form of Japanese physical therapy that involves manual pressure over the body's acupuncture points (Schultz). In the view of eastern medicine, health is related to the flow of energy, or *ki,* throughout the body. This energy flow follows specific pathways or meridians that are related to specific organs and the psychosomatic system. The energy flow is accessed through specific points along the meridians; these points are known as acupuncture points. Stimulation of these points will balance the flow of *ki* throughout the body. Restoration of the energy flow will return the patient to a state of health. Although acupuncture and the various methods of acupuncture point stimulation have gained some acceptance in western medicine, the theoretical basis for the effects of this type of treatment are viewed with a degree of skepticism. Research into the effects of acupuncture has tied it to the endogenous opiate system. Despite the controversy over the actual mechanism of healing, acupuncture point stimulation as a method of treatment has the support of numerous clinical reports, from ancient eastern medicine to the current western practice of allopathic medicine.

In simple translation, *shiatsu* means finger pressure, and that is commonly how it is applied. However, various body parts may also be employed in the treatment techniques. For example, the knuckles, palm, elbows, knees, and feet may be used for specific techniques. Another difference between shiatsu and traditional western massage is that very little stroking or massaging is done in shiatsu. The most frequently used techniques are direct pressure on the acupuncture points or a sustained stretch over large body areas. Because no true massaging is done, no need exists for any type of lubricant, such as oils or powders.

As with all treatment plans, it is inadvisable to treat only the symptomatic regions because you may not be treating the cause of the symptoms. Although it is possible to treat only the involved regions with shiatsu, for the unskilled practitioner some authors recommend that the whole body be treated initially. Others do not consider the whole-body treatment to be necessary for all conditions. Moreover, the treatment for symptoms in one area of the body will involve acupuncture points on various aspects of the body that are removed from the symptoms. Treatment of a headache may include acupuncture points on the head, neck, upper extremity, and abdomen. The recommended sequence for treatment of the whole body is as follows: the back, hips and gluteal region, posterior aspects of the lower extremities, plantar aspects of the feet, scapular regions, head and neck, anterior chest wall, anterior aspects of the upper extremities, hands, abdominal region, and the anterior aspects of the lower extremities. The details of the treatment process for the entire body are beyond the scope of this text; however, the portion of the treatment sequence for the back will be described. The recommended treatment techniques for headaches will also be described.

The technique for applying pressure is similar for all body parts. It is important not to gouge the patient or to apply the pressure with the tip of the fingers or elbows. Thumb and finger pressure should be applied with the pad

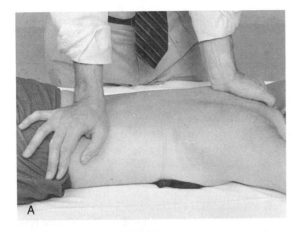

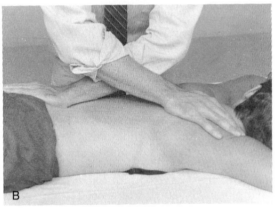

Figure 50-84. (A, B) Diagonal stretch to the back.

THERAPIST: The therapist stands to the side of the patient and places the palm of one hand on the scapula and the other hand on the contralateral gluteal regions (see Fig. 50-84A). While doing this technique, the fingers of the therapist's hands should be abducted to increase the grip and should be pointing away from the other hand.

PROCEDURE: Keeping the elbows straight, the therapist leans over the patient to apply a diagonal stretch to the back. The stretch and subsequent relaxation phases should be synchronized with either the therapist's or the patient's breathing. Ideally, synchronized breathing will develop between both the therapist and patient, with the stretch applied during the patient's exhalation. The stretch is repeated several times along one diagonal. Then the hands are moved to the other scapula and hip, and the process is repeated (see Fig. 50-84B).

The second phase of the back treatment is called the lumbar stretch (Fig. 50-85).

THERAPIST: The therapist stands to the side of the patient. To perform this stretching technique the therapist's arms are crossed, with the palm of one hand placed over the sacrum and the other palm placed on the mid-thoracic region.

PROCEDURE: The therapist leans over the patient and applies a longitudinal stretch to the

of the digit, and not the tip. In addition, when applying pressure with the elbow, the elbow should be partially flexed. This position avoids applying pressure with the tip of the olecranon process, which may be painful. The body part used for the application of the pressure will be determined by the size of the part being treated and the depth of pressure required. The stimulation of each acupuncture point should be held for 10 seconds and repeated three to five times.

The initial phase of treatment for the back is the diagonal stretch (Fig. 50-84).

PATIENT: Throughout the treatment of the back, the patient remains in the prone position with appropriate support.

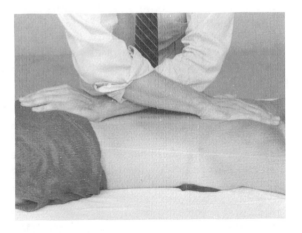

Figure 50-85. Lumbar stretch.

lumbar and lower thoracic spine. As with the diagonal stretch, this technique should be synchronized with the breathing patterns of the therapist and patient, and repeated several times.

The next two steps in the treatment of the back are pressure techniques involving the heel of the hand and the thumbs (Figs. 50-86 and 50-87).

THERAPIST: To apply pressure to the spine with the heel of the hand, the palms are placed on either side of the spine in the mid-thoracic region. The heel of the hand is placed just lateral to the spinous processes, and the palms and fingers lie on the ribs (see Fig. 50-86).

PROCEDURE: Keeping the elbows extended, the therapist leans over the patient, applying pressure to the spine through his hand. When the pressure is relaxed, the therapist moves his hands down to the next vertebral level and repeats the process. In this manner, the treatment will be conducted to the lumbosacral region. The above technique is repeated using the thumbs to apply the pressure (see Fig. 50-87). The thumbs are located paraspinally in the intercostal spaces in the thoracic region and between the adjacent transverse processes in

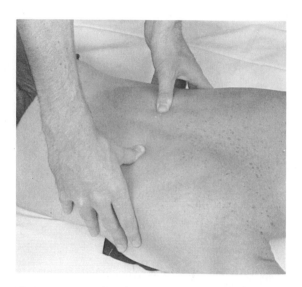

Figure 50-87. Thumb pressure to intercostal spaces.

the lumbar region. As with the stretching techniques, the pressure is applied with the patient's exhalation. The amount of pressure applied to the back should be firm, but it should not reproduce the patient's symptoms.

To finish the treatment of the back, shiatsu may be applied to the sacral and gluteal regions. The treatment sequence for this region consists of thumb pressure over the sacral intervertebral foramen and pressure applied to the gluteal region. Thumb pressure over the sacral intervertebral foramen is applied in the same manner as the thumb pressure to the thoracic and lumbar regions (Fig. 50-88). The first sacral intervertebral foramina are located just superior and medial to the posterior superior iliac spines. The intervertebral foramina at the subsequent levels are located approximately one inch below the preceding level. The foramina are not as easily palpated as the intercostal spaces; consequently, some educated guessing is required. The second portion of this treatment sequence involves pressure applied with the heel of each hand (Fig. 50-89).

THERAPIST: The therapist stands to the side of the patient at the level of the pelvis. The palms are placed on the buttocks with the fingers

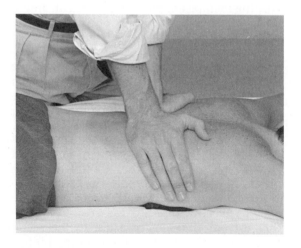

Figure 50-86. Heel of the hand pressure to thoracic and lumbar paraspinal structures.

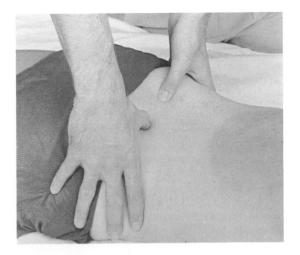

Figure 50-88. Thumb pressure to sacral foramen.

pointing medially and the heel of the hand located just posterior to the greater trochanter of the femur.

PROCEDURE: The pressure is then directed medially through the heel of the hand. As with the other techniques, the pressure is maintained

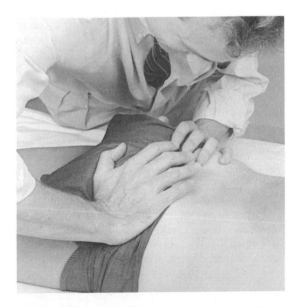

Figure 50-89. Heel of the hand pressure to the gluteal region.

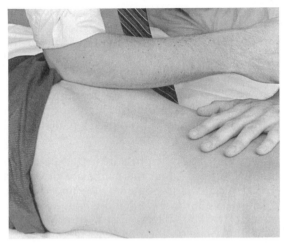

Figure 50-90. Elbow pressure to the gluteal region.

for 10 seconds, repeated three to five times, and coordinated with respiration.

The last portion of this treatment procedure requires elbow pressure to the sacrum and gluteal muscles (Fig. 50-90).

THERAPIST: The therapist places his partially flexed elbow in the sacral sulcus. Following the completion of the sacral pressures, he will position his elbow in the middle of each buttock.

PROCEDURE: With his elbow in the sacral sulcus, the therapist applies pressure in an anterior direction; this is repeated at approximately one-inch intervals to cover the entire length of the sacrum. After treating the sacrum, the therapist will treat the gluteal region. Starting at the iliac crest, the pressure is applied at one-inch intervals inferiorly to the gluteal folds. The sequence is then repeated on the other side.

Comments: In the view of eastern medicine, these techniques will influence the "inner and outer bladder meridians," which are located paraspinally, as well as the "Gall Bladder meridian," which is located posterior to the greater trochanter of the femur. Considering the anatomical structures in this area, recognize that we are applying pressure to the sacral nerve roots, the sciatic nerve, and the piriformis muscle. These structures are often involved in low back pain.

The shiatsu method for treating headaches is a fine example of treating portions of the body that are not symptomatic. Treatment involves pressure applied to the upper extremities, posterior cervical region, and the face. All these regions may be beneficial in the treatment of headaches; however, the acupuncture points on the face are effective in alleviating the symptoms of a sinus headache, and treatment of the posterior cervical region is effective for relieving the pain associated with suboccipital and tension headaches.

Treatment of the upper extremity begins proximally at the shoulder and ends at the web space between the first two digits (Figs. 50-91 to 50-94).

PATIENT: Supine, with the arm abducted slightly and the forearm supinated.

THERAPIST: One hand is placed on the pectoral region to maintain contact with the patient. The therapist's other hand is placed palm down on the arm.

PROCEDURE: Pressure is applied to the patient's arm in a posterior direction. This pres-

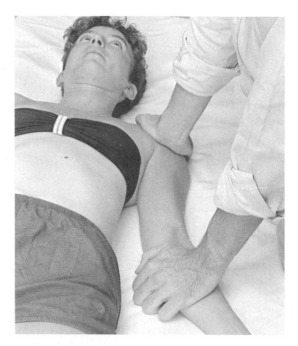

Figure 50-92. Palm pressure to anterior forearm.

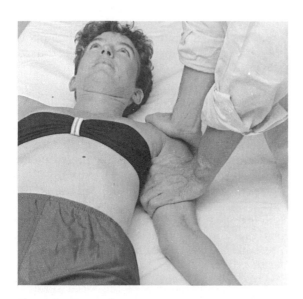

Figure 50-91. Palm pressure to anterior upper arm.

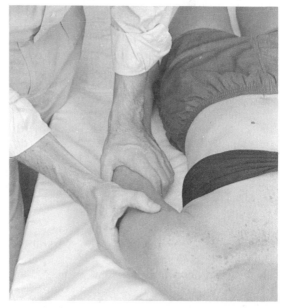

Figure 50-93. Finger pressure to posterior arm.

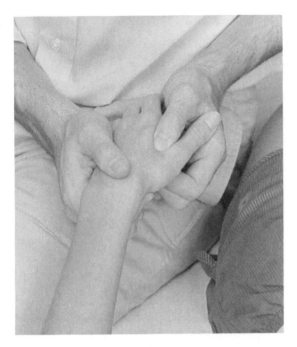

Figure 50-94. Finger pressure to first web space.

sure is applied to the arm from the shoulder to the wrist. The patient will then adduct the shoulder and pronate the forearm. Keeping one hand on the pectoral region, the therapist then holds the arm so he can apply pressure with his fingertips to the posterior aspect (see Fig. 50-93). The posterior portion of the arm is treated in this fashion from shoulders to elbow. The posterior aspect of the forearm is treated with palm pressure from elbow to wrist. Finally, pressure is applied to the acupuncture point located in the web space between the first two digits (see Fig. 50-94). The point is easily located at the proximal end of the crease on the dorsal aspect of the web space. The point is stimulated by pressing it between the therapist's thumb and index finger.
Comments: This sequence of techniques will stimulate the "Small and Large Intestine meridians, Lung meridian, Heart meridian, Triple Heater meridian, and the Heart Protector meridian." The techniques will also be applying pressure along the course of the peripheral nerves in the upper extremity.

The posterior cervical region is treated with finger pressure on various portions of the neck and occipital region.

PATIENT: Supine.

THERAPIST: Standing at the patient's head.

PROCEDURE: Initially, pressure is applied with the middle fingers on either side of the spinous processes from C7 up to the occipital bone. The second portion of the treatment sequence repeats the initial pattern, except that the fingers are positioned just lateral to the cervical paraspinal muscles. In the next part of the sequence, the distal phalanx of one middle finger is placed on top of the contralateral distal phalanx and the pressure is applied between the spinous processes from T1 to C2. The last aspect of the sequence involves applying pressure to the occipital bone, from the suboccipital region out to the mastoid processes. The treatment of the neck can be finished by applying manual distraction to the cervical spine. With each hand cupping the upper cervical spine and occipital region of the head, a gentle distraction force is applied to the neck.
Comments: Again using the terminology of eastern medicine, this sequence will treat the "Bladder and Gall Bladder meridians" and the "Governing Vessel." Pressure is also applied to the cervical nerve roots, the greater and lesser occipital nerves, and over the attachments of the cervical paraspinal and suboccipital musculature.

The initial facial technique applies pressure around the eye (Fig. 50-95 and 50-96).

PATIENT: Supine.

THERAPIST: The therapist places the distal phalanx of either the index or middle finger medial to the inner corner of the eyes.

PROCEDURE: Pressure is applied to these points for three to five seconds. The stimulation is then applied laterally along the supraorbital ridge to the outer corner of the eye. The pressure is then carried medially along the inferior orbital ridge.

The second portion of the facial series is pressure applied to the temples.

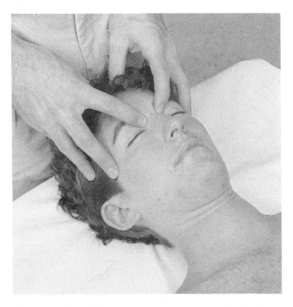

Figure 50-95.   Finger pressure to supraorbital ridge.

PATIENT: Supine.

THERAPIST: The therapist places his fingertips about half an inch superior and lateral to the outer corner of the eye.

PROCEDURE: Pressure is applied to the temporal region by gently rotating the fingertips. The

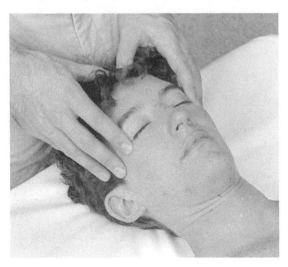

Figure 50-96.   Finger pressure to lateral edge of the orbit.

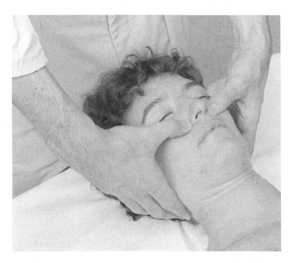

Figure 50-97.   Finger pressure lateral to nasal flares.

stimulation is carried posteriorly to cover the temporalis muscle. Subsequently, a similar technique is performed along the length of the masseter muscles. Lastly, the points just lateral to the nasal flares are stimulated (Fig. 50-97).

Comments: These techniques will stimulate points along the "inner and outer Bladder meridians, Gall Bladder meridian, Large and Small Intestine meridians, and the Stomach meridian." Pressure is also applied to the following anatomical structures: some of the muscles of mastication and facial expression, and portions of the facial and trigeminal nerves.

Acupressure may also be performed in a simpler fashion without following the more involved shiatsu techniques (Schultz). Point stimulation may be performed by stimulating single points along various meridians. As is done in acupuncture, specific points may be selected for treatment of specific conditions, and the stimulation is applied through pressure from various body parts. This pressure is generally performed with either the thumb or finger, but it will vary depending on the size of the person being treated. The selection of points is determined from traditional acupuncture texts, which list the acupuncture points and the expected results.

SWEDISH MASSAGE

Swedish massage includes the traditional massage techniques that are often taught in the physical therapy curriculum. The techniques consist of three generally used strokes: effleurage or stroking, pétrissage or kneading, and friction. The techniques are performed either over the muscle belly or over a portion of the muscle. Because most physical therapists are familiar with the procedures, only a brief description of these techniques will be presented here.

Effleurage is considered synonymous with the term stroking. The effleurage stroke will vary in pressure from slight to firm, which allows tissues to be treated at different levels. Although the direction of the stroke may be either towards or away from the heart with light stroking, when heavy pressure is employed, the stroke should follow the direction of venous flow. Effleurage is usually performed over large anatomical regions or over specific muscles. Whereas no massage medium has been used in the previous techniques, mineral oil, powder, or some other type of lubricant must be used during Swedish massage.

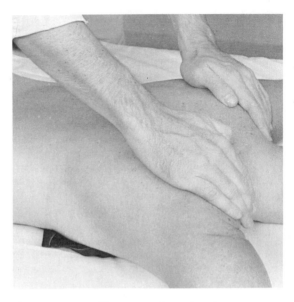

Figure 50-99. Effleurage to thoracic spine.

Using a lubricant decreases the friction between the therapist's hands and the patient's skin during the long stroking techniques. Effleurage to the back and trapezius muscle will be described here (Figs. 50-98 to 50-101).

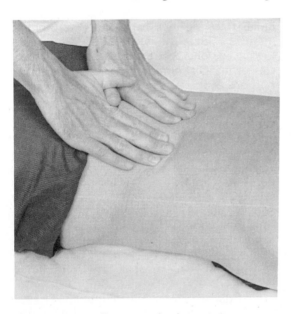

Figure 50-98. Effleurage to lumbar spine.

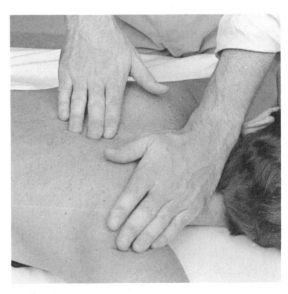

Figure 50-100. Effleurage to upper part of trapezius muscle.

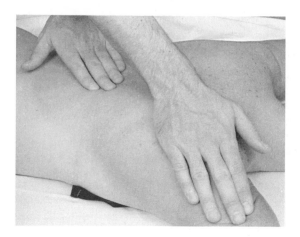

Figure 50-101. Effleurage to lower part of trapezius muscle.

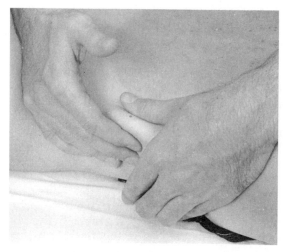

Figure 50-102. Pétrissage to latissimus dorsi muscle.

PATIENT: Prone, with adequate support to the body.

THERAPIST: Standing to one side of the patient, level with the pelvis. The therapist's palms are placed on either side of the lumbar and sacral spinous processes.

PROCEDURE: Effleurage to the entire back is performed bilaterally. The therapist slides the hands along the paraspinal musculature up to the occipital region. From there each hand glides out along the upper trapezius and then back to the midline along the middle trapezius. From this midline position, the hands slide distally to the lumbosacral region. This stroke is repeated three to five times with increasing pressure. Remember that the pressure should be minimal as the hands return to the lumbosacral region from the midline thoracic region.

PROCEDURE: To perform effleurage to the trapezius muscle, the therapist treats first one side and then the other. The stroke is performed along each portion of the trapezius, (upper, middle, and lower) from medial to lateral. The first stroke is performed along the upper trapezius. As this stroke is nearing completion, the therapist's other hand is placed over the middle trapezius. When the stroke to the middle trapezius is nearing completion, the

therapist's other hand is placed over the lower trapezius. This sequence is repeated three to five times on each side.

Pétrissage or kneading is a deeper massage technique performed to individual muscles or portions of these muscles. The technique basically consists of grasping and squeezing a portion of the muscle between the therapist's hands. Pétrissage to the latissimus dorsi muscle will be described here (Figs. 50-102 and 50-103).

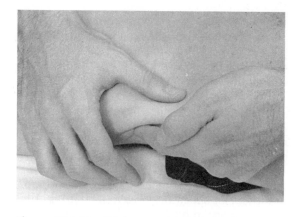

Figure 50-103. Pétrissage to latissimus dorsi muscle.

PATIENT: Prone.

THERAPIST: Standing to the side of the patient, so that the latissimus dorsi muscle may be reached. If the therapist is standing to the left of the patient and is treating the right side of the patient, the ulnar border of the right hand is placed along the lateral border of the muscle. The left thumb is then placed along the medial border of the muscle, in line with the other hand.

PROCEDURE: Using a scooping motion, the therapist grasps the muscle tissue between the two hands and gently squeezes the tissue. As the squeeze is completed, the therapist pronates the right forearm to bring the right thumb along the medial border of the muscle. At the same time, the left forearm is supinated to bring the ulnar border of the left hand along the lateral border of the muscle. The scooping and squeezing technique is then repeated. By repeating this reciprocating motion, the therapist can treat the length of the muscle.

Friction in Swedish massage is a small, circular stroke that is generally performed with firm pressure. The pressure is altered depending upon the patient's condition. The technique is performed sequentially over the entire aspect of the muscle belly. This technique is effective in decreasing fibrotic nodules. Friction to the trapezius muscle will be described here (Fig. 50-104).

PATIENT: Prone.

THERAPIST: Standing at the patient's side, at the level of the thoracic region. The therapist places the treating hand on the patient's upper thoracic region so that the tips of the first and second fingers can be placed in the suboccipital space.

PROCEDURE: Starting just lateral to the spinous process, the therapist performs a small circular stroke over a portion of the upper trapezius muscle. The stroke consists of three to five repetitions over an area about 1.5 inch in diameter. When this small stroke is completed, the therapist slides the fingers laterally to the adjacent portion of the muscle. This sequence is repeated until the therapist reaches the lat-

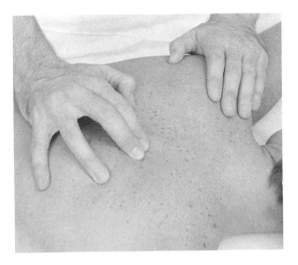

Figure 50-104. Friction to the trapezius muscle.

eral border of the muscle. At that point the fingers are brought back to the midline, and the process is repeated inferior to the previous area.

Although these techniques have been described for specific regions of the back, the strokes can be applied with minimal modification to any specific muscle or anatomical region. As long as the basic principles of pressure and direction are observed, these techniques should be beneficial in reducing muscle activity and increasing muscular mobility.

ANNOTATED BIBLIOGRAPHY

Cyriax J: Textbook of Orthopaedic Medicine: Vol I, Diagnosis of Soft Tissue Lesions, 6th ed. Baltimore, Williams & Wilkins, 1975 (A classic text dealing with differential diagnosis and conservative treatment of musculoskeletal soft tissue lesions.)

Grieve GP: Common Vertebral Joint Problems. New York, Churchill Livingstone, 1981 (The subjective and objective examination at each spinal region is presented in detail. Treatment considerations are presented in reference to pathology and common patterns of clinical presentation.)

Johnson G: Functional Orthopaedics I: Soft Tissue Mobilization, Proprioceptive Neuromuscular Facilitation, and Joint Mobilization. Course notes from the Institute of Physical Art (Detailed description of soft tissue mobilization examination and treatment techniques that were presented in the workshop.)

Kaltenborn F: Manual Therapy for the Extremity Joints, 2nd ed. Oslo, Olaf Norlis Bokhandel, 1976 (Specific joint mobilization treatments based on mechanical principles are illustrated. Especially pertinent are the sections on the wrist and hand and the foot and ankle.)

Lidell L: The Book of Massage. New York, Simon and Schuster, 1984 (Describes traditional massage as well as shiatsu.)

Maitland GD: Peripheral Manipulation. Boston, Butterworth, 1977 (Specific extremity mobilization treatments are illustrated with details about assessment of signs and symptoms. Extremely detailed examination procedures are described.)

Maitland GD: Vertebral Manipulation, 5th ed. Boston, Butterworth, 1986 (Detailed subjective and objective examination methods for the spine are presented. Treatment methods based on assessment of signs and symptoms are illustrated.)

Mennell JM: Joint Pain. Boston, Little Brown & Co, 1964 (Illustrated textbook of extremity manipulation techniques. Differential diagnosis of mechanical joint dysfunction is discussed.)

Mitchell F, Moran P, Pruzzo N: An Evaluation and Treatment Manual of Osteopathic Muscle Energy Procedures. Valley Park, MO, Mitchell, Moran and Pruzzo, Associates, 1979 (Detailed discussion of mechanics, evaluation, and treatment relative to muscle energy procedures. Discusses adjunctive procedures such as correction of muscular length and strength imbalances.)

Mottice M, Goldberg D, Benner EK et al: Soft Tissue Mobilization Techniques. JEMD Co, 1986 (Specific soft tissue mobilization techniques for various anatomical regions are well described.)

Schultz W: Shiatsu: Japanese Finger Pressure Therapy. New York, Bell Publishing Co, 1976 (Provides a clear illustration of the application of shiatsu techniques to various regions.)

Walton WJ: Textbook of Osteopathic Diagnosis and Technique Procedures. St Louis, Matthews Book Co, 1972 (An illustrated textbook of osteopathic manipulative procedures. Differential palpatory diagnosis of acute and chronic spinal segmental lesions is presented.)

Wood CW: Beard's Massage: Principles and Techniques. Philadelphia, WB Saunders, 1974 (A classic text; provides detailed illustrations of traditional Swedish massage techniques to the trunk and extremities.)

Wyke BD: Neurology of the cervical spinal joints. Physiotherapy 65:72, 1979 (Articular mechanoreceptors are discussed with emphasis on their function in cervical pain syndromes. Implications for treatment are presented.)

51 Biobehavioral Techniques

SUSAN J. MIDDAUGH

Biobehavioral treatment procedures apply principles and techniques from behavioral and physiological psychology in patient treatment. This chapter will present information on biofeedback and relaxation training, two biobehavioral treatment procedures that are widely incorporated into physical therapy practice.

Biobehavioral treatment procedures are based on learning principles. They are used to enhance relearning (reeducation) following injury or to enhance acquisition of new therapeutic skills by the patient. In biobehavioral approaches, the patient does not "patiently" await treatment but is always a very active participant, and indeed the primary resource, in the treatment process. The therapist is primarily a teacher whose role is to evaluate the problem, identify what is to be changed, provide learning strategies, monitor progress, and enhance motivation. A close partnership exists between therapist and patient, and the patient takes a large share of the responsibility for his or her own treatment. Biobehavioral treatment approaches also emphasize objective measurement, often through physiological monitoring, as an integral part of the treatment process. This monitoring aids evaluation, guides treatment progression, permits an increased degree of individualization, and provides documentation of treatment outcome. Consequently, biobehavioral procedures lend themselves well to clinical research, and a large body of research supports the use of these relatively new treatment procedures.

EMG MONITORING AND BIOFEEDBACK

One biobehavioral treatment procedure that is highly useful in physical therapy is biofeedback. In clinical biofeedback procedures, physiological recording equipment is used to detect, amplify, and display a physiological response that is to be altered. In electromyographic (EMG) biofeedback procedures, surface electrodes are attached to the skin over a target muscle (or muscle group) and an EMG amplifier is used to record the small electrical signals produced by contracting muscle fibers. These signals are amplified and converted into a visual or auditory signal for display. The patient can then see or hear the muscle contractions and can use this information to guide trial-and-error efforts to contract or to relax the target muscle. An EMG biofeedback device is essentially a teaching tool designed to improve motor learning by providing immediate and accurate information. In therapeutic exercise, a patient may not know whether he is, in fact, contracting the correct muscles or relaxing inappropriate muscles and must rely on the therapist for this information. EMG monitoring can enhance the therapists's ability to provide this vital information.

A strong theoretical basis exists for the use of EMG biofeedback procedures in therapeutic exercise programs. These procedures are based on well-established principles from neurophysiology and learning psychology. In addition, evidence is available, based on a series of controlled experimental studies from my laboratory and the research of other investigators, that EMG biofeedback can improve learning at the level of the muscle. With EMG biofeedback, both normal persons and patients with neuromuscular deficits show (1) improved motor unit recruitment within a muscle when attempting to increase voluntary contraction; (2) improved inhibition of the muscle when attempting muscle relaxation; and (3) improved neuromuscular control when attempting more complex motor tasks. Evidence is also available that EMG biofeedback speeds the motor learning process.

Widespread interest in applying EMG biofeedback in therapeutic exercise programs is justifiably present. However, with biofeedback, as with all treatment methods, it takes considerable time and effort to develop effective treatment protocols and to learn how to carry them out with correct treatment technique. In order to develop optimally effective clinical biofeedback procedures, we need to ask and answer the following questions. What can biofeedback procedures uniquely contribute to the treatment process? Who are appropriate candidates for biofeedback procedures? How should biofeedback sessions be conducted? How should biofeedback be combined with nonbiofeedback procedures to form a total treatment program? Currently, substantial progress is being made in answering these questions in many areas of application, such as stroke and musculoskeletal pain, and EMG biofeedback is recognized as a substantive and important development in therapeutic exercise.

Interestingly, one aspect of EMG biofeedback that is often overlooked is that it has brought EMG recording out of the research laboratory and into the physical therapy clinic. The same EMG equipment that provides feedback for the patient (biofeedback) can also provide feedback for the therapist (muscle monitoring), and the importance of this feedback for the therapist cannot be overestimated. As physical therapists we constantly work with muscles; yet, we often do not know with any

assurance or accuracy what these muscles are actually doing. Surface-recorded EMG, when carried out with appropriate technique, provides valuable information that can be used to evaluate the patient, plan an initial treatment approach, note progress, and alter the treatment plan accordingly. Widespread use of muscle monitoring can only advance our knowledge of neuromuscular function and greatly improve the effectiveness of *all* of our therapeutic exercise procedures, not just biofeedback procedures. The use of EMG monitoring as feedback for the therapist is a major advance with many implications for physical therapy research and practice. Excellent equipment is becoming available at reasonable cost, and the use of EMG monitoring is becoming routine.

EVALUATION AND TREATMENT PRINCIPLES: CHRONIC MUSCULOSKELETAL PAIN

EMG biofeedback and concurrent muscle monitoring procedures have produced significant advances in both the understanding and treatment of chronic musculoskeletal pain, particularly cervical and low back pain. A look at the history and the status of biofeedback applications in this clinical area illustrates how biofeedback concepts have stimulated advances in theory, research, and clinical work. The review also illustrates how these advances have led, over time, to the development of effective biofeedback treatment procedures.

Since the earliest days of biofeedback, considerable interest has been apparent in the use of EMG biofeedback procedures in the treatment of musculoskeletal pain syndromes. However, clinical procedures were initially slow to develop. In addition, effectiveness of early procedures was questionable because of two major assumptions.

The first assumption was that the facial muscles, as muscles of emotional expression, reflected general muscle tension throughout the body. Biofeedback procedures that taught relaxation of these key facial muscles were thought to produce effective relaxation of all other muscles. Because of this assumption,

EMG biofeedback evaluation treatment protocols specified that electrodes be placed on the forehead, over the frontalis muscles bilaterally, while the patient was seated in a recliner.

Investigators have since found that frontalis muscle biofeedback primarily teaches relaxation of the scalp, facial, and jaw muscles, which are all within the actual area of the EMG recording when using forehead electrode placement. One can observe no reliable effect of frontalis muscle biofeedback on other muscles of the body. Investigators have also found that no single muscle reflects general muscle tension and, in fact, no such thing exists as a general level of muscle tension that rises or falls like a tide in muscles throughout the body. When not in use, muscles normally relax completely and rapidly with no motor unit activity. Therefore, no action potentials are present and a constant low level of contraction is not maintained. An individual person may habitually overuse certain muscles and may, for example, frown, clench the jaw, or clench the fists for extended periods of time. However, these habitual muscle contractions are usually localized (hands may be relaxed with jaws clenched) and individualistic (a frowner may not be a fist clencher). As a result of these findings, site-specific electrode placement is used for EMG evaluation of muscles within an area of pain (eg, over the lumbar paraspinous muscles in patients with low back pain). These findings have also stimulated current efforts to develop more appropriate and advanced biofeedback protocols for treatment of patients with chronic musculoskeletal pain (Middaugh and Kee).

The second basic assumption was that sustained muscle contraction was a causative or contributory factor to chronic cervical and low back pain. Pain, often from an initial trauma, was thought to trigger reflexive muscle contractions or "spasms." These muscle spasms, in turn, produced further pain and initiated a continuous pain-spasm-pain cycle. Biofeedback procedures were, therefore, initially designed to teach muscle relaxation in order to eliminate muscle spasm and interrupt this chronic pain cycle.

The search for effective biofeedback treatment procedures has also led to some interesting discoveries about the assumption concerning muscle contraction and pain. The presumed culprit in chronic musculoskeletal pain, the muscle spasm, has proven to be quite elusive. The term "muscle spasm" implies a reflex contraction of muscles surrounding an area of injury. Muscle spasm can be found with acute injury when strong, reflexive muscle contractions can immobilize and protect a painful area. However, multiple studies of lumbar muscle activity in patients with chronic low back pain have produced little evidence that acute muscle spasm actually becomes chronic or that continuous, reflexive muscle contractions are typically present. EMG activity in the paraspinous muscles of a patient with chronic low back pain can be elevated, equal to, or below normal levels. Therefore, one cannot assume a universal, direct, one-to-one causal relationship between muscle tension and pain, design biofeedback treatment protocols accordingly, and expect these procedures to be very effective. Instead, the appropriate course of action is to (1) suspend earlier preconceptions about muscles and pain; (2) develop EMG evaluation procedures that clarify muscle status in the individual patient with pain; and (3) use this information to design truly appropriate EMG biofeedback treatment procedures. This approach has stimulated rapid development of clinically appropriate and effective treatment procedures in the area of chronic pain. A similar approach is needed and is being utilized in many other areas of EMG biofeedback application, such as reeducation of upper extremity muscles following stroke.

CLINICAL APPLICATIONS: CHRONIC MUSCULOSKELETAL PAIN

EMG monitoring is used to evaluate muscles in the area of pain in patients with chronic cervical and low back pain. These evaluation procedures have added substantially to our knowledge of the muscular components of chronic pain and have stimulated the development of biofeedback interventions that are firmly grounded on objective findings. This combination of EMG evaluation and biofeedback has provided rapid advances in understanding and treating chronic musculoskeletal pain. EMG evaluations indicate that muscle involvement exists in many patients with chronic pain. However, EMG findings do not support the prevalent explanation of a reflexive pain-spasm-pain cycle; instead, they indicate that postural problems and poor patterns of muscle use (which can include almost constant muscular bracing and guarding) produce most of the muscular problems found in these patients. EMG evaluation is useful for identifying these problems, and EMG biofeedback is useful for treating these problems when they (1) are based on the EMG evaluation findings, (2) use site-specific electrode placements, and (3) employ dynamic rather than static training procedures.

EMG Evaluation of Cervical or Shoulder Girdle Pain

Patients with pain in the cervical or shoulder girdle areas most frequently report muscle soreness and pain unilaterally or bilaterally in the areas shown in Figure 51-1. These patients are always evaluated bilaterally using one or both of the electrode placements shown in Figure 51-2, according to the area of reported pain. Readings are typically obtained from two sites at a time, usually from the same muscle group on the right and the left. EMG is first recorded during quiet sitting to note muscle activity at rest and then during several repetitions of test movements designed to assess the muscle use during cervical and upper extremity movements and muscle relaxation following contraction. Standard test movements are cervical rotation to the right and left, shoulder shrug, and shoulder abduction to horizontal. Finally, the muscle is observed during quiet standing.

EMG evaluation of patients with chronic cervical or shoulder girdle pain indicates that the majority (65%) do show elevated EMG activity in painful muscles during quiet sitting, but many do not (35%). The most significant finding (in 85% to 90% of patients) is slow or incomplete relaxation of the muscles after use. Painful muscles often take minutes to relax

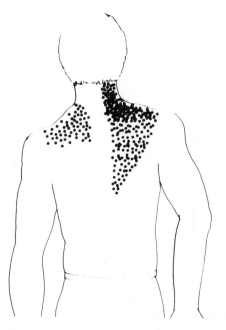

Figure 51-1. Common areas of reported pain in patients with chronic cervical and shoulder girdle pain.

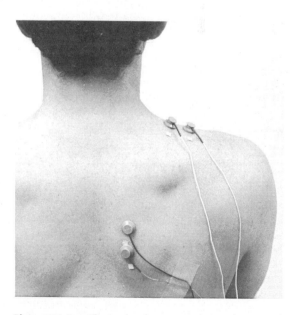

Figure 51-2. Electrode placements for evaluation of patient with chronic cervical and shoulder girdle pain.

after a brief cervical or arm movement; in comparison, nonpainful muscles normally relax rapidly, often in two to three seconds. Painful muscles may contract inappropriately for extended periods of time, and thus, muscle factors are strongly implicated as major contributors to chronic pain in many patients with cervical or shoulder girdle pain. However, this muscle hyperactivity does not have the characteristics of reflexive muscle spasm. No sudden onset of increased pain occurs with increased muscle contractions, and no indications are present by EMG or patient report of muscles grabbing or cramping during the testing. Instead, patients are usually not aware that their muscles are contracting at all, and the pain is unchanged when the muscle relaxes completely. Muscular pain appears to result from excessive use of these muscles for protective guarding and postural bracing that has become habitual and almost continuous. This chronic overuse keeps the muscles sore, and the muscle soreness undoubtedly reinforces the guarding and bracing.

EMG Biofeedback Treatment of Cervical or Shoulder Girdle Pain

EMG evaluation procedures provide information on the individual patient, muscle by muscle, which leads naturally to appropriate treatment with EMG biofeedback. Figure 51-3 shows the raw EMG signal as it appears on an oscilloscope screen. In Figure 51-3*A*, a 64-year-old man with unilateral (right) cervical pain of

many years duration as a result of an industrial accident showed normal, relatively complete relaxation of the right and left upper trapezius muscles during quiet sitting (ECG artifact is present in the left tracing). However, whenever the patient talked (Fig. 51-3*B*), the muscles on the painful right side contracted continuously and strongly. The right upper trapezius muscle also showed excessive contraction and slow relaxation with other activities, such as standing, walking, and upper extremity use. For this patient, the EMG feedback training procedure was obvious. The patient was provided with a single-channel auditory feedback tone that signaled muscle activity in the right upper trapezius muscle. Using this tone as a guide, he practiced (1) relaxing the upper trapezius muscle, reliably and rapidly, following brief cervical and upper extremity movements; (2) maintaining good relaxation while talking, standing, and walking; and (3) developing improved sensory awareness of muscle contraction and muscle relaxation. Muscle soreness subsided gradually as muscle control improved over the course of eight weekly outpatient sessions, with daily practice without biofeedback at home. These sessions also included relaxation training and active exercise (discussed later in the chapter).

EMG Evaluation of Low Back Pain

Patients with chronic low back pain are evaluated using electrode placements over the paraspinous muscles (thoracic or lumbar, according

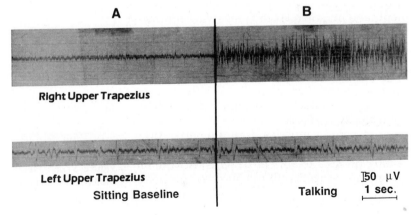

Figure 51-3. EMG recordings from the upper trapezius muscles of a 64-year-old man with right shoulder and cervical pain: (*A*) during quiet sitting, and (*B*) while talking. ECG artifact is present on bottom tracing.

A   **B**

Right Upper Trapezius

Left Upper Trapezius

Sitting Baseline   **Talking**

50 μV
1 sec.

to area of pain) as shown in Figure 51-4. Recording is from two sites at a time, usually over the same muscle group on the right and left. The EMG is recorded while the patient is standing quietly and also during several repetitions of brief test movements (typically, forward trunk flexion, trunk extension, and trunk rotation) designed to assess muscle use during trunk movements and muscle relaxation following contraction. The EMG is also recorded while the patient is sitting with the back supported.

EMG evaluation indicates that a majority (61%) of patients with chronic low back pain have elevated EMG activity in the paraspinous muscles during quiet standing. However, many similar patients (39%) do not. In most patients the paraspinous muscles relax quickly and completely once the patient sits down. Unlike cervical pain patients, only a small minority of low back patients (26%) show retarded muscle relaxation following contraction. The primary finding for these patients has been disruption of the normal, reciprocal pattern of muscle use during trunk rotation. The normal contraction pattern is illustrated in Figure 51-5: When the trunk rotates to the right, the left lumbar muscles contract more strongly; when the trunk rotates to the left, the muscles reverse and the right lumbar muscles contract more strongly. Deviations from this normal pattern

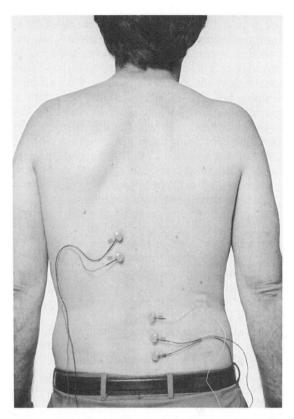

Figure 51-4. Electrode placements for evaluation of patient with chronic low back pain. The ground is the upper lumbar electrode.

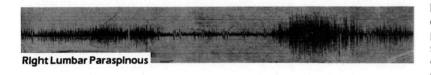

Right Lumbar Paraspinous

Left Lumbar Paraspinous

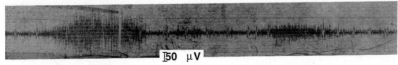

50 μV

Rotation to the Right   2 sec   **Rotation to the Left**

Figure 51-5. EMG recording of lumbar muscles of a normal, pain-free, 40-year-old man showing normal reciprocal contraction of these muscles during standing trunk rotation. ECG artifacts are present on both tracings.

are seen in 87% of the patients. The most common deviation (seen in 65% of patients) is illustrated in Figure 51-6, which shows the lumbar muscles of a 42-year-old woman with a four-year history of low back pain as a result of a serious fall (no surgery). Trunk rotation is guarded and slow. In addition, muscles on both the right and left contracted with rotation in either direction, indicating mass action of the low back muscles. Other patients underused painful muscles on one or both sides during attempted trunk rotation.

Muscle factors do play a role in chronic low back pain; however, as with cervical pain patients, little evidence exists of muscle spasm. Instead, poor posture is the primary cause of elevated EMG while standing. For example, many patients shift weight away from a painful leg or hip, and this posture produces a unilateral contraction of the low back muscles in an effort to stabilize the pelvis. Many patients also stand with the trunk continuously flexed, thus shifting the center of gravity forward of the midline and causing the low back muscles to contract, often forcefully and bilaterally, to counteract gravity. A second major cause of EMG abnormality is protective guarding and bracing, which produces abnormal patterns of muscle use during trunk movements. Most patients with chronic low back pain have a substantial problem with inappropriate and inefficient use of the low back muscle for posture

and movement. These EMG findings are consistent with the clinical observations of Cailliett and others that most patients with chronic low back pain have major postural problems that probably develop in response to the pain, increase musculoskeletal strain, and contribute to pain chronicity.

EMG Biofeedback Treatment of Low Back Pain

EMG evaluation provides a rational basis for EMG biofeedback treatment of individual patients with low back pain. EMG biofeedback is most often used for postural retraining. EMG biofeedback (with a dual-channel visual display) is used to demonstrate the adverse effects of poor standing (or sitting) posture on the low back muscles and to teach correct posture. Although all patients with low back pain are repeatedly told that posture is important, a biofeedback display reinforces this instruction in a way that is concrete and effective. The required postural adjustments can be subtle, and a therapist working with a biofeedback display can often coach the patient in a way that the therapist working alone cannot. For example, a patient can often reduce strong, bilateral lumbar muscle contractions with slight pelvic tilt and slight knee flexion.

A second use of EMG biofeedback, in selected patients who show poor muscle relaxation following movement, is to teach relax-

Figure 51-6. EMG recordings from the lumbar muscles of a 42-year-old woman with bilateral low back pain during standing trunk rotation to the right. ECG artifacts are present on both tracings.

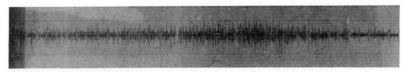

Right Lumbar Paraspinous

Left Lumbar Paraspinous

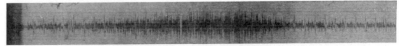

$\overline{J}50$ μV

2 sec

ation of problem muscles following brief trunk and upper extremity movements, both sitting and standing. Portable EMG biofeedback units (with a single audio channel) are often used to encourage frequent practice during daily activities. In all cases, biofeedback practice is interspersed with nonfeedback practice, and training continues until the patient learns the "feel" of the correct response and can perform reliably on nonfeedback trials (verified by EMG monitoring). Such training with objective verification is very practical with EMG biofeedback but difficult, if not impossible, without it.

RELAXATION TRAINING

A second biobehavioral treatment approach is relaxation training. Substantial experimental evidence indicates that emotional stress has physiological effects mediated by neural and humoral systems, and that these effects can be deleterious. Relaxation training is designed to reduce emotional stress and thereby reduce or prevent these stress-related effects.

Emotional stress can affect many systems of the body, including the immune system. Of particular interest to physical therapists are the effects of stress-related physiological arousal on the neuromuscular, respiratory, and circulatory systems. Emotional distress also has cognitive consequences; it can interfere with the patient's ability to attend, learn, and remember, and so can decrease the effectiveness of any therapeutic intervention. Therefore, relaxation training is a versatile tool with many different applications.

One major use of relaxation training is in prevention of health problems. Relaxation training is routinely included in programs designed to promote and maintain health and wellness, and such programs are being offered in many community, school, and business settings. The use of relaxation training is supported by experimental evidence that stress affects the immune system and can increase susceptibility to experimental infections or implanted tumors. Animal studies have shown that corticosteroids are released during stress, and these adrenal hormones can suppress im-

mune function by reducing the number of circulating T lymphocytes. Research has also shown that emotional stress can reduce immunocompetence in humans. Moreover, the stress need not be unusually severe or prolonged to produce such negative effects; a variety of relatively common stressors, such as final exams, have been shown to alter immune system function. Evidence exists that therapeutic interventions that are designed to reduce stress have beneficial effects. Relaxation training has been found to enhance immunocompetence (an increase in natural killer cell activity) in geriatric persons (Kiecolt-Glaser and coworkers). These findings are important because decrements in immunocompetence are normally associated with aging. Therefore, relaxation procedures promise to be particularly valuable for maintaining health and wellness in this "at risk" population.

A second major application of relaxation training is in the treatment of patients with diseases such as diabetes and hypertension. Relaxation training procedures are added to treatment programs for their positive physiological effects. Relaxation training also has many applications in rehabilitation. Such training is routinely included in cardiac rehabilitation, in the treatment of asthma and other respiratory disorders, and in the treatment of headache and chronic musculoskeletal pain. Many other uses of relaxation training in rehabilitation programs are possible for neurological patients. Patients with spasticity (eg, cerebral palsy, cerebrovascular accident [CVA], spinal cord injury) frequently report intensification of this symptom when under emotional stress, and sound neurophysiological reasons can explain why this occurs. Serious consideration should be given to providing relaxation training for such patients to counteract these stress-related effects.

CLINICAL APPLICATION OF RELAXATION TRAINING

Contemporary relaxation procedures are based on the concept that relaxation is a complex psychological and physiological skill that is learned with instruction and practice over time (two to three months or more). Relaxation training procedures are multifaceted and combine several different techniques to train the various major components of the relaxation complex systematically. Most often, these techniques are designed to improve muscle relaxation, reduce sympathetic nervous system arousal, improve the rate and pattern of breathing, and increase mental concentration and control. Physiological monitoring is used to evaluate patients and verify progress in achieving relaxation goals, and biofeedback is often included as an instructional tool.

Relaxation training is most effective when taught as an active coping skill over which the patient can exert personal control, rather than as a passive, escape-oriented procedure. Patients need to learn how to relax, but the acquisition of basic relaxation skills is only the first step. Patients must learn how to *apply* these relaxation skills effectively in the context of their daily activities and under stressful conditions. For this learning to occur, detailed instruction by, and interaction with, a skilled therapist over a period of weeks or months is necessary. Instructional tapes can be helpful, particularly for home practice. Patients who are systematically taught relaxation skills and how to use these skills effectively in a series of weekly sessions with daily homework benefit substantially.

ASSESSMENT OF STRESS-RELATED RESPONSES

EMG is initially recorded over the upper trapezius muscle, because this muscle is frequently involved in muscular bracing and mass action patterns. Other muscles may also be observed as training progresses. Respiration is assessed by counting respiratory cycles and observing the respiratory pattern (chest versus abdominal excursion, and regular versus erratic rate). Hand temperature provides an easily monitored and useful index of autonomic arousal. A reduction in sympathetic nervous system activity reduces peripheral vasoconstriction, and the resulting vasodilation increases skin temperature. These measures are repeated to as-

sess progress in learning the relaxation procedures.

A TREATMENT PROTOCOL

Under stress, patients are often muscularly "on guard" and may show considerable muscle bracing even when sitting still. Mass muscle action is also common, and patients use many more muscle groups than actually needed to perform a given activity. Patients often develop a shallow, rapid, erratic upper-chest breathing pattern that can easily lead to hyperventilation. Signs of autonomic nervous system arousal (sympathetic predominance) can be apparent in gastrointestinal symptoms or cardiovascular signs (blood pressure elevations, cardiac arrhythmias, peripheral vasoconstriction). Mental concentration can be poor, and patients may be easily distracted. Reactions to stress are highly individualistic, and a given patient may show few or many of these characteristics. Stress symptoms may be largely episodic, or may be present almost continuously. Basic relaxation skills include progressive muscle relaxation, diaphragmatic breathing, and guided imagery. The patient must learn how to apply these relaxation skills to everyday situations.

Training goals are (1) maintenance of relatively complete muscle relaxation in the target muscle; (2) regular respiration at 8 to 12 breaths per minute with minimal upper-chest excursion; and (3) hand warming to 94°F (or higher) during a 15-minute relaxation period.

The patient is taught a progressive muscle relaxation (PMR) procedure, with consists of gently tensing, briefly holding, and then relaxing major muscle groups, beginning with the feet and ending with the face, while sitting (not reclining) in a comfortable chair. Homework consists of practicing relaxation with an instructional tape twice a day with attention to (1) recognizing tension and relaxation in each of the muscle groups, (2) tensing only the target muscle group while leaving all other muscles relaxed, and (3) breathing regularly and learning not to hold the breath while tensing. Patients progress from this tense-relax PMR procedure to a think-relax PMR procedure, in which the same muscle groups are relaxed without tensing them first. Patients are encouraged to notice throughout the day whether they are excessively tensing muscles or holding the breath during daily activities.

The patient is also taught diaphragmatic breathing, first supine and then sitting. Once the correct diaphragmatic pattern is established, the patient is instructed to slow the breathing rate to 8 to 12 breaths per minute. Patients should practice diaphragmatic breathing for five minutes at a time several times a day.

Guided imagery is the third relaxation procedure. While relaxing his muscles and breathing correctly, the patient imagines a relaxing scene of his own choosing and maintains a clear mental focus on that scene for 10 to 15 minutes. This process improves mental concentration and control.

The patient also learns to combine relaxation techniques in a brief, 30-second relaxation procedure that can be carried out while sitting, standing, and walking. This procedure consists of taking one deep breath and concentrating on relaxing the muscles (face, shoulders, arms) while breathing out, and then taking four or five slow diaphragmatic breaths, relaxing further with each exhalation. Patients practice this brief relaxation procedure frequently throughout the day. The goal is to establish relaxation as a habit under a wide variety of conditions and to prevent stress reactions before they occur.

Regular practice over a two- to three-month period is essential. In addition, effective stress management usually requires more than learning to relax when faced with stress; it also involves learning to identify and eliminate (when possible) the sources of stress. Alterations in life-style and a reordering of priorities may be necessary, and patients may need concurrent work with a psychologist or other counselor to achieve effective stress management.

This basic relaxation training program can easily be combined with a wide variety of other therapeutic procedures as needed. For example, EMG biofeedback procedures can assist muscle relaxation, and temperature biofeedback training (hand warming) can aid autonomic learning. Frontalis muscle EMG biofeedback can be helpful in improving mental concentration and control.

BIOBEHAVIORAL TREATMENT PROGRAMS

CHRONIC PAIN REHABILITATION PROGRAMS

EMG monitoring, biofeedback, and relaxation training are well-recognized components of multidisciplinary programs for rehabilitation of chronic pain. Patients who have had pain on a daily basis for six months or longer (often cervical or low back pain) that has not responded to standard medical or surgical procedures can benefit substantially from a comprehensive rehabilitation program designed to reduce both the physical disability and the psychological distress that are typically produced by persistent pain.

Medical care is primarily directed toward diagnosis and medication management. Narcotics are systematically reduced and replaced with non-narcotic analgesics and antidepressant medication, if indicated. Physical therapy care emphasizes posture and body mechanics and includes a systematic exercise program to improve strength, flexibility, and endurance. An aerobic exercise component (bicycling, walking, or swimming) has beneficial effects on mood (reducing depression and anxiety), sleep, and fitness. Occupational therapy emphasizes energy conservation and work efficiency to increase tolerance for daily activities at home and on the job. Clinical psychology is directed toward teaching the patient how to understand and manage the physical, emotional, and cognitive effects of persistent pain. Patients are taught to select and pace activities more appropriately to stabilize, and then systematically increase, the amount and range of daily activities. The goal is to resume gradually a more normal and satisfying life-style.

The biofeedback treatment component for

these patients typically includes EMG monitoring for evaluation, site-specific biofeedback, and relaxation training as described in the preceding sections. EMG biofeedback is designed to teach relaxation and appropriate use of muscles in the areas of pain for posture and daily activities (eg, writing, driving, walking). Relaxation training is directed toward reducing the physiological and cognitive effects of pain-related stress.

These treatment components overlap in a deliberate and constructive manner. Emphasis is on patient education, responsibility, and self-help with daily homework. By the end of treatment, the patient should be working effectively with a daily home program and applying the procedures taught in the program. Approximately 50% to 75% of patients treated in multidisciplinary pain programs make substantial improvements, continue a home program, and maintain their gains.

PRE-CHRONIC PAIN AND HEADACHE PROGRAMS

A similar but individualized and streamlined treatment program can be highly effective for two other groups of patients. One group consists of patients with musculoskeletal pain that continues past the acute care stage (longer than two months). These patients have pain that is less severe, less continuous, or less long standing than the patients discussed above, but they are progressing toward the chronic pain stage. A second group consists of patients with muscle contraction or vascular headache. These two groups of patients may benefit substantially from a physical therapy program that combines relaxation training and EMG biofeedback with a therapeutic exercise program. Many of these patients will also benefit from clinical psychology for assistance with stress management, life-style change, and medication reduction. Patients with severe episodic headaches, such as migraine, are particularly likely to require this second component in order to achieve lasting improvements.

CONCLUSION

Biofeedback and relaxation training procedures are versatile, effective, and highly useful new facets of physical therapy practice. These biobehavioral treatment approaches combine behavioral principles and procedures with more traditional practices to enhance treatment outcome. These procedures also encourage use of physiological monitoring for evaluation of patients, individualization of treatment, and documentation of patient gains. These biobehavioral procedures have many different applications in rehabilitation, and make a substantial contribution to treatment of chronic musculoskeletal pain.

ANNOTATED BIBLIOGRAPHY

Bennett RM (ed): Fibrositis and fibromyalgia syndrome: current issues and perspectives. Am J Med, 81(3A), 1986 (This journal supplement contains the proceedings of a symposium on the title topic with papers and discussions by authorities in the field of musculoskeletal pain.)

BMA Audio Cassettes, A Division of Guilford Publications, 200 Park Avenue South, New York, NY 10003 (This catalog lists many widely used cassette tapes for relaxation training including those by T. Budzynski, J. Procter, and M.S. Schwartz.)

Cailliett R: Low Back Pain Syndrome. Philadelphia, FA Davis, 1981 (This book illustrates the contribution of faulty posture in low back pain.)

Davis M, Eshelman ER, McKay M: The Relaxation and Stress Reduction Workbook. Oakland, New Harbinger Publications, 1982 (This workbook contains information on many different techniques for relaxation and stress management.)

Fried R: The Hyperventilation Syndrome: Research and Clinical Treatment. Baltimore, The Johns Hopkins University Press, 1987 (This book contains a wealth of information on the physiological effects of hyperventilation, the role of faulty respiration in clinical syndromes such as migraine, and methods for breathing retraining.)

Kiecolt-Glaser JK, Glaser R, Williger D et al: Psychosocial enhancement of immunocompetence in a geriatric population. Health Psychol 4:25, 1985 (This journal article presents a study of the beneficial effects of relaxation training on immune system function in the elderly.)

Middaugh SJ: Muscle training. In Doleys DM, Meredith RL, Ciminero AR (eds): Behavioral Medicine: Assessment and Treatment Strategies, p 145. New York, Plenum Press, 1982 (This book chapter contains an extensive review of the literature related to biofeedback and relaxation training in rehabilitation.)

Middaugh SJ, Kee WG: Advances in Electromyographic Monitoring and Biofeedback in Treatment of Chronic Cervical and Low Back Pain. In Eisenberg MG and Grzesiak RC (eds): Advances in Clinical Rehabilitation, p 137. New York, Springer Publishing, 1987 (This book chapter contains a review, with references, of studies related to EMG evaluation and EMG biofeedback in patients with chronic musculoskeletal pain. It also contains detailed information on the EMG evaluation and treatment procedures outlined in this chapter.)

Miller NE: Effects of emotional stress on the immune system. Pavlov J Biol Sci 20:47, 1985 (This journal article contains a short, readable review of the title topic.)

Selye H: Stress in Health and Disease. Boston, Butterworths, 1976 (This book is an extensive annotated bibliography on the physiological effects of stress, including effects on muscular function [p 671] and the muscular system [p 704].)

Wall PD, Melzack R (eds): Textbook of Pain. New York, Churchill Livingstone, 1984 (This book contains extensive reviews and current information on theory, research, and treatment in the area of pain.)

52 Prosthetics and Orthotics

DAVID E. KREBS

Prostheses and orthoses (P&O) are mechanical or electrical appliances that permit the neurologically or orthopedically disabled patient to move with maximum freedom and with minimum discomfort and inconvenience. Limb prostheses are commonly known as "artificial limbs," while orthoses are sometimes called "braces."

Physical therapists participate with the clinic team's prosthetic and orthotic effort in prescription of and training with appliances fabricated by prosthetists and orthotists. To do so, physical therapists assess the patient's kinesiological deficiencies prior to provision of the device, review or "check out" the device after fabrication to determine whether it is safe and effective enough to be used permanently as a definitive appliance or only temporarily for training, and finally instruct the patient in use and care of the device.

According to the best available estimates, approximately 400,000 amputees are in the United States, and roughly 10 times that number require an orthosis. Good data describing orthosis users are sparse; however, data concerning the population of persons having major limb amputation (ie, loss of a limb segment proximal to the carpals or tarsals) are fairly reliable. Approximately 70% of the amputee population, the majority of whom are adults, has a lower limb deficiency. Among the 10% of amputees who are under 21 years old, the largest category have below-elbow amputations. Chronologically, then, most individuals with congenital (ie, at birth) amputations have up-per-limb deficiencies; most individuals with acquired amputations to age 21 are either below-elbow, generally from gunshot or heavy-equipment trauma, or above-knee, generally from carcinomas; the incidence of amputation is rather low in individuals from age 21 to 50, and most have amputations at varying anatomical levels and etiologies primarily related to motor vehicle and workplace injuries; and most all individuals after age 50 have amputations of the lower limbs, secondary to vascular diseases.

HISTORY AND CURRENT STATUS

Historically, improvements in materials and technology have augmented prosthetic and orthotic options. Although advances in surgical and pharmaceutical treatment of limb and spinal cord disorders have also contributed to rehabilitation of the neurologically and orthopedically impaired, prosthetic and orthotic care is largely based on biotechnical matching. Articulated, or jointed, limbs were available only to the very wealthy until the Civil War. Leather-lined sockets were used in most prostheses until the advent of thermoplastics in the late 1950s; leather-lined metal orthoses were by far the most common until as recently as the early 1980s. At present, the use of polymer plastics and composite carbon-fiber materials originally developed for the aircraft industry contribute substantially to affording lighter weight and more suitable materials for prosthetic-orthotic devices.

In general, designers of state-of-the-art P&O devices strive to provide the patient with the maximum *comfort, function, and appearance.* These three factors are the dimensions used in both research and clinical assessment of patient acceptance of a given P&O approach. Clearly, patient perceptions of their appliances are affected both by the appliance *per se* and by the psychological factors of each patient. A growing body of literature addresses the psychology of the disabled and P&O patients in particular, so a few common themes may be described.

PSYCHOLOGICAL CONSIDERATIONS

Just as each therapist has a unique personality, so does each patient, and neither amputation nor motor disability negates that fact. Perhaps surprisingly, the psychology of the disabled as a professional discipline began only in the 1940s.

In general, the conclusion of the research is that the process of psychologically dealing with a prosthesis or orthosis parallels that of survivors coping with death: the stages of denial, anger, and so forth ultimately yield to acceptance and a continuation of life.

Furthermore, persons who have well-integrated, "normal" personalities prior to disability onset are better able to cope with the stresses of disease and are on the whole better rehabilitation candidates. Conversely, persons who have poorly integrated personalities or who are excessively neurotic adjust poorly to disability and do not function in society to their maximum potential.

PROSTHETICS

Replacement of a body part with a prosthesis is important to several fields. "False teeth" are replacement teeth; an "artificial hip" is an orthopedic implant, and both are prosthetic devices. Physical therapists are responsible for treating patients with upper- or lower-limb

prostheses (ULPs or LLPs, respectively). This chapter will consider only upper-limb prostheses or lower-limb prostheses.

All limb prostheses have at minimum a socket and a terminal device (TD). The socket juxtaposes the residuum (ie, the residual limb, or "stump") and the prosthesis; the TD connects the amputee and the prosthesis to the external environment. In all cases, the comfort of a prosthesis is chiefly related to socket adequacy, while its function is chiefly related to the weight, position, and ease of operation of the TD.

The socket performs at least three roles: It contains the residuum tissues; provides a means of suspending the limb; and transfers forces from the residuum to the prosthesis and thence to the floor. The TD for an upper-limb prosthesis is a hand or a hook; for a lower-limb prosthesis it is almost invariably a foot.

LOWER-LIMB PROSTHETICS

Virtually all lower-limb amputees wear a prosthesis, and thus are within the scope of treatment of the physical therapist. Unlike the upper-limb amputee who can function rather well with only one sound hand, the lower-limb amputee requires a replacement limb to function with a semblance of normal mobility. Therapists must possess specific knowledge of the mechanical behavior of prostheses and of the biomechanics and functional capacities of lower-limb amputees to generate the best biotechnical match among the various component options and the patient's needs. Therapists then teach the patient to function harmoniously with the prosthesis to effect smooth and safe ambulation and activities of daily living.

Biomechanics

Biomechanical considerations in P&O largely fall into two categories: the biomechanics of tissue and the biomechanics of propulsion. With respect to tissue biomechanics, the means by which loads are transferred to the residuum-prosthesis interface and the behavior of the "pseudoarthrosis" between the prosthesis and residuum are of paramount importance. Apropos of propulsion biomechanics, the alignment of the prosthesis and the mechanical behavior of its components are chiefly of interest. Both categories are interrelated. Changing the socket's alignment will undoubtedly affect tissue load transfer, and changing the socket's shape will often alter the alignment and thus the amputee's gait.

Tissue Biomechanics

The ability of various tissues to accept loading is important in designing a comfortable prosthesis. Patients experience the loading forces as pressures (where pressure=force/area). Pressure-sensitive areas are accommodated prosthetically either by mechanically relieving or eliminating the loading forces or by distributing the forces over a larger area. Pressure-tolerant tissues accept loads with minimal discomfort and thus serve as bulwarks in protecting pressure-sensitive areas of the residuum and in transferring weight and other forces between the amputee and the socket to the ground.

Mechanisms for Achieving Selective Pressure Distribution. Physical therapists must be acutely aware of each tissue's tolerance because prosthetic sockets are designed to exploit fully the various capabilities of residuum tissues. Although a socket that contacts the entire residuum (ie, a "total-contact" socket) is widely accepted as optimal for patient comfort, total-contact sockets require careful and skillful efforts by the prosthetist who makes the device.

Pressure-tolerant anatomical areas are juxtaposed to the socket with greater force by "building up" the socket, and pressure-sensitive areas are relieved by putting less material against the amputation limb. Thus, during check-out of the prosthesis, the therapist must ensure that the entire residuum firmly contacts the socket, that the reliefs and build-ups are appropriate, and that the patient is comfortable before accepting the device as adequate.

Above-Knee Pressure Tolerances. Pressure-sensitive areas of typical above-knee (AK) residua include (in approximately ascending order of

tolerance) the distolateral cut end of the femur, the pubic symphysis, the perineal area, and, rarely, the distal residuum end (Fig. 52-1). Pressure-tolerant AK residuum areas include (in approximately descending order of tolerance) the ischial tuberosity, the gluteal mass,

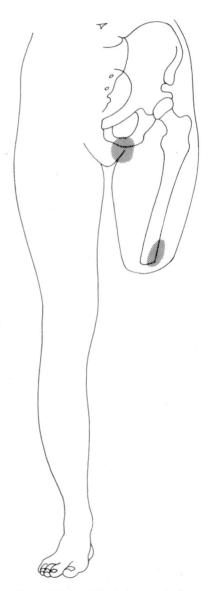

Figure 52-1. Stippled areas indicate typically pressure-sensitive AK residuum tissue.

the vertical residuum walls and the distal end.

Below-Knee Pressure Tolerances. Pressure-sensitive areas of typical below-knee (BK) residua include the anterior distal end of the tibia (sometimes called the kick-point), the anterior tibial crest, the fibular head, fibular neck, the peroneal nerve, and, rarely, the distal residuum end (Fig. 52-2). Pressure-tolerant BK residuum areas include the patellar tendon, the medial tibial plateau, the tibial shaft, the fibular shaft, and the distal residuum end.

As an example of how sockets are made to take advantage of BK tissue tolerances, the BK socket made in the United States virtually always has a protrusion that pushes forcefully on the patellar tendon. By contrast, many European-made BK prostheses have no such protrusion; the sockets merely fit so tightly that they provide an even fit, or "total bearing" surface throughout. With sockets made in the United States, the therapist must carefully ensure that the residuum is in total contact with the appliance, thus preventing edema (Fig. 52-3A) and dermatologic problems (Fig. 52-3B) that result from insufficient socket contact; with European devices, "stump edema" syndrome and related non-total-contact disorders are rare.

Suspension Effects. The type of auxiliary prosthetic suspension influences unit pressures. Thigh corsets for BK amputees, and to a lesser extent pelvic bands for AK amputees, accept some load that would otherwise be borne by the socket. Supracondylar BK suspension effectively elongates the socket and provides a greater vertical support surface, but simultaneously increases the lever arm of ground reaction forces and amplifies the deleterious effects of poor alignment.

Thus, the therapist must recognize the importance of the various reliefs and protrusions within the prosthetic socket that permit a comfortable transition between residuum and appliance. During the check-out session prior to approving the device, the therapist must also ensure that total contact between skin and socket is maintained to prevent dermatologic problems.

Propulsion Biomechanics

The forces that propel the amputee during gait are caused by a combination of muscle activity, gravity (ie, the amputee's weight), and the ground reactions to these forces. Because the prosthesis experiences the forces both from the amputee above and from the ground below, alignment of the device is critical.

Alignment Effects. Prosthetic alignment refers to the relative position of the prosthetic components and the amputation limb; this alignment determines the direction and magnitude of the ground reaction force, which in turn are important in making the prosthesis comfortable and mechanically efficient during walking. If the forces from above and below are not co-

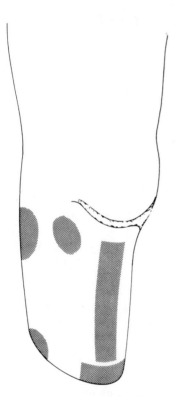

Figure 52-2. Stippled areas indicate typically pressure-sensitive BK residuum tissue.

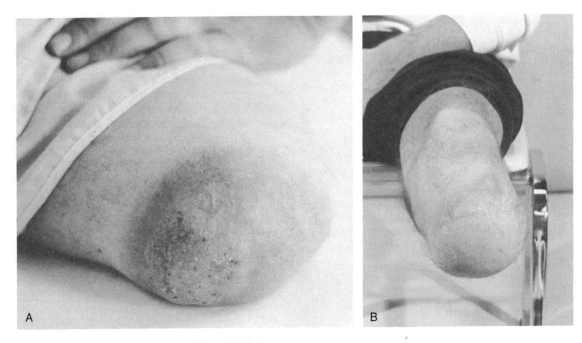

Figure 52-3. (A) Stump edema syndrome and (B) epidermoid cysts result from a poorly fitting, non-total-contact socket.

linear, the prosthesis will tend to rotate at its pseudoarthrosis with the amputation limb. These rotational forces not only cause increased (and inappropriately localized) pressure within the socket, they cause the amputee to walk inefficiently because greater effort must be exerted to prevent the center of gravity from straying too far from its normal sinusoidal path.

The cardinal rule of propulsion biomechanics is that the shortest distance between two points is a straight line. The goal of alignment, then, is to permit the center of gravity (COG) to be transported along as straight a line as possible. The COG normally oscillates about 5 cm* vertically and horizontally, while the normal walking base is about 5 to 10 cm. One therefore attempts to align the prosthesis so that the amputee's gait conforms as closely as possible to normal gait. In practice, correct alignment usually means that the prosthetic heel is di-

*1 in = 2.54 cm.

rectly under the ischial tuberosity during midstance and the limb is comfortable during quiet standing.

Mediolateral Alignment. Normal mediolateral alignment calls for the knee to be in the same sagittal plane as the ischial tuberosity and the foot. Therefore, the BK amputee with preamputation genu varum or valgum will find that a "compromise" prosthetic alignment that places the foot under the residuum end or knee, or both, best balances the forces experienced through the prosthesis. Excessive foot outset in any amputee causes undue mediolateral COG oscillation, and thus increases the energy consumption and increases the distomedial and the proximolateral residuum pressures during stance phase (Fig. 52-4). Excessive foot inset may interfere with the swing phase by causing the prosthetic limb to hit the contralateral limb and may increase the unit pressure (which may increase the discomfort) at the distolateral and proximomedial residuum.

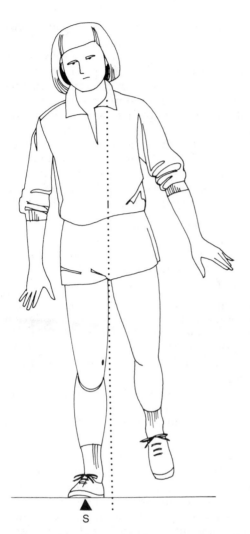

Figure 52-4. Excessive outset of the prosthetic foot causes lateral displacement of the center of gravity (COG) to permit the amputee's weight to be supported by the floor at point S. During gait, the moment of interia (I) at the COG will cause excessive oscillation, consuming more energy than necessary.

Anteroposterior Alignment. Normal anteroposterior alignment occurs when the knee center is in the same frontal plane as the greater trochanter and the ankle. For the BK amputee, the anteroposterior center of the socket should be placed directly above the ankle (ie, it should be vertically above the ankle bolt of a solid ankle-cushion heel [SACH] foot). Aligning the socket too far forward (or the foot too far back) increases the knee flexion moment during stance, which at once causes the COG to dip down and concentrates excessive pressure on the anterodistal kick-point and posteroproximal popliteal tissues. Excessively posterior BK socket placement subjects the knee to hyperextension moments, which must be overcome with increased energy expenditure and concentrates excessive pressure on the anteroproximal and posterodistal residuum aspects.

For the AK amputee, aligning the socket too far forward relative to the prosthetic knee creates an excessively stable limb, which requires greater energy expenditure in late stance. Excessively posterior AK socket placement engenders knee instability. In my experience, sagittal plane linear malalignment is rarely responsible for excessive tissue pressures. Correct sagittal plane AK alignment depends upon the residuum length and muscle strength. The projection of the amputee's weight (which corresponds to the line connecting the ankle—or the center of the bolt attaching the prosthetic foot to the shank—and the trochanter) should fall directly on the knee joint center for all residuum lengths greater than 33% of the contralateral femur. Very short residua generally require the prosthetic knee joint to be 2.5 cm posterior to the trochanter-knee-ankle (TKA) line to permit the knee joint to be stable.

Nonlinear Alignment. Angular relationships of the socket to other components significantly affect the amputee's tissue and propulsion biomechanics. The BK socket is generally flexed about 7 degrees relative to the prosthetic shank both to provide the quadriceps with a slightly more advantageous length-tension relationship and to increase patellar tendon and tibial shaft loading while relieving the kick-point. A slight genu valgus relationship is desirable to prevent excessive lateral thrust and to increase loading on the medial tibial flare. The AK socket is generally flexed about 5 to 10 degrees relative to the prosthetic thigh section to increase the mechanical advantage of the hip extensors and to increase loading on the ischial tuberosity. Adduction to tolerance is advised to increase the mechanical advantage of the hip abductors and to load the lateral aspect of the femur; the proximal medial brim, particularly in men, limits excessive frontal angulation.

Gait

Prosthetic gait differs from normal gait because the mechanical device imposes its own limitations and the amputation itself produces deficiencies. As in normal ambulation, the goal is to transport oneself as smoothly and efficiently as possible.

Kinematics and Causes

Gait kinematics depend upon a variety of factors—from the person's mood and psychogenic factors to the environment surrounding the person. In the context of amputee gait analysis, it should be understood that virtually all gait deviations can be caused by psychogenic factors or habit, but such factors only rarely account for an observed deviation.

The physical therapist must treat the habit or learned compensations and must be able to recognize deviations caused by incorrect or inappropriate prosthetic prescription or fabrication. For example, to spend time teaching the patient not to vault or circumduct a prosthesis that is too long is obviously unproductive. However, unless the therapist can differentiate between prosthetic causes and learned or "motor behavior" causes, the therapist may not recognize this unproductive "teaching."

Prosthetic Causes. Prosthetic causes of gait deviations generally are related to the socket shape or the alignment of the prosthesis. As indicated previously in "Biomechanics," both alignment and socket shape can independently and jointly contribute unfavorably to tissue pressures and thus are often responsible for socket discomfort. Socket discomfort, in turn, causes compensatory gait deviations. Gross kinematic consequences of poor alignment are chiefly detectable in the BK amputee by observing knee motion; in the AK amputee, the observer should be most attentive to hip motion.

Habit. Nonprosthetic causes of gait deviations generally are related to muscle weakness, to proximal residuum joint range-of-motion restrictions, or to memory of a prior experience with a poorly prescribed or fabricated prosthesis that induced a now unnecessary gait compensation. In all but the latter "habit-induced" causes of behavioral gait deviation, the first joint proximal to the prosthesis is again vitally important: for the BK amputee, knee ROM and quadriceps power is paramount; for the AK amputee, hip extensor ROM and abductor/extensor power is paramount.

Below-Knee Amputee Gait

The BK amputee should exhibit near-normal gait kinematics, except for prosthetic ankle motion (Fig. 52-5). The foremost goals of BK prosthetic gait restoration are as follows:

1. optimal comfort for the walking amputee;
2. symmetrical and normal double-flexion knee motion during stance (ie, 10 to 15 degrees knee flexion just after heel-strike and at least 40 degrees knee flexion at toe-off);
3. two to four inches between heel centers in stance phase; and
4. full foot contact with the floor during stance.

A simple summary of BK gait analysis is as follows. The left knee and hip should move like the right knee and hip. Both knees are intact, so sagittal knee motion should be smooth and controlled as in normal gait. Stance and swing durations should be approximately equivalent, because weight-bearing forces and durations should be roughly equal on both limbs. The mediolateral socket brim relationship to the residuum should not vary during stance phase: in particular, the lateral brim should not "thrust" excessively away from the lateral residuum during stance phase. Table 52-1 summarizes the important aspects of BK amputee gait and lists some possible causes for gait deviations.

Above-Knee Amputee Gait

The AK amputee must contend with more inert weight from the prosthesis and must control

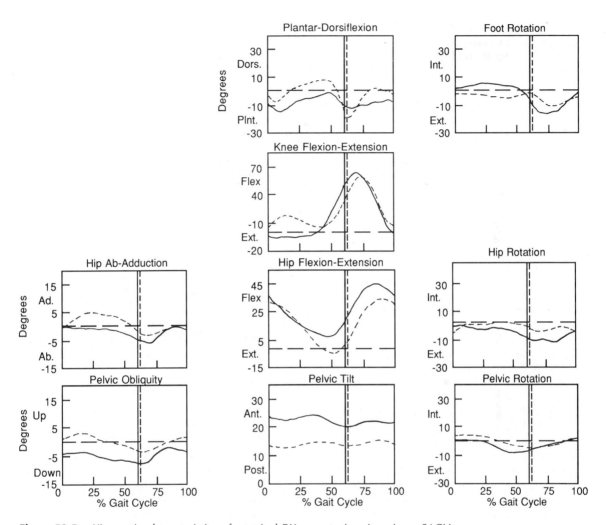

Figure 52-5. Kinematic characteristics of a typical BK amputee's gait, using a SACH foot (*solid lines*) compared with kinematic characteristics of normal subjects (*dotted lines*). (Courtesy of Newington Children's Hospital, Newington, CT)

another prosthetic joint. Thus, the AK amputee's hip extensor and abductor muscles must control not only the prosthetic foot but also the prosthetic knee. Again, prosthetic limb stability must be maintained by alignment if the amputee's hip extensors cannot prevent knee buckling during stance. The foremost goals of AK gait restoration are as follows:

1. optimal comfort for the walking amputee;

2. symmetry of left-right stance durations and loading;

3. minimal energy consumption; and

4. maximal safety and stability.

Note that the goals for AK gait are substantially more modest than those for BK gait, in keeping with the commensurately more modest physiological resources of the AK amputee. As indicated in Figure 52-6, conventional components

Table 52-1. Below-Knee Prosthetic Gait Deviations

GAIT DEVIATION	WHERE; WHEN TO OBSERVE*	POSSIBLE CAUSES
Excessive knee flexion	Sagittal; early stance	1. Excessive foot dorsiflexion or anterior socket tilt 2. SACH heel, or single-axis plantar flexion bumper, too stiff 3. Socket too far forward 4. Knee flexion contracture 5. Excessive posterior placement of tabs in PTB cuff suspension-type sockets
Insufficient knee flexion	Sagittal; early stance	1. Excessive plantar flexion or insufficient socket flexion 2. Excessively soft heel or plantar flexion bumper 3. Posterior socket linear displacement
Forward lurch of head and shoulders	Sagittal; early stance	1. Distal anterior tibia (kick-point) discomfort
Excessive lateral thrust	Frontal; mid-stance	1. Foot placed too far medial or socket too far lateral 2. Socket in abduction
Early knee flexion	Sagittal; mid-stance	1. Excess anterior socket displacement 2. Excess dorsiflexion or anterior socket tilt 3. SACH toe break or keel too far posterior 4. Single-axis dorsiflexion bumper too soft
Delayed knee flexion	Sagittal; mid-stance	1. Socket too far posterior 2. Toe break or keel too far anterior 3. Excessive plantar flexion or posterior socket tilt 4. Dorsiflexion bumper too hard

*"Where to Observe" indicates the optimal plane in which to view the gait deviation; thus, a frontal plane deviation would be best observed from the front or back of the walking amputee.

require that the prosthetic knee joint be fully extended during stance phase. Consequently, the shock absorption and lowering of the COG usually afforded by the intact knee's double flexion wave during stance is absent in the AK prosthesis, thus exacerbating prosthetic stance phase shock and increasing swing phase limb-shortening requirements.

The absence of transverse plane rotation at the single-axis AK prosthetic knee and foot also inhibits gait normalcy. Transverse plane motion insufficiency is typically compensated in the AK amputee by excessive ipsilateral hip, sacroiliac, and spinal rotation. The resultant decrease in pelvic rotation furthermore inhibits arm swing and contributes to left-right asymmetries. Perhaps most importantly, the absence of transverse rotation in the prosthetic limb causes increased shear stresses at the prosthesis-residuum interface (namely, within the socket) and is a major instigator of residual limb skin irritation and discomfort. Installing a rotator unit (ie, a transverse plane limited-motion joint) often both improves the gait ap-

pearance and relieves the residuum discomfort of such amputees.

Probably the most common gait deviations among AK amputees are left-to-right "Trendelenburg" lurch during prosthetic stance and insufficient clearance during prosthetic swing. Mediolateral lurching often results from insufficient hip abductor power or from habitually maintaining the prosthesis in abduction (keeping the feet too far apart). Insufficient prosthetic limb clearance during swing phase is often the result of fear of knee flexion, which effectively creates an excessively long prosthesis during swing phase; the amputee often compensates by vaulting during sound limb stance or circumducting and "hip hiking" during prosthetic swing phase. Table 52-2 summarizes the important aspects of AK amputee and lists some possible causes for gait deviations.

Components

All lower limb prostheses have a socket, a foot, and some material in between. The socket is usually hand-crafted by the prosthetist, but off-

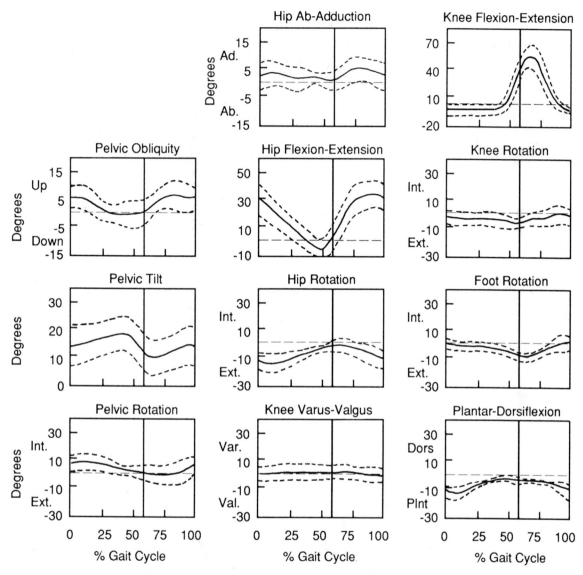

Figure 52-6. Kinematic characteristics of adult unilateral AK amputee gait. Solid lines denote mean, dotted lines denote standard deviation of six healthy subjects. Note especially the constant knee hyperextension during stance because of excessively stable knee alignments, and the wide variation in pelvic tilt because of diversity in lumbosacral and hip contributions to each amputee's prosthetic excursion.

the-shelf components are used for the ankle and foot, and where appropriate, knee and hip joints. Socket characteristics reflect the biomechanical requirements described earlier in "Biomechanics" regarding the particular level of amputation and the resources of the amputee. Each prosthesis must also have a means of suspension to maintain the device securely on the amputee during swing phase. Thus, a proper prescription specifies the type of socket,

Table 52-2. Above-Knee Prosthetic Gait Deviations

GAIT DEVIATION	WHERE; WHEN TO OBSERVE*	POSSIBLE CAUSES
Abducted gait	Frontal; stance	1. Weak abductors 2. Abducted socket or mechanical hip joint in abduction 3. Insufficient lateral wall contact 4. Latero-distal femur pain 5. Habitual walking with too wide a base (due to insecurity, crotch discomfort, or too long a prosthesis) 6. Short prosthesis
Lateral bending of trunk	Frontal; swing	1. Same as abducted gait

Circumduction or vaulting	Frontal; swing	1. Fear of knee flexion
		2. Manual knee lock, or knee too stable
		3. Prosthesis is functionally too long
		  (a) Foot plantar-flexed
		  (b) Socket too small to enter completely
		  (c) Poor suspension, thus pistoning in swing phase
		4. Insufficient knee friction, thus prosthesis not in mid-swing when body is at its highest point during contralateral mid-stance

Medial or lateral whip	Frontal; swing	1. Poor knee bolt alignment 2. Suction socket with flabby muscles or poor socket-stump purchase 3. Prosthesis donned in internal or external rotation 4. Foot is rotated
Rotation of foot on heel contact	Frontal; stance	1. Heel cushion or plantar flexion bumper too hard 2. Excess toe-out
Foot slap	Sagittal; stance	1. Heel or plantar flexion bumper too soft
Uneven heel rise	Sagittal; swing	1. Insufficient knee friction 2. Insufficient or no knee extension aid 3. Fear of knee flexion in early stance, therefore forceful thigh impulse and, usually, terminal swing impact 4. Excess heel rise due to items 1 to 3 above; insufficient heel rise due to mechanical opposites of excess
Terminal swing impact	Sagittal; swing	1. Insufficient knee friction 2. Knee extension aid too forceful 3. Thigh impulse too forceful (usually due to fear) 4. Absent or worn extension bumper in knee
Uneven left-right step lengths	Sagittal; swing	1. Uncomfortable socket; therefore, decreased stance time 2. Insufficient hip extension ROM 3. Poor balance, fear; therefore, decreased stance time 4. Knee not sufficiently stable
Lumbar lordosis	Sagittal; stance and swing	1. Hip flexion contracture 2. Insufficient socket flexion 3. Insufficient anterior brim support 4. Weak hip extensor muscles 5. Weak abdominal muscles

*"Where to Observe" indicates the optimal plane in which to view the gait deviation; thus, a frontal plane deviation would be best observed from the front or back of the walking amputee.

foot, suspension, and where appropriate, knee and hip components, as well as the fabrication materials for all components.

Fabrication

Cast and Check-Socket. At the patient's first visit to the prosthetist, a cast is taken to make a negative mold, or model, of the residuum. Thereafter, plaster of paris is poured into the cast to make a positive residuum image. The plaster model is then modified according to the pressure-tolerant or pressure-sensitive areas, and a socket is constructed to conform to the plaster model. At this point, a transparent check-socket should be fitted to the patient to inspect for proper fit. If the check-socket fit is satisfactory, the prosthetist constructs a definitive socket and mounts this socket on a wood block.

Laboratory Wear. The patient's next visit to the prosthetist is for static and dynamic alignment. The socket and wood block are temporarily bolted to the shank or knee of an "adjustable leg." The adjustable leg permits the foot or knee or both to be positioned during quiet standing (static alignment) and during ambulation (dynamic alignment) in the prosthetic laboratory. Many prosthetists will fit several check-sockets and perform multiple alignments over the course of a week or two to ensure that the finished prosthesis is optimal.

Transfer and Cosmetic Finish. The finished prosthesis is fabricated by transferring the alignment of the adjustable leg to an alignment jig. This jig holds the definitive socket and foot securely in place on a bench while the prosthetist replaces the temporary adjustable leg's distal components with a permanent shank or knee or both. The distal components are usually bolted or glued to the wood block of the socket; once their alignment has been permanently established, the prosthesis is removed from the alignment jig, and the cosmetic shaping and coloring is performed. The external color, of course, should match the amputee's skin color.

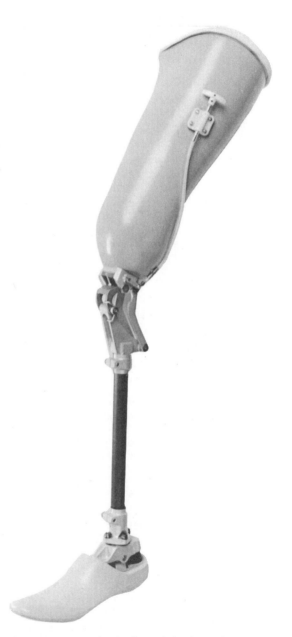

Figure 52-7. Unfinished exoskeletal prosthetic components. Note their overly large shape and rough appearance, which permits contour and color customization for each amputee.

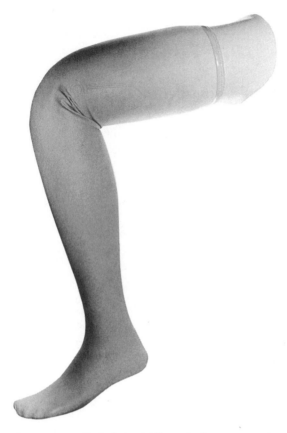

Figure 52-8. Endoskeletal AK prosthetic components. The cosmetic foam cover is shaped to conform to the amputee's sound limb, and covered with a stocking dyed to the amputee's skin color. (Courtesy of Hosmer Dorrance Corp., Campbell, CA 95008)

Basic Component Types

Two basic types of components are commercially available: exoskeletal (Fig. 52-7) and endoskeletal (Fig. 52-8). Exoskeletal, or conventional, components are typically made of wood. There are glued to the socket and foot, and colored by the prosthetist with commercially available dyes applied to the finish lamination to achieve an aesthetically pleasing shade. Endoskeletal components are typically made of metal, and are bolted to the socket and foot. An endoskeletal knee and ankle, for example, are separated by a pipe, or pylon; endoskeletal components are covered by a soft foam

and an external stocking, making them generally more cosmetically attractive than an exoskeletal prosthesis.

Recently, titanium and other high-strength alloys have been introduced to endoskeletal prosthetics to make them mechanically as strong as their exoskeletal counterparts. However, the durability of the endoskeletal cosmetic cover is less than that of the hard plastic laminate of the exoskeletal prosthesis.

Below-Knee Components

Component prescription for the typical BK amputee includes endoskeletal versus exoskeletal construction as described above, and foot, socket, and suspension. A variety of feet are available, but they essentially constitute two groups: energy storing and energy absorbing.

Foot. In addition to having adequate cosmetic appearance, the prosthetic foot must assist the remaining limb musculature in controlling shank kinematics during stance phase. For example, toe-out angle is generally set to be cosmetically identical to the contralateral side. The toe-out angle, however, also affects dorsiflexion and transverse plane kinematics: If the foot is turned out of the plane of progression, less dorsiflexion resistance results. Transverse plane torque absorption is also affected by the foot's constituent materials—softer, better-looking materials sometimes do not withstand the rigors of amputee gait, but their lack of durability may be offset by enhanced shear stress absorption.

Heel durometer (stiffness) is important in determining plantar flexion kinematics. Heavier, fast-walking persons apply greater forces at heel strike and thus find a stiffer heel (more plantar flexion resistance) to be desirable. Lighter, slow-walking persons, especially the elderly, require a softer heel in order to prevent the "rake-handle" effect: If the heel is excessively stiff, excessive knee moments are generated to reach foot-flat, as though the patient were stepping on a face-up garden rake.

Energy-Absorbing Foot. The solid ankle-cushion heel (SACH) foot is by far the most commonly prescribed (Fig. 52-9). The popularity of

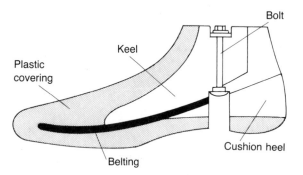

Figure 52-9. SACH foot cross section. Foam rubber composes the cushion heel, and wood or hard plastic composes the solid ankle and keel.

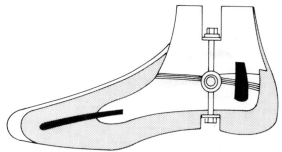

Figure 52-10. Single-axis foot cross section. The anterior and posterior (dorsiflexion and plantar flexion resistance) bumpers are replaceable, and can be made stiffer or softer according to the individual amputee's needs.

the SACH foot stems in part from its durability and in part from its low price. The SACH foot can also permit a limited amount of frontal and transverse plane motion, and it is among the lightest available. The cushion heel comes in a variety of durometers, which accommodate a range of body weights and activities. If excess knee flexion at heel strike is found at prosthesis delivery, the therapist can drill a hole in the foam rubber heel to make it effectively softer. If the foot cannot dorsiflex sufficiently, the cause is usually an excessively long keel; here, the foot must be replaced because the internal keel can be altered only during the manufacturing process.

The second most commonly used foot, the single axis foot, is also energy absorbing and was invented prior to the SACH. The single-axis foot has anterior and posterior bumpers (Fig. 52-10) that limit dorsiflexion and plantar flexion similar to the effect of the SACH foot's anterior keel and foam rubber heel, respectively. The gait deviations effected by excessively soft or stiff bumpers are also similar to the SACH foot. The single-axis foot is advantageous for bilateral and AK amputees because it is slightly more stable, it permits only sagittal plane motion and it reaches foot-flat slightly faster than does the SACH. The single-axis foot makes more noise during gait than the SACH, which is actually an advantage for blind amputees.

The solid-ankle flexible endoskeletal (SAFE) foot (Fig. 52-11) contains both energy-storing and energy-absorbing features. The SAFE foot works essentially like a SACH foot, but permits slightly more nonsagittal plane motion and is somewhat heavier than the SACH foot.

The Seattle (not an acronym!) foot is an energy-storing foot with an internal keel of springy plastic that stores energy during early stance and releases is during late stance to assist push-off (Fig. 52-12). The Seattle foot is slightly heavier than the SAFE, permits roughly the same amount of mediolateral and transverse plane motion, but is externally more lifelike in appearance and is quite sensitive to superincumbent weight. The elasticity of the internal keel must be fine tuned to the amputee's size and activity pattern. This foot was specifically developed for sports and jogging, but many amputees find it preferable for daily use as well.

The Flex-Foot is really not just a foot, but is rather a foot-shank endoskeletal combination device (Fig. 52-13). The carbon fiber laminated interior section acts like a pogo stick or like the leaf-spring suspension on a truck body. Thus, during early stance it stores energy and during late stance it releases energy, resulting in a push-off thrust. This foot is expensive and has had some durability problems. It is particularly

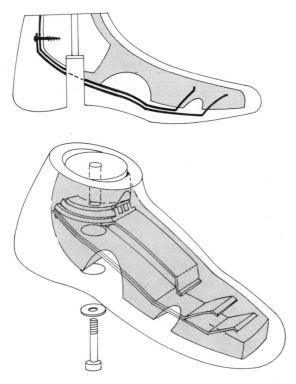

Figure 52-11. SAFE foot cross sections. (Top) standard SAFE foot. (Bottom) adjustable heel-height foot to enable shoe interchange. The internal "ligaments" store energy and add to foot stability. (Courtesy of Campbell-Childs, Inc., Phoenix, OR 97535)

useful for BK amputee runners (particularly marathon participants) and is a real boon to the leaping ability of BK amputee basketball players.

Socket. Socket prescription should be specified by shape and materials. Shape affects prosthetic suspension by altering the socket's purchase (snugness) on the residuum. Materials prescription requires specification of a conventional socket, hard socket, or flexible socket.

The conventional socket is simply a hard socket with a soft liner in it (Fig. 52-14). The liner is usually made of Pelite and is essentially a filler to decrease the problems of residuum volume fluctuation that cannot be accommodated by differing numbers of stump-socks. Hard sockets are popular in the southern United States, because the absence of excessive material helps minimize heat. Flexible sockets are made of a soft, very pliable, thermoplastic material and are supported by a rigid carbon fiber-reinforced frame (Fig. 52-15).

Suspension. Suspension of BK prostheses is accomplished conventionally by a corset, by a leather cuff or a supracondylar socket extension, or by suction. Suction suspension requires the socket to grasp the residuum and seal it with atmospheric pressure to secure the

Figure 52-12. Seattle foot cross section. The internal keel compresses during early stance to "cock" the spring, which provides elastic thrust during mid- to late stance for push-off impetus. (Courtesy of Model + Instrument Development, Seattle, WA 98144)

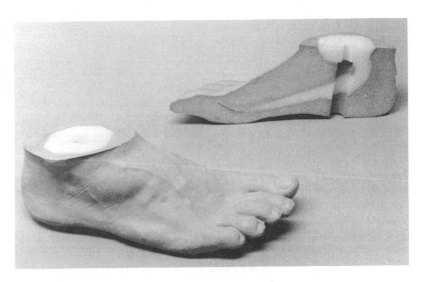

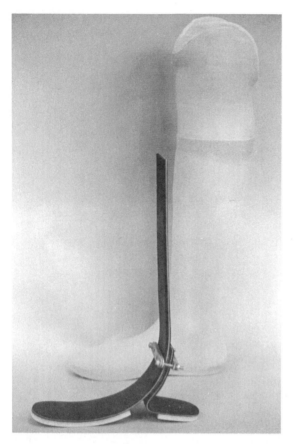

Figure 52-13. Flex-foot. The leaf-spring shank (*fore-ground*) attaches directly to the socket, and therefore must be carefully aligned for each amputee. Both are covered by an exoskeletal-type foam cover. (Courtesy of Flex-Foot, Inc., Irvine, CA 92718)

prosthesis' purchase on the residual limb. Suction is not widely used with current rigid BK sockets because they do not conform sufficiently well to the residuum; however, the flexible socket system may accommodate suction well. The shape of the socket for the other three methods differs primarily in the proximal trim line.

Corset suspension provides a larger surface for weight bearing through the corset applied to the thigh. The prosthetist can thus decrease the amount of material encasing the residuum by lowering the proximal trim line in a corset-suspension BK prosthesis (Fig. 52-16). The corset can furthermore act as an auxiliary knee orthosis, protecting the residuum and anatomical knee from hyperextension or medio-lateral abnormal forces.

Cuff suspension utilizes a leather belt buckled above the femoral condyles to grasp the amputation thigh, with the cuff's distal ends riveted to the prosthesis (Fig. 52-17). Of the methods described, cuff suspensions are most easily fabricated and are most easily adjusted by the patient.

Supracondylar (SC) suspension requires the prosthetist to extend the proximal socket trim lines to encompass the femoral condyles monolithically by the socket. Many amputees prefer SC suspension because of its lack of buckles and straps (Fig. 52-18). If genu recurvatum is present, a suprapatellar (SP) socket extension can provide a counterforce, but otherwise SP extensions merely interfere with good cosmesis during sitting and add weight unnecessarily to the prosthesis.

In general, normal length (15 cm or longer) residua do well with cuff or SC suspension, whereas short residua require SC, SC-SP, or corset suspension to obtain sufficient purchase on the amputation limb during swing phase.

Above-Knee Components

The prescription for the AK amputee specifies the type of foot, knee unit, and suspension in addition to exoskeletal versus endoskeletal construction. Because the latter has already been discussed and because the types of feet available to the AK amputee are identical to those for the BK amputee, the concentration here will be on the knee unit and suspension specifications. A special concern of the AK component prescription is distal segment weight. The double-pendulum action of the AK prosthesis amplifies foot and shank weight according to the distance between the pendulum's hinges at the knee and hip joints, thus amplifying the prosthesis' weight effect on energy consumption much more than in the BK prosthesis.

Knee. Single-axis knee units can be classified according to the type of friction they provide

Figure 52-14. Conventional BK socket. Note the contoured interior of the "hard socket" (*left*) and the soft Pelite liner (*center*). This compressible liner distinguishes a conventional socket from its hard socket worn-alone counterpart. (*Right*) Cross section of socket with liner insert. (Courtesy of J.E. Hanger, Inc., Southeastern Group.)

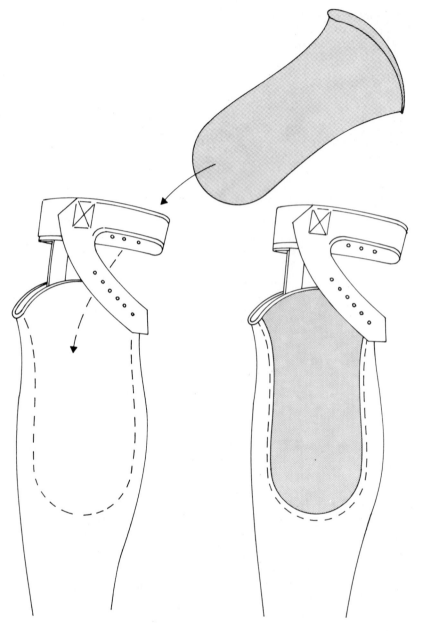

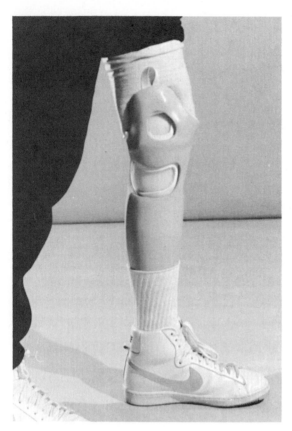

Figure 52-15. The BK socket is a transparent, flexible socket supported by a rigid frame, which may attach to any exoskeletal or endoskeletal shank.

and the presence or absence of a knee lock. The most commonly prescribed knee is a constant-friction device (Fig. 52-19). The constant-friction knee has a "hose clamp" similar to that used for garden hoses. Tightening the screws of the clamp increases the friction, and loosening them decreases knee friction. More friction is needed for an amputee with a fast gait, and less friction is needed to prevent too-rapid extension for an amputee with a slow walking speed.

Hydraulic knee units (Fig. 52-20) automatically adjust to the amputee's walking speed and are therefore indicated for young or energetic persons who frequently vary their walking rate. Hydraulic units are heavier, require

more maintenance, and are much more expensive than constant-friction knees. Because constant-friction knees cannot adjust dynamically to the amputee's cadence, they are prescribed primarily for older patients who cannot be expected to exhibit a wide range of walking speeds.

Knee locks are prescribed for persons who require a constantly locked knee, such as those

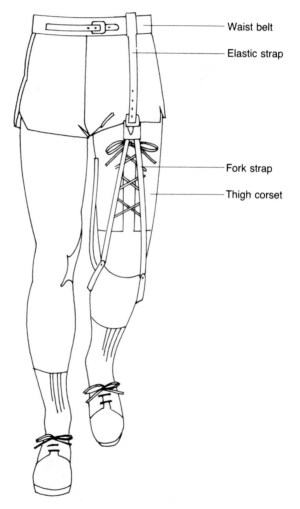

Figure 52-16. Corset suspension. Note the excessive number of buckles the patient must fasten to use this suspension. However, the joint-and-corset combination provides a built-in knee orthosis to help stabilize the anatomical knee joint.

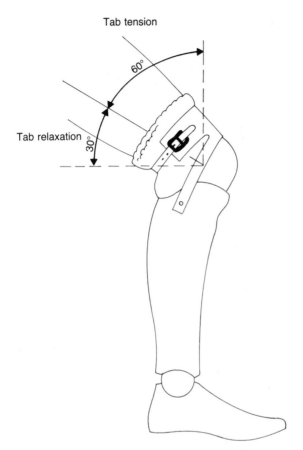

Figure 52-17. Cuff suspension. The cuff tabs are placed on the limb and socket so the patient can sit comfortably, yet maintain minimal pistoning (≤ 1 cm [0.5 in] motion between residuum and socket) during swing phase.

amputees who work on ladders or in otherwise unstable environments, or those who require a locked knee only during stance. This is provided by the Otto-Bock "Safety" constant-friction knee or by the Mauch "Swing and Stance (SNS)" hydraulic knee. Occasionally a knee extension assist, either an internal spring or an external elastic strap, is provided for amputees who need extra swing-phase acceleration of the prosthetic shank.

Alignment and prosthetic stability depend on the type of knee prescribed and the residuum characteristics. Single-axis knee units are so called because they provide a door-hinge-like joint about which the shank rotates during swing phase. Prosthetic knee stability thus results from how far posteriorly they are aligned relative to the projected trochanter-

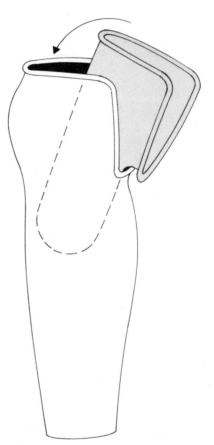

Figure 52-18. Supracondylar suspension. Occasionally, the anterior portion of the socket may also be enclosed by the rigid material (in which case the suspension is called supracondylar-suprapatellar [SC-SP]). The suprapatellar portion is only indicated biomechanically to control knee hyperextension.

length, the knee should be aligned 2.5 to 5 cm posterior to the TKA line; if the residuum is greater than 70% of the normal thigh length and the amputee has sufficient hip extensor power, the knee should be directly on the TKA line.

Multiple axis and other special knee units are in general more stable inherently than single axis joints and are sometimes used for very short limbs or for bilateral amputees. A multiple axis knee joint will also permit a bilateral amputee to sit with the shank in a more cosmetic position because the shank moves linearly beneath the thigh at full flexion.

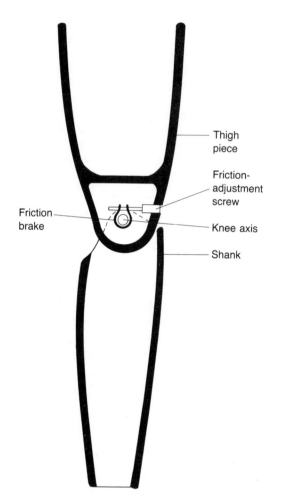

Figure 52-19. Constant-friction knee unit. Set screws increase or decrease friction by adjusting tension of the hose clamp around the knee's single axis.

knee-ankle (TKA) line. If the prosthetic knee axis is more the 2.5 cm posterior to the TKA line, the knee will be very stable and will require little hip extension effort to prevent buckling during stance. However, excessively stable knees impede the amputee's progress, imposing an excessive energy expenditure for each step. The general rule is that if the residuum is less than 30% of the normal thigh

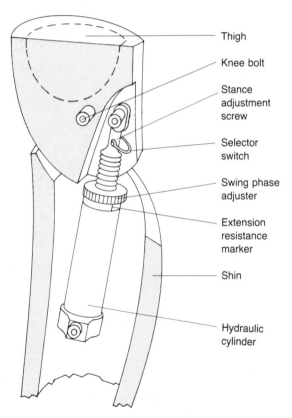

Figure 52-20. Hydraulic knee unit. Cylinder has valves that permit more or less rapid ascent of the middle rod, which damps knee flexion or extension according to the amputee's walking rate.

Suspension. AK socket suspension is accomplished with suction, a Silesian bandage, or a rigid metal pelvic band (Fig. 52-21). Suction suspension achieves maximal prosthesis control and intimacy between the socket and the residuum. Thus, suction should be employed whenever possible, namely, whenever the amputee has sufficient physical resources to don and doff a suction suspension prothesis. The Silesian bandage controls transverse rotation to some extent, but provides little auxiliary suspension, so it is often used only in conjunction with suction or semisuction. The pelvic band is bulky and adds extra weight, but is sometimes the best option for severely debilitated persons because it provides maximum pelvofemoral stabilization.

Other Types of Prostheses

Prostheses for Gritti-Stokes and other long transfemoral amputations, Syme, Boyd, joint disarticulation, and corporectomy amputations are much less standardized (Fig. 52-22). In most cases, prostheses are individually fash-

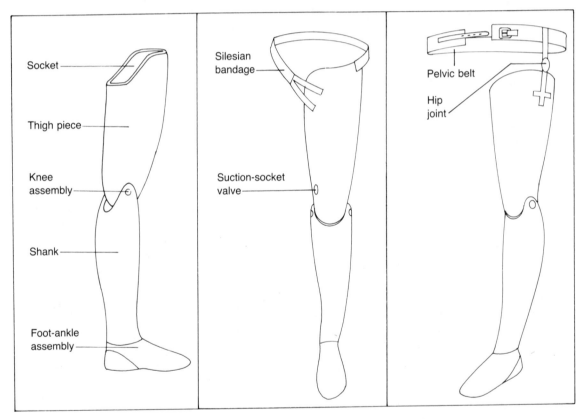

Figure 52-21. AK suspension methods. (*Left*) Suction socket. (*Center*) Silesian bandage. Note the valve at the socket's bottom through which air can escape, but not enter. The Silesian strap is sometimes also used for control of pathological rotatory motions, and is thus sometimes combined with sockless suction suspension, or with semi-suction suspension having a single stump sock. (*Right*) Pelvic band. The rigid portion serves the same kinematic purpose as the pelvic band of a HKAFO, and as such is sometimes used for control of Trendelenburg gait deviations.

Functional Capacities

The ability of amputees to conduct their lives with minimum interference from the prosthetic device and with maximum enjoyment of life is perhaps an overly broad definition of functional capacities, but it sets appropriate goals for the amputee. Functional capacities of amputees are limited by the following:

1. Factors that limit all human beings—the energetics of walking and fighting gravity, the amputee's personal fitness level (cardiovascular efficiency, aerobic capacity, muscle power, and general flexibility), age weight, and psychosocial factors;
2. Underlying disease process and concomitant pathology such as bilateral amputation, cardiovascular disease, or diabetes;
3. Limitations imposed by the prosthesis, including its limited flexibility necessitating excessive center of gravity excursion (which compels greater energy cost with each step); and
4. Loss of "live lift" from the amputated muscles, and in their place the "dead weight" of the prosthesis to be transported with each step, along with the neurological deficits that accompany the amputation of muscle, tendon, joint, and skin receptors.

Pain and poor motivation also limit functional capacity. The most obvious place for the physical therapist to begin searching for causes of less-than-expected functional performance is the fit and comfort of the prosthesis. If the device is satisfactory, the physical discomfort and psychological uneasiness require adjustments that the therapist can facilitate with encouragement and explanations of the prosthetic rehabilitation process and the patient's attendant expectations.

Compensations for Decreased Functional Capacity

For a variety of reasons, amputees respond to their extraordinary mechanical burden by moving more slowly than nonamputees. The shorter the amputation limb, the more energy per unit time is required for functional activi-

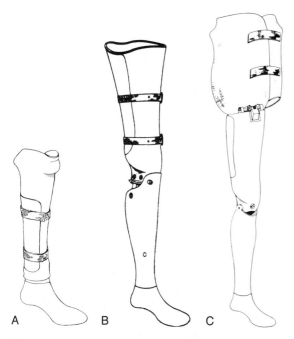

Figure 52-22. Prostheses for (A) Symes, (B) knee disarticulation, and (C) hip disarticulation amputations. Note that in each case the socket must be individually designed. As more of the limb is amputated, the prosthetic replacement becomes more extensive, and component weight commensurately more critical. (Courtesy of Hosmer Dorrance Corp., Campbell, CA 95008)

ioned according to the needs of the given patient. Because these amputations are performed more rarely than AK and BK, the reader is referred to works in the annotated bibliography for further information.

Prosthetic Check-Out

The therapist and clinic team should check out the prosthesis following delivery to ensure that the prescription is correct as written and was properly executed by the prosthetist. A systematic, thorough inspection of the device on and off the patient and during ambulation is mandatory. Forms to assist such efforts are included in the Appendix at the end of this chapter.

ties. Thus, at a given walking speed, AK amputees will consume more energy per unit time than BK amputees; short BK limbs will impose a greater mechanical burden than long BK residua, and thus will require greater energy consumption by the amputee during ambulation. Vascular amputees consume more energy for a given task than do traumatic amputees, even when age matched. Amputees decrease their walking speed to correspond roughly to their increase in energy cost.

For example, unilateral AK amputees consume about 65% more oxygen (measured as mL O_2/kg/sec) than do normal persons during smooth level surface walking, but they compensate by walking slower than normal. Thus, they achieve a normal rate of energy consumption, per unit time, at the expense of walking speed. Traumatic amputees of a given amputation level will generally perform at a higher functional level and will walk at rates more closely approximating normal than vascular amputees. Indeed, an otherwise healthy, young, traumatic mid-shank BK amputee will walk only 5% to 10% (almost imperceptibly) more slowly than normals.

Metabolic factors alone support the dictum that surgeons should "Preserve the knee at virtually all costs; maintain the greatest residuum length possible." Furthermore, the additional support surfaces offered by longer residua not only permit stance phase forces to be distributed over a greater area but also enhance prosthetic suspension.

Aerobic Training. If an amputee's fitness level was increased with an exercise program, aerobic reserves and therefore walking speed should also increase, although little empirical data exist to support the notion. (This assertion, although attractive from an amputee management perspective, would also predict that normal persons with greater cardiorespiratory reserves would walk more quickly than their less-fit peers, which is not the case.) However, at least one study *has* shown that a moderate aerobic training program benefits the amputee both by an improved psychological outlook with feelings of environmental

mastery and by increased walking rate through decreased metabolic cost.

Sports. Often, encouraging the amputee to participate in recreational activities will bring about positive change in functional and psychological outlook. Prostheses specifically designed for running, spelunking, and other sporting activities are now commercially available. However, the therapist should not focus only on the young traumatic amputee when considering amputee sports.

Other recreational activities can enhance prosthetic accommodation and aerobic capacity. Some examples are (1) kicking a ball while seated, progressing to standing "soccer;" (2) rhythmic "dancing" while seated, for increasing durations; and (3) riding a stationary bicycle.

Component Effects. Heavier prostheses cost the amputee more energy. Lightweight component prescription is thus imperative for the elderly or severely debilitated person. Proper component selection and prescription further contribute to metabolic efficiency by permitting prosthetic movement to be as physiologically and kinetically normal as possible. For example, eliminating the articulating knee from an AK prosthesis increases ambulation costs by at least 20%; providing a pelvic band decreases normal frontal plane motion, which decreases movement efficiency; adding a rotator unit or Silesian bandage to control excessive transverse plane motion may also decrease energy costs of activities of daily living.

To decrease energy requirements of walking, the prosthesis should permit the amputee's center of gravity to progress along as straight a horizontal line as possible, with vertical and left-right oscillations limited to about 10 cm.

Vocational Considerations. The functional capacities of a given amputee will vary by many factors, but among the most important is choice of vocation. If the lower-limb amputee worked at a desk premorbidly, little accommodation to the new functional status may be required. But if the amputee was a laborer or was required to function outdoors in rough terrain (eg, supervising construction), the functional capacity of the amputee will need to match the job requirements. Work simulation training programs, vocational counseling (including realistic consideration of the alternatives to the amputee's prior vocation), and proper component prescription are mandatory.

For example, if the AK amputee works on a ladder in a shop stocking shelves, provision of a manual knee lock can permit longer work periods without fatigue, because the lock supplies forces that would otherwise require muscular exertion. A durable prosthesis will improve the functional capacity of a farmer, whereas a lighter-weight device will aid the executive who needs to withstand long hours of low-level physiological activity.

Summary. To increase the functional capacity of lower-limb amputees, the physical therapist must decrease the energy requirements of movement with the prosthesis and increase the energy efficiency of the amputee by maximizing cardiovascular capacity and minimizing gait deviations.

Training and Pre-Prosthetic Care

Perhaps the therapist's most unique contribution to amputee management is the provision of exercise and education immediately following amputation. Although therapy should begin prior to amputation and should include at that time strengthening, aerobic, and flexibility exercises, many facilities only offer physical therapy postoperatively. Whenever begun, the therapist must provide exercise for the entire body, including the amputated and sound limbs, and must teach the patient mobility, ADL, and hygiene.

Pre-Prosthetic Care

Before receiving the prosthetic limb, the amputee should be emotionally and physically prepared for the ensuing life-style changes. These changes include the unfortunate but real social stigma of being an amputee; the extra energy, time, and planning required for accomplishing simple ADL because of the prosthetic encumbrance; and the necessity of learning to cope with having one less appendage. During the immediate postoperative phase, however, many amputees have not yet psychologically accepted their limb loss, so approaching these subjects gently and offering a matter-of-fact acknowledgment of their emotional gravity is helpful.

One excellent means of helping the amputee accept the limb loss is provided as a matter of course during physical therapy. Showing the amputee that he can still walk, can still use the remaining muscles, and can take care of the remaining limb are simple actions that help restore physical and emotional confidence. Instituting "residuum toughening" exercises is a good practice during the pre-prosthetic phase. Having the amputee touch, stroke, press, and hit the residuum not only should speed physiological accommodation to the amputation, but should encourage the patient's psychological acceptance of amputation. The pre-prosthetic phase is an especially good time to emphasize the importance of good hygiene, particularly if the amputation cause was dysvascularity. Instruction in residuum care and monitoring scar healing and edema should be offered at this time.

Bandaging. "Stump bandaging" (Fig. 52-23) is widely practiced in the United States and Europe. Whether bandaging actually accelerates residuum healing and reduces edema is unproven, but it probably plays an important role in shaping and desensitizing the postoperative residual limb, and in helping the amputee learn to handle the limb. Further, the dry bandage padding provides a barrier between the residuum and the environment, which helps to inhibit infection, trauma, and bleeding. Three major methods are employed in bandaging: (1) flexible, or Ace, bandage; (2) semirigid, or Unna Paste, shells; and (3) rigid, or plaster of paris, casts. The methods are listed in approximate order of increasing effectiveness and decreasing convenience. Thus, although rigid dressings are no doubt the most effective means of shaping the residuum and controlling its volume, they are generally opaque and thus

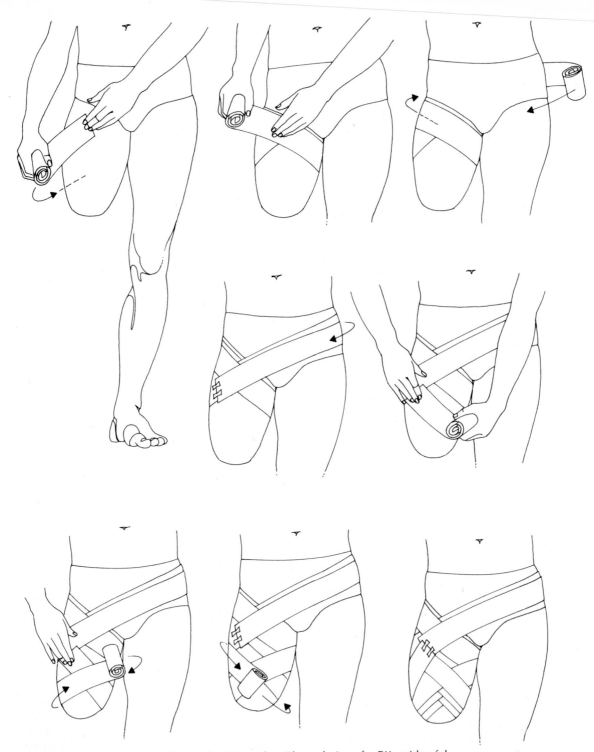

Figure 52-23. Bandaging technique for AK residua. The technique for BK residua follows a similar figure-of-eight pattern, but usually does not require a waistband.

inhibit monitoring of the healing process; furthermore, they are difficult to apply and remove. Rigid dressings with a built-in zipper will probably obviate the latter concern.

Strengthening. Although the prosthesis is designed to be as biomechanically efficient as possible, all prostheses require muscle power for propulsion. The AK amputee depends most heavily upon hip extensors to control the prosthetic knee and prevent excessive forward rotation; the BK amputee depends substantially on knee extensors for ambulation. Because the muscles distal to the amputation site are lost, most stance-phase propulsion must derive either from sound-limb efforts and inertia or from the remaining hip or knee extensors. Good hip abductors are also necessary to maintain mediolateral pelvic stability.

A great deal of emphasis is placed upon strengthening exercises in some facilities, but I am not convinced therapists should continue this excessive emphasis. The amputee needs only slightly more muscle power than does a normal person. If the amputee can arise from a low toilet or chair, stand, and support his weight, I consider muscle power to be satisfactory. In general, if the knee or hip extensors and pelvic abductors are graded as "Good" or better, I emphasize functional and training activities that take at least one to three minutes to complete. Such activities more closely match normal ADL requirements.

Most importantly, when the amputee is first referred to therapy, one most often sees the debilitating effects of bed rest and surgery. Almost any graded activity that eventually permits the amputee to exert normal forces through the remaining limbs is therapeutic. Doing upper extremity exercise, however, may not be time well spent, particularly if the amputee receives the impression that the arm muscles will substitute for the amputated limb. The amputee must understand that upper extremities and assistive devices are to be used only if all else fails. Too often therapists condemn elderly or high-level amputees to using a walker, cane, or crutch despite the fact that no such device was used premorbidly.

Among lower-extremity strengthening exercise choices are "dynamic stump exercises," progressive resistive exercise, and isokinetics. No data exist to guide the therapist wishing to choose among these options.

Dynamic stump exercises are well known because they are so simple. They employ gravity, leverage, and the amputee's weight to provide resistive exercise to the residual limb. A bolster or stool is placed on a plinth under the residual limb and the amputee lies in a supine, prone, or side-lying position upon the plinth. Exercise intensity is graded by increasing the number of repetitions and the therapist's manual resistance.

Progressive resistive and isokinetic exercises can be adapted for amputees in part by providing the means for attaching the residuum to the exercise apparatus. Exercise intensity is essentially symptom limited, but it is probably advisable to encourage the repetitions to be performed at maximum speed and with minimal rest between repetitions to approximate functional activities as closely as possible. Between-set rest periods should be graded according to cardiovascular status.

Mobility. Some therapists emphasize standing and unilateral mobility, including "hopping" on the sound limb, in the pre-prosthetic phase. Although no data exist to support or refute my opinion, I believe unilateral efforts are a poor use of time. Most amputees will learn to hop without instruction; I believe that encouraging weight to be taken by the sound limb inhibits prosthetic training, when most efforts should be directed toward prosthetic limb weight bearing. It is nonetheless true that each amputee needs to be able to move about without a prosthesis in case of emergency; therefore, hopping ability should always be checked before discharging the patient from therapy.

Prosthetic Training

Following delivery of the prosthesis, training should include (1) ADL—donning and doffing, prosthetic care, and personal hygiene; (2) strength and flexibility; and (3) gait training, especially for weight shifting and walking rate.

Activities of Daily Living. The patient must learn to shower, dress, use the toilet, and keep the prosthesis and remaining limb clean.

Donning and doffing training is largely a matter of rote repetition, ensuring that the residuum is introduced into the prosthesis without wrinkling the skin or any socks that intervene within the socket. It is here that the value of prescribing Velcro closures has its greatest merit for all amputees, young and old. When donning a BK prosthesis with corset or lacer suspension, the latter should be secured only when the amputee is standing; if the thigh corset is snug during sitting, it will be too tight for ambulation. When donning a BK prosthesis with SC suspension, the liner is normally donned to the residuum, then the prosthesis to the liner. Suction donning in particular is quite idiosyncratic. Some amputees decrease donning friction with wet cream whereas others use dry powders; some pull the residuum skin into the socket with Ace bandages whereas others use socks or even shoestrings (Fig. 52-24). The important aspect is that all of the residuum—especially the abductor roll in the groin area—must be introduced into the socket with the donning technique.

Most amputees find that dressing the prosthesis first, then donning the device, and finally pulling up the skirt or trousers is most efficient. In particular, it is much easier to tie a shoelace prior to donning a prosthesis than while it is being worn.

Periodic maintenance of the prosthesis prevents premature erosion of parts. Hinges and joints should be checked and oiled every few weeks or months as warranted; the leather and rubber of prosthetic feet and lacers should be inspected for breakdowns. The device should be inspected by a certified prosthetist every year or so.

Hygiene is a particular problem in three areas: (1) the residuum, (2) the prosthetic socket and stump socks, and (3) the perineum of bilateral AK amputees. All amputees need to keep the residuum and the materials with which it is in contact as clean as possible. Stump sock fabric preference (cotton or wool) will vary according to each amputee's personal experience. Cotton socks are said to be more absorbent of body moisture, easier to launder, and less expensive than wool, but the latter are more resilient and feel more cushiony than do cotton stump socks. Like any socks, stump socks should be changed and laundered at least daily. The interior of the socket should be washed with soap and water or alcohol every day, preferably before retiring at night. The residuum should be inspected thoroughly for dermatologic problems or reddened areas. As a rule, if erythematous markings remain for 45 minutes or more, the amputee should see the prosthetist for a socket fitting adjustment.

Finally, apropos of stump socks, one often hears that socket fit is acceptable so long as 15 or fewer plies of socks are worn. The folly of this statement is apparent if you ask yourself how many layers of socks you like to wear within your shoes. The answer in both cases is, "Fewer socks, more comfortable." Flexible sockets, in particular, should be fit with no more than *one* ply of socks, whenever possible.

Strength and Flexibility. Lower-limb amputees demand the highest performance from the extensor muscles of their most-distal joint. Thus, training should include exercises with the prosthesis that encourage hip and knee extension, respectively, for AK and BK amputees. These exercises should be performed in the standing position with the prosthesis in an attitude that approximates that used in gait. Such movement also encourages flexibility.

Flexibility, or ROM, exercises entail maintenance of normal joint mobility and stretching of contractures. The most troublesome joints are the knee and hip, which typically display a capsular pattern of decreased ROM. Prevention, of course, is the best treatment for these problems. However, once acquired, splinting, casting, active ROM, and joint mobilization techniques should all be applied because these contractures are devastating to prosthetic restoration and should be treated with everything available. Five to seven degrees of hip or knee flexion contracture are acceptable, but substantially more limitation requires prosthetic ac-

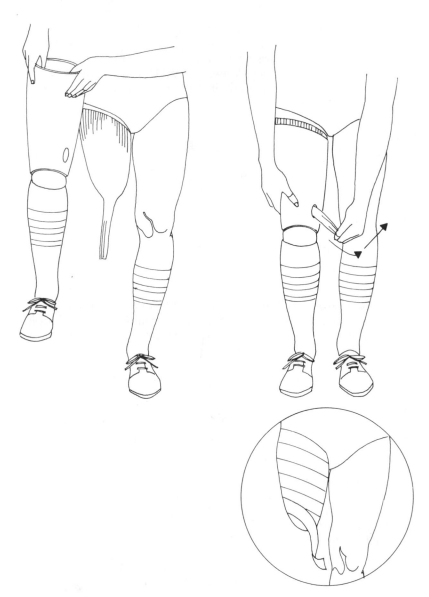

Figure 52-24. Suction donning techniques.

commodation such as an uncosmetic "bent-knee" prosthesis.

Sound limb and trunk flexibility should also be facilitated, because the amputee will use all available resources to compensate for the inherent loss of flexibility engendered by the prosthesis. For example, the amputee may attempt to substitute lumbar lordosis for hip ROM blocked by the prosthesis; pain and dysfunction may result if trunk flexibility is insufficient.

Gait Training. Two types of gait training are currently used in P&O rehabilitation: conventional and biofeedback assisted. Although the method of instruction differs somewhat, the principal goal of both is to assist the patient in (1) accepting weight on the prosthesis during stance, thereby achieving right-left timing and weight-bearing symmetry; and (2) restoring gait speed to as near-normal rates as possible.

No matter what type of training is employed, I feel very strongly that parallel bars should *not* be used. If a patient needs more support than I can manually offer—and the number of such patients is comparatively small—I will employ a walker as a last resort. I find, however, that using parallel bars encourages amputees to pull upward to maintain balance and relieve weight bearing on the prosthesis. Such a technique is not available from other assistive devices and is certainly not a habit to be encouraged.

In conventional gait training, the therapist should concentrate on achieving smooth and complete weight shifting from sound limb to prosthesis to sound limb. One of the easiest and most effective means of accomplishing normal weight shifting is by using graduated-height blocks (Fig. 52-25). The patient is instructed to keep the prosthesis in stance phase and move the sound limb over an initially short vertical and horizontal distance, which requires little weight to be transferred to the prosthesis for a short time. As the blocks become increasingly tall and wide, all the amputee's body weight must be accepted onto the prosthetic side for longer times, approaching the half second or so of unilateral stance required for normal ambulation symmetry. One added advantage of this graduated block approach is that it mirrors the preliminary requirements of stair climbing. Eventually, the blocks should be as high as normal curbs or stair steps (13 to 20 cm), as high as bus steps, whose mastery is required for independent mobility by city-dwellers (28 to 36 cm), and as high as ladder-rung separations. Thus, the amputee learns to master both smooth level-surface ambulation with minimal weight bearing asymmetry and stair climbing.

Bilateral amputees need less work on weight acceptance, because they have little choice but to bear weight through their residua; thus, training time should be directed toward ADL skills, such as arising from sitting or arising from the floor. Syme, Gritti-Stokes, and hip, knee, and ankle disarticulation amputees with their special weight-bearing distal re-

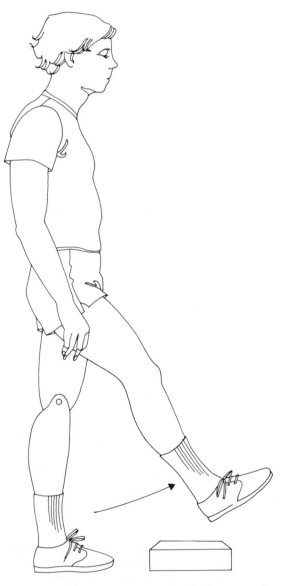

Figure 52-25. Graduated-height blocks are used to encourage increasing weight bearing on the prosthetic limb.

siduum ends need special attention to encourage weight bearing, but they almost always achieve excellent gaits.

Biofeedback-assisted methods can be used with conventional techniques as well. Their unique feature is that they employ electronics. A number of sources document the technical issues involved with kinematic, kinetic, and EMG biofeedback. The conceptual issues are simply, "What are the best means of learning prosthetic gait?" Biofeedback can tell the patient precisely how much weight the prosthetic limb is accepting; how much motion occurs in the amputation limb's knee or other joints; and how much muscle activity the residuum produces—the latter could be used for more physiological suspension or for controlling an externally powered prosthetic component.

Cosmetic and Preparatory Prostheses

Not all prostheses are made for full-time functional ambulation. Cosmetic and preparatory appliances are provided for special purposes, namely to look at or to use temporarily.

Cosmetic prostheses are used to create a visual illusion of limb normality. Of course, the fact that they do not move limits the effectiveness of the use, but for persons who sit in wheelchairs, such as bilateral amputees, cosmetic prostheses are a boon. They are light weight, are easy to care for, and may cost about half the price of a functional device. Cosmetic limbs are often fabricated by nonprosthetists, including (in generally increasing order of cost) surgical supply vendors, therapists, and surgeons.

Preparatory prostheses at one time were a major part of a therapist's pre-prosthetic training program (Fig. 52-26). Preparatory prostheses are available as off-the-shelf items, including several plastic see-through models, but physical therapists often fashion a socket by hand, using plaster of paris. Their popularity has waned recently, both because fiscal pressures encourage early discharge and because the opaque plaster may not permit the patient to take adequate precautions while walking in a plaster-and-pylon "temporary." Certified prosthetists, who are properly trained in fitting prostheses, use clear, rigid plastic materials that are less abrasive than plaster. Under optimal circumstances, the prosthetist fabricates a preparatory prosthesis for training while the patient awaits a definitive device. Where this is not possible, I urge therapists to employ customizable, commercially available temporary prostheses during training.

UPPER-LIMB PROSTHETICS

Because the vast majority of upper-extermity (UE) amputees have unilateral involvement, modest goals should be set for most patients. Compared with a normal UE, the mechanical and sensory limitations of UE prosthetic restoration prevent normal function from being a reasonable goal.

In virtually all patients who have a sound hand, the prosthetic terminal device (TD) is relegated to, at best, an assistive role. A prosthesis would never be used to pick up jelly beans, paper clips, or an egg if a sound hand were available. The goal of therapy is to maximize the *assistive* utility of the prosthesis. Patients with bilateral UE amputations represent the other end of the rehabilitation spectrum: They must maximize their unilateral *and* bilateral functional prosthetic skills.

Acquired UE amputation results in very different problems and clinical presentation than does congenital amputation. Having never developed hand dominance, congenital amputees naturally learn to use the sound limb for most activities and do not experience the psychological trauma of losing a limb. In addition, they may be resistant to wearing a prosthesis because their early body image includes only one hand. The traumatic amputee who loses the dominant limb must learn to transfer dominance to the sound side and to use the once-dominant limb as a nondominant helper.

Thus, the therapist's primary goals are as follows:

1. Clearly establish what role the prosthesis should play in the patient's life-style, and prescribe a device accordingly;

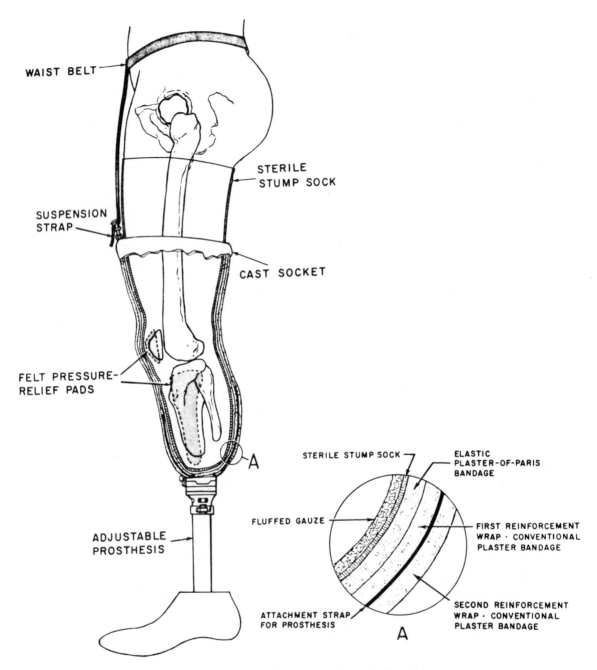

WAIST BELT

SUSPENSION STRAP

FELT PRESSURE-RELIEF PADS

ADJUSTABLE PROSTHESIS

STERILE STUMP SOCK

CAST SOCKET

A

STERILE STUMP SOCK

FLUFFED GAUZE

ATTACHMENT STRAP FOR PROSTHESIS

ELASTIC PLASTER-OF-PARIS BANDAGE

FIRST REINFORCEMENT WRAP · CONVENTIONAL PLASTER BANDAGE

SECOND REINFORCEMENT WRAP · CONVENTIONAL PLASTER BANDAGE

A

Figure 52-26. Plaster-and-pylon preparatory BK prosthesis. *(A)* Detail of circled area.

2. Enhance the dexterity of the contralateral limb and hand; and

3. Instruct the patient in the most appropriate use of the device.

The mechanical purpose of any UE prosthesis is to position in space a clamp that the amputee can open and close at will. This clamp (the hook or hand TD) is connected to the amputee by a socket, perhaps with an elbow intervening, and usually with a harness. Thus, the overall prescription goals are to provide the lightest and most comfortable prosthesis with the strongest clamping force the amputee can control. Overall training goals, in addition to donning-doffing skills and hygiene, are to position the device in space, to control its grasp, and to develop functional skills in prosthetic *control activation* and *object approach, grasp, transport,* and *release.*

Components

All UE prostheses consist of a TD, forearm and wrist, socket, harness system, and in addition for above-elbow (AE) amputees, an elbow and arm (Fig. 52-27). Because there are so few AE amputees and because elbow components are so mechanically simple, this section will focus on the TD, harness, and socket. The socket, forearm, and arm are custom fabricated for each amputee. A great deal of prescription-

writing time is spent considering the merits of powered and conventional devices for each amputee.

Conventional Versus External Power. Conventional or body-powered UE prostheses impart function by transmitting forces from the residual anatomy to a cable-operated elbow, hook, or hand. Bilateral scapular abduction of the shoulder girdles or ipsilateral humeral flexion create cable excursion that pulls the prosthetic component, usually to open a hook or flex an elbow. Externally powered (usually battery-powered) miniature motors can provide a reasonable substitute for forces from the residual anatomy to otherwise conventional components (Fig. 52-28). These motors are controlled either by microswitches activated by the same motions as used for body-powered devices or by EMG detectors (myoelectric devices) that switch the motors on or off.

Little data exist comparing the merits of body-powered and myoelectric hands. Many amputees prefer externally powered devices. The principal objections to externally powered prostheses are their weight, durability, and maintenance. For the AE amputee, prosthetic weight overshadows all other objections. These amputees need external power because their own muscle forces may be insufficient to power a conventional device with a very strong

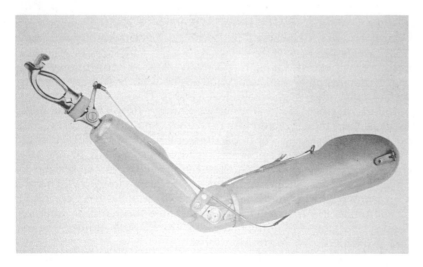

Figure 52-27. Above-elbow prosthesis. (Courtesy of Hosmer Dorrance Corp., Campbell, CA 95008)

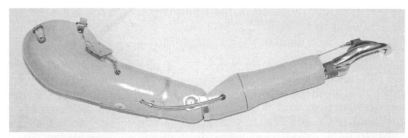

Figure 52-28. NYU-Hosmer electric elbow and prehension actuator. (Courtesy of Hosmer Dorrance Corp., Campbell, CA 95008)

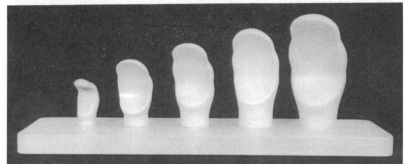

Figure 52-29. Sports terminal devices. (Courtesy of TRS, Inc., Boulder, CO 80303-1797)

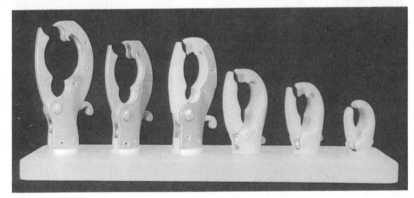

Figure 52-30. Voluntary closing terminal devices. (Courtesy of TRS, Inc., Boulder, CO 80303-1797)

grip or elbow lift, but the extra prosthetic weight negates many advantages of current externally powered components. Lastly, the amputee may require more time to learn to control an externally powered prosthesis, and the amputee does not have the same kind of kinesthetic feedback that is obtained from feeling the tension exerted on a cable.

Terminal Devices. The only commercially available terminal devices in wide use are hooks and hands. Passive TDs and special-purpose sports mitts (Fig. 52-29) are available for extremely appearance-conscious or active pa-

tients, respectively. Among conventional TDs, the major choice is between voluntary opening and voluntary closing TDs.

Voluntary opening (VO) TDs are the most commonly used. A VO hand uses a spring and a VO hook uses one or more rubber bands to provide prehension force (see Fig. 52-28). The amputee must overcome the elastic tension to open the device. Voluntary closing (VC) hands and hooks (Fig. 52-30) usually use a spring to open the TD. To close the hand or hook as tightly as desired, the amputee adjusts the cable tension force.

Externally powered TDs use either a winch

to pull open a VO hand or hook (see Fig. 52-28) or they use a direct-drive motor to both open and close the TD under voluntary myoelectric control. One major advantage of myoelectric hands (Fig. 52-31) is that they can generate much more pinch force than VO hands; furthermore, they require no cumbersome harness. The excess weight of myoelectric hands in comparison with the body-powered TD is particularly a problem in AE amputees, because the distal placement of this extra weight is amplified by its comparatively long distance from the supporting socket and residuum.

Harness. The harness, not used in myoelectric below-elbow (BE) prostheses, usually helps suspend the limb and transmit forces to the cable of a conventional elbow or TD. Typically, the harness is a strip of cloth that loops around the contralateral axilla, crosses the back, and attaches to the arm (figure-of-eight harness) or directly to the socket.

Socket. Socket shape and materials selection follow the same logic as indicated for lower-limb prosthetics with respect to the biomechanics of tissue and force transmission. In the AE residuum, pressure-tolerant tissues are the fleshy portions proximal to the residuum end; pressure-sensitive tissues are bony prominences and distal bone end. In the BE residuum, the pressure-tolerant tissue is usually found over the "handbag" muscles or just proximal to the distal end on the lateral aspect of the radius; pressure-sensitive tissues are the bony distal end, condyles, and olecranon.

Most AE sockets are conical and present no major fitting problems. However, the complex bony anatomy of the BE limb presents several challenges. In general, longer limbs are fitted with flexible hinge suspension and "standard" sockets (Fig. 52-32), whereas shorter limbs are fitted with supracondylar sockets (see Fig. 52-31).

The longer the residual forearm, in general, the more pronation and supination persists after amputation. Thus, a long residual limb would rarely be fit with an SC suspension, because it would block residual forearm transverse motion. Indeed, an amputee with intact carpals may possess full pronation and supination and have prominent radial and ulnar stylii. Such a limb would permit good socket suspension while extending only 2 to 5 cm above the wrist unit, preserving natural pronation and supination.

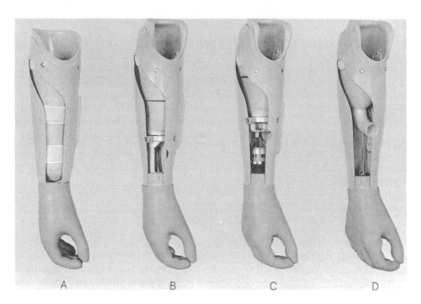

Figure 52-31. Myoelectric BE prostheses, cutaway views. (Courtesy of Otto-Bock, Inc., Minneapolis, MN)

A   B   C   D

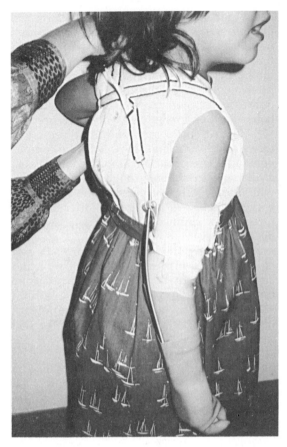

Figure 52-32. Flexible hinge suspension. Note the figure-of-eight harness.

Above-Elbow Amputees

Although only about one third the number of the below-elbow (BE) population, above-elbow (AE) amputees have substantially greater biomechanical deficits. AE amputees have much less sensory apparatus than BE amputees, and AE amputees must not only learn to control a TD, but they must control a prosthetic elbow—a feat only slightly more difficult for some amputees than having to generate sufficient muscle power to control both TD and elbow. Little wonder, then, that the majority of AE amputees do not wear prostheses. Furthermore, although the advent of externally powered elbows has brought some relief to this group of patients (who could most benefit from powered substitutes), they are most negatively affected by the weight of batteries, motors, electronics, and gears.

The principal training goal for AE amputees is to learn to position the TD in space. The conventional elbow is flexed using the same cable that controls the TD, so the TD is first brought to its functional position in space by scapular and humeral motion, then a combination of scapular depression and humeral extension locks the elbow, thus enabling the "split cable" to exert force on the TD. Once control activation is well learned, the therapist should provide functional instruction. Controlling an externally powered elbow is simply a matter of learning when to turn the flexion and extension motors on and off.

Below-Elbow Amputees

The typical BE amputee spends little time on the learning of control activation motions. The therapist directly guides the amputee's shoulders to demonstrate the correct procedure a few times, and the simple motion is acquired. The BE amputee needs to concentrate most on rotating the TD on the wrist unit and on functional activity training.

Pre-positioning the TD prior to approaching the object to be grasped is one key to good BE prosthetic control. With experience, the amputee learns when to pronate or supinate the TD with the contralateral limb to obtain its optimal position before reaching the object. After control activation and pre-positioning skills are acquired, functional training proceeds.

Functional training consists essentially of presenting the amputee with tasks that compel bimanual, repetitive grasp. Table 52-3 lists a variety of such tasks in order of difficulty and expected developmental age skills.

Upper-Limb Prosthetics Summary

To treat an upper-limb amputee optimally, the therapist must prescribe a device that is lightweight and strong; the major training goals are to teach the amputee to position the clamp (the TD) in space, to activate the TD, and finally to perform bimanual functional activities. The

Table 52-3. Suggested Bimanual Activities

TASK

1. Riding ride-on (tricycle)
2. Pull apart toys (eg, Pop-It beads)
3. Stringing large objects: large beads, spools
4. Remove a toy from cloth drawstring bags (eg, separate bubble gum bags)
5. Don/doff mitten to sound hand, fasten Velcro at wrist
6. Open zippered pencil case; remove large felt pen; draw
7. Remove loose clothing (eg, wool sweater or jumper) from a doll
8. Open packages of cereal or raisins
9. Wind up spring-propelled toys
10. Open/close felt-tipped pens
11. Screw/unscrew nested Kittie-in-the-Kegs
12. Take off and put on prosthesis
13. Remove hard candy from wrapper
14. Wrap charm or little toys
15. Screw threaded rod and nut set
16. Blow soap bubbles
17. Grasp and pull up trousers or skirt
18. Grasp trousers and pull belt through loops, buckle
19. Remove and open facial tissue from purse-size package
20. Fill cup with water from low spigot
21. Remove candy wrapper from soft candy (eg, Kit-Kat)
22. "Shopping": push baby cart and pick up items from floor
23. Dry dishes
24. Open a package of potato chips
25. Open and dump contents of 2-inch (restaurant-sized) sugar packages
26. Cut or tear 8½ × 11-inch paper into four pieces
27. Buckle belt mounted on table
28. Open and remove padlock
29. Peel a banana (started by therapist if necessary)
30. Sharpen pencil with hand-held sharpener
31. Grasp small orange and peel
32. Open toothpaste and apply to toothbrush
33. Sewing cards
34. Small bead stringing (macrame)
35. Hammer nails into wood
36. Apply adhesive bandage to doll arm
37. Start and zip zipper
38. Cut 6-inch circle from 8½ × 11-inch paper; paste to another paper
39. Unwrap a stick of gum
40. Put curtains on rod
41. Sweep with brush and dust pan
42. Start and zip zipper of a jacket
43. Cut 6-inch circle from marked 8½ × 11-inch paper
44. Tear many pieces of masking tape off roll
45. Grasp paper container of milk and open
46. Tie a bow with large laces (boot provided) or lace boot on own foot
47. Fold paper, insert in envelope, seal envelope
48. Shell a hardboiled egg
49. Grasp and pull on overshoes
50. Shuffle and deal five cards
51. Erector sets; Meccanno
52. Use safety pin
53. Open a pat of butter, spread butter on crackers
54. Roll paper and put rubber band around it
55. Leather work (lacing)
56. Cut (hotdog or clay) meat with knife and fork
57. Sew on a button: cut length of thread (cotton) from spool, thread needle, attach button to shirt
58. Wrap and tie package
59. Rewire electric plug
60. Unbutton cuff on sound side
61. Open can with hand- and wall-type can openers
62. Chair or stool weaving

amputee must, at a minimum, be able to open and close the TD at waist, mouth, and shoe levels to use the device functionally.

SPECIAL CASES

As indicated previously, bilateral amputees, congenital and child amputees, and multimembral amputees represent only a small segment of the amputee population, but their therapeutic and prosthetic needs are great due to their complexity.

In addition to the several considerations listed in the previous sections, the complex *interaction* of the disabilities of these special cases deserves attention beyond the scope of this chapter. The therapist is referred to the sources indicated in the bibliography, to the various specialty amputee journals such as *Journal of the Association of Children's Prosthetic-Orthotic Clinics* and *Prosthetics and Orthotics International,* and to the specialty amputee clinics around the country for assistance in managing these special cases.

In brief, the unusual and important issues that must be considered for these cases are their atypical mobility and ADL needs. For example, the bilateral UE amputee will probably need special utensils for bottoning a shirt or for bowel and bladder activities. The trimembral amputee may need a special dressing space to facilitate prosthesis donning-doffing. The amputee with congenital bilateral UE absence may well become more adept at ADL with the feet than might ever be realistic with conventional UE prostheses. Conversely, young children with total lower-extremity (LE) deficiency generally become more adept at walking with their hands than with prostheses.

A variety of equipment manufactuers have attempted to solve the problems of the multiply disabled, but in my experience, ingenuity and some mechanical aptitude are critical attributes of the therapist in modifying the usual assistive devices and prosthetic aids for special cases. The therapist who would hope to serve the multiple or congenital amputee community will profit from looking carefully at the experience of therapists worldwide in attempting to solve the varied needs of these special cases.

ORTHOTICS

An orthosis is a device that restricts or increases motion or reduces the body weight transferred to an anatomical lower limb segment. Orthoses are typically constructed from plastic, aluminum, or steel components. In contrast to a prosthesis, an orthosis is designed to supplement, not replace, human anatomy. However, an orthosis may replace a *functional* or physiological loss, such as occurs with muscle or ligament insufficiency. For example, a foot orthosis (FO) can be designed variously to (1) support the arches and thus restrict navicular depression; (2) provide a springy steel shank and thus increase forefoot motion; or (3) transfer body weight away from the metatarsal heads. Because of the enormous variety of orthoses, this chapter will address only the conceptual principles underlying orthotic practice and the major orthosis types.

To assist in concise presentation, the now commonly accepted terminology for orthoses will be adopted: a device is named for the body parts it covers, not for its inventor. Thus, there are lower-limb, upper-limb, and spinal orthoses (LLO, ULO, SO). There is an ankle-foot orthosis (AFO) and a trunk-hip-knee-ankle-foot orthosis (THKAFO). A "Craig-Scott orthosis" is a knee-ankle-foot orthosis (KAFO) with a special thigh cuff and shoe attachment arrangement.

Spinal orthoses will receive brief consideration; they are also named for their function. Thus, the thoraco-lumbo-sacral orthosis controls flexion, extension, lateral bending, and transverse rotation (TLSO-FELR).

THE THERAPIST'S ROLE

In general, the therapist participates in the orthotic clinic team effort by the prescription of and patient training with orthoses. Knowledge of biomechanics, normal gait, ADL, and available prescription options is critical. Orthoses should be as strong, lightweight, simple, and durable as possible and they should be unobtrusive. The prescription should include the joints to be spanned by the device, the materials used for construction, and any special considerations such as springs or stops to increase or limit motion. After checking out the device, the patient should be instructed in its use as it pertains to his vocation and life-style, and finally given advice regarding its maintenance and need for periodic replacement. (See Appendix at the end of this chapter.)

Orthotic training is usually required to use an orthosis effectively. In the case of LLOs, normal gait training procedures are implemented, but the therapist must be aware of the influence the device has on the limb motions available to the patient. Beginning with standing balance and weight-shifting activities, teaching how to control the appliance during sitting, transfers, and donning-doffing is requisite. Choice of gait pattern and assistive device is critical. For ULOs and SOs, donning-doffing, ADL, and maintenance are important considerations. In most cases, patients should be psychologically prepared to spend the rest of their lives with the appliance, so careful planning is vital.

MECHANICS AND BIOMECHANICS

Orthotic prescription should be based on the patient's abilities and needs, and should consider currently available materials and component options. The principles of tissue and propulsion biomechanics outlined above under "Prosthetics" are equally valid for orthotics, with the exception of the principles specifically related to the distal residuum. Thus, to be effective—to apply forces—orthoses must avoid pressure-sensitive areas and limit the areas to which forces are applied to pressure-tolerant structures.

Three-Point Pressure Systems

The basic mechanical principle of orthotic correction is the "three-point pressure system." As indicated in Figure 52-33, three-point pressure systems apply corrective or assistive forces, which are implemented at the surfaces of the orthosis through the skin and are transmitted to the underlying soft tissues and bones. Because no orthosis can replace human anatomical ligaments and joints accurately, perfect fit is impossible; thus, careful consideration of the pressure tolerance of the skin and subcutaneous structures is imperative.

Alignment

The second most important principle of orthotic correction is proper alignment. Correct alignment is the device position that minimizes relative movement between limb and brace ("pistoning") while simultaneously permitting effective orthotic action. In addition to the inability of an orthosis to conform precisely with the contour of the underlying limb, most orthoses use single-axis joints, which cannot track the complex multiaxial underlying joint motions. Thus, the effects of this pistoning motion can be minimized by (1) placing the orthotic joint as close as possible to the skin and to the average center of anatomical rotation, relative to the plane of greatest motion (usually the sagittal plane), and (2) carefully preventing the orthosis from pressing on structures such as the fibular neck or popliteal artery so as to avoid dangerous, if inadvertent, force applications.

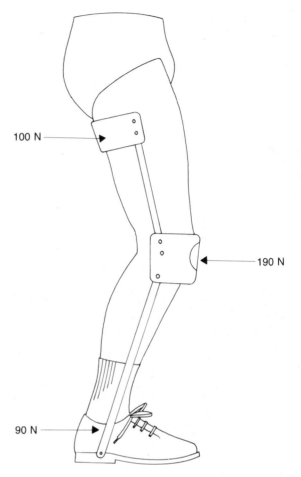

Figure 52-33. Three-point pressure system. Note that one force is directed toward the angulation or deformed area to be corrected, and the other two counterforces are applied distal and proximal to the corrective force.

For example, to prevent excessive valgus knee motion for a patient with arthritis, one must realize that the single-plane, single-axis joints of the knee orthosis (KO) and KAFO cannot accurately track the knee's motion; therefore, some relative motion will occur. That being the case, any attempt to apply forces must consider not only the amount of force required to maintain the knee in a nonvalgus attitude but also the possible damage such forces might impose on the skin and tissues deep to the area of force application, particularly because these forces will continually move proximally and distally as the knee flexes and extends, causing the brace to "piston." The orthosis most likely chosen would spread its mediolateral three-point force system over as great an area as possible, thus decreasing unit skin pressure and at the same time avoiding pressing on the superficial nerves and vessels that supply the popliteal area.

LOWER-LIMB AND SPINAL ORTHOSES

Because they assist the patient in gait, LLOs are the appliances most frequently seen by physical therapists. LLOs must be light enough for patients with weak muscles to transport constantly, but sturdy enough to withstand the rigors of moderate activity. SOs must be well fitting and unobtrusive to be acceptable to most patients with trunk disorders.

Components

Components of LLOs vary by country, and within the United States, by region and patient income. Those areas of the country where there are highly trained orthotists and where the patients can be provided with the best devices use primarily plastic and metal hybrid orthoses; other areas (including most third world countries) use primarily leather and metal LLOs.

The chief advantages of plastic components are that they are lightweight, hygienic because they do not absorb body fluids, more cosmetic because they fit directly on the skin (thus offering a very low profile), and perhaps most importantly, do not require special, "orthopedic" shoes. This last point means that the patient can wear any shoe style so long as the sole and heel heights are within 1 cm of that for which the device was fit and so long as the braced-side shoe is about a half-size larger than normal to accommodate the device. By wearing a dark sock over the exterior of the appliance, relatively little visual attention is drawn to the foot.

Joint Alignment

To minimize relative motion and to maximize the available free orthotic joint motion, the brace should be aligned such that (1) the foot is flat on the floor in midstance and quiet standing; (2) the orthotic hip joint is placed 0.8 cm anterior and superior to the tip of the greater trochanter, and the medial knee joint is vertically midway between the medial joint space and the adductor tubercle (about 2 cm above the joint space in adults) and on the anteroposterior dividing line—with the lateral knee joint parallel to it, and the ankle joints at the tips of the malleoli; (3) the surfaces of the plastic or metal uprights conform as closely as possible to the contours of the limb, and the thigh and calf bands (if any) are horizontal; and (4) there is no undue pressure over superficial nerves, blood vessels, or anesthetic, acutely painful, inflamed, edematous, or dysvascular skin. If no motion occurs about an anatomical or orthotic joint, such as occurs when an orthotic hip, knee, or ankle is locked, joint placement and alignment is unimportant.

Foot Orthoses and Shoe Inserts

The shoe is literally the foundation of most LLOs. Sturdy shoes with a heavy steel shank and a firm sole surface to which ankle uprights are attached is requisite for the leather-and-metal LLO variants. The low quarter Blucher shoe with its wide throat readily admits even stiff or spastic feet, but the same can be said of sneakers. The latter are especially popular for use with plastic AFOs and among children, who cherish the ability to wear the same shoes as their peers.

The major foot problems are in the hindfoot, midfoot, and forefoot. Hindfoot problems such as heel spurs and fractures are generally treated with a soft heel or shoe insert. Midfoot problems, typically described as fallen arches, are generally bolstered with an arch support of varying rigidity. Forefoot problems, primarily metatarsalgia, are treated by supporting the transverse metatarsal arch or by transferring weight posterior to the painful metatarsal heads. All foot problems are interrelated, so if, for example, a patient has a painful metatarsal, one must look for the cause in the remainder of the foot or LE.

Shoe modifications are an important aspect of LLO prescription. If the patient or orthosis has insufficient plantar flexion, a soft SACH-type heel should be substituted for the shoe's off-the-shelf rubber or leather heel. If the patient or the orthosis has insufficient dorsiflexion, a shoe buildup called a "rocker bar" should be added just posterior to the MTP joints to assist rollover in late stance. Other shoe attachments include an array of pads and leather, metal, and rubber arrangements (such as "Thomas" heels and "Morton" toe supports) all of which have their proponents.

Ankle-Foot Orthoses

More AFOs are used than any other type of LLO. All provide some degree of foot and leg support, generally by affecting dorsiflexion and inversion-eversion.

Plastic leaf-spring (PLS) dorsiflexion assist orthoses are perhaps the most widely prescribed device. These unobtrusive braces slip into most patients' shoes easily, and classically, provide little support other than in prevention of plantarflexion or "foot drop." The three-point pressure system of the PLS (Fig. 52-34) can be modified as required to change its function. Bringing the anterior trim lines toward the malleoli increases its resistance to dorsiflexion, whereas raising its foot plate or building a flange into one of its shells can limit inversion and eversion. For example, to raise the longitudinal arch, applying forces that push the arch up, supinate the midfoot, pronate the forefoot, push the medial malleolus medially, and rotate the tibia externally will limit arch depression. As the abbreviated trimlines of the PLS progress anteriorly, it becomes a solid-ankle AFO.

A free single-axis ankle joint does not intentionally limit ankle ROM, but it certainly limits normal hindfoot and forefoot motion.

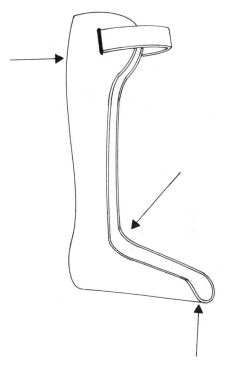

Figure 52-34. Posterior leaf splint (PLS) orthosis. Arrows indicate three-point pressures.

The foot and ankle are encouraged to act as hinges, with rotation occurring only about the orthotic ankle joints. Because the foot will not move in this manner, the normal, complex motion of the foot continues despite the "best" orthotic efforts by pistoning within the AFO and the shoe.

Limited-motion metal ankle joints appear the same externally as a free single-axis ankle joint, but their metal hinges are ground by the orthotist to comply with the prescribed degree of dorsiflexion-plantar flexion restriction. Plastic low-profile "lap joints" have become available to orthotists (Fig. 52-35). These plastic limited-motion joints are promised to provide all the advantages of plastic and metal, and none of the disadvantages. A foam rubber shock absorber can be added where the shank and

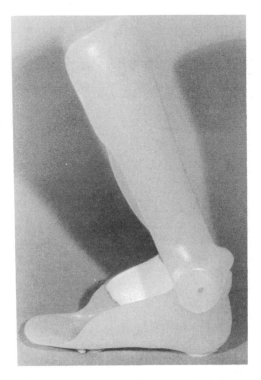

Figure 52-35. Limited-motion overlapping plastic joints. Posterior "lip" at ankle level limits allowable plantar flexion by determining where the proximal and distal pieces meet. The white Pelite pad lining the arch support attenuates the force transition between the foot and the supportive plastic. (Device made by David Huysman, CPO.)

foot pieces meet at the ankle to limit plantar flexion and cushion heel strike.

To eliminate as much foot and ankle motion as orthotically possible, an intimately fitting calf shell and University of California at Berkeley Laboratory (UCBL) foot plate are made of unitary plastic. A "solid-ankle" joint could be made from metal components (as in the Craig-Scott), but it could still permit some nonsagittal motion within the shoe. The term "solid ankle" is usually reserved for plastic AFOs. Like all custom plastic orthoses, solid-ankle AFOs are made from a plaster mold of the patient's anatomy, in a manner similar to that described under "Lower-Limb Prosthetics." Because they allow no ankle motion, a

cushion heel and rocker bar, which may be attached to the brace or shoe, must be prescribed to permit normal heel-toe gait.

Knee-Ankle-Foot Orthoses and Knee Orthoses

Orthoses that control the knee joint are provided for patients with joint malalignment or muscle weakness, and occasionally, for patients with spasticity. Orthotic attempts to prevent knee buckling among patients with paraplegia and quadriplegia are no longer fashionable (except by using the "Reciprocator," described below) because few persons with thoracic or higher lesions will ambulate outside the clinic.

Bracing the weak knee is a challenge not because the three-point pressure system is complex (all that is required is one force directed at the knee and one each below and above the knee) but rather because suspension is difficult. Using a KO to prevent knee flexion during stance might be optimal, but suspending the KO from the femoral condyles is difficult. The device in Figure 52-36 uses a flexible polyethylene material and a special strap arrangement to achieve good suspension, yet still provide anteroposterior and mediolateral

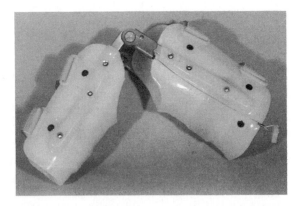

Figure 52-36. Side view of knee orthosis. The posterior cutaways permit full knee flexion in sitting. The lateral upright has a single, spring-loaded knee lock, which can be released by pulling the thigh-level trigger.

orthotic correction. However, in most cases suspension will be insufficient, so a KO will not be satisfactory, thus forcing the prescription of a KAFO. Sports orthoses employ a rubber sleeve or special undergarment to suspend the KO, but few people are willing to wear such tight, binding suspensors more than a few hours during sports; thus, KOs are rarely used for the disabled.

Most KAFOs are prescribed with a knee lock, so little relative motion occurs between the patient and the appliance unless a free ankle joint is also prescribed. KAFOs are often prescribed for unilateral, high-level flaccid weakness, including spina bifida, muscular dystrophy, and polio. They are occasionally prescribed for spastic disorders such as cerebral palsy and hemiplegia, but they are rarely useful in these cases.

Weight-Bearing and Fracture Braces

A weight-relieving orthosis is an orthosis-prosthesis combination designed to transfer weight from some proximal structure to the shoe or floor, bypassing an arthritic joint or fracture site. The proximal portions of the patellar weight-bearing AFO and the ischial weight-bearing KAFO follow the socket designs of their cousins, the BK and AK prostheses, respectively. Distally, they usually terminate in a rigid metal ankle joint attached to a leather shoe. Thus, superincumbent weight is accepted by the orthosis, is transmitted along its uprights or shells, and finally is dissipated into the ground at the heel or at a "Patten" (hoof) bottom that transfers weight directly from the weight-bearing surface to the floor.

Fracture braces may look exactly like any other LLO, but they usually include some encompassing circumferential component, such as calf or thigh shells that are designed to achieve hydrostatic support of the fracture area. Fracture braces may be custom made or they may be purchased as off-the-shelf prefabricated appliances. The latter come in a variety of sizes, which is encouraging therapists and orthopedists to attempt to fit these LLOs themselves.

Hip and Trunk Orthoses

Bracing the hip, pelvis, and above requires the therapist to pay scrupulous attention to the goals of orthotic management and to the weight of the total appliance package. One should question the need for connecting the LLOs to any support above the waist, because few persons who need such extensive bracing will in fact be functional ambulators. The choices for hip joints are straightforward, as are their attachments to a trunk support.

Hip Orthoses

Orthotic control of hip motion requires prescription specification of whether sagittal motion or frontal motion should be restricted. Isolated transverse plane restriction requirements are rarely called for, but the orthotic treatment is simply to apply a Silesian bandage (as described earlier in the discussion of AK prostheses) to limit rotation. Similarly, an AK prosthetic-type pelvic band with a single-axis free sagittal motion joint will limit abduction or adduction. "Hip action" orthoses that permit free abduction but limit adduction (usually to 0 degrees) are often prescribed for conditions of spastic adductor activity. All orthotic hip joints may be attached to thigh cuffs or to KAFOs. In the latter case, they become part of HKAFOs.

Reciprocator

Invented in Toronto and further developed at Louisiana State University, the "LSU Reciprocator" permits paraplegic patients to walk with an alternating gait (Fig. 52-37). The reciprocator essentially attaches the thigh pieces of a THKAFO so that when the patient leans on one limb, forcing it into extension, the free-swinging opposite limb is pushed into flexion. The patient repeats the process, substituting upper extremity power exerted through crutches for paralyzed lower-limb muscles.

Spinal Orthoses

Many back braces are in use. Most SOs have an abdominal support that not only provides counterforces to complete the biomechanical three-point pressure systems, but perhaps more importantly, to increase intracavitary *in-*

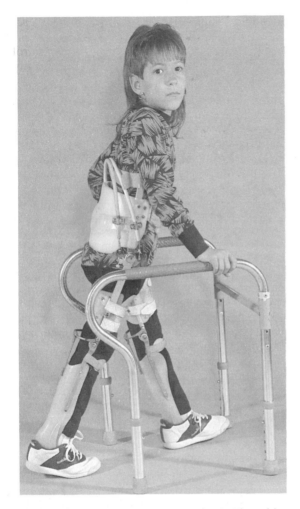

Figure 52-37. Reciprocating gait orthosis. The cables connecting the lower limbs permit contralateral hip extension to drive ipsilateral hip flexion. (Courtesy of Durr-Fillauer Medical, Inc., Chattanooga, TN 37406)

ternal support for the spine. The most commonly provided SOs are soft corsets, sacroiliac binders, and cervical collars, whose greatest physiological effect may be warmth.

Most SOs today are made of lightweight plastic materials, but to some extent metal, leather, and canvas are still used. These older materials permit precise placement of pressure pads and force-applying uprights. Knight-Taylor and Williams SOs (TLSO-FEL and LSO-EL,

respectively) enjoyed immense popularity, probably because they were so mechanically simple. Plastic materials, in addition to being somewhat hotter, spread the forces over a greater area and, at least in scoliosis treatment, permit the prescription of more comfortable, less obtrusive braces.

Orthoses, of course, may provide a variety of other benefits. They provide tactile and other sensory feedback to remind the patient to move in the prescribed manner, they enhance heat retention, and sometimes they provide psychological secondary gains.

Scoliosis orthoses include the classic "Milwaukee" and the now standard "Low Profile" plastic body jacket. The former, because they extend to the neck, may be used for all scoliotic and kyphotic curves, while the latter are said to be useful for mid-thoracic or lower curves of 40 degrees or less.

UPPER-LIMB ORTHOSES

Orthotic treatment of the upper limb more closely resembles ULP than LLO. Indeed, some persons with total UE disability opt for amputation, because the ULP is frequently more functional than the ULO. Most orthotic effort is directed toward creating usable prehension by attaching splints and supports to the fingers and wrist. Attempts to provide the patient with a means of positioning the hand in space are often futile.

Most ULOs are passive positioning devices (Fig. 52-38). A variety of low-temperature plastics, such as Orthoplast and Hexalite, can be applied as temporary splints, but they deform too easily with prolonged use. Many different types of shoulder slings and "subluxation" remedies are commercially available.

Active ULOs are available for patients with prehension dysfunction. Wrist-driven prehension orthoses employ the "tenodesis" effect to permit the wrist extensors to approximate the thumb and forefingers. Various motor-driven ULOs have been attempted, but their weight and complex control systems inhibit current practical applications.

Functional training with the various pre-

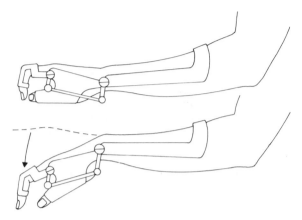

Figure 52-38. Wrist-driven prehension orthosis.

hension orthoses should include the bimanual activities in Table 52-3. As in ULP rehabilitation, unless the therapist finds ways to show the patient that two hands are better than one—even if one hand is encumbered by a mechanical appliance—the orthosis will be underutilized.

FUNCTIONAL ELECTRICAL STIMULATION

Application of electrical stimulation to weakened muscles and nerves is familiar to most physical therapists. Portable stimulators, which can be triggered by an external event such as heel strike, can now deliver enough cycles over the course of a day to permit their use as orthoses.

Differing only in size and control actuation from the clinical muscle stimulators, functional electrical stimulation (FES) devices offer several major advantages over mechanical appliances. FES has been used with limited success with multiple sclerosis patients. In addition, trials with paraplegia, scoliosis, subluxed shoulder, and simple foot drop conditions are proceeding. In brief, FES offers a very unobtrusive profile, is lightweight, and in sharp contrast to the atrophy expected with application of a mechanical orthosis has the possibility of actually improving or hypertrophying the target muscle. However, presently the bother of applying electrodes, allergies to the gel, and

having to get used to the electrical stimulus *per se* are disadvantages that inhibit long-term orthotic substitution. Furthermore, the control actuation mechanisms are not yet sufficiently reliable or physiological for routine clinical use.

CONCLUSION

Physical therapists participating in the clinic team's prosthetic and orthotic rehabilitation efforts are involved in the prescription, check-out, and training phases of this multidisciplinary field. To formulate the prescription, a biotechnical matching process is used to determine pathokinesiological deficits and equip the patient for optimal biomechanical and physiological performance. Check-out procedures ensure that the prescription was correctly formulated and carried out. Training with the accepted device includes instruction related to the prosthesis or orthosis and to the vocation or life-style to which the patient can return. More research is needed to differentiate those orthotic and prosthetic approaches that are valid, useful contributions to clinical practice, from those that have survived because they "have always been used."

ANNOTATED BIBLIOGRAPHY

American Academy of Orthopaedic Surgeons: Atlas of Limb Prosthetics. St Louis, CV Mosby, 1981 (The definitive text on prosthetic components and biotechnical matching criteria.)

American Academy of Orthopaedic Surgeons: Atlas of Orthotics. St Louis, CV Mosby, 1985 (The definitive text on orthotic components and biotechnical matching.)

Engstrom B, Van de Ven C: Physiotherapy for Amputees: The Roehamptom Approach. New York, Churchill Livingstone, 1985 (Well-illustrated, hands-on description of training techniques for lower limb amputees, with one chapter on upper limb amputee training.)

Kostuik J, Gillespie JR: Amputation Surgery and Rehabilitation. New York, Churchill Livingstone, 1981. (Excellent history of prosthetics and surgery. Contains a good section on gait training and on myoelectric prostheses.)

Krebs DE, Fishman S: Characteristics of the child amputee population. J Pediatr Orthop 4:89, 1984 (Describes the demographics of pediatric amputees in the US, and briefly reviews the literature concerning adult populations.)

Krebs DE: Neuromuscular re-education and gait training. In Schwartz, MS (ed): Biofeedback. Englewood Cliffs, NJ, Guilford Press, 1987 (Using amputees and brace wearers as case examples, a biofeedback "how to do it" is provided.)

Mensch G, Ellis PM: Physical Therapy Management of Lower Extremity Amputations. Rockville, MD, Aspen Publishers, 1986 (Well-illustrated text emphasizing exercises and gait training.)

NYU Prosthetics and Orthotics Staff: Lower-Limb Prosthetics; Lower-Limb Orthotics; Upper-Limb Prosthetics; Upper-Limb Orthotics; Spinal Orthotics. New York University Post-Graduate Medical School Prosthetics and Orthotics, 1980 to 1986 (These manuals are perhaps the most widely used technical expositions on their respective subjects.)

Redford JB: Orthotics, ETC. Baltimore, Williams & Wilkins, 1986 (Provides a useful supplement to the AAOS *Atlas* by documenting the many lesser-used orthotic appliances.)

Skinner HB, Effeney DJ: Special review: gait analysis in amputees. Arch Phys Med Rehabil 64:82, 1985 (Reasonably complete literature review describing amputee gait analysis; 28 references.)

APPENDIX*

The patient data summary form is the same for any prosthetic check-out; therefore, it is reproduced only once here.

Date _____

Patient _____

Amputation Type _____

_____

_____

Initial Check-out ☐   Final Check-out ☐

Pass ☐   Provisional Pass ☐   Fail ☐

If the patient needs further attention, please indicate the type of treatment required:

Medical-Surgical _____ ☐   Training _____ ☐

Prosthetic _____ ☐   Other _____ ☐

(Vocational, Psychological, etc.)

Recommendations and Comments _____

_____

_____

_____

_____

Clinic Chief

*(Prosthetic and orthotic check-out forms courtesy of Prosthetics and Orthotics, New York University School of Medicine, Post-Graduate Medical School)

PROSTHETIC CHECKOUT: ABOVE KNEE

_____ 1. Is the prosthesis as prescribed? If a recheck, have previous recommendations been accomplished?

CHECK WITH THE PATIENT STANDING

Fit and Alignment

_____ 2. Is the patient comfortable while standing with the midlines of the heels not more than 6 inches apart?

_____ 3. Is the adductor longus tendon properly located in its channel and is the patient free from excessive pressure in the anteromedial aspect of the socket?

_____ 4. Does the ischial tuberosity rest properly on the ischial seat?

_____ 5. Is the prosthesis the correct length?

_____ 6. Is the knee stable on weight bearing? (Without the patient using excessive effort in pressing backward with his stump.)

_____ 7. Is the brim of the posterior wall approximately parallel to the ground?

_____ 8. Is the patient free from vertical pressure in the area of the perineum?

_____ 9. When the valve of a total-contact socket is removed, does stump tissue protrude slightly into the valve hole and have satisfactory consistency (approximately that of the thenar eminence)?

Suspension

_____ 10. Are the lateral and anterior attachments of the Silesian bandage correctly located?

_____ 11. Does the pelvic band accurately fit the contours of the body?

_____ 12. Is the center of the pelvic joint set slightly above and ahead of the promontory of the greater trochanter?

_____ 13. Is the valve located to facilitate pulling out the pull sock and the manual release of pressure?

CHECK WITH THE PATIENT SITTING

_____ 14. Does the socket remain securely on the stump?

_____ 15. Does the shank remain in good alignment?

_____ 16. Is the center of the knee bolt ½ to ¾ inch above the level of the medial tibial plateau?

_____ 17. Can the patient remain seated without a burning sensation in the hamstring area?

_____ 18. Can the patient rise to a standing position without objectionable air noise from the socket?

(*Prosthetic Checkout: Above Knee continues on next page.*)

CHECK WITH THE PATIENT WALKING

Performance

____ 19. Is the patient's performance in level walking satisfactory? Indicate below the gait deviations that require attention.

____ a. Abducted gait

____ b. Lateral bending of trunk

____ c. Circumduction

____ d. Medial whip

____ e. Lateral whip

____ f. Rotation of foot on heel strike

____ g. Uneven heel rise

____ h. Terminal swing impact

____ i. Foot slap

____ j. Uneven length of steps

____ k. Lumbar lordosis

____ l. Vaulting

____ m. Other

Comments and Recommendations: _____

_____

____ 20. Is suction maintained during walking?

____ 21. With a total-contact socket, does the patient have the sensation of continued contact between the stump and socket in both swing and stance phases?

____ 22. Does the patient go up and down inclines satisfactorily?

____ 23. Does the patient go up and down stairs satisfactorily?

Socket

(Check these items *after* the performance evaluation has been done.)

____ 24. Does the ischial tuberosity maintain its position on the ischial seat?

____ 25. Is any flesh roll above the socket minimal?

____ 26. Does the lateral wall of the socket maintain firm and even contact with the lateral aspect of the stump?

Miscellaneous

____ 27. Does the prosthesis operate quietly?

____ 28. Are the size, contours, and color of the prosthesis approximately the same as those of the sound limb?

____ 29. Does the patient consider the prosthesis satisfactory as to comfort, function, and appearance?

CHECK WITH THE PROSTHESIS OFF THE PATIENT

Examination of the Stump

____ 30. Is the patient's stump free from abrasions, discoloration, and excessive perspiration immediately after the prosthesis is removed?

Examination of the Prosthesis

____ 31. Are the anterior and lateral walls at least 2 inches higher than the posterior wall?

____ 32. Does the inside of the socket have a smooth finish?

_____ 33. Is there satisfactory clearance at knee and ankle articulations?

_____ 34. Are the posterior surfaces of the thigh and shank shaped so that there is minimal concentration of pressure when the knee is flexed fully?

_____ 35. With the prosthesis in the kneeling position, can the thigh piece be brought to at least the vertical position?

_____ 36. In the total-contact socket, is the bottom of the valve hole at the level of the bottom of the socket? (It may be lower, particularly with a soft insert.)

_____ 37. Is a back pad attached to the posterior wall of the socket?

_____ 38. Is the general workmanship satisfactory?

_____ 39. Do the components function properly?

PROSTHETIC CHECKOUT: BELOW KNEE

_____ 1. Is the prosthesis as prescribed? If a recheck, have previous recommendations been accomplished?

_____ 2. Can the patient don the prosthesis easily?

CHECK WITH THE PATIENT STANDING

_____ 3. Is the patient comfortable while standing with the midlines of the heels not more than 6 inches apart?

_____ 4. Is the anteroposterior alignment of the prosthesis satisfactory? (The patient should not feel that his knee is unstable nor should he feel that his knee is being forced backwards.)

_____ 5. Is the mediolateral alignment satisfactory? (The shoe should be flat on the floor and there should be no uncomfortable pressure at the lateral or medial brim of the socket.)

_____ 6. Is the prosthesis the correct length?

_____ 7. Is piston action minimal when the patient raises the prosthesis?

_____ 8. Are the anterior, medial, and lateral walls of adequate height?

_____ 9. Do the medial and lateral walls contact the epicondyles, and with the patellar tendon-bearing variants, the areas immediately above?

Thigh Corset

_____ 10. Do the uprights conform to the flares above the epicondyles?

_____ 11. Are knee joints close to the epicondyles (above ⅛ to ¼ inch)?

_____ 12. Does the thigh corset fit properly, with adequate provision for adjusting corset tension?

_____ 13. Do the length and construction of the thigh corset appear to be appropriate for its intended function of weight-bearing or stabilization?

CHECK WITH THE PATIENT SITTING

_____ 14. Can the patient sit comfortably with minimal bunching of soft tissues in the popliteal region, when the knees are flexed to 90 degrees?

CHECK WITH THE AMPUTEE WALKING

_____ 15. Is the patient's performance in level walking satisfactory? Indicate below the gait deviations that require attention.

_____

_____

_____

_____ 16. Is piston action between the stump and socket minimal?

_____ 17. Does the patient go up and down inclines and stairs satisfactorily?

_____ 18. Are the socket and suspension system comfortable?

_____ 19. Does the knee cuff maintain its position?

_____ 20. Is the patient able to kneel satisfactorily?

_____ 21. Does the prosthesis function quietly?

_____ 22. Are size, contours, and color of the prosthesis approximately the same as those of the sound limb?

_____ 23. Does the patient consider the prosthesis satisfactory?

CHECK WITH PROSTHESIS OFF THE AMPUTEE

_____ 24. Is the patient's stump free from abrasion, discolorations, and excessive perspiration immediately after the prosthesis is removed?

_____ 25. Does the weight bearing appear to be distributed over the proper areas of the stump?

_____ 26. Is the posterior wall of the socket of adequate height?

_____ 27. Do the check strap and fork strap have adequate provision for adjustment?

_____ 28. Is the general workmanship satisfactory?

The patient summary form is the same for any orthotic check-out; therefore, it is reproduced only once here.

Date _____

Patient _____

Diagnosis _____

Disability/Deformity _____

Initial Checkout ☐   Final Checkout ☐

Pass ☐   Provisional Pass ☐   Fail ☐

If the patient needs further attention, please indicate the type of treatment required:

Medical-Surgical _____ ☐   Training _____ ☐

Orthotic _____ ☐   Other _____ ☐

(Vocational, Psychological, etc.)

Recommendations and Comments _____

_____

_____

Clinic Chief

ORTHOTIC CHECK-OUT: ABOVE KNEE (KAFO)

_____ 1. Is the orthosis as prescribed? If a recheck, have previous recommendations been accomplished?

_____ 2. Can the patient don the orthosis without difficulty?

CHECK WITH PATIENT STANDING

Shoe

_____ 3. Is the shoe satisfactory and does it fit properly?

_____ 4. Are the sole and heel of the shoe flat on the floor?

Ankle

_____ 5. Are the mechanical ankle joints aligned so they coincide approximately with the anatomic ankle?

_____ 6. Is there satisfactory clearance between the anatomic ankle and the medial and lateral mechanical ankle joints?

_____ 7. If a varus or valgus strap or shoe insert is used, is sufficient force exerted to produce the desired support without causing significant discomfort?

_____ 8. If a shoe insert is used, is there minimal rocking between insert and shoe?

Knee

_____ 9. Are the mechanical knee joints aligned so they coincide approximately with the anatomic knee?

_____ 10. When the patient stands with most of his weight on the braced leg, is there satisfactory clearance between the mechanical knee joint and the patient's knee on both the medial and lateral sides?

_____ 11. Is the knee lock secure and easy to operate?

Uprights

_____ 12. Do the uprights conform to the contours of the leg and thigh?

_____ 13. Is there satisfactory clearance between the medial upright and the perineum?

_____ 14. Is the lateral upright below the head of the trochanter but at least 1 inch higher than the medial upright?

_____ 15. Are the uprights at the midline of the leg and thigh?

_____ 16. In a child's orthosis, is there adequate provision for lengthening all uprights?

Bands and Cuffs

_____ 17. Are the bands and cuffs of proper width and do they conform to the contours of the leg and thigh?

_____ 18. Are the bands and cuffs comfortable?

_____ 19. Is there sufficient clearance between the top of the calf band and the head of the fibula?

_____ 20. Are the distal thigh band and the calf band equidistant from the knee?

Quadrilateral Brim (When Prescribed)

_____ 21. Is the adductor longus tendon properly located in its channel and is the patient free from excessive pressure in the anteromedial aspect of the brim?

_____ 22. Does the ischial tuberosity rest properly on the ischial seat?

_____ 23. Is any flesh roll above the brim minimal?

_____ 24. Is the brim of the posterior wall approximately parallel to the ground?

_____ 25. Is the patient free from vertical pressure in the area of the perineum?

Hip

_____ 26. Is the center of the pelvic joint slightly above and ahead of the greater trochanter?

_____ 27. Is the hip lock secure and easy to operate?

_____ 28. Does the pelvic band fit the contours of the body accurately?

Special Attachments

_____ 29. If a special attachment, such as a torsion shaft, is used, are the intended forces exerted without subjecting the limb to undesirable force?

Stability

_____ 30. Is the patient stable?

CHECK WITH PATIENT WALKING

_____ 31. Is the shoe flat on the floor during the mid-stance phase of walking?

_____ 32. Is there adequate clearance between the patient's ankle and knee and the corresponding mechanical joints?

_____ 33. Does the varus or valgus strap or shoe insert provide the desired support?

_____ 34. Is the patient's performance in level walking satisfactory? Indicate below the gait deviations that require attention:

_____ a. Lateral trunk bending   _____ i. Lordosis

_____ b. Hip hiking   _____ j. Hyperextended knee

_____ c. Internal (external) hip rotation   _____ k. Knee instability

_____ d. Circumduction   _____ l. Inadequate dorsiflexion control

_____ e. Wide walking base   _____ m. Insufficient push-off

_____ f. Excessive medial (lateral) foot contact _____ n. Vaulting

                                                _____ o. Rhythmic abnormalities

_____ g. Anterior trunk bending   _____ p. Other, including arm motion, noises, etc. (Describe) _____

_____ h. Posterior trunk bending

_____

_____

_____ 35. Is the orthosis sufficiently strong and rigid?

_____ 36. Does the orthosis operate quietly?

CHECK WITH PATIENT SITTING

_____ 37. Can the patient sit comfortably with his knees flexed 90 degrees, and can he flex his knee an additional 15 degrees without undue pressure?

_____ 38. Do the mechanical ankle joints provide the prescribed range of motion?

_____ 39. Are the mechanical knee-joint adjustments adequate?

_____ 40. Are the sole and heel of the shoe flat on the floor?

CHECK WITH ORTHOSIS OFF THE PATIENT

_____ 41. Is the limb free from signs of irritation immediately after the orthosis is removed?

Orthosis

_____ 42. Is the shoe firmly attached to the orthosis, and is the shoe shank strong enough for its anticipated use?

_____ 43. Is the heel flat and firmly nailed to the shoe, and are wedges and lifts as neat and inconspicuous as possible?

_____ 44. Do the ankle and knee joints move without binding?

_____ 45. Do both medial and lateral stops of the ankle and knee joints make simultaneous contact when the joints are fully flexed and extended?

_____ 46. Is the calf band adequately and smoothly lined and padded?

_____ 47. Is there adequate provision for adjustment of the straps and cuffs?

_____ 48. Are the metal parts of the orthosis smooth and free from sharp edges and sharp bends?

_____ 49. Is the leatherwork neat?

_____ 50. Is the general appearance of the orthosis satisfactory?

_____ 51. Does the patient consider the brace satisfactory as to comfort, function, and appearance?

ORTHOTIC CHECK-OUT: BELOW KNEE (AFO)

_____ 1. Are the orthosis and shoe as prescribed? If a recheck, have previous recommendations been accomplished?

_____ 2. Can the patient don the orthosis without difficulty?

CHECK WITH PATIENT STANDING

Shoe

_____ 3. Is the shoe satisfactory and does it fit properly?

_____ 4. Are the sole and heel of the shoe flat on the floor?

Ankle

_____ 5. Are the mechanical ankle joints aligned so they coincide approximately with the anatomic ankle and is there adequate clearance?

_____ 6. Is sufficient force exerted by the varus or valgus correction strap or shoe insert to produce the desired support without causing significant discomfort?

_____ 7. Is there minimal rocking between the shoe insert and shoe?

Uprights

_____ 8. Do the uprights or plastic shell conform to the contour of the leg?

_____ 9. Do the uprights provide adequate clearance and are they at the midlines of the leg?

_____ 10. In a child's orthosis, is there adequate provision for lengthening uprights?

Bands and Brims

_____ 11. Is the band or shell comfortable, of proper width, and does it conform to the contours of the leg?

_____ 12. Is there sufficient clearance or relief for the head of the fibula?

_____ 13. If a patellar-tendon-bearing brim is used, is there adequate reduction in weight bearing at the heel?

Stability

_____ 14. Is the patient stable?

CHECK WITH PATIENT WALKING

_____ 15. Is there adequate clearance between the malleoli and the mechanical ankle joints?

_____ 16. Does the varus or valgus correction strap or shoe insert provide the desired support?

_____ 17. Is the patient's performance in level walking satisfactory? Indicate any gait deviations that require attention:

_____ a. Lateral trunk bending

_____ b. Hip hiking

_____ c. Internal (external) limb rotation

_____ d. Circumduction

_____ e. Abnormal walking base

_____ f. Excessive medial (lateral) foot contact

_____ g. Anterior trunk bending

_____ h. Posterior trunk bending

_____ i. Lordosis

_____ j. Hyperextended knee

_____ k. Excessive knee flexion

_____ l. Excessive genu valgum or varum

_____ m. Inadequate dorsiflexion control

_____ n. Insufficient push-off

_____ o. Vaulting

_____ p. Rhythmic disturbances

_____ q. Other, including arm motion, noises, etc. (Describe) _____

_____

_____

_____

CHECK WITH PATIENT SITTING

_____ 18. Can the patient sit comfortably with his knees flexed approximately 105 degrees?

CHECK WITH ORTHOSIS OFF THE PATIENT

_____ 19. Are the foot and leg free from signs of irritation immediately after the orthosis is removed?

_____ 20. Do the ankle joints move without binding and provide the prescribed range of motion?

_____ 21. Do medial and lateral stops of the ankle joint make simultaneous contact when the joint is fully flexed and extended?

_____ 22. Is the general workmanship of the orthosis satisfactory?

_____ 23. Is the general appearance of the orthosis satisfactory?

_____ 24. Does the patient consider the orthosis satisfactory as to weight, comfort, function, and appearance?

53 Mobility and Ambulatory Aids

JANICE TOMS

One of the major tasks of a physical therapist is selecting equipment and instructing patients in the use of mobility and ambulatory aids. The physical therapist may also be responsible for delegating portions of the treatment activities to support personnel.

The physical therapist will work closely with the patient, the patient's family, community agencies, and members of the health care team in selecting and purchasing equipment. Therefore, it is necessary to be familiar with recent advances in design and function of equipment and with the agencies that may be involved in helping the patient purchase the equipment. To assist and teach the patient the safest, most efficient manner to use the equipment, the therapist must be knowledgeable about the guarding techniques, gait patterns, and transfer techniques appropriate for that patient.

The ultimate goal for the patient is to achieve the highest possible functional level. Some patients will become totally independent in using mobility or ambulatory aids, whereas others may always require some assistance.

This chapter includes a discussion of the types of assistive devices most commonly used for functional mobility (ie, wheelchairs, canes, crutches, and walkers); how to evaluate for appropriate fit; safety factors; guarding techniques; and teaching the patient how to use the device.

SITTING MOBILITY: WHEELCHAIRS

To enhance mobility for the person who has achieved sitting balance but lacks the strength, coordination, and balance to progress to ambulatory activities, a wheelchair is the logical assistive device to select. Other patients who have the balance and coordination to ambulate but who lack endurance may be able to combine a wheelchair and crutches, walker, or cane to provide for maximum functional mobility.

The "standard" wheelchair usually seen in most clinical facilities weighs about 40 lb and consists of a metal, collapsible frame with a vinyl seat and back and padded armrests. The front wheels or casters are small, and the back wheels are large. Most standard chairs are equipped with footrests and hand brakes (Fig. 53-1).

The tires may be narrow and made of hard rubber, or they may be inflatable (pneumatic). The inflatable tires add to the overall width of the chair, but also provide more shock absorption and a smoother ride. The inflatable tires are desirable, particularly for outdoors on uneven or rough surfaces.

Wheelchairs also come equipped with "tilt bars." The tilt bars, one on each side, project from the back of the frame, usually about 2 to 3 inches above the floor. The person pushing the wheelchair uses a foot to press down on the tilt bar, tilting the chair back on the rear wheels to raise the front casters up over a step, mat, or rug.

Footrests support the lower limbs. Many footrests also include heel loops, which keep the feet from sliding off the footrest (Fig. 53-2). To perform a standing transfer safely, it is necessary to fold the footrests up. The footrests are also folded up when the chair is collapsed for storage. It is also possible to get "swing-away" foot and leg rests (Fig. 53-3*A*). This option is necessary if the patient needs to move the chair in close to objects for working or transferring.

An outer rim extending from each wheel enables the patient to propel the chair himself (see Fig. 53-3*B*).

With the proper modifications, manual propulsion of a wheelchair can be performed independently by patients who have the functional use of only one upper limb. This can be achieved by adding another rim to the wheel on the patient's functional side. The two rims

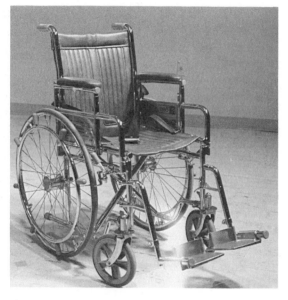

Figure 53-1. Standard wheelchair, with footrests and hand brakes.

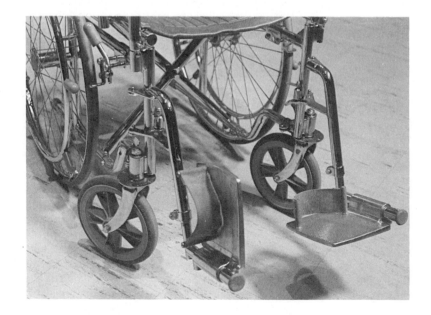

Figure 53-2. Footrests with heel loops.

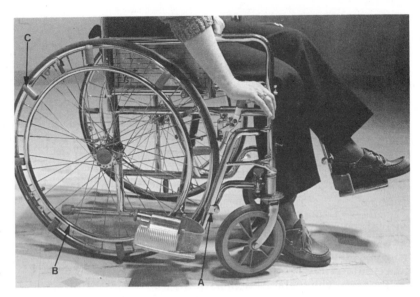

Figure 53-3. (A) Swing-away foot and leg rest. (B) Rim for propelling the chair. (C) Projections on wheel rim for propelling the chair using the thumbs.

on the one side control both wheels. The wheelchair can be propelled forward or back by pushing on both rims simultaneously. Direction can be controlled by pushing or pulling on a single rim (eg, pushing forward on the right rim will turn the wheelchair to the left).

Another common modification, projections on the wheel rim, will allow the patient with weakness of both upper limbs to hook the thumbs over the projections and propel the chair (see Fig. 53-3C). Sometimes taping the palms of the hands makes it possible to get enough traction on the wheel rims to propel the chair without adding projections.

Patients lacking the strength or coordination to propel a wheelchair independently may require a motorized chair. Powered chairs are operated by means of a toggle switch or a mouthstick. Powered chairs are much heavier and more difficult to transport because they require a battery and a holding panel for the battery.

When a patient requires assistance to propel and maneuver the wheelchair, it is important to be familiar with the techniques of descending ramps and ascending or descending curbs or a step. If the ramp does not exceed the required standard of 1 inch per foot of rise or if the patient can help control the speed of the wheelchair, a ramp can be descended in a forward direction. However, if the ramp exceeds the standard angle of rise or if the patient's weight is such that you may not be able to control the speed of descent if the wheelchair is facing forward, the chair should be turned, facing backward down the ramp. The therapist can brace the body against the back of the chair to control the speed of descent.

Descending a curb or a single step in a wheelchair may be performed with or without assistance. The technique is the same regardless of the need for assistance. One method of descending a curb or a single step is performed with the wheelchair facing backward to the curb. With the wheelchair positioned with the back facing the curb, the therapist steps off the curb, gently guiding the chair backward until the rear wheels are over the curb and onto the surface below. The therapist continues to guide the wheelchair until the casters and footrests clear the step. Using the tilt bar, the therapist slowly lowers the front of the chair until the casters are on the lower level. It is also possible to descend a curb by facing the curb. The therapist would push down on the tilt bar until the chair is tilted back on the rear wheels. While the chair is in this position, it is rolled forward and over the step. After the rear wheels are on the lower surface, the front is slowly lowered until the casters are on the same level. This method may be more jarring to the patient and requires more strength to control the speed of descent.

One method of ascending a single step or a curb is performed facing the step. As the wheelchair nears the step, with the casters about 3 to 4 inches away, the therapist pushes down on the tilt bar and tilts the wheelchair back until the casters are high enough to clear the step. From the tilted-back position, the wheelchair is rolled forward until the rear wheels touch the curb. The casters are lowered on the step. The therapist lifts up and pushes forward until the rear wheels are up on the step. Using a backward approach, the therapist tilts the wheelchair onto the rear wheels, then steps up onto the upper level. Keeping the back straight and the knees flexed, the therapist lifts the wheelchair and rolls it backwards until the casters are above the upper surface. The wheelchair is then lowered and turned to resume forward progression.

If a patient is going to be independent in a wheelchair, it will be necessary to learn to do a "wheelie." A wheelie is a technique used to raise the front part of the chair (ie, the casters) in the air, balance on the rear wheels, and propel the chair forward or back while balanced on the rear wheels. This motion is necessary to get the wheelchair up curbs or over objects that would otherwise impede the forward progress of the chair. Performing a wheelie requires a quick backward and forward motion on the rim of the wheels. The hands are placed forward, gripping the hand rims, and the hand rims are moved quickly back, then forward, causing the front casters to lift off the floor. The wheelie position is maintained by balance and a subtle forward and backward motion of the hand rims. While the patient is learning this technique, the therapist stands directly behind the wheelchair in a position to move with the chair,

and the hands are positioned just below the hand grips, ready to "catch" the chair should it tilt backward too far.

The primary safety features found on wheelchairs are the seat belt, the hand bars (grips) that project from the back of the wheelchair, and the brakes. The seat belt prevents the patient from sliding or falling out of the chair. The hand bars, which have plastic or vinyl grips, serve the obvious function of providing a handle to hold while pushing the wheelchair, but also provide protection for the patient's head and neck should the chair tip over backwards. Two types of brakes are used on most wheelchairs, toggle and ratchet brakes. Toggle brakes, which are probably the most common, are applied by pushing forward on the handle and released by pulling back (Fig. 53-4). Ratchet brakes are also applied by pushing forward, but require an additional step of slipping the lever into an appropriate notch to hold the brake in the locked position. In some cases, when a person is unable to reach the brake handle or does not have the strength to operate the brake levers, extensions to the brake handle are added.

Many younger, more active persons are purchasing the lightweight "sport" chairs (Fig. 53-5). As the name implies, these chairs are lighter in weight and have more design options than the standard chair. One design option is the choice of a rigid or folding frame. The rigid frame provides for greater stability and is used more often by active persons who participate in sports and activities on uneven terrain. The major disadvantage of the rigid frame is that it is less convenient to transport because it does not fold. To compensate for this, the wheels can be removed easily and the back comes forward over the seat for storage or transportation. The lightweight chairs are more maneuverable and functional, and provide greater aesthetic quality. The trade-off for these advantages comes in the cost of the wheelchair. The lightweight sport chair is more expensive than the conventional chair.

Regardless of the type of wheelchair, before making a purchase one must consider how

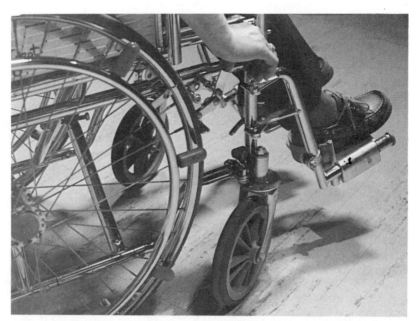

Figure 53-4. Toggle brakes are applied by pushing forward on the handle.

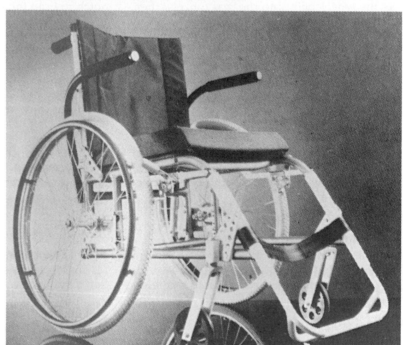

Figure 53-5. A lightweight sport chair.

the chair is going to be used, the quality of the parts and workmanship, the various options available, and the cost.

GUARDING AND TRANSFERS

When guarding a patient who is transferring into or out of a wheelchair the therapist should stand facing the patient, allowing enough room for the patient to move freely between the two surfaces but close enough to assist as necessary. The therapist should be in a semi-crouched position with the feet in a broad stance position (Fig. 53-6). One foot should be in a position to block the wheelchair or the leg of the patient as necessary. When it is not possible to stand in front of the person transferring (eg, wheelchair to car), assistance is given from

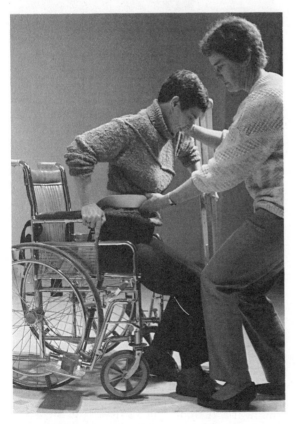

Figure 53-6. Position of therapist while guarding a patient rising from the chair.

behind or beside the patient, whichever provides the most accessibility to the person transferring. The therapist will have to judge how much assistance is necessary when transferring a patient. Always allow the patient to do as much as possible without risking the safety of the patient.

Transferring from the wheelchair may require either a sliding-sitting transfer or a standing transfer. Almost all transfers are done with the wheelchair as close as possible and parallel with or at a slight angle to the other surface. The footrests are swung away and the brakes are locked. Before initiating any transfer, the patient will slide forward or be assisted forward toward the edge of the chair seat.

A sliding-sitting transfer is usually done with a sliding board. With the wheelchair armrest removed, one end of the sliding board is placed under the buttocks of the person transferring, and the other end is placed on the surface of the object onto which the person will transfer. Both feet are removed from the footrests and placed on the floor. By pushing down on the hands, extending the elbows, and depressing the shoulders, the patient slides across the board onto the other surface. Initially, when a patient is learning a transfer technique, maximal assistance and guarding are necessary. As the patient practices and gains skill, balance, and strength, assistance and guarding are withdrawn as appropriate. The therapist guards the patient from the front, placing one hand on the guarding belt at the waist and the other hand on the shoulder of the person transferring. Assistance can be provided by placing both hands under the buttocks, and lifting as the patient depresses the shoulders and slides onto the sliding board.

The standing pivot transfer is another type of transfer that may require maximal assistance by the therapist. This transfer requires the therapist to have enough strength and proper body mechanics to assist the patient to stand, pivot, and sit on the other surface all in one motion. The lift is only high enough to clear the chair and the other surface. The patient supports as much of his own weight as possible. The wheelchair is positioned at a right angle or parallel to the transferring surface. The therapist stands as close as possible to the person transferring, with hips and knees bent and the back held straight, maintaining the normal lordotic curve. The patient's arms are placed around the neck or shoulders of the therapist. The therapist's hands are placed under the buttocks of the patient. Counting aloud will facilitate a synchronized, coordinated movement between the patient and the therapist. As the therapist says "Lift," the patient attempts to stand. In a continuous motion the therapist lifts, pivots, and lowers the patient onto the other surface.

Standing transfers are also performed with the wheelchair at a slight angle from and as close to the other surface as possible. Guarding is usually done from the front, with one hand on the guarding belt and the other on the shoulder to help maintain balance and protect the patient from falling. If the person transferring has one-sided weakness or if one lower limb is involved, the uninvolved limb is usually positioned adjacent to the transferring surface, leading the transfer to the adjacent surface. When transferring from any surface, the patient must get the center of gravity forward to the edge of the surface, place one leg ahead of the other, lean forward, and shift the weight from the buttocks to the lower limbs (Fig. 53-7). Whenever possible, elbow extension and shoulder depression are used to facilitate the weight shift from sitting to standing. When returning to the sitting position, the process is reversed. The person backs up so that the posterior aspect of one leg is touching the seat of the chair, reaches back and places one hand on the armrest, leans forward and flexes the hips and knees until sitting, and transfers weight to the buttocks and thighs. Once sitting, the person pushes down on the armrests and slides back into the chair.

SELECTION AND MEASUREMENT

In today's market the number of wheelchair manufacturers is increasing, and many models exist from which to choose. Knowing what type of wheelchair to order and selecting the

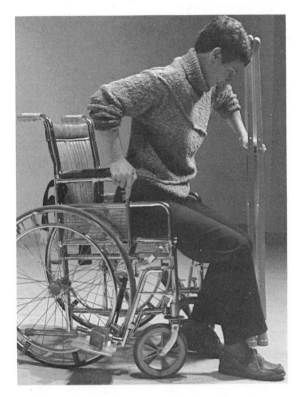

Figure 53-7. Position of the patient with a one-sided weakness when rising from the chair.

appropriate accessories is a major decision. In addition to the therapist applying appropriate knowledge when making these decisions, the patient's goals and wishes also must be taken into consideration. The following dimensions are standard measurements for determining proper wheelchair fit. When taking the measurements, the patient should be sitting in a wheelchair or a straight-back chair, not lying in bed. (Table 53-1 gives the dimensions for wheelchairs purchased direct from the manufacturer.)

Seat Height

Measure the length of the leg from the plantar surface of the foot to the posterior aspect of the thigh. If a cushion will be used, the measurement should be taken with the cushion in place. A 2-inch "safety clearance" exists be-

Table 53-1. Standard Wheelchair Dimensions

TYPE AND DESCRIPTION	SEAT WIDTH (IN)	SEAT DEPTH (IN)	BACK HEIGHT (IN)
Average (standard) adult: Designed for the average person (minimum overall width, 26 in.)	18	16	20
Narrow adult: Developed to fit the full-sized but slender user	16	16	20
Junior: Seat lowered for the small person	16	16	18
Child (13-in, junior chair): For the user with a very small frame	14	13	18
Tiny tot: Scaled down to fit the very young child	12	11.5	17 or 20

(After Palmer ML, Toms J: Manual for Functional Training, 2nd ed. Philadelphia, FA Davis, 1986)

tween the footrest and the ground. The footrest can be adjusted to take pressure off the popliteal area.

Seat Width

Measure from the greater trochanter of one leg to the greater trochanter of the other leg and add 2 inches. Allowing 1 inch on each side of the hips leaves enough room to avoid pressure on the greater trochanters. If the overall width of the chair does not allow the chair to fit through the doorway or if narrow doorways are a problem, it may be necessary to use a narrowing device. Other factors to consider for wheelchair width are the type of armrest and the type of tires.

Seat Depth

Measure from the back of the calf to the posterior aspect of the buttocks. A 2- to 3-inch clearance should exist between the edge of the seat upholstery and the back of the calf.

Arm Height

Measure the distance from the floor to the elbow, with the shoulders relaxed and the forearm parallel to the floor, plus 1 inch. If a cushion is being used, its height should be added to the measurement.

Back Height

Measure from the seat of the wheelchair to the axilla and add 4 inches. Back height will vary depending on the person's disability and stability. For a patient with good balance, the back height will be 1 inch below the inferior angle of the scapula. It will be 1 inch above the inferior angle of the scapula for a patient with poor balance.

When a person lacks trunk and head stability, total support for the trunk is necessary. The measurement is taken from the seat of the wheelchair to the back of the patient's head.

QUAD SYSTEM WHEELCHAIRS*

Improved emergency care is now giving rehabilitation centers many more patients with C1, C2, and C3 spinal cord injuries. Not only are these patients unable to propel a manual wheelchair or perform maneuvers for adequate pressure relief, but with injuries at this level they have no arm function and minimal, if any, head control. Therefore, equipment needs are much more sophisticated. The quad system wheelchair was created to give these persons the ability to propel a wheelchair independently, as well as provide them with an adequate means of pressure relief.

Several companies have put together certain combinations of components and sold

*Section on Quad System Wheelchairs contributed by Vickie Nixon.

them in a package called a "quad system wheelchair." Some companies offer more flexibility than others, but most have options. To ensure that patients receive the most appropriate and useful equipment, physical therapists must be able to evaluate the merits of these packages and so must be familiar with the five basic components: reclining mechanics, inclinator controls, drive systems, switches to operate the controls, and chair construction.

RECLINING MECHANICS

Reclining the wheelchair is not as easy as it might seem. The earlier components that simply let the back down are still available; however, the market is now able to provide other options. These are generally referred to as "low-shear reclining mechanics." No manufacturer has a system that provides *no* shear. Although significantly reduced, some shear will always exist, especially in the first 15 degrees. Basically, three approaches are available to recline the back: moving the back with the patient; moving the seat with the patient; and changing the hinge at the seat angle.

One approach is to use a special hinge, which essentially moves in a C shape. Instead of moving around one point, it rotates around three points, allowing the trunk to move with the back of the wheelchair. This hinge, however, can only be used with wheelchairs made by certain manufacturers.

As a second approach, some have opted to move the back of the wheelchair so the back of the chair actually moves up and down as the chair is reclined.

Finally, another company decided to move the seat. As the chair reclines, the seat moves forward. Like the special hinge, this system will fit only on wheelchairs made by certain manufacturers. In addition, because this movement is accomplished by putting rollers under the seat, the floor-to-seat height is increased by 1 inch. Sometimes a clip-on, drop seat can be used to compensate for this additional height.

All reclining components work best with a high-profile Roho cushion. However, other types of cushions may be used, as long as the patient "settles" to about the same point. Manufacturers assume that as a patient sits, he settles to approximately 2.5 inches above the seat. If the patient settles to a higher or lower point, relationships change and more shear will occur. Some of systems that move the back of the wheelchair with the patient may be able to provide a little more flexibility than others, because they can often adjust the moving range of the chair back.

The older or "high"-shear reclining components are still available and do have some applications. They are extremely durable and have fewer maintenance problems. It also may be easier to fit tall patients in chairs with this component option. However, it will be difficult to capture the trunk to facilitate any positioning, because the relationship of the trunk to the back of the wheelchair will always change as the chair is reclined. In addition, because of this changing relationship, patients may frequently need help with repositioning in the wheelchair after they have returned to the upright position. Finally, because shearing forces will be higher, potential for skin problems exists.

INCLINATOR CONTROLS

Inclinator controls are the electronics needed to operate the reclining mechanics. Only two options exist.

The single-speed control allows the patient to recline at only one speed. It starts somewhat abruptly, which may be a problem for the patient with spasticity.

The adjustable-speed control was developed by some companies to accommodate patients with increased spasticity. In addition to providing a smooth start-up, the speed at which the chair reclines can be adjusted. Some also have a feature that allows the attendant to cancel the remote recliner. Thus, if needed, the patient can be prevented from reclining on his own. Because the demand for this kind of inclinator control is low, it may be a very expensive option.

DRIVE SYSTEMS

The drive system moves the chair from point A to point B. All quad system wheelchairs are modifications of manufacturers' standard wheelchairs. However, because of the sophisticated electronics, different drive systems are needed. In this way, all the electronic components can fit into a small box and be less conspicuous.

Some manufacturers have developed their own quad drive systems to use with their wheelchairs. However, some vending companies put together and sell their own quad system chairs. Such vendors have two options. One is to take the manufacturer's chair, make maximum use of its electronics, and add individual components as needed. This approach is cheaper, because it avoids complete replacement of parts, but it cannot be used with all manufacturers' wheelchair electronics. In cases where a chair's existing components do not allow additions and deletions, the vending companies may use one of the quad drive systems developed by the few companies that specialize in them. These drive systems are more expensive, because they do not use any of the electronics from the chairs upon which they are building.

Proportional control options are available with these drive systems. This option allows the chair to start slowly and pick up speed as more pressure is applied to the control. However, these systems do not interface with sip-and-puff controls.

Most quad drive systems operate under a "latch" system. That is, the drive system will move the chair forward and continue in that direction until it receives another command. Three speeds are available—low, medium, and auto; auto is the fastest. The first puff will set the chair at low speed. The second puff will latch the chair into medium speed, and, if set

on auto, a third puff will put the chair at its top speed of approximately 4.6 miles per hour. (Note: The chair has to be manually set on auto to achieve the highest speed.) Vendors are able to adjust the speed within each of the three settings if necessary.

Some quad drive systems will interface easily with the various reclining mechanics and inclinator controls as well as environmental controls. Others will not be as flexible. Questions about these options should be asked before deciding on a drive system.

SWITCHES TO OPERATE THE CONTROLS

Today's technology can provide almost any type of drive system control, including short throw switches, chin controls, sip and puff controls, and even eyebrow controls. Options are limited only by the available local expertise.

When a latch system is used, a "kill" switch must always be provided for safety. For this reason, the reclining controls often serve the dual function of reclining and shutting down the drive system.

Attendant controls are also available. They allow another person to direct the chair from behind, and are therefore useful when teaching wheelchair controls. Attendant controls will override all other controls.

CHAIR CONSTRUCTION

Quad system wheelchair construction has a few idiosyncrasies, but the basic wheelchair frame should be familiar because systems are built on commercially available wheelchairs. Solid seats and backs can be provided for positioning, if needed.

Headrests used to be fairly big and bulky. However, with the low-shear reclining option, the smaller ones can be used.

Retractable "troughs" are attached to the wheelchair arms to better support the nonfunctional upper extremities. Some systems allow the patient to recline and maintain the arms parallel to the ground. With most systems, however, the arms are inclined up to 45 degrees as the patient reclines back. Arm attachments that are only secured in place at the back (as with some systems that allow the arms to stay parallel to the ground while reclining) may not be as sturdy as others.

The method of swinging legrests off to the side of the chair differs slightly on each system. Most now only require an easy one- or two-step procedure with one hand.

Ventilatory patients no longer require a little wagon trailing behind them with their ventilators. Many quad system wheelchairs now provide space for the ventilator underneath the seat. The respirator tray slides out for easy access and locks in place under the seat.

AMBULATION

A person requiring assistive devices for ambulation will use either crutches, walker, or cane(s). Assistive devices are used to provide support for one or both lower limbs when full weight bearing is contraindicated, when the lower limb(s) are too weak to bear weight, or when additional support is needed to maintain balance.

GAIT PATTERNS

Regardless of the type of assistive device, one of the following gait patterns or a variation of the pattern will be used.

Four-Point Gait

The four-point gait is the most stable of all the gait patterns, providing three points of support while one limb or an assistive device is moving. Usually the person will start by moving one ambulatory aid, such as a cane or crutch, about 12 to 16 inches ahead, followed by moving the opposite foot forward, followed by moving the opposite assistive device forward, and last the other foot is brought forward. The feet always stay about 6 or 7 inches back from the crutch or cane (Fig. 53-8A).

Two-Point Gait

The two-point gait is a natural progression from the four-point gait. It requires more bal-

ance and stability, but has a natural rhythm and arm motion that resembles normal gait. With a two-point gait, the person advances one assistive device and the opposite foot at the same time. One leg and one assistive device always supply two points of support on the floor at the same time. At the beginning of stance on one lower limb, the assistive device on the opposite side makes contact with the floor and provides support for the opposite limb.

Three-Point Gait

The three-point gait is commonly used by someone with involvement of one lower limb. It is used when the affected limb is either non-weight bearing or partial weight bearing (see Fig. 53-8B). During the three-point gait, the assistive device (either crutches or a walker) moves forward with the involved limb. As the unaffected limb begins the swing phase, the body weight is shifted to the upper limbs while the uninvolved limb swings through and is placed on the floor in front of the involved lower limb.

Swing-to Gait

The swing-to gait is best suited for someone with limited use of both lower limbs and instability of the trunk. It is also the logical gait to use in a crowded area. This gait pattern is performed using crutches (either axillary or forearm) or a walker. To perform the swing-to gait pattern, the weight is momentarily borne on both lower limbs as the crutches are moved forward simultaneously. As the weight is shifted onto the hands, both legs are brought forward until the feet are even with or just slightly behind the crutches.

Swing-Through Gait

For the more experienced patient with involvement of the trunk and both lower limbs, the swing-through gait provides a much more rapid means of ambulation than the four-point gait or the swing-to gait. It is the least stable of the gait patterns, and therefore requires strength and balance to perform safely. As in the swing-to gait, the initial step requires bal-

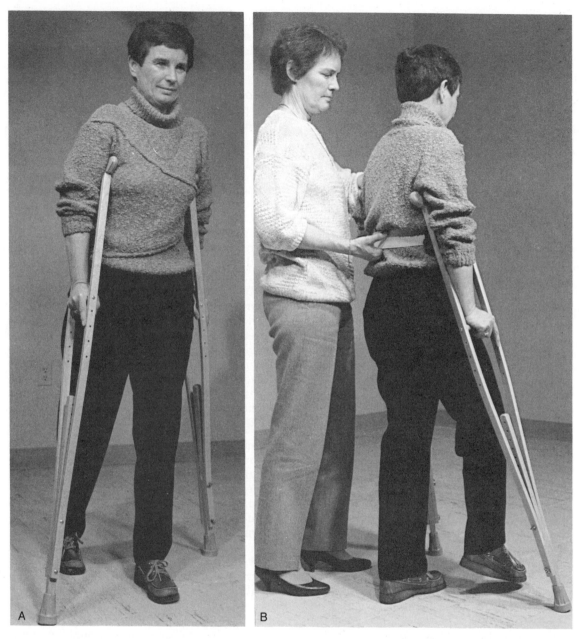

Figure 53-8. (*A*) Position of crutches and feet during four-point gait. (*B*) Position of crutches and the therapist during three-point non- or partial weight-bearing gait.

ancing momentarily on both legs as the crutches are moved forward. This is followed by shifting the weight to the hands and arms, and forcefully depressing the scapula while the legs swing forward and through the crutches, landing on the floor ahead of the crutches.

GUARDING FOR UPRIGHT ACTIVITIES

The position of the therapist while guarding an ambulating patient is from the back and slightly to the side. One hand is placed on the guarding belt and the other is on the patient's shoulder or ready to be placed on the shoulder should the patient's balance be lost. The therapist's feet are positioned to move with the crutch and the foot of the patient. For example, if the therapist is standing to the left side of the patient, the therapist's left leg will be placed forward just behind the patient's left crutch. As the patient's left leg advances, the therapist's right leg is advanced.

ASSISTIVE DEVICES

Walkers

Walkers provide the greatest amount of stability for ambulating, but are less convenient when ascending or descending stairs, maneuvering in crowded areas, and getting around quickly. Basically, walkers consist of a metal frame with four adjustable legs. The hand grips should be at a height that allows for about 20 to 30 degrees of elbow flexion, or about even with the greater trochanter when the person is standing. Many design variations are available, such as the folding walker, which has the same basic design as the standard walker except it is hinged, allowing the sides to fold. The sides swing out and lock into place when opened. When not in use, the sides of the walker fold in, considerably reducing its bulkiness and making it much easier to store or transport. Additional options in design include the rolling walker, the reciprocal walker, and the "hemi" walker.

A rolling walker has small casters on each of the two front legs. Instead of picking up the walker, the user rolls it forward. The reciprocal walker is hinged so that it is possible to move one side at a time. The hemi walker is a modification designed for someone with the use of only one upper limb. The hand grip is placed in the center front of the walker, which allows the person to maneuver the walker with one hand. The patient would be doing a "step-to" gait when using a hemi walker.

Coming to Standing

The patient slides forward in the chair, with one leg slightly ahead of the other. Usually the stronger leg is placed behind the weaker leg so the center of gravity will be over the strongest limb. The exception to this method is with a hemiplegic patient who demonstrates a strong extensor thrust. When extensor thrust is a factor, the involved limb would be slightly behind the uninvolved limb to reduce the possibility of the thrust as the patient comes to standing. When coming to standing with functional strength in both upper limbs, one hand is placed on the arm of the chair and the other on the hand grip of the walker (Fig. 53-9). The patient leans forward and pushes down on the walker and the arm of the chair, extends the knees and hips, and places the hand that was on the arm of the chair on the hand grip of the walker.

Ambulation with a Walker

Ambulation with a regular walker requires enough stability to balance on one or both feet while the walker is picked up and moved forward. The weight is shifted to the hands, pushing down on the walker while the legs move forward. If the patient is non-weight bearing, the walker would be placed 10 to 12 inches in front of the involved lower limb, and the weight would be shifted to the hands as the weight-bearing limb is picked up and moved forward. When it is possible to bear weight on both lower limbs, the most common gait pattern is a "step-to" or a "step-through" pattern. With these patients, the walker is placed 10 to 12 inches in front of the feet, then one foot is placed forward of the other and is brought either parallel to (step to) or slightly ahead of (step through) the opposite foot.

If a person is unable to maintain balance

someone whose balance is good, but whose legs are not equally weight bearing. For this type of patient, the gait pattern would be similar to the two-point gait: The walker and the opposite leg would move forward at the same time, just as the crutch and one leg move together with the two-point gait.

When using a rolling walker, the person shifts the weight from all four legs of the walker to the forward legs with the casters. The walker is rolled forward until the hands are 10 to 12 inches ahead of the feet. The gait pattern used with the rolling walker is a step to or step through.

Some walkers are designed so they can be used on stairs; however, maneuvering a

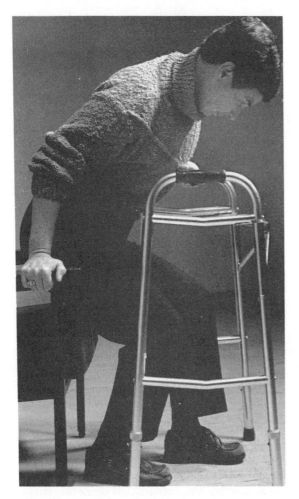

Figure 53-9. Coming to a standing position using a walker.

while the walker is picked up and moved forward, a rolling walker or a reciprocal walker may be more suitable. When using a reciprocal walker, the patient pushes down on one side of the walker while balance is maintained on both feet and one hand, then one side of the walker is moved forward, followed by the opposite lower limb moving forward. When the weight is then balanced on both legs, the opposite side of the walker is moved forward, followed by the opposite leg moving forward (Fig. 53-10). The reciprocal walker can also be used by

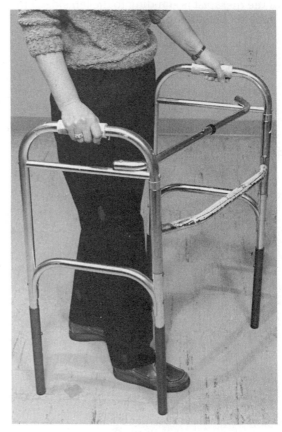

Figure 53-10. Reciprocal walker. The left side of the walker and the right leg move forward together.

walker on stairs is awkward and somewhat unsteady. One method of using a walker on the stairs is to have the patient go up the stairs facing forward with the walker placed sideways. The front of the walker faces the patient. The patient places a hand on the forward hand grip and raises the front legs of the walker up one step. The patient then pushes down on the walker and raises her leg up to the step with the walker. This procedure is repeated until the patient reaches the top of the stairs.

Crutches

Axillary crutches may be constructed of wood or aluminum, and are usually adjustable (Fig. 53-11). Crutches should always be equipped

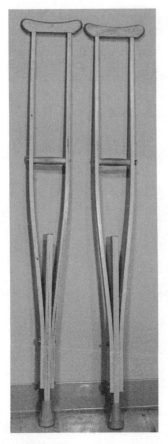

Figure 53-11. A pair of adjustable, wooden axillary crutches.

with rubber tips, which are about 1.5 inch in diameter. The tips provide suction, minimizing the possibility of the crutches slipping on a smooth surface. Many patients prefer axillary pads, which provide a cushion between the top of the crutch and the axilla of the patient. The pads also help keep the crutch tops from slipping out from under the axilla.

When possible, the patient should be standing when fitted for crutches. The crutch tips should be resting on the floor, about 6 to 8 inches lateral to and forward of each foot. If axillary pads are used, they should be in place while measuring. Two or three fingers should fit between the top of the crutch and the axilla. The height of the hand grips is determined by measuring from the floor to the hand with the elbow flexed 20 to 30 degrees and with the shoulders relaxed. The hand grip height is approximately level with the greater trochanter of the femur.

A modification of the axillary crutch is the platform crutch (Fig. 53-12). The platform crutch allows weight to be distributed over the forearm rather than on the wrists and hands. This crutch would be the appropriate choice for a below-elbow amputee, or when weight bearing on the wrist and hand is contraindicated, such as with an arthritic patient.

Forearm, or Lofstrand crutches, resemble a cane except for the presence of cuffs that encircle the forearm (Fig. 53-13). Forearm crutches are adjustable and constructed of metal. These crutches provide less stability than axillary crutches; however, they are better suited for people with good to normal upper limb strength and good balance. With forearm crutches, the person can release the grip of the crutch and free up the hands without having to set the crutches down. They are also less cumbersome and easier to use than axillary crutches, especially on stairs without a railing. Forearm crutches tend to be more expensive than wooden axillary crutches, and it is sometimes difficult to remove the hand and forearm from the cuff. The procedure for measuring the height of the hand grips is identical to the procedure for axillary crutches. The cuffs are also adjustable and should come up as high on the

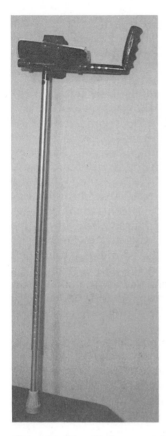

Figure 53-12. Platform crutch.

forearm as possible without restricting elbow flexion. The cuff height is approximately 4 to 5 inches below the epicondyles of the humerus.

Ambulation with Crutches
Regardless of the type of crutches the patient uses, the techniques for transfers and ambulation are similar. Therefore, techniques for ambulation are not described separately.

Coming to Standing
Whenever possible, the surface of the chair from which the person is transferring should be stabilized. If the patient is transferring from a wheelchair, the footrests should be turned up and the brakes locked. The patient slides forward in the chair, with one foot slightly ahead of the other and the stronger leg behind the

weaker leg (Fig. 53-14). Both crutches are placed in one hand. The crutches are gripped with the palms facing down and the fingers grasping the hand grips. The other hand is on the armrest of the chair. Simultaneously, the patient leans forward, pushes down with both hands, extends the hips and knees, and comes to the standing position. The patient reaches across the body and brings one crutch back, under the arm. The other crutch is pivoted around and placed under the other arm. The patient is now ready to begin ambulating.

Sitting from Standing
The procedure for sitting down is the reverse of coming to standing. The patient approaches

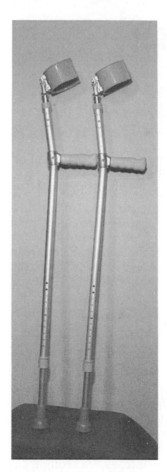

Figure 53-13. Lofstrand or forearm crutches.

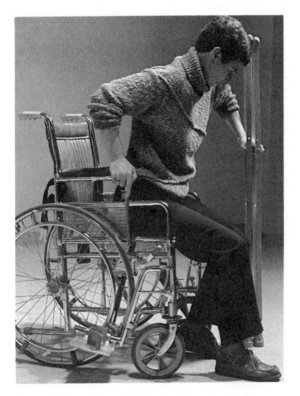

Figure 53-14. Crutch placement and position of patient when rising from the chair.

the chair, turns around, and backs up until one leg is touching the seat of the chair. Both crutches are placed in one hand, and the other hand reaches back for the arm of the chair. In one motion the patient leans forward, bends at the hips and knees, and lowers the weight into the chair.

Ascending and Descending Stairs, One Lower Limb Involved

Ordinarily, patients with involvement of one lower limb do not use the handrail when ascending and descending stairs.

To ascend stairs or curbs, the patient stands facing the stairs or curb. While pushing down on the crutches, the stronger limb is placed on the step above. As the weight is shifted to the stronger limb on the step, the weaker limb and the crutches are brought up and placed on the step. To descend curbs or

stairs, the crutches and the weaker limb are placed on the step below, and the weight is shifted to the crutches and the weaker limb as the stronger limb is lowered onto the step.

Ascending and Descending Stairs with a Handrail, Both Lower Limbs Involved

To ascend stairs, the patient stands facing the stairs, close to the handrail. The hand closest to the handrail grasps the handrail. The other hand reaches across the body and removes the crutch from under the arm at the side of the handrail. Both crutches are placed on the side away from the rail, with the tips of the crutches close to the feet. If the patient finds this method of crutch placement uncomfortable, one crutch would be placed under the arm and the other crutch held in the hand, on the same side, parallel to the floor. Shift the body weight from the feet to the crutches and the handrail, and push down on the handgrips and the rail, lifting the feet and body up to the next step. As the feet land on the step above, the hips are rotated forward so that the pelvis is well ahead of the body, reducing the danger of jackknifing before the crutches can be advanced. Once the balance is reestablished on the step, the crutches are brought up on the same step as the feet.

To descend stairs, the patient stands facing the stairs, close to the handrail with the feet slightly over the edge of the step. Grasp the handrail and position the crutches, using one of the two methods described for ascending the stairs. One or both crutches are placed on the step below. With the head forward, the weight is shifted to the hands, and the elbows are extended, raising the body off the step to the step below. When the feet are placed on the step below, the pelvis is rotated forward to prevent jackknifing.

Canes

Many varieties of canes are available on the market. Canes are the least stable of all the assistive devices for ambulation. However, some are designed to allow for more stability than others. Some models of metal canes have a hand grip that is molded to fit the shape of the hand, providing a more natural, comfortable distribution of pressure when walking. Regardless of the style, most canes are made of aluminum and are easily adjusted by means of a sliding shaft and a locking pin. In addition to the metal adjustable models, standard canes may also be made of wood. Obviously, wooden canes would have to be cut to the proper length for the individual patient.

Cost is a factor to be considered in choosing between a wooden or metal cane. The adjustable metal cane is considerably more expensive than the wooden cane.

A standard cane has a small base of support and, because of its design, the point of support is in front of the hand (Fig. 53-15). Obviously, the standard cane would be appro-

priate only for those patients who have good balance and are not required to put a great deal of pressure onto the cane.

The shafts of some canes may be offset. That is, they are designed in such a way that the point of support is directly below the hand, thus providing slightly more stability than the standard cane (Fig. 53-15).

The quad cane provides a wide base of support through four legs projecting from the base of the cane (Fig. 53-16). The four-point base of the quad cane has two vertical legs on the side closest to the patient and two outer legs that project laterally approximately 45 degrees. The size and shape of the base will vary. The wider base of support provides greater stability; however, with some designs the point of support is

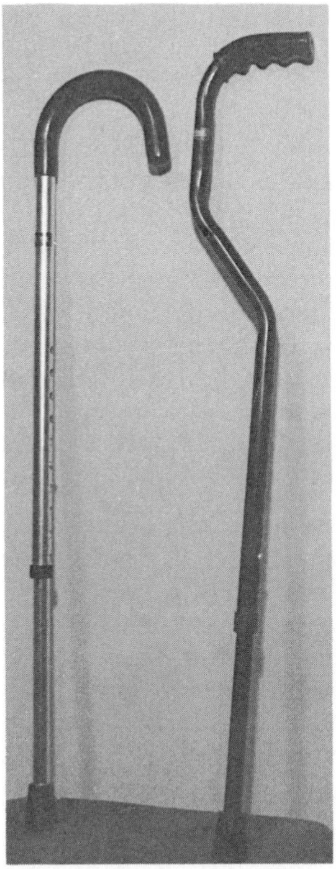

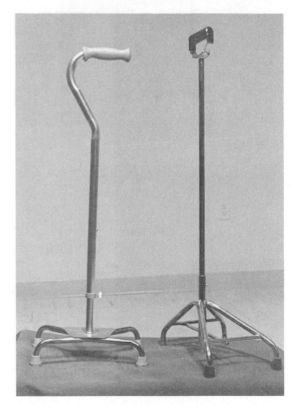

Figure 53-15. (*Left*) Standard cane with the point of support in front of the handle. (*Right*) Cane with the point of support directly below the handle.

Figure 53-16. (*Left*) Quad cane with offset handle, which allows weight to be distributed straight down the handle. (*Right*) Standard quad cane.

not centered. Some cane designs have compensated for this by offsetting the shaft of the cane, which allows the weight to be distributed straight down the shaft (Fig. 53-17). Because of the increased size, a quad cane may have to be turned sideways to fit on stairs; in addition, the quad cane is awkward to carry when using a handrail.

Another device on the market, the Walkane, provides greater stability than a quad cane, and looks like a cross between a cane and a walker (Fig. 53-18). It is lighter and smaller than a walker, more versatile than a hemi walker, and more stable than a cane. The base of the Walkane is too large to be used on stairs, and it would be quite awkward to carry while using a handrail. The angle and height of the Walkane are adjustable. For convenience, the Walkane folds for storage or transporting.

The ability of the patient to use the cane properly is an important consideration in selecting the most appropriate cane. If the quad cane is to be used, it is essential that the patient knows the importance of placing the cane in the proper position so that the legs of the cane, which project laterally from the base, are turned away from the body. If the cane is held incorrectly, the patient's foot may catch on these legs.

Adjusting for proper height and instructions for use are the same regardless of the type of cane. With the patient standing and the tip of the cane placed alongside the toes, the cane height is measured from the floor to the hand with 20 to 30 degrees of elbow flexion and the shoulder in a relaxed position. Another quick method of adjusting cane height is by placing the top of the cane at the level of the greater trochanter of the femur.

Coming to Standing
The patient slides forward to the edge of the chair. If a standard cane is used, it is held in the hand as the patient grasps the armrest of the chair. If the patient is using a quad cane or Walkane, it is placed upright in front of and to the side of the patient. The feet are in a stride position with the stronger foot behind the weaker foot. The exception to the this foot placement is for the hemiplegic patient who demonstrates a strong extensor thrust. When this is a factor, the involved limb would be slightly behind the uninvolved limb to reduce the possibility of extensor thrust as the patient comes to standing.

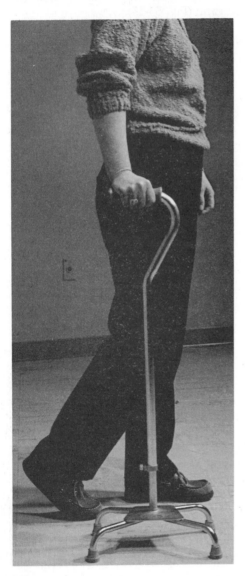

Figure 53-17. Position of cane and limb during gait.

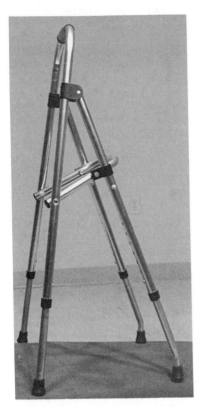

Figure 53-18. The Walkane allows for greater stability than a standard cane or a quad cane.

Sitting from Standing

The procedure for sitting is the reverse of coming to standing. The patient approaches the chair, turns around, and backs up until one leg is touching the seat of the chair. The patient keeps the cane in one hand and reaches back for the arms of the chair with the hands. If a quad cane is used, the patient releases the grip on the cane and reaches back for the arms of the chair. In one motion the patient leans forward, bends at the hips and knees, and lowers the weight into the chair.

Ambulation with a Cane

For ambulation, the cane is held on the side opposite the weaker limb. This position not only provides the greatest base of support and simulates the natural arm motion during nor-

mal gait, but it also distributes the weight through the arm on the opposite side to assist in maintaining the pelvis in a level position during stance on the weaker limb. To use the cane properly, the patient pushes down on the cane during the stance phase on the weaker limb, then swings the cane forward with the involved limb.

Ascending or Descending Curbs or Stairs

When ascending, always lead with the stronger limb; when descending, lead with the weaker limb. To ascend, the patient stands with both feet near the edge of the step. While briefly bearing weight on the weaker limb and pushing down on the cane, the stronger limb is placed on the step above. As the weight is shifted to the stronger limb, the cane and the weaker limb are advanced to the step next to the stronger limb. The procedure is reversed for descending a curb or stairs. The weight of the body is supported on the stronger limb while the cane and the weaker limb are placed on the step below. The weight is then shifted to the cane and the weaker limb as the stronger limb is brought down and placed next to the weaker limb.

Ascending and Descending Stairs with a Handrail

The patient with functional use of both upper limbs could use the cane in one hand and grasp the handrail with the other hand. If only one upper limb is functional, the patient can grasp the cane and the handrail together. The same procedure is followed for ascending and descending stairs or curbs without a handrail.

CONCLUSION

The degree of success experienced by the patient will depend to a great extent upon the physical therapist's ability to select the proper equipment and instruct the patient in the use of mobility and ambulatory aids. The choice of equipment for each patient will require the therapist to be constantly aware of recent developments and changes in technology. It is essential that therapists stay abreast of advances in technology so that the patient will receive maximum benefit from the treatment. A knowledgeable therapist, appropriate and properly fitting equipment, and a patient with the skill and desire to achieve maximum functional independence should result in successfully achieving goals.

ANNOTATED BIBLIOGRAPHY

Minor M, Minor S: Patient Care Skills. Norwalk, CT, Reston Publishing, 1984 (Good photographs and descriptions of procedures.)

Palmer ML, Toms J: Manual for Functional Training, 2nd ed. Philadelphia, FA Davis, 1986 (Comprehensive descriptions for wheelchair and ambulatory activities.)

54 Environmental Modifications

VICKIE NIXON

The problems of access in today's world are, to a degree, the result of improved technology. More lives are being saved at the scene of an accident, more medical complications are being prevented, and the disabled person is being provided with more personal independence than was ever before possible. Great strides have been made in increasing life expectancy. The focus now needs to shift to making life more enjoyable to live.

Rehabilitation hospitals have done much to assist in this shift of focus with their efforts to develop the physical abilities of the individual. However, the process of rehabilitation is not complete unless it also helps the client create an environment in which he can use the personal independence rehabilitation has helped him find and develop. The ultimate outcome of health services should be to maintain or improve an individual's ability to function in *his* environment.

Independence within an environment is not the only requirement in the design of an accessible environment. Because of decreases in coordination, strength, flexibility, sensation, and the like, the disabled person often does not have the same variety of movements available to him as the able-bodied person and is not able to respond as quickly or as accurately to an emergency. Therefore, particular attention should be given to safety concerns. Decreases in physical capabilities will also have an impact on endurance. So, energy expense is also a critical concern for the disabled person in his environment and must be kept at a minimum.

Finally, it should be remembered that each person wants his environment to be comfortable, stimulating, secure, and aesthetically pleasing. The question is, how can the disabled person design an environment that meets all these requirements?

This chapter will approach the problem first in a general way by looking at some overall considerations and then in a more specific way by dealing with the sitting environment, both horizontal and vertical movement within the environment, and aspects of the environment dependent on reach capabilities. The final section will speak to issues surrounding private transportation.

GENERAL CONSIDERATIONS FOR ENVIRONMENTAL MODIFICATION

Physical therapists are often the first information source for the disabled person, and so they need to understand the problems of accessibility, be able to identify other information sources (eg, occupational therapists, social workers, architects, interior designers, human factor engineers), and generally facilitate the problem-solving process.

The decision-making process for environmental modifications is similar to that needed to resolve any problem. Basically the process involves four steps: determining client needs, outlining available finances, establishing priorities, and getting the job done.

DETERMINING CLIENT NEEDS

Creating an environment truly sensitive to a person's specific needs and strengths requires very detailed information about the individual, including balance, strength, mobility, and coordination skills, and the equipment required for various activities. Categories of independence such as those listed in Table 54-1 can give the therapist a starting point in the client evaluation process.

While much of the assessment of an individual's physical capabilities within an environment can be done by trial and error, this method can waste time and is often not complete. Usually, it is both helpful and more expedient to consult some of the available resources.

Local independent living centers and rehabilitation hospitals can frequently provide resources. Vocational counselors and industrial engineers can assist with task analysis in the work setting. In addition to many good books and pamphlets dealing with the subject, several states (many using American National Standards Institute [ANSI] standards) now have their own accessibility codes. These are often free or available at minimal cost to the public. Although most standards are written for public facilities, they are a good reference for employers and can provide initial guidelines for private buildings and homes.

Analysis of the social environment is also essential when determining client needs. If an able-bodied individual is sharing an environment with a disabled individual—particularly if the latter is a full-time wheelchair user—compromises will have to be made. As Goldsmith (1967) points out,

> The assumption sometimes made that a house which is ideal for a person in a wheelchair is automatically suitable for all other disabled people or for nondisabled people is fallacious. The more that a house is planned to suit the chairbound person the less convenient it becomes for the normal person, and equally the more it is planned to suit the normal person the less it is convenient for the chairbound.

The conflict is especially evident when considering placement of work surfaces and storage. While the wheelchair user may be most comfortable with 28-inch-high kitchen counters, the able-bodied person usually works more efficiently with a 36-inch-high counter. The person with arthritis who has difficulty bending or the especially tall person may prefer an even higher kitchen counter.

One of the therapist's major focuses during this period of evaluation should be in helping the person clearly delineate between *wants* and *needs*. The task of establishing priorities will then be much easier.

OUTLINING AVAILABLE FINANCES

Once needs have been defined, the client should be encouraged to determine what fi-

Table 54-1. Categories of Independence

THE AMBULANT DISABLED	THE SEMIAMBULANT WHEELCHAIR USER	THE INDEPENDENT WHEELCHAIR USER	THE DEPENDENT WHEELCHAIR USER
Balance is often the principal problem, especially when walking over uneven surfaces. Has difficulty with stairs, heavy doors, carpeting, etc; therefore, the most important environmental consideration would probably be walking surfaces.	Level surfaces are still important, but circulation space is a much more critical concern. The wheelchair user requires more space to maneuver than someone walking.	Will need the most modifications to the environment. Does not have the luxury of being able to walk even short distances through a narrow door to enter a bathroom, for instance. Stairs cannot be negotiated in a wheelchair, and reach ranges are greatly reduced.	Modification may be more intimately related to the needs and abilities of the caregiver. This wheelchair user may still require a ramp to enter the home. However, he may be able to get by with a little steeper ramp than one who is expecting to negotiate ramps independently.

(After Goldsmith S: Designing for the Disabled, 2nd ed. New York, McGraw-Hill, 1967; and Feuerstein G, Bernard HP: Categories of the disabled and habitation design in practice. Int J Rehabil Res 3(2):225, 1980)

nances will be available. With few exceptions, today's technology can provide viable solutions to almost any accessibility problem. There are stair glides, elevators, adjustable-height kitchen counters, vans with "zero-effort" steering, and elaborate wheelchair systems with environmental controls that can literally be operated with a blink of an eye. The solutions are usually limited by availability of money, not by lack of ideas or technology.

Local independent living centers, rehabilitation facilities, and social workers can all be helpful resources in this step. Although funding may be limited, these people should be able to refer the client to some possible sources. Under certain conditions, some modifications and mechanical devices (eg, ramps and lifts) can be deducted as medical expenses. Such deductions should also be considered in a financial assessment.

ESTABLISHING PRIORITIES

Because most people do not have unlimited financial resources, priorities usually have to be established. If a thorough client and environmental assessment has been done, the therapist should be able to assist the client in setting priorities. The person who will leave the hospital with some walking skills may not need immediate modifications to the bathroom. The same may be true for the person requiring maximum assistance for transfers and hygiene. This individual may opt for a bedpan and a sponge bath in bed, so immediate modifications may be unwise.

Some clients mistakenly assume that all home modifications need to be made before an individual leaves the hospital. In most cases, this assumption is false. In fact, all modifications are not always possible, especially if modifications will be expensive. The environment does have to be usable, but often it will be usable with fairly minor alterations. Ideally, one should wait a year or two before making most major modifications.

Moreover, if decisions are made at the point of hospital discharge, the client will be forced to rely much more heavily on the opinions of health professionals who do not know the specific intimate needs of the disabled person any better than the disabled person knows at that time.

At the point of hospital discharge, most disabled individuals do not truly know the implications of the disability and the impact it will have on the environment. Weekend home visits give a brief experience of what life will be as a disabled person, but cannot give much more.

In addition, functional skills are often still changing at hospital discharge. Modifications made at this point may be more than will actually be needed. For example, the wheelchair user who is familiar with his environment and has achieved a certain degree of expertise may maneuver in less space and through narrower doors.

The process of establishing priorities must focus on both present and future needs and abilities. Is the disease that created the disability progressive? Is further loss of motor function likely? Will fatigue be an important future consideration? If these needs and abilities change, the kinds of environmental modifications required will probably change, too.

Priority determination should also be based on life-style, values, interests, family demands, where the greatest time will be spent, and other considerations. The person interested in gardening and the outside appearance of the house may opt for a less accessible interior and invest more time and money into landscaping an aesthetically pleasing ramped entrance. A two-car garage may be more important than being able to reach all the light bulbs in the house. How are the household responsibilities divided? Who takes out the garbage? If an able-bodied woman does this, it is less urgent that the path to the trash be accessible. On the other hand, the woman who uses a wheelchair and does all the cooking will place a wheelchair-accessible kitchen at the top of the priority list.

Cost, which is also a major consideration in setting priorities, should include the initial investment cost as well as maintenance costs. The money might well be available to build a very spacious dwelling, but the cost of heating such a large, open area may be prohibitive.

GETTING THE JOB DONE

The final step in this problem-solving process involves decisions on specific designs and selecting contractors to do the work. As Laurie (1977) indicated, at this juncture, "Information about existing adaptations, techniques, remodeling plans, and specification is vital, the starting point for individual creativity." At this time, the therapist should be able to refer clients to information sources and may make design recommendations. However, the actual decisions are the primary responsibility of the client. Several organizations and architectural firms exist that specialize in home modifications for the disabled, but they are usually expensive. The disabled person who has done a little reading on the subject or who has thought about the task can often design his own solutions. The following pages should help point to some design options for your clients. Any possible solution should be tested thoroughly by the client to ensure that it will work.

After designs are created, the client will need a carpenter and perhaps an electrician and a plumber. Professional contractors can be hired, but often friends can fill these roles. Clients should look for someone who will listen and be responsive to the specific needs. Familiarity with accessibility codes and available products are helpful, but not absolutely essential. It is only important that the person be able to accomplish the task in a functional, aesthetically pleasing way at the lowest possible cost, meeting all building codes.

THE SITTING ENVIRONMENT

Whether disabled or able bodied, everyone sits to eat, to travel, to work, to see a play, to watch television, and often to socialize.

Indeed, for many of the disabled, all environments seem to revolve around the world of sitting. So optimizing the sitting environment may mean fewer changes in other environments. For example, poor sitting can encourage contractures and pain, which in turn will directly have an impact on reach ranges. Decreases in reach will mean more modifications in locating work surfaces and storage areas. Reach limitations may also decrease the skill with which a wheelchair user is able to maneuver the chair. If turns are less precise, more space will have to be allotted for general movement within an environment.

The best sitting environment is one that will support and encourage the skeletal alignment found in symmetrical standing. Maintaining the lumbar lordosis is particularly important. The question is, how do we do this? How can the environment be changed to encourage this posture?

APPROACHES TO SEATING FOR THE AMBULANT PERSON

The first step in creating a good sitting environment is to find a firm, level foundation for the pelvis—regardless of whether an individual has a head injury and is using a wheelchair full time, or has a back injury but is ambulatory.

Soft, "cushy" seats allow the pelvis to tip to one side or the other and should be avoided. Some seats have a lower rear portion, so the pelvis tends to drop back into a posterior tilt. Without the anterior positioning of the pelvis, the lumbar spine is forced into flexion. Any depressions in the rear portion of a seat should be filled in with towels or magazines. Ideally, the sitting surface should support the anterior position of the pelvis as well as encourage pelvic symmetry.

Hage (unpublished self-help manual for patients with chronic back and neck pain)* believes that the person with good-to-normal trunk strength has two basic sitting-pattern options. She can either sit "back and up" or "forward and up."

---

*Hage MG: Backs for the Future. Available from Physical Therapy Ltd, 448 E. Ontario, Suite 400, Chicago, IL 60611. Discusses pain relief, exercise, and self-care for activities of daily living.

The "back and up" option requires a lumbar support. The exact size and shape of the support varies with each client and is specific to the size and shape of the lumbar cure. To a large degree, the determination is based on trial and error. However, it is often easiest to start by evaluating the size and shape of your client's lordosis in standing. Generally, the more lordosis someone has in standing, the more support for the lordosis she will require in sitting.

Any error in construction, whether the support is overly large, small, firm, short, or long, will eventually result in a movement toward lumbar flexion, as opposed to the desired normal lumbar lordosis. Because it may take a while for this to become apparent, a support should be used for some time before final decisions are made.

Ideally, the client should be able to strap the support in place. Most supports tend to lose their position and slide down the back of the chair. If it is not repositioned, the support will encourage lumbar flexion rather than lordosis.

The concept of lumbar support is not new to the manufacturing world. Many chairs are commercially made with it built in. However, they are usually based on the notion that one size fits all. Therefore, it is difficult to find a ready-made chair with the perfect lumbar lordotic support.

Rather than spending hours looking for the best chair, it is often easier to recommend one with a firm back and seat and then work with the client to create a lumbar support specific to his needs. Again, the client should sit in the chair for a good period of time before any purchase decisions are made.

Sitting "forward and up" is a pattern that many choose quite naturally when they sit on the edge of a seat with their feet tucked under the chair. The foundation requirements for this pattern are the same as those for sitting "back and up." A level, firm seating surface is still needed. However, in this case, instead of directly supporting the lumbar spine, the environmental modification provides support by means of a wedge under the back end of the pelvis. This wedge encourages movement of the pelvis into an anterior tilt, which, in turn, encourages a lumbar lordosis. Anything can act as a wedge—a towel, a rolled-up magazine, of even some of the commercially available lumbar rolls. The size, again, will depend on how much lumbar lordosis is needed.

Some of the newer office chairs allow the seat to tilt forward, creating a very functional pelvic "wedge." This seating option may be particularly appropriate for those who do typing, keypunching, writing, and the like.

The Balans chair was specifically designed with the "wedge" concept in mind (Fig. 54-1). Although those requiring a lot of lumbar lordosis may need to add a wedge to this chair, it basically blocks the pelvis into an anterior tilt, thus encouraging lumbar extension. However, the Balans design chairs can be limiting because they allow only one sitting pattern.

The knee position is another factor that can have a critical impact on the position of the lumbar spine. Brunswic (1984) notes, "When the knees are flexed at 70 degrees or less, the lumbar mechanism is extremely sensitive to any modification in the hip angle." Therefore,

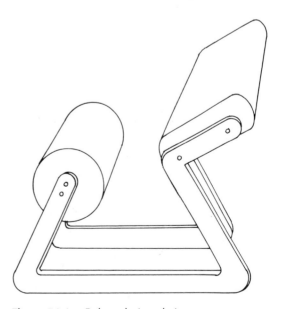

Figure 54-1. Balans design chair.

Brunswic believes that the client whose job requires manipulation of pedals for machinery operation will probably need to have a seat tilted forward 10 to 20 degrees to create the correct spinal alignment.

Cars may present a similar situation. Not only are most car seats tilted back 10 to 15 degrees, which encourages lumbar flexion, but many drivers are forced to stretch their knees to reach the pedals. Moving the seat as far forward as possible creates a better sitting environment by allowing maximum knee flexion. The very short person may need to use a thick back insert to support her even farther forward in the seat. Either a pelvic wedge or a lumbar support may be used to maintain the normal lordotic curve of the lumbar spine.

Sitting is not a static activity. So, it is important that the client be given several sitting options with the appropriate positions and methods to use to achieve these options. Realistically, definitive modifications cannot be made on every chair, but they should be made for the constantly used sitting environments, like those found in the car, office, and home.

APPROACHES TO SEATING FOR THE WHEELCHAIR USER

A good sitting environment is perhaps more critical for the full-time wheelchair user than for the ambulant person, because the former will spend so much time in this posture. However, solutions to many of the seating problems for the wheelchair user can be complex.

Someone with limited trunk strength, for instance, will have trouble maintaining the lumbar lordosis, much less actively moving into it. In fact, until recently many health professionals were opposed to having these individuals sit with the pelvis in an anterior position, not only because of the difficulties in doing so but also because of a belief that this posture would increase ischial pressures, encouraging the development of pressure sores (Noble).

However, Hage (1985) studied the pressures created under the ischial tuberosities of normal subjects when sitting with an extreme anterior pelvic tilt and with an extreme posterior pelvic tilt. His results showed significantly lower pressure readings when sitting with an anterior pelvic tilt than with a posterior tilt. Even the combined pressure under the ischial tuberosities and the thighs was lower in anterior sitting.

Thus, it would seem that even the sitting environment created for the wheelchair user should encourage the normal lumbar lordosis. These individuals, however, will have to rely more heavily on external supports. In addition, solutions will have to be more sensitive to the balance between stability and mobility issues, as well as those of skin integrity.

As with the ambulant person, the first step in designing a proper sitting environment is to obtain a solid back and a solid, nonshifting seat. Upon even a cursory view of a person sitting in a standard wheelchair, one will discover the poor postural support of the sling back and seat (Figs. 54-2 and 54-3).

Cushions can also contribute to poor postural support. However, many wheelchair users require a cushion for sitting to decrease ischial pressures. Inability to readjust posture easily and often decreased blood pressure make them particularly prone to skin breakdown. Using a cushion on a solid seat is usually one of the better compromises.

Once the foundation is laid, the next step is the selection of a lumbar support. Again, the decision regarding size and shape is essentially trial and error. Because evaluation of the lumbar lordosis of these individuals in standing is usually impossible, the therapist must begin by ascertaining the available passive movement into lumbar extension. Evaluating the available movement in several different developmental postures gives a clearer picture of actual limitations and probable causes (ie, muscle activity changes, bony block, etc.).

The person whose injury or onset of disease occurred several years previously may not have enough range in the lumbar spine to sit with any extension. Someone unable to move past a neutral pelvic position will probably have a lower pressure reading under the ischial tuberosities in posterior sitting, and so will

tive seating and positioning can be aggressively approached.

At this point, the solution becomes more complicated by stability issues. The patient with limited trunk strength is often unable to maintain sitting, if forced to use a lumbar support and sit with the normal lumbar lordosis. To resolve this problem, Zacharkow (1984) recommended that the wheelchair back be inclined backward 15 degrees and the seat 10 degrees. These changes can easily be accomplished with wedges or by using clip-on backs and seats with longer hooks at one end. The exact degree of inclination should balance stability against functional needs, with the shoul-

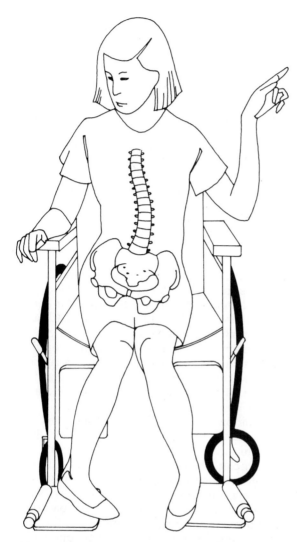

Figure 54-2. The poor postural foundation of the wheelchair sling seat causes the pelvis to lean to one side or the other, creating neck and trunk asymmetries. The legs are often internally rotated and fall into the center.

need to sit with a posterior pelvic tilt. Specific pressure evaluations should be done in the available sitting postures to determine the best option. The person with limited, but not fixed, range deficits will need to receive treatment to increase the lumbar range. After the appropriate range of motion has been obtained, defini-

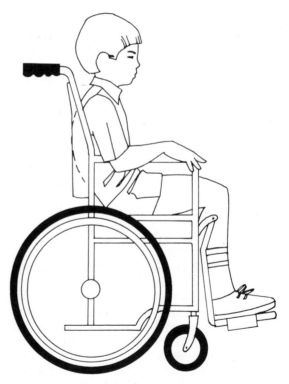

Figure 54-3. The wheelchair sling back allows gravity to pull the pelvis back into a posterior tilt, forcing the lumbar spine into flexion. This decreases the efficiency of breathing and increases the muscle activity necessary for sitting, especially around the neck and shoulders Energy expense for this posture is therefore high.

der position being critical for tabletop activities.

Accessories such as seat belts properly placed across the lap can also be used to encourage an anteriorly titled pelvis. Often, but not always, placing the belt at a 45-degree angle with the seat creates the best support for the pelvis. Abductor rolls and hip blocks can encourage pelvic symmetry and assist in keeping the pelvis centered in the seat. Properly positioned footrests will enable the feet and thighs to support more weight and further decrease the ischial sitting pressures.

Once the pelvis is properly aligned, the trunk asymmetries often seem to correct themselves. However, because of poor trunk musculature or spasticity, it may also be necessary to use external environmental supports to maintain trunk symmetry and alignment. This alignment can be facilitated either distally with lapboards, armboards, and adjustable-height armrests, or proximally with trunk supports. Trunk supports are usually the preferable option because they free the arms for function.

Many different trunk supports exist. Each has its advantages and disadvantages. Most important are their ability to hold a position and the ease with which they are moved out of the way for a transfer. The higher and closer the supports are placed on the trunk, the more stability and support they will provide.

MOVING IN AND OUT OF THE SITTING ENVIRONMENT

Seating modifications should both encourage good sitting positions and allow movement in and out of the sitting environment. Poorly designed modifications may provide good sitting posture, but can make transfers in and out of the chair difficult, if not impossible. Design options that address both issues require more thought and creativity, but are nevertheless possible. Such things as hip blocks and trunk supports, for example, may be fixed to detachable armrests so that they are removed with the armrest in preparation for the transfer. Some trunk supports may be swung out of the way for a transfer. Others may be constructed with a hinge design that allows them to be placed flat against the wheelchair back when not in use.

The height of a sitting surface will also affect transfers. Low surfaces, such as toilets and tubs, present particularly difficult problems. The standard toilet height of 16 inches may be too low for those with stiff joints and decreased strength. Those in a wheelchair (using the average seat height of 19 inches) may not have as much difficulty getting onto this toilet, but neither may they have the strength to transfer "up hill" back into the chair.

The exact toilet height needed will depend to a certain degree on personal preference. Even though easier for transfers, some wheelchair users prefer not to use the 20-inch-high toilet because their feet do not touch the ground. This posture is both uncomfortable and less secure for the person with balance deficits. The 18-inch-seat seems to be the height recommended most often for toilets. Although toilets with higher seats are commercially available, many opt to use one of the portable, raised toilet seats. These are usually less expensive and can be easily removed, if others sharing the environment do not require the raised height.

Commercially available tub shells fit into conventional tubs and raise the tub floor. Even with these shells, transfers in and out of the tub are difficult. Mechanical lifts to assist with such transfers are available, but are expensive and sometimes awkward to use. Most persons opt to shower and use one of many available styles of shower chairs or bath benches in the tub. Shower-hose extensions should be purchased with them. Wheeled shower chairs are also available for those using shower stalls.

A grab bar is another piece of equipment that may be considered to assist with movement in and out of sitting. Special finishes can be used on the bars to make the grip more secure. The exact placement of grab bars will depend on the user. Horizontal bars, which are used to assist in pushing up, are usually placed anywhere from 32 to 37 inches from the floor. They should be placed 1.5 inch from the wall to provide a space that is large enough to allow the hands to grip the bar easily and yet small enough to prevent elbows from falling in between the bar and wall.

Vertical bars are used to assist in pulling up. Angled bars, which can be used for either pushing or pulling up, require a stronger grip and so do not serve either function as well. One must remember that clients will often use anything near them to assist in a transfer. Therefore, all towel racks, sink edges, and the like should be able to support at least 250 pounds.

MOVEMENT WITHIN AN ENVIRONMENT

HORIZONTAL MOVEMENT

General Considerations

According to Goldsmith (1967), a typical ambulatory person, with or without assistive standing and walking devices, can turn in a space only 50% larger than the space he occupies in standing. So, while some minor modifications may be needed, the space modification required for the ambulatory but disabled person will probably be fairly minimal.

The wheelchair user in an average size chair, on the other hand, requires 450% more space than the ambulant person before he even moves. Turning requires a minimum of 800% more space that the ambulant person, or an area 5 × 5 ft.

The actual space needed by the wheelchair user will be specific to that individual and dependent on the width and length of the wheelchair, the techniques used for turning, and the skill of the user. The large, electrically propelled and reclining wheelchairs may require 6 or 7 ft² to turn. The small child-size chair will probably require less than 5 ft². The person who can simultaneously turn one wheel backward and the other forward to accomplish a turn will require less space than the person who has to lock one wheel and push the remaining wheel forward. Clients with head injuries, clients with unequal strength in their arms, or clients who propel the chair with their feet may not be as skilled in wheelchair propulsion and may need more maneuvering space.

In addition to space requirements, the floor treatments must be designed to facilitate horizontal movement within an environment. A slippery floor contributes to falls. Uneven joints or bumps in the floor can be particular problems not only for the wheelchair user but for those using canes and crutches, those with arthritis, and even those with chronic respiratory and cardiovascular problems. Surface firmness will have an impact on energy expense for both the ambulant person and the wheelchair user. Heavily patterned designs may make it difficult to judge distances and delineate the edge of a surface.

The use of carpeting is controversial. Carpets have always been implicated as a source of high energy expense. The area of contact for a crutch tip or a wheelchair tire is much smaller than that of the average human foot, which means that any surface, but particularly carpeting, has to be very resilient before it actually "feels" firm and supportive.

Carpets with dense weaves or deep pile can increase the rolling resistance to the wheelchair two or three times. Propelling a wheelchair on soft surfaces may increase the energy cost of propulsion as much as 37% to 56%, depending on the physical condition of the wheeler (Wolf and co-workers).

If carpeting is desired, dense, low-level pile with a thin but firm padding or no padding at all is recommended. Desmond believes that the combined thickness of the carpet and padding should not exceed 0.5 inch. Shag carpets should be avoided because cane and crutch tips can get caught.

Some recommend cork flooring as a compromise between carpeting and other floor coverings. Cork is easy to clean, provides a firm, non-slip, smooth surface, and is warmer than vinyl.

Halls and Doorways

For those dependent on a wheelchair, maneuverability needs through hallways are based on three measurements: the size of the wheelchair, the size of the hall, and the width of the door openings into the hall.

The average, standard, adult wheelchair is 27 inches wide. At least 2 to 2.5 inches of clearance should be allowed on either side of the chair for the hands. Therefore, the hall should have a minimum width of 32 inches. Wider chairs need more space, smaller chairs less. However, hall width, per se, is not usually a problem, because most houses have 36-inch halls.

Problems arise when the wheelchair user wants to turn off the hall into another room. Hallway width/door width ratios often prohibit this turn. Indeed, hall widths and interior door openings are so integrally related that it is impossible to talk about the two separately.

Illinois standards indicate that a wheelchair cannot make a turn into a doorway with a clear opening of 32 inches unless the hall is at least 42 inches wide. If the door opening is wider—for example, 36 inches—the hall width can be decreased to 36 inches. Cary believes that a hallway has to be 48 inches wide in order for a wheelchair to make a right-angle turn. Obviously, absolute values are not as important as the ratio.

Because widening halls is no small task, most wheelchair users opt to increase the clear opening of doors with fold-back hinges that allow the door to fold back flat against the adjacent wall—usually adding approximately 2 inches to the clear opening—or by removing the doorsill. Sliding doors, either mounted on the wall or in a pocket, are another option.

Pulling a door open can be difficult for the wheelchair user if she has to back up the chair as she opens the door. Providing a space of 18 to 24 inches on the pull side of the door between the hall walls and door gives the wheelchair user a place to park as she pulls the door open.

Even with this additional space, many wheelchair users complain that it is hard to open doors. Many doors, especially many fire doors in work settings, are too heavy for the seated person to open. The person is often forced to lock the chair first before pulling the door open, which adds extra steps to the procedure and makes the task more cumbersome and time consuming. Heavy "push" doors are even more difficult. Sometimes the only way to open these doors is to get a running start and ram them open with the wheelchair.

The door weight can easily be determined by attaching a spring scale to the door handle and pulling on the spring from a seated position until the door opens. The scale reading should not exceed 8 pounds.

If money is not an issue, heavy doors can be modified with automatic door openers. Anything from the more sophisticated, full-sized sliding door to a do-it-yourself radio-controlled system can be used. Openers can be activated with wall switches, photoelectric beams, or floor mat controls. Cary describes a cheaper "ball and cord" option, which is an inexpensive pulley system using venetian blind cord, a small pulley, and a few screw eyes.

People with limited or no use of the hands can find a light door difficult to open if regular doorknobs are used. The easiest door to open is one that is not only light, but can be opened with a clenched fist or a flat hand. Lever or U-shaped handles are usually the best options. Placing an additional handle toward the hinge side of the door will facilitate closing. The wheelchair user can then close the door without positioning the chair in the door path as he reaches for the handle.

Thresholds or doorsills can be a problem for the disabled, particularly so for the wheelchair user who has to manage the threshold in the midst of a turn through a doorway. Given that the function of a threshold is to keep out drafts, it can usually be removed from interior doorways. But if thresholds are needed, they should be beveled and should not exceed 0.5 inch in height.

Bathrooms

In most cases, bathrooms have the narrowest doors and are often the smallest rooms. Therefore, it is frequently an area requiring many modifications for the wheelchair user. The person who is able to walk even very short distances has a significant environmental advantage over the wheelchair user.

As in any small, confined area, the door

should never swing into the room. Swing-in doors subtract space from an already small room. They can also be a safety hazard because an unconscious person lying near a swing-in bathroom door can make entry in an emergency difficult, if not impossible. Doors that swing into the hall require more hall space, and therefore installing sliding doors or even curtains at this room entrance may be a more practical choice. Some wheelchair users may find it easier to transfer into a narrower rolling chair, using grab bars installed near the door to pull themselves into the room, than to change door widths. The shower/commode chairs with 4-inch casters are usually narrower than wheelchairs, and are often able to roll over a standard-height toilet.

The actual amount of space the wheelchair user will need for maneuvering in the bathroom will directly depend on the location of the various fixtures as well as which transfer options are needed. For instance, a transfer that needs to be approached from the side will require more space than one that can be approached diagonally. Those with arthritis or weakness more prevalent on one side of the body may prefer transferring to a specific side.

Although many standards recommend a minimum clear space of 5 × 5 ft within the room, this space may not be necessary if the fixtures can be arranged in such a way that obviates turning and favors transfer preferences. Catlin outlines two options (Fig. 54-4). Choosing wall-hung toilets or ones with receding understructures can also decrease the absolute amount of clear space needed, because footrests will then be able to pass under the toilet in a turn.

Living Rooms and Bedrooms

Living rooms and bedrooms do not usually require major modification for maneuvering. Movement within these rooms is more often related to furniture arrangements. It is more convenient to have one clear 5- × 5-ft area in each room for turning; however, if furniture can be arranged so that full turns are unnecessary, smaller spaces will suffice.

Rooms should be designed and arranged so the user can relax and function with minimum effort. For instance, the person using a wheelchair should have such things as the telephone, a light switch, and the intercom system within easy reach of the bed. Clear, direct travel patterns should be available, because maneuvering around furniture can be both time and energy consuming.

Kitchen

Although the U-shaped kitchen may save steps and energy for the ambulatory person, the L-shaped kitchen provides for the easiest maneuvering of a wheelchair, because this configuration requires the least amount of turning and moving (Cary). U-shaped kitchens will need a 5- × 5-ft turning area in the middle for the wheelchair user. Galley kitchens with doors at each end will also work for the wheelchair user as long as the corridor width is at least 30 inches plus the width of one opened base-cabinet door.

VERTICAL MOVEMENT

A large percentage of the disabled are socially isolated, often the result of difficulties getting in and out of their homes. Those who can get out and around often find that, even though they have good work skills, they are unable to work because they cannot gain access to the building where they might work.

Exterior doors present the same problems as interior doors. They still must have a clear area of 32 to 34 inches for the average wheelchair user. The crutch walker will also appreciate this added width. Revolving doors are impossible for the wheelchair user, and are difficult for the disabled ambulator.

Heavy exterior doors are just as hard to open as heavy interior doors. The only additional complication is that exterior doors often need to be heavier to prevent the wind from blowing them open. Accordingly, automatic door openers may be a necessity, especially in the work setting. Placing shelves both outside and just inside the door will make it easier to handle packages.

Figure 54-4. Bathroom fixtures arranged in these configurations may decrease the absolute circulation space necessary for this room.

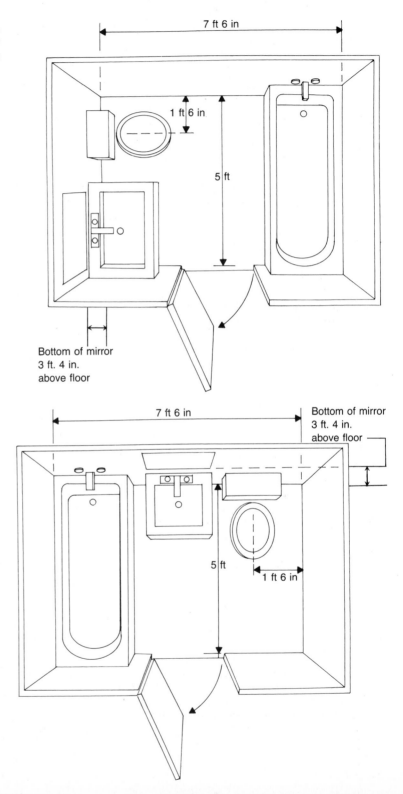

The problem of vertical movement still remains. Unless one is being carried up and down and in and out of buildings, only three options exist—stairs, ramps, or lifts. Lifts are the only option universally acceptable to both the wheelchair user and the ambulatory disabled. Wheelchair users obviously cannot manage stairs very efficiently, and the ambulatory disabled often complain that the ramp incline prevents them from taking a proper step, causing them to trip more easily. Those with cardiovascular problems or general decline in stamina may find ramps too exhausting because of the incline and because of the greater distance traveled.

Installation of a lift—whether a stair glide, an elevator, or a simple platform—is costly. However, unless a high, vertical rise needs to be accomplished in a very small area, lifts are usually not essential in the home. A combination of ramps and stairs or an able-bodied assistant will often enable the client to manage without a lift.

On the other hand, lifts are frequently used in work settings because work environments usually have to meet the needs of both the disabled and the able bodied. In the work setting, lifts are often a more efficient use of space and finances than ramps.

Ramps

Ramps are inexpensive, simple in design, and dependable. (See Table 54-2 for specific construction details.) However, they do require much space. The currently acceptable slope standard is 1:12 (8.3%), which means that for every foot of rise, one needs 12 feet of ramp. A 1:12 slope is fine for those with strong arms or who use an electric wheelchair. (In fact, some may even be able to accomplish a steeper ramp for short distances). But it can be difficult and tiring for others, especially if the ramp is very long.

The Illinois standards recommend a 1:20 (5%) slope. This slope may be especially necessary in inclement weather, when rain, snow, ice, and frost can make a ramp a safety hazard. Minnesota and Michigan have included in their codes a standard slope of 1:20 for exterior ramps.

Ramp design will be based on the total rise (and, therefore, ramp length) as well as location. Pushing up a long ramp is tiring. The descent can be just as difficult. Slowing the wheelchair with the hands to maintain control can cause painful burns. Therefore, any ramp longer than 30 ft should be divided into sections with a 5- × 5-ft platform for resting between sections. Platforms should also be in-

Table 54-2. Ramp Construction Specifications*

Width	36 to 48 inches
Slope	Minimum 1:12; 1:20 is better
Surface	Non-slip (rubber matting, pebble-gravel roofing paper), but not so rough that wheelchair propulsion is difficult.
Curbs	2 × 4-inch strip along edge of ramp to prevent wheels from accidentally rolling off. (A second low handrail can also serve this function.)
Platforms	5 × 5-ft platform needed at both top and bottom of ramp to allow for opening doors, making turns, etc. (If door swings inward, a 3 × 3-ft platform may suffice.) Platforms are also needed every 30 ft and whenever changes in direction are made.
Handrails	Placed 32 inches above ramp surface on both sides and extending at least 12 inches (some prefer 18 inches) beyond top and bottom of ramp. Handrails should be smooth and easy to grip.

*Because ramps are often used as an emergency egress, fire-retardant materials should be used. Ideally, exterior ramps should be protected from inclement weather by a canopy, electric heating coils, etc.

cluded at points where ramps change directions because it is hard to turn a wheelchair on a slope.

Every change in level, inside and out, need not be ramped. Certainly in the home setting, priorities should be set and ramps should be used in those areas where they would be most functional, inexpensive to construct, and aesthetically pleasing.

Ramps come in all sizes and can be made of wood, concrete, or metal. Concrete ramps usually require a contractor, and once made are difficult to remove. If desired, a person can make his own wood ramp. However, wood will decay and can burn, and so may not be the best choice for fire exits. Many of the portable ramps are metal and may be an option, especially if only trying to accommodate one or two steps or for use in temporary situations. However, portable ramps may be a safety hazard because they are not fixed and may move out of place or create joints that can "trip" a wheelchair.

Stairs

The amputee and many other disabled persons who walk may prefer stairs to a ramp. However, if not well constructed, stairs, too, can be hazardous. Open-riser stairs and those with stair lips are not desired because many persons use the back of the step to guide foot placement. Others compensate for balance deficits by wedging the crutch or cane tip against the back of the step. Toes may catch on an open step or stair lip, and the person may trip.

Heavily patterned tiles and carpeting should also be avoided on stairs. Patterns make it difficult to see the step edge, as does the glare of strong lighting. The elderly and those with weaker eyesight have a particular problem seeing the step edge.

Handrails should be placed on both sides of the stairs approximately 30 to 34 inches from the surface and 1.5 inch from the wall. In addition, handrails should project horizontally at least 12 inches over both the upper and lower landing (some codes say 18 inches). Those individuals with walking deficits frequently require the support provided by this extra length to clear the stairs safely.

Square handrails are hard to grip, and therefore, a rounded version approximately 1.5 inch in diameter seems to be the best.

CREATING A COMFORTABLE REACH

How far a person is able to reach will govern the placement of controls (ie, light switches, socket outlets, window openers), storage areas, and work areas. The use of the "eye level" principle will also assist in determining the best location for work areas and, to a certain extent, storage areas.

While anthropometric charts give a general understanding of the various ranges of reach, the client's needs will probably be more readily met by looking at his specific ranges. Strength, flexibility, balance, the equipment used (ie, canes, prosthesis, wheelchairs), and the approach to the object being reached are just a few of the factors that can change the range of reach. These changes are difficult to accommodate in a chart of averages.

Although it may not be important for a therapist to remember the absolute values of specific chart ranges, understanding *why* the various dimensions are considered and *how* they can be applied to the environment can be helpful in guiding clients. A heavy lift, for instance, can usually be accomplished more easily if the object is below shoulder height, especially if it can be brought to the body. Shoulder height also affects maximum forward reach and sideways reach and is often the preferred location for light switches.

Comfortable diagonal reach will give the upper measurement of the storage zone for the articles used most often, while knuckle height (the location of the knuckles when the arm is hanging down at the side) will give the lower measurement. Comfortable forward reach will indicate the needed depth for work areas.

Eye level will help determine where mirrors are hung and front-door peepholes are located, as well as where work areas are placed.

Hands are most efficiently used if activities are performed between shoulder and elbow height. Fine manipulation activities, such as writing, are usually accomplished most efficiently close to elbow height. Therefore, elbow height measurements must be a consideration in the height for counters and tables.

For the seated person, thigh heights and chair armrest levels are important, because these establish a minimum measurement for clearance under work spaces. The wheelchair-seat height will obviously be important in considering transfers within the environment.

Because of the many complex motions available to the human body, maximum reach is usually much greater than comfortable reach. Comfortable forward reach for the wheelchair user, for instance, is not much further than the front edge of the footpedal. However, if the motion of extending the arm is combined with trunk and hip flexion, considerably more reaching range is available. The comfortable reach area is the one in which the items used most often should be stored and the work spaces should be built.

STORAGE

General Considerations

Good storage areas are not luxury items for the disabled, but are important because they improve safety, make maintenance easier, provide better overall movement through an area, and generally make a more organized, enjoyable space.

Raschko outlines several things to consider in storage design:

- Articles should be stored in or near the area where they are first used. If items are used together, they should be stored together.
- Frequently used items should be stored in easy to reach areas.
- Stored articles should be visible. To enhance visibility, lights can be installed in closets, lighter colors can be used to paint

the interiors of storage areas, and shallower shelves can be used (12 inches is usually recommended for shelves above shoulder height). Shelving material used above eye level should be transparent.

- Because it is difficult for the elderly and those in wheelchairs to use deep storage areas in the upper and lower limits of their reach capabilities, pull-out drawers and shelves for storage above and below 32 inches should be used. These drawers and shelves are available at many lumber yards and building centers.
- Shelves should be made of durable, easy-to-maintain surfaces.
- Forward reach for those in wheelchairs is very limited. A side approach should be considered to ensure maximum accessibility.
- Loading the inside of a storage door with heavy objects may make it too heavy to move.
- Heavy, bulky objects should not be stored at levels above the shoulder or below the hips.
- Excessively wide doors may be too heavy to move.
- Operating hardware should be large and easy to manipulate.

Kitchen Storage

Using anthropometric information from Diffrient and his colleagues, Raschko states that the comfortable area of reach or vertical area accessible to most persons will be between 45.5 and 27.3 inches. The top range is for a small woman in a wheelchair; the lower range is for a standing, tall elderly man unable to stoop or bend.

Kitchen counter tops fall in the middle of this comfortable reach area, wasting space that might otherwise be available for storage. Given that wall cabinets are usually placed around 51 to 54 inches, Raschko believes only about 50% of the shelf space is available to a tall man in a wheelchair and only 33% to the ambulatory, small, elderly woman. With these facts and the reality that the kitchen is a high-storage area, one will quickly understand why the kitchen can pose storage problems.

The literature, however, provides a wide array of storage solutions. Base cabinets can be made more functional with compartmentalized drawers (Fig. 54-5). Bulky and awkwardly shaped items are often more easily stored on peg boards. Roll-out bins, racks, baskets, and shelf trays can also be used. Lazy Susans are another frequently used and inexpensive option.

To make the upper cabinets more accessible, some have lowered them to 12 inches above the counter, or installed a shallow shelf or cabinet below the existing ones. However, these modifications decrease the counter space available for such items as canister sets and small appliances.

Many recommend one tall, full-length storage area in the kitchen, because storage space can be so efficiently used (Fig. 54-6). Another frequently used suggestion is the small, mobile, roll-out cabinet or cart (Fig. 54-7). This cabinet is usually combined with a work area on the top and can be fitted with drawer units or one shelf for garbage and cleaning supplies. Rolling cabinets should be sturdy and easy to push. (A wheelchair user should look for one with at least 3-inch swivel, ball-bearing casters.) The ambulatory person should choose one she can push without bending. Foam or bumpers can be placed on corners to protect walls and other furniture.

If a choice is possible, many recommend the two door side-by-side refrigerator/freezer with slide-out shelves. More door storage is available. In addition, the narrower doors reduce the size of the swing and, therefore, decrease the necessary maneuvering space. Sliding shelves allow more efficient use of the space inside the refrigerator. If this is not an option, Harkness believes that the ambulatory

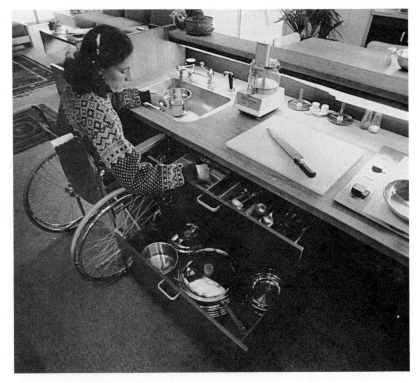

Figure 54-5. Using drawers in base cabinets instead of conventional shelving increases the wheelchair user's accessible storage options. The compartmentalized top drawer makes items easy to find and reach. Note the continuous work surface between the sink and stove, the shallow sink, and the single-lever faucet with spray attachment. (Courtesy of International Lead Zinc Research Organization, Inc)

do better with the freezer on the top and the wheelchair user with the freezer below.

Bedroom Storage

Bedroom closets usually come equipped with a rod for hanging clothes and some shelves. Because the top shelf is often too high to use, Raschko suggests removing it and placing it 10 inches from the floor level. It can then be used to store more efficiently those items ordinarily placed on the floor.

Because so many wheelchair users find it more convenient to dress in bed, Raschko recommends portable, roll-out closet units (Fig. 54-8). These units can also be energy-saving devices for the ambulatory.

If the entire length of an existing closet is not needed for hanging clothes, part of it may be used for full-length, horizontal shelf storage. The many modular shelving and flexible-storage systems commercially available make storage a much simpler task. Closet storage or open storage, set up anywhere, can be both functional and aesthetically pleasing (Fig. 54-9).

Bathroom Storage

Bathroom storage problems are usually fairly simple. Because the wheelchair user has difficulty reaching the medicine chest located over a sink, it is usually better to place the chest on a

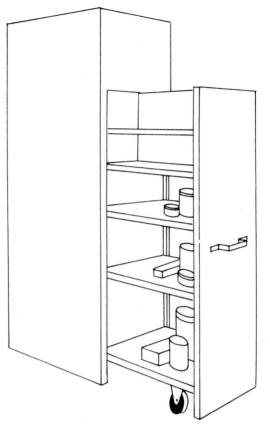

Figure 54-6. Roll-out shelves in a full-length pantry cabinet.

Figure 54-7. Wheeled cabinets or carts can be an energy-efficient means of expanding accessible storage and work surfaces.

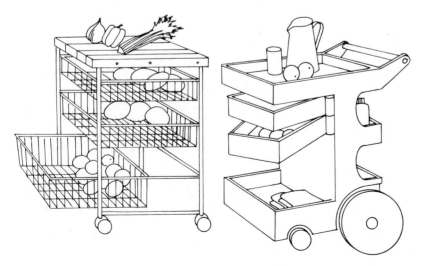

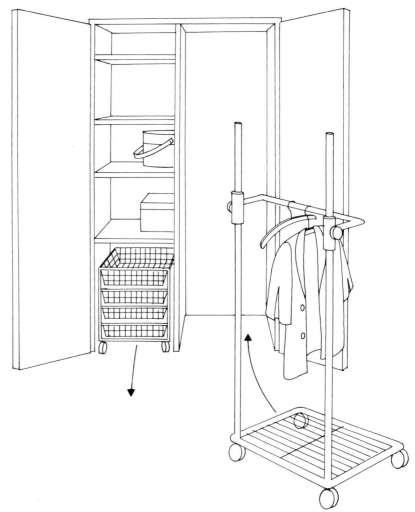

Figure 54-8. A portable clothes rack will save trips to the closet.

PLACEMENT OF WORK SURFACES

side wall. A larger bathroom may easily accommodate the use of a wheeled cabinet. Towels, hair dryers, and shower and other grooming aides may be stored in the cabinet and easily moved to the tub or toilet area whenever needed.

PLACEMENT OF WORK SURFACES

Work-surface heights should be based on the type of work to be done and the posture that will be needed for the work. As posture changes, shoulder heights and reach will change. Whether sitting or standing, many kitchen activities such as mixing, slicing, kneading, and washing are more easily accomplished if performed below the elbow level. Heavy work generally requires a lower work station. Detailed, fine motor work can often be better accomplished with a higher table.

Appropriate placement can greatly reduce energy expenditure. The results of a time study performed at a conveyer belt operation in which the belt was lowered by 2 inches increased production by 10 units/minute (Tichauer).

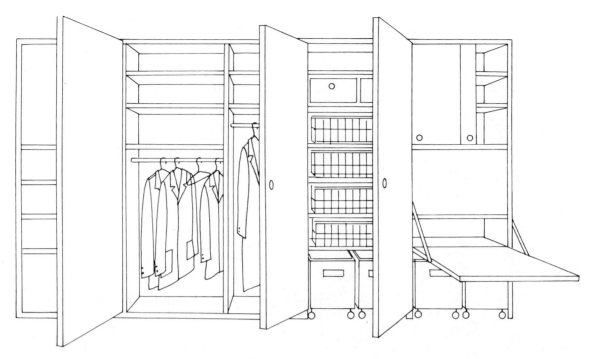

Figure 54-9. A multipurpose storage unit. Seldom-used items can be stored on upper shelves and drawers. Shorter clothes can be hung on the low rod, longer clothes on the high one. Wire baskets make stored items easily visible. Pull-out units below are simple wooden boxes on casters.

For sitting activities, such as writing and dining, the sitting environment needs to be determined first. Raschko recommends that a tabletop be approximately 11 inches higher than the chair seat. Thus, the person using a wheelchair may require higher tables and desks because the seat height is usually a little greater (around 19 inches).

The biggest problems with work-surface placement stem from those activities normally done standing. The standard kitchen counter is 36 inches high, which is well above the elbow level (about 30 inches) of a tall man sitting in a wheelchair and well above the shoulder height of a small woman in a wheelchair.

Those with limited or no lower-extremity function may be able to use standing postures with the assistance of one of many standing aids on the market. Although cheaper options exist, aids like the electrically powered Moto-

Stand, which give the client the ability to move in an upright position as well as easily pick objects up from the floor (Fig. 54-10), are the most convenient. The use of these devices is often limited by the difficulty of getting into them and the cost. An average person usually cannot afford to prioritize the purchase of something like this. However, an exception is found in the work setting, where funds are often more available because a direct link can be made to work productivity.

Because most kitchen work surfaces are designed for standing and most persons using wheelchairs are unable to use standing aids, the wheelchair user is always faced with some difficult decisions in the kitchen, even if planning to live with an ambulatory person. Some opt to leave the kitchen as is and make an "alternate" kitchen work area using a card table or a fold-down table hinged to the wall and sev-

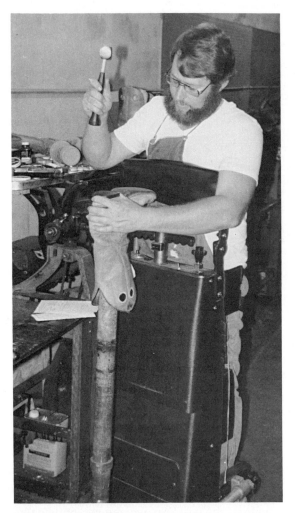

Figure 54-10. The electrically propelled Moto-Stand provides those without the use of their legs the ability to utilize higher work surfaces and shelves. The man pictured has a spinal cord injury at T8 and operates his own boot and shoe repair business. Because he has a Moto-Stand, he did not have to modify his shop in any way. (Courtesy of The Advanced Technology Corp, Kansas City, MO 64141)

eral smaller tabletop appliances (such as hot plates, toaster ovens, and blenders). Although the alternative kitchen is a good option, especially on a temporary basis, the client should be cautioned not to overload the circuits and create a fire hazard.

As mentioned earlier, wheeled cabinets and tables can provide accessible work surfaces. Pull-out shelves (ie, breadboards) and lapboards can also make adequate work surfaces. In addition, pull-out boards can act as a safety feature. When placed under a wall-hung oven door, for instance, they provide an immediate place for hot foods as well as protection for the legs against spills (Fig. 54-11). Pull-out shelves with various cutout holes for holding bowls provide additional stabilization for mixing activities.

With appropriate finances, adjustable-height countertops are available. These can usually be set at 28, 32, and 36 inches. Some of the adaptable housing units being built today already come with this feature. The method of adjustment varies with each model. Countertops that can be easily moved up and down with a crank located at the front are ideal in environments intended to accommodate both the ambulatory person and the wheelchair user. Others require manual adjustment of screws and bolts along a track.

Whether work surfaces are placed to accommodate standing or sitting postures, they should be able to withstand 200 to 250 pounds of pressure, because these surfaces are often used for support as well. Persons with decreased stamina or balance may want to consider textured surfaces, which ensure support and a good grip.

Corner sinks can allow more counter space. Shallower sinks—5 or 6 inches deep—will allow seated persons to reach items at the bottom. If these are not available, raised racks can be used at the bottom of the sink to hold dishes at the proper height.

Wall-hung ovens are preferred, and should be mounted so that the shelves are countertop height. Microwave ovens may be a safety option because they reduce the risk of burns. Stove burners should be easily accessed without having to reach over another burner (Fig. 54-12), which can be accomplished with burners in straight-line or staggered configurations. Electric burners are preferred over gas. Spills may be reduced with ceramic or magnetic induction cook tops, because the heating

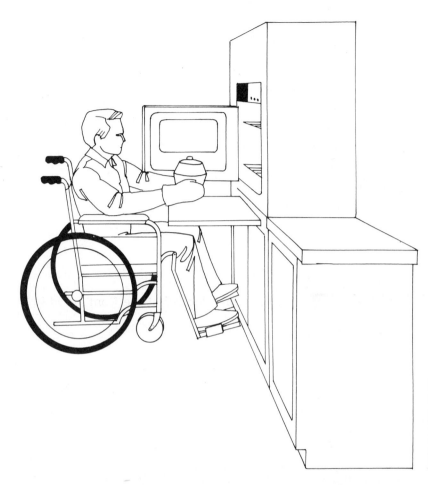

Figure 54-11. The oven door is hinged on the wall side to prevent interference with circulation. A pull-out board underneath provides an immediate place for hot foods and protects legs against spills.

unit is level with the countertop. All controls should be mounted at the front. Mirrors above burners can facilitate seeing into pans.

The wheelchair user must consider not only the height of the work-surface top but the clearance under it, unless he is planning to utilize only a side approach. The space needs to be 28 to 30 inches wide to accommodate the chair's width, 21 to 24 inches deep to provide space for the footrest, and 27 to 30 inches high to allow the knees to fit under the surface. All pipes need to be well insulated to protect against burns.

The tilt of the work surface is another aspect that bears consideration. Tilting a surface may be appropriate for writing, typing, reading, and many other tasks found in a work setting. It often provides the best access to a surface, and, therefore, can decrease the energy expenditure and discomfort that may occur when sitting upright and working at a flat table.

Nation's Business describes a study done by Eickelberg and Less to evaluate the effect of tilting a work surface. They asked 18- to 22-year-old men and women to perform an electrical wiring task on work surfaces titled at various angles. They found that a tilt of 6 to 12 degrees reduced fatigue and improved productivity by 25% to 30%.

The kitchen is an area that usually requires several work surfaces. Thus, as in any multi-

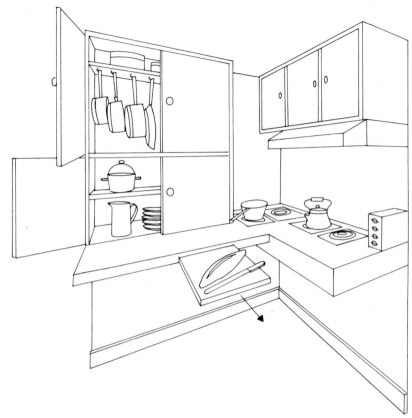

Figure 54-12. Each of the four burners on this countertop stove is easily accessed without reaching over another burner. Straight-line or staggered configurations can also be used to ensure safety. (Note controls mounted on front right wall.)

work area, their placement should depend on work flow. Movement is usually from the refrigerator to the sink to the stove to the table. Therefore, work will be accomplished more efficiently with a work surface between the refrigerator and sink and one by the stove (Fig. 54-13). In addition, a wheeled cart to carry food from the stove to the table is ideal.

PLACEMENT OF CONTROLS

The last area upon which reach capabilities will have an impact is the placement of controls—light switches, electrical sockets, window openers, and the like. The wheelchair user's optimum reach range is approximately a foot less than that of someone who is able to stand and walk. Minimal, if any, modifications have to be made for the disabled person who is able to walk. For wheelchair users, 36 inches seems to be the preferred height for most switches and 18 inches for wall outlets. However, clients should be encouraged to install controls at a height comfortable for them.

Rocker switches or switches easily manipulated with a clenched fist are necessary for those with limited arm and hand function. Cary suggests a light-switch extender, which slips over a standard switch plate and extends down 22 inches, making it easier for someone in a chair to operate. Some suggest illuminating switches, which can be especially helpful at night for the elderly, or for those with visual deficits, or even for those who are a little disoriented. Using an extension cord with its own switch is an inexpensive option for increasing the accessibility of lamp and appliance controls. Low-pressure air switches can also be used to control these items.

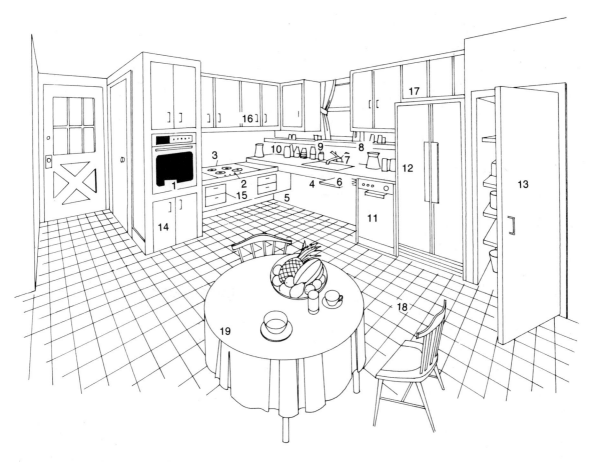

1. Wall oven, for easy access, open at counter height

2. Cooktop controls at the front, to avoid burning

3. Cooktop and counter, height 30 to 33 in

4. Knee space under sink counter to allow sitting in wheelchair at counter

5. High recessed base under cabinets to accommodate wheelchair pedals

6. Pullout work shelf (30 to 33 in) at standard-height counters

7. Mixing faucet at sink, lever handle

8. Cove lighting under wall cabinets, bulb replacement within reach range

9. Shallow shelf over sink counter within reach range

10. Wall space within reach over sink counter, used for hanging utensils

11. Front-loading dishwasher

12. Side-by-side refrigerator doors to allow access to refrigerator and freezer

13. Full height storage closet for easy access

14. Cabinet space under wall-oven within reach range

15. Drawers under cooktop and counter for easier access

16. Easy-grip cabinet door pulls

17. High cabinets (out of reach for the chairbound) for other users

18. Smooth, nonskid flooring, open spaces for wheelchair passage

19. Round table to avoid corners, legs, or pedestal base with no apron to allow for wheelchair

Figure 54-13. This food-preparation area is conveniently located between the refrigerator and sink. Pull-out boards lower than the countertop provide a better height for activities such as mixing and beating. Ingredients and utensils used in preparing food should be stored within easy reach of this area.

Those with very limited or no arm and hand functions can control their environments by means of environmental control units (ECUs). These technical aids come in all sizes and shapes and vary in cost, depending on their functions. Essentially three categories exist—those that interface with the wheelchair; those that can be operated from a wheelchair but will not interface with it; and those that can be operated only from a work station.

ECUs that interface with a wheelchair are the most expensive, costing several thousand dollars. ECUs in this category can operate the television, radio, lights, and telephones; can engage emergency alarms; and can usually be used from any room in a house. Signals are sent from the wheelchair back to the main system, which then sends a signal to the desired appliance or control through the house's electrical wiring. Most systems can also interface with a computer.

ECUs in this category are most often used in conjunction with the quad system wheelchairs. They will interface only with those chairs having four-switch electrical controls. Usually, they will not interface with the basic proportional control electric chair, because the ECU "borrows" switches from the wheelchair for its operation, and the proportionally controlled chair essentially has no switches to borrow.

To operate the ECU, the wheelchair driver first engages the "kill" switch, usually in either the reverse or recline function. Once this is done, the chair controls will not work until the forward switch is again engaged. This arrangement allows the right and left movement switches to be borrowed for ECU controls.

These ECUs use a scanning system; for instance, the right-turn switch would be used to start the scanning and the left-turn switch would then select the desired function in the scanning process.

The systems can be engaged by almost anything, including minimal hand and arm function, air (puff and sipp), or even eye blinks. They come with the ability to interface with 16 to 256 appliances and controls. Most, however, never have more than seven or eight appliances operated by means of the ECU.

A second type of ECU system can be operated from a wheelchair, does not interface with it, and is much less expensive, costing as little as $100. The system is also less complex. Controls are similar to those used in automatic garage-door openers. These only work in the room the person is in and often need to be pointed at the desired appliance.

The third type of ECU has to be plugged into a wall socket, and is also a fairly inexpensive option. It has no remote control and cannot operate telephones or change television channels. Controls are usually push-button, and require some hand function or mouth stick expertise.

GETTING WHERE YOU WANT TO GO

Home and work environments may be created with appropriate maneuvering space, wide doorways, accessible storage, and work areas placed at the best heights, but the disabled person will still be economically dependent and socially isolated without viable transportation.

For the visually impaired, for the poorly coordinated, and often for the elderly, private transportation is not physically possible. For many other disabled persons, it is not economically feasible. Accessible *public* transportation is increasing, but is still far too limited. For further information refer to local independent living centers, rehabilitation hospitals, and the Architectural Transportation Barriers Compliance Board in Washington, D.C.

VEHICLE ACCESS

If private transportation is to be used, access to a vehicle is the first area of consideration. If a person cannot transfer himself or his mobility equipment independently into a car, or does so with great difficulty and energy expense, a van is probably the best option. In addition, a few cars can be driven from a wheelchair.

Wheelchair users and those more skilled at transfers will probably have an easier time entering a two-door car than a four-door model because the door opening is wider, even though the door is heavier. Adjustable steering wheels create a larger space to transfer into, and can provide leverage during the move. Most persons prefer to have the gear shift located on the steering column. Those using wheelchairs have an easier time moving onto a powered bench front seat.

Compact cars can be a real economic temptation. However, because their small size can complicate hand-control conversions and wheelchair loading, very careful evaluation should be made before purchase.

Once the wheelchair driver is in the car, the next consideration is loading the wheelchair. The car trunk is not an option unless the driver has a constant companion. Most opt to load the chair between the front and back seat on the driver's side. Thus, the bottom of the door opening should be as low as possible. It also helps to have a level door sill. Those that slant to the outside cause the wheelchair to roll out of the car if it is not pulled in far enough on the first attempt. Because the average folded width of a wheelchair is between 10 and 12 inches, a powered front seat able to create a 13- to 14-inch opening between the front and back seats is essential. Some find that placing a platform on the back floor to eliminate the change in levels also makes the procedure easier. The chair can also be loaded into the passenger side on the front, but this method is a little more awkward.

The wheelchair can be loaded manually, as described above, or by powered assistance. Powered wheelchair loaders require the user to attach a hook or sling device to the chair. The device then lifts the chair either to a box on the car roof or to the rear passenger area.

Several companies make wheelchair lifts for vans. Selection of the lift should be specific for the individual user. Although portable ramps are a handy item to have when lift doors jam or in an emergency, most persons are unable to use them independently to enter the van. Door openers should also be considered because most wheelchair users are unable to reach and open van doors.

Once in the van, the person can then transfer onto a van seat or drive from the wheelchair. If driving from a wheelchair, however, it is essential that the chair and the driver be separately restrained.

DRIVING EASE

The American Automobile Association's free publication, *The Handicapped Driver's Mobility Guide,* lists several options that will contribute to driving ease and comfort:

- Automatic transmission
- Power steering, brakes, seats (multi-adjustable), and windows
- Remote adjustable outside mirrors
- Two side-view mirrors (especially important for those with limited head and neck movement)
- Rear window defrosters
- Cruise control
- Air conditioning
- A wide-angled mirror

In addition to the factory options available, many companies specialize in modifying the driving mechanics for the more physically involved driver. Modifications can include hand controls, ignition-starting aids, parking brake extensions, "zero-effort" steering, and other features.

To ensure safety during emergencies, disabled drivers should also be encouraged to consider acquiring some sort of attention-getting flag, because they often are unable to raise the car hood. Accessory flashers for the driver's door edge are another option because the disabled usually require more time to enter and leave the car.

PARKING

No discussion of driving is complete without mentioning parking. Whether at work or home, the disabled—especially wheelchair users—need wider parking spaces to allow for transfers. For wheelchair drivers, a minimum of 13 feet is required. The American National

Standards Institute (ANSI) allows 8-feet-wide stalls as long as the stall is next to a 5-feet-wide accessible aisle.

Parking surfaces must be level. Wheelchairs roll out of reach on slopes, and the ambulatory disabled have more difficulty getting a good footing. Surfaces should be firm and slip resistant. Gravel and irregular pavement make wheelchair propulsion and walking difficult.

The distance from the parking lot to the work facility or home should generally be less than 200 feet. Wheelchair propulsion can be exhausting, as can walking with a disability, whether a limp, shortness of breath, or cardiac problems.

CONCLUSION

This chapter has explored basic design concepts for the physically disabled in relation to the home, the work environment, and the car. Tables 54-3, 54-4, and 54-5 summarize key

Table 54-3. Summary of Accessibility Standards

Horizontal Movement	
Clear door width	32 to 34 inches
Door width/hall width	32/42 inches or 36/36 inches
Clear space on side of door	18 to 24 inches
Placement of door levers	36 inches from floor
General circulation need in most rooms	At least 5 × 5 ft (some say 6 × 6 ft) unless furniture/fixtures can be arranged to avoid wheelchair turns and favor transfer preferences
Vertical Movement	
Ramp slope	1:12 minimum; 1:20 preferred
Handrail placement (stairs and ramps)	32 inches from floor; 1.5 inch from wall; projecting 12 to 18 inches into the top and bottom landings
Reach	
Storage	
Low shelves	10 inches above floor
High shelves	48 inches above floor
Depth of shelves	16 inches (12 inches if above shoulder)
Work Surfaces	
Placement	28 to 34 inches
Clear area below	Width 28 inches
	Depth 21 to 24 inches
	Height 27 to 30 inches
Controls	
Light switches	36 to 48 inches
Fuse box	36 to 48 inches
Windowsills	36 to 48 inches
Wall outlets	18 inches
Getting Where You Want to Go	
Parking	12 to 13 ft (8 ft plus 5-ft aisle)

Table 54-4. Energy Conservation Considerations

Sitting Environment	Create a sitting environment that encourages symmetry and normal lumbar
Horizontal Movement	Avoid heavy doors Use door hardware that can be easily manipulated with clenched fist Kick plates on bottom of doors (to decrease maintenance/repairs that may be needed secondary to chips and scratches from wheelchair footrests and canes Pull handle on hinge side of door to facilitate closing Firm surfaces Avoid changes in surface level Clear, direct routes around furniture Choose floor coverings easy to clean and maintain U-shaped kitchens for ambulant; L-shaped kitchens for the wheelchair user
Vertical Movement	Ramps built with slow rise (1:20) Platforms placed on ramps every 30 ft and where direction changes Placement of small shelf by inside and outside of door to set packages while opening door Lifts
Reach	Storage Store items near area where first used Frequently used item should be stored in easy-to-reach places Shelves should be constructed of easy-to-maintain material Avoid excessively wide doors or loading inside of doors with too many items (may be too heavy) Portable roll-out closet for clothes Portable wheeled cabinets Work surfaces Placed at proper height and tilt Arranged according to work flow Continuous counters placed at same height allow sliding of heavy items, decreasing lifting and carrying Burn-proof work area near stove to provide place to slide hot pans off stove Labor-saving devices such as garbage disposals, dishwashers, self-defrosting freezer, self-cleaning oven, etc Long retractable water hose at sink and stove to facilitate filling pans with water Controls Easy to reach and manipulate Two-way switches save steps by allowing lights to be turned on and off at more than one point in room
Parking	Conveniently located

issues. The Paralyzed Veterans of America Association has a book, *Modifying and Designing Accessible Housing*. It is advertised as "an illustrated, how-to-do-it, technical resource manual on accessible housing" and is worth consulting for more specific information.

This chapter has alluded to the many appliances and hardware options available to assist in making an environment accessible. However, other resources, such as the books by Laurie and Hale listed in the Annotated Bibliography, and the ABLEDATA computer search

Table 54-5. Safety Considerations

Sitting Environment	Grab bars placed at appropriate heights with special finishes to facilitate grip and structurally reinforced to withstand 250 pounds of pressure Towel racks, sink edges, etc reinforced to withstand 250 pounds
Horizontal Movement	Non-slip, even surfaces Avoid loose rugs Avoid heavily designed coverings Carpeting may cushion falls Avoid swing-in doors in small, confined areas Avoid sharp, protruding corners and edges on furniture and doors Organize space to avoid fatigue (which can lead to accidents) Bathroom located near bedroom Illuminated light switches to facilitate movement at night
Vertical Movement	Two ways of egress Keep paths free of snow and ice (Hale suggests a specially treated jute mat) Avoid stairs with lips and open risers Stable handrails on both sides of stairs and ramps which extend at least 1 ft onto bottom and top landings Small curbs of low guardrails along the edge of the ramp to prevent a wheelchair from rolling off Adequate lighting Doormats securely fastened or recessed
Reach	Storage Areas and Work Surfaces Easy to reach Able to support 250 pounds of pressure Well-insulated pipes under sinks Wall ovens Microwave ovens Electric stove burners instead of gas Ceramic or magnetic induction stove burners may reduce spills Stove burners staggered or in line at front of counter Heat-proof lap holder for pans Controls Temperature control mixers on water faucets Stove controls located at front of counter Accessible light switches and outlets Avoid overloading circuits with too many small appliances Fuse boxes and circuit breakers in accessible reach Phone jacks in areas where falls might occur (ie, bathrooms)
Fire Prevention	Smoke detectors with warning system Use of fire-retardant furniture, drapes, carpeting, materials used to construct ramps, etc Fire extinguishers in all potentially dangerous areas

should be consulted for more specific information. Quarve-Peterson and Webb's book (see Annotated Bibliography) may also be of assistance.

The Job Accommodation Network, a nationwide computerized service, should be contacted for more information about environmental modifications employers have made for the disabled. To use the network, employers can call a toll-free number and ask for examples of how other employers have solved specific work-accommodation problems. Contact the West Virginia University Rehabilitation Research and Training Center, Morgantown, WV 26505, (800) JAN-PCEH for more details.

Finally, when modifying any environment—whether a house, apartment, mobile home, or place of employment—one should bear in mind the following: "The ultimate objective is that physically handicapped people should be enabled to live meaningful and self-determined lives" (Goldsmith).

ANNOTATED BIBLIOGRAPHY

American National Standards Institute: Specifications for Making Buildings and Facilities Accessible to and Usable by Physically Handicapped People, ANSI A117.1. New York, American National Standards Institute, 1980 (These standards were developed by a committee representing 52 organizations and associations of disabled people, rehabilitation professionals, design professionals, builders, and manufacturers. The original version [1961] formed the technical basis for the first accessibility standards adopted by the federal government and most states. This current edition is based on research funded by HUD and continues to be used as a basis for model state and local building codes.)

Bergen AF, Colangelo C: Positioning The Client with Central Nervous System Deficits: The Wheelchair and Other Adapted Equipment. Valhalla, NY, Valhalla Rehabilitation Publications Ltd, 1982 (A well-illustrated, thorough discussion of seating and positioning. Any study of positioning techniques should start here.)

Brunswic M: Ergonomics of seat design. Physiotherapy 70(2):40, 1984 (The implications for seat design of unsupported sitting are discussed in the light of two experiments. They show the importance of considering seat design as an integral part of task and workspace design rather than in isolation.)

Cary JR: How to Create Interiors for the Disabled. New York, Pantheon Books, 1978 (A practical look at designing environments for the disabled. Basic concepts are presented as well as some product information.)

Catlin J: Adaptable Housing. Chicago, Access Living, 1982 (A 12-page manual providing a concise guide to minimum adaptable housing design. Available from Access Living, 815 W. Van Buren St, Chicago, IL 60606.)

Desmond MG: Modifying the Work Environment for the Physically Disabled: An Accessibility Checklist for Employers. Albertson, NY, National Center on Employment of the Handicapped, Human Resources Center, 1982 (This publication explains in easy-to-understand language both the kinds of modifications that may be required in the workplace as well as the reasons behind them. It is arranged to guide the user from the exterior of the building through the interior. Checklists are provided at the end of each chapter.)

Feuerstein G, Bernard HP: Categories of the disabled and habitation design in practice. Int J Rehabil Res 3(2):225, 1980 (A brief research report on how to improve the living environment for the disabled in Austria. The study tries to point to the wide spectrum of disability as well as provide a numerical analysis of disability in this country.)

Garee B (ed): Ideas for Making Your Home Accessible. Bloomington, IL, Cheever Publishing, 1979 (An overview of what can be done to make the home of a wheelchair user functional and accessible. Illustrations are kept to a minimum but those provided are helpful. Two pages on mobile homes are included as a final chapter. Each chapter includes sources for equipment options outlined in the chapter.)

Goldsmith S: Designing for the Disabled, 2nd ed. New York, McGraw-Hill, 1967 (This fairly technical guide to designing for the disabled is an outcome of the research project Planning for the Disabled done in Norwich, England. The book begins with two sections describing general characteristics of the disabled population and discussing some of the measurements required in designing environments for the disabled [ie, anthropometrics, wheelchair measurements]. Subsequent sections deal with the various aspects of building design, with more emphasis on public building design.)

Hage MG: Ischial and femoral weightbearing during anterior and posterior sitting postures. Thesis. Evanston, IL, Northwestern University Physical Therapy Graduate School, 1985 (This study attempted to determine the effect of various alignments of the pelvis and lumbar spine during sitting on ischial and femoral pressure values. A very complete literature review is included.)

Hale G: The Source Book for the Disabled. New York, Paddington Press, 1979 (An excellent book of tips for the physically disabled seeking to be more independent. It is written in easy-to-read language and illustrated with hundreds of drawings.)

Jones MA: Accessibility Standards Illustrated. Springfield, IL, Capital Development Board, 1978 (A clear explanation of the Illinois accessibility standards and their rationale, highlighted with illustrations. [Available from the Capital Development Board, Third Floor, William G. Stratton Bldg, 401 South Spring St, Springfield, IL 62706.])

Laurie G: Housing and Home Services for the Disabled: Guidelines and Experiences in Independent Living. New York, Harper & Row, 1977 (A comprehensive, where-to-find-it guide to independent living for the disabled. Each chapter includes bibliographies with extensive annotations.)

Luce TP: The Handicapped Driver's Mobility Guide, rev ed. Falls Church, VA, American Automobile Association, Traffic Safety Department, 1984 (A free publication distributed by the American Automobile Association. The first sections in the book deal with such topics as vehicle selection, available factory options, special equipment and modifications, equipment installation, and maintenance tips. Several hand control manufacturers are also listed. The remainder of the book lists, according to state, services and materials provided by various organizations.)

Nation's Business: Can a tilt score a jackpot in productivity? March, 1973 (This article describes research done by Warren B. Eichelberg and Menahem Less with the assistance of Hans Krobath, Research Engineer at the Human Resources Center [Albertson, NY] under a grant from the Insurance Company of North America. Researchers were operating under the premise that backache problems are a result of the high energy expenditure required to maintain an upright sitting position. The study concluded that tilting a work surface would reduce fatigue and increase productivity.)

Noble PC: The prevention of pressure sores in persons with spinal cord injuries. Monograph No. 11. New York, World Rehabilitation Fund, 1981 (Addresses the patient with a spinal cord injury and the associated potential soft tissue problems. Noble gives an overview of the practical approaches to pressure sore management with emphasis on "pressure clinics" and cushions, including the principles of cushion materials, structure, and function; specific criteria for cushion selection; and the construction of a contoured, custom-fitted wheelchair cushion. Chapters include etiological factors, practical measures for prevention, and an assessment of the effectiveness of a clinically based pressure-sore prevention program. An extensive bibliography is included.)

Quarve-Peterson J, Webb LE: 1981 Product Inventory of Hardware, Equipment and Appliances for Barrier-Free Design, 2nd ed. Minneapolis, MN, National Handicap Housing Institute, 1981 (This book was designed to provide the information needed to better select home appliances and equipment for the disabled. Each appliance section begins with some general comments about advantages and limitations of available features. The report contains information on many commercially available products as well as products designed specifically for the disabled. Available through National Handicap Housing Institute, 12 South Sixth St, Suite 1216, Minneapolis, MN 55402.)

Raschko BB: Housing Interiors for the Disabled and Elderly. New York, Van Nostrand Reinhold, 1982 (A very detailed look at accessibility design options in the home. The author moves well past the basic concepts and into such details as the selection of carpeting and fire-retardant upholstery and furniture. A wide variety of illustrations is included.)

Tichauer ER: Human capacity, a limiting factor in design. Institute of Mechanical Engineers, Proceedings, 1963–1964, vol 178, pp 979–990 (Tichauer discusses how the knowledge of anatomical, physiological, and engineering design can be used to create an optimal man-machine task. [Man using a mechanical device is defined as a man-machine task.] He believes that a system can only operate at maximum efficiency if solutions to discrepancies between the optimal performance rates of equipment and man can be found.)

Wolf GA, Water R, Hislop HJ: Influence of floor surface on the energy cost of wheelchair propulsion. Phys Ther 57(9): 1022, 1977 (This study used two surfaces—one concrete and the other concrete covered with indoor/outdoor carpeting—to evaluate the effect of surface on the energy cost of wheelchair propulsion. In addition to energy cost, the authors looked at wheelchair velocity differences between the surfaces and made several comparisons to normal walking.)

Zacharkow D: Wheelchair Posture and Pressure Sores. Springfield, IL, Charles C Thomas, 1984 (Explores very thoroughly wheelchair sitting posture as a major etiologic factor in pressure sore formation. Chapters include discussions on proper sitting posture for able-bodied individuals, inherent problems with the wheelchair as a seat, essential modifications for proper sitting posture, pelvic obliquity and pressure sores, and wheelchair cushion selection. The application of posturing principles to other patient populations concludes the text. The book includes a very complete literature review.)

55 Teaching

JAMES R. MORROW

Skillful teaching is essential to the delivery of quality physical therapy services. It is a prerequisite of professional competence for at least two reasons. First, physical therapists are frequently asked or required to function as teachers. In this role, they are, or may be, involved in planning, implementing, and evaluating structured programs for patient and family education; student education in the clinical or academic setting; staff and professional education through continuing education or in-service programs; and community education in the areas of awareness, health promotion, health maintenance, and illness prevention.

Second, and perhaps more importantly, teaching is a *tool* of therapeutic intervention. It is one of the principal methods for delivering patient care services. For example, physical therapists *teach* patients how to do specific exercise regimens, how to manage their wheelchairs, how to transfer from wheelchair to bed, how to ambulate with assistive devices, how to manage chronic pain, and how to move to avoid injury or reinjury. In each of these situations, teaching is the primary tool of therapeutic intervention. In other instances, teaching may be an important adjunct to therapeutic intervention, such as when the therapist explains the rationale for bronchial hygiene while assisting the patient with deep breathing and coughing.

Based on this brief analysis, it is evident that the achievement of almost all goals of patient care depends to some extent on the therapist's ability to manage the teaching-

learning process and promote active learning on the part of the patient. And yet, in spite of its importance, much of the teaching in physical therapy is done on an ad hoc basis, without regard for the application of concepts, principles, or practices of effective teaching or efficient learning. This disregard is particularly evident in the teaching that occurs as part of therapeutic intervention. As a result, the outcomes of these teaching-learning activities are frequently less than optimal.

Undoubtedly, many reasons exist for therapists' current approach to the teaching-learning process; however, two factors appear to be of particular importance. First, many practicing physical therapists were not exposed to concepts and principles associated with teaching and learning as part of their professional preparation. Second, when the teaching-learning process has been included in the curriculum, the focus has been on teaching as a role rather than as a tool of therapeutic intervention. Teaching as a vital and integral component of almost all other forms of therapeutic intervention has not been stressed. As a result, physical therapists have not recognized that the planning, implementation, and evaluation of patient care activities should be guided by concepts and principles of teaching and learning in the same way that these processes are guided by principles of therapeutic exercise, rehabilitation, and manual muscle testing.

This chapter is designed to introduce physical therapy students and practitioners to basic concepts, principles, and practices of effective teaching and learning. It is intended to provide a framework for the development, implementation, and evaluation of teaching-learning interactions; to help physical therapists integrate teaching into their clinical practices; to help them find practical ways to apply concepts and principles of teaching and learning to the clinical environment; and to create a level of awareness of the importance of skillful teaching and active learning in all aspects of physical therapy. Although the emphasis throughout the chapter is on *teaching as a tool of therapeutic intervention and the patient as the primary learner*, the concepts and principles discussed are applicable to the development, implementation, and evaluation of teaching-learning activities for other clients and for teaching in other environments.

TEACHING AND LEARNING DEFINED

According to Narrow, "Teaching and learning are elements of a single process in which both the teacher and learner are actively involved." Teaching is the intentional and deliberate act of helping people learn. It is a highly complex activity that must be adapted to a vast array of human and environmental conditions. *Skillful teaching* is the ability to create conditions and circumstances that maximize learning with the least expenditure of time, energy, and other resources.

Learning is the means by which humans adapt to the environment and circumstances. To say that a person "has learned" implies that behavior has changed as a result of experience; the change in behavior is related to repeated presentations of a situation and efforts by the learner to respond to the situation effectively.

Learning is a process rather than a product and is a function of motive-incentive conditions. That is, learning occurs when a need, a motive, or a goal exists, and learning will help to reduce the need or to satisfy the motive. The product of learning is the acquisition or modification of cognitive, social, behavioral, or psychomotor skills.

WAYS OF LEARNING

Learning occurs in a variety of ways. People learn through conditioning, trial and error, imitation, and insight. Regardless of the manner of learning, three elements must be present: a learner (in the context of this discussion, a human being); a stimulus or stimulus situation; and a response. Learning has occurred or can be inferred when the learner's response to the stimulus situation has changed as a result of contact with the stimulus situation.

CONDITIONING

In the classical sense, conditioning occurs when a response aroused by a natural stimulus—an unconditioned stimulus—is associated with and evoked by an entirely different stimulus—a conditioned stimulus. The conditioned stimulus-response connection is developed through conscious or inadvertent simultaneous pairing of the unconditioned and conditioned stimuli until the response is associated with the conditioned stimulus.

Many responses of young children are the result of conditioning. For example, children frequently respond to health care workers with obvious signs of anxiety or distress. This response is the result of a learned association between white clothing (a conditioned stimulus) and being sick, painful procedures such as injections, or bad-tasting medicine (unconditioned stimuli). The response to the natural or unconditioned stimulus (pain, discomfort, distress) is evoked by the "new" or conditioned stimulus (white clothing). The conditioned stimulus-response connection is strengthened each time a health care worker dressed in white clothing administers an injection or other unpleasant form of treatment.

In this and many other situations related to conditioned learning, the primary concern of the physical therapist is to "break up" or extinguish the learned stimulus-response pattern. To do so usually necessitates the creation of still another conditioned response. For example, the physical therapist who is gentle, who spends time talking and playing with the child, and who is honest when a procedure will hurt will eventually create a different stimulus-response connection.

Conditioning, in the classical sense, is of limited value in clinical teaching. It is most useful in developing reflexive patterns of behavior, habits, and, in some instances, attitudes. It can be of value in working with young children or adults with impaired cognitive abilities.

Operant conditioning is more useful in the teaching-learning process in physical therapy. It occurs when correct or near correct responses are reinforced and incorrect responses are ignored. As a result of the differential reinforcement, correct or near correct responses are strengthened and incorrect responses are weakened and eventually eliminated.

In practice, operant conditioning is used to *shape* a patient's behavior by rewarding responses that approximate the correct response. Words of praise or encouragement or a pat on the back are used to strengthen the desired responses. As learning occurs, reinforcement is reserved for increasingly more correct approximations of the desired response.

Either classical or operant conditioning is probably involved in all other forms of learning. In all situations where conditioning is involved, the primary concern is to enhance attitudes or behaviors that are to the learner's advantage and eliminate or modify those that are to the learner's disadvantage.

TRIAL AND ERROR LEARNING

Trial and error learning is employed when an individual is faced with a stimulus situation and does not have a readily available response. Trial and error learning is most apparent when the learner has no relevant experience to guide responses, and the benefit of others' experiences are unavailable.

Trial and error learning involves a series of random, hit-or-miss responses that eventually lead to the appropriate response. When placed in a new situation, one for which no response or clues to a correct response are available, the motivated learner will engage in various "trials" to attain satisfaction. Responses that are rewarded by motive satisfaction will be strengthened and other responses will be weakened. In successive encounters with the stimulus situation, the correct response will be achieved faster and the number of incorrect trials will be reduced. Through repetition, the correct response is learned and the incorrect responses are eliminated.

Trial and error learning wastes time and energy because of the number of incorrect responses that must be made before the correct response is learned. Because of this, its use should be minimized. However, it is important to recognize that other forms of learning, namely, imitation and insight learning, involve some degree of trial and error learning.

IMITATION

Imitation is a useful and powerful way of learning. It involves both conscious and unconscious copying of observed behaviors in others. The behaviors that are imitated may be mannerisms, speech patterns, attitudes, or motor skills. The only requirement for learning by imitation is that the learner has the prerequisite skills for the behavior that is to be imitated. For example, if a speech pattern is to be imitated, the learner must possess the ability for speech.

In practice, demonstration and modeling are frequently used to promote learning by imitation. The physical therapist shows the patient how to perform a motor skill or models attitudes, values, or behaviors in the hope that the learner will copy the motor performance, behavior, attitudes, or values.

Because learning by imitation occurs at both the conscious and unconscious levels, the teacher must be aware that the learner may imitate undersirable habits, attitudes, or behaviors as well as those that are desirable. Thus, the teacher must be certain to model only desirable attitudes and behaviors.

INSIGHT

Insight learning is the most efficient way of learning for adults with unimpaired cognitive abilities. It involves providing the learner with as much guidance as possible prior to learning and specific feedback during learning. More specifically, it involves explaining what the learner is going to do, the rationale for doing it, the relationship between parts of the task, and the relationship between current learning and past learning or experience. It also entails providing feedback about what the learner is doing right, what needs to be modified, cues for performance, and the like. The goal of insight learning is to guide the learner to goal achievement in the the shortest possible time by minimizing the need for trial and error learning.

THE TEACHING-LEARNING PROCESS

The teaching-learning process is a comprehensive, systematic approach to organizing and conducting teaching activities that foster active participation and interaction between "teacher" and "learner" and capitalize on their respective roles in the process. Like the patient care process, the teaching-learning process can be described in five interdependent stages. These stages—assessment, planning, implementation, evaluation, and documentation—will be described in the sections that follow.

ASSESSMENT

Like other forms of physical therapy intervention, the first step in the teaching-learning process is assessment. Information about the client's ability to learn, physical and psychological readiness to learn, diagnosis, physical condition, prognosis, treatment regimens, attitudes, values, interests, and motivation are all essential to the development of an adequate description of the client's learning needs and as a basis for structuring the most effective and efficient approach to teaching. These data can be obtained from a variety of sources and by using a combination of methods.

For example, information about the client's diagnosis, physical condition, prognosis, and treatment can be obtained by reading textbooks and journals, reading the patient's medical record, conducting the physical therapy evalu-

ation, and discussing the client's status with other health care personnel involved. Data about the client's ability to learn, readiness to learn, attitudes, interests, and motivation can be gathered through careful observation of the client, discussion with other health care personnel, and interaction with the client and the family. Another useful tool for collecting this information is the structured interview.

Through a series of carefully constructed questions, the physical therapist can obtain information about the client and family, lifestyle, health habits, reactions to disability, current level of knowledge about disability, and plans and concerns about the future. In addition, as the interview progresses, the observant therapist can gain a wealth of information about the client's willingness and ability to communicate, listening skills, level of literacy, memory, question-asking skills, attention span, ability to concentrate, reactions to distractions, and reactions to new situations. Each of these types of information is essential to developing appropriate plans for patient learning.

In addition to assessment of the client, assessment of the characteristics of the physical therapist and the environment is essential to planning effective teaching-learning interactions. The attitudes, values, knowledge, skills, and biases of the physical therapist must be considered in relation to the client's problems and learning needs. In like manner, information about facilities, equipment, personnel, media, materials, and time for teaching needs to be available as planning activities are initiated.

Once the assessment has been completed, the data should be carefully analyzed and used as a guide to planning the teaching-learning activities. Although all the information collected is important to planning the teaching-learning interventions, some aspects deserve particular attention. To assure adequate planning, the therapist should be sure to answer the following questions during analysis of assessment data: (1) What are the client's learning needs? (2) What is the client's perceptual status? (3) What is the client's level of motivation? (4) What is the client's level of readiness for learning?

The Client's Learning Needs

Learning is based on needs. Individuals learn best when they feel a need to learn. Therefore, the client must feel a need to change some aspect of his or her behavior if the outcomes of teaching and learning are to be maximized.

Planning for learning and the implementation of teaching-learning activities should begin with mutually agreed upon learning needs, even if they differ from those that the therapist believes are essential. Over time, the patient will recognize other needs. By focusing on what the patient feels a need to learn, the therapist builds a sense of trust, motivation, and caring, and the outcomes of the teaching-learning interaction are enhanced.

On some occasions, the physical therapist may define learning needs for the patient that differ from those defined by the patient. In these instances, the therapist should employ the technique of *therapeutic seeding* in an effort to create a sense of need in the patient. That is, the therapist should discuss with the patient or suggest possible learning needs in the hope that this discussion will help the patient identify needs or will, in fact, result in the development of need within the patient. The development of need in response to therapeutic seeding may be immediate or it may be delayed.

The Client's Perceptual Status

Perception is the process through which the individual becomes aware of the environment. It is the mechanism through which the individual defines and relates to the world. Perception is absolutely essential for learning. When perceptual abilities are altered or lacking, learning will be slowed or rendered impossible.

Concerns for perception are particularly important when working with patients because many of them will exhibit diminished perceptual abilities. Their perceptual abilities may be decreased, distorted, or completely lacking. Disturbances in patients' perception may be the result of illness, stress, intense emotional

reactions (such as fear or anxiety), or disorientation or confusion caused by the environment; or they may be a function of interruption of the sensory apparatus. Regardless of cause, recognition of and planning for disturbances of perception must be done. Therefore, for the purpose of planning the teaching-learning process, it is very important to assess the patient's vision, hearing, language comprehension, touch, and other sensory modalities. The teaching-learning process must accommodate for distorted or limited perceptions if the patient is to achieve maximal benefit.

The Client's Level of Motivation

Motivation is an internal state, a force within the individual that drives him to action. Motivation is a function of physical or emotional needs, interests, or environmental factors. In most instances, individuals are motivated in the direction of the most pressing need and will act to reduce that need or satisfy that interest. With regard to learning, individuals are motivated to learn when the need to learn is more pressing or stronger than other needs.

Patients are frequently not motivated to learn. This does not mean that they are not motivated, as is sometimes assumed. Rather, it suggests that other needs are stronger and are the primary driving force for the patient at the moment. When these needs have been satisfied or reduced, the patient may be motivated to learn. During periods when the patient is not motivated to learn or attend to other aspects of physical therapy intervention, the therapist needs to try to understand and be supportive, accepting, and nonjudgmental.

A variety of factors serve to motivate patients to learn. These factors include a desire to get well, to understand their illness, to return to work, to be self-sufficient, to feel better, to avoid complications, or even to please others.

The Client's Level of Readiness for Learning

Readiness refers to the learner's willingness and ability to profit from instruction. While it includes motivation, readiness is also affected by the learner's comfort, energy level, and physical, emotional, and intellectual capabilities. Some authors have indicated that skillful teaching and readiness are the two major determinants of learning.

Several factors need to be considered in determining the client's level of readiness. For example, the client's level of physical and psychological comfort, previous learning and experience, developmental stage, physical and intellectual capabilities, and energy level are all determinants of readiness. Because energy levels vary as a function of time of day, medications, hospital routines, stress, and attitude, these factors need to be considered in the assessment of readiness and in planning for instruction. For example, the patient may be ready for learning at 10 AM but unable to profit from learning at 2 PM because of fatigue or confusion caused by medications.

PLANNING

As soon as adequate information has been gathered and analyzed, planning can begin. Planning is a deliberate activity and involves making a series of conscious decisions about *what*, *how*, *where*, and *when* to teach the client and how teaching-learning activities will be integrated with other aspects of therapeutic intervention. Planning to meet the learning needs of the client can and should be incorporated into the process of planning to meet other therapeutic needs.

Although time consuming, the planning process is absolutely essential in that it provides the foundation for all subsequent phases of the teaching-learning process; it helps to assure optimal utilization of often limited resources such as time, space, and equipment; and, if documented, it helps to assure continuity of activity among all health care personnel involved with the patient. Planning for the teaching-learning process involves the identification of goals and objectives, selection of content, determination of priorities, organization and sequential arrangement of learning experiences, and selection of methods to evaluate whether appropriate learning has occurred and the effectiveness of specific teaching-learning activities.

The first step in the planning process involves describing what can realistically be accomplished in view of the client's status, the environment, the available time and resources, and the physical therapist's knowledge and skills. Physical therapists employ this same process to specify goals of patient care.

Goal setting is a fundamental and essential aspect of the planning phase of all physical therapy intervention. Its importance owes to the need for everyone to know what is to be accomplished and when it is to be accomplished. Physical therapists are experienced in the process of setting both long-term and short-term goals. However, they rarely analyze the specified goals for explicit or implicit teaching-learning needs, which represents an important next step!

As patient care goals are articulated, they should be examined for inherent or implied learning needs of the client. Scrutiny of patient care goals will reveal areas of need for new information or knowledge, new or modified attitudes, and new or modified motor skills. As learning needs are identified, they should be translated into behavioral objectives. Although this may seem like a burdensome process, it helps to assure that the patient is provided opportunities to learn that which is necessary for achieving the goals of intervention.

Specifying Behavioral Objectives

Behavioral objectives serve to guide the planning of teaching-learning activities and the evaluation of outcomes. They help to assure that the teaching-learning process is tailored to the unique needs of the client and to the resources and limitations of time and the environment. When objectives are clearly stated, both the physical therapist and the client know what is expected and how to channel their energy.

All behavioral objectives relate to one of three domains of learning: they are either cognitive objectives, affective objectives, or psychomotor objectives. Cognitive objectives are concerned with the acquisition or use of knowledge or the development of intellectual skills.

Affective objectives deal with feelings and emotions as reflected in attitudes, interests, values, and appreciations. Psychomotor objectives are concerned with the development of motor skills and musculoskeletal coordination. Although much of the teaching done in physical therapy is associated with the psychomotor domain, physical therapists are also involved in teaching in both the cognitive and affective domains.

Like long-term and short-term goals of patient care, behavioral objectives should be written in clear, unambiguous, and measurable terminology. They should be written in simple terms; each objective should specify a single behavior; and each objective should describe the following:

1. the learner's behavior—what the learner will be able to do after instruction,
2. the criteria of performance—how well the learner will be able to do it, and
3. the conditions of performance—the conditions under which the learner will perform the desired behavior.

Perhaps the hardest part of writing a clear behavioral objective is the selection of words that describe *what* the learner will be able to do following instruction. The following list provides a sample of action verbs that describe appropriate behaviors for each of the domains of learning.

- *Cognitive:* describe, discuss, state, identify, select, list, explain, explore, compose, teach, analyze
- *Affective:* express, share, listen, relate, conserve, choose, approach, help, modify
- *Psychomotor:* demonstrate, practice, perform, walk, administer, give, construct, assemble, record, use, move

The common characteristic of each of these words is that they describe observable behaviors, which are behaviors that can be seen, heard, or felt. In addition, they are words that are easily understood. Obviously, many other words could be added to each list.

After the learner's behavior has been de-scribed, the conditions and criteria of performance should be specified. Conditions of performance include factors such as time of day, use of special equipment, place, and surfaces. For cognitive and affective objectives, conditions of performance may be stated as "givens." For example, the objective may be worded as follows: "Given a list of health indicators, the learner will correctly identify five of the seven warning signs of cancer." Criteria include factors such as level of independence, accuracy, distance, and frequency or speed of performance. In the example provided, the criterion of performance is accurate identification of five out of seven warning signs of cancer.

Once goals and objectives have been specified and agreed upon by the patient and the physical therapist, a number of other decisions must be made before any significant learning activities can be initiated. These decisions concern content, learning priorities, essential learning experiences, and evaluation procedures. These activities are essential to assure that the specific needs of the patient are met and to maximize the use of available time, resources, and personnel.

Determining and Sequencing Content

Content includes the knowledge and skills with which the learner needs to be confronted in order to achieve the specified objectives. As such, it should be selected according to the patient's learning needs and the mutually agreed upon objectives.

To facilitate the selection of content, each behavioral objective should be considered in relation to two questions: "What steps are necessary to achieve the objective?" and "What knowledge is necessary to accomplish each step?" Although this sounds like a laborious process, it is one of the few methods available to ensure that important content is not omitted.

Once content is selected, it needs to be arranged so that it flows in a logical, integrated, continuous manner. No single correct approach to sequencing content exists, but several factors should be considered. Content should generally be sequenced so that it flows from familiar to unfamiliar, from simple to complex, and from concrete to abstract. Content should be sequenced with consideration given to the learner's previous experience and preparation and with concern for assuring that the learner is prepared for subsequent learning. When skills are being taught, content can be sequenced according to part-whole relationships or according to the manner in which the skill is normally performed.

Setting Priorities

As learning needs and content are identified, serious consideration must be given to establishing teaching and learning priorities. These priorities are essential to (1) assure maximum utilization of available teaching time; (2) accommodate to the client's level of readiness and needs for prerequisite learning; and (3) avoid overloading the learner with too much content, which can be anxiety producing and counterproductive.

Priority setting should be based on consideration of several factors. These factors include what the patient and family see as important, the patient's level of anxiety or concern about a particular topic or skill, the level of need (eg, survival skills) associated with a particular topic or skill, the patient's level of readiness, and the anticipated time available for teaching and learning.

Selecting and Organizing Learning Experiences

Learning experiences are planned combinations of people, materials, facilities, methods, media, and content that are designed to assist the learner to achieve the goals of instruction. In general, appropriate learning experiences should focus on essential objectives, be consistent with principles of learning, reflect cooperative efforts between teacher and learner, maximize flexibility and resources utilization, and provide for vicarious learning. The selection and organization of appropriate learning experiences necessitate decisions about what will be taught, how it will be taught, who will teach it, and when and where it will be taught. As learning experiences are selected and organized, careful attention should be given to specific activities planned for the teacher and the learner. Because effective learning experiences should be based on principles of learning, the selection or organization of activities should:

1. reflect concern for individual differences in readiness, motivation, learning style or preference, and rate of learning;
2. provide for active involvement and participation by the learner;
3. provide for success and knowledge of results;
4. provide ample opportunities for practice of the desired behaviors or skills; and
5. be consistent with the capabilities and limitations of the teacher and the learner.

The selection of appropriate instructional methods and media is an important aspect of organizing effective learning experiences. Instructional methods are teaching formats and include lecture, discussion, demonstration, independent study, simulation, role-playing, and practice. Instructional media are tools that enhance learning or retention. They are generally used in combination with instructional methods to assist the learner to understand, visualize, or retain facts, concepts, principles, or skills. Commonly available media include chalkboards, flipcharts, bulletin boards, overhead projectors, films, videotapes and television, audio materials, photographs, drawings, objects and models, games, and printed materials such as books, pamphlets, or handouts. Any of these media can be used to enhance and reinforce learning and to accommodate individual differences in rate and style of learning. Given the diversity of available instructional methods and media, it is unfortunate that so many physical therapists restrict their choices to lecture-discussion methods augmented by an occasional pamphlet or handout and, in so doing, limit the effectiveness of their teaching-learning efforts.

No hard and fast rules exist for selecting instructional methods or media. In general, selection should be based on consideration of their compatibility with the objectives of learning, the nature of the task and the types of learning required, the strengths and weaknesses of the teacher and learner, and the programmatic requirements, resources, and constraints.

Planning for Evaluation

Evaluation is an integral part of the teaching-learning process. It is a systematic, ongoing process that involves analysis of both teaching and learning. Plans for evaluation of the learner's progress, and teacher's effectiveness, and different aspects of the teaching-learning activities should be developed as plans for other components of the program are developed. These plans should include identification of the types of data to be collected, the sources of the data, and the methodology for collecting and recording the data.

IMPLEMENTATION

The implementation stage of the teaching-learning process encompasses the teaching activities that bring together all of the previous planning and transaction of the learner with the environment. It represents the teaching act itself and involves management of all aspects of the plan for teaching, the environment, and the events of instruction.

Gagne and Briggs have described eight events of instruction. During implementation, the therapist is responsible for the following events:

1. gaining the learner's attention;
2. informing the learner of the objectives and purposes of instruction in an effort to orient the learner to the tasks at hand and provide a "set" for learning;
3. stimulating recall of previous related learning;
4. presenting the stimulus for learning and performance;
5. providing guidance, feedback, and reinforcement to the learner;
6. eliciting performance and providing opportunities for practice;
7. assessing performance; and
8. enhancing retention and transfer of learning.

Throughout the implementation phase, the teacher should monitor and control aspects of the environment or situation that may affect the learner's responses. It is a well-established principle that learner responses are a function of consequences. Therefore, the teacher should endeavor to create situations that are satisfying to the learner. Elements of teacher behavior that tend to result in learner satisfaction include rewarding the learner's responses rather than correctness, providing for success, providing a sense of direction, providing immediate and specific feedback, allowing the learner to control the length of the teaching-learning interaction, and relating learning to past and future activities. Conditions that tend to have a negative effect on learning include pain or discomfort, fear or anxiety, frustration, feelings of failure, humiliation, or embarrassment, and boredom. These conditions should be avoided to the greatest extent possible.

EVALUATION

Evaluation is an essential component of the teaching-learning process. As such, it should be a planned, systematic, ongoing activity and should reflect the joint efforts of the patient, physical therapist, family members, and other personnel involved in the patient's care.

The primary purposes of evaluation are to determine if the learning objectives have been met and to assess the effectiveness of the teaching interventions. To this end, information needs to be collected and analyzed about the patient's performance relative to the objectives and the adequacy and appropriateness of the format, content, teaching-learning activities, media, and resources employed in the teaching-learning process. In addition, data should be collected regarding patient and family satisfaction with the teaching-learning experiences.

The best sources of data for evaluation of the patient's achievement and satisfaction and the effectiveness of specific elements of the process are (1) direct observation of the patient's performance and reactions, (2) written and verbal feedback from the patient and family members, and (3) written and verbal feedback from other personnel involved in the patient's care. These data can be obtained through formal or informal discussion, by asking a limited number of carefully worded questions, or through the use of checklists and questionnaires.

The physical therapist is responsible for initiating evaluation activities, collecting and recording data in a systematic manner, summarizing and documenting findings, and providing constructive feedback to the patient and family. In addition, results of the evaluation should be used to plan learning experiences designed to reinforce learning or promote achievement of objectives not yet accomplished.

DOCUMENTATION

Documentation is the last phase of the teaching-learning process. It is essential to provide for a complete and continuous patient record and to assure continuity of care and accountability.

Documentation of teaching-learning activities should be ongoing and should concentrate on three components of the process. These components are documentation of (1) major elements of the plan for patient learning and any subsequent modifications of the plan, (2) specific teaching-learning activities in progress, and (3) the patient's progress toward achievement of the learning objectives.

CONCLUSION

To facilitate client learning, the teaching-learning process should be structured to begin where the client is and progress at a rate that is comfortable for the learner. Activities should be based on the learner's needs, capabilities, limitations, age, sex, interests, background, and readiness to learn.

The focus of this chapter has been on teaching as a tool of therapeutic intervention and the patient as the primary learner. As indicated at the outset, physical therapists are also involved in planning, implementing, and evaluating structured educational programs for students enrolled in professional preparation programs; for staff or other health care workers through in-service or continuing education programs; and for individuals or groups within the community.

Regardless of who the learner is or how many learners there are, the concepts, principles, and process described in this chapter apply. The learner or learners must be assessed and needs, level of readiness, and motivation must be determined. Systematic planning must occur and should include the identification of goals and objectives, the selection of content, the organization and sequential arrangement of learning experiences, and the selection of methods to evaluate whether learning has occurred and the effectiveness of specific teaching-learning activities. As activities are planned, implemented, evaluated, and documented, principles of teaching and learning should be consistently applied.

The major differences involved in teaching individual patients and other groups of learners relate to the environment, the time available for teaching, and the procedures used for accomplishing certain aspects of the teaching-learning process. In some instances these differences make teaching students, staff, other health care workers, or community groups easier. For example, activities associated with in-service education, continuing education, or community education are usually conducted in classroom-like environments; time for teaching is allotted and scheduled; and, often, more advance information exists regarding the learners, purposes, focus, and scope of the activity. Each of these factors facilitates planning and implementation of effective teaching-learning interactions.

On the other hand, some aspects of the process are more difficult when working with *groups* of learners. For example, assessing learners' needs, interests, and levels of readiness; establishing realistic goals and objectives for all learners; planning appropriate learning experiences; and selecting methods and media to accommodate differences in learners' needs, rates of learning, and styles of learning all become much more complex activities as the number and diversity of learners increases. In general, teaching groups of learners demands increased levels of responsiveness, creativity, and ingenuity on the part of the teacher, and the judicious selection and combination of methods, media, material, and personnel to meet the needs of both the group and individuals within the group.

In all teaching-learning interactions, regardless of audience or environment, the skillful teacher should provide carefully planned learning experiences that recognize that the learner is more apt to attain goals that he has set rather than goals that are imposed on him. Learning experiences should be designed to engage the learner in active participation; to provide for insight, but allow for trial and error exploration and learning by imitation; to provide for practice of the desired response; to provide for specific feedback and reinforcement of the desired responses; to encourage practice in different situations in order to promote response generalization; and to establish a set for learning by helping the learner understand what is to be learned and the reasons for learning it.

ANNOTATED BIBLIOGRAPHY

Bille DA (ed): Practical Approaches to Patient Teaching. Boston, Little, Brown & Co, 1981 (Provides a systematic and practical description of all aspects of developing a comprehensive program of patient education.)

Brookfield S: Understanding and Facilitating Adult Learning. San Francisco, Jossey-Bass, 1986 (Includes a complete and comprehensive analysis of principles and practices related to adult learning.)

Gagne R, Briggs L: Principles of Instructional Design. New York, Holt, Rinehart & Winston, 1974 (Describes a systematic approach to developing teaching-learning activities with emphasis on the relationship between instructional strategies and different types of learning objectives.)

Gronlund N: Stating Behavioral Objectives for Classroom Instruction. New York, Macmillan, 1970 (Provides a concise and practical guide to writing and evaluating objectives. Very useful.)

Hyman R: Ways of Teaching. Philadelphia, JB Lippincott, 1970 (Provides a complete and useful analysis of the most commonly used teaching-learning strategies.)

Kemp J: Planning and Producing Audiovisual Materials, 3rd ed. New York, Crowell, 1975 (An excellent reference on the selection, use, and development of various types of media and their appropriateness to different types of teaching and learning.)

McKeachie W: Teaching Tips: A Guidebook for the Beginning College Teacher. Lexington, MA, DC Heath, 1978 (Provides an excellent background and practical suggestions related to all aspects of the teaching-learning process. The discussion of teaching methods is particularly useful.)

Narrow B: Patient Teaching in Nursing Practice: A Patient and Family-Centered Approach. New York, Wiley, 1979 (Provides a detailed description of the teaching-learning process with many practical suggestions for teaching in the clinical environment.)

Oxendine J: Psychology of Motor Learning, 2nd ed. Englewood Cliffs, NJ, Prentice-Hall, 1984 (Provides a comprehensive analysis of concepts and research findings related to the acquisition and development of motor skills. "Must" reading for physical therapists.)

Rankin J: Patient Education: Issues, Principles, and Guidelines. Philadelphia, JB Lippincott, 1983 (Discusses issues and principles related to patient education with useful suggestions for resolving problems associated with teaching in the context of contemporary health care.)

56 Referral

JACK D. CLOSE
PHILIP PAUL TYGIEL

DEFINITION

The term "referral" may be defined as the process by which a practitioner transfers responsibility either temporarily, permanently, or for part of the patient's care to another practitioner or agency (Froom, 1984). Traditionally, the physical therapist had been involved at the "receiving" end of the referral process. Today the physical therapist is involved in the referral process as a maker as well as a receiver of referrals.

HISTORY

Over the years, a marked change occurred in the physical therapy referral process. Historically, the patient was referred to a physical therapist with a specific order or prescription describing the modalities or procedures that the physician desired the therapist to provide. This referral came from the patient's primary care physician or from a medical specialist. The physical therapist completed this order or prescription in a somewhat similar manner as a pharmacist "filling" a prescription order from a physician (Fig. 56-1).

With the increase in the knowledge base, practice skills, abilities, and expertise of the physical therapist, the physician could not keep up with the rapid advances in medical practice and also the changes and the growth in physical therapy practice. As a result, the vast majority of the physical therapy "referrals" became more general in nature and authorized the physical therapist to utilize appropriate expertise to "evaluate and treat" the referred patient. In this relationship, the physician did not relinquish the "control" of the patient. Rather, the physical therapist was authorized to provide the appropriate treatment for the referred patient for a specific period of time or number of treatments, and to then return the patient to the physician for reevaluation, modification of the treatment program, or discharge.

Even as a participant in this authorization/referral process, several opportunities exist for the physical therapist to be a "referring" practitioner. Usually, this referral would occur in one of the following three circumstances.

1. In treating a patient who had been referred by a physician, the physical therapist found that the patient had a secondary condition that would benefit from consultation with another type of physician, or the patient had a condition that required the skills of another physical therapist or other health care practitioner (eg, speech pathologist, occupational therapist). In the first case, the physical therapist might suggest or recommend to the referring physician that the patient be referred to another physician for specialty consultation (eg, orthopedics, neurology). In some circumstances, the therapist might even feel so inclined to recommend a particular specialist. In either case, the physical therapist

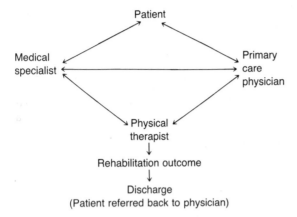

Patient

Medical
specialist

Primary
care
physician

Physical
therapist

↓

Rehabilitation outcome

↓

Discharge
(Patient referred back to physician)

Figure 56-1. Traditional physical therapy referral process.

would make this referral to the patient's referring physician.

2. In treating a patient upon the referral of a particular physician, the physical therapist found that the patient was dissatisfied with the physician and requested that the physical therapist recommend someone else. This scenario almost always places the physical therapist in a rather awkward position. The physical therapist is faced with a decision to ignore the request, inform the referring physician about the problem, or recommend another physician to the patient. Of the three options, usually the most difficult alternative seems to be for the therapist to discuss the problem with the physician and either to facilitate a reconciliation between the patient and the doctor or to receive the doctor's permission to recommend another physician to the patient. If the therapist decides to recommend a new physician for the patient, the clinical facility in which the therapist is employed would usually have some type of procedure to follow. If this procedure provided for the recommendation of a new physician, the therapist would usually provide a list of at least three physicians from which the patient could select a new doctor. However, with this process, the physical therapist would be prudent not to recommend one physician over another.

3. As part of the health care community, the physical therapist finds that friends, relatives, and acquaintances periodically ask the therapist to recommend a physician to take care of a particular medical problem. This request usually occurs at social gatherings, athletic events, and the like. After the acquaintance has provided a brief general description of complaints, but without a detailed history or physical examination, the therapist would usually be asked to recommend a physician. In this situation, the physical therapist might recommend a physician who is best qualified to treat this particular problem, or the therapist would follow the standard rule and provide the patient with a list of three physicians from which the potential patient could select a new physician.

In each of these referral relationships, the therapist served more as a "resource" person than as a referral source. In these circumstances, the therapist was not exposed to malpractice as a result of the recommendation. However, the physical therapist's reputation could definitely be affected—either favorably or unfavorably—according to the results of the recommendation.

MODERN REFERRAL PROCESS

Significant changes have occurred in the traditional role of the physical therapist's participation in the referral process. In June 1979, the American Physical Therapy Association (APTA) declared that in those states where it was "legal," it was ethical for a physical therapist to evaluate patients without a physician's referral. In June 1982, this position was expanded by the APTA's House of Delegates to state that, in those jurisdictions where it was "legal," a physical therapist could ethically practice without referral and could therefore both evaluate and treat a patient's problem within the scope of physical therapy practice. Following these changes, physical therapists in various states sought modifications in their state physical therapy practice acts to allow for evaluation and treatment without referral. Some of the recorded testimony in favor of these changes described such benefits as reduced health care costs, improved health care, an increased opportunity for preventive health care, and a decrease in the delay in providing health care services.

These modifications in the physical therapy practice acts significantly changed the role of the physical therapist in that the physical therapist now became a point of entry into the health care field and the patient had direct access to the physical therapist. As seen in Figure 56-2, the patient would then have a choice of practitioners who could serve as the entry point into the health care system (physician, physical therapist, or other health care specialists). However, this modification in the traditional medical care model did not signify an end to the physician/physical therapist referral relationship; in many cases, this relationship broadened and improved. Following the evaluation of the patient, the entry point practitioner could then freely utilize the expertise of the other members of the health care team by referring the patient for appropriate care and treatment (primary physician to health care specialist, specialist to physical therapist, etc) until the desired rehabilitation outcome is achieved and the patient is discharged. Within this model, the physical therapist could then choose to become an independent practitioner and a true referral source. Because of the natural interrelationship between the physical therapist and the physician, physical therapists may still choose to practice with physician referral. However, in those states where these legisla-

tive changes have occurred, an increasing number of physical therapists are functioning within this health care model and are also taking advantage of the opportunity to serve as consultants to industry, schools, athletic teams, and health clubs. As a result, physical therapists have been able to evaluate a patient's problem before making a referral to a physician.

EVALUATION WITHOUT REFERRAL

In those jurisdictions where a physical therapist evaluates or consults without referral, but still needs a physician's authorization for treatment, the physical therapist is a true referral source. The patient is carefully evaluated and the physical therapist is then able to draw certain conclusions or impressions regarding the patient's clinical problems. The therapist has to determine in accordance with the appropriate expertise and the scope of physical therapy practice the patient's differential or clinical diagnosis. Following this, a decision is made as to whether the patient's problems warranted the implementation of a physical therapy treatment or rehabilitation program. The therapist determines whether he possesses the physical therapy skills needed for this particular patient. After completing this process, the physical therapist refers the patient to a physician for (1) confirmation or additional input regarding the diagnosis; (2) supplementary tests and care; and (3) permission to implement the recommended physical therapy program. In this relationship, the therapist serves as a referral resource; however, the referral of the patient back to the therapist from the physician is still required prior to the initiation of any physical therapy. Ultimate authority for the care of the patient still rests with the physician.

The process a physical therapist might utilize in this "evaluation without referral" environment to select a consultant for the patient will be discussed later in this chapter.

EVALUATION AND TREATMENT WITHOUT REFERRAL

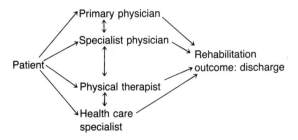

Figure 56-2. Simplified model of direct patient access to physical therapy services.

In those environments where evaluation and treatment can be legally performed without a physician's referral (ie, the patient has direct access to the physical therapist), the physical therapist accepts added options and professional responsibilities and liabilities. In accepting a patient without a physician's referral, the physical therapist utilizes clinical skills that enable functioning at an independent diagnostic level of expertise. As an entry point into the health care field, the therapist must also realize that legal exposure to malpractice increases markedly. In this environment, the therapist in many cases has the ultimate authority for the care of the patient.

When seeing a patient within this direct access model, the therapist carefully records and analyzes the patient's condition based upon an accurate and complete compilation of the patient's history along with the completion of a comprehensive physical examination and evaluation. Following this evaluation, the therapist must form a conclusion or an impression regarding the patient's differential or clinical diagnosis. The therapist might feel that the patient's condition can be clinically diagnosed completely within the scope of the physical therapist's skills, expertise, and training. If this is the case, the therapist determines if she has the skills required to provide the appropriate treatment. If so, treatment is initiated. If not, the patient is referred to a therapist who does possess the skills and expertise to provide the appropriate physical therapy treatment.

If the physical therapist determines that although a provisional clinical diagnosis can be made, the diagnosis needs to be confirmed with further tests (ie, radiological or laboratory studies), the patient is referred to the appropriate physician. With this referral, appropriate communication and correspondence takes place between the physical therapist and the physician regarding this patient's clinical status and the reasons for the referral. The selection of a consultant in this referral process is based upon the criteria that will be described later in this chapter.

The physical therapist might also conclude that the clinical diagnosis or care for this particular patient is beyond the scope of physical therapy practice (eg, visceral pain patterns).

This situation also warrants the referral of the patient to the appropriate physician and is covered in the APTA's "Guide for Professional Conduct" for the physical therapist:

> Principle 3.1 B: When the individual's needs are beyond the scope of the physical therapist's expertise, the individual is to be so informed and *assisted in identifying a qualified person to provide the necessary service.* (Emphasis added.)

With the initiation of the treatment or rehabilitation program, the physical therapist frequently reevaluates the patient's condition during the course of therapy. If the condition resolves in a relatively short period of time, no further consultation is indicated. However, if the patient's condition or problem does not, within a reasonable period of time, respond well to the treatment, or if in fact the patient's condition worsens, the physical therapist refers the patient to a physician or other health care practitioner for consultation and treatment.

In the "direct access" scenario, the physical therapist does not legally require the permission or authorization of the physician to treat the patient. The major goals of referral to the physician are for consultation and augmentation of the patient's care. The consultant may or may not agree with the opinion or recommendations of the physical therapist. In some cases, the therapist may not agree with the consultant's conclusions or recommendations. If this disagreement occurs and it is in the best interest of the patient, the therapist may recommend to the patient that the physical therapy be initiated as indicated by the therapist, or that the patient be referred for another consultation with a different physician.

Another factor that may complicate the referral process is when the patient's health insurance "covers" physical therapy services only on the authorization or referral of a physician. To satisfy this requirement, the therapist must select a physician who is willing to authorize the treatment, or the patient must be willing to assume total financial responsibility for the treatment rendered.

SELECTION OF A CONSULTANT

In either the "evaluate without referral" or the "evaluate and treat without referral" environment, once it is determined that the patient is to be referred to a physician for consultation or supplemental care, it is important that the physical therapist use some type of criteria for selecting a consultant. In this referral process, as in all matters in health care, the patient's best interest should be the most important factor in making the selection. However, several other factors are involved that may influence this selection process.

The physical therapist must realize that a referral has important implications for the cost, utilization, and quality aspects of the care provided. The cost implication is obvious, because it means that two (and possibly more) providers must be paid for services rendered rather than just one. In addition, for a given illness or injury, consultation with a specialist is likely to be more expensive than with a general practitioner. The consultant should be recognized by the physical therapist as being competent in the problem area under consideration. Competence is demonstrated by a high quality of patient management; thoroughness of the evaluation; problem and treatment explanation to the patient or family; thoroughness and efficiency of treatment; and comprehensiveness of treatment. When possible, continuity of patient care is best served by the consultant who is known by the therapist to possess these professional abilities and where some working relationship has been established, including open and ongoing dialogue between the therapist and the physician and *timely* communication. It is also important that the physician to whom the patient is referred has a clear understanding of the knowledge, scope, and practice of physical therapy.

Other patient-related factors that should also be considered in the referral process include (1) in addition to the medical cost of the referral, consider the additional patient costs related to travel expenses, babysitting costs, lost wages, and the like; (2) consider the convenience to the patient in seeing the consul-tant—evaluate the distance the patient will have to travel, how much discomfort will be involved in traveling, the ease in locating where to go, parking, any architectural barriers, the extent of disruption of the patient's and the family's home life, and so on; (3) consider the implicit or explicit desire by the patient or the family to be referred or not be referred; (4) consider any previous use of and satisfaction with the consultant by the patient or the family; and (5) if feasible, attempt to match the patient's and the physician's personalities—the rapport developed between a patient and the consultant can surely affect the end result of the consultation. In spite of all of these factors, a patient's right of free choice of a physician must be maintained.

In the selection of a consultant, the therapist must decide whether to recommend one in a given specialty or to give the patient a choice of several. Some therapists feel that it is always better for "political" reasons (and some feel "ethical" reasons) to provide the patient three names from which to select a consultant. However, others feel that, at least in those situations where it is clear that one physician is better than others at treating this patient's particular problem, only one name should be provided. In the APTA's "Guide for Professional Conduct" for the physical therapist, the following statement is applicable in these situations:

> Principle 3.3 C: When there is no referral, physical therapists are to *refer persons under their care to other qualified individuals* if symptoms or conditions are present which require services beyond the scope of their expertise or for which physical therapy is contraindicated. (Emphasis added.)

Situations in which the referral is not in the best interest of the patient should be avoided, for example, when a physical therapist refers a patient to a consultant solely for the "public relations" or "political" benefits in order to increase referrals, or when the referral is done to "protect" the physical therapist from liability in the unlikely event that the differential diagnosis is incorrect.

SUCCESSFUL REFERRALS

In becoming a referral source, it is a most frustrating experience to refer a patient to a consultant and then never hear of that patient again. In these situations, not only is the referring physical therapist's curiosity and professional concern unsatisfied, but the opportunity for continuing education regarding this patient is lost. If the referred patient later returns from the consultation and no follow-up information has been provided or received, other difficulties and problems will be the end result. The therapist will obviously feel embarrassed about the situation, the relationship between the therapist and the consultant will be impaired, the patient will sense that the care is not being well coordinated, and a subtle weakening of the therapist-patient relationship will occur.

If the referral is to be successful, the following five steps should be accomplished.

1. The need and purpose of a referral must be defined by both the patient and the referring physical therapist. A positive attitude of the referring therapist regarding the necessity of the consultation will greatly influence and facilitate its outcome and contribution to patient care. The referring physical therapist should certainly tell the patient the reason for the referral and approximately what to expect.
2. The need and purpose of the referral must be communicated to the consultant. The use of verbal referrals should be avoided unless the patient's condition is classified as an "emergency." In the correspondence, items that could be included would be the patient's vital statistics, previous history, and the findings or results of the physical therapy clarifying evaluation. The patient should take any clinical studies that have already been accomplished to the consultant. In addition, any nonmedical history that might prove to be helpful to the consultant in evaluating the patient should be included.
3. The consultant should perform a timely and appropriate evaluation.

4. The consultant's findings and recommendations should be communicated to the referring physical therapist in a timely fashion. This report may include such items as additional patient information and history, clinical findings, laboratory results, x-ray films, diagnosis, consultant actions or procedures, follow-up plan, recommendations for future care or treatment, and lastly, *what the patient was told by the consultant.*
5. Secure an understanding by the patient, the consultant, and the referring physical therapist concerning who is taking responsibility for the patient's continued care and treatment.

PROS AND CONS OF REFERRAL

In the referral relationship, the physical therapist must be aware that definite pros (benefits) and cons (negatives) result from the referral process. The most important benefit is the knowledge that the patient is receiving proper care and treatment. In addition, the referral relationship provides for improved and more frequent communication between the therapist and the consultant about the patient's condition and future course of physical therapy. In each of these cases, the primary benefit should be the recovery of the patient. However, the physical therapist will also benefit from the referral relationship by receiving increased awareness in the medical community as a result of the opportunity to demonstrate professional skill and expertise as an entry level (direct access) practitioner. Thus, the physical therapist not only receives the referred patient, but will also probably receive additional referrals from the consultant.

However, some aspects of the referral process may be classified as cons (negatives). Sometimes, in spite of all efforts to select the "correct" consultant, the consultant may provide the patient with an improper or less than optimal evaluation or treatment. Not only is it a disservice to the patient, but it also reflects poorly upon the referring physical therapist.

Another problem arises when the communication between the therapist and the consultant turns out to be less than expected. This problem will certainly affect the rehabilitation and recovery of the patient and may also create a credibility problem between the therapist and the patient. A potential negative aspect of referral may occur if the consultant assumes total care of the patient and the patient becomes permanently "lost" to the physical therapist. This development may have a negative effect on the reputation and the practice of the physical therapist. Another aspect of the referral process that may negatively affect a physical therapist's practice is the loss of patients as a result of professional jealousy (ie, when one physician or medical group determines that you, as the physical therapist, have been referring to other physicians or groups rather than their practice). This happening may occur regardless of the therapist's expertise, and the end result may mean that this medical group might stop referring patients for evaluation or treatment. A final negative aspect of the referral process may occur when a difference of opinion exists between the physical therapist and the consultant. Such a rift not only affects the outcome of the treatment but will also create a great amount of confusion for the patient. In addition, if the disagreement is not handled professionally, the physician/physical therapist working relationship may be permanently damaged.

LEGAL RAMIFICATIONS

Over the years, except for acts of negligence, the therapist has not had a great deal of legal exposure to malpractice claims. Historically, the malpractice insurance premiums for physical therapists have generally been some of the lowest in the country for a health profession. This apparently is due, at least in part, to the fact that in the past the physician had the primary responsibility for the *care* of the patient and was the one who made the *"diagnosis"* of the problem. If either of these were wrong, the physician was determined to be at fault be-

cause it was interpreted that the therapist was functioning under the "order(s)" of the physician. However, with the physical therapist as a primary entry point into the health care field, the physical therapist is as "exposed" as the physician is to malpractice claims.

In addition, because the physical therapist is a "referral source," additional malpractice exposure and liability results from the therapist's "referral" of the patient to a consultant. For physicians, this referral malpractice liability has been linked to the term "concert of action." Wark (1981) stated the following:

> A physician who calls in or recommends another physician is not liable for the other's malpractice where there is no concert of action or common purpose. Concert of action means acts done by two or more people which serve to accomplish a common goal. Also, a physician is not liable for those acts or omissions of another physician who called him or her into the case unless he observed the negligent acts of the other.

It appears that the best course of action to help avoid this malpractice exposure is to select carefully and correctly the consultant for your patient. In addition, progress notes and the referral correspondence must clearly identify the therapist's scope of responsibility with the patient.

GROWING AND FUTURE TRENDS

As the scope of physical therapy practice continues to expand and as the role and the reputation of the physical therapist continues to grow, more opportunities for physical therapists will arise to be involved in the referral process.

Independent physical therapy examinations (IPTE) are being requested more frequently by third party payors. In this event, the physical therapist is called upon to evaluate a patient's condition and the treatment being provided by other practitioners. The therapist can make recommendations to the third party payor that the therapy should continue, be modified, or the like, or can advise that another physician or another type of specialist should be consulted.

In addition, physical therapists are being sought out by patients for second opinions. These requests might be from patients who have not yet received physical therapy, or they may be from a patient who is currently receiving treatment and would like additional input regarding the current condition and treatment. These situations provide the physical therapist with opportunities to become a "referral" source for these patients.

Lastly, the opportunity for the physical therapist to be an "expert witness" in legal proceedings is definitely apparent. In those states that have independent practice, attorneys are referring patients to physical therapists for evaluation and in some cases treatment of the client's condition. Thus, not only is the therapist's expertise tested, but also is the therapist's ability to communicate findings in a legal "courtroom" environment.

CONCLUSION

As the physical therapy profession continues to grow in scope of practice and reputation, opportunities will increase to assist persons incapacitated by injury or disease. Additional skills and abilities will be developed, and with this will come additional professional duties and responsibilities. The referral process is a very important part of this expanded role of the physical therapist, and it must be used wisely, skillfully, correctly, and ethically.

ANNOTATED BIBLIOGRAPHY

American Physical Therapy Association: Guide for Professional Conduct. Alexandria, VA, American Physical Therapy Association, 1985 (Provides the Association's interpretations of its Code of Ethics, and for this subject details the referral relationships.)

Froom J: Risks of referral. J Fam Pract 18(4):623, 1984 (A treatise on the mechanisms of referral and the positive and negative aspects of referral.)

Wark PM: Malpractice liability of referring and consulting physicians. J SC Med Assoc, November 1981, p 563 (Covers the subject of medical malpractice of physicians when they refer to consultants.)

57 Consultation

JAY M. GOODFARB

All consultants play many roles: analyst, auditor, devil's advocate, investigative reporter, trouble shooter, problem-solver, visiting guru, counselor, confessor. How many of these roles consultants play in a given situation depends upon their skill and comfort level in a given role and upon the "image" their clients want or expect them to project. Probably few consultants would appreciate a consulting job that did not have some element of problem-solving in it. Problem-solving provides the necessary challenges and the opportunities for consultants to use their skills.

It is safe to say that physical therapists who assume consulting roles will be primarily problem-solvers. Their highly specialized knowledge of human movement and function, of how to restore function and prevent disability, and of how to prevent injury to the body creates a "problem-solver" image in the minds of their clients. In addition, the entire health care profession and community is geared to this kind of *modus operandi*: identify the problem (disease, injury) and solve it (cure or heal the patient).

Clients expect consultants to know everything within their specialty. What is more, clients expect consultants to do everything well, including all the peripheral skills associated with consulting: speaking, writing, presenting, planning, and formulating strategy. Consultants who are independent business persons must be skilled in marketing and business strategy. One soon becomes aware that consulting presents a special paradox. A consultant must be both a specialist and a generalist at the same time, all in one compact package.

Because of health care economics and other changes in health care practice and because of the nature of their profession, most physical therapists who elect to become full-time or part-time consultants will do so independently rather than become members of a consulting firm. This chapter will focus on the consultant in an independent role.

THE INDEPENDENT CONSULTANT DEFINED

What is an independent consultant? What does one do? Many people in business, including managers who feel that they need a consultant, are not always sure.

For our purposes, however, an independent consultant is a person who accepts a specified fee to use highly specialized knowledge and abilities to solve an out-of-the-ordinary problem or to produce some specified result or product in a limited amount of time on behalf of a client. The client usually cannot afford or cannot find an employee to perform these services.

Generally speaking, an independent consultant should possess several qualities or characteristics in addition to specialized knowledge or expertise:

1. A working knowledge of research techniques.

2. A well-rounded measure of common sense.
3. The ability to anticipate the future.
4. Honesty, and the ability to convey it.
5. A genuine liking for people and a strong concern for their problems and needs.
6. The ability to handle ill-defined or undefined situations and problems with relative ease.
7. The ability to adapt and use feedback and resource information.
8. Self-discipline and mature work habits.
9. A sense of propriety that directs one to know when to speak (and what to say) and when to keep one's own counsel.

Independent consultants must have several other kinds of skills in order to do their job effectively and successfully. First, they must have the same kinds of skills as any other good business person: management, sales, marketing, and accounting. Second, they must have the kinds of skills necessary to perform their consulting work and to communicate the results to their clients: analytical and organizational skills, listening skills, reporting, writing, and presentation skills. The better consultants are able to master these skills, the better they will be able to please their clients. For in the final analysis, good consulting has only one criterion: client satisfaction.

CONSULTING OPPORTUNITIES FOR THE PHYSICAL THERAPIST

Up to this point, we have been discussing independent consulting in general terms. In this section, we will discuss what is "out there" for the physical therapist who becomes a consultant: who are the prospective clients, and what are some of their needs. To assume this role, physical therapists must think of themselves in innovative ways. They must see themselves as "musculoskeletal engineers," "pathokinesiologists" who know when and what to look for in body movement and its relationship to health. The physical therapist must recognize that the biggest new market in health care is not the treatment of sick people, but rather maintaining people in good health. Traditional health care, including physical therapy, has always waited for people to become ill or injured. The role of the physical therapy consultant today is directed toward keeping people well, active, and injury free. Performing these kinds of services constitutes a vast market for the physical therapist. Some of the markets and their consulting opportunities for physical therapists are as follows:

Manufacturing and industry: design ergonomics, wellness program design and implementation, plant design to reduce physical problems and accidents, preplacement muscle evaluation for new employees, pre-work stretching and exercise programs, work hardening programs, postural evaluation, work site evaluation, research to prove cost effectiveness of preventive measures

Architects: residential, office, and plant design

Manufacturers of rehabilitation equipment: exercise equipment design, wheelchair design

Furniture manufacturers: furniture design

Automobile manufacturers: seating and exit design

Airlines: interior design (eg, galleys and other airline personnel work stations), loading and unloading design for passenger carry-on luggage, baggage handling facilities, and equipment.

Attorneys: personal injury cases, disability settlements, accidental death, determining earning power

Insurance: reviewing and evaluating personal injury claims; reviewing and determining disability by using objective testing centers

Industrial commissions: determining work or no-work status for certain injuries (eg, head injuries or those causing paraplegia or quadriplegia)

Medical clinics: design and installation of a physical rehabilitation department

Hospitals: physical therapy department design, employee injury prevention (eg, back and other lifting injuries)

Governmental agencies: designing work stations for employees (eg, office police, postal employees); establishing wellness centers

Sports teams and fitness centers: stretching and flexibility programs, injury prevention, conditioning

Other physical therapists: how to improve practice; new marketing strategies; how to market to physicians and other health care personnel

Vocational rehabilitation and counseling agencies: how to establish degree of disability; determining how to reduce economic burden to individual and society; how to improve daily living conditions for handicapped (eg, the arthritis patient)

Nursing homes and senior living centers: wellness programs, exercise programs, ergonomic designs, family cooperative care planning (training the family to care for seniors)

Health care companies: program design, facility design

Hotels and resorts: designing exercise facilities and programs for travelers; designing injury prevention programs for high-risk sports such as skiing

The brief vignettes that follow are actual representative case studies of an independent physical therapist-consultant.

Case 1

Client   Major hospital in the Southwest

Problem   Very high rate of low back injuries among female employees in a central supply work area in which plastic containers of dirty surgical instruments (weighing approximately 40 lb each) were removed from a conveyor terminal, placed on carts, and moved to instrument washers.

Study   Consultant conducted half-day site visit, observing the workers, their lifting techniques, and equipment installations.

Findings   Conveyor terminal is too high, and does not allow safe lifting for all employees. Taller male employees were less susceptible to back injuries. Load weights were too high. Too few containers made container overloading necessary.

Recommendations   Make necessary architectural changes to lower conveyor terminal to appropriate level. Furnish enough containers so that container loads could be limited by operating room personnel to 25-lb maximum weight. Instruct employees in safe lifting techniques for that particular situation.

Results   Back injuries in that area reduced by 80% within 90-day period.

Case 2

Client   Major airline

Problem   Excessive number of minor injuries among cabin attendants, particularly those who served food to passengers. Many complaints on file from union representatives protesting "poor working conditions."

Study   Consultant boarded "typical" flight and observed attendants preparing food in galley and serving passengers. Attendants exhibited many poor postural techniques in performing their duties. Galley design created several potential causes for injury.

Recommendations   Install customized education program to correct bending, stooping, and stretching techniques. Reconfigure galley layout and storage to minimize strain and awkward lifting situations.

Results   Back injuries reduced by 36%. Better results anticipated when new galley design installations are completed.

Case 3

Client   Major hospital in New York City

Problem   Physical Therapy Department revenues steadily falling over last two years. High employee turnover. Many patient complaints.

Study   Consultant made one-week site visit. Conducted extensive interviews with management and clinical personnel. Examination of department financial reports and clinical records.

Recommendations   Install incentive program for all physical therapy employees (profit-sharing and bonus plans). Develop plan to open four new services within 18-month period. Redesign physical therapy department area, particularly to make patient egress easier and patient waiting areas more comfortable and private. Design better access to parking for outpatients.

Results   Physical plant changes underway. Patient revenues up 8% for last quarter. Most recent Patient Satisfaction Survey shows patients much happier with services. Reduction in employee turnover of 23% during last quarter reported.

THE "HOW-TO'S" OF CONSULTING

ESTABLISHING A CLIENT-CONSULTANT RELATIONSHIP

Clients generally feel that consultants become a part of their institution or firm, even for a brief time. Consultants become privy to company secrets. They know what is behind the company facade. As a result, the consultant's personality and the ability to form good interpersonal relationships quickly are extremely important in establishing the idea in the client's mind that the consultant is competent and trustworthy.

If we could assemble the image of the ideal consultant, we would see someone who does not come on too strong, yet exudes quiet self-confidence. The loud, effusive glad-hander and the bland, timid person usually do not make it as a consultant. Few of us like extremes, especially when we must deal with those extremes over a period of time and listen to their advice. Therefore, at all times, the consultant must give the impression of someone who can be trusted, who knows what he or she is doing, who is dignified and businesslike, and who can listen and observe carefully.

The initial meeting is a critical time for con-

sultants. They must sell themselves and their services, yet maintain the impressions we have just mentioned. Golightly, a management consultant for more than 30 years and author of *Consultants: Selecting, Using and Evaluating Business Consultants*, advises managers who are seeking help from a consultant to "observe the consultant's attitude." If a prospective consultant looks around the room, does not look directly at the manager, or otherwise shows that he or she is not intensely interested in the manager's problem, that is the time, Golightly advises, to "terminate the interview and give the consultant no further consideration."

Many beginning consultants get so wrapped up in selling themselves, convincing the client they are the right person for the job, that they forget they must act, at all times, like a consultant, whether they have been hired or not.

During an initial meeting, good technique dictates that the consultant find out as soon as possible *what the client's needs are*. If you are a beginning consultant and do not have any idea how to find out, it is simple. Do what any experienced consultant would do. Ask tactful, well-phrased questions about the client's operation and the problems involved or about what the client wants to accomplish and what he or she expects in terms of end results. Then state what you know you can do to help the client solve the problem or produce the desired results. Do so quietly, quickly, and without exaggeration.

Remember, in terms of one's own interests as a consultant, the purpose of every initial meeting with a prospective client should be to get that client to tell you what you should propose to do for him or her.

If you read the last two paragraphs carefully, you must realize that a consultant must always be seeking information, analyzing that information, and *relating it to the client's needs*, from the initial meeting until the day the job is completed. Consultants cannot perform this function unless they develop and constantly practice one of the most basic skills in consulting—listening.

Listening is not passive. It is an active process that involves leading or guiding the client by asking questions. Focus all of your attention on the client's answers; within them you will find the client's needs or problems. Perhaps you will not get complete answers; perhaps the client will not disclose the magnitude of the needs or problems. But you must have a very good idea what they are so that you can get what you want out of the meeting. This kind of focus will automatically force you to be a better listener.

Take good notes. Unless you have total recall, you will need them later if you get the job. If you cannot listen, analyze, and take notes at the same time, use a tape recorder, making sure you ask permission first.

As you listen, you should be able to find out not only what the client's needs are, you should also find out what kind of help the client will expect from you. Remember, the most common mistake of the beginning consultant is to try to impress the client during the initial meeting with the wealth of knowledge and experience that the consultant can bring to a situation. If you do that, you are not going to be able to hear and to focus on what the client wants. Put information about your credentials in a small brochure that you can leave with the client, and just *listen and observe!*

SPECIFIC SKILLS

We have mentioned a few general skills other than specialized knowledge required of the successful independent consultant. In this section, we will discuss some specific skills that experienced consultants are expected to possess.

Writing and Reporting

Most clients expect the consultant to develop a "study plan." The plan consists of a written outline or description that tells how the consultant expects to acquire the necessary data to arrive at conclusions and recommendations. In addition, interim reports may be required at various stages of the consult. And of course, a final report is usually expected that lists the rec-

ommendations, solutions, and conclusions made by the consultant. Good consultants write well, simply, and clearly. Consultants who bury their ideas in a mass of charts, big words, and difficult language are not likely to work very often as consultants.

Reporting is not always in the written form. Good verbal communication skills are necessary. For example, it is not uncommon for independent consultants to present their findings and recommendations to full meetings of management people, including boards of directors. Experienced consultants are able to design and to use audiovisual aids skillfully, such as graphs, slides, overhead projector transparencies, and other communication tools to help clarify their ideas.

Analyzing and Researching

Careful analysis includes a complete study of a problem or desired result. This study usually involves research to find a historical perspective, to interpret current trends, and to predict what is likely to happen in the future. The independent consultant should have a good working knowledge of research methods, demographics, and statistical analysis.

Management Skills

Most business problems that require the help of independent consultants involve finances, either directly or indirectly. Independent consultants should have experience in financial management: how to read and interpret financial data, how to determine the degree of productivity and profitability that would result from a recommended course of action, and how to determine whether a particular operation is profitable.

THE BUSINESS END OF CONSULTING

Many consultants, especially those who begin their professional careers as employees of nonprofit institutions, have considerable difficulty in making the mental and philosophical transition required to think in more profit-oriented, entrepreneurial terms. In fact, while we recommend that physical therapists begin their careers in institutional settings, we believe that they need two to three years of independent private practice in order to develop the necessary skills and attitudes to consult for a private, for-profit enterprise. Many physical therapists become middle managers in hospitals, for example. Although they are responsible for departmental business, clinical practice, and budgets, they have little control over major business decisions, even those that may affect them directly. A great deal of difference exists between this kind of business management and the kind in which a manager's decisions may literally make or break a business.

As a result of this institutional conditioning, many new consultants, especially physical therapists new to the entrepreneurial world, find that some of the most difficult tasks facing them are pricing, proposing (bidding), and contracting their services to prospective clients.

Pricing

The simplest way to price your services is to set an hourly rate. Larger jobs can be estimated in terms of hours and priced accordingly. What hourly rate should you set? Some consultants set their rates to correspond with those of accountants and attorneys. As a beginning consultant, however, you will not command the rate of a senior CPA or a partner in a law firm. You may receive the rates of a junior accountant or a new associate with a law firm. That rate can be reviewed and increased as you gain experience and a reputation.

Most experienced independent consultants advise setting an hourly rate and then sticking by it. Do not haggle. The tendency for an inexperienced consultant is to quote a rate, and, if the client's eyes visibly widen or if he gulps, to lower the rate. Do not get into the habit. If you are sure of the quality of your services, be just as sure of the validity of your hourly charges. It may help to keep in mind the benefits you can bring to the client, financial and otherwise.

In some situations, hourly rates may not be the way to price your services. For example, early in his consulting career, a professional

writer and business consultant was asked to quote a price to solve a problem for a large diagnostic imaging firm. The company was having problems collecting radiologists' interpretation fees from patients, fees separate from the cost of performing x-ray procedures in hospitals or clinics. The patients simply did not understand why they should have to pay two separate amounts of money for what was, in their minds, one process. As a result, accounts receivable were well into six figures. Five full-time employees were hired to try to deal with the problem. The new consultant quoted a rate of $75 per hour, although he realized that the solution was simple and would take only a very short amount of his time. He designed an attention-getting flyer that explained in plain language why two charges existed for x-ray services. The flyer was posted prominently in every hospital x-ray department waiting room and in every clinic served by the imaging company. It was also sent to the patients with every first billing. The consultant billed the company $225 for three hours of his time. As the result of his service, the diagnostic imaging company reduced its accounts receivable a quarter of a million dollars in three months and was able to reduce the number of employees dealing with the problem from five to one within two months.

In that situation, an hourly rate was inappropriate. A better approach to the client might have been to say, "I think I can solve your problem. If I can, my fee is $2,500. If I cannot, it will cost you $100 per hour for my attempt." That kind of approach may be a little difficult at first, but if you have confidence in yourself, it may pay off.

In the end, the axiom of "researching the client before pricing the service" may be the best strategy.

Proposing

Many decisions to hire consultants are based on proposals and fixed-fee contracts. A few considerations are basic. One of the most important considerations is to base your proposal on the client's needs: how the present problem can be solved, what benefits your services can bring to the client, how productivity can be increased, how dollars can be saved, and how the employee's lost time will be reduced.

Another basic consideration is that in designing the proposal you give only enough information to sell the client on your ideas, not disclose in detail a step-by-step plan to solve the client's problem. If you do that, the client may simply say "Thank you," keep your proposal, and walk away to follow your advice or have someone else follow your advice, free.

Obviously, proposal writing always involves some risk. Be willing to assume it.

A proposal should describe what your general approach will be (objectives and anticipated results) and the resources you will need to complete the job (remember to include things such as secretarial help and out-of-pocket expenses). If it is appropriate, specify what access you will need to company records and documents in order to do a good job. Finally, include an estimate of the cost to the client. You may want to break the cost down by an hourly rate. What the client wants, however, is a maximum cost figure—your assurance that the cost will not exceed this figure. Remember to be fair to yourself first and to your client. Figure what the job will cost you to perform and build in an appropriate profit. You are entitled to it, and you must make a profit to remain in business. Some experienced consultants compute their costs, add a fair profit, then figure in a "hassle factor." The hassle factor takes into consideration unforseen problems, delays, unavoidable increases in estimated time, and the like. The hassle factor may run from as low as 10% to as high as 25%.

Unfortunately, many clients hire the consultant who submits the lowest bid. Do not mourn if you are passed over for this reason. Clients who select consultants solely on this basis too often get what they deserve. On the other hand, if you lose bid after bid, find out why. You may have to reconsider your bidding structure. However, our advice is to err on the high side of the bidding process. Most new consultants err on the low side.

Earlier in this section, we advised against haggling with clients over an hourly rate. Correspondingly, do not engage in an auction with other bidders for the job. Any client who permits that to happen or who shares bid amounts with competing bidders is unethical, to say the least, and is not worthy of your further involvement.

Contracts

First, be sure you have a contract. Do not begin work without it! You are asking for trouble if you do, even if you know the client well (especially if you know the client well!). The client will respect you for insisting that this detail be completed. Second, keep any contract simple and to the point. Avoid legal mumbo-jumbo—no "parties of the first part" or the like. Leave that kind of talk to attorneys. A contract is perfectly legal and binding when written in simple, common language. Several excellent examples of proposals and contracts are available in the references cited in the annotated bibliography at the end of this chapter.

After some trial-and-error attempts, you may be able to design permanent formats for some of these documents so that you do not have to reinvent the wheel for each prospective client.

MARKETING YOUR SERVICES

Here are some ways that consulting services are marketed. You may think of ways to add to the list.

- Direct mail
- Presenting at seminars
- Brochures
- Charitable services
- Directories
- Networking
- Trade show exhibits
- Display ads in print media
- Client visits
- Public speaking
- Teaching
- Articles; books
- Word of mouth

The only truism that one can safely say about marketing is that one must always do it.

No matter what kind of business, no matter how many years in business, no matter how well known the business, marketing must be an ongoing process in order for any business to survive. For the beginning independent consultant, having a marketing plan is critical. It is very tempting for new consultants to get two or three "bread-and-butter" accounts and then stop marketing themselves. Most experienced consultants try to maintain a list of 15 to 20 consulting prospects as a routine business practice.

Several of the marketing ploys listed above will be reviewed in terms of their effectiveness for the beginning consultant.

A brochure may be given to prospective clients during an initial meeting. It should be professionally done, well designed, printed on quality paper, and create an initial image of professional competence in a client's mind. A good brochure may be expensive, especially in the quantities that you will need, but consider it a good investment.

Direct mail is a good way to get your message out. Again, be sure that it promotes your image as a competent professional. Because writing is a requisite of a good consultant, you may be judged entirely by the content of your mailing piece. This mailing must not contain slipshod, careless writing with misspellings and mechanical errors. If you have some problems in this area, hire a good copywriter.

The drawbacks about direct mail are its cost and the fact that so much competition exists for your prospective clients' attention in this medium. Do not use bulk mail. Do use quality paper and envelopes. Many busy people or their secretaries sort mail by bulk versus first-class markings. Messages printed on the outside of the envelope used to be effective in getting recipients to open the mailing piece. However, this technique has been so widely used recently that it has lost its effectiveness. We recommend a plain, stamped envelope. Direct the primary written message toward the potential client's needs. Your brochure can also be enclosed in case they are interested enough to contact you.

Seminars are a great source of clients. Assess your special knowledge and public speaking abilities, and let various associations and institutions know about your talents and availability to present at seminars. Obviously, your presentations must be knockouts. No one will hire you as a consultant if it is clear that you were unprepared or that you could not gain the interest and respect of your audience.

Networking is more an art than a science, but it is a very productive marketing technique. It requires a considerable investment of time, because it involves making constant personal contacts. One can network through Chamber of Commerce functions, civic and professional clubs and associations, and by swapping business contacts with colleagues and associates by "talking up" your value as a business resource whenever you get the chance. The danger here, of course, is that you become overzealous. Know your limits.

Public speaking involves getting your name out as a speaker to program chairpersons, members, and officers of civic clubs and professional organizations. Remember that preparation for these events takes a great deal of time, and, if you use slides or other audiovisual help, a considerable dollar investment. You also run the risk of the likelihood that only a very small percentage of your audience has any real need for your services.

Use any or all of the techniques listed. Find out which ones work best for you. Get professional help when you need it. If you are weak in writing skills or public speaking, check your local college curriculum. Many schools employ working professionals who can give meaningful help.

You can be the greatest, most innovative physical therapist in the world, but you cannot be a successful consultant in your profession if you cannot sell your ideas and yourself to someone. One successful consultant puts marketing in perspective this way: "Marketing and selling is little more than answering a prospective client's needs. Once you have found out what those needs are, you have a major part of your job completed."

One final word is that at some point in

your consulting business, you may find it necessary to pinpoint your marketing strategy. You can accomplish this by market research. If you are familiar with this technique, do your own. If not, you may find it necessary to employ a market research firm or a marketing consultant with experience in your general area.

ANNOTATED BIBLIOGRAPHY

Golightly H: Consultants. New York, Franklin Watts, 1985 (Valuable because it is written for managers in search of consultants. Tells managers what to look for in a prospective consultant.)

Holtz H: How to Succeed as an Independent Consultant. New York, John Wiley & Sons, 1983 (One of the most thorough treatments of the subject.)

Smith B: The Country Consultant. Cambridge, MA, Consultants News, 1982 (Designed for consultants setting up practice in a rural area. One of the best sources, however, for the beginning consultant anywhere. Considerable information on business practices, budgets, forms, proposals, contracts, and so forth. Excellent reference guide in the Appendix.)

Tepper R: Become a Top Consultant. New York, John Wiley & Sons, 1985 (Good general book on the art and science of consulting. Follows the careers of 10 top consultants in their respective fields.)

OTHER RESOURCES

Private Practice Section of the American Physical Therapy Association, 1030 15th Street, NW, Suite 956, Washington, DC 20005, (202) 842-2555 (Excellent resource for the physical therapist as entrepreneur. Offers research studies, courses, and the like for the therapist in or contemplating private practice. A valuable membership.)

American Demographics (Journal published by Dow Jones. Gives the results of demographic studies in all kinds of American markets, including health care.)

PART VI

Clinical Management Studies

IN THE FIRST FIVE SECTIONS of this text you have been introduced to information that may be considered the essence of physical therapy. Parts I and II included a historic view of the profession and recounted the philosophical, conceptual, and theoretical foundations that underpin the practice of physical therapy. In Part III, various bodily systems were explored with the factors that, should they occur singly or together, give rise to movement dysfunction or physical disability. The techniques by which physical therapists analyze the functioning of the different bodily systems were presented in Part IV. Part V included an array of therapeutic interventions physical therapists utilize in the prevention or treatment of various conditions that may occur in these systems of the body.

This section of the text contains 12 studies of physical therapy clinical management. Each study not only depicts a situation in which a physical therapist interacts with a client from initial meeting and evaluation to intervention, but also allows you to get inside each therapist's head and see her thought processes in action. At times, those thought processes will be analytical in nature and patient information will be methodically gathered, sorted, grouped, and compared to past experiences. At other times, because of the wealth of background and experience, the thought processes will be intuitive in nature and the therapist's mind will seem to leapfrog through his knowledge base, skipping through various combinations of cues until a solution "feels right."

Cheryl Wardlaw writes:

> I put away her chart and, for the first time, I slipped into the back of Jennie's room to watch quietly for a while. Her head was a mass of brown stubbles. Red crescent-shaped scars from her evacuation and shunt arched over each ear. The right eye was expressionless and unmoving, while the left was covered with a patch. Her top teeth rested on her lower lip, giving her the appearance of a large rabbit. Jennie's stocky frame was well muscled. (No sign of disuse atrophy.) The right arm was torqued internally at the shoulder by the weight of the cast. The right hand hung limply from the plaster, indicating a possible brachial plexus injury during the accident. The other extremities rested in a relaxed but decorticate posture. No spontaneous movements occurred.

This is a master clinician at work. Almost before physical therapists greet their patients, their minds are in a whirl, processing nonverbal cues. Does the patient seem in pain as indicated by slowness of movement and facial grimaces on movement or weight bearing? Does the client's posture, speed of movement, and respiratory pattern suggest she is young-old or old-old? Does the family seem to be depressed or to be having difficulty coping with the situation?

As the clinician is identifying clinical etiologies and conditions, she is simultaneously thinking of specific problems and patient care goals. If there is pain, where is it located, why is it there, and what can I do to reduce it? Do I need to intervene with direct treatment or is patient education the most effective way to obtain a long-term goal? These are the decisions physical therapists make in the clinical management of their clients.

The purpose of this section of the text is to present brief sketches of physical therapist clinicians and the methods they utilize in the evaluation and management of their clients' potential and actual problems. The studies demonstrate the mental processes by which these master clinicians decide which cues to look for, which cues are more important than others to interpret when identifying an etiology, and which of many alternative long-term goals should be selected for a given patient. The studies are not to be considered as the only acceptable interventions for the conditions discussed, but simply as representative of the current mode of practice.

58 Chronic Low Back Pain

SUSAN J. ISERNHAGEN

As I prepared for the evaluation of my patient, Roy, I reviewed the brief written history prepared by his rehabilitation consultant. It stated the following:

1. Roy was injured 10 months ago at his place of work while lifting a heavy carton.
2. He has been off work for 9.5 months.
3. Six years ago, he had a back injury that resulted in a laminectomy at the L4-L5 level. After that surgery there was a cash settlement consistent with a 10% disability. He and his family then moved to this city.
4. Roy has worked for the current employer for five years. His work record was satisfactory until 10 months ago when he was injured.
5. The treating physician is Dr. Ryle, a family physician. He has medically approved the necessity for the time off work. When no improvement was noted after eight months of numerous medications, a referral was made to Dr. Ames, an orthopedic surgeon. He confirmed that there was decreased motion in the back, that there was no fracture or dislocation, and that neurological findings were within normal limits. Dr. Ames then made the referral to this occupational medicine program for evaluation and treatment.
6. The employer seeks resolution of this case by return to work. The employer is willing to make some accommodations to facilitate return to the original job. Roy, on the other hand, is seeking another permanent dis-

ability rating and subsequent retraining in a more sedentary job.

PATIENT EXAMINATION

I waited for Roy in our occupational medicine department while he was being admitted. I knew that when he arrived, he would have signed releases of information to his physician, employer, rehabilitation consultant, insurance company, and attorney. This will have prepared him for the idea that my evaluation will be communicated to all of those interested in his employment status and potential return to work.

As Roy entered the department, I noted that he walked slowly with diminished arm swing. As he descended the few steps into our department, he leaned heavily on the railing. He moved stiffly and guardedly.

I introduced myself and asked him to have a seat so that we could review his history and present condition. I told him that I had received and read his medical and work history, but I also would like *his* perspective on his background and present problem.

I began by asking if he knew why he had been referred to our occupational medicine program. He was unclear about the reason, although the doctor had told him that he might have to return to work depending upon what we found. Roy appeared guarded and closed toward me during our conversation.

Roy reviewed his current accident with me. He described a job involving heavy lifting, which had been done for approximately half a day when his "injury" occurred. He stated that he had felt the work was too strenuous for him and that its difficulty caused his accident. For this reason, he did not feel he would be able to return to work. He had to pick up heavy boxes from a ground-level conveyor and load them into a truck. The motion began at waist height and ended at overhead height. His back has been painful during activity since his injury.

In reviewing his medical history, he stated that he had been a construction worker previously and had been hurt on that job while shoveling. He had undergone surgery. After his "back operation," he received a sum of money which allowed him to move himself and his family back to his hometown. Wanting to work, Roy was convinced by his brother to join the factory where he now works. He likes the plant because many of his friends, his father, and his brother work for the same company. They also have a strong union.

At this time, I silently summarized. Roy believed that, for him, his work was physically very difficult. He liked the camaraderie at work, but did not like the stress and strain of the physical work. He has had former experience with an accident, a surgery, and a subsequent settlement. I believe that he is aware of the workers' compensation system and the possibility of another settlement with subsequent retraining. Therefore, I decided that during the rest of my testing I would be neutral in statements regarding return to work. I would mention his ability levels in reference to his current job, but not feed into any antagonism that would indicate that I would "force" him to return to an unsafe job. Nor would I indicate that he was unable to do his job and should expect retraining.

I asked Roy to explain, in his own words, how the past months off work had been and how he felt about his physical functioning. He stated that he had worked for two weeks beyond his initial injury. During those two weeks, he felt that he was becoming progressively more sore and more disabled. The employer had not made an effort to allow "light duty" after the initial injury. When he stopped

work on his own, he was very painful and tired. He then saw his family physician, who immediately put him on strict bed rest for six weeks. Following that, the doctor tried numerous medications to relieve the pain, but none have been successful enough to allow return to work. He stated that he feels weak, is unable to sit for long periods of time, is unable to do exercise at home, and is unable to help with household chores. In general, he sits or lies down most of the day.

Silently summarizing again, I could see that Roy had physical reasons to become debilitated during his period of recovery. I could understand that without job modification or an adequate explanation of abilities and limitations after his initial injury, he could have increased his symptoms by continuing to do the same heavy work.

When I asked about other treatment, he mentioned physical therapy at another hospital for the past seven months. The heat and massage helped him temporarily. He also participated in a back school, which taught him how to lift and carry with safe body mechanics. The suggestions had also helped him to sit and sleep more comfortably.

He told me that his family physician, Dr. Ryle, had indicated that "medicine" had done as much as it could to cure him. This is when he was referred to Dr. Ames, who referred him to us. He didn't know what would happen to him now but hoped that some settlement would be made in the future so he could go on with his life. I noted the "passive role" he had settled into. He did not like the idea of having to "live with back pain" and would like to feel better, as well as go on to another vocation. Roy knew that he could get formal retraining if the doctor found a permanent disability. He liked the idea of a new vocation of computer operator. His wife and children were also tired of having him around the house, and they were hoping that something productive would happen soon. Money problems had surfaced, and his wife had returned to part-time work for financial reasons and partly to "get out of the house."

During this history taking, I noted that Roy sat relatively comfortably, did not shift position much, and maintained a neutral posture. He continued to act in a semiguarded manner toward me, although he also seemed relieved that I would listen.

I explained that he would be evaluated for work function. No recommendations regarding return to work or safety of activities would be made until the end of the second day. I explained that he would be a full participant in the testing, and that I valued his opinions and comments on the tests. I told him that all aspects of the tests were safe. He would be asked to perform some strenuous activities, and his full cooperation was needed. If full effort was not forthcoming, that would be stated in the test report. He could refuse to do any test, but his refusal would also be documented. I told him that the best thing for him to do would be to try as hard as he could, and then if there were a true physical problem it would be documented. Subsequently, that unsafe activity could then be eliminated from work. He seemed open to this and stated that he was surprised that he would be allowed to be part of the system. He said that at one point in his injury six years ago, he had been briefly seen by a physician who said that there was nothing wrong with him and he could return to work. That interaction left a bitter memory about "experts" who try to get you back to work.

I told Roy that while I evaluated his physical functioning, I would be most concerned about physical safety. I asked him what type of discomfort he generally had and told him that we would use that as a baseline during the testing. He stated that he had constant aching in the low back, and that it is worse with movement, walking any long distance, or sitting too long. His knees ached at night and sometimes they swelled. He stated that his knees were worse since he has been off work and seem to be getting stiffer. He also stated that the amount of pain in his low back has been constant for approximately the last four months. He did have some pain in his back and knees upon starting this test. He said that he knew he'd be sore after these activities because he was always sore after trying any activity at home. I mentioned that this would be considered a normal finding, so that if he was sore tomorrow he should think of that as a normal consequence of his activity and not another injury. We would expressly document any discomfort or change in function tomorrow that related to today's work.

At this point, I felt that Roy would be cooperative because he did brighten when I stated that we would not do anything unsafe during the test. I also felt that the symptoms he described were consistent with deconditioning, loss of range of motion through inactivity, and the new observation of knee joint dysfunction bilaterally. I knew that during the preliminary assessment I needed to pay particular attention to his low back mobility, general strength, and knee joint function. He was of stocky, muscular build and looked as if he had done heavy manual work in the past. He had excess weight, which was carried in the abdominal area. I began an assessment of his physical status before beginning the actual test items.

- Height: 5 ft 10 in
- Weight: 205 lb
- Blood pressure: 145/90
- Resting pulse: 96
- Standing posture: slightly forward head, slightly rounded shoulders, flattened lumbar curve

The baseline posture was noted so that any changes can be identified during testing. It was my impression that he has had this type of posture for at least the last six years (since his laminectomy). His posture may have been like this long before. The postural deviations were not strongly abnormal. All in all, his posture looked quite functional.

As I had Roy go through functional active ranges of motion, I watched the quality of motion, the speed of motion, and any facial expressions that might indicate discomfort or tightness at any points in the range. Having Roy stand and then sit, I had him go through active range of motion of the shoulders, elbows, wrists, fingers, and thumb. On the plinth he went through active motions, prone and supine, which included hip flexion, extension, abduction, adduction, internal rotation, external rotation, straight leg raising, ankle motion, and toe motion. He sat guardedly and moved stiffly from prone to supine. He held his trunk in a rigid position. I saw almost no trunk rotation during any of those motions. This was consistent with his gait, in which he also showed very little trunk motion. The guarding appeared to be constant rather than in response to a sudden pain. Again, I knew that this was consistent with someone who has guarded against discomfort for many months or years. Ranges of motion in the upper extremities and lower extremities, with the exception of the knees, were within normal limits. He lacked 5 degrees of full knee extension, and the last 10 degrees of available extension took a few seconds to reach. His knee flexion was 110 degrees. While he was actively performing knee motion, I palpated his knee joint and felt crepitus bilaterally. The crepitus was through the full range of motion along the joint lines laterally and medially. Roy stated that the motion did not hurt him, but he had noted that there had been "crunching" in his knee for approximately the last 10 years. He stated that it had been getting worse with age. He wondered if the back problem could have caused his knee problem. I thought to myself that, most likely, it was the knee problem that contributed to the back problem.

I noted that during the range of motion, the prone position appeared uncomfortable to him. After the functional assessment he would need a more complete workup on total measurement of hip motion and knee motion. I also thought that a potential exercise program should include hip and knee range of motion activities, as well as trunk motion activities. I then filed this information away so I could observe whether the slight hip and knee flexion problems or limitations would be of any functional consequence during our testing. It had been my experience that similar movement limitations were not always a functional problem. Rather, they are something people learn to compensate for over the years. In Roy's case,

however, I wondered if his knee flexion problem was becoming worse as the suspected arthritic changes in his knees progressed. Close observation of the hips and knees would be necessary during functional assessment.

Trunk range of motion was done in the functional position of standing. In forward bending, he had significant discomfort after 30 degrees but could complete 50 degrees of motion. The curves were essentially normal during the flexion motion. His flattened lumbar curve did remain. In further tests, he stated that discomfort was present almost from the beginning of trunk rotation and side bending. This was consistent with earlier findings. As he rotated both to the right and the left, he was able to rotate his shoulders approximately 25 degrees from the neutral position. He was limited to approximately 15 degrees bilaterally of lateral trunk flexion. When asked to do extension from the standing position, he could extend his neck considerably but had very little extension in the thoracic or lumbar spine. This was also consistent with earlier findings.

I documented that trunk rotation, lateral bending, flexion, and extension were significantly limited. This was consistent with debilitated chronic low back patients that I had observed previously. Evidently, Roy had continued to function by using a guarded position for most of his movements. When coupled with difficulty in the knee joints, I could see that the loading and unloading of heavy boxes had put considerable stress on his tight back and his arthritic-like knees. In my observations, I had noticed no limitations in the cervical spine or upper extremities. I felt they were his strongest attribute and had probably helped to compensate for low back and lower extremity dysfunction.

In doing muscle testing of all large muscle groups in the upper and lower extremities and trunk, he exhibited grade 4-5 muscle strength. I felt that it was not his basic strength that precluded him from activity, but that endurance might be affected even though strength was not.

In reviewing functional movement patterns, I noted the following: His gait was similar to the one I observed when he entered the department. I had wondered whether he walked slowly and shuffled somewhat for my benefit in demonstrating that he was disabled. However, when I noted the limitations he had in motion and heard the patterns of activity that he used, I decided that this gait was usual for him. I considered his stair climbing from when he entered the department. He had less difficulty ascending then descending, and used the rail heavily in descending. He was able to do toe rises bilaterally and unilaterally. However, he was not able to stoop to the floor safely. He was able to flex the knees within the ability of his limited range of motion, and the rest of the flexion came from the low back. His hand reached the floor with his back flexed and in a horizontal pattern rather than an upright pattern. This was very uncomfortable for him both in the knees and in the low back. Again, I felt that this was consistent with physical findings. With his eyes open and closed, Roy was able to hold his balance well. When he was asked to reach overhead and behind him, he pivoted rather than rotated at the trunk.

Conclusions of Initial Findings

Roy had suffered his second major back injury during heavy manual activity jobs. He presented as deconditioned with guarded movements. He stated that he has discomfort, which increased with activity.

PHYSICAL FINDINGS

Roy had normal range of motion and strength in the upper extremities and cervical area. However, the low back, hips, and knees demonstrated limitations in motion. He did have crepitus in the knees bilaterally. Overall, three relevant functional problems were present. Areas that should be closely observed during the functional assessment would be any motions, repetitious activities, or strength activities that involved (1) low back and trunk; (2) knees; or (3) aerobic capacity.

I was then ready to begin the functional evaluation. I had reviewed both his job description and my standardized testing procedure to determine test items. The functional abilities that I had chosen to test were lifting from the floor; lifting at table height; overhead lift; weight carry; overhead work; hand coordination; stoop to the floor; repeated bending from the hips and waist; stair climbing; pushing; pulling; and standing tolerance.

In addition, I now decided to add three items that I believed would be necessary considering his physical abilities and his potential future plans. Those items were sitting tolerance, balance, and walking.

I first discussed the lifting items. Roy told me that since he was injured at work, he has avoided lifting anything. He was very fearful of reinjury and did not want to go through the pain and suffering that he has had in the past. If he did, he said "life would not be worth living." I explained that all lifting we would test would be safe for him. If we did not try it, we would never know where his capability levels were and where his limitations began. I told him that we would find out his maximum lift, and that I would make a statement that would indicate that lifting beyond his safe maximum should not be done. This would help protect him upon return to work. Also, it would show him what he could do safely at home. He said he would appreciate that, because he did want to do some things around the house. He didn't want to feel like an invalid forever. He said that he would try, but he hoped it wouldn't hurt him so that he would "pay for it tomorrow."

We began with procedures for lifting weight from floor level. I placed a weight basket on the floor and asked Roy to stoop down to pick it up. As I anticipated, his knee pain, knee dysfunction, and limited range of motion prevented him from maintaining the upright back position needed to prevent stress to the disks. He stated that he had learned correct lifting in his back school. He knew that he should bend his knees and lift with his back straight. He said that one reason he didn't lift from the floor was because he couldn't do it in the position they taught him. It also was very uncomfortable in his low back. Because he did attempt the test, and I could determine that knee dysfunction caused his inability to perform safely,

I documented that lifting from the floor level would be an unsafe activity for him. His condition for lifting from the floor would not change unless his knees changed in both motion and strength.

In a second lifting test, Roy showed ability in lifting from table height. He was able to grasp the weight firmly and bring it in toward his body. He could pivot with his feet and take the weight to another table height position. He continued to use his guarded back posture. But because this activity does not require trunk flexion, extension, or rotation, he had no difficulty performing this task. I noted that Roy's extremely strong upper extremities compensated for some of the other problems. After working Roy up slowly to maximum, I determined that he could lift 60 lb from table height. He did not have an endurance problem in his upper extremities, although he was flushed after the lifting. At the 60-lb limit, Roy stated it was the pressure on his back that kept him from going further. I had observed that he contracted his trunk muscles strongly as he lifted at the higher weight levels. This corresponded with the feeling of intense pressure, which could have been caused by a combination of trunk stabilization effort and the increased compression the additional weight put on his spine. His pulse rate after the last table height lift was 120.

In the overhead lift, from table height to a shelf at eye level, Roy's upper extremities performed well. He had good scapular, deltoid, wrist, and handgrip strength. The difficulty with this position was the increased lordosis that the overhead lift required. When he tried a stance with one foot forward, he was able to lift to a higher weight level, because his lumbar area could remain flat. His maximum weight lift for this overhead task was 35 lb.

The weight carry was done righthanded, lefthanded, and bilaterally. Both of the unilateral lifts increased his low back symptoms and he reported strong, sharp pains in his lumbar area. This correlated with his attempts at stabilizing the trunk through the lateral trunk muscles. On initiation of carry, they were strongly contracted, but as the carry progressed, stabilization was lost and lateral flexion occurred.

This was unsafe and also painful to him. Therefore, both right and left unilateral weight carries were limited to 20 lb for 100 ft. On the bilateral weight carry, he was able to stabilize the weight at midline and keep it close to his center of gravity. Because this required mainly back extensor stabilization, which appeared stronger for him he was able to weight carry 55 lb. This was almost as much as he had been able to lift at table height.

- Therefore, the *lifts that he was able to do safely* were table height lift (to 60 lb), overhead lift (to 35 lb), and bilateral weight carry (to 55 lb).
- *A functionally limited activity* was the unilateral weight carry (to 20 lb), which was limited by inability to tolerate lateral spine flexion and inability to stabilize strongly.
- *Functionally unsafe* was the lift from floor level.

I knew that a strong program of trunk flexibility and strengthening would allow higher poundages and better endurance in several of these lifting capacities. I considered Roy's previous surgery and wondered if he had ever been totally rehabilitated after it. Perhaps the poor trunk flexibility and stability strength had been one of the factors that had contributed to this recent injury. He had been performing repetitious activity, which could have overtired the trunk stabilizer muscles, thus allowing painful stretching and positioning. In his current deconditioned state, return to his old job would also result in poor performance of his stabilizers and put him at risk of reinjury.

In testing another type of overhead work, I had Roy sustain activity at 6 in above eye level. He was able to use a hammer, do simple activities unweighted, and also repeat those simple activities with 10- and 15-lb tools. He appeared to have no difficulty with his cervical extension or deltoid strength and endurance. The only difficulty was the increased lordosis in the low back. Significant weight shifting indicated when the low back discomfort made him less functional. If he used a stool for resting one foot at a time, with the low back flattened, he could do overhead work at a higher weight load and for a longer term.

In the standardized hand coordination test, Roy performed at a normal level for his age. In fact, he excelled at subtests requiring strength and fine finger dexterity. This indicated no deficit in hand coordination and a capacity to work with his hands, which would be necessary in computer programming. I did not make that work translation during testing, but I felt it would be important to include in the summary.

To examine repetitious motions, I had Roy begin with squatting to the floor. Consistent with the earlier assessments during the standup lift, Roy was unable to bring his hands to floor level by bending his knees. When he did reach floor level by bending at the hips and back, he had significant difficulty in rising again. He stated that he had back discomfort after this activity even though he performed it only once. The back discomfort was consistent with the stressful flexed posture previously documented and poor antigravity muscle control necessary to the movement. His inability to perform this movement safely because of back and knee dysfunction would lead to a functional work restriction.

In the repeated activity of bending at the hip and low back, he performed better. Although he had exhibited limitation of motion in forward bending on the preliminary assessment, he was able to carry out some functional repetitions. He automatically resumed full extension after each forward motion, which is typical of patients with back flexion discomfort. However, as the repetitions increased, he began to show less ability for both flexion and extension. This is consistent with diminished trunk range of motion. I concluded that if repetitions were limited, this activity could be performed safely, but it should not be done continuously. Working in a back-flexed position without a frequent opportunity to return to the extended position would be contraindicated because of the muscle tension and increased symptoms consistent with trunk muscle guarding. In thinking ahead to the restorative program that I would recommend, increased trunk

flexibility could lead to increased tolerance for bending.

Roy accomplished stair climbing with heavy use of the rail while descending. He moved in a slow, guarded manner. Lower extremity strength was adequate for this task. However, the restricted knee motion and knee dysfunction were a limiting factor. After three minutes of stair climbing, his pulse rate increased to 135. This increase was consistent with both the high resting pulse rate found at the early assessment and his deconditioning. Aerobic conditioning would be needed.

Push and pull were done using a weight sled. As long as Roy could keep his low back in a relatively upright position and use his upper extremities as the main force, push and pull was accomplished safely to 100 lb. His body mechanics indicated that he had a long-standing method for push and pull that utilized primarily trunk stabilization and the upper extremity muscles. His pace and body mechanics indicated that he would be unable to work with push and pull if either a sudden force or a fast rate were required.

Standing tolerance was excellent, as long as Roy was allowed to shift his weight. He was surprised that he was able to stand so long, and then he recalled that standing jobs at work had never bothered him.

Sitting tolerance was also a pleasant surprise for Roy. If he used a small lumbar support and a table height that allowed 90-degree elbow flexion, he was able to do manipulations with the hand and writing. His sitting tolerance was 45 minutes—enough to allow him to do desk work with frequent breaks. He stated that while sitting at home, he generally was in a recliner or a soft chair and experienced discomfort after 20 or 30 minutes. He did have a chair similar to ours, however, and he would be interested in modifying his sitting to increase his tolerance.

Balance tests indicated that Roy's strong trunk stabilization, although functional for normal walking, was actually a hindrance in balance activities. He did not have the low back-pelvic mobility to allow walking with one foot directly in front of the other without significant discomfort. Forward and backward walking were both difficult for him. As long as he could keep a wide base of support, balance was no problem. However, on a narrow base of support, balance became a definite problem. An additional problem surfaced as I observed the quadriceps muscle function during balance activities. The muscle quivered considerably, indicating difficulty in stabilization at terminal extension. Perhaps the long-term degenerative process in his knees and the lack of full extension much of the time had speeded the terminal extension weakness. Because of his low back discomfort during activities without a wide base of support, compounded by the quadriceps stabilization problem during full extension, activities requiring balance should be carefully selected. Roy stated that he was surprised he had balance problems. Although walking on sand and snow had been difficult for him he had never understood why. The inability to walk on snow had prevented him from getting outside during the winter for recreational walking.

In endurance walking on level surface with a normal base of support, Roy showed no difficulty. Because his pace was slow, the pulse rate increase was small and did not indicate aerobic stress.

Evaluation of Roy's functional items on the first test day showed consistency between his history, his own comments, and the physical examination done prior to the testing. When he left, Roy stated that he was glad he was participating because he found he could do some things that he hadn't tried for nine months. He also stated that his performance on the tests might also indicate that he is still physically restricted and unable to return to heavy work. As he departed, he stated that he would probably have a lot of pain at home and a sleepless night. I encouraged him to return for the second short day of testing, so that we could document increased symptoms if he had them. They would be important in helping us judge whether return to work was possible. Workers' compensation representatives would be looking for physical abilities before any type of retraining could be instituted. A complete re-

port was needed, and his return for the second day of testing was very important.

On the morning of the second day Roy returned, and, true to his earlier comments, he stated he had experienced significant discomfort in the low back and knees overnight. They had "ached" into the evening and had prevented a good night's sleep. Observation of his ranges of motion showed that his trunk motion was the same as the previous day, but his stated discomfort began earlier in all the ranges. Knee flexion was the same bilaterally, but the right knee was slightly swollen medial to the patella. The increased discomfort during the range of motion of both trunk and knees was consistent with the stresses we had placed on them the previous day. Soreness of muscles is natural after they have been used beyond their usual work load. It was encouraging to see that motion had not been lost in the trunk in spite of the restriction on the first day. This indicated that, structurally, the stress on the facet joints and disks did not produce symptoms that would decrease motion. The back extensors and the lateral trunk rotators were sore to palpation. There was no soreness in the knees, except for a general aching, which could not be palpated but was recorded.

There were no other physical signs or symptoms upon the beginning of the second day. Blood pressure and pulse rate were similar to measurements on the first test day.

All of the lifting items were repeated except for the lift from the floor, because it had been determined to be unsafe. Roy was able to lift the same amount of weight as on the first day, except in the unilateral weight carries, where only 10 lb could be carried. During this test, lateral flexion appeared sooner, which correlated with the severe discomfort he felt in his low back. This was also consistent with muscles that are weak and have low endurance and postactivity soreness. It was encouraging that the abilities in overhead lift and bilateral weight carry remained the same, and indicated that physically those activities could be performed repeatedly.

I asked Roy what he did during the last nine months when soreness followed a strenuous activity. He stated that the only treatment he knew was bed rest, which allowed his symptoms to subside. I mentioned that even though he felt better, the muscles and joints of his low back and lower extremities would be weaker and tighter after bed rest. To show him what our treatment program might be, I asked him to do very basic trunk motion exercises with me. He said that he knew they would hurt, and he did not want to try them. I told him that they would not injure him and may help him, and that he had nothing to lose by trying. We stood and did some very mild flexion, extension, rotation, and lateral bending exercises. As he moved gently through the ranges, he began to feel less discomfort. At the end, the range of motion testing was more comfortable even though it had not increased. He stated that he was surprised he could decrease his discomfort by doing more work instead of doing no work.

On this positive note, I sat down with Roy and we went over all the work activities we had tested and the results in regard to activities at home and at work.

I asked him to keep an open mind about physical restoration as we went through the recommendations. I explained that his two problem areas during functional activity (his low back and knees) did not make him completely nonfunctional. We were going to concentrate on what he could do rather than on what he couldn't do.

The first items related to lifting. Because his knees were limited in motion, they did not allow for a safe stoop to the floor needed for that type of lift. He was very happy to hear that, and stated that he knew it all along. He felt it was one of the reasons he was injured during loading on the last day of work.

Moving on to a more positive area, I told Roy that lifting overhead was functionally safe up to 35 lb as long as he could keep his back flat. He agreed that the activity had not caused a problem.

Lifting from table height showed a high level of ability, with no danger of reinjury. The safe limit in this lift was 60 lb.

Unilateral carrying was a problem when the weight exceeded 10 lb because of poor low back stabilization and discomfort with lateral motion. Bilateral weight carrying, however, could be accomplished safely, up to 55 lb, because of good bilateral placement close to the center of gravity and the advantage of strong upper extremity strength.

Overhead work showed his upper extremities were strong in both strength and endurance. His excellent neck motion and tolerance to static positioning were also demonstrated. He agreed that his arms have always been his strongest feature. He stated he had several recreational activities as a young man that were related. He was the arm wrestling champion in his hometown and was able to throw the javelin and shot put well in track. He began to look much more positively upon this report as he recalled his past physical abilities. He appeared to gain hope from the fact that he was an able person, not a disabled person.

We continued with the positive areas of the report. I gave him the results of his hand coordination test, which showed that he had normal hand coordination and actually excelled in the strength and fine dexterity test.

We turned to his repeated activities. Roy accepted the results without the "I told you so" attitude. I emphasized his inability to reach floor level and the need for him to avoid stooping to the floor. I discussed alternative methods of reaching the floor.

As for the repeated bending, he realized that bending was not out of the question, but that he would have to limit the depth and repetition of the activity. This did not elicit a negative response. Instead, he felt that he was well in control of where his abilities lay and where he needed to stop himself when symptoms began.

The stair climbing showed that his legs did have strength and endurance. Although the knee dysfunction was present, he was functional going slowly and using the rail while descending. Because of the inability in unilateral carrying and the need to use the rail, he should not descend stairs while carrying a load.

Roy was also concerned about the rise in

his pulse rate after this activity. He noticed that he would become "winded" earlier than he used to. This brought up the subject of aerobic conditioning and deconditioning. Roy had read a few articles on conditioning in the papers and understood the principle of exercising until the pulse rate was higher. He had never tried it because the activities generally caused him too much discomfort. Further, he felt uncomfortable walking outside in the winter. He did not have the money or the interest to join a health spa, so he stayed away from strenuous activities. He recalled that he used to be in excellent shape and would like to regain the tolerance for bicycling, stair climbing, and walking without feeling so tired afterwards. I was pleased that *he* was now expressing the desire to improve his physical condition.

We continued to the push and pull activities. He could see where he had learned to compensate in body mechanics while doing these activities. His previous job had required pushing and pulling. Because he was able to guard himself so tightly, he knew that he could be as strong as anyone else at work in these activities. I credited him with his ability to stabilize himself while using his full weight in the activity. Again, it pleased him that he had done something in a positive way toward work. He wished his boss knew that. He said that his boss was hard on him because he didn't feel that Roy had tried hard enough during the two weeks following his injury. I pointed out that lifting was entirely different from pushing and pulling activities. Because lifting had caused the injury, perhaps some of the other ability levels had been overlooked. I told Roy that if he returned to work, we would make very clear which activities were safe and which were unsafe. His feeling that he had tried hard at work was reestablished.

He was pleased to hear that his standing tolerance was good. He had felt uncomfortable in the past while standing. Sitting tolerance also appeared to be a positive for him. He stated that he would like to try a different type of chair at home, but he hadn't tried it last night because of the discomfort he felt after the first day of testing.

In discussing the balance activities, he was surprised to hear of a problem. He did remember that in recent years he had difficulty with balance but had not mentioned it to anyone. He thought perhaps the weather conditions had caused it. I explained that a physical reason was at the root of this problem. It was related to back stability and pelvic movement for his low back combined with the weakness of his quadriceps muscles at the straightest position of his knee. We discussed which activities needed the most careful attention.

The last activity, walking, was also a positive experience for Roy. He felt pleased that he could walk indoors for one-half mile without feeling unduly fatigued or uncomfortable.

After hearing the individual results, Roy stated that he was glad to have done the tests. There were many things he could not do as "proven" by the tests. However, he felt that he understood that he could do things to enable him to be more functional. He was tired of feeling sore and fatigued. By understanding the reasons for his physical condition, he felt optimistic about a restorative program.

This was a natural lead-in for discussing the treatment program offered by our occupational medicine department. One option is a graduated work hardening program for specific restoration regarding return to work. In Roy's case, the main limiting factors were decreased mobility in the low back; decreased endurance in low back stabilization; loss of full knee motion; lack of quadriceps muscle strength in terminal extension; and decreased aerobic capacity.

I told Roy that these were activities for which specific programs were designed. A work hardening program could increase his trunk mobility and trunk strength (so lifting and carrying would not be as painful). Furthermore, he could exercise his hips and knees to gain motion. Although we could not affect any arthritic changes that might already have taken place, we could show him how to reduce further stress on the knees by strengthening the muscles of the knees. This would allow functional movement in a restricted range.

Roy initiated discussion of the third area in

which he needed work, aerobic conditioning. Activities that would increase and maintain heart rate would help him to increase his tolerance to heavy activity. This would include stair climbing, walking, swimming, and worklike activities. Most likely it would also, over time, reduce his resting pulse rate and allow him to feel "more in condition."

Roy said he knew he would be sore after the first day of testing and was discouraged that the testing confirmed his disabilities. However, on the second day, he could see that his problems were not totally unsolvable. He did not feel that we could eliminate his back and knee pain, but he was willing to try something to make him feel better and more functional. He still questioned whether a return to work was possible. He had hoped for retraining. But his paramount desire was to continue his life in a healthier fashion.

The assessment report to the physician included a recommendation for a six-week work hardening short program for the following specific purposes.

1. Increase trunk mobility.
2. Increase strength and endurance of the trunk stabilizer muscles.
3. Identify problems in motion of the knees, and secondarily the hips, with concentration on increased mobility of the knees and hips, and increased strength of the muscles affecting the knees and hips. This would correlate with a planned diagnostic work-up of both knees by a physician.
4. Functionally evaluate the job so that work hardening activities could simulate the job tasks. At the end of the program, the job description could then be directly compared with results of work hardening.
5. Increase aerobic capacity.
6. Increase speed and effectiveness of balance reaction.
7. Increase ability to relax the trunk muscles, to counteract the constant "guarding" that has prevailed.

Optionally, psychological consultation regarding the presence of clinical depression might be considered.

At this point, the referring physician, employer, and rehabilitation consultant received results of this functional evaluation, and a conference was called for the four of us and Roy.

At the conference we discussed the physical limitations that led to Roy's work limitations. The mechanism of repetitive trauma injury (repetitive lifting) was identified and discussed as a possible cause of injury. Roy's abilities were highlighted, as well as the efforts he made at work. Because the problem could now be understood on a "physical" level, the mistrust and fears of both sides began to disappear. The orthopedic physician and I felt that maximum physical function was not yet evident. To get a clearer idea of Roy's future physical abilities (pertaining to return to work or a disability settlement and retraining), the physician decided to do a thorough diagnostic workup on Roy's knees and hips, and to refer Roy to the suggested work hardening program for a six-week trial period.

Initally, the treatment regimen would be five times per week, four hours per day, for the objectives stated previously.

Protocol for this specific work hardening program would include the following:

1. Setting goals with the patient to establish a plan of restoration to be accomplished within the given time period. The patient would record his progress daily on a chart.
2. Thorough range-of-motion testing of hips and knees bilaterally, with muscle testing throughout the range of hip and knee musculature. (Isokinetic testing may be appropriate with a restorative program.)
3. Thorough trunk range of motion documentation and individual muscle testing of trunk stabilizers. (Isokinetic testing may be appropriate with a restorative program.)
4. Work simulation of the following: lifting, carrying, bending, stair climbing, and balance activities. Tasks during work hardening should simulate actual work box sizes and heights and repetitions as much as possible.
5. Aerobic conditioning, depending upon the patient's tolerance for exercise equipment, may include swimming, walking, stair

climbing, bicycling, rowing, isokinetic exercise equipment, and pulleys.

6. Balance activities would include balance equipment, gymnastic ball for trunk and lower extremities, stimulation of balance reactions, walking on uneven surfaces, and balance beam.

7. Relaxation techniques, especially of the trunk muscles.

The functional reevaluation at the end of six weeks would indicate the possible types of case resolution for Roy. Monitoring of the work hardening program by the therapist would include changes in weight abilities for the weighted items; degrees of gains of range of motion for the mobility items; ability to do aerobic capacity tasks; changes in balance reaction; and increase in ability to relax trunk muscles at rest.

Roy would also be observed to see whether an increase in functional ability occurs. Learning should accompany the conditioning program; thus, changes in Roy's functioning would be anticipated as his physical capacities increased. Things to watch for would be increase in knee swelling or dysfunction, increase in guarding or muscle spasm in the low back after activity, or lack of ability to progress in any of the areas.

RESULTS OF INTERVENTION

At the end of the six-week period, Roy stated, " I feel so much more competent now than I did when I came here. I am not as afraid of activities, although I realize that I could hurt myself again by doing the wrong things. Now I think I know what I can do safely and what I can't do. I realize that there are things at work that I would be able to handle and things I shouldn't do if I go back. I have started doing exercise at home and my wife has joined me. Working out at home, in addition to working here, has made me feel 10 times better. The amazing thing is that I am not as sore as I was three or four weeks ago. I never believed that by being more active I would have less pain instead of more pain."

A partial functional test was repeated to document changes in functional capacity.

Objectively measured gains in Roy's ability showed that he could perform most job tasks safely. Aerobic conditioning improved. Roy is now on an exercise program that will continue to reduce blood pressure and pulse rate and raise activity tolerance. Measurements of trunk mobility indicate increases in all motions, as well as an increase in the pain-free range. Trunk musculature also increased in strength. Knee extension is now 0 degrees, and flexion is 130 degrees. Terminal quadriceps muscle strength has improved. Balance has improved, but continues to be mildly impaired. New weight capacities are as follows:

- Lifting from table height, 70 lb
- Overhead lifting, 45 lb
- Unilateral weight carry, 25 lb
- Bilateral weight carry, 60 lb

The ongoing restrictions would be as follows: (1) no lifting from floor level; (2) repetition limitation in bending activities; (3) no weights to be lifted over maximum results in second test; and (4) no carrying of objects while climbing stairs.

The physician signed a release to return to work, and referred Roy back to work hardening for rechecks and an updated home program.

The employer modified Roy's work according to ability level and the physical restrictions applied. He met with the foreman and the union representative to formulate an "in-plant plan" to facilitate Roy's safe return to work.

The rehabilitation consultant worked with the insurance company and the workers' compensation system to facilitate this satisfactory case resolution.

During the six-week period the rehabilitation consultant worked with the employer to write a functional job description that can now be matched with Roy's ability level.

1. Roy is required to lift and load boxes onto a truck. However, because there are enough employees, it is possible for Roy to avoid warehouse lifting, which is at ground level. It is possible for Roy to work on the beginning of the assembly line where boxes are taken from table height and

merely lowered slowly to the assembly line. This requires a lesser degree of stooping, and Roy's upper extremity strength should provide the ability to lift and hold up to 60-lb boxes. Therefore, lifting and loading in a limited manner could be done by Roy upon return to work.

2. A second activity necessary at work is stacking shelves. Roy will have no difficulty with the overhead stacking and should be capable of inventory and care of equipment loaded on higher shelves. Table-height shelves should also be possible. As long as the work is restricted to these two heights, Roy is capable of accomplishing it.

3. While at the workbench, Roy is required to make parts, load them into boxes, and then load the boxes into the truck. Because of Roy's excellent hand coordination and upper extremity strength, this assembly process at workbench height produces no difficulty for him.

4. Driving the truck to the customer should be tolerated because Roy's sitting tolerance is good. If the seat could be modified with a lumbar cushion, Roy should be capable of the truck-driving component of his job.

5. In the unloading, Roy can take boxes from truck height and place them at table height for the purchaser. As long as Roy remains at the table and truck bed level, the activity should not cause a problem.

6. Because of Roy's dramatic increase in trunk stabilization during the work hardening program, repetitious activities (up to two hours in duration) of loading and unloading 20- to 40-lb boxes would be safe. However, if he is to work at maximum weight level, repetitious activity should be done for less time. The repetitious activity should not be a problem because of his increased stabilization, but the height of the activity is of greatest importance.

7. Roy's aerobic conditioning is gradually approaching normal but stair climbing, repeated lifting, and overhead lifting should be done only to his tolerance level. His aerobic conditioning will improve over time.

Roy has learned to monitor his own pulse rate so that he can work within his safe limit. The foreman should be apprised of Roy's self-monitoring system and should allow Roy to rest when necessary.

SUMMARY

Because Roy's physical abilities have improved, he is able to return to his original job. The employer has agreed to stay within weight and repetition parameters for his loading and unloading activities. Because of the number of personnel involved, shifting Roy to the beginning of the conveyer belt is not a problem. Although apprehensive, Roy has agreed to return to work provided he is able to rest when his pulse rate reaches a high level. He understands which activities are unsafe. If the opportunity to lift from a lower height than has been shown as safe arises, Roy will refuse that activity.

OUTCOME

Work hardening increased the patient's capacities to an ability level equal to return to work. Roy's employer has agreed to take Roy back with slight modifications of work assignments. Roy returns to work in a safe and reconditioned manner. Roy will continue to be monitored by work hardening specialists, and will continue his home exercise program. It is expected that his return to work will be successful.

CASE VARIATION 1

Frank's case is exactly like Roy's, except for the results of the work hardening program. Work hardening has increased his ability to a certain extent, but long-standing arthritic changes in the lower extremities have not allowed an increase in motion. Therefore, Frank is still unable to stoop to the floor. Work hardening has shown that carrying for short distances and nonrepetitious activities are safe, but carrying for long distances is aerobically stressing, and the weight bearing puts additional stress on his knees. This has been indicated by swelling and temporary loss of range of motion after weighted activities. Although the back stabilizers have increased his strength, the motion of the trunk has not increased. Frank is able to move through the limited range with less discomfort and is able to stabilize, but still maintains a semiguarded and nonmobile positioning of the back.

Aerobic conditioning is somewhat slowed because of extreme discomfort in the low back and knees from activities such as bicycling, and use of rowing machines and other exercise equipment. Therefore, walking, upper extremity exercise, and swimming have been the three main areas of conditioning. Frank states that he continues to feel somewhat sore after exercise each day, but at least the amount of discomfort is not increasing. He feels that he is in slightly better condition and can hold heavier objects with more stability. He is still reluctant to do any activity that involves lifting and carrying because he can feel the tiredness in his low back, and he becomes more symptomatic. The therapist can document that while tolerance to repetitive stabilization during a weighted activity or bending has increased somewhat, full stabilization has not yet taken place.

Frank's employer has stated that if he does not return to work in the near future, the company will be forced to hire a permanent replacement. The company has had more orders for their product. Frank's experience makes him a valuable asset to the company; however, waiting another three or four months is impossible.

The rehabilitation consultant is working with Frank and the employer to obtain a satisfactory job placement through the methods outlined below.

OUTCOME

Satisfactory return to work can still occur with increased cooperation of all interested parties. This case would be resolved by extensive (although not expensive) work modification.

1. Loading from the floor-level conveyer belt is a major problem for Frank. It has been established that he cannot bend to that level. On the other hand, when he tried working at the beginning of the conveyer belt, the repetitious loading of boxes onto the conveyer belt was too much for his low back stabilizers. He was able to do loading for approximately 15 minutes, after which time he noticed that the guarding increased, which decreased active motion. The stabilizers began to fail and caused instability in the back. Therefore, Frank is not able to work at either end of a floor-level assembly line. One solution to this problem would be job-site modification, namely, the placement of permanent risers on the circular assembly line. This would increase the height of the conveyer belt to a constant height of 3 ft throughout the area. The cost of this addition would be $1,000. When the employer compares this cost to the increased cost in workers' compensation premiums (if Frank could not return to work), the alternative appears feasible. This worksite modification will be made.

2. Truck driving is not a problem for Frank because he has a sitting tolerance. However, unloading the truck at the end of the drive continues to have the same effect on him. He can unload the truck to table height. If the load is small, he has enough endurance to complete the entire process. However, if the load is large, he requires assistance or a long rest break between periods of unloading. Because of the cost of long rest breaks, his employer has decided to change the method of operations by having the purchasing company unload the truck with the driver's supervision. This frees Frank from the physical repetitious work, and the purchasing company is pleased by the reduced purchase rate resulting from using their own personnel. The increased efficiency for Frank and the other truck drivers is also beneficial, because their entire work load has increased.

3. Assembly-line work continues to be adequate and is safe because of Frank's abilities shown in the functional assessment.

4. Although his aerobic conditioning is improving, it is not yet at a level consistent with repetitive loading, unloading, or carrying items upstairs. For long periods of time, even overhead lifting can cause considerable fatigue. Therefore, while Frank will continue to do work hardening exercises at home, another work modification has been made. The freight elevator, which was rarely used, has been cleaned so that he and other personnel can use the elevator to bring small items to other floors. The slight increased cost of using the elevator outweighs the workers' compensation cost if he cannot return to work.

Note that the work modifications that allow Frank to return to work will also help prevent injuries to other employees. For example, the elevated conveyer belt will allow all employees to avoid the most strenuous lift from floor level. It should reduce back injuries. The avoidance of unloading freight at the end of a delivery should decrease the risk of injuries. The use of the freight elevator has increased productivity in bringing boxes and items to other floors, and should reduce the risk of injuries that happen while carrying heavy items up and down stairs. The union initially was opposed to changes in the work. However, after an explanation of the physical benefits that Frank could expect, the union then wanted to have the same plant changes made for all employees.

Frank was very happy with the work accommodations. He felt his employer had met him halfway in allowing him to return to work. He only wished the employer had thought of this long before his injury, because he knows he will not be the same again since he was injured. However, I feel strongly that Frank was in a deconditioned and guarded state even before he was injured. Perhaps the work hardening and the change in the work structure will, in fact, allow him many more productive years than he would have had without the injury and subsequent changes in the worksite.

CASE VARIATION 2

George's case is exactly like Roy's, except for the results of the work hardening program. The three weeks of work hardening did improve George's physical condition to some extent. However, he has not improved in motion of the spine, and the orthopedic surgeon believes that George has a permanent disability of the low back. The orthopedist does not have documented evidence regarding his range of motion at the beginning of his job; therefore, he must assume that he had normal range of motion. He will give him a percentage disability based on the lack of mobility in the low back.

George has also been diagnosed with degenerative arthritis in both knees. Again, the physician does not know if this was present prior to the injury, but must document that there is a loss of range of motion in both knees. Roentgenograms do show some arthritic changes. The physician believes that the combination of the knee dysfunction and the low back dysfunction will never allow George to return to a heavy job.

OUTCOME

The physician will give George an additional 10% disability rating of the low back and a 30% disability rating of both knees. This will cause a workers' compensation settlement to be paid and will likely lead to formal retraining. His strong physical areas of sitting, hand coordination, and good upper extremity function will aid the decision. It is possible that computer programming will fit into this plan.

Whether George undergoes retraining or not, he understands his physical ability and limitation levels so that he can apply them in any future work and at home. He is able to do more around the house and is more helpful in areas such as woodworking, carrying in groceries, and the like. Because he will be more financially able after the settlement and will be retrained to return to less strenuous work, the family is returning to a more normal state. George states that a positive outcome is that he has shown he has tried very hard to do the kind of work that he used to do, and the medical field has "backed him up" in his real physical problems. While he realizes that he cannot return to his old job, he also realizes that he can do more in his daily life. In addition, he is aware of exercises and restorative programs that he can do to keep himself in better condition. He may or may not decide to do that, because the settlement is so helpful that he can rest and do a lower-level physical job. He might not need "all the conditioning" in such a job.

I suggested that if George returns to a new type of work after retraining, the result of the functional assessment should be given to his new employer. If his physical condition has changed, he should be retested because his physical problems will not disappear. He will continue to have a low back tightness and possible lack of stability. He will continue to have degenerative changes in the knees, which will change his functional movements there. Balance will continue to be a problem. A new employer should have the benefit of a full functional description regardless of the nature of the work.

59 A Whiplash Injury

SUSAN PAULSEN LAYFIELD

Janice Smith was referred to physical therapy following an auto accident. Her car had been rear ended while stopped at a red light one month prior to the physical therapy evaluation. To prepare for her first visit, I organized a treatment file consisting of an evaluation form (Fig. 59-1) and prescriptions from referring physician and dentist. The referral from the physician read "Diagnosis: status post auto accident, cervical strain. Treatment: evaluate and treat." The dentist's prescription noted "Diagnosis: masticatory myalgia and temporomandibular joint (TMJ) capsulitis. Treatment: evaluate and treat." So that I would be ready to perform the evaluation when Janice arrived, I placed a measuring tape, a millimeter ruler, rubber gloves, a stethoscope, and a small glass of water in a treatment cubicle.

Janice entered the clinic walking slowly and wearing a soft cervical collar. Her posture was stiff and I could see tension in her shoulders, neck, and face (a common observation following a traumatic soft tissue injury). I introduced myself and explained what we would be doing in the evaluation. She was shown into a treatment cubicle and was asked to remove all outer clothing and put on a gown with the opening in the back. (Adequate exposure of all areas to be examined is important. A discrepancy, weakness, or tightness in one area can cause dysfunction in another area and could be missed if all areas are not visible.)

I like to divide the evaluation into several sections so that I can collect the information in an organized fashion. I chose to include the cat-egories of subjective examination, planning the objective examination, objective examination, assessment, and treatment plan in this evaluation. Through observation, specific movements, and palpation I believed I could thoroughly assess Janice's problems and design an appropriately individualized treatment plan.

To begin the subjective examination I asked Janice to describe the location and nature of her symptoms, beginning with the most severe. She indicated four major problems:

1. pain in the entire upper back, beginning at the inferior border of the scapulae,
2. headaches that traveled up the posterior aspect of the head and into the forehead and lateral regions of the head,
3. facial pain concentrating in the TMJ and masseter region, left greater than right, and
4. anterior cervical soreness.

I then asked Janice to describe the kind of pain she felt. She described it as dull, but severe, aching at rest, and sharp if she made quick movements of the head or jaw. I also asked Janice to indicate her symptoms on the diagram on the evaluation form. (Diagrams make the patient's description of symptoms easier for me to report to other health care providers and easier for them to interpret.)

Then, I asked Janice a series of questions about the behavior of her symptoms. (These questions are helpful in deciding how aggressively to begin treatment.) When asked if the symptoms were constant or intermittent, she

(Text continues on p. 1157.)

Name _____

Diagnosis _____

Date _____

Dentist _____

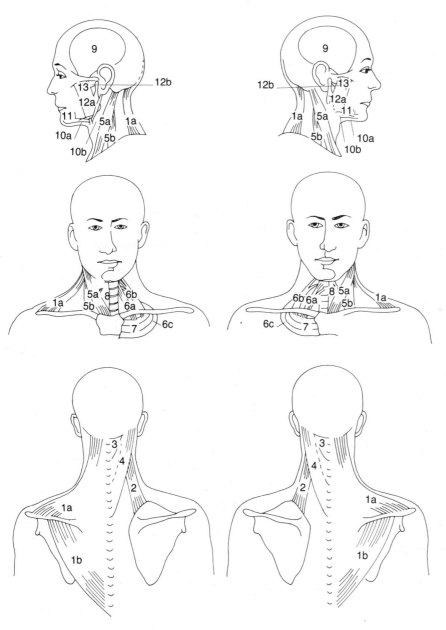

Location

Key: Chief complaint (cc): circled
Symptoms in
decending intensity:
P_1, P_2, P_3, etc.
Palpation: (x) mild
      x definite
      # severe
Headache (HA): / / /
Clear: + +

Palpation

1. Trapezius
   a. Upper/middle
   b. Lower
2. Levator scapulae
3. Cervical paraspinals
4. Splenius capitis
5. Sternocleidomastoideus (SCM)
6. Scaleni
   a. Anterior
   b. Middle
   c. Posterior
7. Upper intercostals
8. Longus colli
9. Temporalis
10. Digastricus
   a. Anterior
   b. Posterior
11. Mylohyoideus
12. Masseter
   a. Superficial
   b. Deep
13. Coronoid process

Figure 59-1. An upper-quarter evaluation form. *(Figure continues.)*

Behavior of Symptoms

Provocation:

Eases:

Night symptoms (sx):
    Sleeping position
    Pillow

Morning sx:

Day sx:

Occupational posture:

History

Current:

Previous:

Relevant medical history:

Objective

Negative

- [ ]   Observation

     Posture

- [ ]   Standing:
- [ ]   Leg length (LL):
- [ ]   Sitting:

     Facial symmetry

- [ ]   Horizontal plane:
- [ ]   Vertical plane:

     Rest position

- [ ]   Lips:
- [ ]   Tongue:
- [ ]   Mandible:

Special Questions

Negative

- [ ]   General health
- [ ]   Nutrition:
- [ ]   Medication:

     Oral habits:

- [ ]   Bruxism:
- [ ]   Chewing pattern:
- [ ]   Swallowing pattern:
- [ ]   Gum chewing:
- [ ]   Smoking:
- [ ]   Clenches:
- [ ]   Dentures, orthodontics,
           appliance:

Active Range of Motion (AROM)

- [ ] Upper extremity (UE):
- [ ] Cervical spine (C/S):
- [ ]   Forward bending (FB) _____ cm (chin → sternal notch)
- [ ]   Backward bending (BB) _____ cm (chin → sternal notch)
- [ ]   Rotation right (ROT[R]) _____ cm (chin → acromial clavicular
           joint [A/C jt])
- [ ]   Rotation left (ROT[L]) _____ cm (chin → A/C jt)
- [ ]   Side bending right (SB[R]) _____ cm (tragus → A/C jt)
- [ ]   Side bending left (SB[L]) _____ cm (tragus → A/C jt)

Figure 59-1. *(Continued.)*

Objective

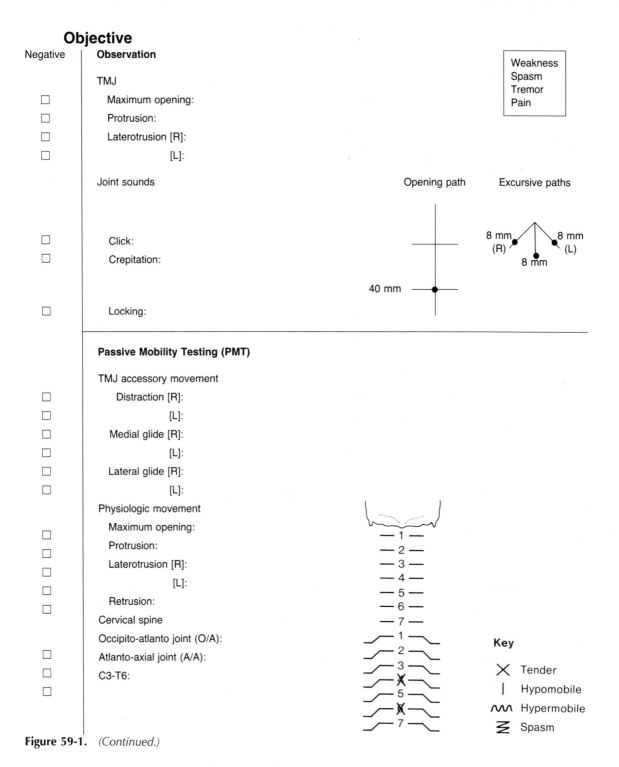

Figure 59-1. *(Continued.)*

Negative	**Static Tests (Isometric)**
	TMJ
☐	Laterotrusion [R]:
☐	[L]:
☐	Closing:
☐	Opening:
☐	Protrusion:
	Cervical spine
☐	FB:
☐	BB:
☐	ROT [R]:
☐	ROT [L]:
☐	SB [R]:
☐	SB [L]:

Assessment (quality, intensity, progressivity, disability, chronicity)

Treatment Plan

Estimated Cost

_____ **P.T.**

replied that they are constant, but of varying intensity. She indicated that head or upper extremity movement, wearing the cervical collar for longer than 30 minutes, and fatigue all aggravated the upper back area. Fatigue and upper back symptoms increased the headaches. Talking, chewing, and yawning caused more facial pain. Swallowing was uncomfortable because of pain in the anterior cervical area. Rest decreased the upper back pain and aspirin lessened the intensity of headaches. Janice found she reduced the facial and anterior cervical soreness when she ate foods that were soft and easy to chew.

I then asked Janice about the position in which she slept and its effect on her symptoms. She said she usually slept prone with one polyester pillow. In the morning she awoke with significant stiffness, neck pain, and soreness in the TMJ area. I was concerned about Janice sleeping on her stomach. In this position, the neck is exposed to extreme rotation, sidebending, and extension. The mandible is also placed in a position of abnormal stress. A new sleeping position would have to be included in her treatment program.

We then focused on symptoms in a "typical" day. She said that the symptoms always increased in intensity as the day progressed and often prevented her from falling asleep. Janice worked as an office manager for a large furniture manufacturing company. Most of her working hours were spent sitting. In addition, she drove a half hour each way to and from work. This closely resembled backgrounds of other patients I had treated whose upper back and neck symptoms were aggravated with prolonged sitting. At this point in the subjective examination I wanted to find out what happened during the auto accident. Janice said she was driving a small car and was rear ended by another while stopped at a signal light. The other car was traveling about 25 mph. Her seat belt was fastened; however, her headrest was positioned very low and did not provide protection for her head, which was thrown backward and forward. Upper back and anterior neck pain began immediately after the accident.

This kind of whiplash injury in a deceleration accident throws the head and neck into extension as the seat accelerates forward, taking the lower parts of the body with it. The neck is then forced into excessive flexion because of a reflex muscular contraction of the stretched anterior cervical muscles. The mandible is also forcibly moved posteriorly and then anteriorly, often traumatizing the TMJ area as well.

Janice's symptoms had decreased about 10% since the accident. The headaches developed one or two days later and had continued unchanged. Her facial symptoms began approximately one week after the accident, and their intensity had steadily increased. Her physician had believed that the facial symptoms would subside within a short period of time. When they did not, Janice was referred to a dentist specializing in the treatment of TMJ-related disorders. Janice had not experienced any TMJ symptoms prior to the auto accident. If she had, the cause and course of previous episodes would have been of importance. If the TMJ symptoms had been preexisting, it would assist in determining predisposing factors and possibly affect prognosis for the present symptoms.

I asked Janice the following questions to identify more specifically the nature of her problems.

1. *Have you experienced dizziness since the accident?* Janice said she suffered occasional dizziness with quick movements of her head. Referral from soft tissue trigger points or autonomic disturbances could cause this symptom.

2. *Have you experienced tingling in your feet or hands?* She said no. This question helps rule out central cord symptoms.

3. *How would you describe your general health?* Janice indicated her health was excellent.

4. *Are you taking any medication?* Janice answered that she takes two aspirin four times a day (QID). I think medication can be important when looking for an objective indicator of progress. When patients begin to feel better, they usually reduce their medication.

I then asked some specific questions regarding her facial symptoms.

1. *Have you modified your diet because of the symptoms?* Yes, she was unable to eat foods that required much chewing.
2. *Do you grind your teeth (bruxism)?* She did not think so. A person who bruxes may not be aware of it, but will exhibit a "wearing" or flattening of areas on the teeth.
3. *Do you prefer to chew on one side?* She felt the left side was more comfortable. It is common for a patient to chew more comfortably on the more painful side because this "unloads" the joint and therefore allows for more comfortable chewing.
4. *Do you chew gum?* Yes, before the accident, but she stopped afterwards because of the jaw pain. I have found it common for gum chewing to overwork the masticatory muscles, which leads to fatigue and increases the symptoms.
5. *Do you smoke?* She said occasionally. I ask this question because of the protrusion of the mandible that is necessary to position the cigarette. This can aggravate the soft tissue already traumatized by the accident.
6. *Do you clench your teeth?* She said that she did when she was under stress. I strongly believe that clenching is a major contributing factor to facial pain and must·be corrected for optimal rest and healing of this area. Clenching is quite common, and most patients are unaware of how much they clench until they are made aware of the correct resting position of the jaw. With this position maintained, the muscles of mastication are properly aligned and clenching is significantly reduced.
7. *Are you wearing an orthotic appliance (splint)?* She recently received an acrylic appliance from the dentist that she wore over her top teeth. She wore the appliance all the time except when eating (Fig. 59-2).

I wanted to observe her swallowing pattern, so I asked her to drink some water. The pattern was normal. During the act of swallowing the tongue moved up onto the palate, her

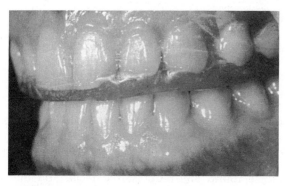

Figure 59-2. A maxillary appliance designed to decrease both TMJ and facial symptoms.

teeth came together, and her lips gently touched.

The physician's report noted that the roentgenographic findings showed mild reversal of the cervical lordosis and normal TMJ bilaterally. It is not unusual to find normal TMJ roentgenograms in patients immediately following an accident.

As Janice finished drinking the water, I mentally compiled all the subjective information and began to plan the objective examination. I have found that planning the objective examination phase is very important. Planning requires extra time, but it results in a more organized, concise, and efficient examination, I decided to examine the following areas:

1. Joints
   - Occipitoatlanto-C7
   - T1-T6
   - glenohumeral joints
   - TMJs
2. Muscles
   - trapezius
   - rhomboids
   - levator scapulae
   - thoracic paraspinals
   - splenius capitis
   - cervical paraspinals
   - sternocleidomastoideus
   - scaleni
   - upper intercostals
   - longus colli
   - digastric

- mylohyoid
- masseter
- temporalis
- medial pterygoid
- lateral pterygoid

3. Test for vertebral artery insufficiency. I elected to perform this test because Janice complained of dizziness. It was performed to ensure that movement of the cervical spine would not interfere with circulation of the vertebral artery.

As I planned the objective examination, I kept in mind the factors that would affect treatment. Because Janice's symptoms were constant and the result of traumatic injury, caution was indicated in the initiation of treatment. Contraindications for treatment would include any treatment that reproduced Janice's symptoms. The intensity and frequency of symptoms described by Janice further indicated caution when administering the movement and palpation phases of the objective exam. These symptoms also suggested what I could find through palpation and movement that would reproduce the symptoms.

Based on these considerations, I selected the movements to be tested. They included active and passive movements of the cervical spine (forward bending [FB], sidebending [SB], backward bending [BB], and rotation [ROT]) and active and passive movements of the mandible (depression [opening], elevation [closing], laterotrusion, protrusion, and retrusion). Another appropriate area for examination was leg length. Uneven leg length is a frequent perpetuator of soft tissue irritation. The postural muscles are affected secondary to their attempt to maintain the head and shoulder balanced over the feet.

Now that the planning phase was completed, I moved on to the actual objective examination. The objective tests are done to define the client's described symptoms in terms of muscles, joints, and nerves that might cause the symptoms. I also wanted to determine the physical factors that could have contributed to the onset of the symptoms. My objective examination of Janice consisted of ob-

servation, palpation, and testing for movement.

The first thing I did was ask Janice to stand. I wanted to observe how easily she moved and what posture she assumed. I then evaluated her posture from the posterior, anterior, and lateral views. I noticed her head was in a forward position. This was a result of BB of the head and upper cervical spine and FB of the lower cervical and upper thoracic spine to maintain the head level. (This position is common following a cervical strain and seems to be a major cause of symptoms in the chronic stages.) I also noticed there was a 7-in distance between the medial borders of her scapulae (4 in is desirable) and a decrease in her lumbar lordosis. Her sitting posture was an exaggeration of the above. Standing leg length was equal.

Next, I checked Janice for facial symmetry from a horizontal and vertical perspective to rule out any visible anatomical factors that might contribute to the symptoms. No asymmetry was observed. When at rest, her lips were comfortably touching as they should be. (This ensures efficient nasal breathing and relaxation of the facial muscles.) When I asked Janice to describe her tongue position, she said her tongue was resting on the floor of her mouth. This finding is common in patients who clench their teeth. When the tongue is not resting on the palate, the muscles of mastication are active and will fatigue, contributing to symptoms in the area. She also said that her teeth were positioned together, another contributing factor to facial symptoms.

Remembering the significant tenderness Janice expressed, and the considerations I made as I planned the objective exam, I expected to find many tender trigger points. I therefore proceeded with caution to palpate for myofascial trigger points. Myofascial trigger points are small points of hypersensitivity within a muscle that are locally tender and can give rise to referred pain and tenderness.

With each muscle relaxed and on a slight stretch, I palpated the muscles I identified in my planning. I palpated with a flat finger positioned transverse to the direction of the muscle fibers. As I palpated, I asked Janice to describe the intensity of discomfort in terms of a number from 0 to 3 (0 described no discomfort and 3 described significant discomfort). I also asked her to tell me if the discomfort was in the spot I was palpating or was felt elsewhere (referred pain).

I used the head and upper trunk chart on the evaluation form to record Janice's responses. The symbols recorded were 0=0, 1=(x), 2=x, and 3=#. If she described referred pain, an arrow was used to map the direction and area of the referred pain.

I then asked Janice to open her mouth. I placed my little finger into each auditory meatus and had her close her mouth slowly. This evaluated each TMJ's ability to withstand additional mechanical stress. It was very painful for Janice, another indication of joint capsulitis.

In summary, significant (#) tenderness was present in the following muscles bilaterally, some more pronounced on the left:

- thoracic paraspinals (#)
- trapezius (#)
- rhomboids (#)
- levator scapulae (#)
- cervical paraspinals (#)
- upper intercostals (#)
- longus colli (#)
- scaleni (#)
- sternocleidomastoideus (#)
- external auditory meatus (##)
- digastric (###)
- mylohyoid (###)
- masseter (####)
- temporalis (####)
- medial pterygoid (####)
- lateral pterygoid (####)

#: These findings support the complaints of headaches and upper trunk pain.

##: External auditory meatus symptoms support the impression of capsule irritation.

###: Tenderness in these muscles supports the complaint of soreness in swallowing.

####: Tenderness in these areas supports the mandibular complaints.

Before testing movements of the cervical spine, I performed the vertebral artery test. Janice was positioned supine and her neck was positioned in full backward bending with rotation and held for 30 seconds. She was asked to report any tinnitus, dizziness, nausea, throbbing, or unusual sensations. Her pupils were observed for constriction or dilation that lasted for any length of time after the head was brought back to neutral. The procedure was then repeated with rotation to the opposite side. The results were negative.

I progressed to testing specific movements. Active, passive, and resisted tests made up this section of the examination. I looked for joint mobility, general flexibility, and movements that reproduced Janice's symptoms. Because of the amount of pain she had described earlier in the examination, I expected to reproduce symptoms without much effort and proceeded carefully. I corrected her posture and looked for a change in symptoms. She reported less strain across the upper back.

She was then instructed to bend her head forward as far as she could. Active tests provide information on the quantity and quality of movement. I watched for the quality of movement and measured the distance with a tape measure. (See Figure 59-1, evaluation form, for landmarks.) FB was painful throughout the full range and was also painful on return to neutral. This reflected both joint and muscular origin of symptoms. BB was painful, limited in range, and painful on return to neutral. SB was restricted bilaterally and painful on the side opposite the direction of movement. Tenderness was also reported throughout the range of rotation. Upper extremity (UE) range was within normal limits (WNL) bilaterally, but Janice expressed general soreness throughout the range of all movements.

I then focused on the mandible. I examine the TMJ of all patients following cervical trauma. It takes only a brief examination to rule out involvement. The examination consists of measuring the jaw opening, which should be at least 40 mm. This movement should be pain free, in midline, and silent. If one or more of these indicators is positive, a more detailed exam should follow. Observing the quality of movement and placing my index finger gently over each TMJ, I asked Janice to open her mouth as far as she could. The movement was very guarded and was significantly restricted at 17 mm because of bilateral pain. Her jaw "wiggled" from right to left, indicating incoordination of the masticatory muscles. Capsular irritation could also restrict mandibular movement.

I went on with the more detailed TMJ exam in which each movement is measured in millimeters. Protrusion was limited to 7 mm because of pain in the left TMJ. (Normal is 8 to 10 mm.) Laterotrusion was 7 mm bilaterally, and pain was experienced in the left TMJ with movement both to the right and left. (Normal range for laterotrusion is also 8 to 10 mm in each direction.) Retrusion was extremely painful, further supporting the diagnosis of joint capsulitis. Retrusion of the mandibular condyle imposes on the majority of blood vessels and nerves supplying the TMJ.

Passive movements were 20 mm opening, no difference in laterotrusion, 8 mm for protrusion, and no difference in retrusion. An empty end-feel was noted, which is common in conditions where pain is the predominant complaint.

With a stethoscope I listened to each TMJ during all movements and found the joints to be silent. No clicking or locking was evident and Janice did not report experiencing either symptom. Clicking has numerous causes. Some that are more common include a mild displacement of the articular disk and incoordination of movement between the disk and condyle. The most common cause of joint locking is a displacement of the disk. When this occurs, opening is limited to less than 40 mm, protrusion is limited with deflection to the ipsilateral side, and laterotrusion is limited to the contralateral side. Most disk displacements occur anteriorly and medially, which accounts for the pattern of movements most often found.

Passive mobility tests evaluate the specific range of motion available in joints. If these tests reproduce symptoms, then noncontractile tissue such as the capsule, ligament, bursae, nerves, nerve sheaths, cartilage, disks, and dura mater are involved. Full, pain-free passive mobility movements are essential for normal joint movement. Passive mobility tests of both TMJs were painful, further indicating capsular irritation. Distraction, medial glide, and lateral glide are the passive mobility tests for the TMJ. The movements were performed intraorally, noting restriction and pain.

With Janice prone, I tested for quality and quantity of movement of the joints from the occipitoatlanto (OA) joint through T6. The OA, C5-C6, and C7-T4 joints were very tender to palpation and restricted in mobility. I used resisted (isometric) testing to find muscular involvement in the mandibular and cervical areas. The tests were done in a comfortable position. The contractile elements of the area, including muscles, tendons, and their attachments, were stressed by the tests. Because trauma had been experienced, I was not surprised to find a generalized soreness when these tests were performed on both the mandibular and cervical movements. Janice was asked to sit, and I tested FB, BB, SB, and ROT. Mandibular testing included opening, closing, laterotrusion, and protrusion. She was then asked to lie prone, and the middle and lower trapezius and rhomboids were tested.

I strongly believe that the assessment component is one of the most important parts of the evaluation process. During this phase, the subjective and objective information is summarized and the symptoms are analyzed for their severity. From this, the appropriate selection of treatment techniques may be outlined. As I complete an assessment, I typically look at (1) the quality of the symptoms, (2) the intensity of the symptoms, (3) the extent of the disability caused by the accident, (4) the chronicity of the symptoms, (5) the progressive nature of the symptoms, and (6) a prognosis based on the above.

Janice was a 35-year-old female. Her chief complaint was constant, varying back pain in the posterior and anterior cervical areas. She also complained of bilateral facial and TMJ pain (left greater than right) and headaches. The upper back symptoms, cervical symptoms, and headaches were aggravated by active movement and fatigue. The facial symptoms were aggravated by mandibular movements such as chewing and yawning. All symptoms were decreased with rest and gentle massage.

The symptoms were the result of an auto accident one month ago in which Janice's car was rear ended while stopped at a red light. Following one week of rest at home, she returned to work on a part-time basis for five hours daily. The symptoms prevented her from playing tennis or hiking, activities she enjoyed and participated in regularly.

The symptoms in the upper back and cervical areas had decreased 10%. However, the intensity and frequency of the headaches and facial pain had increased. Factors that contributed to the persistent symptoms included poor posture in sitting, standing, and lying, incorrect fitting of the cervical collar, and habits such as jaw clenching and occasional smoking.

Several tests reproduced her symptoms. These tests included palpation of the myofascial trigger points throughout the upper quarter, active and passive cervical and mandibular movements in all directions, and joint mobility testing of OA, atlanto-axial (AA), C6, C7-T6, and both TMJs.

Because Janice had not experienced any of the above symptoms prior to the accident, I concluded that the symptoms were a result of the trauma she sustained. The intensity of the symptoms appeared significant enough to indicate caution when initiating treatment and home instruction. They indicated that early treatment would be focused on treating the pain.

Janice appeared to have sustained multiple soft tissue and joint injuries involving the entire upper quarter. The trauma resulted in masticatory, cervical spine, and mid-upper thoracic spine myalgia, TMJ capsulitis, and joint restriction at OA, AA, C6, and C7-T6, most likely resulting from local muscle spasm and joint irritation. The prognosis for Janice returning to work full time, playing tennis, and hiking was very good, although the progress would probably be slow with a treatment duration of several months.

Based on the above assessment, I divided the treatment plan into a home program and a treatment section. The goals of the home program were to obtain the correct postural position, restore the normal resting length of the muscles, achieve normal joint mobility, and achieve normal body balance. To meet the goals I designed a home program that was divided into four phases. Phase I included rest and use of the cervical collar, instruction in correct posture for sitting, standing, and lying, gentle ROM exercises for the upper back and mandible, instruction in correct body mechanics, and instruction in the use of ice.

As Janice responded to Phase I of the home program and treatment in the clinic, she would progress through Phases II, III, and IV. Phase II would include general body stretching and additional ROM exercises for the upper quarter. Phase III would include instruction and guidance in a general conditioning program. In Janice's case, this would be stationary bicycling and walking. Phase IV would be the follow-up phase, in which Janice would be reassessed at 1, 3, 6, and 12-month periods after therapy was ended.

I began the home instruction with emphasis on the importance of rest. The cervical collar was turned around "backwards" and found to fit Janice's neck well and comfortably. Because she was experiencing quite a bit of pain, I asked her to wear the collar except when sleeping. I instructed her to avoid quick movements of the head and jaw and to limit active movements to the range of comfort.

It was important at this time to emphasize the importance of various postural relationships. These included the head to the upper cervical spine, all aspects of the cervical spine to the shoulders, and the mandible to the maxilla. I believe the patient's understanding is important because the correction of posture is the foundation for all further exercises and treatments.

Correction of Janice's posture in standing, sitting, and lying followed. Sitting in a firm, upright seat with a lumbar support was emphasized. The use of a lumbar support ensured the maintenance of the lumbar lordosis, served as a reminder to sit up straight, and placed the muscles of the middle and upper back under less tension because the lumbar lordosis was maintained. Janice was instructed to sleep on her side or supine with a pillow in place to support her head correctly. The rationale for avoiding the prone position was explained again for reinforcement.

The correct resting position of the tongue (comfortably resting against the palate) was discussed and demonstrated. An exercise was designed to restore muscular balance during mandibular opening. Janice was instructed to place the tip of her tongue on the palate and open her mouth in midline, maintaining contact of the tongue on the palate. Gentle ROM exercises for the upper back consisted of shoulder girdle elevation with shoulder flexion, performed within a pain-free range of motion (Fig. 59-3). Janice was also given a diaphragmatic breathing exercise. It was taught in the supine position. Patients seem to learn this exercise more easily in this position with the knees flexed.

I counseled Janice to begin a semisoft diet. This meant avoiding foods that required aggressive chewing, such as raw vegetables, tough meat, hard or sticky candy, gum, and bread such as bagels. I also instructed Janice to cut her food into bite-sized pieces to minimize stress on her jaw.

As Janice progressed, phase II was added. It consisted of a set of general body ROM exercises. This involved 18 exercises, requiring 15 minutes to perform daily. A contract-relax exercise for the head and neck was also added.

Other instructions included facial and scalp massage, isometric exercises for jaw strengthening and coordination, and an isotonic proprioceptive neuromuscular facilitation (PNF) neck flexion pattern. Only one exercise was added at a time, and all exercises were reviewed with Janice during each treatment session until each was performed correctly and smoothly. Correct posture, tongue resting position, and the diaphragmatic breathing pattern were expected to become "new habits" within several weeks and replace the former "poor habits." I instructed Janice to repeat each exercise six times and to perform the series six times daily to ensure the new habits developed.

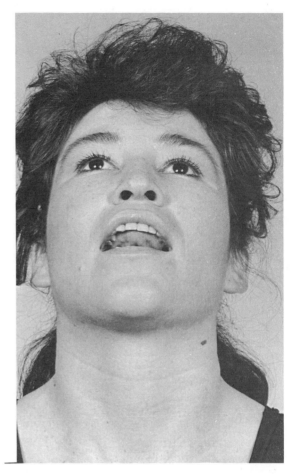

Figure 59-3. Correct position of the tongue against the palate.

The goals of treatment were to reduce pain through manual techniques and modalities, restore functional ROM, improve strength of the upper quarter, and improve general endurance. The techniques and modalities I chose to use for treatment were:

1. Massage to the posterior thoracic and cervical areas, anterior cervical region, and facial and cranial soft tissue.
2. Continuous ultrasonography at 6 to 8 W for three minutes to the masseter, distal temporalis, and suprahyoid areas using a rubber glove filled with water (Fig. 59-4).

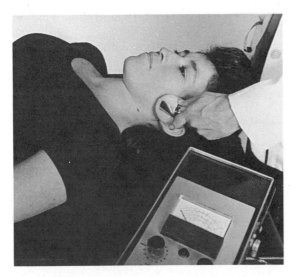

Figure 59-4. Ultrasound administered through a surgical glove filled with water.

3. Fluoromethane stretch and spray to restore the muscles to their normal resting length.
4. Gentle manual traction. I prefer this form of traction to mechanical traction because of its effectiveness, the greater degree of control, and the ability to grade the amount of pull. Mechanical traction has not proven effective in treating soft tissue dysfunction.
5. The joint mobilization technique of gentle cervical rotation.
6. ROM exercises consisted of scapular patterns and hold-relax neck patterns. Upper extremity and upper trunk patterns were added as tolerated. This included the PNF activities of chopping, lifting, bilateral upper extremity patterns, and isotonic neck patterns.
7. Cold packs to the upper back, neck, and cheeks for 15 minutes.

As soon as the acute symptoms eased, stationary bicycling was begun and progressed from 5 to 30 minutes per session. As healing and relaxation of the muscles took place, Janice's dentist made several adjustments of her oral appliance.

The long-range goal of treatment was to have Janice achieve a level of comfort at which she could function, and return to her full-time job and the activities that she enjoyed prior to her injury. Because of the nature of whiplash injuries, periodic exacerbations of the symptoms may be experienced.

The intention of the home instruction was to educate Janice in exercises and modalities that would be helpful when she experienced a flare-up. In such cases, she could then reduce the symptoms quickly. The rationale for the general conditioning program was to improve her endurance, assist in the healing process, and correct poor habits present prior to the accident.

This case is a typical example of a whiplash injury that involved the entire upper quarter. Because of the complex neurological and soft tissue relationship of the upper quarter system (the shoulder girdle, cervical spine, cranium, and mandible) this entire area must be evaluated and treated for optimal results. Although various combinations of treatment techniques and modalities are quite useful, I believe the most important aspect of treatment in the long run is patient education. The patient should know the ways she can prevent further recurrences, methods of self-treatment for mild exacerbations, and when to seek short-term treatment if symptoms continue. This approach instills confidence in the patient and further supports the fact that we as physical therapists are a vital part of the team treating patients with upper quarter dysfunction.

POSSIBLE VARIATIONS OF SYMPTOMS

CASE VARIATION 1

Tom was referred to me for treatment with the diagnosis of anterior disk displacement with reduction, left TMJ. This situation differs from Janice's in that clicking was present with mandibular opening, protrusion, and laterotrusion to the right. Because a displaced disk most often is positioned anteriorly and medially, Tom's pattern of clicking is understandable.

Tom did not complain of upper back or facial pain, as Janice had, but only referred to soreness around the left TMJ, most likely the deep fibers of the masseter, lateral pterygoid, capsule, and posterior attachments within the capsule (Fig. 59-5).

Goals

The goals for Tim consisted of (1) avoidance of joint noise; (2) restoring coordination of the muscles related to the movement of the mandible; and (3) decreasing stress on the joint.

Treatment

1. The hinge axis exercise is designed to limit mandibular opening only to the rotation phase of opening to correct any tendency for early translation, and to reposition the condyle comfortable within the joint fossa. By maintaining this limited opening, the joint will be protected against excessive stress such as clicking. I instructed Tom to place his index fingers over his TMJs and position the tip of his tongue on the palate (roof of the mouth). When opening his mouth, he was to keep the tip of his tongue on the palate. No joint sound should occur. This exercise is then progressed to where the mouth is opened without the tongue on the palate, thus allowing translation to occur. Again, clicking should not accompany this movement.

2. As with all conditions involving the upper quarter, posture was corrected in standing, sitting, and sleeping.

3. I then instructed Tom to cut all food into bite-sized pieces to limit stress on the joints when chewing.

4. He was asked to keep the tip of the tongue on the palate when yawning for the same reason as above.

5. His dentist fitted Tom with an appliance that assisted in the reduction of muscle guarding and helped restore normal intracapsular function.

6. I selected modalities and techniques such as ultrasonography and cold packs initially to decrease accompanying muscular and joint soreness. I used moist heat and spray-and-stretch techniques to restore pain-free ROM to the jaw. I have found that by incorporating high-voltage gal-

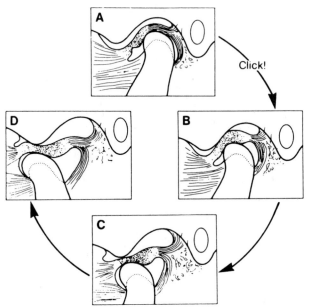

Figure 59-5. Click evident with mandibular opening due to disk-condyle dysfunction. (*A*) TMJ with mouth closed. (*B*) As the condyle rotates and begins to translate forward, it must move over the thicker, posterior portion of the disk onto the central, thinner part of the disk, causing a click. (*C*, *D*) Normal joint motion resumes to complete opening.

vanic stimulation with the intraoral probe near the lateral pterygoid, coordination of mandibular movements is improved.

7. Tom was discharged from therapy after 14 treatments. The TMJ and soft tissue symptoms had resolved. He continued to wear the appliance at night because of his tendency to brux when sleeping.

CASE VARIATION 2

Sarah was referred for treatment with the diagnosis of a disk displacement without reduction. This indicated that the joint had "locked." There was no audible joint noise, but pain and a pattern of reproducible movement restrictions were present during movement of the mandible (Fig. 59-6). These symptoms differ from Janice's in that Sarah's articular disk is actually displaced. Sarah's symptoms did not follow an acute trauma. Rather, they began insidiously, and developed following a long history of nonpainful joint clicking. This progressed to joint soreness, and finally to the point where the clicking ceased. Instead, she was left with an inability to move her mandible freely to open, protrude, or move laterally to the opposite side.

Figure 59-6. Anterior displacement of the disk resulting in the inability of the condyle to complete translation (locking). (*A*) Mandible in the rest position. (*B*) As the mandible begins to open, condylar translation is prevented by the displaced disk. (*C, D*) Full translation (full jaw opening) is blocked.

Goals

Based on the above findings, I set the following goals: (1) restore the normal disk-condyle relationship and (2) relieve soft tissue symptoms.

Treatment

1. The technique used to recapture a displaced disk is distraction of the condyle in a downward direction, followed by the condyle being pulled anteriorly and medially. Once the disk is "recaptured," as verified by the return of normal mandibular movements, an appliance was made to maintain the disk-condyle position. The appliance positioned the mandible forward, and was made by a dentist who was knowledgeable in TMJ dysfunction.

2. I instructed Sarah in the hinge axis exercise and also in a diet of soft foods.

3. During treatment, Sarah was asked to wear the appliance. The length and amount of time a patient will wear the appliance varies, depending on the diagnosis and philosophy of the treating dentist. When treating for a disk displacement, the appliance is worn 24 hours a day. Sarah's appliance was adjusted frequently by her dentist. As

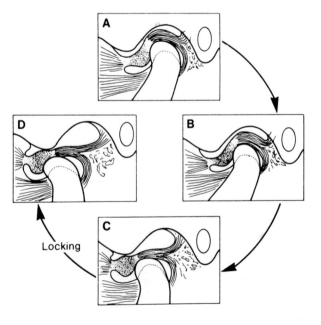

the symptoms diminished and joint movement was restored, she wore the appliance fewer hours during the day and eventually was able to function well without it.

4. I chose treatment modalities and techniques to decrease the soft tissue and joint pain. These included ultrasonography, cold packs, massage, and gentle joint mobilization techniques. I then progressed to the techniques and modalities that improved range of motion, such as spray and stretch, moist heat, and contract-relax exercises.

5. Because of the influence that head and cervical posture can have on the position of the TMJ, Sarah was instructed in proper posture in standing, sitting, and sleeping.

6. Sarah was discharged from therapy after two months of treatment. At this time she was free of pain, and functional ROM of the mandible was restored. She continued to wear the splint, but was undergoing regular adjustments as her symptoms and jaw movements improved. It is possible, in a situation similar to Sarah's, for the disk to remain displaced. In this event, treatment would be directed toward reducing the acute symptoms. The patient would then continue to monitor the diet and avoid mandibular movements that caused pain. These movements usually are toward the end of the rotation phase of movement. If a situation such as this continues to interfere with function and is painful, surgery may be necessary to correct the problem.

CASE VARIATION 3

John was evaluated for treatment of constant, varying headaches in the area of the posterior head and the temples. He also reported a history of mild posterior cervical soreness. His symptoms were a result of a fall down 13 concrete steps two months previous to the physical therapy examination. John did not demonstrate nor did he complain of TMJ pain or dysfunction. He did not complain of neck soreness, but demonstrated tightness at the end of the range of cervical movements. My conclusion, based upon the examination, was that I would be treating cervical joint and soft tissue hypomobility more so than pain. The initial soft tissue and joint irritation had subsided, but John was left with joint and soft tissue tightness. Following the treatment plan listed below, John was discharged from physical therapy with restored range of motion and the absence of headaches after eight treatments.

Goals

The goals for John were to restore joint and soft tissue mobility of the upper, middle, and lower cervical spine.

Treatment

1. Deep soft tissue massage to the upper back and posterior cervical areas.

2. Joint mobilization techniques were applied to the upper cervical spine at the end of the range of motion.

3. Soft tissue range of motion techniques were used with the part to be stretched at the end of range.

4. Cold packs were applied to the upper back while John was positioned in static cervical traction. The upper cervical spine was gently distracted.

5. A combination of ultrasonography and high-voltage galvanic stimulation was used, usually before stretching.

6. John was instructed in home exercises for correct posture in sitting, standing, and lying down, self-mobilization techniques for the cervical spine, stretching exercises for the entire body, and modalities for home use, such as static traction, cold packs, or moist heat, whichever he found to work best.

ANNOTATED BIBLIOGRAPHY

Bell W: Clinical Management of Temporomandibular Disorders, 2nd ed. Chicago, Year Book Medical Publishers, 1985 (Chapter 7 outlines and describes symptoms of masticatory dysfunction. A good reference book.)

Maitland G D: Vertebral Manipulation, 5th ed. London, Butterworths, 1986 (This book is an excellent reference for evaluation and treatment techniques for the cervical spine.)

Rocabado M: Diagnosis and treatment of abnormal craniocervical and craniomandibular mechanics. In Solberg W, Clark G (eds): Abnormal Jaw Mechanics: Diagnosis and Treatment. Chicago, Quintessence, 1984 (Chapter 7 offers a good overview of factors contributing to abnormal craniocervical and craniomandibular mechanics.)

Saunders D H: Evaluation, Treatment, and Prevention of Musculoskeletal Disorders. Minneapolis, Viking Press, 1985 (This book contains many clear illustrations of evaluation and treatment techniques. The chapter on the temporomandibular joint is an informative description of TMJ anatomy and dysfunction.)

Travell J, Simons D: Myofascial Pain and Dysfunction: The Trigger Point Manual. Baltimore, Williams & Wilkins, 1983 (This book is an excellent source for the examination, diagnosis, and treatment of the individual muscles of the head and cervical areas. The authors describe referred pain patterns that the therapist must know to treat symptoms related to the upper quarter.)

60 Knee Trauma

STEVEN R. TIPPETT

Tom is a 22-year-old white male collegiate basketball player with a diagnosis of quadriceps tendinitis of the right leg. He is 6 ft 7 in tall and weighs 215 lbs. Currently, Tom is a red-shirted junior majoring in business at a private university with an enrollment of 4000 students.

HISTORY

The initial onset of right superolateral quadriceps tendon discomfort was approximately 16 months ago. Physician orders of rest and cryotherapy were progressed to quadriceps muscle strengthening exercises; quadriceps, hamstring, and gastrocnemius-soleus stretching exercises; and ultrasonography, which all proved unsuccessful. A subsequent injection of hydrocortisone in the involved area also afforded no relief. The patient was taken to surgery after eight months of conservative measures had failed. Arthroscopic examination revealed a small radial tear of the lateral meniscus as well as grade II and III chondromalacia patellae with minimal degeneration of the lateral tibial plateau. Open exploration of the quadriceps and patellar tendons revealed a normal patellar tendon, but gross evidence of quadriceps tendon inflammation and fatty infiltration. Microscopic examination disclosed broad bands of heavy, poorly cellular tendinous material and areas of cartilaginous tissue with marked focal variation in chondrocyte arrangement. Fatty tissue infiltration without histologic abnormality was found along with vascular proliferation of varying sizes.

EVALUATION

The patient was referred to me after six months of routine postarthroscopic rehabilitation. After talking to Tom in my initial evaluation, he impressed me as being genuinely concerned, desiring my help to get back into competition, but having a moderate degree of skepticism. After all, he had been around the block with this knee problem. He had already missed one year of basketball and was only weeks away from the scheduled start of the present season. Tom appeared well informed regarding his situation and possessed semirealistic expectations. Motivation did not seem to be a problem. In fact, he seemed very eager to begin whatever it took to get back on the court; however, the exact how and what specifically pertaining to this latest rehabilitation effort was definitely an uncertainty.

The subjective portion of my evaluation was very enlightening in a few areas. Complaints of pain in terms of location, exacerbating factors, and the like were as I expected. When pressed for a chief complaint Tom responded, "I have less than 20% deficits in quad

1169

strength but still can't jump." Certainly, Tom's past experiences in physical therapy had rubbed off. His answers gave me the subjective information on which to build a treatment program; more important, however, were the answers that gave me insight into Tom himself.

Of vital concern to me were the physical therapy programs Tom received before and after surgery. In order to treat the patient adequately I needed to know specifically what he had done regarding his injury. I found that Tom had essentially done everything asked of him by the two previous therapists, and then some. It was the "and then some" that got him into trouble. He did indeed comply with the formal treatment program outlines while in the physical therapy department as well as at school and, when applicable, on the basketball court. However, in addition to the prescribed exercises and activities, Tom usually did more. At the outset, when instructed to rest, he did so for a few days but every so often tested the knee to check the effectiveness of the rest. Testing the knee usually involved stationary jumping drills or attempts to dunk the basketball. When instructed in an eccentric loading program he performed the modified knee drops as instructed, but commonly did two to three times the specified number, usually with quadriceps tendon pain.

Tom was very matter of fact when recounting his past rehabilitation. It was obvious that he did not understand that his willingness to do more to get better actually made him worse. Tom was well motivated and eager to cooperate. However, his overzealous cooperation had resulted in his not playing basketball yet. He would require reassurance from me that rest and "listening to the pain" were as important a part in his rehabilitation as quadriceps strengthening. Also, judging from Tom's past performance, my reassurance would have to be constant.

The objective information gathered from the initial visit was as follows.

GAIT

Tom walked without an assistive device. No limp was noted, nor were any gross gait deviations observed.

RANGE OF MOTION

Active range of motion of the lower extremities was bilaterally symmetrical and grossly within normal limits with the following exceptions: long-sitting active dorsiflexion with knees at 0 degrees flexion was symmetrical bilaterally at 0 to 7 degrees; active knee extension in the supine position with the hips flexed to 90 degrees, noninvolved left side −25 degrees from the neutral position and on the involved right side −30 degrees from neutral. Passive hamstring flexibility, resistance to stretch was felt at −45 degrees from neutral on the left and −50 degrees from neutral on the right side. Passive stretch of the quadriceps was symmetrical bilaterally with both heels easily moved to the buttocks.

MUSCLE STATE

The noninvolved quadriceps muscle was normal in that there was good visual definition throughout the muscle group individually and palpation of the quadriceps showed firm muscle mass. The involved right quadriceps was visually defined only at the vastus medialis. Palpation of the vastus medialis muscle revealed soft muscle mass. Bilateral measurement of the circumference of the quadriceps was taken 3 in and 6 in proximal to the joint space. The measurement revealed a 3/8-in atrophy of the right side at the 3-in site and no difference 6 in proximal to the joint space.

RELATED AREAS

Visual inspection of the knee showed well-healed superolateral and inferomedial arthroscopic wounds as well as a longitudinal scar centered over the patella extending from approximately 1.5 in proximal to the superior pole of the patella to approximately 1 in distal to the tibial tubercle. The scar area was not hypersensitive, but was not pliable, suggesting the presence of subcutaneous adhesions. No signs of increased temperature or abnormal skin color was noted.

KNEE EVALUATION

No intra-articular effusion or periarticular swelling was evident. No tenderness at the tibial tubercle, patellar tendon, or inferior pole of the right patella was noted. No tenderness at the medial or lateral joint line was noted. There was moderate lateral patellar facet discomfort to palpation on the right side and minimal medial facet tenderness. Palpation of the superior pole revealed marked tenderness at the center, greater than the lateral aspect of the superior pole. An area approximately 1.5 in proximal to the superior pole and approximately ¾ in lateral to the midline of the patella was exquisitely point tender. Deep palpation of this area was painful and revealed a small oblong mass (3 × 7 mm) in the quadriceps tendon. This area was located superolateral to the superolateral arthroscopic scar.

Bilateral examination of the lateral and medial collateral ligaments by means of varus and valgus stress, respectively, was negative for asymmetry or instability at 0 degrees and 30 degrees of flexion. Posterior cruciate laxity was absent as measured by the posterior drawer test, and again bilateral symmetrical findings were noted. Anterior cruciate stability was symmetrical bilaterally as measured by the Lachman test and anterior drawer test with the tibia externally rotated, internally rotated, and at neutral. Meniscal signs of rotation with hyperflexion as well as extension were absent. Medial parapatellar plicae were palpated bilaterally with no asymmetrical enlargement or tenderness noted. Q angles were symmetrical bilaterally at 16 degrees.

MUSCLE STRENGTH

Isokinetic testing on the Kin-Com* to assess both concentric and eccentric muscle strength was performed. Initial Kin-Com measurements were as follows: At 60°/sec the uninvolved left side produced an average of 264 ft·lb per repetition for five consecutive concentric repetitions and 161 ft·lb for eccentric contractions. The involved right side was able to generate an average of 163 ft·lb per repetition for five consecutive concentric repetitions and 110 ft·lb for the eccentric contractions. Concentric quadriceps output to body weight ratio was evaluated as 122% on the left side and 75% on the right

side. Concentric strength was 61% of eccentric output on the left side and 67% on the right. The involved right quadriceps muscle was 38% weaker than the left side concentrically and 32% weaker eccentrically.

At 210°/sec, the noninvolved left side produced an average of 166 ft·lb per repetition for 10 consecutive concentric repetitions and 134 ft·lb for 10 eccentric contractions. The involved right side was able to generate an average of 175 ft·lb per repetition for 10 eccentric repetitions. Concentric strength was 82% of eccentric output on the left side and 84% on the right side. Side-to-side deficit was 23% eccentrically.

ADDITIONAL SUBJECTIVE INFORMATION

Tom was able to dunk the basketball from a stationary start using only the uninvolved left side to push off. Any attempt to use the right leg to provide propulsion in vertical jumping was painful. Sprinting speed was estimated by Tom to be about one-half normal, and any attempts to stop or start quickly were simply not possible. Jogging was tolerated well in a straight-ahead pattern but figure eights, straight, and crossover cutting were painful, especially when planting off the right leg attempting to move left. Present basketball drills consisted of free-throw shooting and jump shots limited to about 2 to 3 in off the floor. While off the court, Tom would ride the stationary bike, picking out a player on the floor and riding hard when the player was sprinting and slowing down when the player slowed down. Tom also used a rowing machine; did knee flexion and extension on an Orthotron* with a velocity spectrum workout; and performed positive and negative work knee extension on an N-K table.[†] Inconsistently, he performed modified knee drops, step ups, and line jumps.

After the initial visit, I checked with the university's athletic trainer and the physical therapist who had been seeing Tom during the summer while the patient was at home. Rehabilitation efforts in the summer consisted of

---

*Chattecx Corp, Chattanooga, TN

*Cybex, Division of Lumex, Inc, Ronkonkoma, NY
†N-K Products Company, Soquel, CA

isokinetic concentric and eccentric velocity spectrum training of the knee. The rehabilitation programming at the university was essentially as Tom had related to me. However, the trainer at the university was unaware that Tom was continuing eccentric loading away from the training room as well as inconsistently performing practice drills that were painful. The program at the university consisted of 8- to 10-lb weights on the N-K table with emphasis through the last 30 degrees of extension. The velocity spectrum workout on the Orthotron was appropriate, as were stretching exercises for the hamstrings. Gluteal strengthening was also being done to provide secondary backup for muscles used in jumping. Endurance training was being done in the form of pool running for 20 to 30 minutes three times a week.

Overuse injuries are graded on the athlete's perception of pain or lack of pain, as it relates to activity. Tom was still having pain with athletic activity. Pain had progressed to the point that it was affecting his level of play, but had not yet significantly affected activities of daily living. My impression of the patient's condition concurred with the clinical and arthroscopic diagnosis of quadriceps tendinitis, specifically stage 3.

TREATMENT

After initial evaluation and speaking with others involved in Tom's care, the following goals were established.

1. Increase muscle strength of the involved quadriceps both concentrically and eccentrically, as well as normalize the ratio of concentric to eccentric strength on the uninvolved left side.
2. Normalize muscle tone, which should occur if strength increases. For patellar tracking, my main area of concern here was the atrophied right vastus medialis muscle.
3. Decrease tenderness and pain, specifically the superolateral quadriceps tendon discomfort.
4. Improve bilateral flexibility of the hamstrings and gastrocnemius-soleus.

5. Improve function in a progressive manner to return Tom to basketball.
6. Maintain strength of noninvolved body parts as well as maintaining cardiovascular condition.

In addition to the physical goals, I hoped to gain Tom's trust. It was important for him to know that I also wanted him back in basketball as soon as possible. But at the same time, he needed to know that I was the boss, that I knew the best way to get him back on the court in as short a time as possible. A secondary psychological objective was to help to establish realistic goals.

Priority number one in implementing Tom's treatment program was to streamline my efforts and those of the trainer. It was important to reach an early mutual understanding of what I would do in the clinic and what the trainer would do in the training room. Discussions were held to lay down the groundwork for treatment emphasis and role delineation. This left no questions of expectations from Tom while in my presence, while in the training room, and what he could do at home.

I believed the most important area to emphasize was the lack of quadriceps strength, especially the eccentric strength, in this jumping athlete. Concentric strengthening was being addressed at school and would be continued. To focus on eccentric strengthening, I took Tom off all modified knee drops and concentrated on controlled, low-force, slow-speed eccentric loading on the Kin-Com. Strengthening work on the Kin-Com would address the decreased eccentric strength on the involved left side as well as both concentric and eccentric strength on the right side.

Coupled with the goal of increasing the muscle strength was the goal of increasing muscle tone. Concentric strengthening work on the N-K table through the last 30 degrees of extension was encouraged with simultaneous use of functional electrical stimulation. Abnormal muscle length existed in the form of tight hamstrings and gastrocnemius-soleus as well. In addition to stretching before and after workouts in the sit and reach position, prolonged wall stretches were added. Prolonged stretching of the calves was also done using a slant-board to supplement the forward leaning against the wall, which was done before and after workouts. Effective warm-up or the use of hot packs to the areas to be stretched was encouraged also.

The key to decreasing the pain and tenderness of the peripatellar area was activity modification. Prior to implementing the program, the trainer and I established who would do what, thereby minimizing the potential for overuse in the treatment program. More importantly, Tom had to understand that any activity that produced pain was making the knee worse and should be avoided. All jumping and tipping drills would be initially avoided, pain-free jogging was allowed, set shots were allowed, but small-scale jump shooting was not allowed if painful.

The area superior and lateral to the patella was treated with ultrasonography, continuous to tolerance, followed by deep massage (both transverse cross friction and longitudinal release as tolerated).

All functional progression drills were supervised by the trainer and were developed by the trainer and me. Tom would continue weight training of the upper body and lower body, with the exception of the quadriceps muscles. Gluteal strengthening and gastrocnemius-soleus strengthening were emphasized. Both aerobic and anaerobic conditioning work was also stressed, by use of the bike, rowing machine, and work in the pool.

After three weeks of isokinetic strengthening two to three times a week, another Kin-Com test was performed. At 60°/sec, noninvolved quadriceps strength (both concentric and eccentric) was 284 ft·lb. Therefore, eccentric strength was approximating normal in terms of eccentric to concentric ratio. The quadriceps to body weight ratio was still above normal at 132%. At 210°/sec, concentric to eccentric ratios were appropriate.

The involved right concentric quadriceps output for repetition at 60°/sec increased to 230 ft·lb, while eccentric strength was 159 ft·lb. Quadriceps to body weight ratio concentrically was now an acceptable 107% but still 19%

weaker than the opposite side. The concentric to eccentric strength ratio was still subpar, with eccentric strength 70% of concentric strength. Deficits of 15% were still present concentrically and eccentrically at 210°/sec.

Isokinetic training continued two to three times a week. As strength improved, forces were raised; if the knee was particularly sore on a given day, then forces were lowered. Forces were varied in a progressive resistive exercise (PRE) manner during the workouts. Strengthening continued less frequently on the noninvolved side. Concentric work on the involved right side was emphasized early in the workout at a velocity spectrum of 60, 90, 150, and 210°/sec, and later in the workout eccentrics were emphasized. The motions to be emphasized were easily controlled by the velocity settings, which are also capable of being adjusted independently of one another. For example, early in the workouts when eccentrics were de-emphasized, the speed of the unit was adjusted through the velocities previously mentioned on the upswing of the knee only and forces were kept high; the downswing (eccentric component) speed was kept consistently low, as were the forces, thereby requiring virtually no energy expenditure on eccentrics. As the emphasis changed to stressing eccentrics later in the workout, concentric speed was kept consistently low, with low forces required to move the lever arm. A slight pause was added in the workout after completing each concentric repetition, then varied forces were used at slow velocities to work the eccentric component of knee extension. As discomfort decreased with slow-speed eccentric loading, speeds were gradually increased, placing more stress on the tendon. Adjustments in force and velocity varied daily as dictated by patient tolerance.

Two weeks after the first retest, another Kin-Com evaluation was performed. At 60°/sec, output on the involved right side increased to an average 262 ft·lb per repetition concentrically and 222 ft·lb eccentrically. Concentric deficit comparing the involved right side to the left side was now 8% and eccentric deficit was 22%. Concentric to eccentric ratio had improved, with eccentrics 16% weaker than concentrics. The velocity and force spectrum workouts continued for concentric and eccentric work for another two weeks, at which time final measurements were recorded as follows. Concentric output at 60°/sec and eccentric work per repetition were less than 5% weaker than the left side. Eccentric strength improved at 60°/sec until it was actually 8% stronger than concentrics. A final test of the noninvolved left side showed eccentrics 12% stronger than the concentrics. Results at 210°/sec showed no deficit from side to side concentrically or eccentrically, with concentric to eccentric ratios also similar side to side.

Functional electrical stimulation with simultaneous quadriceps setting and terminal knee extension were stressed on the days Tom did not see me in the clinic. Weights were kept low, with emphasis placed on maintaining a firm contraction of the quadriceps with superimposed quadriceps setting and terminal extension on the N-K table, with the arm of the N-K table offset approximately 60 degrees. Definition of the vastus medialis muscle improved. Bilateral palpation of the vastus medialis muscle revealed that tone on the right was still decreased compared to the left. There was no difference in circumferential measurements at the termination of the treatment.

Active dorsiflexion of both ankles in the long-sitting position improved to 0 to 9 degrees, and I encouraged Tom to continue. Hamstring flexibility showed an increase of 18 to 20 degrees bilaterally, but continued vigorous work was encouraged here as well.

Knee extension work did not cause patellofemoral discomfort throughout the full range of motion. The patient received a total of six ultrasonography treatments to the superolateral quadriceps tendon. He was gradually able to tolerate increased pressure to this area when both he and I did deep friction massage to the quadriceps. Size of the mass diminished to approximately 3 × 3 mm.

It appeared to me that Tom complied with activity restrictions. During our treatment program, I believed he was honest with me regarding discomfort at the superior pole of the patella during eccentric loading. However, at the termination of treatment, he entered a game situation and attempted to block a shot. During the jump up and forward he noted significant discomfort at the quadriceps tendon. After this incident, his activity was reduced greatly for two weeks and he was allowed back into competition slowly. Rehabilitation after the incident was managed well by the trainer. As a result of the incident, Tom was not allowed to enter a game situation without aggressive warm-up and vigorous stretching.

Tom evaluated a variety of neoprene sleeves both during rehabilitation as well as in competition. Superior buttresses were incorporated into the sleeve, but were not tolerated. Nylon-lined interior sleeves were discarded in favor of nonlined neoprene. Tom said that the neoprene next to the skin felt warmer and gave uniform support, and that he did not have to work as hard to get the knee warm prior to activity.

Tom was progressed from forward and lateral step ups off a 3-in platform to an approximately 8-in platform. At the termination of our treatments, he was gradually eased into an eccentric loading program consisting of the modified knee drops. Jogging on the court was advanced to one-half speed sprinting, to three-quarter speed, and finally to full speed. The sprinting progression began by jogging into the sprint and slowing down slowly, and progressed to the point where sprinting was performed from a stationary position. Quick stops were then added. Tipping and jumping drills were kept pain free, and performance varied from day to day. Jump shots were progressed from bilateral support at take off and landing, gradually increasing the height of the jump, to unilateral take off and landing, to unilateral work while off balance. Vertical jump had improved, but not yet to the point of preinjury level.

During the first retest a small problem presented itself. As a safety feature of the Kin-Com, if excessive force is applied to the load cell, the machine will shut itself down to protect itself from damage. Originally, the force settings were low, and as Tom got stronger he was able to exert too much force at these low settings and shut the machine down. Tom seemed fascinated by his ability to overcome the machine, and suddenly began to show interest in which force settings were used.

CASE VARIATION 1

Tom shared some similarities with other athletes I have seen. Pat was a talented senior volleyball player at one of the local Catholic high schools. She also had an involved case of jumper's knee, which presented itself early in the season when a weight training program was added to regular training by an enthusiastic graduate student. However, Pat also had vague peripatellar pain, pain on ascending stairs, and pain after sitting for a prolonged period of time (movie sign). She also had marked medial patellar facet tenderness, and decreased vastus medialis definition both by palpation and visual inspection. Eccentric loading was too painful to be performed. Pat required a different program because of the impression of patellofemoral pain syndrome and possibly chondromalacia patellae. Initial efforts were directed at decreasing patellofemoral symptoms. All full knee extension exercises were stopped, and heavy concentration was given to hamstring flexibility. Active knee extension with the hips flexed to 90 degrees was 45 degrees from complete knee extension. All concentric weight training was done through the last 30 degrees of knee extension. Spiking drills as well as blocking drills at the net were stopped. Pain gradually decreased over the course of three weeks to allow a pain-free eccentric loading program. The program was gradually progressed to allow a safe return to all jumping activities. Pat recovered completely. She led her team to a conference championship and won all-conference honors herself.

CASE VARIATION 2

Dick was also another patient with a stubborn case of extensor mechanism overload. Most of Dick's symptoms involved the patellar tendon versus the quadriceps tendon. He was a recreational volleyball player in a men's league that played competitively twice a week. Dick thought that the sun rose and set over his volleyball activities, and he had an even tougher time than Tom did in modifying his activity level at a pain-free stage. Dick also did a lot of "doctor shopping," that is, he sought numerous opinions until he heard what he wanted to hear. Early in Dick's rehabilitation, he inquired about an injection into the area that would let him play without pain. I explained to Dick that this was indeed done, but only as a last resort. I also tried to impress upon Dick the need for absolute rest after a steroid injection. Finally, Dick fell by the wayside, and failed to keep his last scheduled appointment. The last time I saw him he was still experiencing pain when playing volleyball, but he would not quit. His painful knee caused him missed time from work as a truck driver, which, he confided to me, was also causing problems in his marriage. The pain was so bad that he was unable to ascend or descend stairs or rise from a chair without assistance from his arms. Needless to say, his vertical jump was nonexistent, he was not happy with his volleyball capabilities, and he wanted to have something done. Dick returned two weeks after missing his last scheduled appointment with me, "feeling like a new man." He had received a cortisone injection the previous day from yet another physician. "You think I can play tonight?" he asked. With a vehement "*No!*," I explained for what seemed like the hundredth time the need for absolute rest after an injection. Two weeks later, I saw Dick's name on the surgery schedule for repair of a ruptured patellar tendon.

CASE VARIATION 3

John was a basketball player at a local high school. He was a junior who started varsity as a sophomore. John's summer vacation was no vacation, because he spent it at three national-level basketball camps. The last camp was cut short when he developed quadriceps tendon pain, which was exquisite when he first saw me. Hamstring and gastrocnemius-soleus flexibility were adequate. Rest and ice did not significantly decrease John's pain. Friction massage was also of no benefit. John underwent five treatments of phonophoresis with 10% hydrocortisone, which decreased his pain significantly. After completing the course of phonophoresis treatments, John began quadriceps setting exercises and straight leg raising for another two weeks, and returned for a baseline isokinetic evaluation. Concentric to eccentric ratios were normal, and the deficit of the involved right knee was less than 5% compared to the noninvolved left side both concentrically and eccentrically after three weeks of rehabilitation. John's quadriceps definition was outstanding and quadriceps to body weight ratios were both over 110%. However, hamstring to quadriceps ratio was a pitiful 30%. All weight training at the school had emphasized the quadriceps (ie, knee extension, vertical and horizontal leg presses, and squats.) The only hamstring work was one set of 10 repetitions of bilateral knee flexion. This was increased in intensity and unilateral work was begun. John was able to play his next season without symptoms.

CONCLUSION

The role of the extensor mechanism of the knee is vital in sports, especially in those requiring jumping. I consider all of these problems a true professional challenge. What makes them interesting is not only the individual personalities involved, but also the specific clinical presentation and management of each case.

61 Head Trauma

CHERYL WARDLAW

The picture grew worse as I read through Jennie's chart. The active life of this 22-year-old woman had been rudely interrupted a month ago in a car accident. Her friends were already out of the hospital. Jennie wasn't as lucky. A CT scan had confirmed the suspected left subdural hematoma in the parietal region. A left craniotomy had been performed to evacuate the hematoma and reduce the damage from its pressure.

Jennie had remained unresponsive to all but the deepest pain since the accident. Initially ventilator dependent, she quickly regained her respiratory control. Now, a month later, she was transferred to our facility for further evaluation and care.

The problem list grew as the medical evaluations took place. A subsequent CT scan at our facility revealed a hydrocephalic condition and a right temporal enhancement of a hematoma. (Jennie's motor problems could involve all extremities!) A ventriculopuncture (VP) shunt was placed on the right. Her left eye was infected with *Candida,* and a vitrectomy was performed. (We didn't know if her vision would return.) The right elbow fracture, sustained in the accident, would require a joint replacement "eventually." (Frankly, none of the medical staff thought she would wake up enough for the elbow to matter.) For now, the elbow remained cast in 100 degrees of flexion.

I put away her chart and, for the first time, I slipped into the back of Jennie's room to watch quietly for a while. Her head was a mass of brown stubbles. Red crescent-shaped scars from her evacuation and shunt arched over each ear. The right eye was expressionless and unmoving, while the left was covered with a patch. Her top teeth rested on her lower lip, giving her the appearance of a large rabbit. Jennie's stocky frame was well muscled. (No sign of disuse atrophy.) The right arm was torqued internally at the shoulder by the weight of the cast. The right hand hung limply from the plaster, indicating a possible brachial plexus injury during the accident. The other extremities rested in a relaxed but decorticate posture. No spontaneous movements occurred.

A lab assistant entered the room and began to draw a blood sample. Jennie curled tighter into her decorticate posture. Only the right arm and hand remained limp. Her teeth chewed her bottom lip savagely and Jennie's neck arched into extension. The response to pain was obvious.

After the lab assistant left, I walked over to Jennie. As I began to handle her, I talked to her and told her what I was doing. She again resumed her posturing and lip biting. Any contact at this point was noxious to her. Any passive motion of the right arm evoked the strongest response. I felt certain that poor positioning had allowed the weight of the cast to torque the right shoulder during turning. This continued abuse to the shoulder must have caused soft tissue and capsular damage. Attempts to assess the range of motion of the right shoulder beyond the neutral range appeared cruel. The long finger flexors and extensors of the right hand were slightly contracted. Passive movement of the right hand did not evoke a mass response, which told me that there was no sensation in the hand.

It took considerable strength to break the spastic posturing of Jennie's body. Her neck remained rigidly in extension. Attempts to open the jaw and reposition the lips were unsuccessful. Because of the spasticity, accurate range measurements were impossible. Clearly, however, the neck and right shoulder were severely limited in range. The flexor spasticity in her left upper extremity and the extensor spasticity in her lower extremities was almost impossible to move against. However, with the exception of a dorsiflexion contracture 10 degrees from neutral in the right ankle, the joints were at least functionally flexible. A positive response to the Babinsky test could be elicited bilaterally. I assumed by her response to pain that at least crude sensation was present.

Jennie's family was intelligent, caring, and eager to carry out any activity. With rare exception, someone was always with Jennie. I assumed that Jennie had been just as intelligent as the other members of her family. I asked them about her likes, dislikes, and life-style. I discovered that Jennie had been caring, fun loving, hard working, sarcastic, and an avid football fan. She preferred the company of a few friends to large parties, and was extremely close to her family. She worked as a computer operator in the family business. Country and western music was her favorite, but not the "moaning and groaning" kind. All this information would help our team tailor a positive, familiar environment that could coax Jennie from the dark world of her coma. We surrounded her with the smells and sounds she would recognize. We kidded with her as if we had been longtime friends, even though she could not respond at this time. Finally, the family brought in a picture of Jennie—she was lovely. I asked the family if I could post the picture in Jennie's room, because I wanted everyone to know her better.

I estimated that Jennie was at level 2 on the Rancho Los Amigos Cognitive Scale (Table 61-1):

Patient reacts inconsistently and nonpurposefully to stimuli in a nonspecific manner. Responses are limited in nature and are often the same regardless of the stimulus presented. Responses may be physiological changes, gross body movements and/or vocalizations. Often the earliest response is to deep pain. Responses are likely to be delayed.

At this point, our diagnosis, goals, and treatment for Jennie's traumatic head injuries were as follows.

Diagnosis

- Left parietal subdural hematoma
- Hydrocephalus
- Right temporal hematoma
- Level 2 cognitively

Goals

1. Alter the patient's perception of contact from negative to selective.
2. Reduce decorticate posturing.
3. Promote some purposeful movement.

Treatment

1. Campaign of positive input: familiar sounds (family talking to her about family happenings, music to drown out the hospital noises); familiar smells (favorite powders, perfumes, her own pillow from home); familiar tactile input (using Jennie's own hand to touch her face and body; stroking; gentle and nonpainful touch); explain what was going on and why, whenever a painful procedure had to be used.
2. Perform gentle ranging, with emphasis on rotation and activities with the distal segment fixed (eg, hook lying). Concentrate on head position; use gentle soft tissue mobilization techniques to elongate muscles, then use approximation to stabilize the neck in a neutral position, progress to short range rotation of the neck (place patient's hand behind her head and use her hand to rotate the head). Use the sidelying position to flex Jennie and reduce tonic influence. Perform tilt tabling with careful positioning to fix the distal segments (right upper extremity in sling during this proce-

Table 61-1. Levels of Cognitive Functioning

1. No response	Patient appears to be in a deep sleep and is completely unresponsive to any stimuli presented to him.
2. Generalized response	Patient reacts inconsistently and nonpurposefully to stimuli in a nonspecific manner. Responses are limited in nature and are often the same regardless of stimulus presented. Responses may by physiological changes, gross body movements and/or vocalization. Often the earliest response is to deep pain. Responses are likely to be delayed.
3. Localized response	Patient reacts specifically but inconsistently to stimuli. Responses are directly related to the type of stimulus presented as in turning head toward a sound, focusing on an object presented. The patient may withdraw an extremity and/or vocalize when presented with a painful stimulus. He may follow simple commands in an inconsistent delayed manner such as closing his eyes, squeezing or extending an extremity. Once external stimuli are removed, he may lie quietly. He may also show a vague awareness of self and body by responding to discomfort by pulling at nasogastric tube or catheter or resisting restraints. He may show a bias toward responding to some persons (especially family and friends) but not to others.
4. Confused-Agitated	Patient is in a heightened state of activity with severely decreased ability to process information. He is detached from the present and responds primarily to his own internal confusion. Behavior is frequently bizarre and nonpurposeful relative to his immediate environment. He may cry out or scream out of proportion to stimuli even after removal, may show aggressive behavior, attempt to remove restraints or tubes or crawl out of bed in a purposeful manner. He does not, however, discriminate among persons or objects and is unable to cooperate directly with treatment efforts. Verbalization is frequently incoherent and/or inappropriate to the environment. Confabulation may be present; he may be euphoric or hostile. Thus gross attention to environment is very short and selective attention is often nonexistent. Being unaware of present events, patient lacks short-term recall and may be reacting to past events. He is unable to perform self care (feeding, dressing) without maximum assistance. If not disabled physically, he may perform motor activities such as sitting, reaching and ambulating, but as part of his agitated state and not as a purposeful act or on request necessarily.
5. Confused, inappropriate nonagitated	Patient appears alert and is able to respond to simple commands fairly consistently. However, with increased complexity of commands or lack of any external structure, responses are nonpurposeful, random, or at best fragmented toward any desired goal. He may show agitated behavior, but not on an internal basis (as in level 4), but rather as a result of external stimuli, and usually out of proportion to the stimulus. He has gross attention to the environment, but is highly distractable and lacks ability to focus attention to a specific task without frequent redirection back to it. With structure, he may be able to converse on a social-automatic level for short periods of time. Verbalization is often inappropriate; confabulation may be triggered by present events. His memory is severely impaired, with confusion of past and present in his reaction to ongoing activity. Patient lacks initiation of functional tasks and often shows inappropriate use of objects without external direction. He may be able to perform previously learned tasks when structured for him, but is unable to learn new information. He responds best to self, body, comfort and often family members. The patient can usually perform self-care activities with assistance and may accomplish feeding with maximum supervision. Management on the ward is often a problem if the patient is physically mobile, as he may wander off either randomly or with vague intention of "going home."

(Hagen C, Malkmus D, Durham P: Communication Disorders Service, Rancho Los Amigos Hospital, Downey, CA, 1972. Revised 11/15/74 by Malkmus D, Stenderup K)

continued

Table 61-1. Levels of Cognitive Functioning (continued)

6. Confused-Appropriate	Patient shows goal-directed behavior, but is dependent on external input for direction. Response to discomfort is appropriate and he is able to tolerate unpleasant stimuli (as NG tube) when need is explained. He follows simple directions consistently and shows carryover for tasks he has relearned (as self care). He is at least supervised with old learning; unable to be maximally assisted for new learning with little or no carryover. Responses may be incorrect due to memory problem, but they are appropriate to the situation. They may be delayed to immediate, and he shows decreased ability to process information with little or no anticipation or prediction of events. Past memories show more depth and detail than recent memory.
	The patient may show beginning immediate awareness of situation by realizing he doesn't know an answer. He no longer wanders and is inconsistently oriented to time and place. Selective attention to tasks may be impaired especially with difficult tasks and in unstructured settings, but is now functional for common daily activities (30 min. with structured). He may show a vague recognition of some staff, has increased awareness of self, family and basic needs (as food), again in an appropriate manner as in contrast to level 5.
7. Automatic-Appropriate	Patient appears appropriate and oriented within hospital and home settings, goes through daily routine automatically, but frequently robot-like, with minimal-to-absent confusion, but has shallow recall of what he has been doing. He shows increased awareness of self, body, family, foods, people and interaction in the environment. He has superficial awareness of, but lacks insight into his condition, decreased judgment and problem-solving and lacks realistic planning for his future. He shows carryover for new learning, but at a decreased rate. He requires at least minimal supervision for learning and for safety purposes. He is independent in self-care activities and supervised in home and community skills for safety. With structure he is able to initiate tasks as social or recreation activities in which he now has interest. His judgment remains impaired; such that he is unable to drive a car. Prevocational or avocational evaluation and counseling may be indicated.
8. Purposeful and appropriate	Patient is alert and oriented, is able to recall and integrate past and recent events and is aware of and responsive to his culture. He shows carryover for new learning if acceptable to him and his life role, and needs no supervision once activities are learned. Within his physical capabilities, he is independent in home and community skills, including driving. Vocational rehabilitation, to determine ability to return as contributor to society (perhaps in a new capacity), is indicated. He may continue to show a decreased ability, relative to premorbid abilities, in abstract reasoning, tolerance for stress, judgment in emergencies or unusual circumstances. His social, emotional and intellectual capacities may continue to be at a decreased level for him, but functional in society.

(Hagen C, Malkmus D, Durham P: Communication Disorders Service, Rancho Los Amigos Hospital, Downey, CA, 1972. Revised 11/15/74 by Malkmus D, Stenderup K)

dure. Improve lip closure and swallowing (use Rood's three-point jaw control with stroking and use of icing around lips to improve closure).

3. Provide appropriate amounts of vestibular stimulation (rocking with Jennie resting against us in bed, and rocking in sidelying position, as well as the head and neck work listed earlier). Create a kinesthetic awareness of movement (place Jennie in a variety of positions and "teach" her how to get out of the positions through the use of approximation, quick stretch, tapping, quick icing, as well as the techniques of rhythmic initiation and repeated stretch at the beginning of the range). Sessions were kept short to avoid overstimulation.

I was also convinced that she had sustained soft tissue or capsular damage in the right shoulder. Diagnosis, goals, and treatment for the shoulder were as follows.

Diagnosis

- Soft tissue and capsular damage to right shoulder

Goals

1. Reduce pain in shoulder.
2. Increase range of motion.

Treatment

1. Grade 2 joint mobilization; soft tissue mobilization; moist heat; careful positioning (family assigned to be "watchdogs" to see that the arm was always in a good position; arm in sling whenever Jennie was out of bed).
2. Use of positioning to maintain range as above methods reduced pain and more range could be obtained.

During this time, the occupational and speech therapy departments were pursuing similar goals. Each group provided a different emphasis, yet all overlapped to provide Jennie with a plan of coordinated care. This teamwork was Jennie's only hope. The occupational therapist approached our goal of improving Jennie's perception by providing pleasant tactile input through identifying textures Jennie appeared to like and training the family how to use them. The occupational therapist also developed visually stimulating activities for Jennie. Proper sling selection and splint fabrication assisted in the goal of improved range and joint protection. The speech therapist concentrated on the development of Jennie's lip closure and swallowing. The development of the ability to take foods orally would move Jennie that much farther from the darkness she was living in.

At this point, ask yourself what you would do if the patient stayed at this level? How long would you continue with the same treatment before you would try something else? How long would you treat the patient before terminating the treatment?

It took weeks for our treatment plan to pay off, but slowly Jennie's posturing and lip biting diminished. I'll never forget the day Jennie began vocalizing. My mind must have been miles away as I overstretched Jennie's right heelcord. The leg flew up into flexion. Jennie screamed animalistically. I apologized profusely, and it seemed to me that the leg began to relax. (Were we finally communicating? Had she reached a higher level of cognitive functioning?) I stroked Jennie's face and talked to her gently to calm her. For an instant, her vacant stare seemed to focus.

Jennie began using grunting and nonspecific yelling to communicate her displeasure. Left alone, she was quiet. We couldn't be sure she was responding verbally to us until the day her mother entered the room with a cheery "Hi, Jen," and Jennie stopped howling and looked towards her mom. Finally, Jennie was beginning to vary her response to match the stimulus presented! This type of behavior gave us our first undeniable clue that Jennie's coma level was improving. Tracking gradually improved as well. Occasionally, I was sure Jennie intentionally smiled or refrained from smiling! One day during rolling activities, Jennie turned her head to help roll back. I was certain at that point that Jennie was now at level 3 on the cognitive scale:

> Patient reacts specifically but inconsistently to stimuli. Responses are directly related to the type of stimuli presented. . . . The patient may withdraw an extremity and/or verbalize when presented with painful stimulus. He may follow simple commands in an inconsistent delayed manner such as closing eyes, squeezing or extending an extremity. Once external stimuli are removed, he will lie quietly. He may show a vague awareness of self and body by responding to discomfort by pulling at nasogastric tube or catheter or resisting restraints. He may show a bias towards responding to some persons (especially family and friends) but not to others.

Our goals and treatment for cognitive level 3 functioning were as follows.

Goals

1. Facilitate righting and balance reactions.
2. Independent head control.

3. Sit independently for brief periods.
4. Promote purposeful communications.

Treatment
1. While Jennie was in supported sitting or on the tilt table, the left hand was positioned so that irradiation would promote weight bearing and righting response. Tracking activities were carried out by the family (often using pictures of loved ones or personal belongings). Approximation was used to facilitate stabilization, then Jennie would be moved slightly off center so that she would either "fall" (a feeling Jennie hated), or catch herself.
2. Use of approximation was followed by placing Jennie slightly off center to promote balance reaction from head (and trunk).
3. Two therapists were required to position Jennie appropriately for sitting. The therapist in front would keep Jennie's hips abducted and flexed, and approximate through the heels to promote balance reactions (a treatment block was placed under the right heel because of contracture). The therapist in back would prevent Jennie from throwing herself back into extension (neck and trunk) and keep her pelvis in an anterior tilt. Following massive yelling on Jennie's part and energy expenditure on our parts, Jennie would "rest" in a good sitting position. Approximation was used to "teach" her the position kinesthetically.

   The Indian sitting position in bed was also used when Jennie was too agitated to safely sit on the side of the bed. We would use the electric bed to bring her into sitting, block her with our bodies, and then lower the bed.
4. We would explain simply what Jennie must do, and explain that we expected her to do it or we couldn't leave. (This posture was not carried out to an extreme; any sign of fear or anger on Jennie's part ended the session.) Encouragements were made for Jennie to speak instead of just scream when she wasn't happy. Often we would ask her, "Tell us if you are tired. Are you tired? Say 'yes' and you can stop. Tell us what hurts," and so on.
5. In addition, all activities relating to care of Jennie's right shoulder were continued.

The occupational therapist stressed the faciliation of motor function for the left upper extremity, using many of the same techniques outlined earlier. Stimulation activities, splint modification, and positioning aides were stressed. The facilitation of righting reactions were a major team effort. The speech therapist was able to progress her bulbar program as Jennie's bite diminished. Swallowing and lip closure continued as key emphasis areas.

At this point, once again ask yourself how long you should give the treatment a try before changing treatments. What other treatments could you try if Jennie stayed at the same level?

For a while, the therapists were getting all the exercise. I often believed that Jennie knew how to use her spasticity to "work us over." Regardless, we stayed the course for the treatment plan. One day the fighting stopped, and Jennie pulled herself up onto a balanced sitting position. Her left arm pushed to help her balance (she had only demonstrated a flexion synergy until then). Then Jennie relaxed back against me. The therapy sessions were less of a battle and more of a team effort from then on. On some days Jennie's headstrong nature won out, but we now had a better picture of what was possible. Until then, we were not certain of what physical limitations to expect as a result of her closed head injury. After several repeats of Jennie's sitting performance, we were reasonably sure that she had the potential functionally to use all but her right arm. The right arm remained motionless, even with the cast now removed.

Attempts at meaningful communication took a dramatic turn for the better. I entered Jennie's room to take her to the physical therapy department. Jennie looked exhausted, as did her mother. I asked "Jennie, you look tired. Are you up to exercising?" Jennie looked towards me and simply said "No." All eyes focused on Jennie's face. We were completely silent, doubting what we had heard. Her mother rushed to Jennie's side, begging her to speak. The answer was a garbled but beautiful ''Maaa.'' Jennie's level was on the rise!

The ability to use purposeful, one-word responses increased, as did Jennie's ability to follow simple commands, although the latter was inconsistent. Until now, we had been limited to activities that evoked automatic responses. Jennie's growing ability to understand and follow simple commands allowed us to emphasize higher-level skills. We quickly progressed to standing activities, but not without a fight. Pushing activities were refined into reaching activities. The occupational therapist could now begin training Jennie for activities of daily living. The speech therapist continued to develop Jennie's swallowing, but began to work on development of speaking skills.

We transferred Jennie to the rehabilitation center shortly after that. Our two-month relationship saw Jennie progress from a cognitive level 2 to a cognitive level 4:

Patient is in heightened state of activity with severely decreased ability to process information. He is detached from the present and responds primarily to his own internal confusion. Behavior is frequently bizarre and nonpurposeful relative to his immediate environment. He may cry out or scream out of proportion to stimuli even after removal, may show aggressive behavior, attempt to remove restraints or tubes or crawl out of bed in a purposeful manner. He does not, however, discriminate among persons or objects and is unable to cooperate directly with treatment efforts. Verbalization is frequently incoherent or inappropriate to the environment. Confabulation may be present; he may be euphoric or hostile. Thus gross attention to environment is very short and selective attention is often nonexistent. Being unaware of present events, patients lacks short-term recall and may be reacting to past events. He is unable to perform self care without maximum assistance. If not disabled physically, he may perform ambulating, but not as a purposeful act or on request necessarily.

For cognitive level 4 functioning, the following goals and treatments were implemented.

Goal
1. Minimal assistance with coming to stand and standing.
2. Equal weight bearing; ability to weight shift.
3. Increased sitting balance.
4. Increased ability to process commands.
5. Promotion of purposeful communications.

Treatment
1. On tilt table, manually bend Jennie's knees within her ability to straighten the knees. Progress to resisting knee straightening. In bars, use therapists to maintain trunk in flexion as Jennie pushes herself up into standing. Once in standing, use approximation with feet even first. Progress to feet uneven.
2. Same activities as above, plus assisting weight shift, followed immediately by approximation. Use of rhythmic initiation, progressing to resistance. Mat activities emphasize terminal extension and posterior depression of the pelvis.
3. Same procedures as in treatment for level 3. Progress with use of resistance as Jennie tolerated (first in static posture, then to dynamic changes). Fixed left upper extremity was used as key point of control.
4. Simplify commands, and repeat them slowly. Give plenty of time for processing. Gestures are helpful.
5. Reward Jennie for talking, not screaming (eg, give her popsicles following treatment; take her outside).

Throughout our care for Jennie, several concepts were basic to our approach. The first concept was that physical limitations result from cognitive impairment as well as from neurologic and orthopedic trauma. Second, despite limitations, the patient remains a human being, deserving the same dignity and caring that any other human being receives. Third, controlling the nature of all stimuli is critical, with the emphasis on providing positive and well-proportioned stimuli. Fourth, pain must be avoided. Fifth, the constructs of simple to complex, and reflex to purposeful certainly apply.

Jennie continued to improve after her transfer to the rehabilitation center. While there, she progressed through levels 5 and 6 on the cognitive scale. Use of the right arm did not return. The elbow was for all intents fused, the hand motionless, and the shoulder moved only as a response to the movement of the rest of her body. As to our hypothesis that the bra-chial plexus had been injured, no tests were ever performed to confirm or refute the possibility. Upon discharge, Jennie was able to ambulate, dress, and feed herself. The skills of cooking, money changing, and community transportation eluded her. Jennie could carry on a limited conversation and follow two-step commands. With the assistance of the hospital social service department, Jennie was placed in a community center for persons with closed head injuries. I am convinced that she had no idea who I was when I visited her there.

62 A Spinal Cord Injury

MARION B. SCHONEBERGER

Shortly after I arrived at work this morning, my supervisor told me that I would be assigned a new patient who was being transferred from another state. From the preadmission referral I learned that Robert Smith was a 19-year-old male who was injured 2 weeks ago when he fell while swinging on a rope. The preadmission referral gave a diagnosis of paraplegia secondary to T12 compression fracture. The patient underwent posterior Harrington rod instrumentation and spinal fusion from T9 to L3. He had no medical complications following surgery and was being transferred in stable condition. I would have to wait until he arrived with his complete medical history to get more information, but it appeared that the patient was appropriate for a comprehensive rehabilitation program.

It was late morning by the time Mr. Smith arrived. I wondered if I would be able to see him today to begin my evaluation. A patient is quite busy for the first several days of his admission because of the many different team members who must meet and evaluate him: physician, nurse, physical therapist, occupational therapist, social worker, psychologist, orthotist, and recreation therapist. As I walked by his room I noticed that the curtain was drawn around his bed and the physician was taking a history and doing a physical. I decided that now would be a good chance to review the medical record for more detailed information about him and his injury.

As I reviewed his chart I looked for the date and location of the vertebral fracture, as well as the date and type of surgery done. This information tells me whether the spine is stable and gives me evaluation and treatment guidelines (Table 62-1). Because Mr. Smith's T12 compression fracture was reduced with Harrington rod instrumentation and a posterior fusion performed from T9 to L3, his spine was considered stable. However, because it was less than three weeks since the injury, I would need to avoid motion of the pelvis and spine, which might interfere with healing of the fracture and surgery. Specific activities to avoid are stretch to the hips when measuring range of motion and manual resistance to trunk and hips when muscle testing. I also looked for other fractures or medical problems that might interfere with the initiation of treatment or influence the type of rehabilitation program to be planned. I read that he had a small, superficial sacral pressure sore, which I would look at when I evaluated him. This meant that he would probably not be permitted to sit until the sore was healed. Pressure sores sometimes can delay a full rehabilitation program for weeks to months, and may even require surgical closure of the wound.

The medical record contained other information that helped me know Mr. Smith better, such as educational background, employment status, family situation, and life-style. At the time of his accident, Mr. Smith was attending college and was a sophomore majoring in Communications. He also had worked for three years as a stock boy in a grocery store. His parents live nearby, which explains why he was transferred here from another state for

Table 62-1. Guidelines for the Treatment of Patients with Paraplegia

	PARAPLEGIA WITH SPINE STABILIZATION (FUSION, RODS, SPRINGS)		
TIME	*Treatment*	*Evaluation*	*Activity level*

Onset or post-op	LE: ROM—no stretch to hips
	UE: resistive exercise, bilateral
	Respiratory Program
	    Postural drainage
	    Deep breathing
	    Coughing
	    IPP
	    Reeducation/strengthening
		X-rays: AP and Lateral
		MMT: no resistance to
		    trunk and hips
			Log roll—min. 2 man turn
			Body jacket when upright
			Wheelchair sitting/propulsion
			Self raise
			Dependent sliding board transfer

3 weeks	Hamstring stretch
	Abdominal and back
	    strengthening—
	    symmetrical and isometric
	LE: resistive exercise, bilateral
	UE: resistive exercise, unilateral
		X-rays: AP and Lateral
		MMT: minimal resistance
		    to trunk and hips.
			Prone
			UE: dressing
			Wheelies
			Transfers—straight depression total
			    assist with legs
			Walking (minimal functional loss)
			Self application of external
			    catheter—Sidelying or upright
			    with body jacket

6 weeks	LE: Resistive exercise, unilateral
	Active sitting balance exercise
	Self ROM
		MMT: no limitations	Log roll—1 man with patient
			    assist
			Self bowel program in body jacket
			LE dressing in body jacket
			Transfers—bed, toilet and car
			Gait training—complete injury
			Unrestricted upper extremity
			    activity (eg, driving, household,
			    sports)

3 months	Mat Work
	    Scooting
	    Rolling
	    Coming to Sitting
	    Resistive Balancing
	    Abdominal and Back
	    Strengthening—Resistive
		X-rays: Flexion and
		    Extension
			DC log roll
			DC body jacket
			Self-positioning and lying prone
			Self skin inspection
			Self intermittent catheterization
			    (Females)
			Self ROM
			LE dressing
			Transfers: floor, tub
			Wet bath
			Wheelchair into car
			Curb jumping
			Ambulation with elevation and
			    falling
			Wheelchair sports

(Courtesy of Rancho Los Amigos Medical Center, Downey, CA 90242)

rehabilitation. His family, which includes four brothers, was described as very supportive. His recreational activities included playing baseball and basketball. As I thought about this patient's educational level, his previous active life-style, and his supportive family, I was an-ticipating that he would be a good rehabilitation candidate and was looking forward to meeting him.

As I headed toward the patient's room, I passed the physician in the hall, and asked if he had additional information that would affect my evaluation or program. As I suspected, Mr. Smith was not cleared to sit until his pressure sore was healed. The physician had requested that the orthotist check the fit of the thoracolumbosacral orthosis (body jacket), which is worn for three months to prevent spine motion, especially trunk rotation, while the fusion heals.

I walked up to Mr. Smith's bedside and noticed he was positioned on his right side. The evaluation is more easily performed in the supine position, but this position should be avoided for healing a sacral pressure sore. I introduced myself, and explained that I was a physical therapist who would be working with him during his rehabilitation. I asked what name he liked to be called, to which he replied "Rob." I explained that I needed to test such things as the strength of his muscles and how much feeling he had in his legs. As I was saying this, he nodded his head and said with a smile, "I have already been poked by quite a few people, but go ahead." I returned the smile and was impressed by the patient's sense of humor and cooperation. These qualities would be pleasant for me to deal with during the next few months. More importantly, these qualities indicate a patient who will benefit maximally from a rehabilitation program.

I began with the sensory testing, which included light touch sensation carried through the anterior spinothalamic tract and dorsal columns, superficial pain sensation carried through the lateral spinothalamic tract, and joint proprioception carried through the dorsal columns. Other sensory tests can be performed (ie, vibratory sense, deep pressure, and temperature); however, the ones I chose not only test the function of different tracts in the spinal cord and help to determine the level and extent of neurologic injury, but also have functional importance in projecting goals for the patient. Although Rob was guessing during the sensory testing (he sometimes responded even when I did not touch him), I found all sensation to be absent below the T12 dermatome, including that in the sacral segments. It is especially important to test sacral sensation carefully because its presence indicates an in-

complete lesion, and therefore an improved prognosis for neurologic recovery. The skin is very susceptible to breakdown or pressure sores when superficial pain sensation is impaired. Education about skin care needed to begin immediately with Rob, because he already had a small sacral pressure sore. Rob's absent sensation was also going to affect other functional areas, such as sitting balance, general body handling skills, transfers, and ambulation potential. Even in the absence of volitional motor control, light touch, superficial pain sensation, and proprioception help compensate for motor loss, resulting in improved balance and body-handling skills. The sparing of sensation also can be extremely significant in personal relationships.

Next, I evaluated passive range of motion, looking for obvious contractures or limitations that would interfere with functional activities. All was within normal limits except for straight leg range (SLR). He had only 80 degrees of easy SLR. (Remember, no stretch to the hips is allowed until three weeks after surgery.) The goal is for 110 degrees of SLR, which allows adequate range of motion to long-sit for dressing, self range of motion, and certain wheelchair depression transfers without stretching out the trunk muscles. If the trunk muscles become stretched or elongated, it is more difficult to clear the trunk from the sitting surface in a depression or push-up type of transfer. I also evaluated "fast" range of motion to see if I could elicit spasticity and at what point in the range it "catches." It is important to note when spasticity interferes with positioning or functional activities. Rob had no spasticity, which means either that he was still in spinal shock or had a cauda equina injury. Range of motion in the upper extremities was normal.

The results of manual muscle testing help determine the functional neurologic level as well as establish realistic goals. When performing the muscle testing I kept in mind Rob's orthopedic restrictions: no motion of the trunk, stretch to the hips, or resistance to the trunk and hips. I asked Rob to do an isometric contraction and palpated for trunk flexion, extension, and all hip motions. For abdominal flexion I felt the quality of contraction on both the right and left sides and looked for any deviation of the umbilicus to determine if both the upper and lower abdominals were present. Because trunk motion was not allowed, I was able only to indicate that the abdominals were present, and would not be able to determine a grade until he was cleared for that motion (usually three months after surgery).

For the hips, where no resistance was allowed, I again palpated for an isometric contraction and felt none. Even though Rob repeatedly told me he "could not move his legs," I still tested each muscle for a palpable contraction, focusing on those innervated by the sacral segments, such as toe flexion. Voluntary motor control in muscles supplied by sacral segments indicates an incomplete lesion and an improved prognosis for neurologic recovery. Because Rob had no sensation, it would be possible for him to have a trace contraction that he was not able to feel. I did not palpate any muscle contractions in Rob's legs, and because he had no spasticity I felt confident with my evaluation results. When spasticity is present, it can be more difficult to separate voluntary motor control from a spastic contraction, especially because some patients can voluntarily set off their spasticity. When voluntary motor control is present, the patient should be able to contract and relax the muscle on command. If I am still in doubt I will retest the muscle in question the next day. Voluntary motor control, even a trace contraction, should be reproducible from one day to the next. Testing the strength of Rob's upper extremities was restricted to bilateral resistance to avoid unilateral trunk motion, but I anticipated them to be normal. Once he was three weeks postsurgery and cleared to be up in his chair, I could selectively grade the strength in his arms.

With the sensory and motor testing completed I was able to establish Rob's functional neurologic level. This is defined as the lowest segmental level with intact sensation and at least fair-plus strength. This was at the T12 dermatome level for Rob. Even though I was not able to test his abdominals for fair grade, in my opinion, the quality of his isometric contraction

was obviously better than poor, and I anticipated it to be fair-plus or greater. Rob's lesion was also defined as complete because he had no sensation or voluntary motor control in his sacral segments. Rob's diagnosis was T12 complete paraplegia. A question that remained in my mind was whether he had sustained an injury to the cord or to the cauda equina. Distinguishing between a spinal cord injury (upper motor neuron) and a cauda equina injury (lower motor neuron) is important, especially to the patient. The rate of neurologic recovery in incomplete injuries, the type of paralysis (spastic versus flaccid), the amount of muscle atrophy, and bowel, bladder, and sexual function are different for upper and lower motor neuron injuries and may affect the treatment goals and program.

I completed the evaluation by looking at his respiratory function to make sure there were no problems that needed to be addressed. He had a normal breathing pattern, a functional cough, and a forced vital capacity that was 68% of normal for his age. The decreased vital capacity was not unusual because he had undergone surgery and had been in bed for nearly three weeks. I expected it to return to normal once he was allowed out of bed and began his rehabilitation program.

I was unable to test Rob's functional status in body handling skills, transfers, or wheelchair mobility because of his restriction to bed rest, but I would be able to project goals without this information based on his functional neurologic level (Fig. 62-1). As I concluded my evaluation, I explained that several more people needed to evaluate him. Following this, we would have a team conference where all the members would report their evaluations and projected goals and treatment. Following the team conference, we would schedule a conference with Rob and his family to discuss goals, treatment, and estimated length of stay, and any questions he or his family might have. Family conferences would be scheduled as needed throughout the rehabilitation program, with one usually occurring prior to discharge.

I thanked Rob for being so patient and cooperative during the evaluation session and

☒ INITIAL
☐ MONTHLY
☐ DISCHARGE
☐ FOLLOW-UP

SPINAL INJURY EVALUATION

☐ OP   ☒ IP

PATIENT'S NAME LAST	FIRST		RLAMC #	UNIT	AGE	ADM. TO P.T.	D.C. FROM P.T.
SMITH	ROBERT						

DIAGNOSIS		ONSET	EST. TIME FOR PROG.	DISCHARGED TO
T-12 Complete Paraplegia				

GENERAL INFORMATION

T-12 compression fracture with posterior displacement 2° fall
S/P Harrinston rod and posterior spinal fusion T-9 - L-3.

MUSCULOSKELETAL EVALUATION

		STRENGTH		SLOW ROM		SPAS.	
		L	R	L	R	L	R
NECK	Flexion	N	N	0-30	0-30		
	Extension	N	N	0-30	0-30		
SCAPULA	Elevation	N	N				
	Add. Down Rot.	N	N				
	Abd. Up. Rot.	N	N				
SHOULDER	Flexion	N	N	0-180	0-180		
	Extension	N	N	0-60	0-60		
	Abduction	N	N	0-180	0-180		
	Adduction (Horiz)	N	N	0-30	0-30		
ELBOW	Flexion	N	N	0-150	0-150		
	Extension	N	N				
WRIST	Flexion	N	N	0-80	0-80		
	Extension	N	N	0-70	0-70		
FINGER	Flexion	N	N	WNL	WNL		
	Extension	N	N				
TRUNK	Flexion	Present		NT	NT		
	Extension	Present		NT	NT		
HIP	Flexion	O	O	NT-90	NT-90		
	Extension	O	O				
	Abduction	O	O	0-45	0-45		
	Adduction	O	O	0-35	0-35		
	Int. Rotation			0-45	0-45		
	Ext. Rotation			0-45	0-45		
	SLR			NT-80	NT-80		
KNEE	Flexion	O	O	0-135	0-135		
	Extension	O	O				
ANKLE	Dorsiflexion	O	O	0-15	0-15		
	Plantar √ supine	O	O	0-45	0-45		
	Plantar √ stand.	O	O				
SUB-TALAR	Inversion	O	O	0-35	0-35		
	Eversion	O	O	0-35	0-35		
TOE	Flexion	O	O	WNL	WNL		
	Extension	O	O	WNL	WNL		

FAST R.O.M. LIMITATIONS

NONE

EQUIPMENT

Elastic stockings,
Manual W/C sliding board

SENSORY EVALUATION

N=Normal —=Impaired O=Absent

	SUPERFICIAL PAIN		LIGHT TOUCH	
	L	R	L	R
C2	N	N	N	N
3	N	N	N	N
4	N	N	N	N
5	N	N	N	N
6	N	N	N	N
7	N	N	N	N
8	N	N	N	N
T1	N	N	N	N
2	N	N	N	N
4	N	N	N	N
6	N	N	N	N
8	N	N	N	N
10	N	N	N	N
12	N	N	N	N
L1	O	O	O	O
2	O	O	O	O
3	O	O	O	O
4	O	O	O	O
5	O	O	O	O
S1	O	O	O	O
2	O	O	O	O
3	O	O	O	O
4	O	O	O	O

PROPRIOCEPTION

	L	R
SHOULDER	N	N
ELBOW	N	N
WRIST	N	N
THUMB	N	N
HIP		
KNEE	O	O
ANKLE	O	O
GR. TOE	O	O

UPRIGHT CONTROL

N.A.

	FLEX		EXT	
	L	R	L	R
HIP				
KNEE				
ANKLE				

RESPIRATORY EVALUATION

BREATHING PATTERN ☐ Neck ☒ Chest ☒ Diaph. ☐ Abdom.

COUGH ☐ Functional ☐ Weak Func. ☐ Non-Func.

DIAGHRAGM FUNCTION   NORMAL

VC (supine)		VC Ē GPB		CHEST EXP. (Xiphoid)	
3100	ml	NA	ml	Active N.T.	
68	% N	NA	% N	Ē Air Shift N.A.	

FUNCTIONAL EVALUATION   (+) = Increase   (—) = Decrease
U = Unable   A = Assisted   S = Supervised   ! = Independant

Body Handling Skills	Initial	Current	Goals
Come to sitting	NT		I
Rolling	NT		I
ROM	NT		I
Raise: Type depression	NT		I
Transfers			
Mat	NT		I
Bed	NT		I
Car	NT		I
Toilet	NT		I
Bathtub/Shower	NT		I
Floor	NT		I

W/C Mobility (Man/Elec)	M	E	M	E	M	E
Level Propulsion					I	N
Rough Terrain	NT				I	N
Ramp	NT				I	N
Curbs: Height 4-6"	NT				I	N
W/C into Car	NT				I	N

Walking			
Come to standing	NT		N.A.
Level	NT		N.A.
Rough	NT		N.A.
Stairs	NT		N.A.

Velocity NT M/min   % N   ☐ W/C ☐ Walking

TORQUE   N.A.

	Ī			FES	
	ft/lbs		% N	ft/lbs		% N
	L	R	L	R	L	R	L	R
HIP EXT								
HIP ABD								
KNEE EXT								

PROGRAM: Frequency   6/week

MAJOR PROBLEMS/CHANGES

-Untrained wheelchair mobility

-Untrained transfer skills

-Respiratory dysfunction - decreased vital capacity

-Decreased body handling skills

-Respiratory program
-Lower extremity range of motion
-Hamstring stretch
-Upper extremity strengthening
-Mat activities
-Transfer training
-Wheelchair mobility training
-Patient and family teaching
-Equipment order

M.D. Date_____

R.P.T. Date_____

RANCHO LOS AMIGOS MEDICAL CENTER

Figure 62-1. Evaluation of patient with T12 complete paraplegia. (Courtesy of Rancho Los Amigos Medical Center, Downey, CA 90242)

returned to my desk to determine the treatment goals and program.

After reviewing all of my evaluation results, I identified the following treatment goals for Rob:

1. Maintenance of joint range of motion and prevention of contractures
2. Independence in body handling skills: coming to sit, sitting balance, rolling, ischial pressure relief
3. Independence in wheelchair transfers to mat, bed, car, toilet, bathtub, floor
4. Independence in wheelchair mobility: level surfaces, rough terrain, ramps, curbs (4 to 6 in), putting wheelchair into car
5. Independence in preventive measures: self skin inspection; self lower extremity range-of-motion exercises
6. Identify therapeutic equipment needs: manual wheelchair, bathroom equipment, ramp
7. Plan for discharge

Even though he was limited to bed rest, I initiated lower extremity passive range-of-motion exercises, bilateral upper extremity exercises, and incentive spirometry to encourage deep breathing and improve his vital capacity.

The team conference was scheduled within Rob's first week of admission. After I reported my goals and program, I reminded the team that there might be a need for an interim discharge, possibly after two months, until his body jacket was removed. I was anticipating that Rob was going to be motivated and progress quickly toward his goals, but would be limited by the postsurgical guidelines. Once his fracture and fusion were healed, usually around three months after surgery, he would be readmitted to finish the remainder of his program. It is helpful to bring this up early so that the team, the patient, and the family can plan for the interim discharge. All the team members were impressed with Rob's positive attitude and his sense of humor, and were anticipating him to be a good rehabilitation candidate. The psychologist reminded us that this could be Rob's way of coping with his loss.

Once he was out of bed and involved in an active program and reminded of things he used to be able to do, we might see some depression, anger, or fear. These emotions are all part of adjusting to a disability.

At the family conference, following all the team members' reports, Rob and his parents were asked if they had any questions. Rob's parents asked whether the spinal cord was completely severed. This is a typical question. We explained that such is rarely the case—it is usually stretched or bruised. Sometimes both the patient and family are so overwhelmed by the crisis that they have few questions and may absorb little of what was said by the team. Therefore, we try to make ourselves available to answer questions as they occur, and we plan on repeating much of what was said at the conference when the patient is ready to hear it. (The patient often initiates questions when he is ready to hear the answers.) I had not discussed walking as a goal for Rob, and I wondered when this would come up for discussion with either Rob or his parents.

Because of Rob's functional neurologic level (T12), and the absence of all sensation (especially proprioception at the hips) and voluntary motor control below the level of the lesion, ambulation was not a functional goal at this time. Patients with injuries at this neurologic level are capable of walking with bilateral knee-ankle-foot orthoses (KAFOs) and crutches, but the energy demand is very high. It is not realistic to expect a patient with an injury at this level to be a functional ambulator. Therefore, I did not discuss ambulation as a goal for Rob, and waited for him to initiate discussion of this activity.

Rob was cleared by the orthopedist to be out of bed during the next week, and he began working on sitting tolerance. Because some patients experience the symptoms of postural hypotension when they first get out of bed, I issued Rob a pair of elastic stockings. I provided him with a 4-in foam cushion with an ischial cutout to sit on. He sat 30 minutes the first day and progressed 30 minutes each day after that. He had some complaints of nausea during the first few days. After he had two hours of tolerance, I initiated more aggressive upper extremity strengthening, specifically shoulder depression, in preparation for transfer training and ischial pressure relief. Within a week he was capable of relieving pressure from his ischial tuberosities (a "raise") while sitting in the wheelchair. The cutout in the cushion helps eliminate tissue pressure over the bony prominences, but does not eliminate the need to perform raises. I instructed him to do a raise for 15 seconds each 15 minutes, or for 1 minute each hour. We also worked on wheelchair propulsion on level surfaces.

By the time Rob had four hours of sitting tolerance, we began to work on pretransfer activities such as short-sitting balance with and without hand support, trunk weight shifting forward and back, and side to side, and shoulder depression to raise his buttocks off the mat. After a few days Rob developed confidence in his ability to balance his trunk and shift his weight easily using his upper extremities for support, and he was ready to begin sliding board transfers. Because Rob had gained skill and strength from the mat work, he learned to do a sliding board transfer from the wheelchair to the mat with little difficulty. With each practice session he became more independent with all the steps of the transfer, including positioning his transfer board and the wheelchair. I continued to provide assistance with his legs to avoid trunk rotation, which was still contraindicated. He continued with his upper extremity strengthening program, which I coordinated with occupational therapy so as to avoid duplicating treatment. I then introduced bed and car transfers, which are somewhat more difficult because of the difference in height between the wheelchair and the transfer surface. After several days of practice, he was able to perform both of these transfers with standby assistance for his trunk balance and assistance with his legs. I cleared him and instructed the nurses for assisted transfers on the unit, to provide additional practice getting in and out of bed. I also instructed his family in assisting him with a car transfer so he could leave the hospital if he wanted to go on an outing. (This is just one part of the patient/family

instruction that is required before the patient can leave on a day or overnight pass.)

By the end of Rob's first month he was independent in manual wheelchair propulsion on level and rough surfaces, assisted in sliding board transfers to the mat, bed, and car, and independent in ischial pressure relief. His family had learned how to assist with Rob's car and bed transfers, how to fold a wheelchair, and how to get the wheelchair in and out of the car and up and down curbs. They were eager to take him to a restaurant in the area. In addition to daily functional activities training, Rob continued with upper extremity strength and endurance training, and static hamstring muscle stretch. (SLR was now 90 degrees bilaterally.) He needed greater than normal strength and endurance in his arms because he had to rely on them for most of his functional activities.

During the next month Rob began working on long-sitting balance in preparation for learning self lower extremity range-of-motion exercises and lower extremity dressing (taught by the occupational therapist). We also began working on more difficult transfers, that is, to the tub and toilet. Rob was spending between four and five hours a day in his physical therapy program. During this time I began to notice some changes in Rob's behavior. He was arriving late to some of his treatments, and several times I had to go to the unit and find him. When I asked him about his tardiness he always seemed to have an excuse for being late: the nurse did not help him with his transfer out of bed, or he had to wait for his medication. Initially his excuses seemed legitimate, and I decided not to make too much of his tardiness, but asked him to please be on time. He continued to be late for some appointments and even missed some treatment sessions. When he did arrive, he was less cooperative and began challenging why we were spending so much "time with my arms and doing nothing for my legs." He asked how he was going to be able to walk again if we didn't do some therapy for his legs. This was the first time he had brought up walking with me, although he had told other team members that he was going to walk out of here. I explained to him that we needed to work with the muscles he had, which were in his arms and trunk, and that, at least for now, he would have to rely on his arms for doing most things. My explanation did not seem to satisfy him. When I approached him about ordering his wheelchair he told me he wasn't going to need one. I decided to consult with the psychologist for help in handling the situation.

The psychologist reminded me that Rob had suffered a terrible loss, and the behaviors I was seeing (anger, hostility, tardiness) were his way of coping with this loss and part of the process of adjusting to his disability. The psychologist told me to try to be understanding and supportive of Rob during this stage, to acknowledge his feelings of anger, fear, and sadness about his loss, and to try not to take his attacks personally. He said he would also see the patient for support.

Even though I knew that with Rob's current neurologic picture, functional independent ambulation was unlikely, I was not going to be able to convince him of this and he needed to discover it for himself. I decided it would be a good time to introduce the criteria for an ambulation trial so that he knew what was required of him (Fig. 62-2). The decision to pursue an ambulation trial would become his. Because ambulation is so difficult both physiologically and as a skill, I waited until the patient expressed the desire to walk. I did not want Rob to feel that walking was an expectation I had for him and that he had failed if he did not accomplish it. Rob seemed pleased that we had

---

These criteria must be met before you may try to stand with braces. Your physical therapist will explain to you all of the details.

1. No range of motion limitations (hip flexion, plantar flexion contractures)
2. SLR 0 to 110 degrees, 120 degrees
3. 50 continuous dips in the parallel bars
4. Independent in all of your transfers
5. Attend all of your PT appointments
6. You need to take a Maximum Exercise Test. Your maximum $\dot{V}o_2$ should be at least 20 ml O_2/kg·min
7. If your results for the Maximum Exercise Test are below 20 ml O_2/kg·min, you must participate in the Endurance Class.

   If you have satisfied all of the above criteria, your therapist will fit you with temporary braces. You need to perform each skill within the set time limit. In case you are unable to complete each skill, the ambulation trial will be postponed until you can fulfill each skill requirement.

The ambulation trial consists of the following:

1. You need to stand for five minutes without holding onto anything. There will be three 1-hour sessions to complete this.
2. You need to stand up and walk through the parallel bars independently with your hands open (you may not grip the bars). There will be one 1-hour session to do this.
3. You must be able to stand up with crutches by yourself and balance with your crutches off the ground. There will be one 1-hour session to complete this.
4. You need to walk with crutches, supervised by your therapist, for 20 continuous steps. There will be one 1-hour session to do this.

   If you are able to complete all of these skills, your therapist will order you your own braces and crutches.

   Estimated time limit for ambulation trial is six days.

   You may be reevaluated in three months.

Figure 62-2. Guidelines for ambulation trial for complete paraplegia. (Courtesy of Rancho Los Amigos Medical Center, Downey, CA 90242)

reviewed the criteria. He commented that he was finally going to be working on walking and I anticipated that I would see improved cooperation with all his treatment, because one of the requirements for an ambulation trial is regular attendance at all scheduled therapy.

At our weekly team meeting, where we discuss the patient's progress and problems, I shared Rob's change in behavior. I reviewed Rob's current status: independent in wheelchair propulsion on level surfaces and rough terrain, supervised on ramps; independent in mat, bed, and car transfers except for requiring assistance with his legs; supervised in tub bench and toilet transfers (6-inch raised toilet seat) for trunk balance as well as assisted with his legs; and independent in ischial pressure relief. I had also completed all of the teaching with Rob and his family for a day and overnight pass. Because of his postsurgical restrictions and the limitations imposed by the body jacket, Rob was limited in the progress he could make toward his long-term goals. I suggested an interim discharge until the body jacket was off and he was cleared for all activities. I was also thinking he might return more ready emotionally to resume his program. The occupational therapist mentioned that Rob was unable to progress in his bathing and dressing skills until the body jacket was off, and might be more ready to begin home and community skills after some time at home. The psychologist and social worker agreed that an interim discharge could be very beneficial in Rob's adjustment to his disability and he could return more "ready" to complete his goals. A family conference was scheduled to discuss this with Rob and his family and to make arrangements for his discharge. I gave him a home program for upper extremity strengthening and endurance. Rob was scheduled to return to outpatient clinic in one month.

When Rob returned, a roentgenogram was taken of his spine, and it was determined that his fusion was healed and he no longer required the body jacket. He was admitted to complete his rehabilitation program.

My complete reevaluation showed that Rob had lost some hamstring muscle range (decrease from 90 to 80 degrees of hip flexion with knee extended), but his sensory and motor picture were unchanged. I also noted bilateral 20-degree hip flexion contractures, which could pose a problem for his ambulation. At the team conference, I presented Rob's goals and recommended that one month would be sufficient to accomplish them.

Rob began working on trunk balancing because he felt insecure without the body jacket. It took several days to rebuild his confidence, but he quickly progressed to his remaining body handling skills, transfers, and wheelchair skills. He also was on an aggressive program for stretching his hamstring muscles (he needed 110 degrees for tub and floor transfers, lower extremity dressing, and ambulation) and stretching of his hip flexion contractures. During the next two weeks he learned to roll, come to sit, and do his own lower extremity self range-of-motion exercises. I instructed him to sleep prone at night for both skin care and hip flexion stretch. He perfected his bed, car, tub bench, and toilet transfers without using a sliding board. He also learned to balance independently on the rear wheels of his wheelchair and was working on negotiating curbs and getting the wheelchair in and out of the car independently. Although he talked about walking, he was very cooperative with all parts of his program.

Rob achieved all of the criteria for an ambulation trial. It was obvious he had worked on his arm strength and endurance at home. He was fit with bilateral KAFOs and began balancing activities in the parallel bars. As I anticipated, the combination of his limited lumbar motion (secondary to insertion of Harrington rods from T9 to L3) and his 20-degree hip flexion contractures made it difficult for Rob to balance independently in the KAFOs without leaning forward and holding onto the parallel bars. His hip flexion contractures were pulling his trunk forward (in front of his center of gravity) and he was not able to compensate with increased lumbar extension. Rob and I worked for two sessions on balancing and he asked if he could try "walking in the bars." I agreed, and with much assistance he walked down the parallel bars with a swing-to gait pattern. He requested to stop for the day and was very quiet as we took the braces off.

Before our next ambulation session, Rob sought me out and told me he did not wish to continue working on ambulation. I could imagine that telling me this was very difficult for Rob. I told him that the opportunity for an ambulation trial was always available and that he could request one at a later date through the outpatient clinic. He smiled and seemed relieved by his decision. He then asked when his own wheelchair would be delivered and when we would be making a home visit in preparation for his discharge.

After Rob made the decision to discontinue his ambulation trial, he really concentrated on perfecting his other skills. Once the flexibility of the hamstring muscle allowed 110 degrees of hip flexion, he learned to do wheelchair to floor and wheelchair to bottom of tub transfers. He was able to become independent in the tub transfer, but still required assistance with the floor transfer. This is a particularly difficult transfer, but I was sure that Rob would be able to perfect it with more practice. As I reviewed his other goals, the only one he had not yet achieved was curb jumping. This also is a difficult skill, but I was sure he would master it after he went home. The team scheduled a discharge planning conference with Rob and his family one week prior to his discharge. All the team members reviewed the goals that Rob had achieved and what remained to be accomplished.

During his last week he was more involved with his occupational therapy program, completing his dressing, bathing, home and community skills, and driver's training. The occupational therapist and I took Rob on a home visit to recommend adaptations and determine final equipment needs. His family had already made some changes during his previous discharge. Fortunately, the bathroom was wheelchair accessible, and I checked him out on toilet transfers. He preferred to use the shower stall instead of the tub for bathing, and I made a note to order him a shower transfer bench. We also discussed which entrance to the house

would most easily accommodate a ramp, and I measured the height of the two steps into the house so I could determine the length of ramp I would order.

On Rob's discharge day I checked his cushion for excessive ischial pressure and issued him a new cushion. I told him to plan to come to outpatient clinic for a new cushion at least every four to six months. I gave him his shower transfer bench, and reminded him to come back to outpatient clinic for his scheduled re-evaluations. I had really enjoyed working with Rob, and I looked forward to seeing him in outpatient clinic as he became more involved in his own life again.

From Rob's clinical picture, many of the concerns and components in the physical therapy management of a patient with paraplegia can be identified. However, each patient presents unique problems. Consider the following examples.

CASE VARIATION 1

Sue is a 24-year-old woman who was injured in an automobile accident. She was living in an apartment and working as an elementary school teacher at the time of the accident. She is engaged to be married in one month. Her family includes an older brother who lives in the area and parents who live several hundred miles away. The wedding is scheduled to be in her parent's home. Her goal is to "walk down the aisle" at her wedding. Her fiancé and parents are reported to be very supportive.

Sue's evaluation revealed an incomplete T12 paraplegia. Her sensation was normal through the T12 dermatome, and impaired to light touch and superficial pain through all the lumbosacral dermatomes. Joint proprioception was normal through the hips, impaired at the knees, and absent at the ankle and great toe. The results of her manual muscle test included fair-plus hip flexion, poor-minus knee extension, and trace dorsiflexors and toe flexion bilaterally. Mild clonus was noted at the ankles. No limitations were noted in range of motion. Her upper extremities appeared normal. Her neurologic picture has improved during the week and a half since her injury.

Functional goals for Sue were identical to Rob's with the addition of ambulation in bilateral AFOs. Joint range of motion, selective muscle strength and control, sensation, the influence of spasticity and upper extremity strength are factors in determining ambulation goals. Minimal goals include independence in getting braces on and off, coming to stand, walking on level surfaces and rough terrain, negotiating stairs and ramps, and getting up from the floor. Velocity helps determine how practical walking is, and if it will be used in addition to or instead of wheelchair propulsion.

Sue's treatment involves the same progression described for Rob. Modifications are made in body handling and transfer techniques if the lower extremities can be used. Lower extremity strengthening is included, as well as gait training. Neuromuscular electrical stimulation may be appropriate to use for both lower extremity strengthening, muscle reeducation, and as an adjunct to gait training. If Sue has further neurologic recovery, her functional goals are modified appropriately. If her strength and sensation improve so that she is able to ambulate with bilateral AFOs, her potential for independent community ambulation is greatly improved.

CASE VARIATION 2

Tom is a 16-year-old boy who sustained a gunshot wound to the back, resulting in a complete L1 cauda equina injury. He is the oldest of six children living at home with his mother. His mother depends on him to help care for the younger children in the family because it is necessary for her to work. He has completed the sixth grade and was not attending school at the time of the accident. His goal is to get out of the hospital as soon as he can. His family has been unable to visit him in the hospital because they do not have a car.

Tom's sensory evaluation showed intact sensation through the L1 dermatome and absent sensation below. Joint proprioception was intact through the hips and absent below. Muscle testing revealed fair-plus hip flexion with absent voluntary motion below. No spasticity was noted and range of motion was normal. The upper extremities appeared normal.

Tom's functional goals are similar to Rob's, including ambulation. Tom is capable of walking with bilateral KAFOs, but the energy demand is very high. I would wait for Tom to initiate discussion of this activity. Additional education concerning skin care may be necessary because the atrophy is more profound in injuries resulting in flaccid paralysis.

Tom's treatment progression is the same described for Rob. Tom's youth, his limited educational level, and his family situation are all factors that will influence his goals and treatment.

CASE VARIATION 3

Joe is a 54-year-old man who was involved as a passenger in an automobile accident. He has been married for 30 years and has two adult sons. Joe underwent coronary artery bypass surgery five years ago. He has continued to smoke and is overweight. His wife has been visiting daily and appears quite anxious. He owns his own company and reports working very long hours. Since his admission he has spent many hours on the phone with business calls. He says he needs to get out of the hospital as soon as possible to return to work. His wife has told the team that she wants him to stay for several months because he needs the rest.

Joe's evaluation revealed an incomplete cauda equina injury. Sensation was intact through the L3 dermatome with impairment below. Joint proprioception was normal at the hips and knees, and impaired at the ankle and great toe. Manual muscle testing revealed good hip flexion, fair-plus knee extension, and poor dorsiflexion, hip extension, and abduction bilaterally. Range of motion was within normal limits except for 20-degree hip flexion contractures. Upper extremities were within normal limits.

Joe's goals are similar to Rob's, with the addition of ambulation. Modifications are made in body handling and transfer techniques to utilize his lower extremity function. Orthotic management and ambulation goals are determined from the same factors mentioned earlier (except spasticity), and are adjusted as the neurologic picture changes. Neurologic recovery is usually slow and occurs over a long time.

Joe's treatment progression is the same as for incomplete paraplegia. Protection of weak muscles from overuse or overstretching is important in lower motor neuron injuries. Neuro-muscular electrical stimulation is not used when the peripheral nerve is not intact. Initial orthotic prescription is for bilateral AFOs. Joe has the potential for becoming independent in community ambulation*; however, with his obesity and preexisting heart disease he will need to be carefully monitored to determine if he is physiologically capable of meeting the energy demand for walking.

---

*Our criteria for defining independent community ambulation are 350 m at 40% to 50% of normal walking velocity, and the ability to manage curbs, ramps, and steps.

63 Pregnancy

DIANE U. JETTE

Nancy Edwards had called last week for an appointment to talk about exercises that would be appropriate for her during her pregnancy. I looked forward to talking to her and helping her determine a good exercise program. We had met a couple of times at aerobics class, but I had not seen her since my schedule had changed.

Nancy looked quite healthy and fit as she walked into the office. She is about 5 ft 8 in, I would guess, and average weight. Observing her posture, I noticed a slightly increased lumbar lordosis and thoracic kyphosis. I considered these postural changes normal because of the increased weight of the breasts and uterus, as well as increased ligamentous laxity; however, I thought a little education and correction could prevent any future complaints of back discomfort. There was no awkwardness to her gait, or movement as she sat down, that might indicate pain in the joints of the lower extremities, pelvis, or spine.

In response to my questions, Nancy told me that she was 30 years old and had a 4-year-old boy at home. I felt that there would be no significant risk in exercising because of her age, and believed she would have some knowledge of what pregnancy entailed in terms of physical changes. She also told me that she worked for the local home health agency as a registered nurse. I felt confident that I would be working with an intelligent woman with good background knowledge. Knowing this, I could address her questions at the appropriate level. I

also expected her to be able to relate an accurate medical history.

She had made an appointment with me, she said, because she was interested in continuing with her exercise regimen, including running and aerobics, throughout her pregnancy. She said she was unsure of the precautions she should take, but she felt strongly about maintaining her fitness level. I sensed that her body image might also be an important consideration. Nancy also felt that she needed some help to improve her ability to relax. Her job, she explained, was very often psychologically stressful and her case load was quite large.

I now turned to questions about Nancy's pregnancy and previous medical and obstetrical history. Nancy said that she was in the 20th week of her pregnancy and had experienced no significant problems. In fact, she said she felt great! She had gained 7 lb thus far, and had been eating quite well and exercising. She had not been bothered much by nausea or vomiting. I asked her if she had had a blood test for alpha-fetoprotein levels, because significantly low or high levels might indicate fetal abnormalities. She said that the value was within normal limits. Any fetal abnormality would mean that the fetus might be in jeopardy during vigorous maternal exercise, and would affect the type of exercise I would later prescribe. Nancy told me that there was no indication of cervical incompetence or placenta previa during this pregnancy. These conditions would be contraindications to exercise. Later, I would confirm that her pregnancy was proceeding normally with a phone call to Nancy's obstetrician.

During her previous pregnancy, Nancy had gained about 30 lb, but had returned to her average weight within nine months. Excessive weight gain during pregnancy, or failure to lose weight postpartum, might indicate a tendency toward gestational diabetes. Nancy said that she had felt very well throughout the previous pregnancy, but had experienced thrombophlebitis in the right lower extremity. The problem had resolved with a few days of bed rest. I told Nancy that it would be important for her during this pregnancy to pay attention to any persistent calf pain that might seem like a muscle cramp. Of course, exercise would be contraindicated in the presence of thrombophlebitis. The previous delivery had been a bit difficult, with a prolonged second stage; and her son, who weighed 8 lb 5 oz, had been delivered with forceps. Following the delivery, she had been dismayed to find that she was somewhat incontinent. Although this problem had resolved, it had lasted about six weeks postpartum, and even now she knew she had to empty her bladder before performing activities such as running or aerobics. I made a note to emphasize strengthening the pelvic floor musculature in her exercise program. It was quite likely that the increased pressure on the pelvic diaphragm during pregnancy and delivery had caused overstretching and laxity of the muscles and connective tissue. I also thought that it was possible that Nancy had incurred a partial bladder denervation from pressure on the pelvic nerves during the second stage of labor. This was a point about which I might want to consult with her obstetrician, especially if stress incontinence became a problem as this pregnancy progressed.

Nancy's medical history was uneventful: no metabolic disorders, cardiopulmonary disease, or urinary tract disorders. She did not have anemia, a common problem for women, especially pregnant women. The condition might affect fetal oxygen supply during vigorous maternal exercise. Her alcohol use was minimal and she had never smoked. Because both excessive alcohol and tobacco consumption would place the fetus at risk, it was important for me to establish its usage. Knowing that Nancy was actively engaged in a regular exercise program, I had not expected her to be a smoker. If Nancy had indicated any medical or previous obstetrical problems, I would have contacted her obstetrician for consultation before making any exercise recommendations.

I now began to question Nancy about any specific musculoskeletal problems she might be experiencing with the pregnancy. One of the more common complaints during pregnancy is backache. Ligamentous laxity and a shift in the center of gravity contribute to changes in posture. These changes can affect the sacroiliac joint or other vertebral joints. Nancy had no complaints of any discomfort in the back. She did mention, however, that she had occasional cramping and pointed to the right buttock in the area of the sciatic notch. She couldn't identify any specific activities that caused this discomfort. My thought was that she perhaps was experiencing spasm or cramping of her piriformis muscle, and I made a note to check further. Nancy also said that sudden movements sometimes caused pain in the inguinal area, and mentioned that she had had the same experience with her last pregnancy. She said the midwife had told her that it was from stress on the round ligaments of the uterus, a common problem in pregnancy. Nancy said she was able to prevent this problem by avoiding sudden movements.

One problem that Nancy was having difficulty coping with was muscle cramping in her calves, especially at night. I told her that this was another common complaint in pregnancy. Some clinicians suggest increasing calcium intake, but that might not be the answer. I recommended that she try always stretching her legs with the foot flexed rather than extended so as to avoid extreme cramping. If a cramp should occur, she should stretch the muscles by strongly dorsiflexing her foot or by standing on the foot and leaning forward over the foot with the knee extended.

I then asked Nancy if she had experienced

any numbness or tingling in the extremities. Some pregnant women experience neurological signs associated with pressure on the brachial plexus, or intervertebral disk protrusion, or even carpal tunnel syndrome. Nancy stated that she had none of these problems.

Although I knew Nancy was actively engaged in an exercise program, I needed more specifics about her level of activity. She told me that she exercised at least three, usually four, times per week. Depending on the weather, she would either run or go to the health club for an aerobics workout. She tried to make enough time so that her exercise sessions lasted at least 45 minutes. She had been faithful to this regimen for the past two years. She had even done some recreational road racing. Whereas before her pregnancy she had been running six to seven miles, she now found it difficult to cover that distance in the amount of time she had been doing it. She planned to continue working throughout her pregnancy; but, although the job was not physically difficult, she was tired after an eight-hour day. I reminded her of the importance of sufficient rest during pregnancy.

At this point I asked Nancy to remove her dress and put on a gown. I carefully observed her posture. The shoulders, ASIS and PSIS, greater trochanters, and iliac crests were level, suggesting no sacroiliac dysfunction (Fig. 63-1). The patient stood with slightly rounded shoulders, forward head (Fig. 63-2), and protracted scapulae (Fig. 63-3). Nancy assumed the supine position and I asked her to lift her head off the table as I palpated along the midline of the abdomen to check for any diastasis of the rectus abdominis muscle (Fig. 63-4). There was a separation of about two-fingers breadth. I asked Nancy to palpate her abdomen in the same way to demonstrate the problem to her. I then explained that diastasis recti is not uncommon in women during or following pregnancy, but that she would have to alter her abdominal exercises and avoid any bilateral leg lifting to protect the muscles. She said that she had not noticed the diastasis, and admitted that she had been vigorously performing sit-ups. She had thought, she explained, that hav-

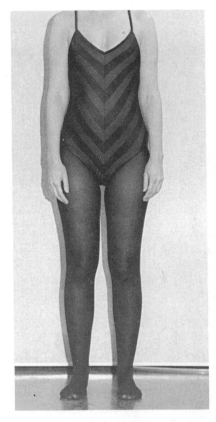

Figure 63-1. Anterior view of posture. The shoulders, ASIS, iliac crests, and greater trochanters are level.

ing her knees bent would protect her from problems.

Continuing my examination, I hoped to determine the cause of the cramping Nancy had described in the right buttock. I palpated the right piriformis muscle with the hip in adduction and internal rotation (Fig. 63-5). Nancy said that there was some discomfort right under my fingertips. The same palpation on the left caused no discomfort. There was no tenderness over the symphysis pubis; and, in both right and left sidelying positions, pressure on the iliac crests in a downward direction caused no discomfort. These findings confirmed my belief that there was no pelvic arthropathy. With the patient now sitting, I resisted hip abduction with external rotation.

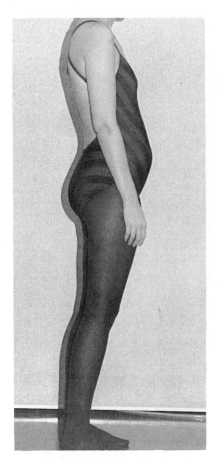

Figure 63-2. Lateral view of posture. The shoulders are rounded, and thoracic kyphosis and lumbar lordosis are slightly increased.

The maneuver also elicited some discomfort in the area of the piriformis muscle. I told Nancy that the findings led me to believe that she probably had some irritation or spasm of the piriformis muscle on the right side and no sacroiliac dysfunction. I showed her how to perform a gentle contract-relax technique, with the help of her husband, to relieve the spasm. I explained that maybe if she tried to avoid twisting while standing or standing too long in awkward positions, she might be able to prevent the cramping.

I next determined Nancy's resting heart rate in order to use it as a determinant of a rec-

ommended exercise target heart rate. Her radial pulse was 76. Her blood pressure was 100/70—no indication of hypertension. Hypertension, a sign of preeclampsia, would preclude exercise. Nancy stated that her blood pressure was always quite low, but her pregnancy had increased her resting heart rate slightly.

My impression was that Nancy was a healthy woman with an above-average fitness level. Although she was experiencing a normal pregnancy, Nancy had the problems of a weakened pelvic diaphragm, a rectus diastasis, and a history of thrombophlebitis. These areas would need special attention. Because she was an aerobically fit person who regularly exer-

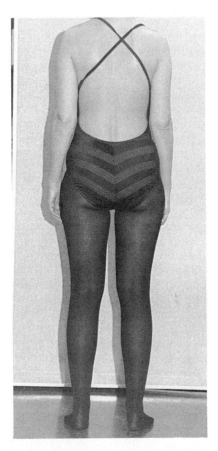

Figure 63-3. Posterior view of posture. The scapulae are protracted.

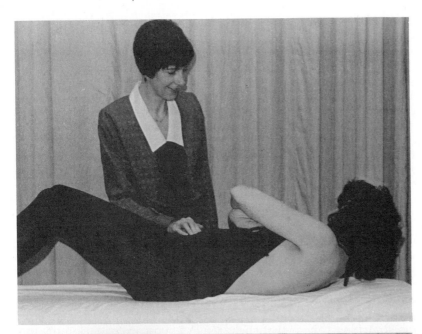

Figure 63-4. Palpating for diastasis of the rectus abdominis muscle.

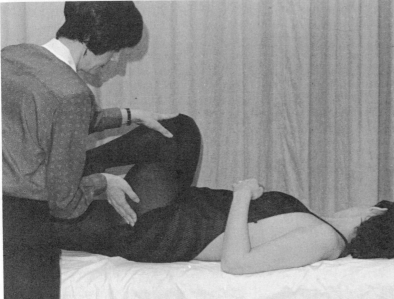

Figure 63-5. Palpating the piriformis muscle.

cised, there was no reason that she could not continue to perform aerobic exercise throughout her pregnancy. She should have relatively strong ligamentous support of her joints and be quite coordinated in the activities she regularly performed. However, the repetitive stress on the joints from running and aerobics might create some problems in joints that are naturally hypermobile from hormonal influences.

I explained to Nancy that in addition to

helping her meet her goals of controlling stress, maintaining her fitness level, and being educated on safe exercise practices, I also wanted her to improve her pelvic floor strength, protect the rectus abdominis muscle from added stress, and improve her posture. I felt it was quite realistic for her to expect to continue with some form of exercise until her delivery.

The emphasis of my treatment plan was on education. I expected Nancy would be very capable of following through with my instructions. I reminded her always to warm up with slow, rhythmic, active exercises and gentle stretching before beginning her aerobic activity. The warm-up period allows changes in the cardiovascular system, associated with exercise, to proceed slowly. Therefore, there is less initial stress on this system. Vigorous stretching is not indicated for a pregnant woman, because her joints may be hypermobile, but many women find that gentle stretching can improve comfort. I told Nancy that stretching of the pectoral muscles would be especially important for her, as indicated by her posture.

I then recommended an exercise target heart rate that was lower than the one she probably reached prior to pregnancy. In order to calculate her target heart rate, I determined her age-predicted maximum heart rate, 220 minus age, or 190 for Nancy. I then subtracted her resting heart rate from this value: 190 minus 76, or 114. I multiplied 114 by 0.60 and added the result to the resting heart rate $[(114 \times 0.60) + 76 = 144]$. I told Nancy that a combination of walking and jogging would be a good form of exercise. As her pregnancy progressed, however, she would probably find that the walking time increased and the jogging time decreased during her exercise session. Her target heart rate might also decrease, depending upon how she felt. I recommended that she continue at the same frequency and duration of exercise, although the intensity should decrease as the pregnancy progressed. I reminded her to pay attention to any signals from her body that she might interpret as being signs of excessive exercise. She should not feel

that she was working or breathing harder than she did when exercising in the nonpregnant state. I felt comfortable in saying this to Nancy because she had had a previous pregnancy and also had been exercising for the past two years. She should have, I believed, a good sense of her own capabilities. I suggested to Nancy that she not engage in competitive road races during her pregnancy simply because of the tendency to overdo in the competitive spirit.

I emphasized to Nancy the need for added calories in her diet, above and beyond that normally recommended in pregnancy, because exercise creates added demand for calories. Most persons who exercise regularly balance caloric intake with energy expenditure fairly well, and Nancy indicated that she ate very well. I also explained the importance of adequate fluid intake, even above that needed to quench her thirst, to compensate for losses during exercise and to prevent hyperthermia. I recommended that she carefully choose exercise clothing that would help her to avoid becoming overheated during exercise, and well-cushioned, supportive shoes to help prevent stress on the lower extremity joints.

Nancy and I also discussed her continuing her aerobics classes, cutting down on some of the jumping, bouncing, and very vigorous arm movements to protect her joints and pelvic diaphragm. Again, she could use a target heart rate to help maintain a safe level of exertion, and should follow the same precautions as when running.

During the part of the aerobics class that emphasizes specific muscle strengthening, I recommended that Nancy be cautious in protecting her back by avoiding bilateral leg lifting in the supine position, or full sit-ups. I explained that these exercises would also increase the diastasis. In order to preserve the health of the abdominal musculature, I showed her how to perform a posterior pelvic tilt and hold it while breathing in and out normally. I also taught her partial curl-ups in the supine position while protecting the abdomen with pressure from the hands. I recommended that she emphasize curling up on the diagonal, shoulder moving toward the opposite knee, to emphasize contraction of the external oblique muscles. I told her that the curl-up would be fine for a short period of time; however, as the pregnancy progressed and the size of the abdomen increased, putting the abdominal muscles at a mechanical disadvantage, she should modify the exercises by starting from the sitting position with knees bent, leaning her trunk back on the diagonal to a comfortable point, and then returning to the upright position (Fig. 63-6). I suggested that in the last few weeks of her pregnancy, she should just concentrate on the pelvic tilt exercise rather than curling up or leaning back to exercise the abdominal muscles. I urged Nancy to avoid holding her breath while exercising, because a Valsalva maneuver both increases pressure on the pelvic diaphragm and causes fluctuations in venous return to the heart. We also talked about the need to avoid exercises that required a knee-to-chest position because of the potential for air emboli.

Nancy had told me that she was very aware of performing pelvic floor exercises following her last pregnancy. However, I felt that

with her previous postpartum difficulty, she needed to review the exercises again with me. I emphasized the necessity of performing only a few contractions at a time, while performing them frequently during the day. I felt that the technique of performing a graded contraction with periodic hold would both increase strength and improve control over the pelvic floor muscles. This technique has been referred to as the "elevator" exercise. I explained to Nancy that it was just as important to learn to relax and control the pelvic floor as it was to contract it. We tried to think of some good cues to serve as reminders for her to do these exercises. Because she drove her car from one patient to the next all day, good reminders might be red lights and stop signs. In the office, phone calls might be good, frequent reminders. The plan was for her to perform three to five graded contractions each time.

Although Nancy's posture was not grossly abnormal and she was not experiencing any back pain, I felt that correction of the increased thoracic kyphosis and lumbar lordosis might help her avoid problems as the pregnancy pro-

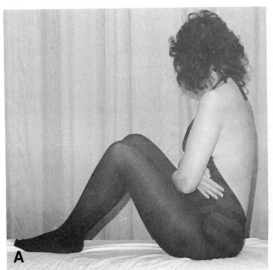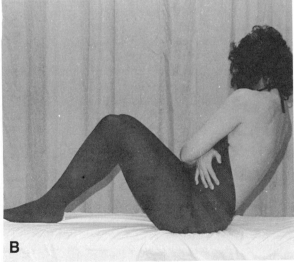

Figure 63-6. (*A*) Exercise of the external oblique muscle starting from the shortened position of the muscle. The rectus abdominis is supported. (*B*) Leaning the trunk back on the diagonal to a comfortable point.

gressed. I demonstrated to her the change I was noticing in her posture and showed her how to correct it. Using a mirror, I had her practice retracting her scapulae, pulling her chin back, and assuming a normal lordotic curve. I explained to her the need to preserve the lordotic curve, and to keep the weight of her abdomen pulled in, back over her feet, rather than giving in to the tendency to "let it all hang out." I gave her a good hand-out depicting examples of good and poor body mechanics. Because I knew she did a lot of driving, I referred her specifically to the section concerned with posture while driving, and recommended a lumbar support cushion for her car.

Lastly, Nancy and I talked about her need for relaxation training. She stated that she had not really practiced any specific relaxation techniques since taking prenatal classes during her last pregnancy. In addition, she had not felt very well prepared to be able to relax during her previous labor. I suggested that she could either purchase an audio tape to use at home to help her with progressive relaxation or she could combine the use of the tape with visits to the clinic for training with biofeedback, and rent a biofeedback unit to use at home. Nancy opted for the biofeedback training, saying she believed that the ability to relax well would be important to her beyond this labor and delivery. I decided to use temperature biofeedback, because increasing fingertip temperature is a good indication of decreasing sympathetic nervous system activity, and relaxation. We set up a schedule for visits three times during the following week to allow her to learn the technique and practice with supervision. At the end of the week, I could assess her progress and decide on a future schedule.

Nancy dressed and she and I set up our appointment schedule for the next week. In addition to starting the biofeedback training at the next visit, I wanted to use that opportunity to check on any problems she might be having with the exercise program, such as finding the appropriate exercise intensity, protecting the diastasis, or maintaining good posture. I also suggested to her that she consider enrolling in a childbirth class that would give her and her husband an update on labor and delivery procedures. As she left my office, I anticipated a rewarding experience working with a woman who was well motivated and had every chance of success in meeting her goals.

CASE VARIATION 1

Not all pregnant women seen by the physical therapist have Nancy's personal and medical background. Because Debbie was not a participant in a regular exercise program, but a sedentary person, and had referred herself to begin an exercise program during her pregnancy, my treatment approach was different. Although many women, because of a changing body image and shape, begin to think of exercising for the first time during pregnancy, I would not recommend starting a new regimen of any strenuous exercise then. Rather than designing a program consisting of jogging and aerobics classes with a target heart rate to meet, I would suggest to Debbie that she engage in a regular program of walking for 15 to 20 minutes daily. She should walk briskly and feel that the exercise was somewhat hard. I would explain to her that in addition to being less stressful on the cardiovascular system than the more strenuous jogging or aerobics program, a walking program does not involve a high level of skill or coordination on the part of the participant. In the early stages of learning a new physical activity, lack of skill and coordination contributes to increased energy expenditure and increases the potential for injury. Therefore, I would not recommend that a pregnant woman, who has a changing center of gravity and hypermobile joints, begin a new exercise program. I would tell Debbie that a reasonable goal would be to maintain her current level of fitness, not improve her fitness level during the pregnancy. I would encourage her to see me postpartum so that we could set up a program to help her meet her goal of improving her aerobic fitness.

Other exercises, recommended for Nancy for the pelvic diaphragm and abdominal muscles, as well as gentle stretching exercises, would be recommended for Debbie to maintain muscle activity, improve pelvic floor control, and increase comfort. Education of the patient would also follow along the same lines, with emphasis on good posture and body mechanics in order to prevent problems with her back during the pregnancy or postpartum.

CASE VARIATION 2

A different problem may exist for a woman with a history of incontinence following her last delivery in that she could have persistent stress incontinence. In this case, I might recommend that we evaluate the strength of the pelvic floor muscles using a perineometer. The perineometer could also be used during pelvic floor exercise as a form of feedback to demonstrate to the woman that she was performing pelvic floor muscle contraction correctly and to document her progress. If the weakness continued postpartum, I would consider instituting a program that included high-voltage DC stimulation to assist in increasing the strength of the pelvic floor musculature. The electrical stimulation would not be used during the pregnancy because its effects on the fetus are unknown.

CASE VARIATION 3

For a woman like Sandy who had type 1 diabetes, yet participated in a regular exercise program, my first action would be to contact her obstetrician. Although physical activity is an important component in maintenance of the health status of the diabetic person, the disease in a pregnant woman places the fetus at risk. The risk is especially great if the woman has difficulty maintaining her blood glucose value at a reasonable level or has diabetes that is complicated by vascular problems. Under these conditions, strenuous exercise could further increase the risk to the fetus by causing fluctuations in blood glucose values or compromising maternal-fetal oxygen exchange. I would ask the physician for an assessment of the patient's level of diabetic control, vascular status, and course of her pregnancy. If Sandy demonstrated good control of blood glucose and had no indication of vascular complications, I would suggest a daily walking program of about 20 minutes duration. I would recommend that she not try to continue her running or aerobics program during her pregnancy. I would explain to her that, to the best of my knowledge, there is not a lot of scientifically proven information on the best way to incorporate exercise in the daily routine of a pregnant, diabetic woman with her obvious level of fitness. Walking would seem to be a safe activity for both her and her baby as long as her blood glucose levels and blood pressure were within reasonable limits. Her goal of maintaining her aerobic fitness program might not be realistic; however, pregnancy itself seems to contribute to an increase in maximal aerobic capacity. Maintaining good diabetic control through a careful balance of diet, insulin, and activity should be her major goal. I would encourage exercises for strengthening the pelvic diaphragm and maintaining abdominal muscle tone, as well as gentle stretching exercises. When done properly, these exercises would not place a large stress on the cardiovascular system of the mother; therefore, they are not likely to cause fetal distress. I would emphasize the need for good posture and body mechanics. Relaxation training to reduce stress would be particularly important, because psychological stress can contribute to poor diabetic control.

CASE VARIATION 4

Another situation that I might encounter would be one in which the obstetrician referred a patient to me immediately postpartum for the first time.

Reading her medical record, I learned that Joan was a healthy 30-year-old woman who delivered her second child 18 hours ago. The delivery was by cesarean section because of cephalopelvic disproportion and nonprogression of labor. She had had a spinal anesthesia and a transverse incision. The baby was a healthy boy with a five-minute Apgar score of 9. The patient was having an uncomplicated postoperative course; her temperature was 37.0°C, and her blood pressure was 115/80 in the supine position. She had no signs of pulmonary infection, atelectasis, hypertension, or other complications. I entered Joan's room. She was partially sitting in bed, combing her hair. The baby was asleep in the bassinet next to her bed. She looked well, smiling as I introduced myself. In answer to my questions, she said that she was quite comfortable, except for some incisional pain. She was trying to take a minimum of pain medication and had been using active relaxation techniques. She was experiencing some minor uterine contractions, which, she said, did not really bother her. She said the nurse had helped her to the bathroom this morning. She had felt a bit lightheaded, but had managed well. She was glad to have the catheter removed. The baby was nursing well, but it was difficult to get into a comfortable position for nursing him because of the incision. She had no breast discomfort.

I told Joan that I would like to listen to her lungs and make sure she was aerating her lungs and coughing well, then I would like to show her some postpartum exercises. She agreed. Joan had normal vesicular breath sounds. Her deep breathing and coughing were adequate, with the abdominal incision supported. I was careful to check because small tidal volumes or poor, weak cough are natural consequences of abdominal incision pain, and can result in pulmonary complications following surgery. Joan laughingly said that every doctor and nurse that had walked in the room had been after her to breathe and cough! I also checked for any deep calf tenderness that might indicate thrombophlebitis. Thrombophlebitis is a possible complication of immobility during anesthesia, and Joan had a history of this problem during her last pregnancy. There was no indication of a problem now.

My impression was that Joan was having a normal recovery from her surgical procedure. Both she and I agreed that the recovery from a cesarean delivery would take longer than the recovery from her previous vaginal delivery because of the stress of major surgery. She would also be caring for two children, one of whom might be inclined to "act out" in this situation! Joan told me that she had been quite active, working at her job as a community health social worker and exercising at her aerobics class up until the time of delivery. She said she would like to avoid getting "too out of shape" while she was recovering. I told her that I would show her some exercises to start now, and before her discharge I would show her how to progress with them in a safe manner.

I explained to her that reasonable goals for the early postpartum period would be to make sure that (1) her lungs remained clear; (2) she was able to schedule enough rest periods for herself; (3) she had good posture in all her activities so that her back was protected; and (4) she was able to perform abdominal muscle exercises and pelvic floor exercises correctly. I told her that probably after six to eight weeks, she could begin to think of performing more vigorous exercises and an aerobics program.

With Joan lying supine, I checked for a diastasis of the rectus abdominis muscle. I found a diastasis of slightly more than two-fingers breadth. I explained my finding to her and showed her how to protect the rectus abdominis muscle by crossing her hands across her abdomen when doing any exercise for abdominal strengthening. With her knees flexed and her hands across her abdomen supporting the abdominal wall, I asked Joan to perform a posterior pelvic tilt, holding it while breathing in and out. I then instructed her to flex her neck while holding the pelvic tilt (Fig. 63-7). This exercise, I explained, caused the contraction of the upper abdominal muscles. Then I asked her again to hold a pelvic tilt, and extend one leg at a time, sliding her heel down the bed. This exercise caused the lower abdominal muscles to contract. I told her that these exercises for the abdomen would be sufficient until she came to my office after her discharge from the hospital. I then reviewed with her the necessity of pelvic floor exercises, explaining that even

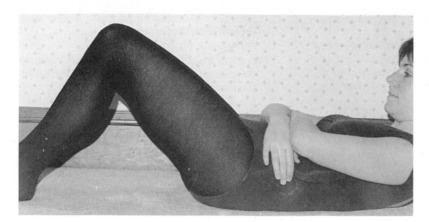

Figure 63-7. Postpartum abdominal strengthening begins. The patient supports the rectus abdominis muscle.

though she had not had a vaginal delivery, the pelvic floor structures could still be overstretched from the effects of pregnancy. I also recommended that as soon as she no longer felt dizzy upon standing, she should take walks in the hallway. Until then, she should point and flex her feet frequently to ensure good venous flow. I demonstrated good posture in the standing and sitting positions, and reviewed proper body mechanics with Joan. I told her that at the moment her posture would be affected by her incisional pain, enlarged breasts, and overstretched abdominal muscles. I felt that it would be appropriate for me to look more closely at her standing posture in a day or two when incisional pain and postural hypotension would not be factors. I gave Joan a booklet with information on exercise, posture, body mechanics, and comfort measures following cesarean delivery. I told her I would check back with her in the morning, and said goodbye.

The foregoing examples demonstrate the different exercise needs of individual women during and following pregnancy. Even apparently healthy pregnant women should be evaluated before recommendations for exercise are made by the physical therapist. Although there are some general guidelines to follow in prescribing exercise for a pregnant woman, programs should be individualized to meet each woman's unique needs.

ANNOTATED BIBLIOGRAPHY

Exercise During Pregnancy and the Post-Natal Period. Washington, DC, American College of Obstetricians and Gynecologists, 1985 (This publication contains conservative recommendations for exercise for the average sedentary pregnant woman. It may be a common source for obstetricians to use in making recommendations to their patients about exercise.)

Lotgering FK, Gilbert RD, Longo LD: The interactions of exercise and pregnancy: A review. Am J Obstet Gynecol 149:560, 1984 (This article is a good review of recent scientific research concerning the effects of maternal exercise on the fetus and mother during pregnancy. The bibliography is extensive.)

Noble E: Essential Exercises for the Childbearing Year: A Guide to Health and Comfort Before and After Your Baby Is Born, 2nd ed. Boston, Houghton Mifflin, 1982 (This book is written in an understandable, informative manner for the average pregnant woman. It is written by a physical therapist who is well respected for her contributions in the area of obstetrics.)

Shangold M, Mirkin G: The Complete Sports Medicine Book for Women, pp 125–133. New York, Simon and Schuster, 1985 (The chapter on exercise during pregnancy recommends aerobic exercise for the fit, pregnant woman. It presents reasonable precautions for exercise.)

Shearer M: Teaching prenatal exercises: Part 1. Posture. Birth and the Family Journal 8:105, 1981 (This article gives an excellent description of the function of the abdominal musculature during pregnancy, and makes recommendations for exercise. It is written by a physical therapist.)

Shrock P, Simkin P, Shearer M: Teaching prenatal exercises: Part 2. Exercises to think twice about. Birth and the Family Journal 8:167, 1981 (The authors discuss some commonly prescribed exercises for pregnant women and explain why they might be poor choices. The authors are physical therapists.)

Woodward SL: How does strenuous maternal exercise affect the fetus? A review. Birth and the Family Journal 8:17, 1981 (This review of the literature lends support to the belief that the physically fit woman with a low-risk pregnancy can exercise safely. The bibliography is good.)

64 Cystic Fibrosis

SUSAN A. LISKA

I entered the pediatric wing of the medical center where I worked to find my new patient, Stephanie Smith, an 8-year-old girl with a diagnosis of cystic fibrosis. My first stop was the chart rack where the patients' medical records were kept. By reading Stephanie's medical record, I would be able to learn some things about my new patient before meeting her. The first thing I learned about Stephanie was that she was an only child and a student in the third grade.

She had been diagnosed as having cystic fibrosis (CF) at 3 months of age by a positive sweat test after having failure to thrive and malabsorption. She was started on Pancrease, a digestive enzyme, at the time and had done well until age 2, when an onset of mild wheezing was noted. She was given theophylline (Slo-Phyllin), a bronchodilator, which seemed to help.

Stephanie was now entering the hospital for her first admission with a pulmonary exacerbation and complaints of increased cough and decreased activity. There had also been a slight decline in her arterial blood gases and pulmonary function tests, both of which are commonly monitored on an outpatient basis. The results of these tests six months ago as compared to the present results are illustrated in Table 64-1.

I was hopeful that with the use of bronchodilators to dilate her airways, antibiotics to fight the infection, and chest physical therapy to mobilize the excess secretions, her pulmonary function tests would improve. More severe cases have less chance for improving these values because of nonreversible airway destruction.

We hoped to be able to raise her arterial oxygenation (PaO_2) by mobilizing the excess secretions in her lungs. I was pleased to find that Stephanie's arterial carbon dioxide ($PaCO_2$) was within normal limits. With progression of the disease, CF patients begin to "trap air" because of destruction of alveoli, and premature closure of the airways. The inability to exhale adequately results in a chronic elevation in $PaCO_2$.

I was also able to look at my patient's chest roentgenograms. Her most recent film was somewhat different in appearance from one taken six months ago. The heart size was normal, but there was a slight increase in interstitial markings, especially in the right upper lobe, compared with previous films. From this, I could assume that the right upper lobe might have greater secretion retention and would require special attention during treatment. There were no focal areas of consolidation or pneumonia. Her lungs were mildly hyperinflated with a slight flattening of the diaphragm.

Also listed in the chart were the medications that Stephanie took routinely at home. These were as follows:

1. *Pancrease* was taken by mouth to provide enzymes necessary for digestion. Cystic fibrosis results in fibrosing of the pancreatic

Table 64-1. Comparison of Pulmonary Function and Arterial Blood Gas Tests

	SIX MONTHS AGO	PRESENT
Pulmonary Function Tests		
Vital capacity (VC)	131	124
Residual volume (RV)	203	282
Peak flow rate (PFR)	121	77
Forced expiratory volume in 1 second (FEV$_1$)	118	114
Mid-maximal flow rate (MMFR)	89	72
Arterial Blood Gases		
PaO$_2$	84	81
PaCO$_2$	34	36
pH	7.41	7.42
Bicarbonate level	21	22

ducts. Therefore, the digestive system does not receive the enzymes necessary to digest fats and proteins.

2. *Multivitamins, vitamin E, and vitamin B* were also necessary because of her problems with malabsorption, which results in a loss of most of the vitamins in her food.

3. *Dicloxacillin and cephalexin (Keflex),* two oral antibiotics, were used to fight the chronic infection in her lungs.

4. *Theophylline (Slo-Phyllin) and albuterol* are an oral medication and an inhaler, respectively. Both are bronchodilators to decrease or reverse the bronchospastic component of her airways.

The plan for Stephanie's admission was for a "clean-out" and family teaching. A "clean-out" for a CF patient generally consists of intravenous antibiotic therapy and intensive chest physical therapy for approximately 10 days to two weeks. In order to determine which IV antibiotic would best benefit Stephanie, a sputum culture would be needed to find out what organisms were in her sputum and what antibiotics these organisms would be sensitive to. *Staphylococcus aureus* and *Pseudomonas aeruginosa* are most commonly associated with pulmonary infection in CF.

By now I had some information that would be helpful in the evaluation and treatment of my new patient. Because this was her first admission, I suspected that she might be a bit apprehensive. From the results of her arterial blood gases and pulmonary function tests, I surmised that she was relatively mild in severity. Because CF is a progressive disease, this would not always be the case. Therefore, it would be important to make sure that my patient and her family were doing all they could to prolong her life and state of wellness.

I keyed into the element of bronchospasm that Stephanie had. Bronchospasm is often present in CF. It would be important to keep this in mind for both her chest physical therapy and exercise program. Also valuable to my assessment was the information that Stephanie was a full-time student in the third grade. Her treatment at home would therefore have to be worked into her school schedule.

Various questions that I kept in mind included: Does her school have physical education? Is Stephanie limited in any way from participating? Does her school have physical therapy services? Is this something that might be relevant in Stephanie's case?

The fact that Stephanie had no siblings was good because her parents would not have to divide their time among several children. However, it also meant that they would have no other diversions. All of their thoughts, concerns, and worries would potentially be on Stephanie. An only child with a chronic, terminal illness can be spoiled as well as overprotected.

I tried to keep my evaluation objective, storing the information I had already received. I also kept in mind that the hospital admission is a good time to get to know a patient and her family, when working with them on a program suitable for home. In this situation, the therapist has more time to develop a rapport with the patient compared to a single outpatient visit.

As I entered the room, I found my patient and her mother both sitting on the bed working on what appeared to be math homework. I introduced myself as one of the chest physical therapists, and said that I would be Stephanie's primary therapist throughout her hospital admission. Mrs. Smith appeared tense and was quick to ask what I would be doing with Stephanie. I told her that initially I would perform an evaluation to formulate an appropriate treatment program and also to establish a baseline to work from. I would then be working with Stephanie daily, performing two to three postural drainage treatments and possibly involving her in group exercise. I made it a point to try to address Stephanie, as well as her mother, because it would be important for her to assume some responsibility for her own care, even at this age. Her mother did not hesitate to inform me that Stephanie would be having a tutor, so as not to fall behind in her schoolwork.

"She's an 'A' student, you know," Mrs. Smith said.

I wondered if Mrs. Smith knew that her daughter had been admitted for medical treatment, and not an extension of her academic work. A certain amount of denial is common in some parents of CF children. This autosomal recessive disorder also promotes some guilt, because both parents are carriers, and in their eyes, are responsible to some degree for the child's illness. This guilt is not deserved, however, because there is seldom a family history, and parents usually have no idea that they are carriers (although approximately every 1 in 20 whites is a carrier) until they have a child diagnosed with cystic fibrosis.

I was not surprised to find that Stephanie was a bright student. Although her digestive and respiratory systems were affected by her illness, her intellect was that of any normal child. Often parents of children with physical disabilities will dwell on other talents, whether musical, artistic, or academic. Therefore, I was not surprised at Mrs. Smith's emphasis on Stephanie's straight-A performance.

Although Mrs. Smith appeared tense and kept looking nervously at her daughter, Stephanie seemed quite friendly and relatively at ease in her new surroundings. My evaluation had begun before I entered the room and continued from the moment I set eyes on my patient. I noticed her petite stature. Although most children with CF are receiving digestive enzymes, many of them still remain small in size compared to their peers. Her extremities were thin. Visual examination of her thorax revealed a very slight increase in anterior-posterior diameter, and her abdomen appeared slightly distended. I noticed an IV in Stephanie's right forearm. She would receive her antibiotics this way while in the hospital.

The nails of her fingers and toes were slightly clubbed. I looked for cyanosis in her nailbeds as well as around her lips. However, they were reasonably pink, which was not surprising with Stephanie's PaO_2 in the 80s. Her respiratory rate at rest was 24, with a good diaphragmatic breathing pattern. Inspiratory to expiratory ratio was 1:3. I did not observe her using accessory muscles to breath while at rest.

Continuing my evaluation, I asked Stephanie to relax and breathe normally while I placed my hands on her lower lateral ribs. I noted good lateral costal expansion and a relatively flexible rib cage. This would be a good time to begin working on thoracic mobility exercises, I thought, in order to maintain this flexibility for as long as possible. With progression of her disease, Stephanie's lungs would become hyperinflated. This, in turn, would lead to an increase in the anterior-posterior diameter of her thorax with a potential decrease in thoracic mobility.

I placed my hand on her diaphragm to

assess its ease and degree of movement. A good diaphragmatic breathing pattern was demonstrated, with nearly full excursion. I palpated her thorax. There was normal tactile fremitus throughout.

"Now, Stephanie, I'd like to take a listen to your breath sounds."

Placing my stethoscope on the areas of her chest over the corresponding lung segments, I asked Stephanie to open her mouth and take some deep breaths. All lung segments were well aerated and free of any adventitious sounds, except the right upper lobe region. Although these segments were free of rales, rhonchi, and wheezes, aeration was mildly decreased. Recalling the findings on chest roentgenogram, I thought we should definitely concentrate on Stephanie's right upper lobe when doing her chest physical therapy.

Throughout all this Stephanie was pleasant and cooperative. After my auscultation of her lungs, she requested a repeat performance on her Cabbage Patch doll, Sandra Ella. I let her borrow my stethoscope and assisted her with the evaluation. I knew from past experience that children are better able to endure a variety of procedures when a favorite doll or stuffed animal shares in the activity. I couldn't help detecting some negative feelings from Mrs. Smith. Perhaps this was directed not so much at me but at the reality of her daughter's illness represented by the present hospitalization.

With a sterile cup in hand, I asked Stephanie to show me how well she could cough. Eager to comply with my request, she demonstrated a strong, yet congested-sounding cough, productive of a small amount of pale green sputum. Her cough was slightly paroxysmal, something we would need to work on, I thought. I was pleased to find Stephanie so cooperative when asked to cough. Many children suppress their coughs, often because they are unable to control it once they get started. These paroxysms of coughing often lead to vomiting.

The oxygen saturation monitor that I brought along seemed to fascinate Stephanie. "Put your finger in here and watch the numbers in lights," I instructed her.

I obtained a resting O_2 saturation of 90%. This would serve as a good baseline for future reference as well as for evaluating exercise tolerance. We then evaluated Sandra Ella's O_2 saturation, a number we both needed a good imagination to obtain.

I decided to save the remainder of my evaluation for the next day, and get on with Stephanie's postural drainage treatment. The staffing levels in our department, unfortunately, did not allow us unlimited time with each patient. The six-minute walk test, posture evaluation, gross manual muscle test, and range-of-motion evaluation would have to wait.

When I asked Stephanie and her mother if they did chest physical therapy at home, they answered at nearly the same time. Mrs. Smith said that it was done regularly, and Stephanie stated simultaneously that they did it "sometimes" or when she "had a cold." These mixed answers did not surprise me. Although most parents are extremely compliant with their child's care at home, there are a few that, for one reason or another, are not. Children, however, usually give an accurate account of what goes on at home. I wondered why the discrepancy in this case? Was time the problem? Could it be denial? Or was Mrs. Smith perhaps just not convinced of the benefits of doing chest physical therapy at home? I hoped that I would be able to be of some assistance.

At this point in my evaluation, my goals were as follows: (1) mobilize excess secretions; (2) improve aeration; (3) work on controlled cough; (4) teaching and instruction (as needed) for chest physical therapy at home; and (5) maintain thoracic mobility.

As we started Stephanie's postural drainage treatment, I was disappointed but not surprised when her mother said she would "go and grab a bite of lunch." I had hoped to review with Mrs. Smith the positions and techniques that I would be using when performing Stephanie's postural drainage treatments. Perhaps she would be available tomorrow.

Stephanie's nurse had previously given her isoetharine (Bronkosol), a bronchodilator, to be inhaled through her aerosol setup. We watched a TV show of Stephanie's choice

("The Brady Bunch"), and talked and laughed while we did her therapy. The ability for a child to enjoy a TV show during therapy many times can help improve compliance of treatment. Her treatment consisted of the use of 11 bronchial drainage positions, percussion, deep breathing with inspiratory hold, vibration during slow, pursed-lip exhalation, huffing, and coughing. I had Stephanie practice coughing twice after each round of percussion and vibration. She tried to stop the cough before it became uncontrollable.

We concentrated on her right upper lobe, anterior and posterior segments. Her cough was slightly more productive in the positions appropriate to drain these areas. We repeated a series of percussion, vibration, and coughing until her cough was nonproductive in each position. Stephanie raised a total of 10 cc of pluggy, pale green secretions.

At times she found her cough difficult to control. "Huffing" seemed to work well by moving secretions high enough to require less work with coughing. Also, premature airway closure is less likely with huffing, compared to coughing; therefore, huffing is especially helpful for someone with reactive airways.

The treatment lasted approximately 45 minutes. Upon auscultation at the end of treatment, all lung segments were well aerated, including the right upper lobe. Scattered high-pitched end-expiratory wheezes were noted throughout. No rales or rhonchi were heard. There had been no significant change in Stephanie's respiratory rate, color, or breathing pattern.

The following morning I was able to complete Stephanie's evaluation. Posture evaluation, gross manual muscle test, and range-of-motion evaluation were all within normal limits. Even though she was without abnormalities in her posture at the present time, this was something we would need to work on to maintain. Many CF patients display the following deviations in posture as the disease progresses: forward head, an increase in thoracic kyphosis, and rounded shoulders.

I took Stephanie up to the chest physical therapy department for the six-minute walk test. The test results would serve as a baseline for Stephanie's exercise tolerance. Her resting respiratory rate was 24, resting pulse was 110, and resting O_2 saturation was 90%. I asked Stephanie to walk up and down a quiet premeasured hallway as many times as she could in six minutes. She seemed pretty excited at the challenge. Mrs. Smith expressed some concern, however, that her daughter not overexert herself. I told Mrs. Smith that aerobic exercise was good for CF patients because it improved endurance as well as trained the ventilatory muscles.

Stephanie was able to complete 24 lengths of the premeasured hallway, which I would calculate into meters. I asked her to rate the task she had just completed using Borg's scale for rating perceived exertion. She gave it a 15. Her respiratory rate was 30 and heart rate was 130 immediately following the walk test. Her O_2 saturation was 87%. She showed no signs of increased bronchospasm.

"What sort of exercise do you do at home, Stephanie?" I asked.

Apparently her parents had discouraged her from "running around too much and getting tired out." In fact, she had been excused from gym class because of her illness. This was an issue I hoped to work on during this admission.

With the remainder of the evaluation complete, my additional goals were as follows: (1) maintain good posture; (2) improve endurance; (3) home instruction to assure Stephanie's regular participation in some form of aerobic exercise; and (4) incorporating thoracic mobility/posture exercises into her program.

Stephanie's mother was still visiting that afternoon. She stayed to observe her daughter's chest physical therapy treatment, and we were able to review the positions and techniques. I was not surprised that Mrs. Smith remembered only 5 of the 11 positions. Her percussion technique was good, but she needed some help with the vibration. Fortunately, she was receptive to my suggestions.

We discussed the importance of daily chest physical therapy at home, even when Stephanie was doing well. I compared it to dusting furniture daily as opposed to waiting for the dust to be two inches thick. Mrs. Smith said that she would prefer her daughter's therapy to be done at home, rather than have her singled out at school for it.

"There are physical therapists available through community agencies who could visit your home to provide Stephanie's therapy," I said. "I think it's best, however, when the child's parents are able to provide the treatment themselves."

I preferred to save community referrals for those situations where it was extremely difficult or impossible for the parents to provide the treatments. Examples of such situations are (1) a single parent with disabling arthritis; (2) both parents working full time in addition to caring for several children; and (3) two or more children with CF in the family, each requiring one or more treatments per day.

I was pleased that Mrs. Smith preferred to do Stephanie's therapy herself. Provided Stephanie's secretion production decreased by the time of discharge, I felt one treatment per day would be sufficient at home. They would be able to increase this if Stephanie had a cold or was more congested than usual.

"Is one time of the day better than another?" I asked. "Well, I suppose in the morning before school would be the easiest," Mrs. Smith said, "Then it would be over with for the day. Maybe my husband wouldn't mind getting breakfast ready while I did therapy."

I arranged to have Mr. Smith come in for a chest physical therapy review so they could alternate. Mrs. Smith asked if they needed to purchase a special postural drainage table. She was concerned about cost and also indicated that she was not very happy about having a piece of medical equipment "in the middle of the house." I told her that a beanbag chair or a foam wedge pillow could do just as well and would probably fit in with the furnishings very nicely. Neither of these was very expensive and could be purchased at a local department store.

The following day I brought Stephanie to the physical therapy department to exercise with some of the other CF patients. Her resting respiratory rate was 22, heart rate was 100, and O_2 saturation was 92%. She started with some warm-up stretches for her lower extremities, including the hamstrings, heelcords, and hip flexors and adductors. I had her ride on one of the stationary bikes we had converted from a regular child's bike. She rode for five minutes without resistance to "warm up." Her respiratory rate was 25, heart rate was 102, and O_2 saturation was 92%.

Gradually adding resistance, I asked her to pedal faster, until it felt like a 13 on Borg's scale of perceived exertion. She continued at this pace for 20 minutes. As she began to work harder, she maintained a good diaphragmatic breathing pattern, showing no signs of accessory muscle use. Monitoring her heart rate and O_2 saturation on the pulse oximeter, her heart rate remained around 125 and her O_2 saturation around 90% throughout the 20 minutes. The resistance was then decreased, and Stephanie pedaled easily for a five-minute "cool down," followed by a repeat of the lower extremity stretches. The exercise had stimulated several productive coughs, which we continued to work on controlling.

Stephanie came to the physical therapy department daily to exercise along with the other CF patients throughout her hospital stay. In addition to the warm-up stretches, I incorporated a few exercises to help maintain good posture. These included trunk rotation (Fig. 64-1) and lateral flexion (Fig. 64-2), thoracic extension (Fig. 64-3), and scapular adduction (Fig. 64-4).

I learned that Stephanie had a bicycle at home and that she loved to ride it. I wrote up the stretching and posture exercises for her. I asked Mrs. Smith to be sure that Stephanie also rode her bike at home for around 20 minutes at least three times a week when the weather was nice. I cautioned her to keep a close watch on Stephanie when exercising in very hot weather. The increased loss of sodium in the sweat of CF patients can have serious effects and can lead to heat prostration. Making sure she had plenty of fluids and increasing the salt in her diet would help.

Before Stephanie was discharged, I made a

(Text continues on p. 1218.)

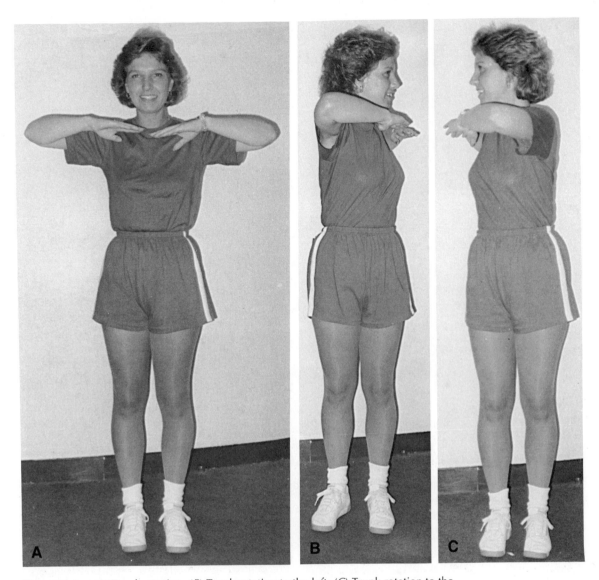

Figure 64-1. (*A*) Trunk rotation. (*B*) Trunk rotation to the left. (*C*) Trunk rotation to the right.

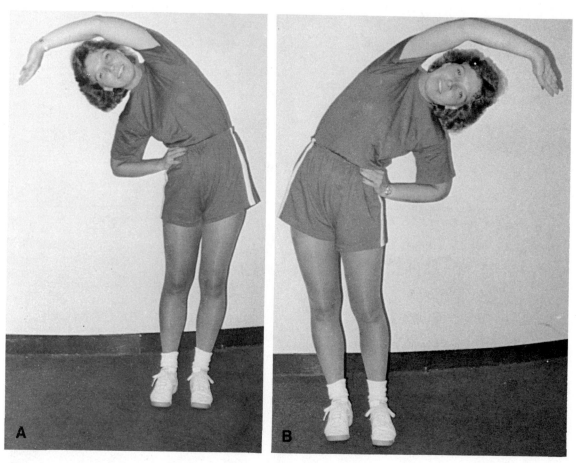

Figure 64-2. (A) Lateral flexion to the right. (B) Lateral flexion to the left.

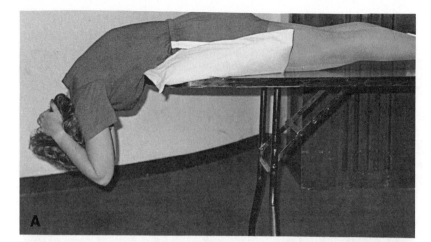

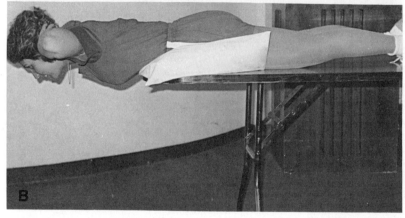

Figure 64-3. (*A*) Thoracic extension from flexed position. (*B*) Thoracic extension to neutral.

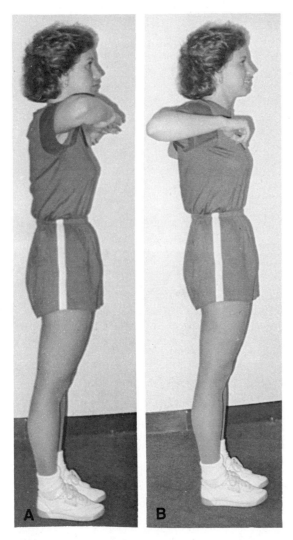

Figure 64-4. (*A*) Slight scapular abduction. (*B*) Scapular adduction.

point of contacting her physical education instructor. I assured her that there was no reason for Stephanie not to participate in gym class. She could run and exercise right along with her classmates. I told her that exercise may lead to coughing, which was nothing to be alarmed about. "Stephanie may just need to step aside a moment in order to keep her cough under control," I said.

Stephanie's two weeks in the hospital seemed to pass very quickly. She was an entertaining child, and at most times, a joy to treat. By the time of her discharge I felt we had done a great deal towards achieving our goals. Stephanie's secretion production had decreased to approximately 2 cc or less. (Table 64-2 lists the discharge pulmonary function tests and arterial blood gases.) A follow-up appointment was made for me to see Stephanie and both her parents during her return visit to the physician in three months.

Table 64-2. Discharge Pulmonary Function and Arterial Blood Gas Tests

	% PREDICTED
Pulmonary Function Tests	
Vital capacity (VC)	133
Residual volume (RV)	132
Peak flow rate (PFR)	120
Forced expiratory volume in 1 second (FEV_1)	119
Mid-maximal flow rate (MMFR)	112
Arterial Blood Gases	
PaO_2	83
$PaCO_2$	35
pH	7.45
Bicarbonate level	24

65 Myocardial Infarction

MARLENE L. BONHAM

I received an order to see a new patient. The rehabilitation department clerk received the following information by phone: *Name,* Jack Bradley; *Diagnosis,* MI; *Therapy,* cardiac rehab; *Physician,* Dr. James; *Room,* 511A; *Date,* 12/10/88. Armed with this, I went to the nursing area where Mr. Bradley was assigned. My first stop was the daily patient summary (DPS), which is located on the main nursing desk. This large sheet of paper briefly summarizes the main points about each patient in that area and indicates the tests that are scheduled for each day. Other information is also noted, such as whether the patient is blind or does not speak English. By glancing over the DPS, I can gather some key information before I study the patient's chart. The DPS contained nothing of special note concerning Mr. Bradley, so I proceeded to read his medical chart.

The first thing I usually check is the admission sheet to determine where and with whom the patient lives, and who to contact in case of emergency. This information gives me an initial sense of the patient's potential support system or lack thereof. Because I know our city well, the street address will alert me to considerations that may affect the design of my home program.

Our facility is a teaching hospital, so gaining quick access to the chart can be a trial. Interns, residents, attending physicians, cardiologists or other specialists, allied health professionals, or any of their students may be reading or adding to the chart. Some of these staff people have completed and documented a history and physical examination; however, many times the data are conflicting. Generally, I start with the most legible history.

The things I look for are general state of health prior to the cardiac event, medical and surgical problems and history, cardiac risk factors, and other information about the patient's social circumstances. (This last item, unfortunately, is usually covered very briefly, if at all.) I also look for electrocardiographic results and any other cardiac studies and their results. I briefly review the medicine sheet to see the general categories of cardiac medication the patient is taking, because some cardiac medicine can alter response to exercise. They all have potential side-effects of which I have to be aware.

I found that Mr. Bradley was the chief executive officer of a small computer firm in the financial district. He had many responsibilities and a very stressful job. He was married, was 57 years old, and had smoked one pack of cigarettes per day for the past 35 years. He drank only socially. He had an appendectomy as a child, and pneumonia 10 years ago. His history was otherwise unremarkable. Motor, sensory, and other basic functions were within normal limits. He was mildly (15 lb) overweight. His mother died of coronary artery disease (CAD) at age 75 years, and his father was alive and well. His two siblings had no know CAD.

Mr. Bradley was in his usual state of health until the morning of his admission to the hospital. On that morning, before leaving for work, he noted a sudden onset of diaphoresis and persistent pain in his left arm. His wife dialed 911 for an ambulance, which brought him to the emergency department. An ECG was immediately performed, and a diagnosis of acute myocardial infarction (MI) of the inferior wall was made.

Mr. Bradley was admitted to the cardiac care unit (CCU) where he was connected to a monitor. Nitroglycerin (NTG) was administered intravenously to control the chest pain and possibly reduce the amount of damage. Diltiazem, a calcium-channel blocker, was started to reduce coronary artery spasm. He was also given propranolol (Inderal), a beta blocker, to control the heart rate and thus reduce the work of the heart.

By the time I reviewed his chart, Mr. Bradley had shown no cardiac symptoms for 24 hours, that is, no chest pain, diaphoresis, lightheadedness, nausea, arrhythmias, or evidence of congestive heart failure (CHF). Enzyme changes, as well as serial ECGs, confirmed a moderate-sized MI of the inferior wall.

As I entered Room 511, I saw a well-groomed middle-aged man wearing his own pajamas and lying quietly in Bed A, reading the *Wall Street Journal*. His nightstand held several containers of flowers and books for light reading. The bulletin board on the wall next to his bed displayed about a dozen get well cards. I introduced myself by my first and last names and my department. I briefly explained to him the purpose of cardiac rehabilitation and physical therapy intervention. Mr. Bradley expressed great interest in all facets of the program. He stated that his cardiologist told him the "cardiac team" would be working with him. He demonstrated a very positive attitude about the program and a desire to learn what he could do to modify his life so as to improve his chance for recovery. I then discussed cardiac rehabilitation, referring to Phases I through IV (inpatient through long-term programs). I told him that in the rest of this session I would interview him to gather baseline information, and perform some objective testing. We would finish with some easy exercises and walking, if tolerated. Mr. Bradley appeared genuinely interested, calm, and focused.

As I began my detailed interview, I looked for more than just the answers to my questions. Besides getting Mr. Bradley's personal assessment of his physical state and limitations, home and community environment, activities, and support system, I also wanted to get a sense of how Mr. Bradley related to me and how he processed and responded to my questions. Mr. Bradley responded quickly and with candor, and appeared to grasp the explanations about the cardiac rehabilitation program. He asked relevant questions at appropriate times. He appeared relaxed, calm, and attentive, and he maintained appropriate eye contact with me throughout the interview. Attending to both the patient's nonverbal and verbal communication enables me to modify my interview style, content, and time to attempt to match the person's responses. This attention also applies to the objective phase of the evaluation, as well as to each treatment.

Mr. Bradley told me that he had injured his knees many times in the past while skiing or playing football, and that he had not participated in either sport for several years. He had never had any corrective surgeries. He tried jogging five years ago, but his knees started to bother him so he gave it up. He stated that he did no form of systematic exercise, but that he occasionally walked to work (downhill, approximately one mile).

His main occupation, preoccupation, and avocation for many years had been the development and running of his company. He stated that he was not involved in many other leisure activities. Periodically, he bowled and played golf, using a cart.

He noted that his wife worked full time and that his 16-year-old son and 14-year-old daughter went to school in the neighborhood. The whole family was very interested in aiding Mr. Bradley's recovery and learning about cardiac rehabilitation and how to live for a healthy heart.

In summary, this is what I now knew about Mr. Bradley that was significant for me. He was very goal oriented, and very involved with his business. Stress was an important risk factor. The cardiac team psychologist needed to be involved directly with the patient, and would have to instruct the rest of the team on how to reinforce stress-reduction techniques. Mr. Bradley had been generally sedentary for many years, but was interested in doing interventions necessary to modify his risk factors. In his case, that meant a progressive exercise program leading eventually to a long-term aerobic exercise program. Lastly, and very importantly, he had a good support system at home.

Now I began my objective testing so that I could gather baseline data to help me design an exercise program and track progress. As with any other patients, I wanted to assess Mr. Bradley's range of motion, strength, posture, gait, judgment, motor planning, and the like— essentially the basic physical therapy information. However, I also needed to monitor Mr. Bradley's cardiac system because of his recent MI. This will tell me if he responds abnormally to exercise, or if he is so unstable that activity will have to be modified or even withheld. Should the latter be true, Mr. Bradley would be re-evaluated before being allowed to begin an exercise program. The parameters I use for basic indicators are heart rate (HR) or pulse, blood pressure (BP), and subjective symptoms. Heart rate should rise with increasing activity; however, activity level in the hospital is very mild, so we don't expect to see much of a rise in HR. If there is a great increase in HR, it may be a sign of severe cardiac damage, deconditioning, or other underlying problems. Twenty beats above the resting rate is generally a parameter used in the inpatient Phase I exercise/ activity program. Systolic blood pressure should rise when work (exercise/activity) is increased. Again, Phase I work is at a low level, so we expect little or no increase in BP. The parameters in Phase I for BP are usually a 10- to 20-mm rise in systolic and a ±10-mm change in diastolic BP. Subjective symptoms such as diaphoresis, shortness of breath (SOB), dyspnea on exertion (DOE), chest pain (CP), and rate of perceived exertion (RPE) are also useful indicators. These can be used serially so that changes in subjective response from one day to the next may be noted. This is useful, for example, when a patient is taking beta-blocking medica-

tion and the HR parameter is no longer totally valid.

The first measurements I took were Mr. Bradley's pulse and blood pressure while he was lying in bed, in the semi-Fowler's position. His pulse was 84 and regular, and his blood pressure was 125/85. These values become the baseline for comparison with future measurements. Next, as a gross inspection of ROM, I asked Mr. Bradley to move his limbs in the bed. At this time, I also did a spot-check of his overall strength. He had no specific deficits in either bilateral knee ROM, girth, strength, or stability.

For efficiency's sake, the first evaluation can also be a treatment session. Therefore, I had Mr. Bradley do some easy, active ROM exercises in bed in the semi-Fowler's position. This is a good starting position because it is less stressful on the cardiac system. He did seven repetitions of shoulder flexion, horizontal abduction, knee to chest, and knee extension movements. He counted out loud with the exercise to control his breathing. There was no undue DOE; HR was 90 and BP was 125/85. Next, I had him sit on the edge of the bed. HR and BP remained the same, and he did not complain of dizziness with the change in position. When he stood up, HR and BP were the same, so we walked 300 feet at an easy pace. I checked the HR and BP every 100 feet using a BP cuff that remained on Mr. Bradley's arm to expedite the procedure. The HR remained at 90 and the BP rose to 130/85. We returned to the room, and he sat on the side of the bed. After three minutes of recovery while sitting and chatting, his HR had returned to 84 and BP to 125/85. No undue DOE or other symptoms were noted.

With my baseline data, I set up a progressive Phase I (inpatient) exercise/ambulation program. Mr. Bradley did light calisthenics, starting in the semi-Fowler's position, progressing to unsupported sitting, and eventually to standing. He also did a moderately paced walking program. This regime was done four to six times a day. Initially, when a person is debilitated or limited because of an acutely damaged cardiac system, the intensity of the exercise is low because that is all that is tolerated. In order to regain stamina slowly with low-level exercise, the frequency of the daily exercise sessions is increased. Stamina can be initially regained in this manner because frequency of exercise sessions is inversely related to the intensity of the exercise sessions. The in-hospital program is coupled with ongoing education about exercise physiology related to cardiovascular (aerobic) conditioning, short- and long-term effects of aerobic exercises, and pacing of activities and exercise so as to balance "resting" and "doing" during recovery. The in-hospital education also helps to reinforce functional stress management techniques.

Mr. Bradley seemed very intent on following the prescribed program and was conscientious about monitoring his pulse and subjective symptoms. He maintained a bedside flow sheet on his daily progress. Again, he seemed appropriately interested in learning and applying these new skills, but not unduly apprehensive about the modification of his life-style. He also did not deny the extent of the problem he faced or refuse to take steps to control the risk factors that were controllable.

Other members of the cardiac rehabilitation team who worked with Mr. Bradley were the occupational therapist, psychologist, social worker, dietitian, and staff nurse. The common goal we all share is to have any patient functioning as completely as possible in the community while trying to cope with and assimilate the positive health habits that it is hoped will reduce the risk of further cardiac events. Generally, the occupational therapist works on modified activities of daily living (ADL) using principles of energy conservation and work simplification. This is especially important in the first few weeks of recovery. The psychologist works with the patient and his support structure (family or significant others) in managing stress and establishing coping mechanisms to deal with a catastrophic illness. Methods to reduce stress and possibly modify "Type A" behavior are also addressed. The dietitian helps the patient and family to set up new diet plans, which may be low fat, low salt, low sugar, or a combination thereof. The social worker may be needed if there are disposition problems or if referrals are needed for community resources. The social worker may also be the connection to other providers, such as a vocational rehabilitation counselor, who may be needed on a case-by-case basis. The nurse is the member of the team who is closest to the patient and his daily activities. She is useful in orchestrating and pacing the patient's daily schedule. She also instructs the patient and his family about medications and basic cardiac anatomy, physiology, and pathology.

All staff members deal with specific techniques and education on risk factor modification. All have a sense of the other members' roles and tasks and are able to reinforce each other's messages.

By the time Mr. Bradley was discharged, he was walking for 10 to 15 minutes at a time at a 2.5-mph pace, which was a comfortable pace for him. He took a low-level stress test (treadmill) while he was still on propranolol (Inderal), and was stopped when his HR reached 120. Mr. Bradley remained on the treadmill for five minutes and no chest pain or ischemic changes were noted.

Mr. Bradley returned to the outpatient center several days after discharge to continue with his Phase II cardiac rehabilitation. His goals for the next four to six weeks were to continue to progress from low- to moderate-level exercise and activity and continue his education by various members of the cardiac team. We continued to monitor his HR, BP, and other subjective symptoms to make sure the cardiac system was responding appropriately to increased work loads and, if not, to notify the physician for further workups and intervention procedures.

Mr. Bradley came to Phase II three times a week for two months. By the end of this time, he was walking (at home) three times a week at a 3-mph pace for 45 minutes a session. His heart rate increase with walking was 20 to 25 beats above resting. In the outpatient program, he was on the stationary bike for 25 minutes and the arm ergometer for 15 minutes. He progressively built up the intensity and duration on each modality, and maintained his HR 30 beats above resting. Systolic blood pressure rise was 15 mm and diastolic BP was stable on the bike and the arm ergometer. He had begun to do some work at home starting in Week 2 and by Week 4 went to his office three afternoons a week. He took a taxi, public transportation, got a ride, or walked until Week 4 when his doctor allowed him to drive again.

Throughout Phase II, Mr. Bradley continued to approach his life-style changes very positively and made every effort to figure out ways to handle his work load with less stress. He began delegating tasks to his staff that he previously had always done himself. His family was extremely supportive of all these efforts. His wife started to exercise with him. The entire household switched to a "healthy-heart diet" and his son stopped smoking.

Mr. Bradley's ultimate goal was 30 to 45 minutes of aerobic-level exercise plus warm-up and cool-down three to five times a week, which would be accomplished as he moved into Phase III cardiac rehabilitation. This usually happens 8 to 12 weeks after the cardiac event without complications, and is a generally accepted guideline in the medical community.

Ten weeks passed and Mr. Bradley returned to work full time. He had an uneventful recovery. He was taking no medication, but had NTG to take as needed. He had diligently worked on exercise and stress management, he had stopped smoking, and the family had converted to a "healthy-heart diet" (low fat, low salt). He had lost 12 pounds.

He was given a maximal stress test without propranolol (Inderal). He got halfway through stage IV of the Bruce protocol and stopped because of fatigue. Heart rate at stopping was 145 and BP was still rising. Recovery after the treadmill test was unremarkable.

Mr. Bradley entered our after-work aerobic exercise program (Phase III) three times a week. We set his exercise prescription using the above mentioned treadmill data as a baseline. Our method of figuring out his target heart rate was Korvonen's, or heart rate reserve, formula:

$$(\text{Maximum HR} - \text{Resting HR} \times 60\% \text{ to } 80\%) + \text{Resting HR} = \text{Target HR}$$

This gave Mr. Bradley target values to achieve and maintain during the aerobic phase of his exercise program. Because Mr. Bradley had been successful with walking and the stationary bike, and he enjoyed both forms of exercise, we continued to use them as the major part of the aerobic component. He continued with the arm ergometer and some light resistive arm pulleys for general toning and strengthening.

Mr. Bradley stayed in Phase III for six months. He had no further sequelae and decided he could continue to ride his recently purchased stationary bike and do a walking program at home. This, then, became his long-term community program (Phase IV). He continued to walk to or from work several days a week. He also rode his stationary bike or walked four times a week for 30 minutes each time, with 10 minutes of light calisthenics for warm-up and a five-minute cool-down. A list of community resources was given to Mr. Bradley by the physical therapist and the nurse who manage the Phase III program. He and his wife joined a cardiac support group at the local chapter of the American Heart Association, and continued to go to its discussion and education sessions once a month.

CASE VARIATIONS

1. *If* in Phase I, Mr. Bradley had chest pain with no or low-level activity, the physician would have been notified. Cardiac catheterization probably would have been used in an attempt to locate correctable lesions. Balloon angioplasty then would have been done, and, if that failed, aortocoronary bypass surgery (ACB). The physician might have elected to do the ACB as the initial intervention. After the therapeutic interventions, Mr. Bradley would have come to

the cardiac team for progressive cardiac rehabilitation, because his underlying CAD and risk factors still remained.

2. *If* Mr. Bradley had more than an occasional ventricular arrhythmia or an increase in arrhythmias with exercise, the physician would be notified immediately. The patient probably would be put on an antiarrhythmic medication, and we would continue to advance exercise carefully and monitor closely because the medication often needs to be adjusted or changed.

3. *If* Mr. Bradley had post-MI congestive heart failure, poor ejection fraction (less than 40%, indicating significant damage to the left ventricle, ie, the main pump), worsening rales after exercise (ie, increased backup of fluid into the lungs secondary to the pump being unable to keep up with the work load), or a drop in BP with exercise, we would reduce our expectations. We would move very cautiously, and monitor his subjective and objective symptoms closely. Ultimately, we want to enable the person to be as mobile and functional as possible within his physiological limits.

4. *If* Mr. Bradley physically was proceeding with an uneventful course after the MI, but he refused to stop smoking or modify his diet, continued to argue with his family and business associates, and became very agitated every time they came to visit, the staff would have to take a different approach. The psychologist would become a key figure both in dealing directly with Mr. Bradley (if the patient let him) and in keeping the staff unified on an approach that might be more reasonable and consistent. Our obligation as health care providers to Mr. Bradley is to provide him with current information and treatment interventions that, to the best of our scientific and medical knowledge, will modify his cardiac risk factors and (it is hoped) reduce his morbidity (length of illness) and extend his longevity.

When a patient is resistant, it seems that the more you push information and suggestions, the more you have to push against. In such cases, backing off and reducing the amount of input and initial expectations might have a positive effect. In our profession, we often see that the messages do not go through the first time around. However, if we keep our lines of communication open, remain nonjudgmental, and keep our services available, often the patient will return after he sorts out his problem and what it means to him.

If a person chooses to ignore all interventions offered, then it is his choice in the end. We still keep the lines of communication open and move on.

In summary, these are my basic assumptions about working with patients who have suffered an MI. The role of physical therapy is to help a person progress in activity and exercise systematically from bed rest, to minimal activity, to aerobic-level exercises.

The more work you do, the more work you become capable of doing. Therefore, a major goal of treatment is to increase the person's endurance no matter what his underlying problem. Even patients with severe cardiovascular (central) damage can train the peripheral vascular system and increase the oxygen utilization in the exercising muscles. This allows higher levels of endurance and functional activities within a safe training heart rate and blood pressure range that does not stress the damaged cardiovascular system. This will enhance a person's quality of living and the control of his environment. Becoming educated regarding the reasons and methods of our program enables a client to understand, value, and habituate a life-style that is considered healthy and safe for the patient with heart problems.

By taking specific steps to help reduce or modify the risk factors that Mr. Bradley could control, such as stopping smoking, he was able to go back to work and regain his place in the community with a forward-looking, yet reasonable, attitude and mind set. His quality of life was enhanced because he was taking active steps to remain in control of his life and destiny. He didn't become a "cardiac cripple" and stop all the activities that he cherished. He didn't ignore the situation and plow ahead as if he never had a heart attack at all, and let what would happen, happen.

After a cardiac event, if the client is lucky, there are no sequelae. The person modifies the risk factors and remains stable for many years. If the person has continuing ischemia and blockage, ACB or angioplasty may correct the blockage but not the underlying coronary artery disease. If the client has congestive heart failure or significant arrhythmias, prognostically these problems may not be good signs. Medical control is sought. This does not mean that there is no place for progressive rehabilitation. However, it does mean that goals and expectations may have to be more modest or different.

In any event, improving the quality of life by helping the patient gain some personal control of his own destiny is still a major reason to begin a graded, progressive exercise and activity program.

As therapists, whether a person will achieve total health or return to the premorbid baseline is not our ultimate concern. Getting a person to cope with whatever remaining function he has, helping him to get back whatever function he can, and making the best of it should be the focus of our training and our philosophical approach to the person suffering from a disability. We must bear in mind that, from a rehabilitation standpoint, cardiac dysfunction is really no different from any other disability.

66 Well Elderly

TIMOTHY L. KAUFFMAN

As I waited to be introduced to the group of senior adults, I thought about what I was going to say about aging, declining mobility, and exercising. I reflected upon the meaning of "aging," its definitions in literature as well as in science, and the paintings and sculptures devoted to the subject. I recalled the delineation of the seven ages of man by Shakespeare in As You Like It, act II, scene VII: "Last scene of all, That ends this strange eventful history, Is second childishness and mere oblivion, Sans teeth, sans eyes, sans taste, sans everything." This description teased my sense of humor, but made my professional self recoil. Not all elderly persons decline to that level of oblivion. In fact, many continue to contribute greatly to society. The names of Michelangelo, Ben Franklin, Arthur Rubinstein, and Claude Pepper quickly flashed across my mind. Philosophically, what is aging? Only the passage of time, which affects each of us by bringing its requisite experience and change, but not necessarily degradation.

My thoughts returned to the meeting room. I observed how persons moved so that I could present examples from the group to support my presentation and possibly motivate them to exercise. Without surprise, I noticed that most of the older women—those over 75 years—and a few of the men had increased kyphotic curves of the thoracic spine. One person even had a kyphosis of his lumbar spine that I could see through his shirt. Two persons were using walkers, and three had canes. One person was wearing a bilateral metal upright ankle-foot orthosis (AFO) and another had a molded AFO. I estimated that nearly one fourth of the group was wearing hearing aids, and it was apparent that several persons had very poor vision.

My observations poignantly demonstrated that all humans age as individuals. Their movement and postures become part of their living history. I recalled my excitement at listening to a former patient talk about life in czarist Russia, and another relate her father's stories about the Battle of Gettysburg. My thoughts were interrupted when one of the women from the group introduced herself to me. "Hi, I'm Emily Wade," she said. "I see that you are watching us closely. What are you looking for?"

I introduced myself and explained that I was the guest speaker for that day. I admitted my enthusiasm for geriatric care, especially for persons like herself who were essentially well elderly and living in the community independently or with some social service help. I told her of my dislike for the negative stereotypes of older persons, and pointed out that most persons over the age of 65 lived in the community and not in nursing homes or hospitals. And yes, lots of older people forget things, but so did younger persons. (I estimated myself to be half of Emily's age, which I guessed was between 78 and 83.) I confessed to her that that morning I had forgotten not only my directions to the senior center but also what time I was supposed to speak.

She laughed and asked if I thought I could help with her problem. She said that she was

1226

81 years old. Since her husband's death two years previously, she had been living alone and doing well until the last six months. At that time, she had fallen and fractured her right wrist. It was healed now, but she still had pain occasionally and continued to drop things. However, since her fall she had become scared of walking and she found herself doing less and less. This concerned her because she was going out with her friends less frequently.

I thought quietly to myself of the activity and the disengagement theories of aging. Persons who are physically, socially, and mentally active generally have greater life satisfaction than persons who have less social interaction. These disengaged persons become isolated and have lower life satisfaction.

Before Emily had introduced herself, I had noticed her helping some of the others, and she seemed to be well liked. However, I had also noticed that she carried her right upper extremity in a somewhat protected position (elbow flexed and close to her thorax). Also, she walked with some of the gait changes typical of aging. She was slightly unsteady; her strides were short, and her feet hardly left the floor during swing phase.

Emily went on to say that her problem was that she had "a little rheumatism" in her back, right shoulder, and knees, especially when it was cold and damp, but her biggest concern was that she was "just slowing down. I can't get around as well as I used to and I'm terribly afraid of falling." She had fallen twice since fracturing her wrist. "Am I too old?" she asked. "Am I over the hill?" I replied, "From my perspective on geriatric rehabilitation, life has value at any age. Persons who live to be 100 years old have all suffered one or more pathological conditions, just as you have. But, it is essential to maintain independent living with the highest level of functioning, although it is difficult to determine what the highest level is. In rehabilitation it is better to fail by trying than to fail without trying."

It was time for me to start my presentation, so I got Emily's and her physician's phone numbers. I told her that I would be happy to

see her the next afternoon in my office, and that I would call her physician.

Dr. Shrum was pleased that I contacted her, because she was concerned about Emily's decline over the past 12 to 18 months. Dr. Shrum related that Emily had a history of degenerative joint disease (DJD) in her knees and spine, and had had one transient ischemic attack (TIA) three years ago from which she had fully recovered. Besides her recent wrist fracture, Emily had suffered compression fractures of the eighth and ninth thoracic vertebral bodies nine years ago. At that time she had been started on estrogen and calcium in an effort to treat her osteoporosis. In addition, Emily had atherosclerotic cardiovascular disease (ASCVD).

I explained to Dr. Shrum that outpatient physical therapy (PT) under Medicare Part B had guidelines that required a proper diagnosis and a decision that the PT was reasonable and necessary treatment for the condition. I suggested that the PT should be reimbursable under Medicare for the diagnosis of DJD with multiple recent falls and a history of TIA, ASCVD, and fractures of the wrist and vertebral bodies. I informed Dr. Shrum that I would get back to her after I evaluated Emily Wade. I suggested that Medicare might pay for several weeks of PT, after which Emily had indicated that she was willing to pay privately.

Emily had already filled out our office intake form when I greeted her in the waiting room. Besides what she had told me the previous day, I noticed that her father died at age 93 from colon cancer and her mother died at 97 from pneumonia. Her weight was 102 lbs and she was 5 ft, 3 in tall. In addition to the complaints she had told me about, she indicated that she had difficulty putting on her stockings sometimes because of right hip and knee pain. I noted that on the human body diagram she had indicated that she had some numbness in her anterolateral right thigh. I made a mental note that this area is the L2-3 dermatomes and may be related to an entrapment of the lateral femoral cutaneous nerve, known as meralgia paresthetica.

In order to assess her mental abilities

quickly, I asked Emily the following questions: When is your birthday? What is today's date? When is the next holiday? Who is the President? What is his name? Add 5 + 8; 92 + 11. Close your eyes, turn around, and raise your hands over your head five times.

Emily responded to all of the questions quickly and had no difficulty even with the three-stage command. She was able to follow directions and her hearing did not seem to be a problem with normal speech. Overall her affect was pleasant, sincere, motivated, confident, and capable. This woman had a lot of poise. I thought she was a good candidate for a rehabilitation program to regain some function and to retard any further loss, especially in mobility.

As Emily stood to go back to a treatment table, I noticed that she pushed up with both hands on the chair armrests. On her first step, she lost balance slightly to the right, but recovered easily. As we proceeded down the hallway, Emily had a little difficulty negotiating around a stool that was jutting into the hallway. Wondering if that was due to visual or motor problems, I asked her if she had any visual problems. She replied, "Yes, I'm developing a cataract in my left eye. But it isn't too bad." She was wearing glasses.

"What is the color of my tie?" I asked. "What color are the curtains? How many fingers am I holding up?" I quickly checked her peripheral vision and her oculomotor ability by moving my fingers and asking Emily to respond each time they entered her visual field and to follow my fingers with her eyes. She responded correctly to these questions and tests, although her left visual field and depth perception were slightly decreased. This could mean a higher risk of stumbling over objects, or falling on steps, especially if there is no handrail.

I left the treatment area and Emily changed into gym shorts and a T-shirt. Upon reentering, I explained what I was going to do in this evaluation. "I will talk and think out loud. Do not worry about the terms I use or things I say. I'll draw my conclusion at the end and then I'll

explain everything. But stop me at any time if you have questions. You go ahead and talk while we are doing this. Your input is important."

I continued, "I usually say so much that most patients are unable to understand everything. So when you go home tonight and questions pop into your mind, please write them down. I think it is very important for you to understand as much as possible. One final thing before I forget it: You may be a little stiff or sore after what I do because I may ask you to do things that you haven't done for a long time. If you do get sore, use a little pain medication—whatever you normally use."

"First, I want to look at your posture. Over the years, because of habit, injury, or disease, the alignment or configuration of our bodies changes. Some of these are common to most older persons and some are idiosyncratic or personal. Some changes may cause pain or contribute to declining mobility; some can be corrected."

While Emily was sitting, I observed her from the front, back, and sides. I noted that her right shoulder remained in that protected position, with the elbow flexed and tight against the thorax and the scapula protracted. Her head was forward and her trunk was sidebent slightly to the right.

In the standing position her head was forward; the thorax was kyphotic; and the lumbar spine was flat. Both shoulders were rounded (scapulae protracted). The feet were equally spaced and weight bearing appeared to be symmetrical. The iliac crests and gluteal folds were level. There was no scoliosis. There was a normal arch in the feet, and the Achilles tendon and calcanei were perpendicular to the floor.

I asked Emily to bend forward, backward, to the left, to the right, and then to rotate left and right. Her trunk range of motion (ROM) was fairly good in that she got her hands to her ankles in forward bend and her shoulders rotated almost 90 degrees left and right; she was able to touch her fibular heads when sidebending each way; and the backbend was at least 30 degrees from the erect perpendicular posture. I did note that when she rotated there was very little motion at the thoracolumbar levels. Most of the rotation occurred in the middle and upper thoracic levels. This is not uncommon.

I asked Emily to perform the same motions with her neck, but I warned her not to hyperextend because of the potential harm of kinking the vertebral arteries. I warned her to be careful of this motion at home in situations such as looking upward to place something on a high shelf or tilting her head backward when drinking something. I explained to her that some experts in aging believe that this simple motion may be why some older persons fall and break their hips when they really were not doing anything to cause a fall.

In the standing position, her head was forward and her shoulders were rounded, so the typical plumb line position of the acromion and the mastoid was not too far off. Her neck was flexed in the lower cervical spine, and hyperextended at the upper cervical spine. This was an important compensation because it maintained the eyes on a horizontal plane.

Emily was able to touch her chin to her chest and extend her neck to neutral. I measured her rotations (70 degrees left and right) and sidebending (60 degrees left and right) with the goniometer. She had the typical shortened and prominent sternocleidomastoids bilaterally and tight pectoralis muscles. I pulled her shoulders back (as a figure eight clavicular splint would) and she responded, "That feels good, but I can really feel the pulling across my chest and neck." Before having her sit down, I asked Emily to walk on her heels, and then on her toes. She did fine for 12 to 15 steps.

With Emily sitting on a treatment table, I observed her posture. It was essentially unchanged from the standing and seated positions in an armchair. I checked her balance by sitting down beside her, then giving her a quick shove. She responded well with appropriate righting responses of upper and lower extremities. After I apologized to her, I explained that I was checking her balance mechanism. Then I checked her equilibrium by

gently pushing her from side to side in the seated position with her eyes open, then with her eyes closed (somewhat like using a tiltboard with a child).

Because she responded so well to these maneuvers when sitting, I made a mental note to assess the same maneuvers when she is standing. I suspected that her falling problem originated in a lower extremity.

Her ankle and knee joints were symmetrical and normal. Both knees were fusiform. Her extensor hallucis longus strength was good. There was no clonus, and I felt no inappropriate muscle activity or resistance to movement at the ankles, knees, or hips.

Next, I asked Emily to lie down on the table. I observed her skin, color, muscle definition, posture, joint alignment, and shape. There was a hallux valgus on the left. The posterior tibial pulse was 72 and strong on the left, but it was a little more difficult to find and was weaker on the right. The dorsalis pedis pulse could not be located on either foot, but capillary filling appeared to be fine and the feet and toes were warm to touch.

Proceeding in a cephalad direction, I saw that her right lower extremity was slightly abducted and shorter by approximately 1.5 cm. I adducted it, and saw that the legs appeared equal in length. After I released the right lower extremity, it abducted once again. I measured the amount of abduction to be 15 degrees from neutral on the right, and 0 degrees on the left. She appeared to have a tightness of the right tensor fasciae latae, hip flexors, and possibly the quadratus lumborum.

On sensory evaluation of the lower extremities, I noted hypoesthesia over the right L2-3 dermatome. Again, I thought of the lateral femoral cutaneous nerve. In all other areas of the lower extremities, Emily responded appropriately to light tactile, pain, and thermal stimuli. Knowing that vibratory sense is associated with balance, I thought to myself, "I wish that tuning fork that I ordered were here. Perhaps Dr. Shrum can check this out."

Emily's straight leg raise was negative at 95 degrees bilaterally. Her lower extremity ROM was essentially within normal limits, except in the following: ankle dorsiflexion was only 5 degrees bilaterally, and her right knee flexion was tight at 120 degrees. There was no marked tenderness with palpation of the lower extremities, except at the iliotibial band, and there was increasing tenderness over the tensor fascia latae and the rectus femoris where they attach at the iliac spine; hypertrophy of these muscles was also present.

I asked Emily to turn onto her left side, and I performed the Ober test to assess TFL tightness. The test was positive. Then still with her on her left side, I kept Emily's hip at 0 degrees extension and I measured her knee flexion. It was limited to 100 degrees on the right, indicating tight quadriceps. In the right sidelying position, the left knee flexed to 130 degrees; my suspicion of meralgia paresthetica (entrapment of the lateral femoral cutaneous nerve) was growing. But was the entrapment at the L2-3 nerve roots? Was there a mass in the right lower quadrant impinging upon the nerves? Was the nerve entrapped on the inguinal ligament, or as it crosses the anterior superior iliac spine (ASIS)? Was this problem the cause of her falling? It was not likely to be a major reason for her falling, because it was not a motor but a sensory nerve; yet, sensation is important for balance, and this entrapment has been associated with back pain, which can contribute to falls.

On a manual muscle test, no asymmetrical weakness was found on any of the lumbar or sacral levels; strength was graded Good (4). However, I did find the hip extensors to be Fair-minus (3−) bilaterally in the prone position. When testing hip extension in the seated position, with a concentric contraction from 90-degree hip flexion to approximately 30-degree hip flexion, I found her hip extension strength was Good (4). I thought of the length tension curves that I learned in physiology and of the concept of stretch weakness as described by Kendall.

Also in the sidelying position, Emily, like most elderly persons, used her TFL and quadratus lumboram in lieu of her gluteus medius.

In the sidelying position her strength was Fair-minus for hip abduction because she had, in essence, forgotten or lost the gluteus medius. I felt these weaknesses were major contributing factors to the shuffling gait and shortened strides.

Before proceeding to the upper extremities, I noted that Emily had no difficulty with the functional tasks of rolling over, turning side to side, and moving from sitting to supine and supine to sitting. I then examined the ligamentous stability of both knees, and found them to be slightly lax (hypermobile) when testing the medial collateral ligaments and the anterior cruciate ligaments. This did not surprise me, but I thought that this slight instability might contribute to balance problems and to the unsteadiness of gait.

When she was prone, I examined Emily's back and found no areas of tenderness, hot or cold spots, or skin problems. However, the fascia over the right lumbar spine and iliac crest was tight, the spinous processes of T4-12 were prominent, and the scapulae were protracted bilaterally.

I quickly went through a passive ROM test of her upper extremities, after which I asked Emily to perform the same motions actively. During the passive test, I did not feel any clonus or marked change in tone or resistance to movement. The right wrist (the fractured side) had functional ROM at 50 degrees flexion, 45 degrees extension, 20 degrees radial deviation, and 30 degrees ulnar deviation. There was no marked tenderness. The skin and circulation to the hand appeared to be good. The web space of the right hand was decreased slightly in comparison to the left, but Emily was able to oppose her thumb to each finger and she could make a tightly closed fist. She appeared to have no difficulty manipulating coins or marbles in her hands. Her stereognosis was satisfactory. Her only complaint was that she occasionally dropped things from her right hand. On a manual muscle test, the strength of her wrist and finger flexors and extensors was Good-minus (4−). Right shoulder strength was Good-plus (4+). I noted atrophy in the thenar and hypothenar eminences as well as in the forearm. I suspected that she had not regained full strength of her right hand.

As I worked on her hand, I assessed her light tactile sensation and position sense by moving her fingers and wrist into flexion and extension and her thermal perception by placing objects of different temperatures into each hand. To check pain perception, I gently pushed her index finger to her palm but I immediately stopped when she withdrew and said, "That hurts!" Her deep tendon reflexes were symmetrical and normal, and her tactile sensation was appropriate in the C2-T1 dermatones. I thought it probable that her hand complaint was not a cervical radiculitis, even though the vast majority of persons over 60 years of age have DJD of the cervical spine on roentgenograms.

I asked Emily to stand up, but warned her to sit for a moment "until your head clears." I cautioned her about sudden movements and especially changes of position, such as standing up, which may cause dizziness because the circulatory and balance control mechanisms may be slow to respond. Once standing, I checked her unilateral stance, sidestepping, and crossover stepping. I also checked her standing balance with her eyes closed. Emily could not stand on either foot longer than five seconds with her eyes open and less than two seconds with her eyes closed. Her crossover steps and sidesteps were unsteady and uncoordinated except when she held on to the parallel bars.

I could see that Emily was getting tired from all of the activity so I decided not to go any further in my evaluation at that time. I summarized Emily's problems for her as follows:

1. The problem with falling is probably caused by some muscle weakness, knee instability, and arthritis. There definitely is some nerve impingement, which causes the numbness of the thigh. Some of the nerves (joint mechanoreceptors and proprioceptors) that help to balance the body are probably less effective than they used to be. (I also think to myself that changing muscle fiber types may contribute to balance, strength, and coordination problems.)
2. The problem with dropping things is most likely caused by weakness and easily fatigued muscles in the hand and wrist.
3. The "rheumatism" in the back is probably caused by osteoporosis and declining flexibility of the disks, joint capsules, ligaments, and other connective tissues. Also, the muscle weaknesses and imbalances, particularly the right hip, may cause abnormal pulling across the back.
4. The old TIA does not show up as much of a problem; however, it may be a factor in slowness and uncoordinated movement and balance and dizziness problems.
5. The heart disease (ASCVD) may be a factor in the fatigue and may possibly cause arrhythmias that result in falls.

I contacted Dr. Shrum and discussed my findings. She agreed to test Emily's vibratory sense. I suggested that a submaximal $\dot{V}O_2$ test be performed in our office to assess her aerobic capacity because of her complaints of fatigue and history of ASCVD. In conjunction with this, I suggested a vital capacity and forced expiratory volume test because of her kyphosis, compression fractures, and fatigue. I also suggested a grip strength measurement for peak force and a power measurement for 10 seconds. An isokinetic evaluation of the knees and hips would also be helpful. Finally, a home evaluation would be in order.

Dr. Shrum informed me that she had been treating Emily's ASCVD for two years now and that it was well-controlled. She agreed that a submaximal $\dot{V}O_2$ test would be fine. Emily had no cardiac arrhythmias. The other tests that I suggested were also acceptable to Dr. Shrum.

At her next visit, I asked Emily, "How did you feel after all the work I put you through last time?" She replied, "I was pretty sore that night, but it went away the next day after I got up and got moving."

After Emily changed into her shorts and T-shirt, I observed her gait from the front, rear, and sides. I asked her to walk at slow, normal, and fast paces. I made the following observations:

1. The gait was reciprocal, without a gluteus maximus or gluteus medius limp.
2. Strides were approximately 15 to 20 cm.
3. Stance phase was essentially symmetrical for each lower extremity.
4. Toe off and foot clearance from the floor were minimal.
5. The base of support was about shoulder width.
6. Arm swing of the right was decreased.
7. Turning around usually caused a loss of balance.
8. The faster pace increased the use of the upper extremities in an apprehensive gait.

After a brief rest, I tested Emily on our computer, following the protocol for group strength. Her results corroborated my findings in the normal muscle test. The peak force generated was 57 lb on the left and 42 lb on the right for a deficit of 26%. The power was 510 lb on the left and 317 lb on the right for a deficit of 38%. (The protocol for this program is to express power as pounds because it is more comprehensible than an expression of power in terms of foot-pounds/second or watts.)

We then proceeded to the spirometer evaluation, which showed Emily to be above average for her age. We moved on to the submaximal $\dot{V}O_2$ test, which was programmed to stop when Emily's heart rate reached 85% of her estimated maximum—in her case, 118 ($220 - 81 = 139 \times 85\% = 118$). Emily performed well, although she had difficulty keeping her feet on the pedals, and she asked to stop the test before she reached 118 because she was exhausted. Her submaximal $\dot{V}O_2$ is 1.1 L, which is average to good for her age.

We decided not to do any more exercise that day, but I put some moist heat on her anterior and lateral right hip and thigh, and on her anterior and posterior right knee. High-voltage electrical stimulation was applied for 20

minutes, with two pads, to her right anterolateral hip and to the right medial and lateral knee joint line. I explained that the heat and electrical stimulation would help increase her blood flow, might reduce her pain, and possibly would make it easier for me to stretch her quadriceps and iliotibial band.

As Emily was receiving her moist heat and electrical stimulation, we chatted about what had been done and what we can do about it together. We established an overall goal: Improve Emily's function by increasing her strength, balance, coordination, ROM, flexibility, and exercise tolerance, and by decreasing the soreness around the right hip and knee. To reach the goal, we established the following objectives:

1. Increase the strength of her hip extensors and abductors so she can properly lift 5 lb against gravity 20 times.
2. Maintain balance in unilateral stance for each leg. Stand for 10 seconds two out of three trials with eyes open, without assistance or losing balance.
3. Perform a cross over step in front and in back for a distance of 20 ft in each direction, without manual assistance or stumbling.
4. Ride three miles in 15 minutes on an exercise bicycle, with minimal resistance.
5. Flex the right knee to 120 degrees or greater with assistance, with the hip at 0 degrees extension in the sidelying position.
6. Reduce the pain so that dressing activities are not difficult.

On Emily's next visit to physical therapy, we completed the computerized isokinetic evaluation of the quadriceps and hamstrings, at 180°/sec and 90°/sec. She was unable to attain a velocity of 180°/sec. This did not surprise me, because there is a greater loss of type II (fast-twitch) muscle fibers with age than type I (slow-twitch) fibers. There were no marked deficits when I compared the two sides. Weakness did not appear to be a major problem, which again corroborated my manual muscle test; however, speed was a problem. I wondered if Emily was a little slow in getting her foot out to catch herself when she stumbles because of this deficit. Her peak torque was 32% of her body weight for her left quadriceps and 30% for her right quadriceps.

I set the speed for 90°/sec for the hip abduction test. There are no norms established for this test, so I was not upset when Emily generated only a peak torque of 12 ft lb on the right and 15 ft lb on the left. I did think that hip abduction needed to be strengthened.

Realizing that older persons can improve strength and that motor learning is a major factor in early strength improvement, I decided not to push her too hard. I warned her not to expect tremendous improvements in one or two weeks, but as she improved we would push harder.

We established the following treatment regimen:

1. ROM to the cervical spine, trunk, and right lower extremity.
2. Strengthening exercises with a progressive resistive routine for the right upper extremity and right hip.
3. Manual resistive exercise for all four extremities, with high velocity, less resistance and slow velocity, heavy resistance, plus an emphasis on working with the terminal ranges of motion. Resistance is applied in cardinal movements as well as in proprioceptive neuromuscular facilitation (PNF) patterns.
4. Stationary bicycling, starting with five minutes and increasing to 20 minutes.
5. Balance exercises, including unilateral stance, sidesteps, high steps, crossover steps, and backward steps. Occasionally we use a foot placement ladder.
6. Weight shift is practiced in the unilateral and bilateral stances to simulate rocking onto heels, then toes, then lateral and medial aspects of feet.
7. Moist heat and electrical stimulation are followed by manual stretch and myofascial release to the lower back, right hip, right thigh, right lower quadrant, and adjacent areas.
8. General conditioning exercises are added

to strengthen her trunk extensors, scapular retractors, and latissimus dorsi.

I scheduled my next visit with Emily to be at her house. As I drove up I noticed that a bus stop was located only one-half block from her door. The sidewalks were level and in good repair. There was a level entranceway into her house through the garage and four steps up to the front door. There was no handrail, but the outside lights were well-placed.

Emily greeted me at the door. As I walked through her home, I was pleased with what I saw. The carpets were not too thick. Only one small throw rug was not well secured. Emily's grandson would fix it with two-way tape. The lights were placed so that she had good illumination without too much glare. The cupboards were not too high and she had a small footstool with an armrest for reaching the top shelf. The kitchen chairs had armrests, and the living room sofa and chairs were not too low for Emily. The steps to the second floor were not worn or slippery, but the landing at the bottom needed a handrail. The bathroom was easily accessible from the bedroom, and there were lights available. I noticed a night-light in the bathroom and the bedroom. The bed was sufficiently firm and not too low. Emily was able to get up from bed and to roll over without any difficulty. There were no electrical cords sticking out to trip her. Emily's husband had a grab bar installed in the bathroom several years ago. There was a nonskid bath mat. I checked the hot water, and estimated it to be only about 130°F. This temperature is good, because sensory changes, medication, or illness often make older persons more likely to get burned from hot water, which is usually at a temperature of 160°F.

We reviewed Emily's exercises (see Appendix), and I pointed out that the kitchen counter and the dining room table were good places for her to practice her high steps and crossover steps.

After several weeks, Emily was progressing well, making good gains in strength, coordination, pain reduction, balance, and endurance. When she arrived for PT on Monday morning of the fourth week, however, she was complaining of a great deal of pain. She had missed the bottom step coming down on her way to church and bumped into the wall, but she had not fallen.

I examined her painful right hip, and it was indeed moderately tender to touch. However, her gait was not grossly affected, and weight bearing was not too bad. I recalled that when I originally evaluated Emily, her responses to pain stimuli were appropriate. Regardless, she was too sore and tender to do much exercise. We changed to ice and electrical stimulation around the hip. The area was only slightly ecchymotic, but perhaps it was a little too soon after the injury to show a lot of ecchymosis. We did a little exercise for her lower extremity, trunk, and both upper extremities, being careful not to strain too much, because she could also have injured her viscera in the accident.

Concerned about the possibility of an impacted fracture of the trochanter, I called Dr. Shrum, who ordered roentgenograms and approved the home use of transcutaneous electrical nerve stimulation (TENS) to ease Emily's pain.

Two days later, Dr. Shrum called back to tell me that there was no fracture but the roentgenograms revealed a marked increase of DJD at the L1-3 levels on the right. I wondered if this was the cause of her meralgia paresthetica. Perhaps not, because she was improving with the increased flexibility she was gaining. I also wondered about microfractures of her femur, pelvis, and lumbar vertebrae. These fractures would not show up in roentgenograms, but they could cause pain. I decided not to stop, but to progress slowly. After two weeks of TENS at home, and moist heat (we switched back after one week) and electrical stimulation, Emily was feeling better and we started to exercise harder again. We had even resumed the endurance and isokinetic training.

We had been working together for six weeks and had come to joke with each other and to know each other well. Emily's fall set her back, but she did not regress to her initial level. While we were working together one day, I noticed that Emily was not as sharp mentally as she usually was. She had not re-

sponded to several comments that I had made, which was not like her. She actually seemed a little confused.

Not wanting to upset her with a straight-forward comment about her confusion, I said, "Emily, you don't seem like yourself today. Is there anything wrong?" She replied that she hadn't "been feeling so good the past few days." "Do you have any idea what is causing you to feel this way?" I asked her. "No," she said.

Realizing that a plethora of factors can cause Emily's symptoms—which, if not remedied, may obviate further progress in rehabilitation—I asked a series of questions, searching for a possible cause of this change in Emily's affect. "Do you have a cold? A cold can make you feel lousy by upsetting your diet, dehydrating your body, and reducing your rest. Each of these problems alone, without a cold, can cause confusion." But no, she had no signs or symptoms of a cold, her diet was unchanged, and she was drinking enough.

"Do you have heart or chest tightness or pain?" Her pulse was 72 and regular. Her respiration was 18 per minute and there was no change in breathing sounds. Her blood pressure was 135/82. There was no increased ankle edema. Her skin color and skin temperature were normal. If any of these measurements had been irregular, I would have contacted Dr. Shrum to discuss it before proceeding. Changes in blood pressure or pulse may cause confusion, but more importantly, they may be indicative of more serious pathology.

"Have your medications changed?" If Emily had said that her medications had been changed three weeks ago by a specialist, I would have checked out the medication in the *Physician's Desk Reference* and called Dr. Shrum's office. A few of the adverse reactions to common hypertensive drugs are muscle weakness, cramps, dizziness, and postural hypotension.

"Are you sleeping enough?" If Emily had said that she had not been sleeping well, I would have reviewed her sleeping position and surface. Further, I would have assured her that alterations in sleep are not abnormal as persons age. If her sleep disturbances were related to cramping in her leg, I would suggest doing Buerger-Allen exercises, wearing leg warmers, and possibly simply walking to stop the cramping. Also, I would encourage her to decrease or stop napping during the day, and tell her that a little exercise or walk in the evening may help. Some persons benefit from a glass of wine or beer as long as there is no social or medical problem with that. However, one major factor to consider is that sleep disturbance is also associated with respiration difficulty, including sleep apnea. If this were Emily's situation, I would refer her back to her physician. Regardless, I would mention Emily's sleep problem in a letter to her physician.

"Has anything in your life changed recently? Has anyone moved away? Are any friends or relatives ill? Are you depressed or upset about anything? These events can cause stress, which can affect your thinking." Again, my questioning was fruitless.

"When was your last bowel movement? Do you have any change or burning with urination?" At last she responded to one of my questions with something that might be causing her to be confused and different in her interaction. She admitted to having a little burning with urination. I checked her oral temperature; it was 99.1°F. That was certainly not high, so I asked Emily, "What is your normal oral temperature?" She replied, "I don't know."

Because core body temperature tends to decrease slightly with increasing age, it is not uncommon for elderly persons to have an oral temperature of less than 98.0°F. I suspected that she might have a slight fever and a urinary tract infection. Emily also admitted that her back pain had been a little worse the past few days. I telephoned Dr. Shrum and advised Emily to go straight to her physician's office after I finished treating her. I thought that we could complete some exercise, but I wanted to be careful not to push Emily too hard.

After several days, Emily's urinary tract infection was under control and her affect was back to normal. She showed renewed enthusiasm, especially because her great-granddaughter was getting married in three months and

Emily must be there. I thought to myself that this was wonderful. Emily was regaining confidence in her abilities, and was reaching out socially.

Three weeks later, after nine weeks of physical therapy, Emily's back pain and thigh pain had decreased so that she had no difficulty with dressing. She had attained all of the other objectives that we had set for her except one. Her unilateral balance on the right (the side she bumped in the near fall) could not be maintained for longer than five seconds because of pain. I encouraged Emily to continue to do all of the home exercises, including number 1 (see Appendix), but she was not to push herself if her pain worsened. I told her that she might need to use a cane in her left hand at times, or possibly all the time, in the future.

The weather was conducive to increased walking outside, and I encouraged Emily to continue to walk at the mall during bad weather. If she could continue her own exercises at home, she could maintain her new found improvements in strength, coordination, balance, ROM, and endurance.

I suggested that I recheck her in three weeks. If there was no regression in her pain control and other abilities, we would discontinue physical therapy. At the time of the recheck, Emily did well, but she expressed an interest in my reevaluating her in six to eight weeks and again in three to four months. After that, treatment would be discontinued if all was going well.

I informed her that these rechecks are not within the guidelines for reimbursement for physical therapy under Medicare Part B. She stated that she was willing to pay privately. She wanted to maintain these functional gains, she told me, because she planned to live at least another 20 years.

APPENDIX: EXERCISES FOR PERSONS 55 YEARS OR OLDER

These exercises are to be started gradually. Work at your own pace and level of ability. Start with 5 or 10 repetitions, fewer if you must or more if you can. Slowly increase by adding two to four or more repetitions every five to ten days. Progress until you can do approximately 15 to 25 repetitions of each. Do these exercises at least three times weekly.

HIGH STEP

Hold on to a chair for balance, and stand up straight. Raise one foot off the floor so that the knee is as high as your hip. Lower your foot. Alternate legs. Try not to lean on the chair too much. As you get stronger, you may be able to raise your leg higher, hold for count of 5 (less if necessary), and decrease the amount of leaning on the chair.

Purpose: Increase hip and leg strength and balance.

SIDESTEP

Hold on to a chair for balance, and stand up straight. Raise one leg out to your side and hold it in the air. Don't bend at the waist. Hold your leg out to the side for five seconds, less if necessary. Then do the same with your other leg. At first, you may be unable to hold your leg in the air. In that case, simply move your foot out to the side.

Purpose: Increase hip and leg strength and balance.

STAND UP-SIT DOWN

This exercise is the key to being independent. Simply stand up, and then sit down. To do this, you must get your feet under the front of the chair. Move your center of gravity forward, and then move your center of gravity up. If necessary, use the armrest of the chair. As you get stronger, decrease the amount of push that you need from your arms.

Purpose: Improve strength, balance, coordination, and joint motion.

SHOULDER SHRUG

Sit up or stand up straight. Shrug the shoulders up high, and then release. Pull the shoulders back. You should feel your shoulder blades (scapulae) pull together.

Purpose: Strengthen back, stretch chest muscles, and improve posture.

CERVICAL RANGE OF MOTION

Sit up or stand up, with head erect but not forward. (1) Turn your chin to the left shoulder, and then to the right. (2) Lean your ear to the left shoulder, and

then to the right. (3) Lightly place your finger on your chin and push your chin backwards.

Do *not* roll your head backwards as if looking up at the ceiling.

Purpose: Improve posture, balance, and range of motion.

WALKING

Walking should be continued at whatever level of ability you have. If you can walk only 50 feet, start at that level and try to increase distance and improve gait speed. Avoid sudden stops and starts. If you are walking longer distances, such as a half mile or longer (5 to 10 minutes), do a little stretching before starting. When finishing, cool down a little by simply walking slowly, stretching, and doing a few of the above or your favorite exercises.

Purpose: Enhance overall health of mind and body: muscles, bones, joints, circulation, heart, lungs, digestion, and bowels.

REMINDER

If you need help getting started, or if you have any concerns about your health, show these exercises to your physician.

Good luck!

ANNOTATED BIBLIOGRAPHY

Jackson O (ed): Physical Therapy of the Geriatric Patient. New York, Churchill Livingstone, 1983. (This excellent text provides many charts and evaluation forms for geriatric physical therapy as well as excellent review papers on biological aspects of aging and drugs that create obstacles to rehabilitation of the elderly.)

Lewis CB (ed): Aging: The Health Care Challenge. Philadelphia, FA Davis, 1985 (This superb text is loaded with treatment suggestions for providing rehabilitation to geriatric patients. Many illustrations, graphs, and tables are included, along with chapters dealing with systems physiology, pathology, stress, drugs, sexuality, research, dying, and finances.)

Topics in Geriatric Rehabilitation 1:1, 1985 (This entire journal volume is highly recommended. All the articles not only describe the age-related changes in physiology and function, but they also provide treatment considerations and principles.)

Villaverde MM, MacMillan CW (eds): Ailments of Aging from Symptom to Treatment. New York, Van Nostrand Reinhold, 1980 (This text presents the symptoms or pathology reported by patients and the treatments to be rendered by the practitioner. It is heavily oriented toward drug therapy.)

67 Neonate with Cerebral Palsy

CAROLYN B. HERIZA

Physical therapy practice in the neonatal intensive care unit (NICU) is a highly specialized, advanced level of pediatric practice. Knowledge and skill requirements in neonatal medicine, infant assessment and intervention, parent education, and interdisciplinary interaction go beyond that of entry into the advanced level of pediatric physical therapy practice. The following case study is used as an introduction to this area. Therapists who wish to pursue this subspecialty of pediatric physical therapy must continue their education through the postgraduate level or continuing education coursework. A supervised clinical internship with a neonatal physical therapist is also advisable. If such a physical therapist is not available, a supervised practicum with a neonatal nurse is strongly recommended.

INTRODUCTION

Mark, born on May 18, 1985 with an estimated gestational age of 30 weeks and weighing 1260 g (2 lb, 12.5 oz), was immediately referred to physical therapy as a result of a previously established protocol based on risk for developmental delay or neurological dysfunction. He was seen for initial physical therapy evaluation on the third day of life (72 hours). This time period of three days allows the physiological impact of the birth process to subside. Before evaluating the infant, I reviewed the infant's chart as well as the mother's to form a picture of this baby; what I may suspect the baby will look like; what evaluation tool I will use; what precautions I will use in addition to common problems that are generally encountered; and what special equipment I may encounter with respect to mechanical ventilators, oxygen therapy, intravenous lines, radiant warmer, or incubator.

CHART REVIEW

The mother's chart revealed that she was 17 years of age, single, and living with her 80-year-old great grandmother in the inner city. Cynthia, Mark's mother, had finished the eighth grade but planned to return to school. Her income was $343 per month from social security. She had received prenatal care at a city clinic, but did not seek this care until April. On May 14, 1985 Cynthia was admitted to a central medical center for treatment of hypertension with blood pressure in the range of 150 to 190/100 to 110. She was treated with bed rest, anticonvulsants, and antihypertensive drugs, with no improvement. She subsequently was transferred to the city hospital where she was admitted and also treated with anticonvulsants and antihypertensive drugs, with no improvement. A cesarean section was performed under general anesthesia.

The infant was intubated after one minute because he was limp and did not respond to bagging with a mask. The Apgar score at one minute was 4, and at five minutes was 6. He was immediately transferred to NICU, where he was placed in a radiant warmer with nasal continous positive airway pressure (CPAP). A lung roentgenogram on May 18 revealed mild to moderate hyaline membrane disease. He did well on the mechanical ventilator and a plan was made to wean him off the CPAP on May 20. On May 21, he developed hyperbilirubinemia and was placed under phototherapy. A cranial ultrasonogram on this day revealed an intraventricular hemorrhage with dilatation of the ventricles (grade III). According to the Ballard, Kazmaier, and Driver Assessment of Gestational Age, Mark was 30 weeks gestational age. He was appropriate for size with respect to head circumference (28.5 cm), length (35.5 cm), and weight (1260 g).

INTERPRETATION OF DATA
FROM CHART REVIEW

What did this information tell me? Mark's mother was at environmental/social and biological risk for having a premature infant because of her educational level; low socioeconomic status; lack of prenatal care until the sixth month of pregnancy; and pregnancy-induced hypertension.

Mark was at high risk for developmental delay or neurological dysfunction because of biological and environmental/social risk factors. He was born premature by 10 weeks (a full-term infant is born at 40 weeks gestation). I know that babies born at 32 weeks gestation or less are at greater risk for developmental or neurologic problems than babies born after 32 weeks. However, he was appropriate for physical size with respect to his head circumference, weight, and length. This tells me that although he was born early, he was not small for his age, indicating that he probably did not suffer intrauterine malnutrition. Although Mark was the correct size for his age, he is considered to be a very low birth weight baby. These babies are defined as having a birthweight less than 1500 g (3 lb, 5 oz). Very low birth weight babies are at increased risk for neonatal and postneonatal mortality and morbidity with poor neurological outcome.

Apgar scores at birth reflect the infant's immediate adaptation to the extrauterine environment. The highest total score that a baby can receive on the Apgar is 10, with 2 points each for the following five measures: heart rate, respiratory effort, muscle tone (degree of flexion and resistance offered to straightening of the extremities), reflex irritability, and color. Mark's scores of 4 at one minute and 6 at five minutes indicate that he may be at high risk for neurological problems. At one minute, Mark received a 2 for heart rate (over 100 beats per minute; 0 for respiratory effort (absent); 1 for muscle tone (some flexion of the extremities, some resistance to movement); 0 for reflex irritability (no response); and 1 for color (cyanotic). At 5 minutes, he received 1 for respiratory effort (slow, irregular, gasping) and 1 for reflex irritability (cry, some motion) in addition to the same scores in the other areas. Since Mark had to be intubated and mechanically ventilated at birth because of inadequate oxygenation, he is also at risk for perinatal asphyxia, which may result in apnea, seizures, and poor neurological outcome.

Hyaline membrane disease, a respiratory problem seen in preterm infants, is caused by lack of surfactant, which interferes with the normal cardiopulmonary transition to extrauterine life. This is an additional reason why Mark needed mechanical ventilatory support. I know that hyaline membrane disease can predispose preterm infants to central nervous system pathology. A complication of hyaline membrane disease in the small premature infant is intraventricular hemorrhage, which is the most common serious neurologic complication of prematurity. Infants with documented grade III intraventricular hemorrhage are at high risk for developmental delay; a variety of neuromotor handicaps including spastic hemiplegia and spastic quadriplegia; and hydrocephalus. Hyperbilirubinemia (neonatal jaundice) is a common problem with preterm babies. If untreated, the baby could also be at risk for later neurological problems.

Because of the clusters of perinatal problems exhibited by Mark in combination with his mother's educational level and suboptimal environmental conditions, I knew that Mark was at risk for poor long-term development. I needed to evaluate him in order to ascertain his current functional status, which would serve as a baseline for documentation of his neurologic recovery on subsequent evaluations. Because early evaluations are questionable with respect to predicting future outcome, I knew that repeat or serial evaluations would provide better indications of CNS insult and recovery. I also needed to choose an evaluation instrument that had been developed for preterm infants and that had the capacity to differentiate neurobehavioral deviations from individual differences in normal neonatal behavior and to identify those deviations most likely to result in significant impairment of future functioning.

KNOWLEDGE BASE: DEVELOPMENT OF PRETERM INFANTS

In order to make clinical judgments regarding evaluation outcome and responses to therapeutic intervention, I must have knowledge of the neuromuscular developmental course of preterm infants and how the infant handles the experiences of the world around him. With respect to neuromuscular development, I rely on Saint-Anne Dargassies' (1977) studies of premature development. Her classic descriptions of sensory responses, neurovegetative responses, primary reflexes, resting postures, joint extensibility, righting reactions, and motility are the nearest thing we have for norms for the developing premature infant. With respect to behavioral and social attributes of the preterm infant, I rely on Als' (1982) theory of synactive development. In this model, the baby is continuously interacting not only within herself but also with the environment. The baby organizes around subsystems that are developmentally sequenced. The baby first organizes the physiological or autonomic system (respirations, color, visceral responses); then the motor system (spontaneous movement, postures); next the state organizational systems (range of alertness, transitional patterns); then the attentional interactive system (visual and auditory responses); and last the

capacity to self-regulate or to use the environment to assist in regulation of responses.

OBSERVATION OF MARK

Before selecting the evaluation tool, I wanted to talk with the nurse who cares for Mark to determine if I needed to take any special precautions when planning for the evaluation, and to learn of any new changes in medical status that have not yet been recorded in the chart. I also wanted to observe how the baby responded to being handled, which would give me information as to how to structure the evaluation so that I would not fatigue him or compromise his physiological, motoric, or state organization.

I observed the morning care of Mark by the nurse. Before going into the nursery, I removed my watch and rings and scrubbed my hands and arms to the elbow for one minute; cleaned my fingernails; scrubbed again for one minute; and put on a sterile gown so that I would not carry any bacteria into the nursery. These babies are sick and very vulnerable, so I do not want to spread infection. I noticed that Mark was lying in an open radiant warmer (Fig. 67-1). This piece of equipment offers nurses and physicians good accessibility to the infant if he needs care immediately, but it also places the baby in an open environment that is noisy, bright, and very active. His temperature was monitored through a sensor attached to his skin and connected to an overhead radiant heating unit. Ultraviolet lights were also overhead for treatment of the hyperbilirubinemia. His eyes were covered to protect the retinas from the UV lights. Surface electrodes attached to Mark were connected to the monitoring cable of a neonatal monitor that was equipped to give digital and oscilloscope readouts of heart and respiratory rates. Mark was supine and receiving continuous positive airway pressure with nasal prongs. A resuscitation bag was positioned on the mattress as backup in case of respiratory failure. An intravenous line was positioned in the left leg.

Before handling by the nurse, Mark was in

Figure 67-1. A typical radiant warmer used in the care of sick infants. Mark's temperature is monitored through a sensor attached to his skin and connected to an overhead radiant heating unit. Surface electrodes are attached to Mark and connected to a monitor cable for digital and oscilloscope readouts of heart and respiratory rates. Mark is receiving continuous positive airway pressure with nasal prongs. A resuscitating bag is positioned on the mattress as backup in case of respirator failure. The UV lights are not shown. (Reproduced by permission from Pernoll ML, Benda GI, Babson SG: Diagnosis and Management of the Fetus and Neonate at Risk: A Guide for Team Care, 5th ed, p 121. St. Louis, 1986, The CV Mosby Co)

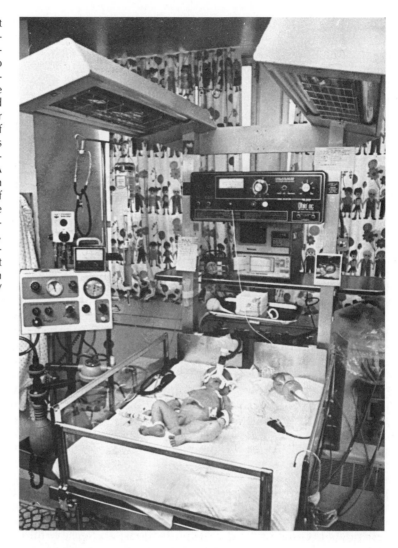

a light sleep. He showed a low activity level with a few twitches. During his morning care, Mark maintained physiological stability. His color did not change during handling and he was able to maintain appropriate cardiac and respiratory rates. However, he was not able to maintain his motor or state organization. His movements became disorganized as he uncontrollably flung his arms and legs out in all directions. At times his movements became frantic. This diffuse movement was accompanied by grimacing and distressed facial expression. He

seemed to have no way to organize himself. At the end of the morning care, he was exhausted and tuned everything out.

INTERPRETATION OF OBSERVATION

From these observations, I knew that Mark had the ability to organize himself physiologically, which was a good sign. I also knew that he became greatly disorganized with respect to his motoric and state organization and was unable to organize himself independently. His solution to the problem was to habituate out all external stimulation. I knew that I would have to be careful not to stress him during my evaluation. I might have to use techniques such as providing my finger for Mark to hold onto or suck, or placing my hand gently but firmly on his head and trunk to help organize him if he became disorganized. There was a strong possibility that I might not be able to complete my evaluation at one time, and I might have to see him over a number of days. I also knew that I did not want to examine him before or after his routine nursery care, in order to avoid fatigue. I decided to evaluate him in midafternoon, which would be a quieter part of his day. He would be rested from routine care, and would be less likely to become fatigued during my evaluation. I must remember that if Mark is in a deep sleep when I come to evaluate him, I will not wake him but will return later. Many preterm infants spend more time in light sleep than they do in deep sleep. I know that babies in light sleep have lower arterial oxygen saturation than they do in deep sleep. Therefore, I do not want to arouse Mark if he is in deep sleep. I would come back later, at a time that would allow me to evaluate him optimally. I know that state or arousal level is a major component of and contributor to an infant's performance. Therefore, it is very important to evaluate Mark in an optimal state. Because of Mark's ability to organize himself physiologically, he was not too ill or unstable to tolerate an initial evaluation. Responses that I observed would reflect his current condition and would provide a baseline for later serial evaluations.

KNOWLEDGE BASE: INFANT ASSESSMENTS

Based on these observations and my knowledge of premature development and behavior, I chose the *Neurological Assessment of the Preterm and Full-term Newborn Infant* (NAPI) by Dubowitz and Dubowitz (1981) because it includes both neurological and behavioral items. Although there is no completely satisfactory reliable and valid clinical tool for the neurological

and behavioral assessment of the preterm infant, valuable information can be obtained by using one of four evaluations. The *Neurological Maturity Sequence* by Amiel-Tison (1968) can be used in serial examinations, but it primarily focuses on the neurological aspects of development with respect to reflex development, passive muscle tension measured by joint angle and resistance offered by the extremities to passive movement, and antigravity movements. *Neurological Development in the Full-Term and Premature Neonate* by Saint-Anne Dargassies (1977) also focuses on neurological development of the preterm infant. This assessment indicates the current neurological age of the preterm infant and can also be used to follow the maturation of the CNS. *The Assessment of Preterm Infant Behavior* (APIB) by Als, Lester, Tronick, and Brazelton (1982) is primarily a behavioral test. The APIB is an excellent tool that documents systematically the premature infant's behavioral organization along five dimensions: physiologic, motor, state, interactional, and attentional and self-regulatory. However, it is lengthy and not feasible for routine clinical use. Best used for research purposes, it requires specialized training for administration and interpretation.

The NAPI combines both neurological and behavioral items and is intended for use by health professionals with limited background in neonatal neurology. The test was developed to assess premature and term infants in serial format. Administration time is relatively brief and recording is systematic, making it clinically feasible for use by physical therapists. The test can be administered at 3 days of life or less, and portions of it can be used with sick infants. The test is divided into four sections and provides information on habituation; posture, passive and active motor activity; reflexes; and interactional behavior.

In addition to this test, I also observe the following postures and movements: active head turning from side to side; head in midline; hands to midline and to mouth; antigravity postures and movements of legs and arms; ability to roll from supine to sidelying; tolerance of prone, supine, and sidelying; and general organization of movement. Because I do not want to stress the infant, I will be watchful for signs of stress reactions. Autonomic stress signals include respiratory pauses, tachypneic respiration, color changes, gagging, spitting, hiccupping, coughing, sneezing, yawning, and sighing. Motor stress signals include motoric flaccidity or "tuning out"; motoric hyperextensions or hyperflexions; and frantic, diffuse activity. State stress signals include diffuse sleep or awake states; strained fussing or crying; staring; active averting; panicked or worried alertness; glassy-eyed, strained alertness; irritability and diffuse arousal; or crying.

PHYSICAL THERAPY EVALUATION

Now that I had a plan for my evaluation, I was ready to assess Mark. Before going into the nursery, I scrubbed my hands and donned a gown to prevent propagation of infection. As I stood by the open radiant warmer, I noted that Mark was supine with extremities extended and head supported in midline to ensure that the nasal prongs were not displaced. He was in a light sleep. I watched him for a few minutes. The digital readouts from the cardiorespiratory monitor indicated that the heart and respiratory rates were fairly regular. He made a few twitching movements. Before beginning the evaluation, I turned off the UV lights and removed the "blindfold." The nurse told me that Mark could tolerate being off the continuous positive airway pressure for short periods of time. She removed the ventilatory assistance. I was very gentle in all of my handling so as to avoid stressing the infant.

The results of my evaluation on the NAPI are noted in Figure 67-2. Mark had a variable response to the light, which made light habituation difficult to interpret. He did not respond to the rattle. His posture showed extension of the extremities. There was no recoil in the arms, some in the legs, and no resistance to traction. The popliteal angle was 180 degrees. Antigravity movements were absent (head control on pull to sit and in sitting; midline

head position from supine; hand to mouth behavior; and trunk extension from ventral suspension). Some tremors and startles were noted. There were no rooting or sucking responses. The Moro reflex was not tested. He did attempt to take steps when held upright. Because Mark was in a light sleep or drowsy during the exam, some of the neurobehavioral items were not administered. During the evaluation Mark did maintain physiological and motoric organization.

Generally, I considered Mark to be an inactive infant who showed extensor posturing, and minimal responses to passive and elicited movements. These findings were not wholly inconsistent for an infant with a gestational age of 30 weeks. It was of interest to note that during this evaluation Mark did not demonstrate motor disorganization, as seen previously during his morning care by the nurse. Although Mark was functioning appropriately for his age, his medical and social history placed him at very high risk for developmental delay and movement dysfunction. Based on my findings, observations, and knowledge of his medical status, I identified two potential problems that Mark might develop as he matured:

1. Extensor posturing of the neck, trunk, and extremities, as a result of being placed supine, and
2. Continued shutdown or excessive reaction to environmental stimuli.

Because Mark needed time to rest, conserve energy, and grow, I established a therapeutic program to be implemented by the nurses. The program would accomplish the following:

1. Promote optimal positioning and normal movement patterns, and
2. Provide a supportive environment to decrease stress behavior and increase self-regulatory behaviors.

Specific treatment activities and their rationales are listed in Table 67-1. If Mark had been older and if he had not been so small, I would have initiated a specific physical therapy treatment program along with a program to be implemented by the nurses. He would have

(*Text continues on p. 1248.*)

NAME *Mark*

HOSP. NO.

RACE SEX ♂

D.O.B./TIME
5-18-85

DATE OF EXAM
5-21-85

AGE
3 days CA

WEIGHT
1260 gms

HEIGHT
35.5 cm

HEAD CIRC.
28.5 cm

E.D.D.
L.N.M.P.

E.D.D.
U/snd.

GESTATIONAL SCORE WEEKS
ASSESSMENT
30 wks

STATES
1. Deep sleep, no movement, regular breathing.
2. Light sleep, eyes shut, some movement.
3. Dozing, eyes opening and closing.
4. Awake, eyes open, minimal movement.
5. Wide awake, vigorous movement.
6. Crying.

						STATE	COMMENT	ASYMMETRY

HABITUATION (≤ state 3)

LIGHT
Repetitive flashlight stimuli (10) with 5 sec. gap.
Shutdown = 2 consecutive negative responses

| No response | A. Blink response to first stimulus only. B. Tonic blink response. C. Variable response. | A. Shutdown of movement but blink persists 2-5 stimuli. B. Complete shutdown 2-5 stimuli. | A. Shutdown of movement but blink persists 6-10 stimuli. B. Complete shutdown 6-10 stimuli. | A. Equal response to 10 stimuli. B. Infant comes to fully alert state. C. Startles + major responses throughout. | 2 |

RATTLE
Repetitive stimuli (10) with 5 sec. gap.

| No response | A. Slight movement to first stimulus. B. Variable response. | Startle or movement 2-5 stimuli, then shutdown | Startle or movement 6-10 stimuli, then shutdown | A. B. Grading as above C. | 2 |

MOVEMENT & TONE
Undress infant

POSTURE
(At rest — predominant) *

| | | | | (hips abducted) | (hips adducted) | Abnormal postures: A. Opisthotonus. B. Unusual leg extension. C. Asymm. tonic neck reflex | 3 |

ARM RECOIL
Infant supine. Take both hands, extend parallel to the body; hold approx. 2 secs. and release.

| No flexion within 5 sec. | Partial flexion at elbow >100° within 4-5 sec. | Arms flex at elbow to <100° within 2-3 sec. | Sudden jerky flexion at elbow immediately after release to <60° | Difficult to extend; arm snaps back forcefully | 3 |

ARM TRACTION
Infant supine; head midline; grasp wrist, slowly pull arm to vertical. Angle of arm scored and resistance noted at moment infant is initially lifted off and watched until shoulder off mattress. Do other arm.

| Arm remains fully extended | Weak flexion maintained only momentarily | Arm flexed at elbow to 140° and maintained 5 sec. | Arm flexed at approx. 100° and maintained | Strong flexion of arm <100° and maintained | 3 |

LEG RECOIL
First flex hips for 5 secs, then extend both legs of infant by traction on ankles; hold down on the bed for 2 secs. and release.

| No flexion within 5 sec. | Incomplete flexion of hips within 5 sec. | Complete flexion within 5 sec. | Instantaneous complete flexion | Legs cannot be extended; snap back forcefully | 3 |

LEG TRACTION
Infant supine. Grasp leg near ankle and slowly pull toward vertical until buttocks 1-2" off. Note resistance at knee and score angle. Do other leg.

| No flexion | Partial flexion, rapidly lost | Knee flexion 140-160° and maintained | Knee flexion 100-140° and maintained | Strong resistance; flexion <100° | 3 |

POPLITEAL ANGLE
Infant supine. Approximate knee and thigh to abdomen; extend leg by gentle pressure with index finger behind ankle.

| 180-160° | 150-140° | 130-120° | 110-90° | <90° | 3 |

HEAD CONTROL (post. neck m.)
Grasp infant by shoulders and raise to sitting position; allow head to fall forward; wait 30 sec.

| No attempt to raise head | Unsuccessful attempt to raise head upright | Head raised smoothly to upright in 30 sec. but not maintained | Head raised smoothly to upright in 30 sec. and maintained | Head cannot be flexed forward | 3 |

HEAD CONTROL (ant. neck m.)
Allow head to fall backward as you hold shoulders; wait 30 secs.

| Grading as above | Grading as above | Grading as above | Grading as above | | 3 |

HEAD LAG *
Pull infant toward sitting posture by traction on both wrists. Also note arm flexion.

| | | | | | 3 |

VENTRAL SUSPENSION *
Hold infant in ventral suspension; observe curvature of back, flexion of limbs and relation of head to trunk.

| | | | | | 3 |

HEAD RAISING IN PRONE POSITION
Infant in prone position with head in midline.

| No response | Rolls head to one side | Weak effort to raise head and turns raised head to one side | Infant lifts head, nose and chin off | Strong prolonged head lifting | 3 |

ARM RELEASE IN PRONE POSITION
Head in midline. Infant in prone position; arms extended alongside body with palms up.

| No effort | Some effort and wriggling | Flexion effort but neither wrist brought to nipple level | One or both wrists brought at least to nipple level without excessive body movement | Strong body movement with both wrists brought to face, or 'press-ups' | 3 |

SPONTANEOUS BODY MOVEMENT
during examination (supine). If no spont. movement try to induce by cutaneous stimulation.

| None or minimal Induced | A. Sluggish. B. Random, incoordinated. C. Mainly stretching. | Smooth movements alternating with random, stretching, athetoid or jerky | Smooth alternating movements of arms and legs with medium speed and intensity | Mainly: A. Jerky movement. B. Athetoid movement. C. Other abnormal movement. | 1 2 |

TREMORS
Mark: Fast (>6/sec.) or Slow (<6/sec.)

| No tremor | Tremors only in state 5-6 | Tremors only in sleep or after Moro and startles | Some tremors in state 4 | Tremulousness in all states | |

STARTLES

| No startles | Startles to sudden noise, Moro, bang on table only | Occasional spontaneous startle | 2-5 spontaneous startles | 6+ spontaneous startles | |

ABNORMAL MOVEMENT OR POSTURE

| No abnormal movement | A. Hands clenched but open intermittently. B. Hands do not open with Moro. | A. Some mouthing movement. B. Intermittent adducted thumb | A. Persistently adducted thumb. B. Hands clenched all the time. | A. Continuous mouthing movement. B. Convulsive movements. | |

1244

REFLEXES

TENDON REFLEXES
Biceps jerk
Knee jerk
Ankle jerk

Absent | (Present) | Exaggerated | Clonus

STATE: 3

PALMAR GRASP
Head in midline. Put index finger from ulnar side into hand and gently press palmar surface. Never touch dorsal side of hand.

(Absent) | Short, weak flexion | Medium strength and sustained flexion for several secs. | Strong flexion; contraction spreads to forearm | Very strong grasp. Infant easily lifts off couch

STATE: 3

ROOTING
Infant supine, head midline. Touch each corner of the mouth in turn (stroke laterally).

(No response) | A. Partial weak head turn but no mouth opening. B. Mouth opening, no head turn. | Mouth opening on stimulated side with partial head turning | Full head turning, with or without mouth opening | Mouth opening with very jerky head turning

STATE: 3

SUCKING
Infant supine; place index finger (pad towards palate) in infant's mouth; judge power of sucking movement after 5 sec.

(No attempt) | Weak sucking movement: A. Regular. B. Irregular. | Strong sucking movement, poor stripping: A. Regular. B. Irregular. | Strong regular sucking movement with continuing sequence of 5 movements. Good stripping. | Clenching but no regular sucking.

STATE: 3

WALKING (state 4, 5)
Hold infant upright, feet touching bed, neck held straight with fingers.

Absent | (Some effort but not continuous with both legs) | At least 2 steps with both legs | A. Stork posture; no movement. B. Automatic walking.

STATE: 3

MORO
One hand supports infant's head in midline, the other the back. Raise infant to 45° and when infant is relaxed let his head fall through 10°. Note if jerky. Repeat 3 times.

No response, or opening of hands only | Full abduction at the shoulder and extension of the arm | Full abduction but only delayed or partial adduction | Partial abduction at shoulder and extension of arms followed by smooth adduction — A. Abd>Add B. Abd=Add C. Abd<Add | A. No abduction or adduction; extension only. B. Marked adduction only.

ASYMMETRY: J / S

NEUROBEHAVIOURAL ITEMS

EYE APPEARANCES

Sunset sign. Nerve palsy. | Transient nystagmus. Strabismus. Some roving eye movement. | (Does not open eyes) | Normal conjugate eye movement | A. Persistent nystagmus. B. Frequent roving movement C. Frequent rapid blinks.

AUDITORY ORIENTATION (state 3, 4)
To rattle. (Note presence of startle.)

(A. No reaction. B. Auditory startle but no true orientation.) | Brightens and stills; may turn toward stimuli with eyes closed | Alerting and shifting of eyes; head may or may not turn to source | Alerting; prolonged head turns to stimulus; search with eyes | Turning and alerting to stimulus each time on both sides

STATE: 3 ASYMMETRY: S

VISUAL ORIENTATION (state 4)
To red woollen ball

Does not focus or follow stimulus | Stills; focuses on stimulus; may follow 30° jerkily; does not find stimulus again spontaneously | Follows 30-60° horizontally; may lose stimulus but finds it again. Brief vertical glance | Follows with eyes and head horizontally and to some extent vertically, with frowning | Sustained fixation; follows vertically, horizontally, and in circle

ALERTNESS (state 4)

Inattentive; rarely or never responds to direct stimulation | When alert, periods rather brief; rather variable response to orientation | When alert, alertness moderately sustained; may use stimulus to come to alert state | Sustained alertness; orientation frequent, reliable to visual but not auditory stimuli | Continuous alertness, which does not seem to tire, to both auditory and visual stimuli

DEFENSIVE REACTION
A cloth or hand is placed over the infant's face to partially occlude the nasal airway.

No response | A. General quietening. B. Non-specific activity with long latency. | Rooting; lateral neck turning; possibly neck stretching. | Swipes with arm | Swipes with arm with rather violent body movement

PEAK OF EXCITEMENT

(Low level arousal to all stimuli; never > state 3) | Infant reaches state 4-5 briefly but predominantly in lower states | Infant predominantly state 4 or 5; may reach state 6 after stimulation but returns spontaneously to lower state | Infant reaches state 6 but can be consoled relatively easily | A. Mainly state 6. Difficult to console, if at all. B. Mainly state 4-5 but if reaches state 6 cannot be consoled.

IRRITABILITY (states 3, 4, 5)
Aversive stimuli:
Uncover   Ventral susp.
Undress   Moro
Pull to sit   Walking reflex
Prone

No irritable crying to any of the stimuli | (Cries to 1-2 stimuli) | Cries to 3-4 stimuli | Cries to 5-6 stimuli | Cries to all stimuli

CONSOLABILITY (state 6)

(Never above state 5 during examination, therefore not needed) | Consoling not needed. Consoles spontaneously | Consoled by talking, hand on belly or wrapping up | Consoled by picking up and holding; may need finger in mouth | Not consolable

CRY

No cry at all | (Only whimpering cry) | Cries to stimuli but normal pitch | Lusty cry to offensive stimuli; normal pitch | High-pitched cry, often continuous

NOTES
✱ If asymmetrical or atypical, draw in on nearest figure
Record any abnormal signs (e.g. facial palsy, contractures, etc.). Draw if possible.

Record time after feed:

EXAMINER: *CBH*

Figure 67-2. Neurological assessment of the preterm and full-term newborn infant for Mark at 30 weeks gestational age. (Reprinted with permission from Dubowitz L, Dubowitz V: The Neurological Assessment of the Preterm and Full-term Newborn Infant, pp 12–15. © 1981, MacKeith Press, 5A Netherhall Gardens, London NW3 5RN)

Table 67-1. Problems, Therapeutic Goals, and Treatment Strategies for Mark at 30 Weeks Gestational Age

PROBLEMS	GOALS	TREATMENT	RATIONALE
Extensor posturing compounded by supine position	Promote optimal positioning and normal movement patterns; promote flexion.	Provide suggestions to nurses for positioning and handling Mark.	Positioning supports developing perceptual and sensorimotor abilities and counteracts abnormal postures and movements. The supine position contributes to extension posture. If Mark has to be supine, a blanket roll should be placed under the head to promote neck flexion and neck extensor elongation and under the knees to promote knee flexion and posterior pelvic tilt.
		1. Position prone; sidelying with support	1. *Prone:* improves oxygenation, respiration, heart rate, quiet sleep, and flexion. (If Mark had also shown too much flexor posturing when prone, I would have emphasized sidelying positions with minimal time in prone and supine.) *Sidelying with frontal support:* promotes flexion, with neck flexion facilitating elongation of neck extensor muscles; hands to midline promoting shoulder protraction; trunk flexion; and hip flexion and adduction.
		2. Handling—bathing, diapering, other care giving activities; picking up and carrying	2. Handling provides a time of sensory interaction with infant. Touch and movement should be slow and gentle. Handling must be carefully planned. (If Mark had not shown motoric disorganization, I would have encouraged fast, but gentle, movements to promote more active movement.) When picking up and carrying, promote flexion. One way to do this is to roll Mark to his side, place one hand on

continued

Table 67-1. (continued)

PROBLEMS	GOALS	TREATMENT	RATIONALE
			his abdomen to promote flexion, move him to prone, pick him up, and rotate into the crook of your arm. Carry him with neck flexed, shoulders depressed and protracted, and pelvis flexed. Reverse procedure when lying Mark down.
		3. Swaddling	3. Swaddling encourages flexion and symmetry, increases tactile experience, promotes quieting, and helps self-regulatory behavior. (If Mark had shown too much flexion and if he had not demonstrated motor disorganization, swaddling would not be necessary.)
Shut down to environment or excessive reaction to environment	Provide supportive environment to decrease stress behaviors and increase self-regulatory behaviors.	No treatment by physical therapist.	Too much handling during this time is contraindicated because the infant needs rest and energy conservation. Mark either tunes out all environmental stimulation or reacts excessively to it.
		Provide suggestions to nurses to facilitate supportive environment.	Nurses interact with Mark continuously. They are in the best position to provide a consistent environment for him.
		1. Establish regular and consistent times for nursing and medical care.	1. Promotes organization of sleep and waking hours.
		2. Avoid waking Mark if in deep sleep.	2. Preterm infants often do not have the opportunity to go into deep sleep. This type of sleep provides better oxygenation and quieting.
		3. Reduce noise and light levels.	3. Bright lights and noise can interfere with establishment of sleep/wake cycles and deep sleep.

continued

Table 67-1. (continued)

PROBLEMS	GOALS	TREATMENT	RATIONALE
		4. Become aware of stress signals and provide specific aids to facilitate self-regulation	4. Mark shows the following motoric stress signals: (a) motor flaccidity or "tuning out"; (b) frantic, diffuse, uncontrollable motor activity.
			Aids to decrease stress and influence self-regulatory behavior: (a) "suckle"—a nipple attached to a terry cloth strap placed across shoulders is always available for Mark and helps promote oxygenation, flexion, and quieting; (b) opportunity to grasp at hands and feet (finger rolls, foot rolls); (c) swaddling

been able to handle the "extra" therapeutic intervention. However, Mark was already being overstimulated, as observed by his habituation or his excessive reaction to his environment. I know that I must avoid the danger of overloading Mark; this could delay his development.

INTERPRETATION OF FINDINGS TO MOTHER

Because Cynthia, Mark's mother, was still in the hospital, I talked to her about my findings. I took a Polaroid picture of Mark since she had not been able to see him because of an infection she had. Cynthia was worried about her baby and wanted to know how he was doing. When I showed her the picture, she was concerned that he was so tiny. She wanted to know about the wires that were attached to him and whether they hurt him.

In response to her questions, I confirmed that Mark was small but that for his age, he was not too tiny. I described the wires and other pieces of equipment. I told her how Mark behaved when I saw him, that he became upset with lots of movement and noises, tired easily, and then shut everything out. I explained that these responses were normal for his age and that he was conserving his energy to grow. Moreover, I would not be treating him until he grew larger. I also told her that I talked with the nurses on ways to place him on his tummy and side, how to move him so as not to upset him, what he does to show that he is overstimulated, and things they can do to calm him. I assured Cynthia that when she was able to see Mark, I would go with her and show her the activities that I had instructed the nurses to do; that way, she can help with her baby's care.

I asked Cynthia if she had any questions. She said no, but then went on to say how frightened she was that the baby might die. This is a normal feeling to have. I made a note to discuss this conversation with the social worker. When she comes to talk with Cynthia about finances and care of Mark when he goes home, she can continue to explore her feelings. This does not mean that I will not listen to Cynthia and acknowledge her feelings, but I also want to let other members of the team (social worker, nurse, and physician) know that she is beginning to discuss her feelings about the baby. She may also want to talk about her fears, and the experiences of delivering a baby early and having a cesarean section. We often only attend to the baby and may not attend to the parent. We must remember that Cynthia and Mark's father have their own feelings that may need to be discussed.

DISCHARGE PLANNING

Discharge planning began with Mark's admission to the NICU. In addition to determining Cynthia's economic status, the social worker began to contact community agencies that provide financial or other support for infants and their families. Mark qualified for Medicaid and needed to be enrolled to ensure financial support for him and his mother. They also qualified for the Women, Infant, and Children (WIC) food program. This program will provide milk and nutritional information for Cynthia and the baby. The community health nurse also talked with Cynthia to ensure a smooth, functional referral system between the NICU and the community. In this community, two programs provide programming for infants and families: (1) the public school system under Public Law 94-142, the Education for Handicapped Children's Act, and (2) the Association for Retarded Citizens. Both offer parent-infant programs that teach the parents how to work with their baby. Because the school system does not have a physical therapist, I work closely with the teaching staff and provide programs for babies, which they carry out. There is a physical therapist consultant with the Association for Retarded Citizens. One issue that will determine which facility to refer to is transportation. Cynthia did not have a car, and she would have to rely on friends, public transportation, or a taxi.

One of the major concerns with Mark and his mother was that only one agency should coordinate services. In this city, we also have an agency that assists families in the coordination of services. A caseworker works with the mothers to ensure that the appropriate programs are fulfilling their needs. Because Cynthia has expressed an interest in continuing her education, this also should be included in program planning for this family.

PARENT EDUCATION

Because I saw Mark and his mother daily, I knew when Cynthia's infection was better. I checked with her to see when she was going to the nursery so that I could be there with her. A very important aspect of the care of the premature infant is the role of the parents. Usually the first visit to the NICU to see the baby is very stressful. They are overwhelmed by the sights and sounds of the medical equipment and how small the baby is. The anxiety level may be so high that the parents do not correctly perceive the full reality of the situation. Some parents respond by keeping a safe distance from their baby at first, and upon each visit they stand a little closer until it feels "safe" to reach and touch the baby.

It was important for Cynthia to feel that she could participate in the care of her baby. It is common for parents to grieve for their baby and feel that they can offer nothing to the baby. They believe that the doctors, nurses, and therapists know what is best. As a result of this belief, they often see no role for themselves in their baby's care and may not come to visit the baby because they feel they have nothing to offer. It is important to promote early parental involvement to help establish parent-infant bonding.

This attachment helped establish the confidence Cynthia needed to participate in the care of Mark. I wanted her to be comfortable seeing and touching him, and to begin knowing him and eventually caring for him. I remembered not to involve Cynthia in the care of her infant too quickly. Each mother has her own timetable for when she feels comfortable touching and caring for the baby. I needed to be aware of behavioral cues from Cynthia that would let me know she was ready to do more. I could facilitate this process by scheduling my time to see Mark when Cynthia visited the baby. I could build Cynthia's confidence by teaching her how to observe Mark's behavior, what it meant, and activities to do with Mark when she came to see him.

She was awkward when she began to interact with Mark, but this did not harm him. While Cynthia was interacting with Mark, not me, I could describe how he was responding to being touched and moved, and I could indicate things he liked and did not like. I could tell her what to do to calm him if he became upset. When he responded to these actions, I praised her. The confidence of parents needs gentle and continuous building. Cynthia needed to have a sense of success in handling Mark, and needed to take pride in what he could do. Often it helps to have a parent plan like the one shown in Figure 67-3. This can be placed near the incubator to help the parents and health personnel remember what the baby can do, and what he likes and dislikes.

What I can do:
I quiet if you place your hand on my head gently but tightly.

Things that stress me:
Bright lights and loud noises
Being moved quickly
Being on my back

Signs of stress:
Frantic, diffuse movement
Limpness
Grimacing
(If you see these signs, give Mark some time out to recover; provide a quiet, calm time.)

What I like to do:
Be on my tummy or side
Suck on my "suckle"
Grasp mommy's finger

How you can help me:
Place me on my tummy or side.
If I am on my side, place a blanket roll on my tummy and at my back.
Talk to me softly.
Give me your finger to suck.
When you hold me, hold me gently but tightly.

Figure 67-3. A parent plan for Mark.

REEVALUATION

When possible, it helps parents to understand their baby, his special sensitivities, and emerging strengths and personality by observing evaluations. When I next evaluated Mark, I let Cynthia know so she could come. (I had been evaluating Mark weekly since his initial evaluation, using the NAPI to document changes in neuromuscular development and organizational capabilities.)

My next evaluation of Mark with the NAPI was at 5 weeks chronological age, or 35 weeks corrected age. It is important to correct for prematurity in order to interpret evaluative findings with reference to biologic or corrected age rather than chronological age. At this time, Mark was in an incubator, having been moved from the open radiant warmer five days earlier. I again washed my hands and donned a gown before entering the NICU. When I had seen Mark earlier, he had been in the warmer, and I evaluated him there. Now, I would conduct part of my evaluation in the incubator. When I opened the portholes, I was careful not to jar the incubator or open them too rapidly, because these noises might cause Mark to startle, jerk, or jump. I also did not put my clipboard and pen on the top of the incubator, because this causes noise that penetrates the incubator more clearly and loudly than my voice. Mark was in a sidelying position (the nurses have been positioning him well), so I gently rolled him to his back and began the test. Because he was awake, I did not do the habituation items. I also wanted to see how he responded to being handled, so I asked the nurse if he could maintain his body temperature if taken from the incubator for a few minutes. He could, so I swaddled him so that he would not lose heat. Loss of body heat may cause an infant to use more calories to maintain body temperature, and may inhibit adequate weight gain. Therefore, I want to make sure that he is warm during my evaluation. After completing my evaluation, I returned Mark to the incubator and placed him prone. The movement startled him and he began to whimper. I placed my hand on his head to console him and offered my finger for him to hold onto. He became quiet, so I gently removed my hand and finger and closed the door. (I never leave a baby without first facilitating a calm state.)

The results of this evaluation are shown in Figure 67-4. Mark now showed some flexion of the legs in the supine position. Leg recoil had not changed from his initial evaluation, but asymmetry was noted, with the right leg being more delayed than the left. Some resistance to extension was now evident on leg traction. The popliteal angle showed greater tightness (120 to 130 degrees). This angle is not inappropriate for his age, but is of concern when compared with the responses of the legs to recoil and traction. No postural flexion, limb resistance, or recoil were present in the arms. There was some improvement in neck flexor muscles on pull to sit. However, when he attempted to right his head once seated, his head fell forward. Spontaneous movements had increased slightly since his initial evaluation, but they were disorganized, becoming more so when he was upset. Tremors were noted when Mark was agitated and crying. A startle was elicited during the Moro test.

Rooting and sucking responses, although present, were insufficient. The Moro test showed arm abduction only, which was asymmetrical (the right arm movement was delayed). In standing, he kept his legs in flexion and did not bear weight. This leg position is in contrast to that seen at 3 days chronological age, when he bore some weight and attempted to take steps. He visually fixated on an object briefly and began to track, but did not respond to auditory stimuli. Lack of auditory orientation was also noted on the initial evaluation.

Mark became very upset with changes in position during the evaluation. His movements became disorganized. He did try to console himself (a good sign) by bringing his hand to his mouth three times when the head was turned to the side (he did not have antigravity arm movements), but he did not insert his finger or suck. He was difficult to console. He responded best to being swaddled with a finger or pacifier placed in his mouth. In this position, he did quiet down and begin to interact with his environment.

His weak sucking and rooting responses prompted me to talk to the nurses about his feeding. He was started on nipple feeding three days ago. The nurses indicated that Mark had difficulty feeding, and was very slow. I decided to do an oral-motor assessment at his morning feed the next day. He was a slow feeder. He needed some assistance in sucking and some jaw control to facilitate mouth closure and swallowing. Because of his inability to control arm and leg movements, I tried swaddling him to see if his feeding improved. It did. Also, positioning him in a semireclined sitting position helped.

Generally, I felt that Mark was slowly developing, but he was functioning more like a 32- to 33-week-old infant rather than a 35-week-old infant. He was developing a flexed posture in the supine position; antigravity movements; and the ability to focus briefly on objects. He was also attempting to console himself. Of concern, however, were (1) decreased responses to limb recoil and resistance to traction for corrected age; (2) a disproportionately tight popliteal angle compared to the angle of the knee during leg traction; (3) asymmetry; (4) decreased motility for corrected age; (5) irritability resulting in frantic diffuse movement; (6) difficulty feeding; and (7) no orientation to auditory stimuli. These clinical signs have been observed in other 35-week-old preterm infants with documented intraventricular hemorrhage. The early developmental delay with the suspected abnormal neurological and behavioral signs indicate that Mark is at high risk for neuromuscular dysfunction.

We would have to follow him closely over the next weeks and months to document his progress, revise his intervention program, and reinstruct his mother in the updated therapeutic program. Only with serial evaluations will we be able to monitor Mark's development and modify, when appropriate, Mark's therapeutic and supportive care to maximize his potential. At this age, it is not possible to predict long-term outcome. Mark's ultimate level of functioning will be determined by the dynamic, continuous interplay of his physiologic, motor, state, and interaction systems and his interaction with the environment. The prognosis for survivors of intraventricular hemorrhage is (Text continues on p. 1254.)

NAME Mark	D.O.B./TIME 5-18-85	O.D. L.M.P.	E.D.D. U/snd.	**STATES**		

STATES
1. Deep sleep, no movement, regular breathing.
2. Light sleep, eyes shut, some movement.
3. Dozing, eyes opening and closing.
4. Awake, eyes open, minimal movement.
5. Wide awake, vigorous movement.
6. Crying.

HOSP. NO. DATE OF EXAM 6-24-85 HEIGHT

RACE SEX ♂ AGE 4 weeks 6 days CA HEAD CIRC. GESTATIONAL SCORE WEEKS ASSESSMENT 32-33 wks

						STATE	COMMENT	ASYMMETRY
HABITUATION (≤state 3)								
LIGHT Repetitive flashlight stimuli (10) with 5 sec. gap. Shutdown = 2 consecutive negative responses	No response	A. Blink response to first stimulus only. B. Tonic blink response. C. Variable response.	A. Shutdown of movement but blink persists 2-5 stimuli. B. Complete shutdown 2-5 stimuli.	A. Shutdown of movement but blink persists 6-10 stimuli. B. Complete shutdown 6-10 stimuli.	A. Equal response to 10 stimuli. B. Infant comes to fully alert state. C. Startles + major responses throughout.	4		
RATTLE Repetitive stimuli (10) with 5 sec. gap.	No response	A. Slight movement to first stimulus. B. Variable response.	Startle or movement 2-5 stimuli, then shutdown	Startle or movement 6-10 stimuli, then shutdown	A. B. C. Grading as above	4		
MOVEMENT & TONE Undress infant								
POSTURE (At rest — predominant) *			(hips abducted)	(hips adducted)	Abnormal postures: A. Opisthotonus. B. Unusual leg extension. C. Asymm. tonic neck reflex	4		
ARM RECOIL Infant supine. Take both hands, extend parallel to the body; hold approx. 2 secs. and release.	No flexion within 5 sec.	Partial flexion at elbow >100° within 4-5 sec.	Arms flex at elbow to <100° within 2-3 sec.	Sudden jerky flexion at elbow immediately after release to <60°	Difficult to extend; arm snaps back forcefully	4		
ARM TRACTION Infant supine; head midline; grasp wrist, slowly pull arm to vertical. Angle of arm scored and resistance noted at moment infant is initially lifted off and watched until shoulder off mattress. Do other arm.	Arm remains fully extended	Weak flexion maintained only momentarily	Arm flexed at elbow to 140° and maintained 5 sec.	Arm flexed at approx. 100° and maintained	Strong flexion of arm <100° and maintained	4		
LEG RECOIL First flex hips for 5 secs, then extend both legs of infant by traction on ankles; hold down on the bed for 2 secs. and release.	No flexion within 5 sec.	Incomplete flexion of hips within 5 sec.	Complete flexion within 5 sec.	Instantaneous complete flexion	Legs cannot be extended; snap back forcefully	4		✓
LEG TRACTION Infant supine. Grasp leg near ankle and slowly pull toward vertical until buttocks 1-2" off. Note resistance at knee and score angle. Do other leg.	No flexion	Partial flexion, rapidly lost	Knee flexion 140-160° and maintained	Knee flexion 100-140° and maintained	Strong resistance; flexion <100°	4		
POPLITEAL ANGLE Infant supine. Approximate knee and thigh to abdomen; extend leg by gentle pressure with index finger behind ankle.	180-160°	150-140°	130-120°	110-90°	<90°	4		
HEAD CONTROL (post. neck m.) Grasp infant by shoulders and raise to sitting position; allow head to fall forward; wait 30 sec.	No attempt to raise head	Unsuccessful attempt to raise head upright	Head raised smoothly to upright in 30 sec. but not maintained.	Head raised smoothly to upright in 30 sec. and maintained	Head cannot be flexed forward	5		
HEAD CONTROL (ant. neck m.) Allow head to fall backward as you hold shoulders; wait 30 secs.	Grading as above	Grading as above	Grading as above	Grading as above		5		
HEAD LAG Pull infant toward sitting posture by traction on both wrists. Also note arm flexion. *						5		
VENTRAL SUSPENSION Hold infant in ventral suspension; observe curvature of back, flexion of limbs and relation of head to trunk. *						5		
HEAD RAISING IN PRONE POSITION Infant in prone position with head in midline.	No response	Rolls head to one side	Weak effort to raise head and turns raised head to one side	Infant lifts head, nose and chin off	Strong prolonged head lifting	5		
ARM RELEASE IN PRONE POSITION Head in midline. Infant in prone position; arms extended alongside body with palms up.	No effort	Some effort and wriggling	Flexion effort but neither wrist brought to nipple level	One or both wrists brought at least to nipple level without excessive body movement	Strong body movement with both wrists brought to face, or 'press-ups'	5		
SPONTANEOUS BODY MOVEMENT during examination (supine). If no spont. movement try to induce by cutaneous stimulation.	None or minimal Induced	A. Sluggish. B. Random, incoordinated. C. Mainly stretching.	Smooth movements alternating with random, stretching, athetoid or jerky	Smooth alternating movements of arms and legs with medium speed and intensity	Mainly: A. Jerky movement. B. Athetoid movement. C. Other abnormal movement.	1 2		
TREMORS Fast (>6/sec.) Mark: or Slow (<6/sec.)	No tremor	Tremors only in state 5-6	Tremors only in sleep or after Moro and startles	Some tremors in state 4	Tremulousness in all states			
STARTLES	No startles	Startles to sudden noise, Moro, bang on table only	Occasional spontaneous startle	2-5 spontaneous startles	6+ spontaneous startles			
ABNORMAL MOVEMENT OR POSTURE	No abnormal movement	A. Hands clenched but open intermittently. B. Hands do not open with Moro.	A. Some mouthing movement. B. Intermittent adducted thumb	A. Persistently adducted thumb. B. Hands clenched all the time.	A. Continuous mouthing movement. B. Convulsive movements.			

1252

REFLEXES

TENDON REFLEXES
Biceps jerk
Knee jerk
Ankle jerk

Absent		Present	Exaggerated	Clonus	STATE
					4

PALMAR GRASP
Head in midline. Put index finger from ulnar side into hand and gently press palmar surface. Never touch dorsal side of hand.

| Absent | Short, weak flexion L>R | Medium strength and sustained flexion for several secs. | Strong flexion; contraction spreads to forearm | Very strong grasp. Infant easily lifts off couch | 4 | | L |

ROOTING
Infant supine, head midline. Touch each corner of the mouth in turn (stroke laterally).

| No response | A. Partial weak head turn but no mouth opening. B. Mouth opening, no head turn. L>R | Mouth opening on stimulated side with partial head turning | Full head turning, with or without mouth opening | Mouth opening with very jerky head turning | 4 | | L |

SUCKING
Infant supine; place index finger (pad towards palate) in infant's mouth; judge power of sucking movement after 5 sec.

| No attempt | Weak sucking movement: A. Regular. B. Irregular. L>R | Strong sucking movement, poor stripping: A. Regular. B. Irregular. | Strong regular sucking movement with continuing sequence of 5 movements. Good stripping. | Clenching but no regular sucking. | 4 |

WALKING (state 4, 5)
Hold infant upright, feet touching bed, neck held straight with fingers.

| Absent | | Some effort but not continuous with both legs | At least 2 steps with both legs | A. Stork posture; no movement. B. Automatic walking. | 6 |

MORO
One hand supports infant's head in midline, the other the back. Raise infant to 45° and when infant is relaxed let his head fall through 10°. Note if jerky. Repeat 3 times.

| No response, or opening of hands only | Full abduction at the shoulder and extension of the arm | Full abduction but only delayed or partial adduction | Partial abduction at shoulder and extension of arms followed by smooth adduction A. Abd>Add B. Abd=Add C. Abd<Add | A. No abduction or adduction; extension only. B. Marked adduction only. | 5 | J S |

NEUROBEHAVIOURAL ITEMS

EYE APPEARANCES

| Sunset sign Nerve palsy | Transient nystagmus. Strabismus. Some roving eye movement. | Does not open eyes | Normal conjugate eye movement | A. Persistent nystagmus. B. Frequent roving movement C. Frequent rapid blinks. | 4 |

AUDITORY ORIENTATION (state 3, 4)
To rattle. (Note presence of startle.)

| A. No reaction. B. Auditory startle but no true orientation. | Brightens and stills; may turn toward stimuli with eyes closed | Alerting and shifting of eyes; head may or may not turn to source | Alerting; prolonged head turns to stimulus; search with eyes | Turning and alerting to stimulus each time on both sides | 4 | S |

VISUAL ORIENTATION (state 4)
To red woollen ball

| Does not focus or follow stimulus | Stills; focuses on stimulus; may follow 30° jerkily; does not find stimulus again spontaneously | Follows 30-60° horizontally; may lose stimulus but finds it again. Brief vertical glance | Follows with eyes and head horizontally and to some extent vertically, with frowning | Sustained fixation; follows vertically, horizontally, and in circle | 4 |

ALERTNESS (state 4)

| Inattentive; rarely or never responds to direct stimulation | When alert, periods rather brief; rather variable response to orientation | When alert, alertness moderately sustained; may use stimulus to come to alert state | Sustained alertness; orientation frequent, reliable to visual but not auditory stimuli | Continuous alertness, which does not seem to tire, to both auditory and visual stimuli | 4 |

DEFENSIVE REACTION
A cloth or hand is placed over the infant's face to partially occlude the nasal airway.

| No response | A. General quietening. B. Non-specific activity with long latency. | Rooting; lateral neck turning; possibly neck stretching. | Swipes with arm | Swipes with arm with rather violent body movement | 4 |

PEAK OF EXCITEMENT

| Low level arousal to all stimuli; never > state 3 | Infant reaches state 4-5 briefly but predominantly in lower states | Infant predominantly state 4 or 5; may reach state 6 after stimulation but returns spontaneously to lower state | Infant reaches state 6 but can be consoled relatively easily | A. Mainly state 6. Difficult to console, if at all. B. Mainly state 4-5 but if reaches state 6 cannot be consoled. | |

IRRITABILITY (states 3, 4, 5)
Aversive stimuli:
Uncover Ventral susp.
Undress Moro
Pull to sit Walking reflex
Prone

| No irritable crying to any of the stimuli | Cries to 1-2 stimuli | Cries to 3-4 stimuli | Cries to 5-6 stimuli | Cries to all stimuli | |

CONSOLABILITY (state 6)

| Never above state 5 during examination, therefore not needed | Consoling not needed. Consoles spontaneously | Consoled by talking, hand on belly or wrapping up | Consoled by picking up and holding; may need finger in mouth | Not consolable | |

CRY

| No cry at all | Only whimpering cry | Cries to stimuli but normal pitch | Lusty cry to offensive stimuli; normal pitch | High-pitched cry, often continuous | |

NOTES ✳ If asymmetrical or atypical, draw in on nearest figure
Record any abnormal signs (e.g. facial palsy, contractures, etc.). Draw if possible.

Record time after feed: 2 hours

EXAMINER: CBH

Figure 67-4. Neurological assessment of the preterm and full-term newborn infant for Mark at 35 weeks postconceptual age. (Reprinted with permission from Dubowitz L, Dubowitz V: The Neurological Assessment of the Preterm and Full-term Newborn Infant, pp 12–15. © 1981, MacKeith Press, 5A Netherhall Gardens, London NW3 5RN)

variable. Often, definitive diagnosis of cerebral palsy is not possible before 8 to 10 months corrected age.

Based on my current findings and observations, my revised problem list included:

1. Continued extension posture, with pelvis in anterior pelvic tilt,
2. Excessive reaction to the environment,
3. Decreased antigravity movement,
4. Difficulty feeding, and
5. Decreased response to visual stimuli; no response to auditory stimuli.

I modified the current plan of care to include direct physical therapy intervention along with continued activities to be implemented by the nurses. My revised goals were as follows:

1. Promote optimal positioning and normal movement patterns.
2. Provide a supportive environment to decrease stress behavior and increase self-regulatory behavior.
3. Promote antigravity movements of the head and the extremities.
4. Increase strength of sucking and amount of fluid intake.
5. Enhance responses to visual and auditory stimulation.

Specific activities and their rationales are shown in Table 67-2.

Table 67-2. Problems, Therapeutic Goals, and Treatment Strategies for Mark at 35 Weeks Postconceptual Age

PROBLEMS	GOALS	TREATMENT	RATIONALE
Continued extension posture; pelvis in anterior pelvic tilt	Promote optimal positioning and normal movement patterns; promote flexion, posterior pelvic tilt.	1. Position prone; sidelying with frontal roll; sitting in infant seat.	1. *Prone:* improves oxygenation, respiration, heart rate, quiet sleep, and flexion. Because Mark is now in an incubator, he should be positioned against blankets next to walls or corners of the incubator. Infants tend to gravitate on their own to the sides of the incubator to maintain contact with a stable surface. This provides proprioceptive input as well as "security." Also in prone, flexion is promoted because the extremities are positioned under the body. Side-to-side rocking in this position will promote sensation of weight bearing. *Semireclined, sidelying with frontal support:* promotes flexion, with neck flexion facilitating elongation of neck extensor muscles; hands to midline, promoting shoulder protraction; trunk flexion, hip flexion and abduction.

continued

Table 67-2. (continued)

PROBLEMS	GOALS	TREATMENT	RATIONALE
			Sitting: Promotes flexion with neck flexion, protraction of shoulders, flexion of hips with pelvic retraction (posterior pelvic tilt).
		2. Handling	2. *Bathing, diapering:* do in sidelying or prone position to promote flexion.
			Picking up and carrying: want to promote flexion. Roll to side, place one hand on abdomen to promote flexion, move to prone, pick up, rotate into crook of arm, carry with neck flexion, shoulders depressed and protracted , pelvis flexed, legs dissociated (one flexed, one extended). Reverse procedure when lying down.
Excessive reaction to environment.	Provide supportive environment to decrease stress behaviors and increase self-regulatory behaviors.	1. Establish regular and consistent times for therapeutic intervention.	1. Promotes organization of sleeping and waking hours.
		2. Move slowly and gently	2. Fast movements disorganize; slow movements decrease irritability.
		3. Rock slowly	3. Rocking slowly helps to calm infant; can be done any time baby becomes upset.
		4. Swaddle	4. Provides tactile/proprioceptive input, warmth, comfort, decreases tremulousness and overshooting movements.
		5. Suckle	5. Nonnutritive sucking has been shown to reduce excessive movement while enhancing a quiet alert state.
		6. Talk softly	6. Encourages alerting and decreases frantic movement.

continued

Table 67-2. (continued)

PROBLEMS	GOALS	TREATMENT	RATIONALE
Decreased antigravity movement.	Encourage head movement from side to midline; hands to midline, and hand to mouth; posterior pelvic tilt with hip flexion and adduction.	Position sidelying with frontal roll; semiflexed position in sitting.	Encourage flexion, hand to mouth, and hands to midline. They are important for self-consolation and self-generated tactile stimulation.
Difficulty feeding.	Increase strength of suck, amount of fluid intake.	1. Provide nonnutritive sucking (pacifier, finger); hand-to-mouth activities.	1. Nonnutritive sucking stimulates the sucking reflex.
		2. During feeding, position in semiupright and flexed position (may or may not swaddle).	2. Flexed position promotes sucking and swallowing,
		3. Provide jaw control.	3. Jaw control promotes mouth closure and swallowing.
Decreased response to visual stimuli; no response to auditory.	Enhance responses to auditory and visual stimulation.	1. Request audiological evaluation.	1. Mark has not responded to auditory input since initial evaluation; rule out primary hearing problem.
		2. Swaddle	2. Mark has difficulty organizing movements. Swaddling helps contain movements for him so that he can use his energies for interactive activities.
		3. Maintain alert state and provide visual and auditory stimuli.	3. To encourage awake state fast movement may be used, also rocking vertically or putting up to shoulder vertically will increase alertness. If Mark becomes irritable, slow rocking will help calm him. A rocking chair is helpful.
			Visual: Use your face and smile gently to get attention. If Mark looks away, do not follow him, wait for him to come back to you. Your face and smile may be too stimulating for him. Let him take the lead. If he does this well, you can move your face and let him follow. If he continues to be responsive, you can add your voice. If he looks away, do not talk; wait for him to come back to you.
			Auditory: Speak softly to Mark on one side and then the other. Wait for him to turn his head to see you. Remember to keep the arms flexed and swaddle him to decrease movements if needed.

ANNOTATED BIBLIOGRAPHY

Als H: Toward a synactive theory of development: Promise for the assessment and support of infant individuality. Infant Mental Health Journal 3:229, 1982 (Reviews the synactive model of development. Provides an assessment procedure to identify behavioral disorganization of the neonate, and provides examples of environmental structuring.)

Als H, Lester BM, Tronick EZ et al: Toward a research instrument for the Assessment of Preterm Infant's Behavior (APIB). In Fitzgerald H, Lester BM, Yogman MW (eds): Theory and Research in Behavioral Pediatrics, Vol I, p 35. New York, Plenum Press, 1982

Amiel-Tison C: Neurological evaluation of the maturity of newborn infants. Arch Dis Child 43:89, 1968

Campbell SK: Clinical decision making: Management of the neonate with movement dysfunction. In Wolf SL (ed): Clinical Decision Making in Physical Therapy, p 295. Philadelphia, FA Davis, 1985 (Discusses management of the neonate with movement dysfunction with respect to determining which infants require evaluation and treatment; when and how to assess movement; and how to plan intervention programs. Text supplemented with two case studies.)

Dubowitz L, Dubowitz V: The Neurological Assessment of the Preterm and Fullterm Newborn Infant. Clinics in Developmental Medicine, No. 79. Philadelphia, JB Lippincott, 1981

Fiterman C: Physical therapy in the NICU. In Connolly BH, Montgomery PC (eds): Therapeutic Exercise in Developmental Disabilities, p 29. Chattanooga, Chattanooga Corp, 1987 (Covers basic information that therapists need to know when working in the NICU. Reviews three case studies.)

Pape KE, Wigglesworth JS: Haemorrhage, Ischaemia and the Perinatal Brain. Clinics in Developmental Medicine, No. 69/70. London, William Heinemann, 1979 (Classic that integrates histopathological and clinical findings of hemorrhagic and ischemic conditions of the developing brain with anatomical and physiological considerations.)

Pernoll ML, Benda GI, Babson SG: Diagnosis and Management of the Fetus and Neonate at Risk: A Guide for Team Care, 5th ed. St Louis, CV Mosby, 1986 (A concise source of information for health care providers who care for the high-risk pregnant mother and the at-risk fetus-neonate.)

Saint-Anne Dargassies S: Neurological Development in the Full-Term and Premature Neonate. New York, Excerpta Medica, 1977 (Classic, comprehensive analysis of neurological development in a complete range of neonates with emphasis on practical applications.)

Sweeney JK: Neonates at developmental risk. In Umphred DA: Neurological Rehabilitation, p 137. St Louis, CV Mosby, 1985 (Provides clear descriptions of neonates at developmental risk and focuses on appropriate treatment strategies and techniques for high-risk infants and their parents. Follows a pathokinesiological model of clinical practice.)

Sweeney JK (ed): The high-risk neonate: Developmental Therapy Perspectives. Physical and Occupational Therapy in Pediatrics 6 (3, 4) 1986 (Classic work on theoretical framework of neonatal behavioral organization; neonatal neuropathology and pathophysiologic complications; assessment of neonates, families, and the environment; and management and outcome of physical therapy of the high-risk infant.)

Wilhelm JJ: The neurologically suspect neonate. In Campbell SK (ed): Pediatric Neurologic Physical Therapy, p 107. New York, Churchill Livingstone, 1984 (Focuses on the management of newborn infants at high risk for central nervous system dysfunction. Provides in-depth background on these infants; critically reviews research on assessment and intervention strategies; and provides suggestions for physical therapists entering the NICU.)

68 Adult with Rheumatoid Arthritis

CAROLEE MONCUR

It is 7:30 AM. I like to review my patients' charts early in the day while my mind is uncluttered with other things. Today I will be seeing an old friend, Ellen Carson, whom I have not seen for a year. She tells me that she is having pain in her left foot and it will not hold her up as it should. Ellen and I go back almost 20 years to the time I first saw her and her husband Bill in the clinic. She had just been told that she had rheumatoid arthritis (RA) and that she needed to take a lot of aspirin, get lots of rest, and go to physical therapy. Then she was 42 years old and had three teenage children to raise. She is now 62. Bill was an accountant for a local hotel firm before he retired.

I'll never forget the first time I saw her. Her face looked tired, anxious, and somewhat cushingoid; she sat with her winter coat and rubber boots on in the waiting room. It was winter outside; however, everyone else in the waiting room seemed to be comfortable without coats on. Bill had a kind-looking face, but his forehead was wrinkled with what seemed to be concern. Rightly so, he was probably wondering what all of this meant in terms of his own future role as the breadwinner.

My usual method of introducing myself to the patient is formal in nature. I extended my hand for greeting. "Mrs. Carson, I presume?" "Yes, I am" she said.

I had a fleeting glimpse of fear in her eyes as she timidly extended her hand toward me. I surmised what must be going through her mind at that time: "Will she squeeze my hand too hard?" I guessed she'd likely had some experience with that before. I placed the palm of my right hand under the palm of her right hand and cradled it while placing my left hand on top of hers in a protective fashion. As I gently held her hand, I said: "I'm very happy to meet you. Is this gentleman accompanying you?" Her face brightened and I could see relief in it as she said, "Yes, this is my husband, Bill."

I introduced myself and *very gently* pressed her hand between mine and then let her slide it away. I observed that she had very swollen metacarpophalangeal joints of her index and middle fingers as well as all of her proximal interphalangeal joints. The dorsum of her hand was also swollen and warm to the touch.

One may wonder why I would take her hand when I observed Ellen was fearful and concerned that her hand might be squeezed too tightly. Let's just call it trust. If I could convey to her at that initial greeting that I understood about rheumatoid arthritis, that I wouldn't be like others she might have to deal with, then we were on our way to sharing the responsibility for the management of her disease.

I extended my hand to Bill and made the assumption he had the same last name as hers. "Mr. Carson, I'm also very happy to meet you. I consider it very important for you to be here with your wife."

"Mrs. Carson," I continued, "Unless your hands are too painful, I need to have you fill out both these insurance forms and this form that asks you questions about how well you are doing today and about your medical history."

I handed her a clipboard with the forms and a pen that had been padded with refrigerator tubing made of spongy foam rubber. The padding was to protect the joints of her thumb and forefinger while writing. (Most of the data to support the rationale of joint protection in this fashion is anecdotal.)

"If you have trouble, Mrs. Carson, perhaps Mr. Carson would be kind enough to write for you."

The forms I asked Ellen to fill out were her insurance forms, a history form, and a functional assessment form. Various functional assessment instruments have been produced, and have had both validity and reliability studies completed on them. The Arthritis Impact Measurement Scale (AIMS) was created at the Robert Breck Brigham Multipurpose Arthritis Center and has undergone extensive reliability and validity studies (Meenan and co-workers, (1980; 1982). The Health Assessment Questionnaire (HAQ) is a product of the Stanford Multipurpose Arthritis Center Fries (1983). The Functional Status Index (FSI) was created by Jette and co-workers (1980) at the University of Michigan, and a less known instrument is the Convery Arthritis Assessment Chart from the University of California at San Diego (1977). Asking the patient to respond in her own words about how well she functions with arthritis will give you baseline data about the patient's perception of her ability. I then ask the patient throughout the days or weeks I see her to demonstrate some of these activities to validate what she has reported.

Ellen filled out the AIMS, from which I determined her functional status from her point of view. While I walked to my office, I wondered (as I automatically do with all my RA patients regarding their social support system) what kind of relationship Bill and Ellen had. Was their bond strong enough to withstand the problems that might lie ahead? Could Bill accept and manage the fact that there might be a

role change ahead for him? Could Ellen allow him to be the homemaker if necessary without feeling guilty? Where were the phone numbers of Jim Manwaring, my clinical psychologist colleague, and Eve Smith, the social worker? And who is Ellen's physician, Dr. Martin? I know all the rheumatologists in town, and he isn't one of them. Her referral says he is an internist, and the order is for heat therapy. On the registration form is the question: "How did you hear about our clinic?" Ellen wrote: "I went to a talk at the Arthritis Foundation and someone recommended you. I asked my doctor if he would refer me and he did." There is a lot of work to do here, but it does sound as if Ellen is willing to take charge of her arthritis.

I prefer to evaluate a patient without the significant other present, and then go over the results and discuss a treatment plan with them together. I want my initial contact with the patient to be such that the patient has my undivided attention. My philosophy is that you cannot do the entire evaluation on the first day. First of all, most new patients with RA are coping with both pain and fatigue. Doing the entire evaluation just wears out the patient and produces spurious results. Evaluation and re-evaluation are ongoing, and form part of the plan of care each time I see the patient. I pay close attention to the nonverbal as well as the verbal messages I get from patients and their perceived social support persons.

As Ellen prepared to come into the treatment area, I made a point of observing how she got up out of the chair, which was with moderate effort. As she walked to the treatment room, her velocity was slower than normal for her age, and her step length was uneven. Her left step length was shorter than her right step. Stance phase on the left side was shorter than on the right. She was not swinging her arms, but held them close to her body. She did not roll off her toes at terminal stance, but walked with a footflat step. I did not observe a wobble about her knees or an extensor thrust.

As we entered the booth I asked her if she would have trouble getting into a gown and the pajama bottoms we used. She said she would be fine as long as she did not have to raise her arms above her head to tie the gown at her neck.

While Ellen dressed, I quickly jotted down what I had observed thus far—mental notes on paper.

1. She sat in the waiting room with her coat and boots on.
2. Her husband was here with her and appeared supportive.
3. She seems interested in taking action regarding her illness.
4. Her right hand hurts, and it is likely that her left one does also.
5. She probably does not know a lot about RA and wants to know more; she appears educable.
6. She is having trouble with her shoulders.
7. She is having trouble with the joints of her lower extremities, and her left lower extremity appears to be worse than her right. I must check all the joints of the kinetic chain.
8. I do not know her doctor.
9. I must talk to her about target joints, rest, and fatigue.
10. At least she knows what kind of arthritis she has.

Today, upon further review of my 20-year-old original assessment, I see where I noted that she believed her onset of illness began 14 years earlier during her last pregnancy. At that time she experienced soreness and swelling in her hands, wrists, and ankles that lasted about one month and then went away. However, after delivery of her son she had recurrent episodes several times in those same joints. These would last two or three days and then subside. It wasn't those symptoms that drove her to see a doctor, but rather an episode with acute back pain. Because of her history of joint complaints, her internist ran an erythrocyte sedimentation rate (ESR) and found it to be elevated. Based on her morning stiffness, pain on motion of her joints, synovitis, symmetric in-

volvement of the joints, x-ray findings of erosions in the bones of her hands, and the presence of rheumatoid factor, the diagnosis of rheumatoid arthritis was made. She was treated with aspirin and prednisone whereupon she noted that her back and other joints began to feel better. However, she never felt substantially better. That's when she searched for the Arthritis Foundation.

As to her internist, I remember how difficult it was for me when she asked about her doctor (the one who had referred her to me). She was concerned that he did not know what he was doing, because she was not getting better. When she began feeling bad, he just had her increase her prednisone to 20 mg twice a day. Then she gained weight, and her face looked fat to her. She was worried because of the things she had heard about steroids. She wanted to know to whom I would suggest she go, which made it easy to launch into my discussion on the patient-doctor relationship. I took the opportunity to impress upon Ellen that she, her doctor, and I may be together for a lot of years, so she should be comfortable with whomever she chose for her health care. That included me. She had never heard of a rheumatologist. (In fact, I find a significant number of patients do not know that rheumatologists exist. It is harder these days, with all the preferred provider schemes and third-party payment arrangements, to get a patient from the primary care provider to a rheumatic disease specialist. If the patient does have the good fortune of being referred to one, it might be for one consult, and the follow-up care has to be done by the primary care physician.)

Anyway, because I firmly believed that my plan of care would be enhanced if Ellen had her disease under control medically, I needed to work closely with her physician. I would prefer it be a rheumatologist who believes physical therapy is a part of the total treatment plan. So I gave her the name of three rheumatologists in whom I have great confidence (who also, by the way, referred to me).

The overview of her musculoskeletal examination 20 years ago was as follows:

1. Skin over the proximal interphalangeal (PIP) and metacarpophalangeal joints (MP) of both hands was hot and cyanotic.
2. The PIPs were tender, swollen, and painful on motion. Both hands lacked 10 degrees to full extension and flexed to 90 degrees in all of the PIPs on active motion. They could accomplish full passive range with a painful arc of motion.
3. The MPs were swollen, tender, and painful on motion.
4. Wrists bilaterally were swollen, tender, and painful on motion. Hyperextension was limited to 20 degrees and flexion was limited to 45 degrees in both with active motion. There was full passive range of motion.
5. Right elbow was tender with pain on motion (with no loss of motion in flexion, extension, or at the radioulnar joint in supination and pronation).
6. There was swelling and tenderness in the left elbow. Extension was −15 degrees; flexion was 110 degrees. Radioulnar jont supination was 70 degrees; pronation was 45 degrees; she had full passive range of motion.
7. There was pain on motion of the right shoulder. Abduction was 110 degrees; flexion was 95 degrees; hyperextension was 30 degrees; external rotation was 50 degrees; and internal rotation was 45 degrees. She was unable to touch the back of her head with her hands.
8. The left shoulder was more painful than the right. Active range of motion was limited by pain. Abduction was 80 degrees; flexion was 90 degrees; hyperextension was 45 degrees; external rotation was 45 degrees; and internal rotation was 50 degrees.
9. All of the motions of her shoulder could be accomplished passively in the presence of pain.
10. There was tenderness on palpation of the paracervical region of C4-C6 bilaterally, and in the suboccipital region bilaterally. She occasionally had headaches and a feeling of heaviness of the head.
11. There was snapping and clicking of the right temporomandibular joint on opening of the mouth. There was no deviation of the jaw.
12. She complained of pain on palpation of the sternoclavicular and costochondral joints.
13. Hip motion was without loss and was pain free bilaterally.
14. Marked synovitis and bogginess was present in both knees. There was tenderness and pain on motion of both knees, with the left greater than the right. Both knees lacked 10 degrees to full extension; right active flexion was 110 degrees; left active flexion was 100 degrees; and right and left passive flexion were within normal limits.
15. Both ankles were tender and swollen; dorsiflexion and plantar flexion were normal.
16. Tenderness was present on palpation of the heels bilaterally.
17. The subtalar joint on the left was painful on motion, and pressure in the sinus tarsi elicited moderately severe pain. Passive inversion was 20 degrees; passive eversion was 7 degrees. The right subtalar joint was painful on motion, but was less than the left. Mild pain was elicited on pressure in the sinus tarsi with the thumb. Passive inversion was 23 degrees; passive eversion was 8 degrees.
18. The metatarsal heads were painful bilaterally both to palpation and squeezing.

Because I prefer to leave manual muscle testing to a time when joints are not so inflamed and painful, I didn't do any that day. Rather, I had her do the following functional activities: walk 100 yards and timed her; walk while I observed her; ascend and descend three stairs; sit down and get up from a chair with arms and no elevated seat; sit down and get up from a toilet; wring out a wash cloth; comb her hair; pick up a quarter and a dime; and write with a pencil.

Based on my observations that day, I

Table 68-1. Classification of Functional Capacity in Rheumatoid Arthritis

CLASS	FUNCTIONAL CAPACITY
I	Complete, with ability to carry on all usual duties without handicaps
II	Adequate to conduct normal activities despite handicap of discomfort or limited mobility of one or more joints
III	Adequate to perform only a few or none of the duties of usual occupation or self-care
IV	Largely or wholly incapacitated with patient bedridden or confined to wheelchair, permitting little or no self-care

(Steinbroker O, Traeger CH, Batterman RC: Therapeutic criteria in rheumatoid arthritis. JAMA 140: 661, 1949)

noted that she was in the Functional Class III according to the American Rheumatism Association criteria (Table 68-1). I also guessed that she would be in the Stage II classification in terms of the progression of her RA on roentgenograms (Table 68-2). I developed a list of problems.

1. Decreased range of motion of hands, wrists, left elbow, shoulders, and knees.
2. Pain in all of above plus right elbow, paracervical region, suboccipital region, knees, sternoclavicular joint, heels (left greater than right), metatarsal heads (left greater than right).

Table 68-2. Classification of Progression of Rheumatoid Arthritis

Stage I: Early

1. No destructive changes on roentgenographic examination.*
2. Roentgenologic evidence of osteoporosis may be present.

Stage II: Moderate

1. Roentgenologic evidence of osteoporosis, with or without slight subchondral bone destruction; slight cartilage destruction may be present.*
2. No joint deformities, although joint mobility may be limited.*
3. Adjacent muscle atrophy.
4. Extraarticular soft tissue lesions, such as nodules and tenosynovitis, may be present.

Stage III: Severe

1. Roentgenologic evidence of cartilage and bone destruction, in addition to osteoporosis.*
2. Joint deformity, such as subluxation, ulnar deviation, or hyperextension, without fibrous or bony ankylosis.*
3. Extensive muscle atrophy.
4. Extraarticular soft tissue lesions, such as nodules and tenosynovitis, may be present.

Stage IV

1. Fibrous or bony ankylosis.*
2. Criteria of stage III.

*These criteria are those that must be present to permit classification of a patient in any particular stage or grade.
(Steinbroker O, Traeger CH, Batterman RC: Therapeutic criteria in rheumatoid arthritis. JAMA 140:661, 1949)

3. Decreased strength assessed functionally: quadriceps femori bilaterally; upper extremity musculature throughout.
4. Gait abnormalities consisted of painful gait during stance phase; decreased velocity; increased cadence; uneven step length (right greater than left); decreased single-stance time (left greater than right); increased knee flexion at initial contact, loading response, midstance, and terminal stance (bilaterally); no roll off; increased ankle dorsiflexion during terminal stance; decreased pelvic rotation; and decreased arm swing.
5. Decreased endurance.
6. Increased fatigue level.
7. She was not resting adequately during the day.
8. Morning stiffness lasting more than 3 hours.
9. Sleep interrupted with pain in shoulders.
10. Sexual activity decreased because of pain and fatigue.
11. Her husband is supportive, but is struggling with role reversal.
12. Her teenaged children continue to be demanding and not entirely understanding of Ellen's illness.
13. Ellen has been programmed to be "super-mom" and feels guilty about not being able to fulfill her role.
14. Ellen is depressed.

I knew we were not going to be entirely successful if Ellen did not get her disease controlled medically. Ellen and I talked first about her medical care, then about the problems, and finally about long- and short-term goals that she and I could realistically work on. We also discussed her role as manager of her arthritis and my role as educator and facilitator.

Since that time Ellen has found a great rheumatologist. She and Bill have a workable, supportive relationship, and her children have grown up and found out what it's like to be parents. But her arthritis has not been as kind as it could be. Ellen has not changed from a Stage II, Class III classification, but she has been an exemplary patient and has made every effort to manage and cope with her disease. My working relationship with her rheumatologist has been such that when Ellen determines she needs help from me, she simply calls my office for an appointment. Because her third-party payer and supplementary insurance company require a referral from a physician, I begin treatment and contact her rheumatologist for coverage.

Bill has been conscientious about making their home accessible for Ellen to get around in and allowing her to carry on some of the home-making responsibilities. The bathroom was modified so she could independently get on and off the toilet with grab bars and an elevated toilet seat. He also had the tub modified with a shower head and grab bars. The washer and dryer were installed in a room next to the bathroom so she wouldn't have to climb up and down stairs to the basement. A ramp was made from the back door to the carport so she could get to the car easily. The kitchen has been equipped with an electric can opener, bottle openers, large faucet handles at the sink, and modifications in utensils and cupboard contents were made so that Ellen could have easy access to those items she routinely uses. These kitchen modifications were based on suggestions from an occupational therapist.

Ellen and Bill also found they had to make adjustments and modifications in their family life. Their children had to become more independent and realize that neither Mom nor Dad was going to be able to cater to their needs. It took some sessions with my clinical psychologist associate to put that all in perspective. There were ups and downs because old "mental tapes" are difficult to erase. Fortunately, Bill had a stable job and health insurance through his employer.

Last year, Ellen's concern was her left shoulder. It interfered with her sleep and she was not able to move it very much. I hadn't seen her for two years previous to that, when she was having trouble with her feet. At that time she needed adjustment of her orthoses and her extra depth shoes had been worn out, particularly her left one. Her left foot has been a problem from the beginning of her disease.

The situation with her shoulder last year wound up being a real disappointment for Ellen. The results of my examination of her shoulder were as follows.

1. Patient history—Functional assessment: patient was unable to touch the back of her head with her left hand. Characteristics of her shoulder pain: dull, boring pain that was worse at night. Movements that bothered her: anything she had to get from a shelf with both hands. Ellen's age: 61 years. Pain relief: holding the arm in neutral flexion, neutral rotation, and slight abduction helped. Taking more prednisone and Tylenol 3 also helped. No complaint of numbness and tingling in the arm. Shoulder musculature appeared atrophied. There was no precipitating injury to the shoulder. The patient demonstrated considerable apprehension to passive motion of the shoulder. The shoulder has been bothering her for about six months. Ellen is right handed.
2. Active movements—elevation through forward flexion of the arm and 70 degrees (painful arc began about 60 degrees, and she hyperextended the trunk to try to get more motion); elevation through abduction of the arm and 80 degrees (painful arc began about 60 degrees, and she shrugged her shoulder to try to get more motion); medial rotation, 70 degrees; lateral rotation, 50 degrees; adduction in front of body, 25 degrees; she could not accomplish horizontal adduction and abduction, and circumduction.
3. Passive movements of forward flexion, abduction, and lateral rotation achieved approximately 5 degrees more in each range, although painful. The end-feel in each case was bone to bone.
4. Resisted isometric movements in supine position elicited pain in the shoulder.
5. Joint play maneuvers elicited pain in the shoulder.

6. The Drop Arm test was positive.
7. Ellen demonstrated a reverse scapulohumeral rhythm.
8. Palpation revealed that the greater tuberosity of the left humerus rode higher against the acromion than on the right.
9. Limitation of motion is in capsular pattern.

To confirm my suspicions, I would need to have roentgenographic information. Ellen had not had roentgenograms of her shoulders for over five years, so we mutually decided that she should see her rheumatologist before I did anything too aggressive. The following conditions needed to be ruled out:

1. Degenerative joint disease
2. Calcium deposition in the tendons
3. Adhesive capsulitis
4. Rotator cuff tear
5. Superior migration of the humerus
6. Impingement syndrome
7. Osteoporosis of the shoulder
8. Rheumatoid arthritis flare requiring medication adjustment or change
9. Frozen shoulder

Until I knew what we were dealing with, our goals were to protect the joint by resting the joint, gentle range of motion and isometric exercises, superficial heat (Ellen preferred that to ice), and transcutaneous electrical nerve stimulation (TENS) for pain control. Our goals for mobility would have to wait for the roentgenograms. We rested the joint by giving Ellen a sling to wear between exercise sessions. She was instructed to do her exercises lying in a supine position with her elbow flexed to reduce the compressive forces on the glenohumeral joint. Our immediate short-term goal was to maintain what motion and muscle strength she had. It is indeed unfortunate that third party payers don't realize that maintaining one's status in rheumatoid arthritis is a success.

The medical insurance system poses the moral dilemma in which I've found myself upon numerous occasions. Do I continue to show progress by the patient, on the side of beneficence? Or, do I comply with the stipulation, particularly in the case of Medicare, and discontinue treating the patient when no progress is being made? Lying would be easy but serves no one well, particularly myself. My choice is to make sure Ellen knows how to manage the problem we are working on, and that she has support from Bill. By that I mean he has seen what she has to do, I have written it down in simple, explicit instructions, and she has demonstrated that she knows what is expected of her. I follow her until I'm convinced she can do what she is supposed to, and then discharge her with a home program that can be readily translated from the clinic to her environment.

Following the roentgenograms, the diagnosis for Ellen's shoulder was osteoporosis, a rotator cuff tear, and superior subluxation of the humeral head. She and her rheumatologist discussed the possibility of having a Neer shoulder arthroplasty, but she has not done so as yet. Like a lot of persons with arthritis, Ellen puts up with a lot of pain because she gets tired of being in and out of the health care system. However, she has been feeling a lot better since her rheumatologist changed her medication to methotrexate.

The diagnosis regarding Ellen's shoulder resulted in a change in my treatment program and goals. With that much damage, and in the face of constant pain caused by the roughened joint surfaces, it was unlikely that anything I did would increase her range of motion. In fact, therapeutic exercises could exacerbate her symptoms. There was no point in putting her through the effort when it was doomed to fail. Rather, the goals would be changed to pain relief, in the form of modalities such as TENS, heat or cold, and maintenance of the motion and muscle strength she had. Ellen had to modify her manner of getting out of a chair. Some of her symptoms were probably due to her habit of using her upper extremities to push up from a sitting position. We elevated the sitting surface of her favorite chairs with 4-in. foam rubber cushions. We also raised her bed so she could get in and out easily.

Here they were today, Bill with his kind face and now white shock of hair and Ellen smiling even though it was immediately obvious that she had rheumatoid arthritis. She had a ''Z'' deformity of the right thumb, nodules in the MCPs of the index and long fingers (bilaterally), Bouchard's nodes (bilaterally), slight ulnar drift of both hands, and a 20-degree flexion contracture of the left elbow. She also wore extra-depth shoes, but was fortunate enough not to have to wear a contour last. That would have made an extra-wide toe box in addition to the extra depth of the shoe. She was able to ambulate without the use of any assistive devices.

"Okay, you two, come on back here and let me see what kind of trouble you've been in." We have been at this so long that Bill comes along, too. He is a reliable source of information to verify what Ellen has been doing. My plan of care will be designed based on the information I get from an evaluation of Ellen's ambulation or transfer status, joint range of motion, joint deformity or instability, muscle strength, swelling or synovitis, pain status, fatigue or endurance, morning stiffness or joint gelling, knowledge of her problem, ability to fulfill her occupational role, personal care, home conditions, and skin and vascular conditions.

"Ellen, could you describe for me exactly what seems to be the problem that brought you here today?"

"I have a new sharp pain in my left foot that has just come on the last two weeks. It happened when I was getting ready for bed. I turned on my left foot to get into bed and felt something 'pop' in my ankle. Now my right ankle is beginning to hurt, too. Of course, I've had more to do the last two weeks, so I have been on my feet more."

The results of my evaluation are depicted in Figures 68-1 to 68-5. In addition to these data forms, my notes on the workup are depicted in Figure 68-6.

(Text continues on p. 1273.)

Name *Ellen Carson*

ID# *6858179*   M/F Age *62*

Diagnosis *RA*

Date *Dec. 18, 1988*

Test Period

Physician *Carroll*

I. Hip

Range of Motion	R	L	Muscle Examination	R	L
Flexion (120°)	WNL	WNL	Flexors		
Extension (0°)			Iliopsoas	3	3
Hyperextension (10°)	−10°	−10°	Rectus femoris		
Abduction (45°)	WNL	WNL	Extensors		
Adduction (15°)	—	—	Gluteus maximus		
Internal rotation (45°)	—	—	Hamstrings		
External rotation (45°)	—	—	Abductors		
			Gluteus medius		
			Gluteus minimus		
			Tensor fascia latae		
Leg length	—	—	Adductors		
Femoral torsion	—	—	External rotators		
Longsitting IR/ER	—	—	Internal rotators	↓	↓

Comments:

II. Knee	R	L	Ligamentous Tests	R	L
Flexion (130°)	120°	120°	Medial collateral l.	—	—
Extension (0°)	−5	−10	Lateral collateral l.	—	—
			Drawer sign	—	—
Genu valgus (slight)	—	—	Lachman's sign	not	done
Genu varus	—	—			
Q angle	WNL	WNL	Muscle Examination	R	L
Patellofemoral:					
Crepitus (slight)	+	+	Flexors		
Pain (compression)	+	+	Biceps femoris	4	4
Subluxing	—	—	Medial hamstrings	4	4
Excessive motion	—	—	Extensors		
Restricted motion	—	+	Quadriceps femoris	3	3
Tibial torsion	—	—			

Comments: Did not do a "break test" on muscle exam. Tested muscles in 3 (fair) position. Pt. ambulatory and able to climb and descend stairs with handrail, one foot at a time.

Figure 68-1. Lower extremity evaluation.

Name *Ellen Carson*   Date *Dec 18, 1988*

ID# *6858179*   M/(F) Age *62*   Test Period

Diagnosis *RA*   Physician *Carroll*

I. General Ankle, Foot, and Toes Evaluation

Visual Inspection	R	L	Muscle Evaluation	R	L	
Calcaneal varus	—	—	Plantar flexors			
Calcaneal valgus	+	+	Gastrocnemius	3	3	⟩ with ↑ pain
Pes planus	+	+	Soleus	3	3	
Pes cavus	—	—	Dorsiflexors			
Plantar tenderness	s ee below		Anterior tibialis ?	4		unable to test/pain
Midfoot pronation	+	+	Invertors			
** Midfoot supination	—	—	Posterior tibialis	3+	3−	
Forefoot varus	—	—	Evertors			
Forefoot valgus	+−	+	Peroneus longus	4	4	
Hallux valgus	+−	+	Peroneus brevis	4	4	pain Ⓛ
Hallux varus	—	—	M. P. Flexors			medial
Hallux rigidus	—	+	Lumbricales	4	4	midfoot
Morton's toe	—	—	Flexor hallucis br.	4	4	
Hammer toes 4th toes	+	+	I. P. Flexors			
Claw toes	—	—	Flexor digitorum long.	4	4	
Tender MTH see below	+	+−	Flexor hallucis long.	4	4	⟩
Subluxing MTH	—	—	M. P. Extensors			
✶ Morton's neuroma	—	−?	Extensor hallucis br.	4	4	
✶↑ tenderness between			Extensor digitorum br.	4	4	
Balance 2 & 3 mT	R	L	I.P. Extensors			
Eyes open	—	+	Extensor digitorum long.	4	4	
Eyes closed	+	+	Extensor hallucis long.	4	4	
Sensation wNL	—	—				
Synovitis (+) see below	+	+				

Comments: 1) Pain on √ of Ⓛ Hallux (15°); Ⓡ hallux √ = 20°
   2) Hammer toe bilat 4th toe   4) Plantar tenderness
3) Tender MTH   Ⓛ severe pain @ origin
    Ⓛ long −mild   Ⓡ mild t −1 thru   of plantar fascia
    4th↳ mild t 5th −mild   5th toes

Range of Motion	R	L	Ⓡ mild/moderate pain @
			origin of plantar fascia
Plantar flexion	WNL	WNL	
Dorsiflexion	−5°	−5°	lacks 5° from getting to neutral

** Subtalar joint
  Ⓛ pain in sinus tarsi − lateral and medial side (moderate)
  Ⓡ pain in sinus tarsi − lateral and medial side (severe)
  Ⓛ lateral and medial malleolus − synovitis, ↑ temperature

Figure 68-2.   Ankle, foot, and toes evaluation.

Perform gait analysis with least possible bracing and support.
Place a check (√) in appropriate box; with bilateral involvement, use (R) or (L) instead of check.
To indicate a sustained posture, place a (P) in the appropriate box.

		SWING			STANCE				
		INITIAL SWING	MID-SWING	TERMINAL SWING	INITIAL CONTACT	LOADING RESPONSE	MID-STANCE	TERMINAL STANCE	PRE-SWING
TRUNK:	Backward Lean								
	Forward Lean								
	Lateral Lean (R or L)								
	Rotates Back								
	Rotates Forward								
PELVIS:	Hikes								
	Symphysis Up								
	Symphysis Down								
	Lacks Forw. Rotation								
	Lacks Backw. Rotation								
	Excess. Forw. Rot.								
	Excess. Backw. Rot.								
	Ipsilateral Drop								
	Contralateral Drop								
HIP:	Flexion: Limited								
	Absent								
	Excessive								
	Inadequate Extension							(L)✓	
	Past Retracts								
	External Rotation								
	Internal Rotation					(L)✓	(L)✓		
	Abduction						(L)✓		
	Adduction					(L)✓	(L)✓		
	Wobbles								

STEP: (Relationship of heel to opposite foot)

R Heel | L Heel

c̄ shoes

WALKING AID: none

Dependent [ ]

EXCESSIVE U.E. WEIGHT BEARING:
Body Lean [ ]
Shld Elevation [ ]

STANCE RATIO: [ ]
Unequal

HEAD CONTROL:
Extraneous Motion
Abnormal Posture [ ]

ARM SWING:
Diminished [✓]
Absent
Abnormal Posture

1268

KNEE:						
Flexion: Limited						
Absent						
Excessive			ⓛ ✓		ⓛ ✓	
Inadequate Extension			ⓛ ✓	ⓛ ✓		
Wobbles						
Hyperextends						
Extension Thrust						
Valgus			ⓛ ✓	ⓛ ✓	ⓛ ✓	
Varus						
Excess. Contral. Flex.						
ANKLE: Forefoot Contact						
& Foot Flat Contact						
FOOT: Foot Slap						
Excessive Planter Flexion						
Excessive Dorsiflexion			✓ ⓛ	✓	✓	
Varus			✓ ⓛ	✓	✓	
Valgus						
Wobbles						
Heel Off				✓	✓	
No Heel Off					✓	
Drag						
Contralateral vaulting						
TOES: Up						
Clawed						

LIST MAJOR PROBLEMS AND CAUSE(S):

SWING:

STANCE:

NAME _Ellen Carson_   RLAH# _____   DATE _12/18/88_

DIAGNOSIS _RA_   RPT _____

Figure 68-3. Full body gait analysis. (Courtesy of Professional Staff Association, Rancho Los Amigos Hospital, Downey, CA 90242)

Figure 68-4

	ABSOLUTE		%NORMAL F
VELOCITY	44.3	M/MIN	55
CADENCE	1.03	STEP/MIN	87
STRIDE LENGTH	0.866	METERS	63
GAIT CYCLE	1.17	SEC	115
STRIDES	5		

	-R-	-L-
SINGLE LIMB SUPPORT		
(SEC)	0.43	0.41
(%NORMAL F)	73	69
(%GC)	36.8	35.0
SWING (%GC)	35.0	36.8
STANCE (%GC)	65.0	63.2
DOUBLE SUPPORT		
INITIAL (%GC)	14.6	13.7
TERMINAL (%GC)	13.7	14.6
TOTAL (%GC)	28.3	28.3

Name Carson, Ellen

Number 6858179

SEX (M OR F)

EVALUATION DATE 12-18-86

REASON FOR TEST
Free Cadence
with shoes and no orthoses
Evaluation

```
L
E  5 5
F           H H H H H H H H H H
T  1 1 1
      T T T T        T T T T T T T T T T
R            T T T T T  T T T T
I              1 1 1 1 1 1 1 1
G  H H H H H H H H H H H H H
H  5 5 5 5 5 5 5 5 5 5
T                                    1

                                     S
                                     E
                                     C
```

Figure 68-4. Sample printout from the Cosmac Foot-switch Stride Analyzer. The patient was walking at her normal walking speed (designated as free cadence) with her extra-depth shoes on and no orthoses inside. One can determine that she is walking at 44 m/min, which is 55% of normal velocity. Her steps per minute (cadence) were calculated as 103, or 87% of normal. Her stride length was 0.866 meters, or 63% of normal. Single limb support time is less than the usual 40% of the gait cycle. The percentages of swing phase and stance phase in the gait cycle are depicted, as is double support time.

Figure 68-5

	ABSOLUTE		%NORMAL F
VELOCITY	56.8	M/MIN	70
CADENCE	119	STEP/MIN	101
STRIDE LENGTH	0.960	METERS	70
GAIT CYCLE	1.01	SEC	99
STRIDES	5		

	-R-	-L-
SINGLE LIMB SUPPORT		
(SEC)	0.38	0.37
(%NORMAL F)	75	73
(%GC)	37.6	36.6
SWING (%GC)	36.6	37.6
STANCE (%GC)	63.4	62.4
DOUBLE SUPPORT		
INITIAL (%GC)	12.5	13.1
TERMINAL (%GC)	13.1	12.5
TOTAL (%GC)	25.6	25.6

Name Carson, Ellen

Number 6858179

SEX (M OR F)

EVALUATION DATE
12-18-88

REASON FOR TEST
Fast Cadence
with shoes and no orthoses
Evaluation

```
L
E                         5 5 5 5 5 5
F      H H H H H H H H H H H H
T                          1 1 1 1 1 1 1 1
        T T T T T T T T T T T T
R        T T T T
I        1 1 1 1
G                                        H
H        5 5 5
T
```

Figure 68-5. Sample printout from the Cosmac Foot-switch Stride Analyzer. The patient's gait parameters during fast cadence when wearing shoes and no orthoses. Mrs. Carson was unable to ambulate successfully barefoot. As in Figure 68-4, the data indicate that she spends less time on the left foot in stance phase compared to the right foot.

Staff Notes

Carson, Ellen
6858179

DATE	Physical Therapy
18 Dec '88	Patient is a 62 y/o white ♀ c̄ a 21-year hx of RA. She has been followed medically by various
	physicians in the Division of Rheumatology. Currently she is followed by Dr. Carroll. Mrs.
	Carson was a participant in our hindfoot study during the month of October. Subsequent to that
	time she had an episode of trauma at her home while getting ready for bed in the evening. She
	turned on her Ⓛ foot to get into bed and felt something "pop" in her Ⓛ ankle. She went to
	Dr. Carroll c̄ a cc: "I am not able to walk like I used to." She presents today for assessment and
	treatment. She was not x-rayed. Her husband is accompanying her. She is wearing new extra-
	depth shoes that contain custom-made semirigid foot orthoses bilaterally.
	S: "I have pain in my left foot that came on suddenly two weeks ago."
	O: 1. Joint tenderness
	a) Sinus tarsi Ⓡ and Ⓛ = Ⓛ =2; Ⓡ =3
	b) Plantar tenderness of MTH bilateral = 2
	c) Plantar tenderness at origin of plantar fascia Ⓛ = 3, Ⓡ = 2
	2. Joint pain on motion
	a) √ of hallux Ⓛ = 1
	b) Inversion/eversion of subtalar joint Ⓛ = 2
	c) Dorsi and plantar √ Ⓛ = 2
	3. Swelling: Ⓛ = 2 (lat. and med. malleolus)
	Ⓡ = 1
	4. Deformity/midfoot Ⓛ = 1
	5. MMT: see attached form
	6. Balance: " " "
	7. ROM: " " "
	8. Gait: See Cosmac Stride strips
	9. Meds: Prednisone 5 mg/day
	Feldene, A.S.A. Buffered, Darvon Compound prn
	(no longer on methotrexate)

Figure 68-6. The physical therapist's notes about the patient. These were incorporated into her chart in the physical therapy department. (*Figure continues.*)

DATE	
	10. ADLs
	a) Walking in home has ↓ in last 2 weeks
	b) Can fix meals
	c) Walks to church less
	d) Not a community ambulator
	A: Problem list
	1. RA active in feet
	2. ↓ strength of Ⓛ posterior tibialis
	3. ↑ tenderness in plantar fascia
	4. ↑ ″ of MTHs
	5. Pronation of the midfoot Ⓛ
	6. Valgus of forefoot Ⓛ
	7. Valgus of hindfoot Ⓛ
	8. Gait:
	a) Free cadence c̄ shoes and no orthoses equal 55% of normal
	b) Fast cadence c̄ shoes and no orthoses equal 70% of normal
	c) Stance phase abnormalities by observation
	d) Single limb support time ↓ Ⓛ>Ⓡ
	9. ↓ muscle strength/functionally assessed
	10. Morton's neuroma?
	11. Metatarsalgia
	12. Talonavicular joint ligamentous and capsular strain?
	13. Deltoid ligament tear?
	14. Fracture of talus?
	15. Avulsion of posterior tibialis tendon from sustentaculum tali?
	P. 1. Refer back to Dr. Carroll for x-ray to rule out fracture of talus and to assess joint integrity.
	2. If fracture or ligamentous tear RTC for gait training, depending on status of UEs
	3. If avulsion of posterior tibialis, then
	a) Modify Ⓛ shoe by medially stabilizing it to ↓ pronation forces.
	b) Institute an aggressive exercise program for posterior tibialis and calf mm.
	c) Continue quadriceps femoris strengthening program
	d) Assess muscle strength, gait, and changes in feet
	e) Institute home program

Figure 68-6. *(Continued.)*

Staff Notes

DATE	
	f) RTC every 2 weeks for 2 months for re-evaluation of her
	progress. When no further progress is made, modify plan of care or d/c.
	4. If Morton's neuroma, may need orthopedic consult.
	5. If metatarsalgia, then modify orthoses and shoe as necessary.
	Overall goals:
	1. ↑ walking velocity without assistive devices to 60% in one month.
	2. Protect joints of the foot with orthoses and shoes, thereby decreasing pain in the foot.
	3. ↑ muscle strength of knees and feet as demonstrated by Ellen
	walking step over step on the stairs, ascending and descending.

Figure 68-6. *(Continued.)*

ANNOTATED BIBLIOGRAPHY

Convery FR, Minteer MA, Amiel D et al: Polyarticular disability: A functional assessment. Arch Phys Med Rehabil 58:494, 1977 (This article describes the use of the Convery Functional Assessment instrument for polyarticular disease, and discusses the reliability of the instrument.)

Fries JF: Arthritis: A Comprehensive Guide. Menlo Park, Addison-Wesley Publishing Co, 1983 (This book is written so that patients may gain a better understanding of the type of arthritis they have in order to be a better consumer and manager of the disease.)

Fries JF: Toward an understanding of patient outcome measurement. Arthritis Rheum 26:697, 1983 (This article describes the use of the Health Assessment Questionnaire created at Stanford University to measure the functional status of patients with rheumatic disease.)

Jette AM: Functional status index: Reliability of a chronic disease evaluation instrument. Arch Phys Med Rehabil 61:395, 1980 (This article describes the reliability and validity of the Functional Status Index measure of function. Furthmore, it describes the dimensions of the instrument.)

Long K, Fries FJ: The Arthritis Helpbook: What You Can Do For Your Arthritis. Menlo Park, Addison-Wesley Publishing Co, 1980 (This book is written for patient education purposes. It describes exercises, self-help devices, dietary needs, medications, and coping mechanisms patients might use to manage the disease.)

Meenan RF, Gertman PM, Mason JH et al: Measuring health status in arthritis: The Arthritis Impact Measurement Scales. Arthritis Rheum 23:146, 1980 (This article provides the original data of the reliability and validity of the AIMS on a small sample of patients.)

Meenan RF, Gertman PM, Mason JH et al: The Arthritis Impact Scales: Further investigation of a health status measure. Arthritis Rheum 25:1048, 1982 (This article is a reexamination of the reliability and validity of the AIMS on a large sample of patients based on clinical data. The report attempts to estimate the clinical applicability of the AIMS instrument.)

69 Brain Tumor

JOYCE L. ADCOCK

As per the policy in this comprehensive cancer center, a written consultation for inpatient rehabilitation was sent to the department. The patient was identified as a newly admitted 24-year-old white female. The only information the consult included was "grade IV glioblastoma, evaluate and treat." Brain tumors are classified by cell type, the location in the brain, and the degree of malignancy. This particular brain tumor is an aggressive one that is rapid growing and highly malignant. It generally requires radical medical intervention including, at least, surgery and radiation treatment. Both the tumor and the treatment can severely impair functional abilities. In light of the diagnosis and not knowing the immediate status of the patient, she was scheduled for an evaluation at bedside.

Once on the nursing floor, my first step is to review the chart for pertinent medical and social information. The identification form indicated that Mrs. Allen was a 24-year-old, white, Jewish female. She was married to an attorney and had two sons, ages 2 and 4. The admissions sheet provided additional information. Mrs. Allen had a craniotomy six days ago. The purpose of surgery is not "curative." The surgeon may be able to debulk the tumor, that is, remove some of the mass. Doing so may decrease some of the symptoms and enhance the effect of radiation treatment. Surgery also provides for an exact diagnosis, which aids in determining the best treatment program. In this case, surgery was to be followed by whole-brain radiation. Mrs. Allen had already received three treatments.

The chief functional problem of Mrs. Allen was a left-sided hemiplegia. Treatment plans were for inpatient radiation and rehabilitation. The usual protocol is six weeks of whole brain radiation, five days a week at 200 rad per day. During the last few days of treatment, the radiation is directed specifically at the tumor site. With this basic information in mind, I then reviewed the remainder of the chart in detail.

Past medical history did not contribute to Mrs. Allen's current problem. The only other hospitalizations she had were for the births of her children. Social history was significant, in that the patient's mother lived out of state, and was staying with relatives while her daughter was hospitalized. She would not provide her daughter with childcare, and insisted on being consulted regarding every aspect of her daughter's medical care. She indicated that she wished to bring her daughter home immediately, and seek a second opinion in her home state. This family situation alerts me to be prudent in conversation, to document all intervention clearly, and to utilize the primary physician as the spokesman for the team caring for this patient. Interfamily relationships, particularly in times of stress, can be explosive. The social services and home care service departments had also been consulted.

Other material in the chart helped to clarify early treatment of Mrs. Allen's current condition. She initially had a seizure several days ago. She was taken to a community hospital, and was evaluated through the emergency service. A computed tomographic (CT) scan showed a large tumor of the right frontal and parietal lobes. At her husband's request, she was transferred to the comprehensive cancer center for further workup and treatment. Phenytoin (Dilantin) therapy was started to reduce the possibility of further seizures. Dexamethasone (Decadron) therapy also was started to aid in decreasing tissue edema in the brain. Within 24 hours of her admission, Mrs. Allen underwent a craniotomy. She developed a profound left hemiplegia following the surgical procedure. All other tests indicated that no disease was evident in other organs or areas of the body. She continued on a medication regimen of anticonvulsants and corticosteroids. In the last two days, the hemiplegia had been slightly resolved, but Mrs. Allen remained nonambulatory and unable to participate in self-care activities. Daily physical and occupational therapy were ordered.

When I entered the room, Mrs. Allen was lying supine in bed, listing slightly to the left. She was immediately aware of my presence and followed my movement with her head. Because she moved only her head, one might assume she had some problem with visual tracking. While introducing myself to the patient, I was already making some initial observations about Mrs. Allen. In terms of appearance, she had good color and normal body weight. It appeared that she had been in good health prior to the illness. She had an intravenous line in her unaffected right upper extremity. The right side of her head was cleanly shaven. A large, healing incision extended from about 2 cm above the right eye and traversed down towards the right ear in the shape of a "C." She also showed evidence of radiation intervention, because there were purple marks along the head and neck for identification of the treatment area. As a result of the radiation treatments, early hair loss about the head and neck was also evident. Mrs. Allen was starting to show a fullness about the face, which was indicative of the large doses of steroids she had already received. It is important for the therapist to understand the role steroids play in the management of the patient with a brain tumor. Because steroids decrease brain edema, functional problems related to in-

creased intracranial pressure can resolve spontaneously. However, long-term administration of high doses of steroids can contribute to proximal muscle weakness and steroid-induced diabetes. Both of these problems can affect the overall outcome of the physical therapy program. Mrs. Allen's general behavior showed her to be fairly bright and able to communicate verbally. I explained who I was, that I was there to evaluate her, how I might be able to help her, and what the possible outcome of rehabilitation may be.

First, I asked Mrs. Allen to recount as much as she could regarding her present hospitalization. This information is critical because it helps the therapist to see how the patient perceives the situation and if that perception is appropriate. She stated that she was on an outing with her family when she suddenly smelled fried chicken. She recalled falling to the ground, and waking up in the emergency room. She stated she was informed she had a seizure. Incidentally, the sensation of smelling fried chicken was a prodrome to Mrs. Allen's seizure. Patients frequently notice a visual, auditory, or olfactory warning signal before a seizure. Mrs. Allen reported that while in the emergency room she developed an unremitting frontal headache. The combination of headache, nausea and vomiting, and papilledema are usually indicative of increased intracranial pressure. The patient who experiences any, or all, of these symptoms combined with seizure leads one to suspect tumor, as opposed to stroke. Mrs. Allen went on to say that, prior to this event, she did not notice any functional problems, changes in mentation, or general malaise. It is possible that she either did not experience any changes in these areas, or she did experience changes and did not recognize them. This is a question that must be reserved for family members or friends.

Mrs. Allen's chief complaints at this time were an inability to walk and trouble using her left arm. She also complained of some residual headache and visual disturbance. She stated that she had not been out of bed since her admission. She had been transported to other departments on a gurney. The nurses were doing most of her care, and she was using a bedpan. Mrs. Allen stated that she had always been healthy and never had any medical problems in the past. She reported that she was married while in college. At the moment, a friend had her two sons, and she had not seen them since her admission. She made no mention of her mother, but stated that her husband comes to the hospital as soon as he leaves work. She was concerned about his welfare. During the course of this interview, I decided that Mrs. Allen was fairly cognizant of her immediate situation on a superficial level. It was not apparent if she understood the serious nature of her disease or her overall prognosis. Because she did not make direct inquiries about this, one might assume that she was not able, or not willing, to discuss these issues at this particular time. Had Mrs. Allen not been able to relate this information, I would have needed to use other sources such as family, nursing staff, and visitors to obtain it.

My next step was to make some assessments of Mrs. Allen's physical and cognitive status. Knowing the site of the tumor, one can anticipate some symptoms and check for specific dysfunction. Because the frontal lobe was involved, I paid particular attention to memory. Judgment and problem-solving ability should be assessed. I also needed to acquire more information regarding her premorbid personality. With the parietal lobe also being involved, I must look for sensory changes, motor problems, and speech problems. Increased intracranial pressure can accentuate functional and cognitive problems. It can also contribute to symptoms that one might not expect to see with this tumor site, that is, behavioral and functional problems associated with diffuse brain involvement. With these things in mind, I began my evaluation of this patient. All systems should be reviewed, including cardiovascular, respiratory, neurological, and musculoskeletal, as well as functional capabilities and cognitive skills.

Mrs. Allen had no previous history of heart disease. Her presurgical electrocardiogram showed no abnormalities. Her resting pulse in supine was 74 beats per minute and regular.

She had no history of respiratory diseases. Her lungs were clear by chest roentgenogram as well as auscultation. She was primarily an upper chest breather. Breaths were 22 per minute in the resting position.

Neurological evaluation revealed a number of significant findings. I first examined the cranial nerves. Two common items usually available in the patient's room are alcohol and soap, which can be used to test the olfactory nerve. It is important to test each side of the nose separately. This is an important test when the patient has a frontal lobe lesion, because the olfactory pathways run under that lobe. It is not unusual for the patient to experience anosmia. It was determined that Mrs. Allen had a good sense of smell bilaterally. It is significant to note that not only could she recognize the presentation of an odor, but also was able to identify it.

I then tested the optic nerves. I examined both visual acuity and visual fields. Mrs. Allen did not wear corrective lenses. There was no evidence of central visual problems. Because the parietal lobe was involved, I checked for contralateral blindness in the corresponding lower quadrants of both eyes. Gross visual fields seemed to be intact. With an opthalmoscope, the optic disks may be examined for papilledema, which is indicative of increased intracranial pressure. The oculomotor, trochlear, and abducens nerves demonstrated good visual tracking. My first impression that Mrs. Allen could track using only head movement proved incorrect. There was no ptosis of the eyelids. There was no evidence of nystagmus. Pupillary light reflex was intact. She did complain of double vision in the extreme left visual field. This was alleviated by covering one eye, indicating that the lens and the retina were intact. The trigeminal, facial, acoustic, glossopharyngeal, vagus, and accessory nerves did not reveal any significant deficits that would clinically impair Mrs. Allen. On testing of the hypoglossal nerve, her tongue deviated slightly to the left, although it did not significantly affect speech or swallowing.

I then tested for primary forms of sensation. Light touch was diminished only in the left extremities, as were pain and temperature. Vibration, deep pressure, and proprioception all were decreased on the left side. Cortical and discriminatory sensation were then tested. She showed deficits in two-point discrimination, localization, texture discrimination, graphesthesia, and extinction, particularly in the left upper extremity. Results of this sensory evaluation are quite interesting. There was a disturbance only in the cortical and discriminatory sensations, with the primary sensations intact. I could assume that she had parietal lobe involvement. Because the primary forms of sensation are also affected, one might guess that the sensory cortex was involved. Brain tumor patients can exhibit diverse symptoms. Considering the degree of insult and the edema in the brain tissue, this type of finding is not completely unexpected. Deep tendon reflexes on Mrs. Allen's left side were markedly hypoactive, but they were normal on her right side. There was no evidence of clonus. The testing of superficial reflexes was deferred at this time because there was no reason to suspect a problem with the corticospinal tract. Babinski reflexes were negative bilaterally. One other pathologic reflex test that should be done on a brain tumor patient is the Brudzinski test. She exhibited neck pain on passive neck flexion, again indicating diffuse brain involvement.

Cerebellar functions were tested on Mrs. Allen's right side. She had no difficulty performing finger to nose, rapid alternating movements, or sliding her heel along her shin. One would not expect coordinated movement to be a problem for her because the cerebellum and basal ganglia chiefly govern these functions. Because of Mrs. Allen's hemiplegia, her left side could not be tested. I made an educated guess that coordinated movement would be intact in light of the patient's diagnosis and physical findings thus far.

Musculoskeletal examination also revealed some significant findings. There was no evidence of tremor, muscle fasciculations, or extraneous movements. Inspection of Mrs. Allen's muscles showed fairly good symmetry and contour. There was no evidence of atrophy. Palpation of the left shoulder revealed early subluxation, although the musculature about the shoulder girdle was in the poor to fair range. She could initiate left shoulder shrug as well as protraction and retraction. The remainder of the left upper extremity was flaccid. She could passively be taken through full range of motion of the left extremities. To conserve energy, trunk and neck range of motion would be evaluated when the patient was sitting up. Gross power in the right extremities was well within normal limits. Mrs. Allen could initiate left hip flexion and abduction. I could induce a visible contraction of the quadriceps through a Marie-Foix reflex. This is significant because if I can elicit movement through this reflex, she may eventually be able to introduce a voluntary effort, which can then be reinforced.

Further evaluation yielded some information about Mrs. Allen's functional skills. When I elevated the head of the bed to 70 degrees, she suffered no ill effects. She required maximal assistance for me to bring her legs over the edge of the bed and come to a sitting position. Mrs. Allen could not maintain static sitting balance without support. I determined that she had good passive range of motion of the neck and trunk. After being up for about three minutes, she started to become short of breath and pale. Blood pressure was 102/66. She was returned to the supine position and these signs resolved spontaneously. Mrs. Allen was experiencing postural hypotension relieved by positioning.

During the course of this evaluation, I had already started to make some assessments regarding Mrs. Allen's cognitive skills, intellect, and the like. However, each of these needs to be looked at individually. In terms of general behavior, Mrs. Allen was amazingly appropriate and congenial. She seemed most anxious to cooperate. I should not automatically believe, however, that she is coping well and understands her situation. I must remember that a great deal has happened to her in a very short period of time. Decisions had to be made immediately, and many were made for her. I anticipate that as Mrs. Allen has time to consider her present situation, she will have many questions regarding her prognosis, physical capabilities, discharge, ability to care for her family, and a host of other psychosocial issues.

With continued radiation treatment, one may expect to see a change in the level of consciousness. Mrs. Allen may become less attentive and more drowsy. These changes should be subtle. If Mrs. Allen were to experience these changes quickly (eg, within a 24-hour period), it may indicate increased intracranial pressure, and the physician should be advised. Usually an increase in the steroid dosage will quickly alter the level of consciousness. If the lethargy persists regardless of steroid administration, these effects may be related to radiation and secondary edema.

When assessing intellectual performance, I must consider the patient's educational and socioeconomic level to make an accurate assessment. Clearly, Mrs. Allen has good recollection of her life premorbidly and some recollection of the first signs of her tumor. To assess her memory for past events, I asked Mrs. Allen the names of her children, her husband's occupation, and other pertinent data about her home and family. Short-term memory was tested by asking Mrs. Allen to repeat two-, three-, and four-digit numbers backwards and forwards. She was able to repeat two and three digits forward and two-digit numbers backwards. Mrs. Allen was then asked to do some mathematical calculations without the use of pen and paper. She could do one- and two-digit addition and subtraction and one-digit multiplication and division. All other calculations were too sophisiticated for her. She was able to count backwards from 100 by threes until 91, and then could not continue.

When orientation was checked, Mrs. Allen knew her name and knew that she was in a hospital, but did not know its name or the current date. I then assessed her ability to solve problems. A situation was presented to Mrs. Allen in which she was to put events into a sequence. When asking a patient to solve a problem, we are looking not only for a reasonable resolution but also for a coherent and viable step-by-step process. She was able to solve the most simplistic problems, but when the

solution required four elements or more, her answers became less cohesive and less reasonable. I also asked some questions dealing with current events, general knowledge, categorizing items, and explaining short maxims. All of this was achieved with some hesitation and Mrs. Allen responded to questions with short answers or "yes" and "no" answers. Her thought content did not lack structure, but it did lack sophistication. She showed some memory loss, particularly short-term memory, and some orientation problems. Mrs. Allen's deficits and behavior, intellectual performance, and thought content should not be surprising. The frontal lobe helps to govern behavior and intellectual performance. One would be most surprised if she did *not* show some changes in these areas.

The evaluation would not be complete, nor could a treatment program be designed, without testing specific cerebral functions. Visual and auditory skills had already been completed. Tactile interpretation, right-left discrimination, and recognition of body parts were, unexpectedly, intact. The willful ability to carry out a motor task requires that a person understand what he is to do, remember what he is to do, and then perform the act. This is critical in order for a patient to participate in a rehabilitation program. Mrs. Allen had no measurable or observable deficits in this area.

The last part of this assessment is language and the ability to communicate. Mrs. Allen was asked to repeat a series of sounds, then words, and finally short sentences. Her speech was clear and she had no difficulty with automatic speech. Volitional speech was decreased. She did not initiate conversation, nor did she attempt to elaborate on her rsponses to questions. Considering her tumor site, one would expect more impairment than was demonstrated. Because the ability to initiate speech and to write are primarily a frontal lobe function, one would expect to have problems, but, in fact, her deficits were minimal. In considering the results of Mrs. Allen's evaluation, her most pronounced deficit is hemiplegia. Her mental capacities and cognitive skills are strong enough so our approach to therapy will not be hampered by an inability to follow instructions or act on those instructions.

There are three significant functional differences between the patient with brain tumor and the patient with a stroke. First, radiation plays a significant part in the patient's physical and cognitive abilities. The patient makes rapid progress in the first three to four weeks. The patient will then start to show signs of increasing lethargy, poor appetite, and decreased attentiveness, which may last for several weeks. Then, the patient starts to improve again for another six to eight weeks, and the functional level will reach a plateau. Second, unlike the patient with a stroke, the patient with a brain tumor does not develop spasticity, but progresses from flaccid muscles to some, if not all, volitional movement. Third, steroids have a marked impact on the patient's overall functional abilities, changing the patient's status not only from day to day but sometimes from hour to hour. These changes require the therapist to be extremely flexible and able to alter the patient's program in accordance with the changing status.

Mrs. Allen's physical therapy program was designed to her tolerance. As she progressed with treatment, she was seen several hours a day in the rehabilitation department. Priorities in the treatment plan were based on the patient's functional skills. Short-term and long-term goal planning were difficult because of the wide variations in skills on a day-to-day basis. My immediate goal was to maintain strength and range of motion of the right extremities, while maintaining range of motion in the left extremities. I also wanted to be cognizant of the patient's skin condition because of her sensory changes. I had to attend to both the cognitive and physical level of the patient, because these vary considerably with corticosteroids and radiation treatment.

Initially, Mrs. Allen was treated at bedside. I started with some active and passive exercises, bed mobility, some self-care, and some intellectual challenges. These included review of current events, problem solving, recall, and the like. When these skills were accomplished without significant problems, Mrs. Allen was put on the tilt table. My purpose was to acclimate her to the upright position without inducing hypotension. She was also able to bear weight on her affected extremity without fear of falling or jeopardizing her safety. When this aspect of her care was well tolerated, the tilt table chest strap was released to permit us to work on trunk stability. She could also work on eye-hand coordination, visual tracking, and other perceptual tasks in this upright position.

It was also appropriate to work on facilitating muscle activity, particularly the left shoulder girdle. I expected to see volitional movement occur from proximal to distal. Once Mrs. Allen tolerated the tilt table and had achieved some trunk control and a sense of the vertical, she started to work on sitting balance. Initially she sat with support, then she progressed to unsupported sitting, and then sitting with challenges. Next I worked on bed, toilet, and chair transfers. A transfer board was necessary only for a short time. Mrs. Allen was fitted with a wheelchair and instructed in its use. I was alert for subtle signs of left-sided neglect, which would make wheelchair activity more difficult for this patient. While the wheelchair afforded her a temporary means of mobility, I continued with exercises and cognitive retraining, and started to get Mrs. Allen up on her feet. In standing, I first worked on static balance in the parallel bars. Then I worked on dynamic standing balance, leading up to gait reeducation. She progressed, but one must be aware that she could have plateaued well before the gait training stage.

Some critical issues exist in terms of the overall management of patients with brain tumors. If the patient were to require any type of orthosis for ambulation, an inexpensive or temporary device should be used early in the program. The expense and time of fabricating an orthotic device might later prove to be premature and unnecessary. With brain tumor, one can expect to see functional changes up to two months after radiation treatment. Another issue is the importance of considering what the patient thinks is necessary. As best as possible, the patient's goals and the therapist's goals should be parallel. We must remember that it is the patient's right to decide what she wants to do, and it is our job to help her do those things if possible. We can try to temper her goals with reality if they are unrealistic, but we cannot set goals devoid of the patient's expectations. Please remember that you are dealing with a patient who is gravely ill, and whose life expectancy is probably less than a year. Our job is to provide practical, expedient treatment that enhances the quality of the person's life.

During the course of Mrs. Allen's rehabilitation, I worked closely with the social worker to help to resolve the family situation. As mentioned earlier, Mrs. Allen's mother wanted to take her home. However, Mr. Allen wanted his wife to remain with him at their home. To ease this conflict, the social worker assisted Mr. Allen in acquiring household help for childcare and day-to-day chores. The social worker also helped Mr. Allen to prepare the children to see their mother, and they started to discuss childcare options if Mrs. Allen should die. Mrs. Allen's mother was allowed to participate in family meetings, but was encouraged to take a more passive role, allowing Mr. Allen to make the final decisions on issues. Mrs. Allen's opinions and decisions were taken into account because childcare was one of her chief concerns.

Schedules were adapted to allow Mr. Allen to participate in the rehabilitation program. I started to introduce the family members to the rehabilitation program, and encourage them to assist as much as possible. I also instructed the family in the use of cues that would be helpful to the patient, such as putting objects in her visual field but far enough away that she really has to scan to find the desired object. Discharge plans were not made until well into the fourth and fifth weeks of Mrs. Allen's radiation treatment. At that time, we had more information on which to base an overall functional prognosis.

With a patient like Mrs. Allen, outcome of treatment can follow several scenarios. First, there is the remote possibility of full physical and cognitive recovery for an indefinite period of time. The second scenario is partial or complete recovery for a short period of time. Third, there is some degree of recovery, but death is imminent.

Chances of a complete recovery and extended survival for a patient with this type of tumor and degree of malignancy are highly unlikely. Prior to discharge, this patient would be tested for independence in ambulation, transfers, and self-care. Overall endurance and gross power would also be assessed. If the patient required further physical therapy after discharge, outpatient visits would be arranged for her. Aggressive therapy is usually stopped when the patient's functional level has plateaued. She would return to the clinic for periodic checkups. Such visits are scheduled to coincide with visits to other services to minimize repetitive trips to the center.

Mrs. Allen's case is an example of the second scenario. She had partial recovery and was discharged to her home. Mrs. Allen was able to transfer independently, and required the use of a walker to ambulate. She was provided with self-care items. Her family and friends were instructed in range-of-motion exercises for her extremities, guarding her during ambulation, and cueing in self-care. Prior to discharge, a home evaluation was performed to provide necessary equipment and make recommendations regarding the removal of architectural barriers from the home. Arrangements were made for childcare as well as household assistance. Nursing care was also provided for Mrs. Allen. Throughout the course of her illness, Mr. Allen continued to see their social worker on a regular basis. This was directed at preparing him to be a single parent without neglecting his business obligations. Mrs. Allen's recuperation was punctuated with repeated hospital admissions. She developed steroid-induced diabetes and deep vein thrombosis of the right lower extremity, and her functional capacities deteriorated. She survived for a year and a half, becoming bedridden, suffering painful headaches, and eventually losing her eyesight—all the result of continued insult from this aggressive tumor. She died at home surrounded by her family and friends.

Cancer patients are special people who

value their lives, who are better motivated than any other patient population, and whose time is a gift. It is our responsibility to provide them with the best possible care. At times, cancer rehabilitation goes against everything we are taught as physical therapists. In most education programs, we are taught to rehabilitate, to restore, to make new, to return the patient to the maximal functional level. Unfortunately, as with Mrs. Allen, the therapist sees the patient on repeated hospital admissions. Chances are that with each admission, the patient's functional level is slowly deteriorating; thus, the therapist is always backstepping. There is nothing wrong with that therapeutic approach. You have to think about the patient as he is *now*, not as he was. It is the therapist's responsibility to see that the patient can be as functional as possible, to maximize his level of independence, and to help him meet realistic goals.

It is critical for the therapist to realize that, although some of the symptoms exhibited by brain tumor patients mimic those of a stroke patient, both the etiology and the outcome are quite different from a stroke. If one is not cognizant of that, and uses the same approach as for a stroke patient, the result of the rehabilitation program will be far less promising. Often, by the time a cancer patient's function is impaired to the point where he requires rehabilitation, there is a good chance that he is already in the final stages of his disease. This may mean a life expectancy of perhaps a year or less. One does not have the luxury of following the textbook, with all the lead-up activities and nuances of therapy. The patient's problems and goals must be identified and a streamlined therapy program implemented to meet those goals as best as possible.

ANNOTATED BIBLIOGRAPHY

DelRegato J, Spjut H: *Cancer Diagnosis, Treatment and Prognosis.* St Louis, CV Mosby, 1977 (This is an older general cancer text. Although there is little mention of rehabilitation, it is an excellent resource. It reviews the incidence and etiology of many cancers as well as their treatment. A new edition [6th] was published in 1985.)

Essentials of the Neurological Examination. Philadelphia, Smith Kline Corp, 1968 (This booklet is available free on request from Smith Kline Corporation. It outlines the essentials of a neurological examination including cranial nerves, reflexes, and sensory test. It is very brief, but is well organized.)

Friedberg S: Tumors of the Brain. *Clin Symp* 38 (4):1986 (This fairly recent issue of Clinical Symposia is a general overview of the most common types of brain tumors, their symptoms, and treatment. It can be acquired at a minimal cost from CIBA.)

Goldberg S: *The Four-Minute Neurologic Exam.* Miami, MedMaster, 1984 (This brief, but comprehensive text covers the basic neurological workup including basic neuroanatomy, how to take a history, the neurological exam itself, and laboratory tests. It also has an appendix regarding use of the ophthalmoscope. Although brief, it helps the therapist evaluate an individual in an orderly manner.)

Segal G: *A Primer of Brain Tumors.* Chicago, Association for Brain Tumor Research, 1978 (This is one of several publications of the Association for Brain Tumor Research in Chicago. Geared for the patient and family, it explains what a tumor is, how certain tumors affect certain parts of the brain, and their diagnosis and treatment. A glossary defines some of the more technical terminology. These booklets, as well as other material, can be requested with a donation to this organization.)

Siev E, Freishtat B, Zoltan B: *Perceptual and Cognitive Dysfunction in the Adult Stroke Patient.* Thorofare, NJ, Charles B. Slack, 1986 (Written by occupational therapists, this book is quite specific in identifying functional deficits, related lesion sites, and testing. Although it is directed towards a stroke population, many patients with brain tumor have similar site involvement and related dysfunction. This text also expands the physical therapist's basic knowledge of perceptual and cognitive dysfunction.)

Index

Page numbers followed by *f* indicate figures; page numbers followed by *t* indicate tabular material.

ISBN 0-397-50798-4

90000

**This book is to be returned on or before
the last date stamped below.**

SCULLY, R.M. and
BARNES, M.R.
Physical Therapy

SCULLY, R.M. and
BARNES, M.R.